A COLOUR ATLAS OF
HUMAN ANATOMY

SECOND EDITION

R. M. H. McMinn

MD, Ph.D, FRCS (Eng.)
Emeritus Professor of Anatomy,
Royal College of Surgeons of England
and University of London

R. T. Hutchings

Freelance Photographer
Formerly Chief Medical Laboratory
Scientific Officer, Royal College
of Surgeons of England

Wolfe Medical Publications Ltd

Copyright © R.M.H. McMinn and R.T. Hutchings, 1977, 1988
First edition published in 1977 by Wolfe Medical Publications Ltd
Printed by Royal Smeets Offset, Weert, Netherlands

ISBN 0 7234 1526 9

A CIP catalogue record for this book is available
from the British Library.

This book is one of the titles in the series of Wolfe
Medical Atlases, a series which brings together
probably the world's largest systematic published
collection of diagnostic colour photographs.

For a full list of Atlases in the series, plus
forthcoming titles and details of our surgical,
dental and veterinary Atlases, please write to
Wolfe Medical Publications Ltd, 2-16 Torrington
Place, London WC1E 7LT, England.

Contents

Preface

In preparing this completely revised second edition of *A Colour Atlas of Human Anatomy* we have been guided by comments and suggestions made over the past ten years by many teachers and students—especially students, for it is for them that the book has been written. Apart from well over one hundred new illustrations, the most important innovation is the inclusion of a short commentary on individual specimens.

When learning a new area, the student comes across a mass of structures and it is difficult to know where to begin the process of sorting things out. The commentary draws attention to the most significant features (giving their key numbers so that they can be identified immediately in the picture), and gives guidance on the important things to look for (and the kind of things that examiners pick out!).

For a number of specimens there are comments and sometimes small diagrams to assist in orientation.

There is more surface anatomy, and selected cross sections of the trunk and limbs have been introduced, together with examples of modern imaging techniques which now supplement traditional radiological methods. We believe it is useful to include not only bones and dissections of soft parts including the brain but surface anatomy and radiology as well, at least in selected areas that have particular medical importance.

The object of this atlas is to assist undergraduates and postgraduates in the study of human anatomy. Of course, good textbooks and atlases already exist and by colouring arteries red and nerves yellow, for example, they are justly popular as aids to learning. But so often, and especially for newcomers to the subject, the interior of the body seems to look very different from the neat diagrams in the book, and we believe it is helpful to show body structures as they actually exist in suitably prepared specimens of the kind that students see in the dissecting room and meet in examinations. In this way we hope to bridge the gap between the description of the textbook and the reality of the body.

Introduction

The body is made up of the head, trunk and limbs. The trunk consists of the neck, thorax (chest) and abdomen (belly). The lower part of the abdomen is the pelvis, but this word is also used to refer just to the bones of the pelvis. The lowest part of the pelvis (and lowest part of the trunk) is the perineum. The central axis of the trunk is the vertebral column, and the upper part of it (cervical part) supports the head.

The main parts of the upper limb are the arm, forearm and hand. Note that in strict anatomical terms the word 'arm' means the upper arm, the part between the shoulder and elbow, although the word is commonly used to mean the whole of the upper limb.

The main parts of the lower limb are the thigh, leg and foot. Note that in strict anatomical terms the word 'leg' means the lower leg, the part between the knee and foot, although the word is commonly used to mean the whole of the lower limb.

For the description of the positions of structures in human anatomy, the body is assumed to be standing upright with the feet together and the head and eyes looking to the front, with the arms straight by the side and the palms of the hands facing forwards. This is the 'anatomical position' (see the illustrations), and structures are always described relative to one another using this as the 'standard' position, even when the body is, for example, lying on the back in bed or on a dissecting room table.

The 'median plane' is an imaginary vertical, longitudinal line through the middle of the body from front to back, dividing the body into right and left halves. The adjective 'medial' means nearer the median plane, and 'lateral' means farther from it. Thus, in the anatomical position, the little finger is on the medial side of the hand and the thumb is on the lateral side; the great toe is on the medial side of the foot and the little toe on the lateral side.

In the forearm where there are two bones, the radius on the lateral (thumb) side and the ulna on the medial side, the adjectives 'radial' and 'ulnar' can be used instead of lateral and medial. Similarly in the lower leg where there are two bones, the fibula on the lateral side and the tibia on the medial side, 'fibular' and 'tibial' are alternative adjectives.

'Anterior' and 'posterior' mean nearer the front or nearer the back of the body respectively. Thus on the face the nose is anterior to the ears, and the ears are posterior to the nose. Sometimes 'ventral' is used instead of anterior, and 'dorsal' instead of posterior (terms from comparative anatomy which are appropriate for four-footed animals).

The hand and foot have special terms applied to them. The anterior or ventral surface of the hand is usually called the palm or palmar surface, and the posterior or dorsal surface is the dorsum. But in the foot the upper surface is the dorsal surface or dorsum, and the undersurface or sole is the plantar surface.

'Superior' and 'inferior' mean nearer the upper or lower end of the body respectively; the nose is superior to the mouth and inferior to the forehead (even if the body is upside down; the upright 'anatomical position' is always the reference position).

'Superficial' means near the skin surface, and 'deep' means farther away from the surface.

'Proximal' and 'distal' mean nearer to and further from the root of the structure: in the upper limb, the forearm is distal to the elbow and proximal to the hand.

The words 'sagittal' and 'coronal' describe certain planes of section, most often used in the head and brain. The 'sagittal plane' is any front-to-back plane that is parallel to the median plane, and the 'coronal plane' (sometimes called the frontal plane) is a vertical plane at right angles to the median plane. ▷

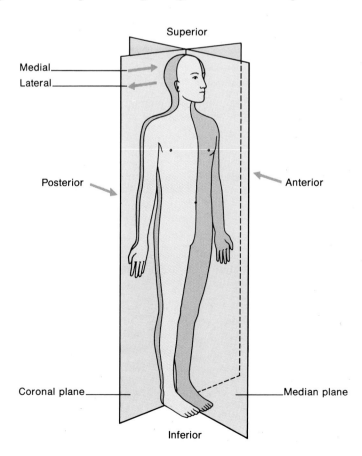

5

The book is arranged in the general order 'head to toe'—head and neck (including the brain), followed by the vertebral column and spinal cord, thorax, upper limb, abdomen and pelvis, and lower limb. In each section the bones are considered first, followed by dissections and other illustrations.

Structures are labelled by overlying numbers which are identified in the key lists. The numbers on the pictures are generally arranged in a clockwise order starting at the top of the picture, although it has not always seemed appropriate to stick rigidly to this pattern. Sometimes in crowded areas or for small structures, leader lines are necessary; an arrowhead at the end of a leader indicates that the item is just out of view beyond the tip of the arrow. Self-testing can be carried out by covering up the key.

For bones, the parts of each are first named, and then the pictures are repeated indicating the sites of attachments of muscles and ligaments. Although the details of individual skull bones are included, for most students knowledge of the skull as a whole is much more important.

Dissections and other items are introduced by a short commentary which draws attention to the most significant features, so helping to sort out 'the wood from the trees'. The commentary is supplemented by notes which again emphasize the more important features or help to explain difficult topics, but they are not intended to give a comprehensive description of everything seen. The book is designed to supplement existing texts, not to substitute for them.

The Appendix at the back of the book contains reference lists of vessels, nerves, muscles and skull foramina, with illustrations of the whole skeleton and of the principal vessels and nerves. The diagram of the arteries, for example, shows at a glance which are the main vessels of the upper limb, and in the reference lists their branches are named.

Acknowledgements

For the preparation of new material for this edition we are most grateful for the help given by Dr Colin Chumbley, St George's Hospital Medical School, and Bari Logan, Prosector in the University of Cambridge. For making us so welcome in their Departments and for assistance in many ways we express our sincere thanks to Professor J.W.S. Harris, Tjeu Gysbers and John Norton of the Royal Free Hospital School of Medicine; Professor K.E. Webster, Peter Brinck and Donald Farr of King's College London; and Professor P.N. Dilly, John Fish and Frank Simpson of St George's Hospital Medical School. For the generous provision of radiographic material we are much indebted to Dr Oscar Craig and Dr Paul Grech of St Mary's Hospital and Medical School, and to Dr Kim Fox and Dr Richard Underwood for the MRI scan of the thorax.

We renew our thanks: to all those who over many years contributed specimens to the Anatomy Museum of the Royal College of Surgeons of England, and especially to Dr D.H. Tompsett who also prepared the corrosion casts (full details of the methods used can be found in his book *Anatomical Techniques*, 2nd edition, 1970, Livingstone), and to the late Sir Edward Muir who as President of the College allowed us to reproduce the illustrations of museum specimens; to Dr J.L. Cordingley, formerly of King's College London, Professor T.W. Glenister of Charing Cross and Westminster Medical School, and Professor F.R. Johnson, formerly of the London Hospital Medical College, for the loan of osteological material; to Mr V.H. Oswal of the North Riding Infirmary, Middlesbrough, for the coloured dissections of the ear; and to our models.

To the memory of Peter Wolfe

Head, neck and brain

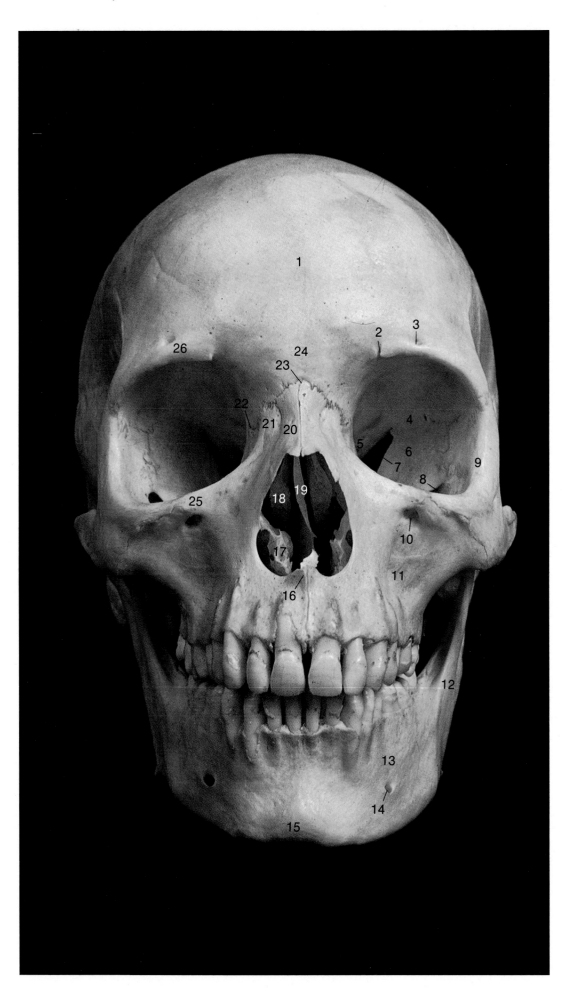

Skull, from the front

 1 Frontal bone
 2 Frontal notch
 3 Supra-orbital foramen
 4 Orbit (orbital cavity)
 5 Lesser ⎫
 6 Greater ⎭ wing of sphenoid bone
 7 Superior ⎫
 8 Inferior ⎭ orbital fissure
 9 Zygomatic bone
10 Infra-orbital foramen
11 Maxilla
12 Ramus ⎫
13 Body ⎭ of mandible
14 Mental foramen
15 Mental protuberance
16 Anterior nasal spine
17 Middle ⎫
18 Inferior ⎭ nasal concha
19 Nasal septum
20 Nasal bone
21 Frontal process of maxilla
22 Lacrimal bone
23 Nasion
24 Glabella
25 Infra-orbital margin
26 Supra-orbital margin

● The term 'skull' includes the mandible, and 'cranium' refers to the skull without the mandible, but these definitions are not always strictly observed.
● The calvaria is the vault of the skull (cranial vault or skull-cap) and is the upper part of the cranium that encloses the brain.
● The front part of the skull forms the facial skeleton.
● The supra-orbital, infra-orbital and mental foramina (3, 10 and 14) lie in approximately the same vertical plane.
● Details of individual skull bones are given on pages 23 to 32, of the bones of the orbit and nose on page 18, and of the teeth on page 20.

A Skull, from the front. Muscle attachments

1	Temporalis
2	Masseter
3	Orbicularis oculi
4	Procerus
5	Corrugator supercilii
6	Levator labii superioris alaeque nasi
7	Levator labii superioris
8	Zygomaticus minor
9	Zygomaticus major
10	Levator anguli oris
11	Nasalis
12	Buccinator
13	Depressor labii inferioris
14	Depressor anguli oris
15	Platysma
16	Mentalis

• The attachment of levator labii superioris (7) is above the infra-orbital foramen and that of levator anguli oris (10) is below it.
• The attachment of depressor labii inferioris (13) is in front of the mental foramen and that of depressor anguli oris (14) is below it.

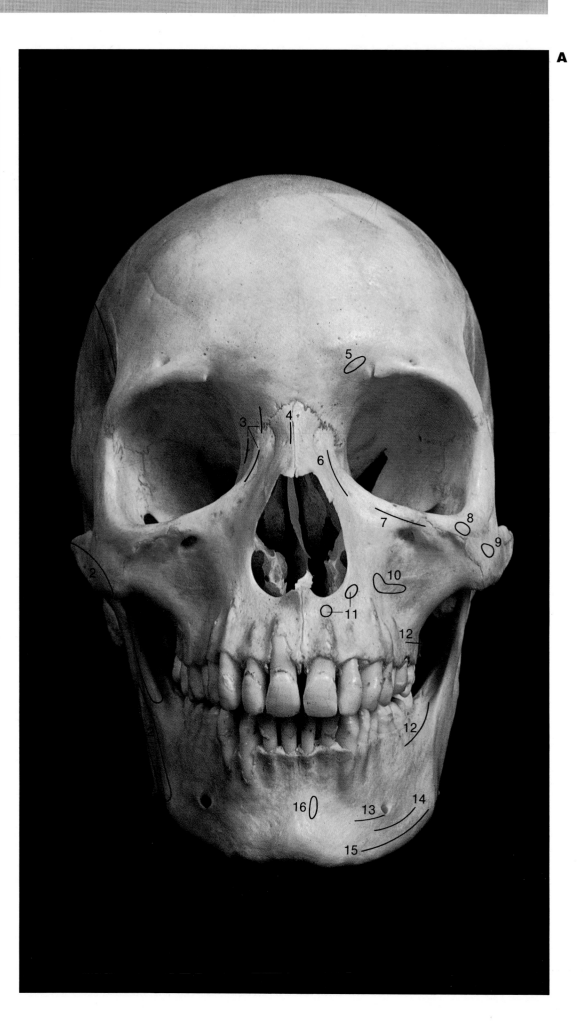

A

B

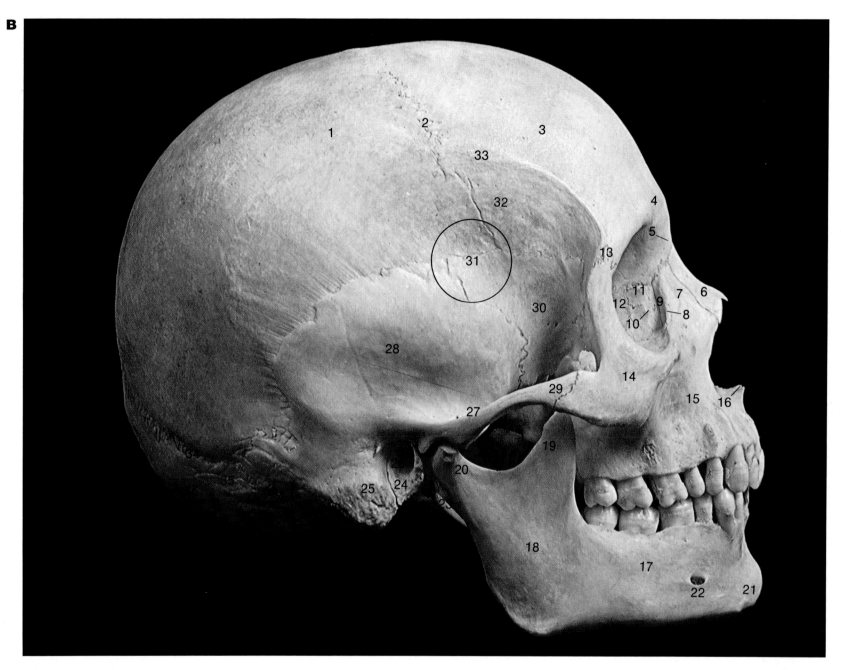

B Skull, from the right

1	Parietal bone	21	Mental protuberance
2	Coronal suture	22	Mental foramen
3	Frontal bone	23	Styloid process
4	Glabella	24	Tympanic part
5	Nasion	25	Mastoid process
6	Nasal bone	26	External acoustic meatus
7	Frontal process of maxilla	27	Zygomatic process
8	Anterior lacrimal crest	28	Squamous part
9	Fossa for lacrimal sac	29	Zygomatic arch
10	Posterior lacrimal crest	30	Greater wing of sphenoid
11	Lacrimal bone	31	Pterion (encircled)
12	Orbital part of ethmoid	32	Inferior
13	Frontozygomatic suture	33	Superior
14	Zygomatic bone	34	Lambdoid suture
15	Maxilla	35	Occipital bone
16	Anterior nasal spine	36	External occipital protuberance (inion)
17	Body		
18	Ramus		
19	Coronoid process		
20	Condyle		

23–28 of temporal bone

32–33 temporal line

17–20 of mandible

● Pterion (31) is not a single point but an *area* where the frontal (3), parietal (1), squamous part of the temporal (28) and greater wing of the sphenoid bone (30) adjoin one another. It is an important landmark for the anterior branch of the middle meningeal artery which underlies this area on the inside of the skull (page 22, 45).

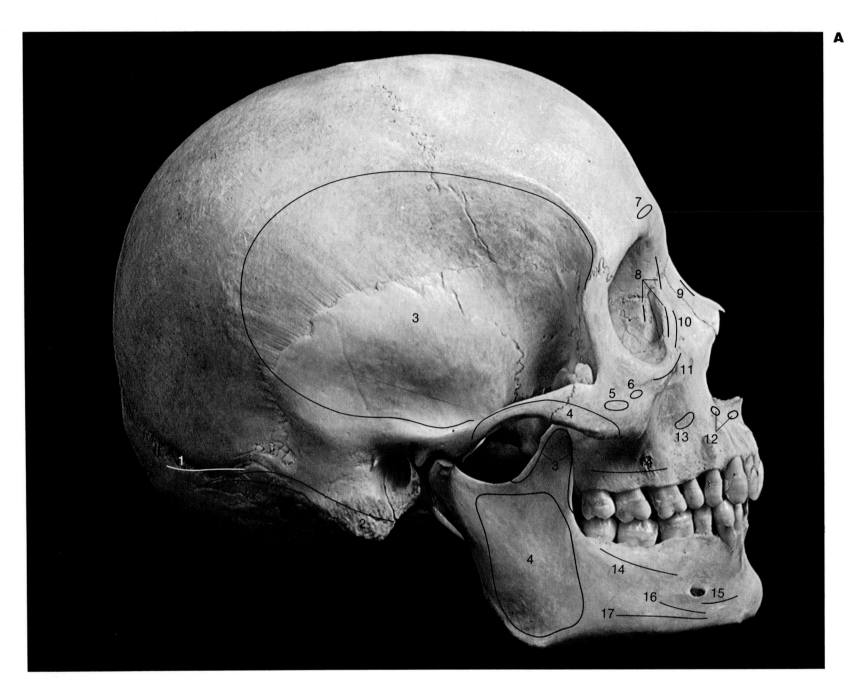

A

A Skull, from the right. Muscle attachments

1 Occipital part of occipitofrontalis
2 Sternocleidomastoid
3 Temporalis
4 Masseter
5 Zygomaticus major
6 Zygomaticus minor
7 Corrugator supercilii
8 Orbicularis oculi
9 Procerus
10 Levator labii superioris alaeque nasi
11 Levator labii superioris
12 Nasalis
13 Levator anguli oris
14 Buccinator
15 Depressor labii inferioris
16 Depressor anguli oris
17 Platysma

● The bony attachments of the buccinator muscle (14) are to the upper and lower jaws (maxilla and mandible) opposite the three molar teeth. (The teeth are identified on page 20, A.)
● The upper attachment of temporalis (upper 3) occupies the temporal fossa (the narrow space above the zygomatic arch at the side of the skull). The lower attachment of temporalis (lower 3) extends from the lowest part of the mandibular notch of the mandible, over the coronoid process and down the front of the ramus almost as far as the last molar tooth.
● Masseter (4) extends from the zygomatic arch to the lateral side of the ramus of the mandible.

B

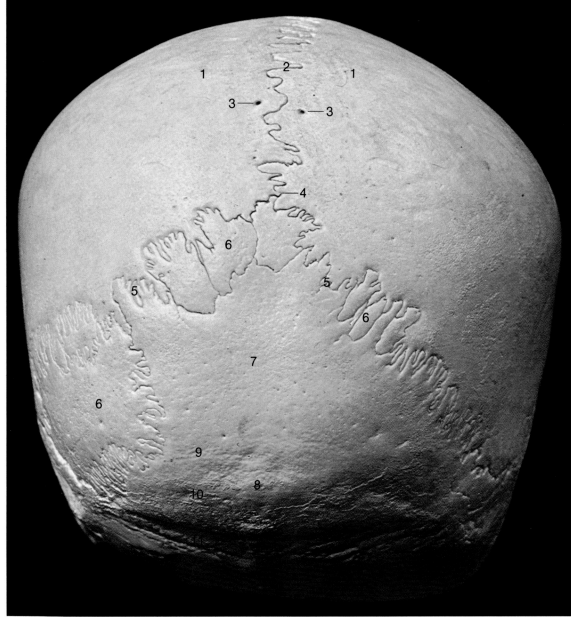

B Skull, from behind

1	Parietal bone
2	Sagittal suture
3	Parietal foramen
4	Lambda
5	Lambdoid suture
6	Sutural bone
7	Occipital bone
8	External occipital protuberance (inion)
9	Highest
10	Superior } nuchal line
11	Inferior

● This cranium shows several sutural bones (6) in the lambdoid suture (5) and one of them (lower left) is unusually large.

C Skull. Right infratemporal region, obliquely from below

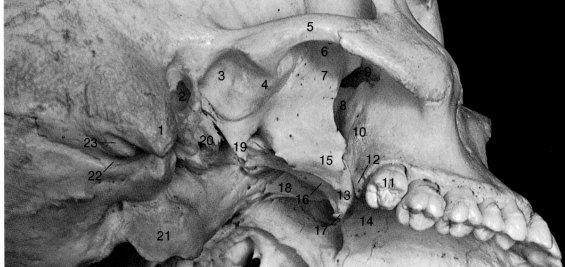

1	Mastoid process
2	External acoustic meatus
3	Mandibular fossa
4	Articular tubercle
5	Zygomatic arch
6	Infratemporal crest
7	Infratemporal surface of greater wing of sphenoid bone
8	Pterygomaxillary fissure and pterygopalatine fossa
9	Inferior orbital fissure
10	Infratemporal (posterior) surface of maxilla
11	Third molar tooth
12	Tuberosity of maxilla
13	Pyramidal process } of palatine
14	Horizontal plate } bone
15	Lateral
16	Medial } pterygoid plate
17	Pterygoid hamulus
18	Vomer
19	Spine of sphenoid bone
20	Styloid process and sheath
21	Occipital condyle
22	Occipital groove
23	Mastoid notch

A

B Skull. Internal surface of the cranial vault, central part

1 Parietal foramen
2 Depressions for arachnoid granulations
3 Groove for superior sagittal sinus
4 Sagittal suture
5 Parietal bone
6 Frontal bone
7 Frontal crest
8 Coronal suture
9 Grooves for middle meningeal vessels

● The arachnoid granulations (page 62), through which cerebrospinal fluid drains into the superior sagittal sinus, cause the irregular depressions (2) on the parts of the frontal and parietal bones (6 and 5) that overlie the sinus.

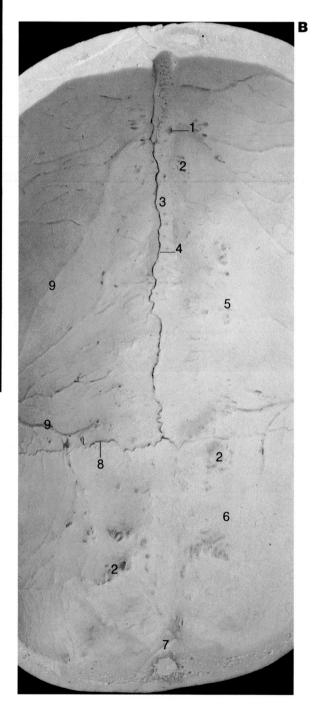

B

FRONT

A Skull, from above

1 Occipital bone
2 Lambda
3 Lambdoid suture
4 Parietal bone
5 Sagittal suture
6 Parietal eminence
7 Coronal suture
8 Frontal bone
9 Bregma
10 Parietal foramen

● In this skull the parietal eminences are prominent (6).
● The point where the sagittal suture (5) meets the coronal suture (7) is the bregma (9). At birth the unossified parts of the frontal and parietal bones in this region form the membranous anterior fontanelle (page 19, D5).
● The point where the sagittal suture (5) meets the lambdoid suture (3) is the lambda (2). At birth the unossified parts of the parietal and occipital bones in this region form the membranous posterior fontanelle (page 19, C19).
● The label 8 in the centre of the frontal bone indicates the line of the frontal suture in the fetal skull (page 19, A6). The suture may persist in the adult skull and is sometimes known as the metopic suture.

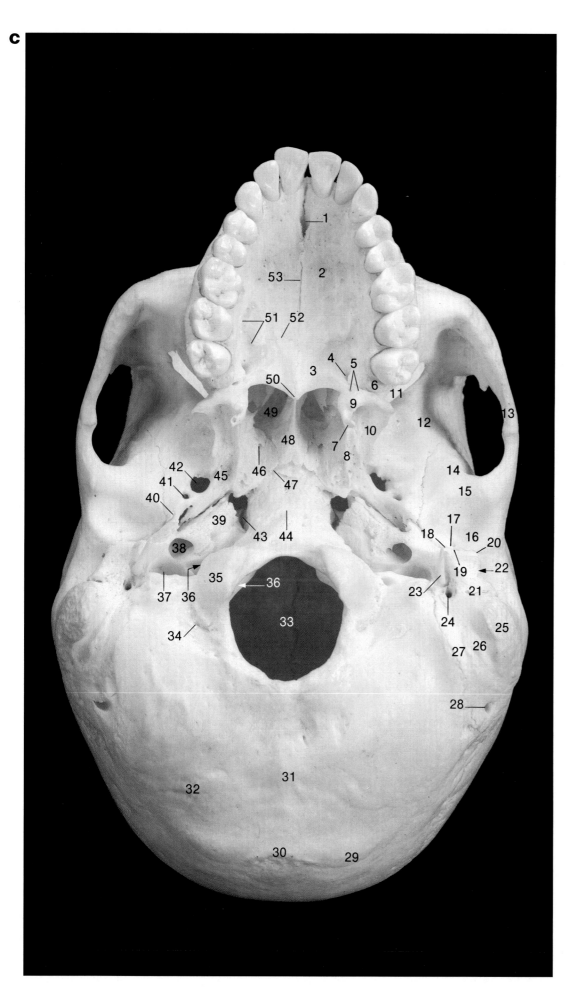

C Skull. External surface of the base

1	Incisive fossa
2	Palatine process of maxilla
3	Horizontal plate of palatine
4	Greater palatine foramen
5	Lesser palatine foramina
6	Tuberosity of maxilla
7	Pterygoid hamulus
8	Medial pterygoid plate
9	Pyramidal process of palatine
10	Lateral pterygoid plate
11	Inferior orbital fissure
12	Infratemporal crest of greater wing of sphenoid
13	Zygomatic arch
14	Squamous part of temporal
15	Articular tubercle
16	Mandibular fossa
17	Petrosquamous fissure
18	Edge of tegmen tympani
19	Petrotympanic fissure
20	Squamotympanic fissure
21	Tympanic part of temporal
22	External acoustic meatus
23	Styloid process
24	Stylomastoid foramen
25	Mastoid process
26	Mastoid notch
27	Occipital groove
28	Mastoid foramen
29	Superior nuchal line
30	External occipital protuberance
31	External occipital crest
32	Inferior nuchal line
33	Foramen magnum
34	Condylar canal
35	Occipital condyle
36	Hypoglossal canal
37	Jugular foramen
38	Carotid canal
39	Apex of petrous temporal
40	Spine of sphenoid
41	Foramen spinosum
42	Foramen ovale
43	Foramen lacerum
44	Pharyngeal tubercle
45	Scaphoid fossa
46	Palatinovaginal canal
47	Vomerovaginal canal
48	Posterior border of vomer
49	Posterior nasal aperture (choana)
50	Posterior nasal spine
51	Palatine grooves and spines
52	Transverse palatine suture
53	Median palatine suture

● The palatine process of the maxilla (2) and the horizontal plate of the palatine bone (3) form the hard palate (roof of the mouth and floor of the nose).
● The spaces on either side of the vomer (48) leading forwards into the nasal cavity are the posterior nasal apertures or choanae (49).
● The gap medial to the zygomatic arch (13) indicates the lower part of the temporal fossa, where it merges with the upper lateral part of the infratemporal fossa.
● The carotid canal (38), recognized by its round shape in the inferior surface of the petrous part of the temporal bone, does not pass straight upwards to open into the inside of the skull but takes a right-angled turn forwards and medially within the petrous temporal to open into the back of the foramen lacerum (43).
● For the contents of skull foramina see page 339.

A Skull. External surface of the base. Muscle attachments

1 Masseter
2 Upper head of lateral pterygoid
3 Deep head of medial pterygoid
4 Superficial head of medial pterygoid
5 Superior constrictor
6 Tensor veli palatini
7 Palatopharyngeus
8 Musculus uvulae
9 Levator veli palatini
10 Pharyngeal raphe
11 Longus capitis
12 Rectus capitis anterior
13 Rectus capitis lateralis
14 Styloglossus
15 Stylohyoid
16 Stylopharyngeus
17 Posterior belly of digastric
18 Longissimus capitis
19 Splenius capitis
20 Sternocleidomastoid
21 Occipital part of occipitofrontalis
22 Trapezius
23 Semispinalis capitis
24 Superior oblique
25 Rectus capitis posterior minor
26 Rectus capitis posterior major
27 Capsule attachment of atlanto-occipital joint
28 Capsule attachment of temporomandibular joint

● The medial pterygoid plate has no pterygoid muscles attached to it. It passes straight backwards, giving origin at its lower end to part of the superior constrictor of the pharynx (5).
● The lateral pterygoid plate has both pterygoid muscles attached to it: medial and lateral muscles from the medial and lateral surfaces respectively (3 and 2). The plate becomes twisted slightly laterally because of the constant pull of these muscles which pass backwards and laterally to their attachments to the mandible (page 24).
● For the contents of skull foramina see page 339.

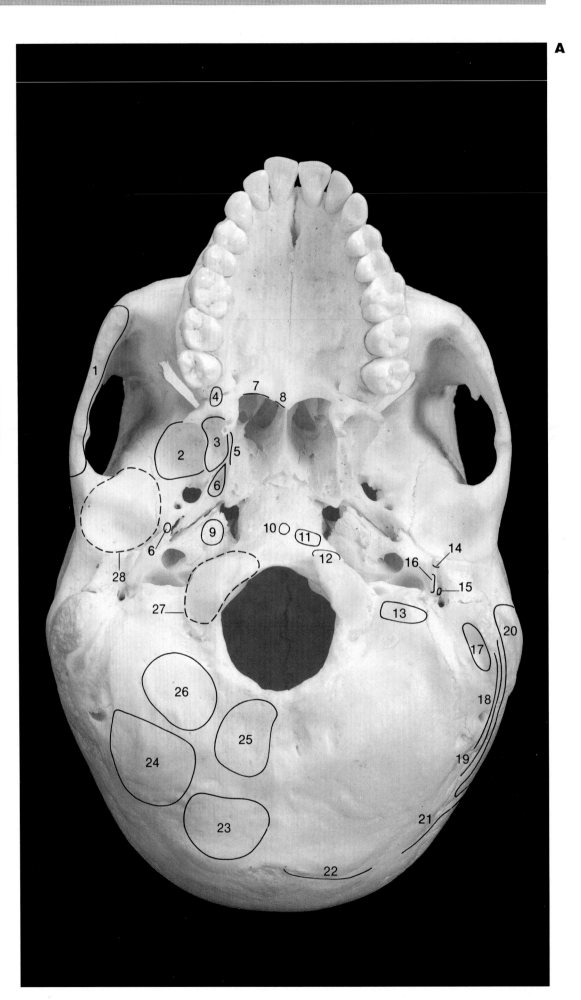

A

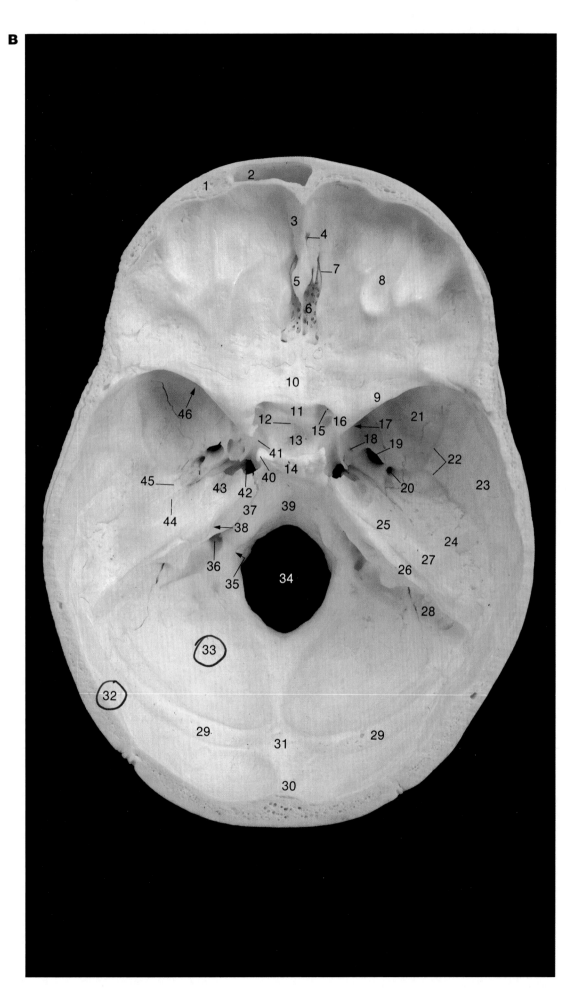

B Skull. Internal surface of the base (cranial fossae)

1 Diploë
2 Frontal sinus
3 Frontal crest
4 Foramen caecum
5 Crista galli
6 Cribriform plate of ethmoid
7 Groove for anterior ethmoidal nerve and vessels
8 Orbital part of frontal
9 Lesser wing of sphenoid
10 Jugum of sphenoid
11 Prechiasmatic groove
12 Tuberculum sellae
13 Pituitary fossa (sella turcica)
14 Dorsum sellae
15 Optic canal
16 Anterior clinoid process
17 Foramen rotundum
18 Venous foramen
19 Foramen ovale
20 Foramen spinosum
21 Greater wing of sphenoid
22 Grooves for middle meningeal vessels
23 Squamous part of temporal
24 Tegmen tympani
25 Petrous part of temporal
26 Groove for superior petrosal sinus
27 Arcuate eminence
28 Groove for sigmoid sinus
29 Groove for transverse sinus
30 Groove for superior sagittal sinus
31 Internal occipital protuberance
32 Parietal bone
33 Occipital bone
34 Foramen magnum
35 Hypoglossal canal
36 Jugular foramen
37 Groove for inferior petrosal sinus
38 Internal acoustic meatus
39 Clivus
40 Posterior clinoid process
41 Carotid groove
42 Foramen lacerum
43 Trigeminal impression
44 Hiatus and groove for greater petrosal nerve
45 Hiatus and groove for lesser petrosal nerve
46 Superior orbital fissure

● The anterior cranial fossa is limited posteriorly on each side by the free margin of the lesser wing of the sphenoid (9) with its anterior clinoid process (16), and centrally by the anterior margin of the prechiasmatic groove (11).
● The middle cranial fossa is butterfly-shaped and consists of a central or median part and right and left lateral parts. The central part includes the pituitary fossa (13) on the upper surface of the body of the sphenoid, with the prechiasmatic groove (11) in front and the dorsum sellae (14) with its posterior clinoid processes (40) behind. Each lateral part extends from the posterior border of the lesser wing of the sphenoid (9) to the groove for the superior petrosal sinus (26) on the upper edge on the petrous part of the temporal bone.
● The posterior cranial fossa, whose most obvious feature is the foramen magnum (34), is behind the dorsum sellae (14) and the grooves for the superior petrosal sinuses (26) are on the upper edges of the petrous parts of the temporal bones.

A Skull. Bones of the left orbit

The bones forming the roof, lateral wall, floor and medial wall of the orbit are indicated in the list below by being bracketed together

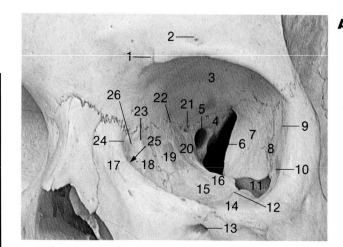

1	Frontal notch	
2	Supra-orbital foramen	
3	Orbital part of frontal	} forming roof
4	Lesser wing of sphenoid	
5	Optic canal	
6	Superior orbital fissure	
7	Greater wing of sphenoid	} forming lateral wall
8	Zygomatic	
9	Marginal tubercle	
10	Zygomatico-orbital foramen	
11	Inferior orbital fissure	
12	Infra-orbital groove	
13	Infra-orbital foramen	
14	Zygomatic	
15	Maxilla	} forming floor
16	Orbital process of palatine	
17	Frontal process of maxilla	
18	Lacrimal	} forming medial wall
19	Orbital plate of ethmoid	
20	Body of sphenoid	
21	Posterior ethmoidal foramen	
22	Anterior ethmoidal foramen	
23	Posterior lacrimal crest	
24	Anterior lacrimal crest	
25	Nasolacrimal canal	
26	Fossa for lacrimal sac	

● The fossa for the lacrimal sac (A26) is formed partly by the lacrimal groove of the frontal process of the maxilla (A17) and partly by the similar groove on the lacrimal bone (A18).

● When covered by mucous membrane, the ethmoidal bulla (B8) and the uncinate process of the ethmoid (B10) form the upper and lower boundaries respectively of the semilunar hiatus (page 48, A7).

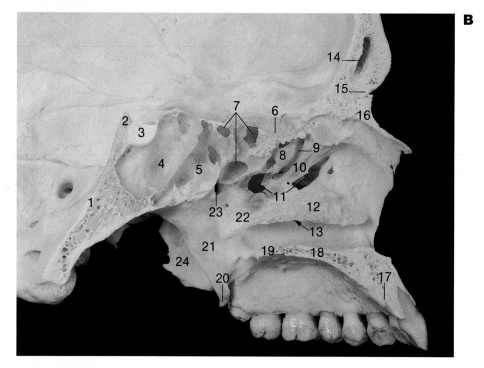

B Lateral wall of the left nasal cavity

In this midline sagittal section of the skull, with the nasal septum removed, the superior and middle nasal conchae have been dissected away to reveal the air cells of the ethmoidal sinus, in particular the ethmoidal bulla (8). Compare this bony background with A on page 48

1	Clivus
2	Dorsum sellae
3	Pituitary fossa (sella turcica)
4	Right sphenoidal sinus
5	Left sphenoidal sinus
6	Cribriform plate of ethmoid bone
7	Air cells of ethmoidal sinus
8	Ethmoidal bulla
9	Semilunar hiatus
10	Uncinate process of ethmoid bone
11	Opening of maxillary sinus
12	Inferior nasal concha
13	Inferior meatus
14	Frontal sinus
15	Nasal spine of frontal bone
16	Nasal bone
17	Incisive canal
18	Palatine process of maxilla
19	Horizontal plate of palatine bone
20	Pterygoid hamulus
21	Medial pterygoid plate
22	Perpendicular plate of palatine bone
23	Sphenopalatine foramen
24	Lateral pterygoid plate

● The roof of the nasal cavity consists mainly of the cribriform plate of the ethmoid bone (B6) with the body of the sphenoid containing the sphenoidal sinuses (B4 and 5) behind and the nasal bone (B16) and the nasal spine of the frontal bone (B15) at the front.

● The floor of the cavity consists of the palatine process of the maxilla (B18) and the horizontal plate of the palatine bone (B19).

● The medial wall is the nasal septum (page 22) which is formed mainly by two bones—the perpendicular plate of the ethmoid and the vomer—and the septal cartilage.

● The lateral wall is the most interesting and complicated, consisting of the medial surface of the maxilla with its large opening (B11), overlapped from above by parts of the ethmoid (B7, 8 and 10) and lacrimal bones, from behind the perpendicular plate of the palatine (B22), and below by the inferior concha (B12).

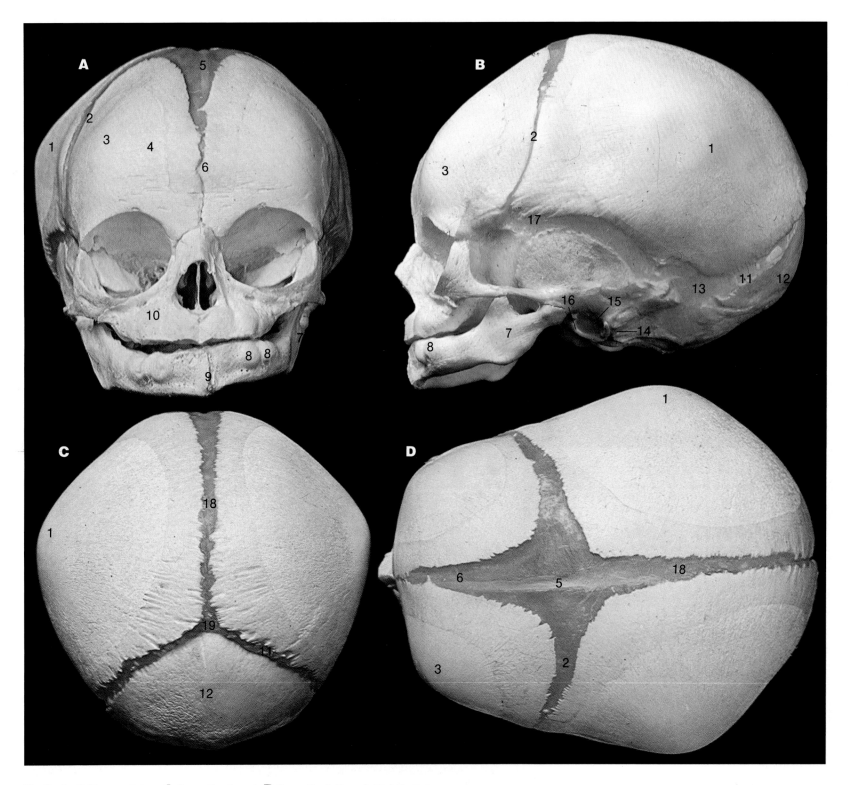

Skull of a full-term fetus, A from the front, B from the left and slightly below, C from behind, D from above

1	Parietal tuberosity	10	Maxilla
2	Coronal suture	11	Lambdoid suture
3	Frontal tuberosity	12	Occipital bone
4	Half of frontal bone	13	Mastoid fontanelle
5	Anterior fontanelle	14	Stylomastoid foramen
6	Frontal suture	15	External acoustic meatus
7	Ramus of mandible	16	Tympanic ring
8	Elevations over deciduous teeth in	17	Sphenoidal fontanelle
	body of mandible	18	Sagittal suture
9	Symphysis menti	19	Posterior fontanelle

● The face at birth forms a relatively smaller proportion of the cranium than in the adult (about one eighth compared with one half) because of the small size of the nasal cavity and maxillary sinuses and the lack of erupted teeth.
● The posterior fontanelle (C19) closes about two months after birth, the anterior fontanelle (A5, D5) in the second year.
● Due to the lack of the mastoid process (which does not develop until the second year) the stylomastoid foramen (B14) and the emerging facial nerve are relatively near the surface and unprotected.

A

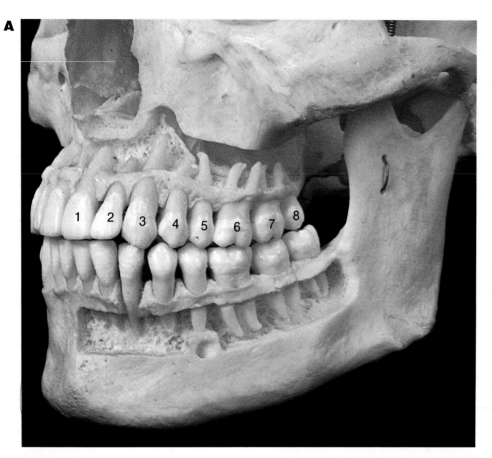

B

C

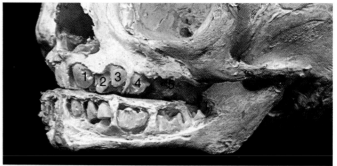

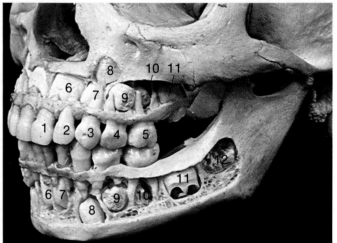

A Skull.
Permanent teeth,
from the left and in
front

The alveolar bone
has been partially
removed to show the
roots of the teeth,
which are numbered
and named on the left
side

1	First (central)	} incisor
2	Second (lateral)	
3	Canine	
4	First	} premolar
5	Second	
6	First	} molar
7	Second	
8	Third	

• The corresponding teeth of the upper and lower jaws have similar
names. In clinical dentistry the teeth are often identified by the
numbers 1 to 8 (as listed here) rather than by name.
• The third molar is sometimes called the wisdom tooth.

Skull. Upper and lower jaws from the
left and in front, B in the newborn
with unerupted deciduous teeth, C in
a four-year-old child with erupted
deciduous teeth and unerupted
permanent teeth

• The deciduous molars occupy the positions
of the premolars of the permanent dentition.

1	First (central)	} incisor	
2	Second (lateral)		of deciduous
3	Canine		dentition
4	First	} molar	
5	Second		
6	First (central)	} incisor	
7	Second (lateral)		
8	Canine		
9	First	} premolar	of permanent
10	Second		dentition
11	First	} molar	
12	Second		

D Skull.
Edentulous
mandible in old
age, from the left

1	Ramus
2	Angle
3	Body
4	Mental foramen

• With the loss of teeth the alveolar bone becomes absorbed, so that
the mental foramen (4) and mandibular canal lie near the upper
margin of the bone.
• The angle (2) between the ramus (1) and body (3) becomes more
obtuse, resembling the infantile angle (as in B and C, above).

D

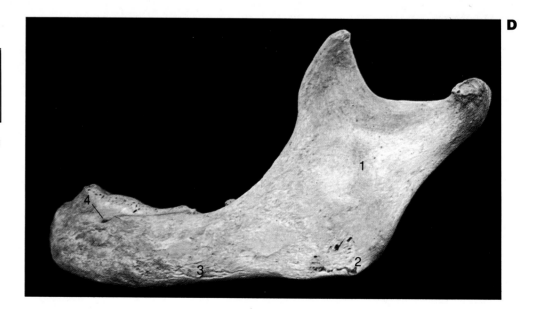

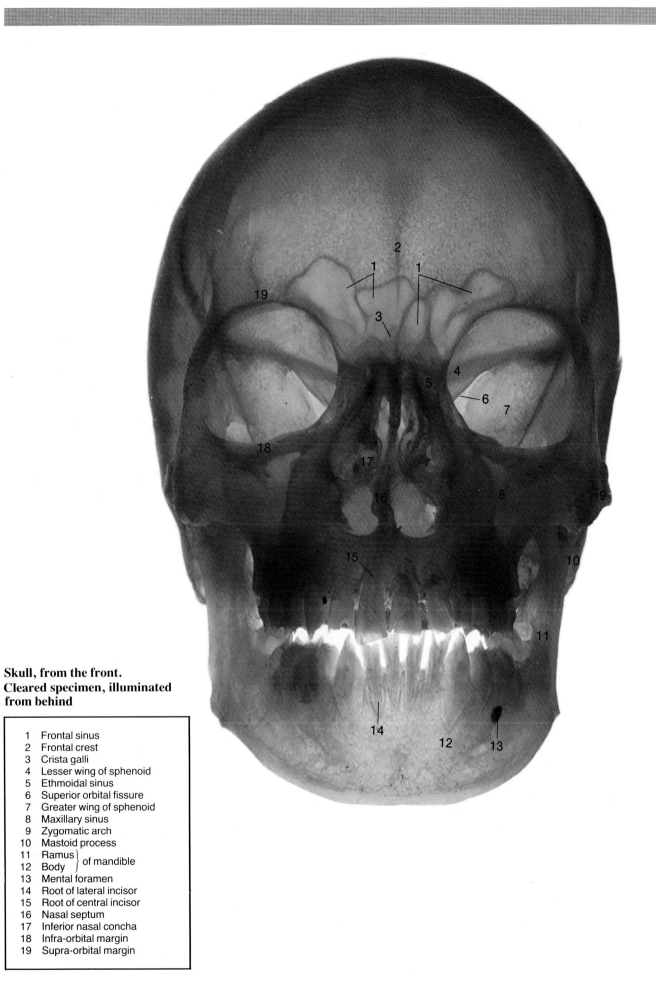

**Skull, from the front.
Cleared specimen, illuminated
from behind**

1	Frontal sinus
2	Frontal crest
3	Crista galli
4	Lesser wing of sphenoid
5	Ethmoidal sinus
6	Superior orbital fissure
7	Greater wing of sphenoid
8	Maxillary sinus
9	Zygomatic arch
10	Mastoid process
11	Ramus ⎫ of mandible
12	Body ⎭
13	Mental foramen
14	Root of lateral incisor
15	Root of central incisor
16	Nasal septum
17	Inferior nasal concha
18	Infra-orbital margin
19	Supra-orbital margin

● Compare with the skull on page 9 and
with the radiograph on page 73.

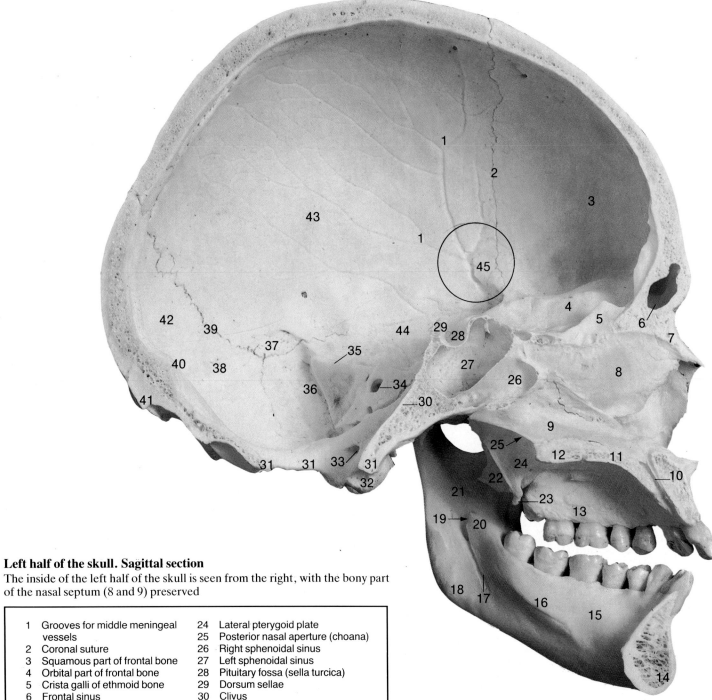

Left half of the skull. Sagittal section

The inside of the left half of the skull is seen from the right, with the bony part of the nasal septum (8 and 9) preserved

1	Grooves for middle meningeal vessels	24	Lateral pterygoid plate
2	Coronal suture	25	Posterior nasal aperture (choana)
3	Squamous part of frontal bone	26	Right sphenoidal sinus
4	Orbital part of frontal bone	27	Left sphenoidal sinus
5	Crista galli of ethmoid bone	28	Pituitary fossa (sella turcica)
6	Frontal sinus	29	Dorsum sellae
7	Nasal bone	30	Clivus
8	Perpendicular plate of ethmoid bone	31	Margin of foramen magnum
9	Vomer	32	Occipital condyle
10	Incisive canal	33	Hypoglossal canal
11	Palatine process of maxilla	34	Internal acoustic meatus in petrous part of temporal bone
12	Horizontal plate of palatine bone	35	Groove for superior petrosal sinus
13	Alveolar process of maxilla	36	Groove for sigmoid sinus
14	Mental protuberance	37	Mastoid (posterior inferior) angle of parietal bone
15	Body of mandible	38	Groove for transverse sinus
16	Mylohyoid line	39	Lambdoid suture
17	Groove for mylohyoid nerve	40	Internal occipital protuberance
18	Angle of mandible	41	External occipital protuberance
19	Mandibular foramen	42	Occipital bone
20	Lingula	43	Parietal bone
21	Ramus of mandible	44	Squamous part of temporal bone
22	Medial pterygoid plate	45	Pterion (encircled)
23	Pterygoid hamulus of medial pterygoid plate		

- The bony part of the nasal septum consists of the vomer (9) and the perpendicular plate of the ethmoid bone (8). The anterior part of the septum consists of the septal cartilage (page 47, B6).
- The palatine processes of the maxilla (11) and the horizontal plate of the palatine bone (12) form the hard palate. Its lower surface is the roof of the mouth; its upper surface is the floor of the nasal cavity.
- In this skull the sphenoidal sinuses (26 and 27) are large, and the right one (26) has extended to the left of the midline. The pituitary fossa (28) projects down into the left sinus (27).
- The internal acoustic meatus (34) is in approximately the same vertical plane as the hypoglossal canal (33).
- The grooves for the middle meningeal vessels (1) pass upwards and backwards. The circle (45) marks the region of the pterion, and corresponds to the position shown on the outside of the skull on page 11, B31.
- The groove for the transverse sinus (38) on the occipital bone (42) extends on to the mastoid angle (37) of the parietal bone (43), and then curls downwards on the temporal bone as the groove for the sigmoid sinus (36) to reach the jugular foramen (page 17, B36).
- The external occipital protuberance (41) is not on the most posterior part of the back of the skull but some distance below and in front of it.

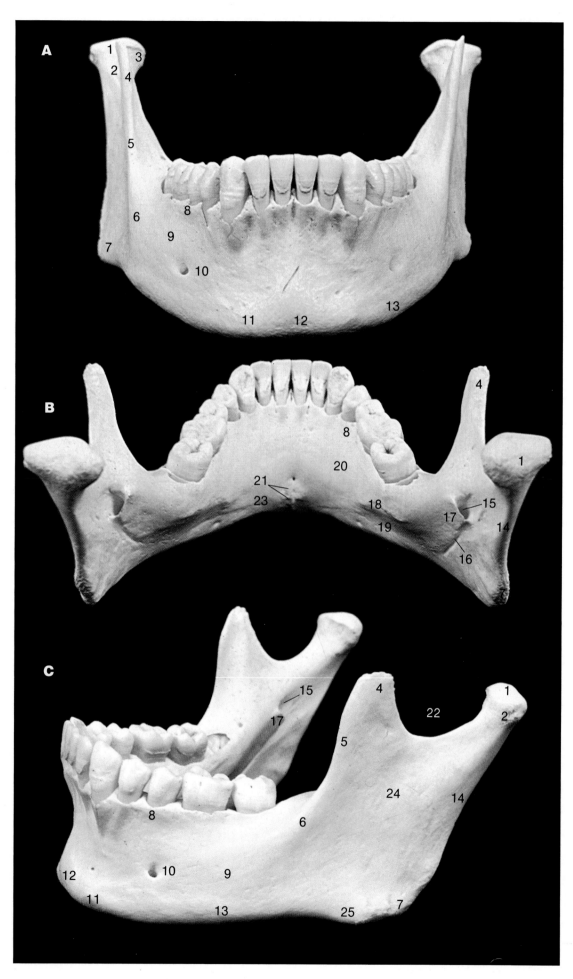

Mandible, A from the front, B from behind and above, C from the left and front

1	Head
2	Neck
3	Pterygoid fovea
4	Coronoid process
5	Anterior border of ramus
6	Oblique line
7	Angle
8	Alveolar part
9	Body
10	Mental foramen
11	Mental tubercle
12	Mental protuberance
13	Base
14	Posterior border of ramus
15	Mandibular foramen
16	Mylohyoid groove
17	Lingula
18	Mylohyoid line
19	Submandibular fossa
20	Sublingual fossa
21	Superior and inferior mental spines
22	Mandibular notch
23	Digastric fossa
24	Ramus
25	Inferior border of ramus

● The head (1) and the neck (2, including the pterygoid fovea, 3) constitute the condyle.
● The alveolar part (8) contains the sockets for the roots of the teeth.
● The base (13) is the inferior border of the body (9), and becomes continuous with the inferior border (25) of the ramus (24).
● In this mandible (also shown with muscle attachments on the next page) the third molar teeth are unerupted.

23

Mandible, A from the front, B from behind and above, C from the left and front.
Muscle attachments

Interrupted line = capsule attachment of temporomandibular joint; dotted line = limit of attachment of the oral mucous membrane

1	Temporalis
2	Masseter
3	Lateral pterygoid
4	Buccinator
5	Depressor labii inferioris
6	Depressor anguli oris
7	Platysma
8	Mentalis
9	Medial pterygoid
10	Pterygomandibular raphe and superior constrictor
11	Mylohyoid
12	Anterior belly of digastric
13	Geniohyoid
14	Genioglossus
15	Sphenomandibular ligament
16	Stylomandibular ligament

● The lateral pterygoid (A3) is attached to the pterygoid fovea on the neck of the mandible (and also to the capsule of the temporomandibular joint and the articular disc—see page 37, B).
● The medial pterygoid (B9, C9) is attached to the medial surface of the angle of the mandible, below the groove for the mylohyoid nerve.
● Masseter (C2) is attached to the lateral surface of the ramus.
● Temporalis (C1) is attached over the coronoid process, extending back as far as the deepest part of the mandibular notch and downwards over the front of the ramus almost as far as the last molar tooth. Note that in this mandible the last molar has not erupted.
● Buccinator (C4) is attached opposite the three molar teeth, at the back reaching the pterygo-mandibular raphe (C10).
● Genioglossus (B14) is attached to the upper mental spine and geniohyoid (B13) to the lower.
● Mylohyoid (11) is attached to the mylohyoid line.

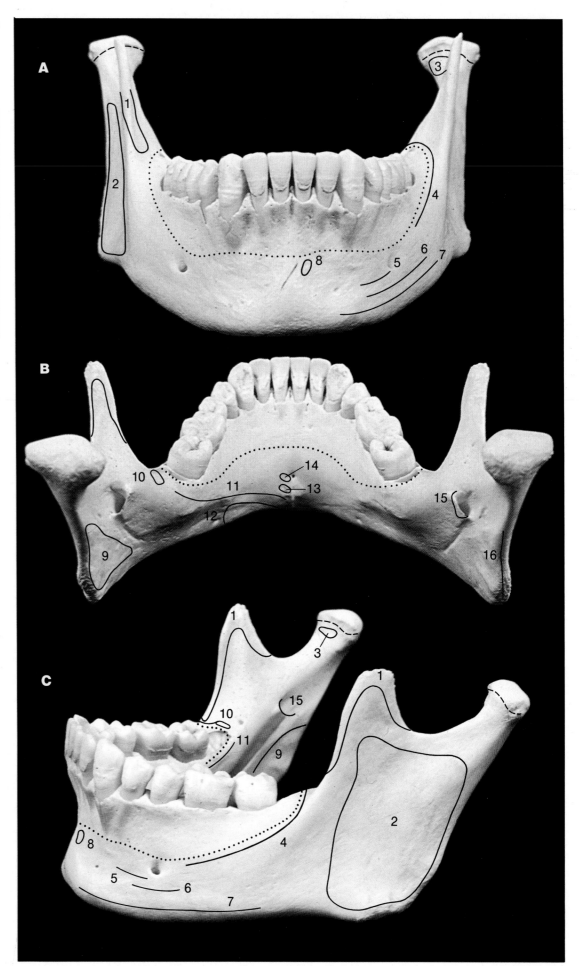

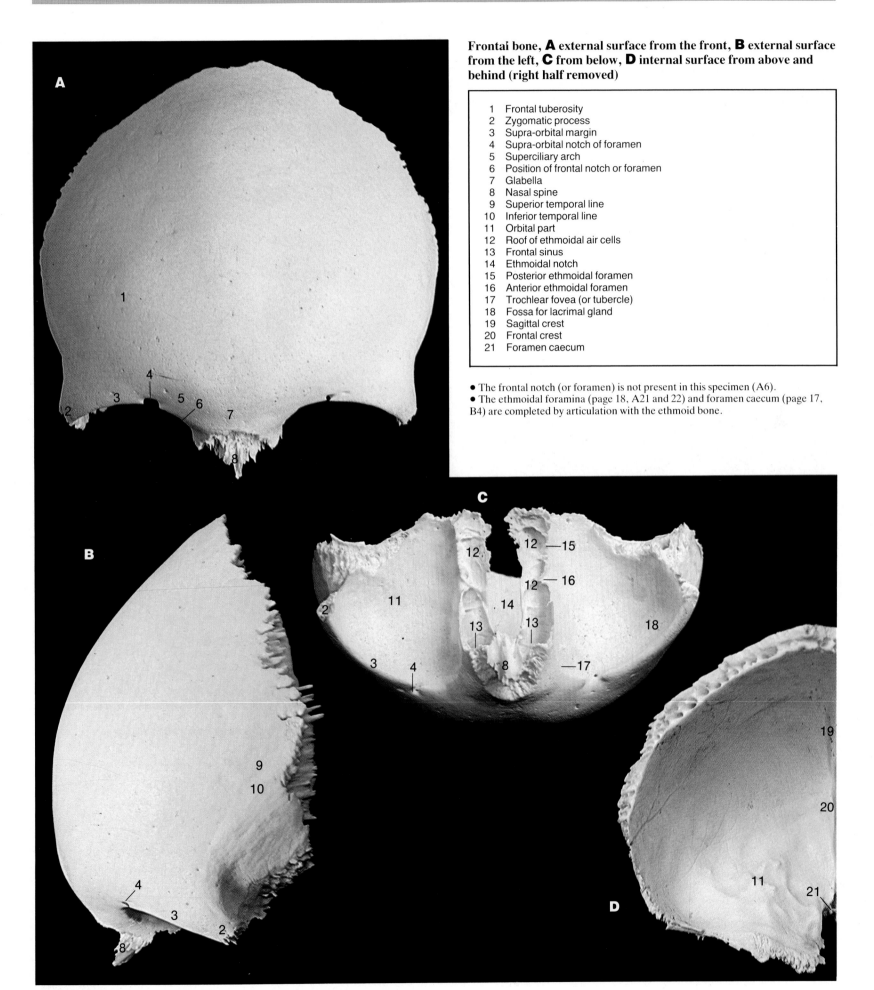

Frontal bone, A external surface from the front, B external surface from the left, C from below, D internal surface from above and behind (right half removed)

1	Frontal tuberosity
2	Zygomatic process
3	Supra-orbital margin
4	Supra-orbital notch of foramen
5	Superciliary arch
6	Position of frontal notch or foramen
7	Glabella
8	Nasal spine
9	Superior temporal line
10	Inferior temporal line
11	Orbital part
12	Roof of ethmoidal air cells
13	Frontal sinus
14	Ethmoidal notch
15	Posterior ethmoidal foramen
16	Anterior ethmoidal foramen
17	Trochlear fovea (or tubercle)
18	Fossa for lacrimal gland
19	Sagittal crest
20	Frontal crest
21	Foramen caecum

● The frontal notch (or foramen) is not present in this specimen (A6).
● The ethmoidal foramina (page 18, A21 and 22) and foramen caecum (page 17, B4) are completed by articulation with the ethmoid bone.

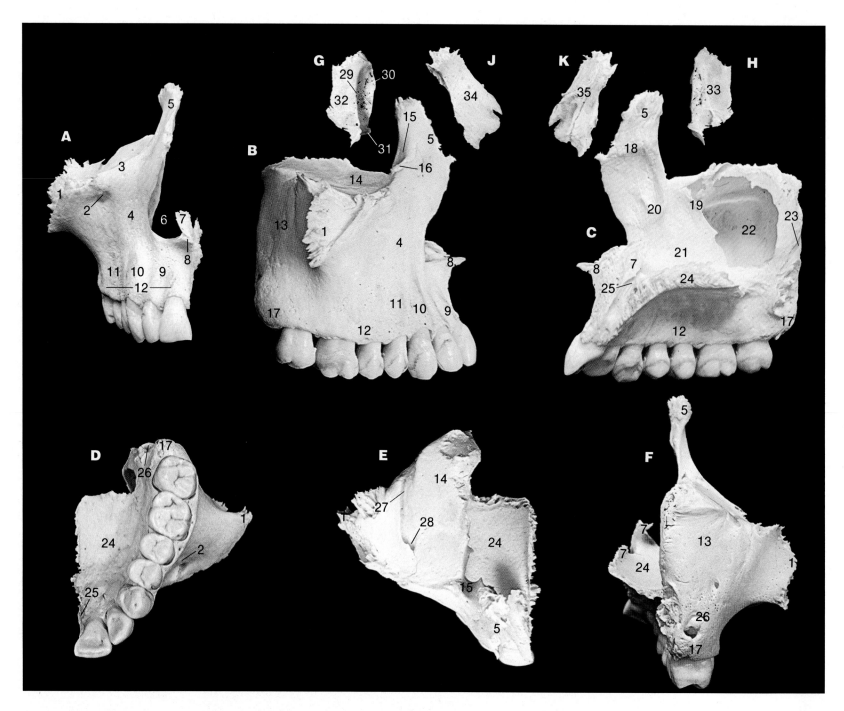

Right maxilla, A from the front, B from the lateral side, C from the medial side, D from below, E from above, F from behind

1	Zygomatic process	15	Lacrimal groove
2	Infra-orbital foramen	16	Anterior lacrimal crest
3	Infra-orbital margin	17	Tuberosity
4	Anterior surface	18	Ethmoidal crest
5	Frontal process	19	Middle meatus
6	Nasal notch	20	Conchal crest
7	Nasal crest	21	Inferior meatus
8	Anterior nasal spine	22	Maxillary hiatus and sinus
9	Incisive fossa	23	Greater palatine canal
10	Canine eminence	24	Palatine process
11	Canine fossa	25	Incisive canal
12	Alveolar process	26	Unerupted third molar tooth
13	Infratemporal surface	27	Infra-orbital groove
14	Orbital surface	28	Infra-orbital canal

Right lacrimal bone, G from the lateral side, H from the medial side

29	Posterior lacrimal crest
30	Lacrimal groove
31	Lacrimal hamulus
32	Orbital surface
33	Nasal surface

Right nasal bone, J from the lateral side, K from the medial side

34	Lateral surface and vascular foramen
35	Internal surface and groove for anterior ethmoidal nerve

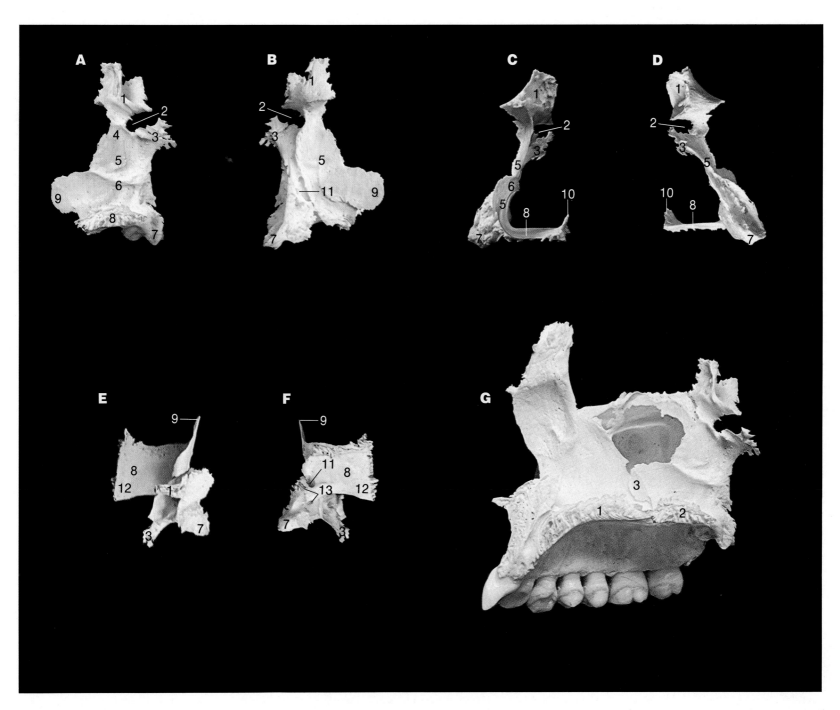

Right palatine bone, A from the medial side, B from the lateral side, C from the front, D from behind, E from above, F from below

G **Articulation of the right maxilla and the palatine bone, from the medial side**

1	Orbital process
2	Sphenopalatine notch
3	Sphenoidal process
4	Ethmoidal crest
5	Perpendicular plate
6	Conchal crest
7	Pyramidal process
8	Horizontal plate
9	Maxillary process
10	Nasal crest
11	Greater palatine groove
12	Posterior nasal spine
13	Lesser palatine canals

1	Palatine process of maxilla	
2	Horizontal plate	} of palatine
3	Maxillary process	

● Compare with C, opposite.

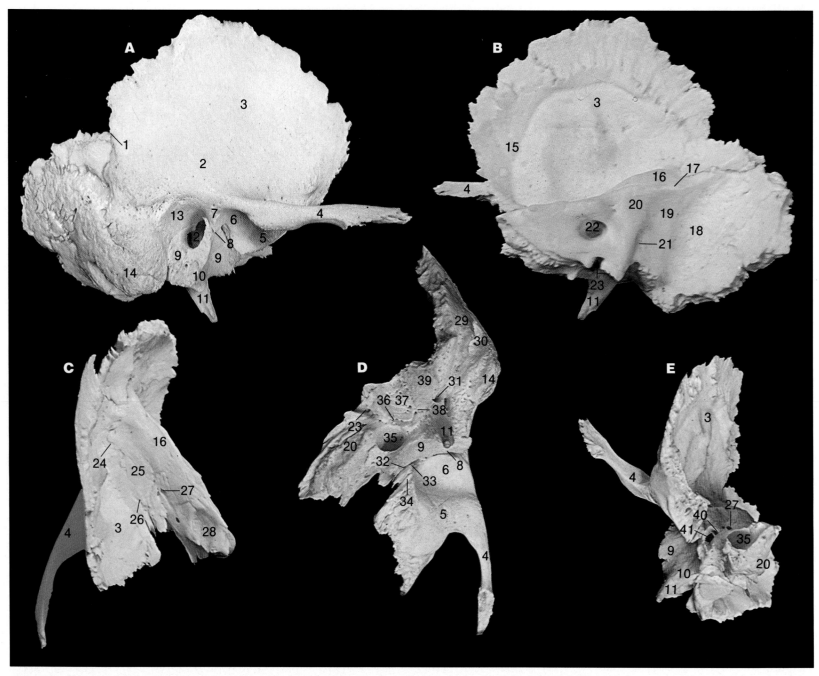

Right temporal bone, A external aspect, B internal aspect, C from above, D from below, E from the front

1	Parietal notch	16	Arcuate eminence	31	Stylomastoid foramen
2	Groove for middle temporal artery	17	Groove for superior petrosal sinus	32	Petrotympanic fissure
3	Squamous part	18	Groove for sigmoid sinus	33	Edge of tegmen tympani
4	Zygomatic process	19	Subarcuate fossa	34	Petrosquamous fissure (from below)
5	Articular tubercle	20	Petrous part	35	Carotid canal
6	Mandibular fossa	21	Aqueduct of vestibule	36	Canaliculus for tympanic branch of
7	Postglenoid tubercle	22	Internal acoustic meatus		glossopharyngeal nerve
8	Squamotympanic fissure	23	Cochlear canaliculus	37	Jugular fossa
9	Tympanic part	24	Petrosquamous fissure (from above)	38	Mastoid canaliculus for auricular branch of
10	Sheath of styloid process	25	Tegmen tympani		vagus nerve
11	Styloid process	26	Hiatus and groove for lesser petrosal nerve	39	Jugular surface
12	External acoustic meatus	27	Hiatus and groove for greater petrosal nerve	40	Canal for tensor tympani
13	Suprameatal triangle	28	Trigeminal impression on apex of petrous part	41	Auditory tube
14	Mastoid process	29	Occipital groove		
15	Grooves for branches of middle meningeal vessels	30	Mastoid notch		

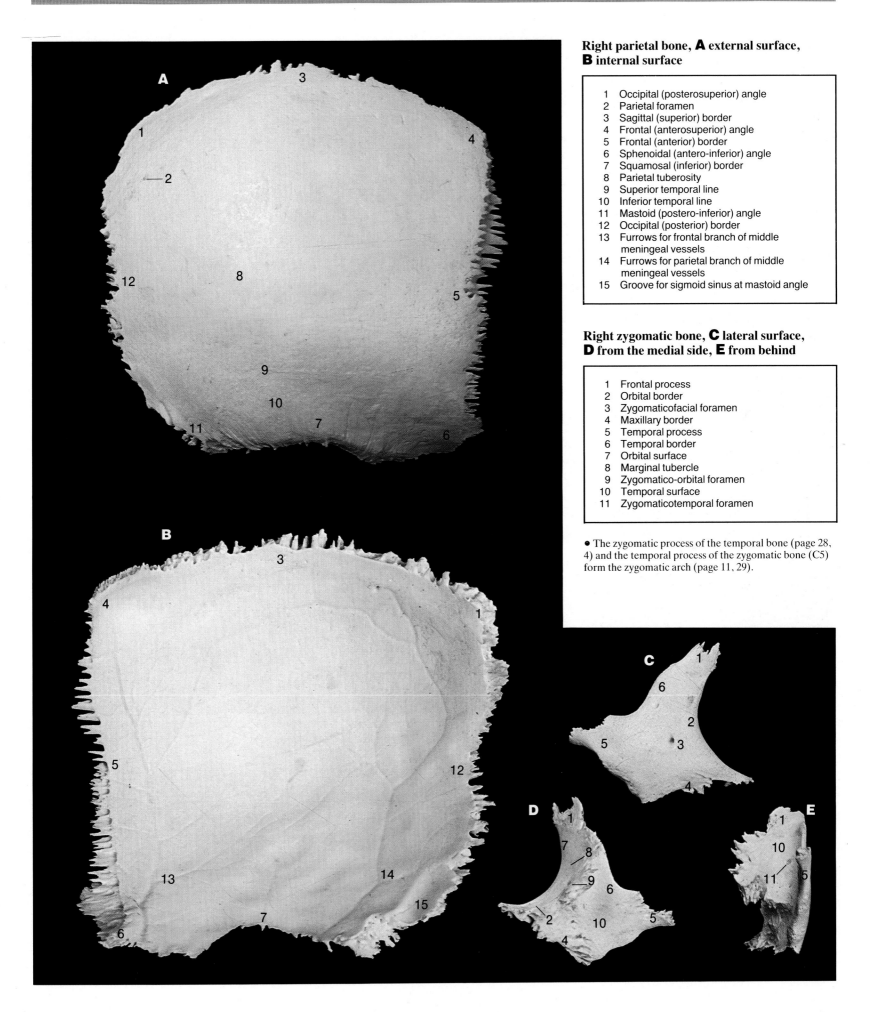

Right parietal bone, **A** external surface, **B** internal surface

1	Occipital (posterosuperior) angle
2	Parietal foramen
3	Sagittal (superior) border
4	Frontal (anterosuperior) angle
5	Frontal (anterior) border
6	Sphenoidal (antero-inferior) angle
7	Squamosal (inferior) border
8	Parietal tuberosity
9	Superior temporal line
10	Inferior temporal line
11	Mastoid (postero-inferior) angle
12	Occipital (posterior) border
13	Furrows for frontal branch of middle meningeal vessels
14	Furrows for parietal branch of middle meningeal vessels
15	Groove for sigmoid sinus at mastoid angle

Right zygomatic bone, **C** lateral surface, **D** from the medial side, **E** from behind

1	Frontal process
2	Orbital border
3	Zygomaticofacial foramen
4	Maxillary border
5	Temporal process
6	Temporal border
7	Orbital surface
8	Marginal tubercle
9	Zygomatico-orbital foramen
10	Temporal surface
11	Zygomaticotemporal foramen

● The zygomatic process of the temporal bone (page 28, 4) and the temporal process of the zygomatic bone (C5) form the zygomatic arch (page 11, 29).

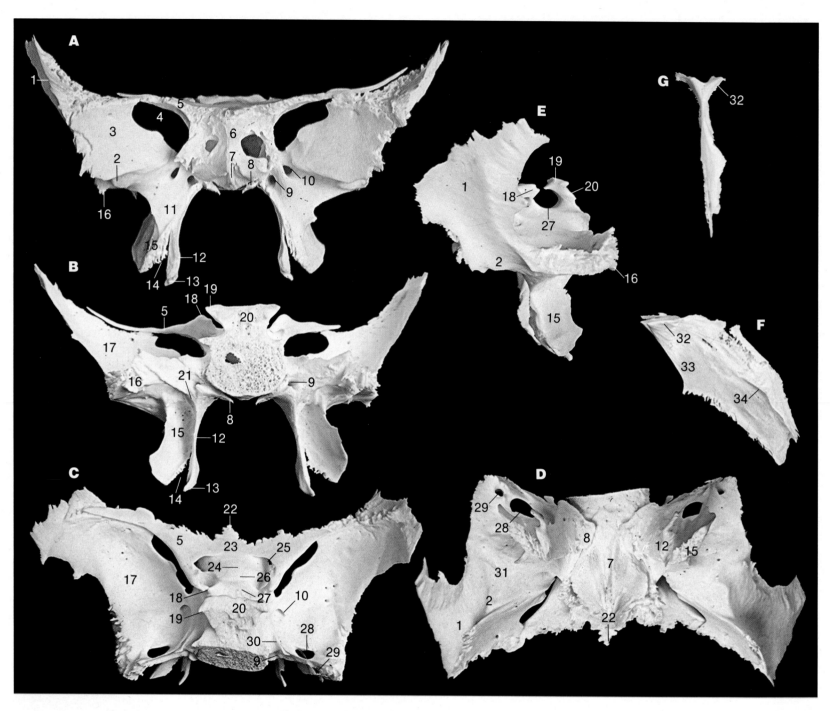

Sphenoid bone, **A** from the front, **B** from behind, **C** from above and behind, **D** from below, **E** from the left.
Vomer **F** from the right, **G** from behind

1	Temporal surface	} of greater wing
2	Infratemporal crest	
3	Orbital surface	
4	Superior orbital fissure	
5	Lesser wing	
6	Body with openings of sphenoidal sinuses	
7	Rostrum	
8	Vaginal process	
9	Pterygoid canal	
10	Foramen rotundum	
11	Pterygoid process	
12	Medial pterygoid plate	
13	Pterygoid hamulus	
14	Pterygoid notch	

15	Lateral pterygoid plate
16	Spine
17	Cerebral surface of greater wing
18	Anterior } clinoid process
19	Posterior
20	Dorsum sellae
21	Scaphoid fossa
22	Ethmoidal spine
23	Jugum
24	Prechiasmatic groove
25	Optic canal
26	Tuberculum sellae
27	Sella turcica (pituitary fossa)
28	Foramen ovale

29	Foramen spinosum
30	Carotid groove
31	Infratemporal surface of greater wing
32	Ala
33	Posterior border
34	Groove for nasopalatine nerve and vessels

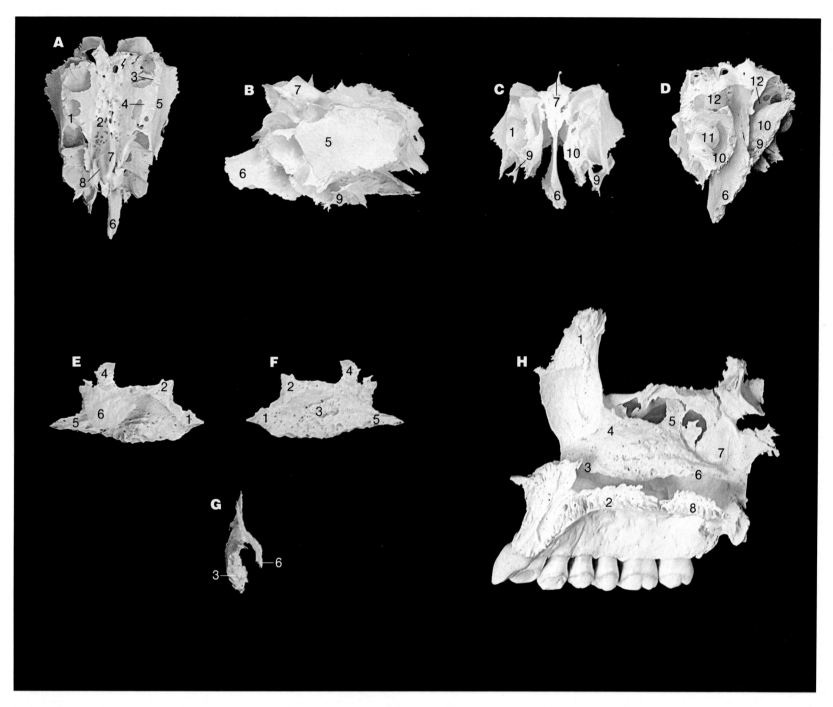

Ethmoid bone, A from above, B from the left, C from the front, D from the left, below and behind

1	Ethmoidal labyrinth (containing ethmoidal air cells)
2	Cribriform plate
3	Posterior ⎫ ethmoidal groove
4	Anterior ⎭
5	Orbital plate
6	Perpendicular plate
7	Crista galli
8	Ala of crista galli
9	Uncinate process
10	Middle nasal concha
11	Ethmoidal bulla
12	Superior nasal concha

Right inferior nasal concha, E from the lateral side, F from the medial side, G from the front

1	Anterior end
2	Lacrimal process
3	Medial surface
4	Ethmoidal process
5	Posterior end
6	Maxillary process

H Articulation of right maxilla, palatine bone and inferior nasal concha, from the medial side

1	Frontal process ⎫ of maxilla
2	Palatine process ⎭
3	Anterior end
4	Lacrimal process
5	Ethmoidal process of inferior nasal concha
6	Posterior end
7	Perpendicular ⎫ plate of palatine
8	Horizontal ⎭

● Compare with G on page 27 and C on page 26.

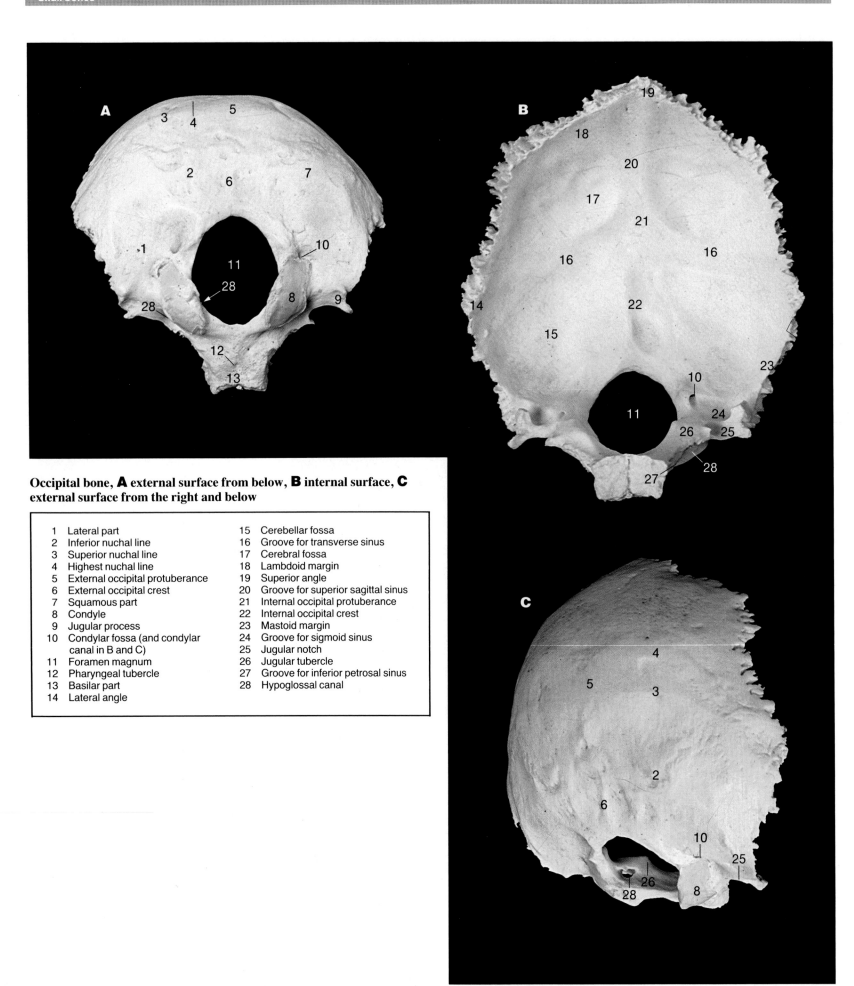

Occipital bone, **A** external surface from below, **B** internal surface, **C** external surface from the right and below

1	Lateral part	15	Cerebellar fossa
2	Inferior nuchal line	16	Groove for transverse sinus
3	Superior nuchal line	17	Cerebral fossa
4	Highest nuchal line	18	Lambdoid margin
5	External occipital protuberance	19	Superior angle
6	External occipital crest	20	Groove for superior sagittal sinus
7	Squamous part	21	Internal occipital protuberance
8	Condyle	22	Internal occipital crest
9	Jugular process	23	Mastoid margin
10	Condylar fossa (and condylar canal in B and C)	24	Groove for sigmoid sinus
11	Foramen magnum	25	Jugular notch
12	Pharyngeal tubercle	26	Jugular tubercle
13	Basilar part	27	Groove for inferior petrosal sinus
14	Lateral angle	28	Hypoglossal canal

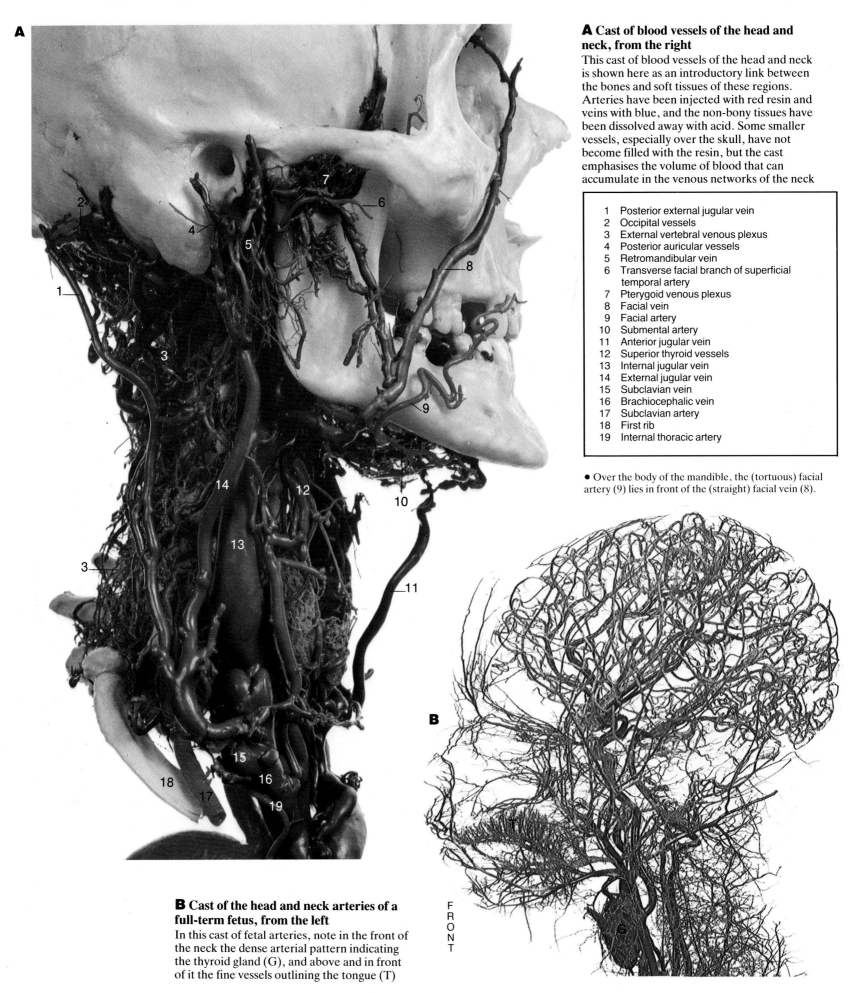

This cast of blood vessels of the head and neck is shown here as an introductory link between the bones and soft tissues of these regions. Arteries have been injected with red resin and veins with blue, and the non-bony tissues have been dissolved away with acid. Some smaller vessels, especially over the skull, have not become filled with the resin, but the cast emphasises the volume of blood that can accumulate in the venous networks of the neck

1	Posterior external jugular vein
2	Occipital vessels
3	External vertebral venous plexus
4	Posterior auricular vessels
5	Retromandibular vein
6	Transverse facial branch of superficial temporal artery
7	Pterygoid venous plexus
8	Facial vein
9	Facial artery
10	Submental artery
11	Anterior jugular vein
12	Superior thyroid vessels
13	Internal jugular vein
14	External jugular vein
15	Subclavian vein
16	Brachiocephalic vein
17	Subclavian artery
18	First rib
19	Internal thoracic artery

● Over the body of the mandible, the (tortuous) facial artery (9) lies in front of the (straight) facial vein (8).

B Cast of the head and neck arteries of a full-term fetus, from the left

In this cast of fetal arteries, note in the front of the neck the dense arterial pattern indicating the thyroid gland (G), and above and in front of it the fine vessels outlining the tongue (T)

FRONT

A Face. Superficial dissection, from the front and the right

The facial muscles are displayed but platysma, which extends from the mandible into the neck, has been removed with the skin. The largest facial muscles are orbicularis oculi (3), orbicularis oris (13) and buccinator (20). The facial artery and vein (18 and 19) pass from the neck on to the face at the lower anterior angle of the masseter muscle (23), and branches of the facial nerve (25, 24, 20 and 17) fan out from below the anterior margin of the parotid gland (27). This gland has an unusually large accessory part (22) which extends forwards over the masseter and obscures the parotid duct (which can be seen on page 36, A15)

1	Auriculotemporal nerve and superficial temporal vessels
2	Anterior branch of superficial temporal artery
3	Orbicularis oculi
4	Frontalis part of occipitofrontalis
5	Supra-orbital nerve
6	Supratrochlear nerve
7	Procerus
8	Nasalis
9	Levator labii superioris alaeque nasi
10	Levator labii superioris
11	Zygomaticus minor
12	Levator anguli oris
13	Orbicularis oris
14	Depressor labii inferioris
15	Depressor anguli oris
16	Body of mandible
17	Marginal mandibular branch of facial nerve
18	Facial artery
19	Facial vein
20	Buccinator and buccal branches of facial nerve
21	Zygomaticus major
22	Accessory parotid gland overlying parotid duct
23	Masseter
24	Zygomatic ⎫ branches of
25	Temporal ⎭ facial nerve
26	Temporalis underlying temporal fascia
27	Parotid gland
28	Great auricular nerve
29	Sternocleidomastoid

● The facial artery (18) is tortuous and lies anterior to the facial vein (19) which is straight. Both vessels pass deep to the zygomaticus muscles (21 and 11).

● The facial expression group of muscles, which includes those of the mouth, eyelids, nose and scalp (except the occipitalis part of occipitofrontalis) (see Appendix, page 338), is supplied by the facial nerve.

● The muscles of mastication, which include masseter (23), temporalis (26) and the medial and lateral pterygoids, are supplied by the mandibular branch of the trigeminal nerve.

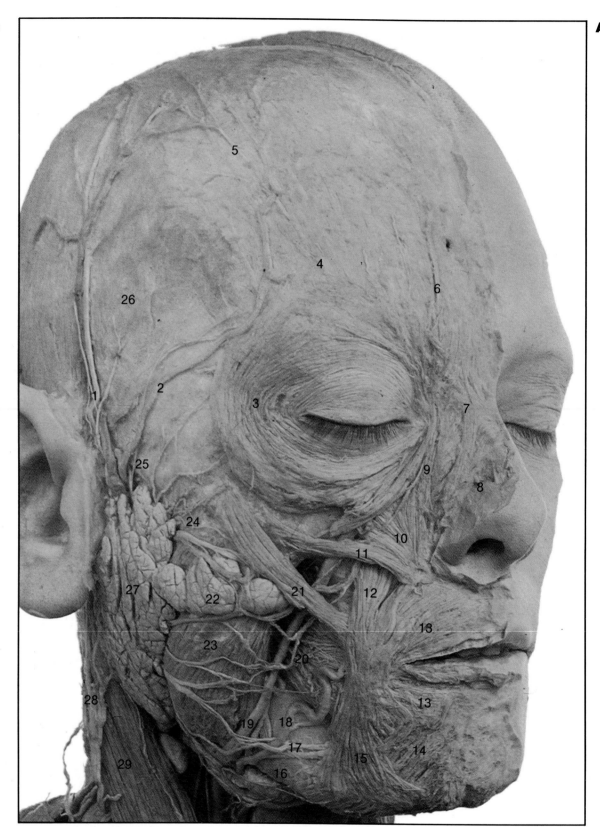

A

B Face. Surface markings on the front and left side

Compare many of the features noted here with the dissection opposite. Details of the eye are given on page 56, and of the ear on page 58. For surface markings of the neck see page 42

1	Glabella
2	Root
3	Dorsum
4	Apex
5	Septum } of external nose
6	Ala
7	External aperture
8	Alar groove
9	Frontal notch and supratrochlear nerve and vessels
10	Supra-orbital notch (or foramen), nerve and vessels
11	Lateral part of supra-orbital margin
12	Medial palpebral ligament in front of lacrimal sac
13	Infra-orbital margin
14	Infra-orbital foramen, nerve and vessels
15	Zygomatic arch
16	Head of mandible
17	Auriculotemporal nerve and superficial temporal vessels
18	Tragus
19	Parotid duct emerging from gland
20	Parotid duct turning medially at anterior border of masseter
21	Angle of mandible
22	Lower border of ramus of mandible
23	Anterior border of masseter and facial artery and vein
24	Lower border of body of mandible
25	Mental foramen, nerve and vessels
26	Lateral angle of mouth
27	Philtrum

● The external apertures of the nose (B7, the nares) are commonly called the nostrils.
● The inner end of the eyebrow overlies the supra-orbital margin (as at B9 and 10) but the outer end lies above the margin (B11).
● The pulsation of the superficial temporal artery (A1, B17) is palpable in front of the tragus of the ear (B18).
● The parotid duct (A22, B19 and 20) lies under the middle third of a line drawn from the tragus of the ear (B18) to the midpoint of the philtrum (B27).
● The pulsation of the facial artery (A18, B23) is palpable where the vessel crosses the lower border of the mandible at the anterior margin of the masseter muscle, about 2.5 cm (1 in) in front of the angle of the mandible (B21).
● The infra-orbital foramen (B14) is about 0.5 cm below the infra-orbital margin (B13).

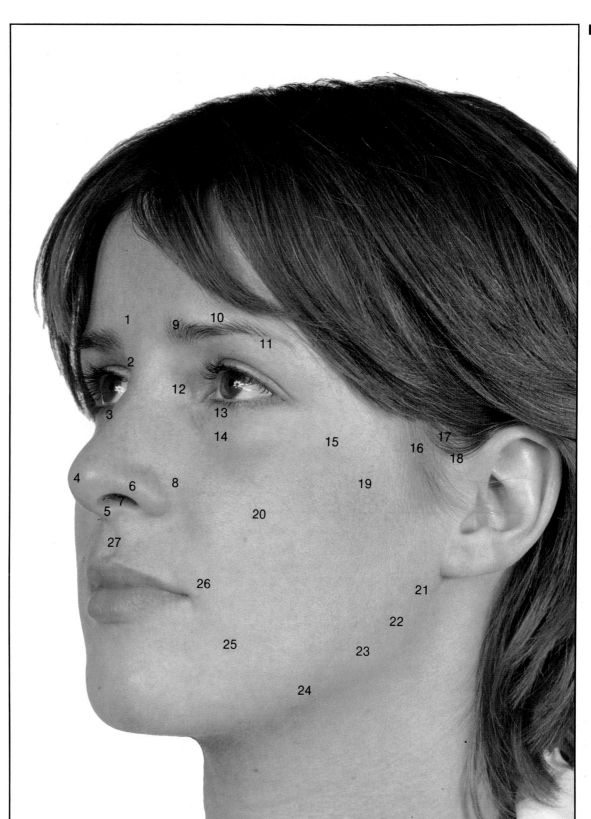

B

Right lower face and upper neck, **A** parotid and upper cervical regions, **B** submandibular region

All fascia has been removed, together with part of platysma in A and the whole of it in B. In A the various branches of the facial nerve (see note) emerge from beneath the anterior border of the parotid gland (11). The parotid duct (15) crosses the masseter muscle (16) before piercing the buccinator (18), and a large accessory parotid gland (14) lies just above the duct. In B the facial vein (17) has formed a plexus as it crosses the lower border of the mandible and overlies the submandibular gland (31). The facial artery (19) has been deep to the gland and appears at its upper border to run on to the face in front of the vein. On the face the facial vessels are superficial to buccinator (18) but deep to other facial muscles such as zygomaticus major (20)

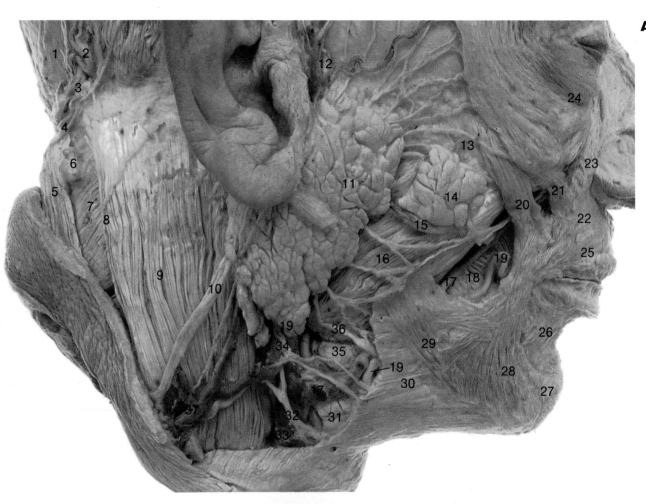

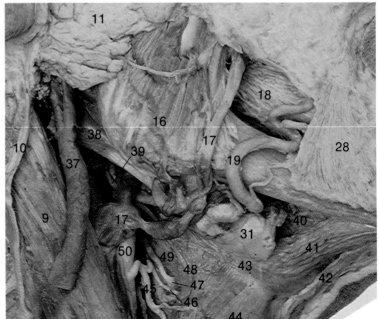

1	Occipitalis part of occipitofrontalis	26	Depressor labii inferioris
2	Occipital artery	27	Mentalis
3	Greater occipital nerve	28	Depressor anguli oris
4	Third occipital nerve	29	Risorius (aberrant)
5	Trapezius	30	Platysma
6	An occipital lymph node	31	Submandibular gland
7	Splenius capitis	32	Transverse cervical nerve
8	Lesser occipital nerve	33	Internal jugular vein
9	Sternocleidomastoid	34	Cervical branch of facial nerve
10	Great auricular nerve	35	Submandibular lymph nodes
11	Parotid gland and facial nerve branches at anterior border	36	Marginal mandibular branch of facial nerve
12	Superficial temporal vessels and auriculotemporal nerve	37	External jugular vein
13	Transverse facial vessels	38	Posterior belly of digastric
14	Accessory parotid gland	39	Hypoglossal nerve
15	Parotid duct	40	Mylohyoid
16	Masseter	41	Anterior belly of digastric
17	Facial vein	42	Anterior jugular vein
18	Buccinator	43	Greater horn of hyoid bone
19	Facial artery	44	Superior belly of omohyoid
20	Zygomaticus major	45	Superior thyroid artery
21	Zygomaticus minor	46	Superior laryngeal artery
22	Levator labii superioris	47	Internal laryngeal nerve
23	Levator labii superioris alaeque nasi	48	Thyrohyoid
24	Orbicularis oculi	49	Thyrohyoid membrane
25	Orbicularis oris	50	External carotid artery

● The risorius muscle (29) has no bony attachment. It normally passes from the parotid fascia to the skin at the angle of the mouth, but is at a lower level in this specimen.

● The five branches of the facial nerve on the face fan out from below the anterior border of the parotid gland (A11). The first three are usually multiple. Several temporal and zygomatic branches are seen between labels A12 and 13. Buccal branches overlie the masseter muscle (A16), and the marginal mandibular and cervical branches are separately labelled (A36 and 34).

● The marginal mandibular branch (A36) of the facial nerve sometimes runs just below the lower border of the mandible for part of its course instead of just above it, and so may overlie the submandibular gland (B31).

● Embedded within the parotid gland are the facial nerve (A11), the retromandibular vein, the external carotid artery and its terminal branches (maxillary and superficial temporal, page 37, B35, 9 and 24), filaments from the auriculotemporal nerve (A12) which convey to the gland secretomotor fibres from the otic ganglion (page 49, D29), and lymph nodes.

A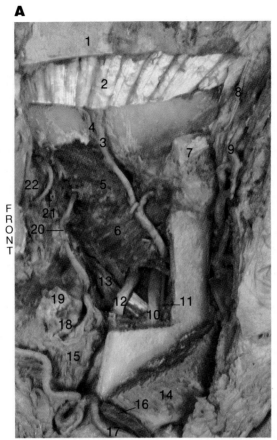

B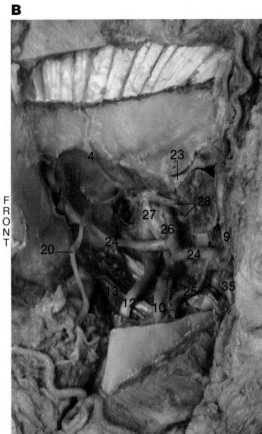

C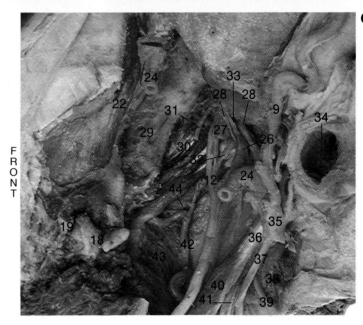

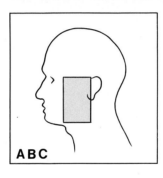

ABC

Left infratemporal fossa, **A** with the pterygoid muscles intact, **B** after removal of the lateral pterygoid, **C** after removal of the lateral and medial pterygoids

In A the zygomatic arch and the lower part of the temporalis muscle (2) with the coronoid process and part of the ramus of the mandible have been removed to display the two pterygoid muscles (5 and 6, 13), with the inferior alveolar and lingual nerves (10 and 12) emerging between the lateral and medial pterygoids, and more anteriorly the buccal nerve (20) emerging between the two heads of the lateral pterygoid (5 and 6). In B, removal of the lateral pterygoid reveals the maxillary artery (24) and two of its largest branches—the inferior alveolar (25) passing downwards to the mandibular foramen and the middle meningeal (26) passing upwards between the roots of the auriculotemporal nerve (28) to the foramen spinosum. In C (a different specimen from A and B) both pterygoid muscles and the mandible have been removed to show the lateral pterygoid plate (29), with tensor veli palatini (30) behind it and the chorda tympani (32) joining the lingual nerve (12) superficial to the muscle. The styloid process (36) is also seen with its three attached muscles—stylohyoid (37), styloglossus (40) and stylopharyngeus (41)

1 Temporal fascia
2 Temporalis
3 Deep temporal artery
4 Deep temporal nerve
5 Upper head ⎫ of lateral
6 Lower head ⎭ pterygoid
7 Capsule of temporomandibular joint
8 Auriculotemporal nerve
9 Superficial temporal artery
10 Inferior alveolar nerve
11 Nerve to mylohyoid
12 Lingual nerve
13 Medial pterygoid
14 Masseter
15 Buccinator
16 Facial vein
17 Facial artery
18 Molar glands
19 Parotid duct
20 Buccal nerve
21 Posterior superior alveolar artery
22 Infratemporal surface of maxilla
23 Articular disc
24 Maxillary artery
25 Inferior alveolar artery
26 Middle meningeal artery
27 Mandibular nerve
28 Roots of auriculotemporal nerve
29 Lateral pterygoid plate
30 Tensor veli palatini
31 Nerve to medial pterygoid
32 Chorda tympani
33 Accessory meningeal artery
34 External acoustic meatus
35 External carotid artery
36 Styloid process
37 Stylohyoid
38 Internal jugular vein
39 Accessory nerve
40 Styloglossus
41 Stylopharyngeus and glossopharyngeal nerve
42 Ascending pharyngeal artery
43 Superior constrictor of pharynx
44 Levator veli palatini

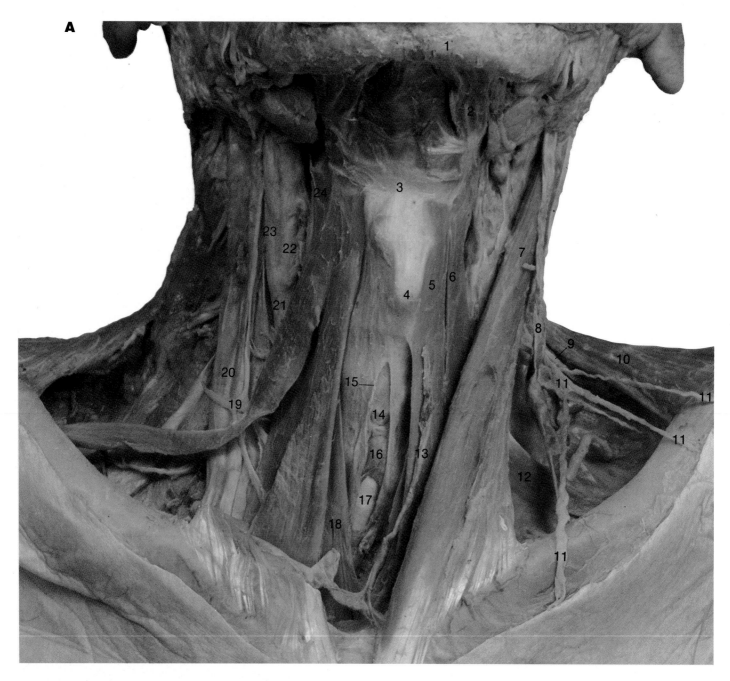

A Front of the neck. Superficial dissection

The right sternocleidomastoid, carotid sheath and the investing layer of deep cervical fascia have been removed. The pretracheal fascia (15) is being incised to show the isthmus of the thyroid gland (16)

● Midline landmarks in the neck include the body of the hyoid bone (3), the laryngeal prominence (Adam's apple, 4), the arch of the cricoid cartilage (14) and the trachea (17). Many of the features shown here can be seen again when looking at the neck from the side (pages 40 to 44).
● Sternocleidomastoid (7) completely overlaps the internal jugular vein (20) but the bifurcation of the common carotid artery (21) into the internal and external carotids (23 and 22) is just in front of the anterior border of the muscle (between labels 6 and 7, where the connective tissue of the carotid sheath is

1	Lower border of mandible	13	Anterior jugular vein
2	Anterior belly of digastric	14	Arch of cricoid cartilage
3	Hyoid bone	15	Pretracheal fascia (cut edge)
4	Laryngeal prominence (Adam's apple)	16	Isthmus of thyroid gland
5	Sternohyoid	17	Trachea
6	Superior belly of omohyoid	18	Sternothyroid
7	Sternocleidomastoid	19	Ansa cervicalis
8	External jugular vein	20	Internal jugular vein
9	Accessory nerve	21	Common carotid artery
10	Trapezius	22	External carotid artery
11	Supraclavicular nerve	23	Internal carotid artery
12	Inferior belly of omohyoid	24	Thyrohyoid

intact; on the other side the sheath has been removed).
● The site for feeling the carotid pulse (pulsation of the common carotid artery) is in the lower front part of the neck, between the anterior border of sternocleido-mastoid and the side of the larynx, as indicated on page 42, A12. In this specimen the bifurcation of the common carotid is lower than usual; it is often level with the hyoid bone (3).
● Sternohyoid (5) and the superior belly of omohyoid (6) lie superficial to sternothyroid (18) and thyrohyoid (24).

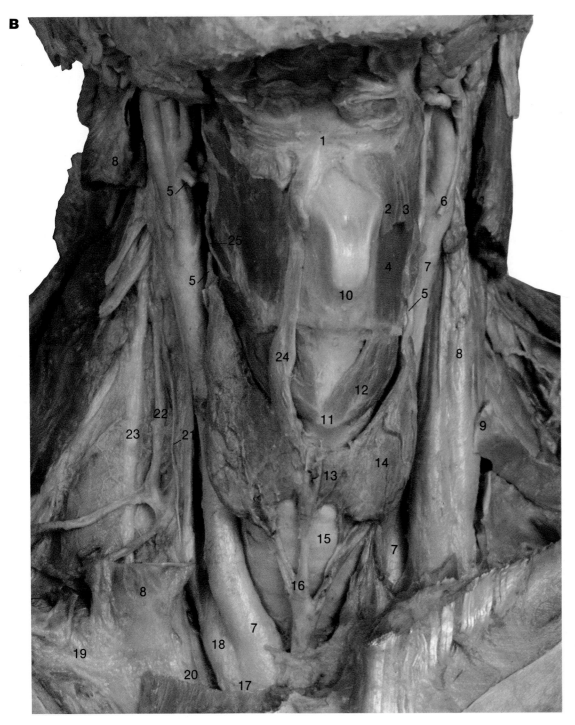

B Front of the neck. Superficial dissection

Most of both sternocleidomastoids, the right internal jugular vein (8) and part of the right clavicle have been removed. The lateral lobes of the thyroid gland (14) overlap the common carotid arteries (7), and a pyramidal lobe is present (24). The inferior thyroid veins (16) run down in front of the trachea (15). On the right side a segment of the superior thyroid artery (5) has been cut out to show the external laryngeal nerve (25) which runs down immediately behind the artery. On the left the artery has an unusually high origin

1	Body of hyoid bone
2	Sternohyoid
3	Superior belly of omohyoid
4	Thyrohyoid
5	Superior thyroid artery
6	Upper root of ansa cervicalis
7	Common carotid artery
8	Internal jugular vein
9	Tendon of omohyoid
10	Laryngeal prominence (Adam's apple)
11	Arch of cricoid cartilage
12	Cricothyroid
13	Isthmus of thyroid gland
14	Lateral lobe of thyroid gland
15	Trachea
16	Inferior thyroid veins
17	Brachiocephalic trunk
18	Subclavian artery
19	Subclavian vein
20	Right brachiocephalic vein
21	Carotid sheath (cut edge)
22	Ascending cervical artery
23	Phrenic nerve behind prevertebral fascia
24	Pyramidal lobe of thyroid gland
25	External laryngeal nerve

● The upper end of the brachiocephalic trunk (17) divides into the right common carotid and right subclavian arteries (7 and 18).
● The phrenic nerve (23) runs down over scalenus anterior under cover of the prevertebral fascia.
● The internal jugular vein (8) and the subclavian vein (19) unite (behind the sternoclavicular joint) to form the brachiocephalic vein (20).
● The tendon of omohyoid (9) is a guide to the underlying internal jugular vein (8).
● The pyramidal lobe of the thyroid gland (24) is more common on the left side than on the right, as here. It represents the remains of the thyroglossal duct from the pharynx, from which the gland develops. The duct may also form cysts or a fibrous cord; if muscle fibres are present in the latter they constitute the levator of the thyroid gland.
● Cricothyroid (12) is the only intrinsic muscle of the larynx to be seen on the outside of the larynx.
● For the back of the thyroid gland see page 50.

A Left side of the neck, from the left and front

In this superficial dissection, platysma and most of the investing layer of the deep cervical fascia have been removed. The accessory nerve (9) emerges from within the substance of sternocleidomastoid (2) to pass beneath the anterior border of trapezius (8). It must be distinguished from cervical nerves to trapezius (10) which emerge from behind sternocleidomastoid

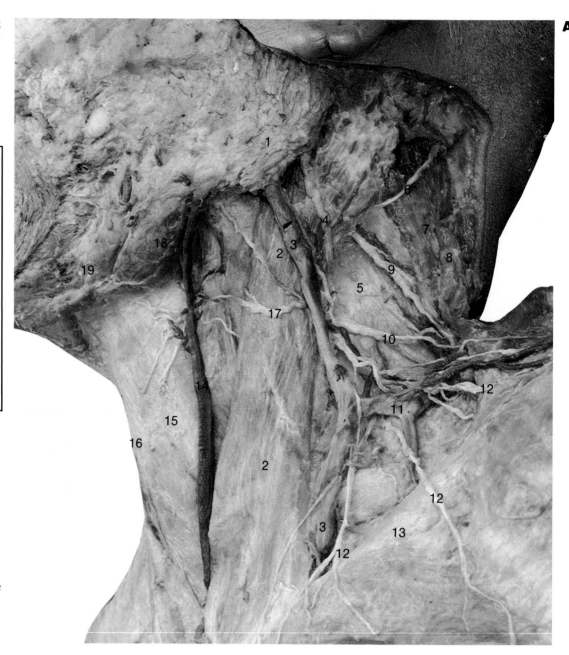

A

1	Parotid gland
2	Sternocleidomastoid
3	External jugular vein
4	Great auricular nerve
5	Prevertebral fascia overlying levator scapulae
6	Lesser occipital nerve
7	Splenius capitis
8	Trapezius
9	Accessory nerve
10	Cervical nerves to trapezius
11	Superficial cervical vein
12	Branches of supraclavicular nerve
13	Clavicle
14	Anterior jugular vein
15	Investing layer of deep cervical fascia
16	Laryngeal prominence (Adam's apple)
17	Transverse cervical nerve
18	Submandibular gland
19	Lower border of mandible

● The nerve commonly known in English as the accessory nerve (or spinal part of the accessory nerve) is in official anatomical nomenclature the ramus externus of the truncus nervi accessorii. The cells of origin are in the anterior horn of the upper five or six cervical segments of the spinal cord, and the fibres supply sternocleidomastoid and trapezius. (The cranial part of the accessory nerve, ramus internus of the truncus nervi accessorii, is derived from the nucleus ambiguus in the medulla oblongata and joins the vagus nerve to supply muscles of the soft palate and larynx.)
● The motor nerve supply of trapezius (8) is usually the accessory nerve (9), with the branches from the cervical plexus to the muscle (10) being afferent only, but in some cases the cervical branches do appear to be motor.
● The motor nerve supply of sternocleidomastoid (2) is the accessory nerve (9). The cervical branches to the muscle (10) are afferent.

B

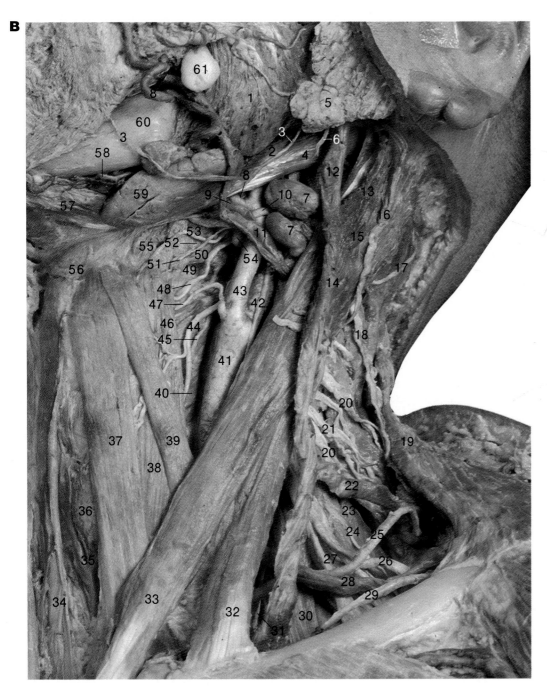

1	Masseter
2	Stylohyoid
3	Marginal mandibular branch of facial nerve
4	Posterior belly of digastric
5	Parotid gland
6	Cervical branch of facial nerve
7	Jugulodigastric lymph nodes
8	Facial artery
9	Lingual vein
10	Hypoglossal nerve
11	Facial vein
12	Posterior branch of retromandibular vein
13	Posterior auricular vein
14	External jugular vein
15	Sternocleidomastoid
16	Great auricular nerve
17	Lesser occipital nerve
18	Accessory nerve
19	Trapezius
20	Cervical nerves to trapezius
21	Supraclavicular nerve (cut upper edge)
22	Superficial cervical vein
23	Scalenus medius
24	Dorsal scapular nerve
25	Superficial cervical artery
26	Suprascapular nerve
27	Upper trunk of brachial plexus
28	Inferior belly of omohyoid
29	Suprascapular artery
30	Scalenus anterior
31	Phrenic nerve
32	Clavicular head } of sternocleidomastoid
33	Sternal head
34	Anterior jugular vein
35	Inferior thyroid vein
36	Thyroid gland
37	Sternohyoid
38	Sternothyroid
39	Superior belly of omohyoid
40	Inferior constrictor of pharynx
41	Common carotid artery
42	Internal carotid artery and superior root of ansa cervicalis
43	External carotid artery
44	Superior thyroid artery
45	External laryngeal nerve
46	Thyrohyoid
47	Superior laryngeal artery
48	Internal laryngeal nerve
49	Thyrohyoid membrane
50	Greater horn of hyoid bone
51	Nerve to thyrohyoid
52	Hyoglossus
53	Suprahyoid artery
54	Lingual artery
55	Mylohyoid
56	Body of hyoid bone
57	Anterior belly of digastric
58	Submental artery and vein
59	Submandibular gland
60	Body of mandible
61	Buccal fat pad

B Left side of the neck, from the left and front

Platysma and the deep cervical fascia have been removed. The external jugular vein (14) crosses sternocleidomastoid (15) to pass behind the clavicle near the front corner of the posterior triangle and the brachial plexus (27), and the accessory nerve (18) emerges from the muscle to cross the posterior triangle and enter trapezius (19) about 5 cm above the clavicle. The common carotid artery (41) divides into the external and internal carotids (43 and 42) below the level of the greater horn of the hyoid bone (50), and at about this same level the internal laryngeal nerve (48) and the superior laryngeal artery (47) pierce the thyrohyoid membrane (49). The lower pole of the parotid gland (5) lies behind the angle of the mandible covered by masseter (1), and the submandibular gland (59) is below the mandible and crossed by the marginal mandibular branch of the facial nerve (3)

● The external jugular vein (14) is formed by the union of the posterior branch of the retromandibular vein (12) and the posterior auricular vein (13).

● The accessory nerve (18) emerges into the posterior triangle from within the substance of sternocleidomastoid (15); the cervical nerves to trapezius (20) and other cervical plexus branches emerge from behind the muscle.

● The dorsal scapular nerve (24) emerges from scalenus medius (23); the suprascapular nerve (26) is a larger nerve arising from the upper trunk of the brachial plexus (27).

● The suprascapular artery (29) runs across the lowest part of the posterior triangle (often behind the clavicle) at a lower level than the superficial cervical artery (25).

● The external laryngeal nerve (45) is found immediately behind the superior thyroid artery (44).

● The internal laryngeal nerve (48) and the superior laryngeal artery (47, a branch of the superior thyroid) pierce the thyrohyoid membrane (49) to enter the larynx.

● Sternohyoid (37) and the superior belly of omohyoid (39) overlie sternothyroid (38) and thyrohyoid (46).

● In 20 per cent of faces, as in this specimen, the marginal mandibular branch of the facial nerve (3) arches downwards off the face for part of its course and overlies the submandibular gland (59).

A Neck. Surface markings of the front and right side

Compare many of the features noted here with the dissection opposite, and with those on pages 40 and 41

1 Mastoid process
2 Tip of transverse process of atlas
3 Sternocleidomastoid
4 External jugular vein
5 Lowest part of parotid gland
6 Angle of mandible
7 Anterior border of masseter and facial artery
8 Submandibular gland
9 Tip of greater horn of hyoid bone
10 Hypoglossal nerve
11 Internal laryngeal nerve
12 Site for palpation of common carotid artery
13 Anterior jugular vein
14 Body of hyoid bone
15 Laryngeal prominence (Adam's apple)
16 Vocal fold
17 Arch of cricoid cartilage
18 Isthmus of thyroid gland
19 Jugular notch and trachea
20 Sternal head   ⎫ of sterno-
21 Clavicular head ⎭ cleidomastoid
22 Sternoclavicular joint and union of internal jugular and subclavian veins to form brachiocephalic vein
23 Clavicle
24 Pectoralis major
25 Infraclavicular fossa and cephalic vein
26 Deltoid
27 Inferior belly of omohyoid
28 Upper trunk of brachial plexus
29 Accessory nerve passing under anterior border of trapezius
30 Accessory nerve emerging from sternocleidomastoid

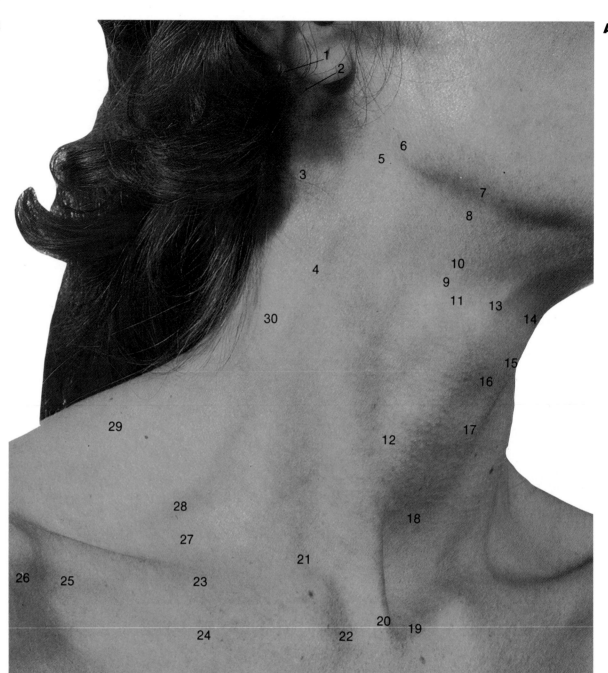

● The accessory nerve (B58) emerges from the posterior border of sternocleidomastoid (A30) at about the junction of the upper and middle thirds of the muscle and crosses the posterior triangle to pass beneath the anterior border of trapezius (A29) at a point 5 cm (2 in) above the clavicle (A23).
● The hypoglossal nerve (A10, B24) curves forwards just above the tip of the greater horn of the hyoid bone (A9), and the internal laryngeal nerve (A11, B34) runs downwards and forwards just below it.
● The pulsation of the common carotid artery (A12, B38) can be felt by backward pressure in the angle between the lower anterior border of sternocleidomastoid and the side of the larynx and trachea.
● The cricoid cartilage (A17) is about 5 cm (2 in) above the jugular notch of the manubrium of the sternum (A19).

● The lower end of the internal jugular vein (B42) lies behind the interval between the sternal (A20) and clavicular (A21) heads of sternocleidomastoid (when viewed from the front), just above the point where it joins the subclavian vein to form the brachiocephalic vein (A22).
● The external jugular vein (A4) passes obliquely downwards and backwards over the upper part of sternocleidomastoid (A3), and then crosses the posterior triangle to enter the subclavian vein below and behind the clavicle (near the label 23).
● The uppermost part of the brachial plexus (A28, B49) can be felt as a cord-like structure in the lower part of the posterior triangle.

B Right side of the neck. Deep dissection

Parts of the mandible, the parotid and submandibular glands, mylohyoid and sternocleidomastoid have been removed. Key features of this dissection are the posterior belly of digastric (64) and the posterior border of hyoglossus (18). For further dissection of this specimen see page 44

1	Auriculotemporal nerve
2	Superficial temporal artery
3	Capsule of temporomandibular joint
4	Zygomatic arch
5	Temporalis
6	Ramus of mandible
7	Buccinator
8	Molar glands
9	Parotid duct
10	Facial artery
11	Inferior alveolar nerve
12	Nerve to mylohyoid
13	Styloglossus
14	Glossopharyngeal nerve
15	Ascending palatine artery
16	Stylohyoid ligament
17	Lingual nerve
18	Hyoglossus
19	Deep part of submandibular gland
20	Mylohyoid and nerve
21	Submandibular duct
22	Sublingual gland
23	Deep lingual artery
24	Hypoglossal nerve
25	Geniohyoid
26	Anterior belly of digastric and nerve
27	Hyoid bone
28	Sternohyoid
29	Superior belly of omohyoid
30	Thyrohyoid and nerve
31	Sternothyroid
32	Stylohyoid
33	Thyrohyoid membrane
34	Internal laryngeal nerve
35	Superior laryngeal artery
36	Superior thyroid artery
37	External laryngeal nerve
38	Common carotid artery
39	Superior thyroid vein
40	Lateral lobe of thyroid gland
41	Middle thyroid vein
42	Internal jugular vein
43	Upper root ⎫ of ansa cervicalis
44	Lower root ⎭
45	Inferior belly of omohyoid
46	Scalenus anterior
47	Superficial cervical artery
48	Scalenus medius
49	Ventral ramus of fifth cervical nerve
50	Roots of phrenic nerve
51	Cervical nerves to trapezius
52	Levator scapulae
53	Trapezius
54	Splenius capitis
55	Lesser occipital nerve
56	Sternocleidomastoid
57	Great auricular nerve
58	Accessory nerve
59	Sternocleidomastoid branch of occipital artery

60	Occipital artery
61	Vagus nerve
62	External carotid artery
63	Linguofacial trunk
64	Posterior belly of digastric
65	Posterior auricular artery

• The hypoglossal nerve (B24) curls forwards round the sternocleidomastoid branch (B59) of the occipital artery (B60) to run forwards into the tongue superficial to hyoglossus (B18) and deep to mylohyoid (B20).

• The lingual nerve (B17) lies superficial to hyoglossus (B18) and at this level is a flattened band rather than a typical round nerve, with the deep part of the submandibular gland (B19)

below it. The nerve crosses underneath the submandibular duct (B21), lying first lateral to the duct and then medial to it.

• Omohyoid (B29, B45) is of little functional importance, but the tendon joining the two bellies (adjacent to the label 45) is a useful landmark in dissections and operations—it overlies the lower part of the internal jugular vein (B42).

• The deep lingual artery (23) is the name given to the lingual artery distal to the anterior border of hyoglossus (18).

• The thyrohyoid membrane (33) is pierced by the internal laryngeal nerve (34) and the superior laryngeal artery (35).

• Apart from supplying muscles of the tongue, the hypoglossal nerve (24) gives branches to geniohyoid (25) and thyrohyoid (30) and forms the upper root of the ansa cervicalis (43). These three branches consist of the fibres from the first cervical nerve that have joined the hypoglossal nerve higher in the neck; they are not derived from the hypoglossal nucleus.

A

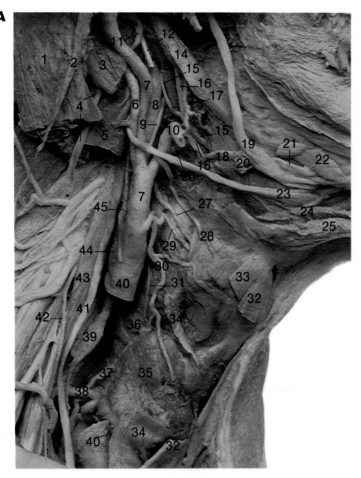

B

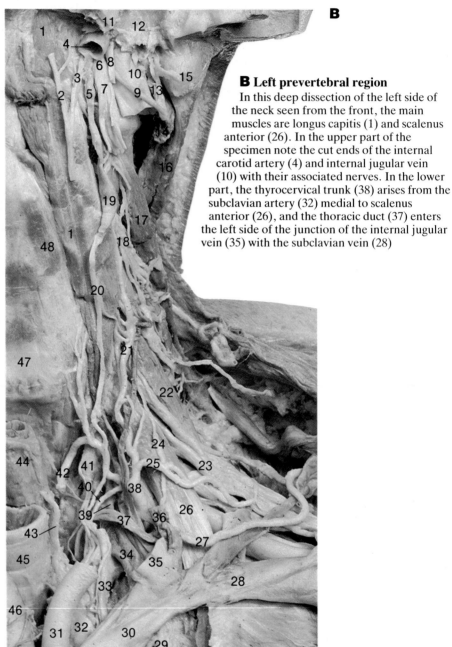

A Right side of the neck. Deep dissection

This dissection is similar to B on page 43 but after the removal of parts of the great vessels, posterior belly of digastric, stylohyoid and infrahyoid muscles. The lingual (26) and facial (10) branches of the external carotid artery (7) arise from a common trunk. The hypoglossal nerve (23) hooks forwards round the occipital artery (6), and the glossopharyngeal nerve (15) curls round stylopharyngeus (13)

B Left prevertebral region

In this deep dissection of the left side of the neck seen from the front, the main muscles are longus capitis (1) and scalenus anterior (26). In the upper part of the specimen note the cut ends of the internal carotid artery (4) and internal jugular vein (10) with their associated nerves. In the lower part, the thyrocervical trunk (38) arises from the subclavian artery (32) medial to scalenus anterior (26), and the thoracic duct (37) enters the left side of the junction of the internal jugular vein (35) with the subclavian vein (28)

1	Sternocleidomastoid	24	Mylohyoid
2	Great auricular nerve	25	Anterior belly of digastric
3	Posterior belly of digastric	26	Lingual artery
4	Accessory nerve	27	Internal laryngeal nerve
5	Internal jugular vein	28	Thyrohyoid and nerve
6	Occipital artery	29	Superior laryngeal artery
7	External carotid artery	30	Superior thyroid artery
8	Internal carotid artery	31	External laryngeal nerve
9	Ascending pharyngeal artery	32	Sternohyoid
10	Facial artery	33	Superior belly of omohyoid
11	Posterior auricular artery	34	Sternothyroid
12	Stylohyoid (cut end displaced medially)	35	Lateral lobe of thyroid gland
13	Stylopharyngeus	36	Inferior constrictor
14	Styloglossus	37	Recurrent laryngeal nerve
15	Glossopharyngeal nerve	38	Inferior thyroid artery
16	Stylohyoid ligament	39	Middle cervical sympathetic ganglion
17	Ascending palatine artery	40	Common carotid artery
18	Hyoglossus	41	Vagus nerve
19	Lingual nerve	42	Phrenic nerve
20	Submandibular ganglion	43	Scalenus anterior
21	Submandibular duct	44	Carotid sinus
22	Sublingual gland	45	Upper root of ansa cervicalis
23	Hypoglossal nerve		

● The glossopharyngeal nerve (A15) passes downwards and forwards, curling round the lateral side of stylopharyngeus (A13).
● The vagus nerve (A41) runs straight downwards between the internal jugular vein (A5) laterally and the internal (A8) and common carotid (A40) arteries medially.
● The accessory nerve (A4) passes downwards and backwards behind the posterior belly of digastric (A3) and (usually) in front of the internal jugular vein (A5) before entering sternocleidomastoid (A1).
● The hypoglossal nerve (A23) passes forwards by hooking underneath the sternocleidomastoid branch of the occipital artery (A6); this unlabelled branch overlies the cut end of the internal jugular vein (A5).
● Lying superficial to hyoglossus (A18) are, in order from above downwards, the lingual nerve (A19) with the attached submandibular ganglion (A20), the submandibular duct (A21) and the hypoglossal nerve (A23).
● Passing deep to the posterior border of hyoglossus (A18), in order from above downwards, are the glossopharyngeal nerve (A15), the stylohyoid ligament (A16) and the lingual artery (A26).
● The removal of parts of the sternohyoid (A32), omohyoid (A33) and sternothyroid (A34) displays the lateral lobe of the thyroid gland (A35). Note the inferior thyroid artery (A38) behind the lower part of the lobe, with the recurrent laryngeal nerve (A37) passing deep to this looping vessel to enter the pharynx beneath the inferior constrictor (A36). The nerve may lie behind or in front of the artery or pass between branches of it.

1 Longus capitis
2 Ascending pharyngeal artery
3 Meningeal branch of ascending pharyngeal artery
4 Internal carotid artery
5 Internal carotid nerve
6 Vagus nerve
7 Inferior vagal ganglion
8 Glossopharyngeal nerve
9 Accessory nerve
10 Internal jugular vein
11 Spine of sphenoid bone
12 Tympanic part of temporal bone
13 Occipital artery
14 Posterior belly of digastric
15 Mastoid process
16 Sternocleidomastoid
17 Levator scapulae
18 Ventral ramus of third cervical nerve
19 Superior cervical ganglion
20 Sympathetic trunk
21 Ascending cervical artery and vein
22 Scalenus medius
23 Upper trunk of brachial plexus
24 Phrenic nerve
25 Superficial cervical artery
26 Scalenus anterior
27 Suprascapular artery
28 Subclavian vein
29 Internal thoracic artery
30 Left brachiocephalic vein
31 Left common carotid artery
32 Left subclavian artery
33 Vagus nerve
34 Vertebral vein
35 Internal jugular vein
36 Jugular lymphatic trunk
37 Thoracic duct
38 Thyrocervical trunk
39 Vertebral artery
40 A large oesophageal branch of inferior thyroid artery
41 Middle cervical ganglion
42 Inferior thyroid artery
43 Recurrent laryngeal nerve
44 Oesophagus
45 Trachea
46 Brachiocephalic trunk
47 Anterior longitudinal ligament
48 Longus colli

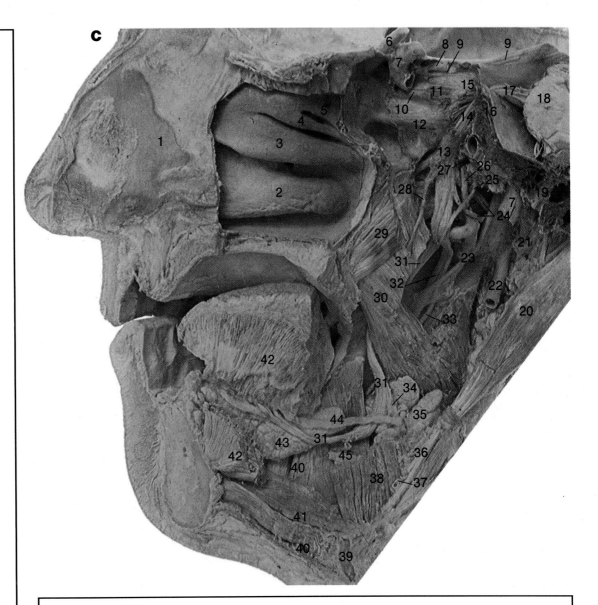

C Right trigeminal nerve branches, from the left

This dissection of right-sided structures (in a sagittal section of the head) is seen from the left side after removal of part of the base of the skull (mainly the petrous part of the temporal bone), so giving an unusual view of the medial or deep aspect of the ophthalmic (11), maxillary (12) and mandibular (13) branches of the trigeminal nerve (17) which are usually seen and dissected only from their lateral sides. Part of the medial pterygoid (30) has been cut away to show the lingual nerve (31) lying in front of the inferior alveolar nerve (32); compare with the lateral view of these structures on page 37, 10 and 12. In the mouth, where much of the tongue has been removed, the lingual nerve (31) is seen curling under the submandibular duct (44). The cut ends of the hypoglossal nerve (45) and lingual artery (37) are separated by hyoglossus (38)

1 Nasal septum
2 Inferior
3 Middle
4 Superior } nasal concha
5 Supreme
6 Optic nerve
7 Internal carotid artery
8 Oculomotor nerve
9 Trochlear nerve
10 Abducent nerve
11 Ophthalmic } branches of
12 Maxillary } trigeminal
13 Mandibular } nerve
14 Motor root of trigeminal nerve
15 Trigeminal ganglion
16 Petrous part of temporal bone
17 Trigeminal nerve
18 Pons
19 Jugular bulb
20 Posterior belly of digastric
21 Parotid gland
22 External carotid artery
23 Sphenomandibular ligament and maxillary artery
24 Roots of auriculotemporal nerve
25 Chorda tympani
26 Middle meningeal artery
27 Marker in auditory tube
28 Nerve to medial pterygoid
29 Tensor veli palatini
30 Medial pterygoid
31 Lingual nerve
32 Inferior alveolar nerve
33 Nerve to mylohyoid
34 Submandibular ganglion
35 Submandibular gland
36 Stylohyoid ligament
37 Lingual artery
38 Hyoglossus
39 Body of hyoid bone
40 Mylohyoid
41 Geniohyoid
42 Genioglossus
43 Sublingual gland
44 Submandibular duct
45 Hypoglossal nerve

● The occasional supreme (highest) nasal concha (5) is present in this specimen.
● The chorda tympani (25) leaves the skull through the petrotympanic fissure and joins the posterior aspect of the lingual nerve (31) about 2 cm below the skull.
● The right cavernous sinus has been opened up from the medial side, so revealing from this aspect the nerves that lie in the sinus—the ophthalmic (11), maxillary (12), oculomotor (8), trochlear (9) and abducent (10).
● The lower end of the lingual nerve (31, in the mouth) is seen hooking under the submandibular duct (44), lying first lateral to the duct and then medial to it.

● The mandibular nerve (13) is labelled just after it has passed through the foramen ovale and where it divides into its various branches. Note the inferior alveolar nerve (32) entering the mandibular foramen after giving off the nerve to mylohyoid (33), with the lingual nerve (31) anterior to it and being joined by the chorda tympani (25).
● The middle meningeal artery (26) runs upwards between the two roots of the auriculotemporal nerve (24) to reach the foramen spinosum.

A

A Right half of the head, in sagittal section, from the left

The section has been cut slightly to the left of the midline and shows the right half of the head with the nasal septum intact. The hard palate (31) forms the roof of the mouth and the floor of the nose, and is a little below the level of the foramen magnum (17). The pons (14), medulla oblongata (16) and cerebellum (11) are on approximately the same level as the nose. The inlet of the larynx (23) is below and behind the epiglottis (26), in the front of the laryngeal part of the pharynx (22)

1	Left frontal sinus
2	Left ethmoidal air cells
3	Falx cerebri
4	Medial surface of right cerebral hemisphere
5	Anterior cerebral artery
6	Corpus callosum
7	Arachnoid granulations
8	Superior sagittal sinus
9	Tentorium cerebelli
10	Straight sinus
11	Cerebellum
12	Great cerebral vein
13	Midbrain
14	Pons
15	Fourth ventricle
16	Medulla oblongata
17	Margin of foramen magnum
18	Cerebellomedullary cistern (cisterna magna)
19	Posterior arch of atlas
20	Spinal cord
21	Intervertebral disc between axis and third cervical vertebra
22	Laryngeal part of pharynx
23	Inlet of larynx
24	Thyroid cartilage
25	Hyoid bone
26	Epiglottis
27	Vallecula
28	Oral part of pharynx
29	Tongue
30	Mandible
31	Hard palate
32	Soft palate
33	Nasopharynx
34	Dens of axis
35	Anterior arch of atlas
36	Pharyngeal tonsil
37	Opening of auditory tube
38	Choana (posterior nasal aperture)
39	Nasal septum
40	Sphenoidal sinus
41	Pituitary gland
42	Optic chiasma

• The falx cerebri (3) separates the two cerebral hemispheres. The tentorium cerebelli (9) separates the posterior parts of the cerebral hemispheres from the cerebellum (11).
• The hard palate (31, floor of the nose, roof of the mouth) lies in approximately the same horizontal plane as the foramen magnum (17).

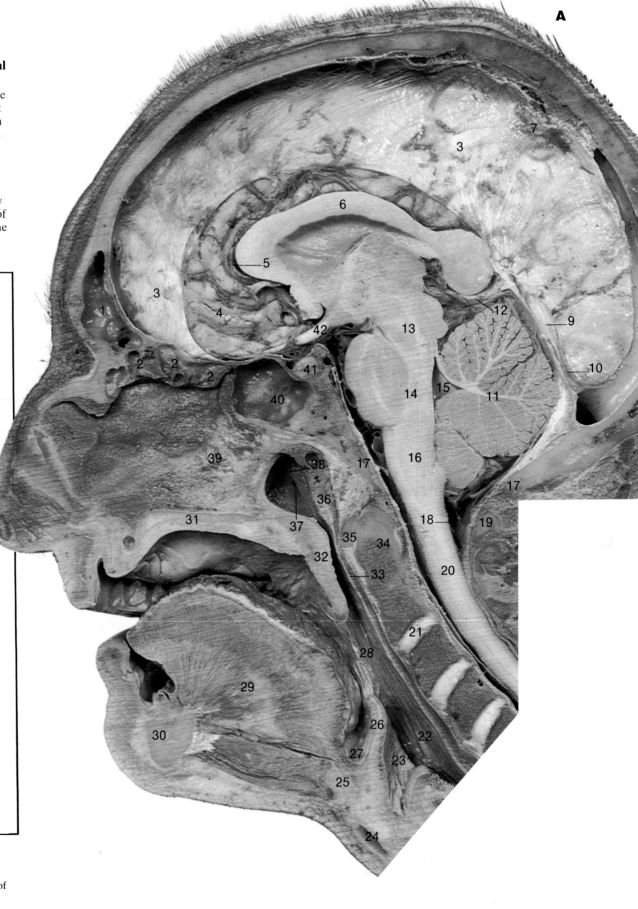

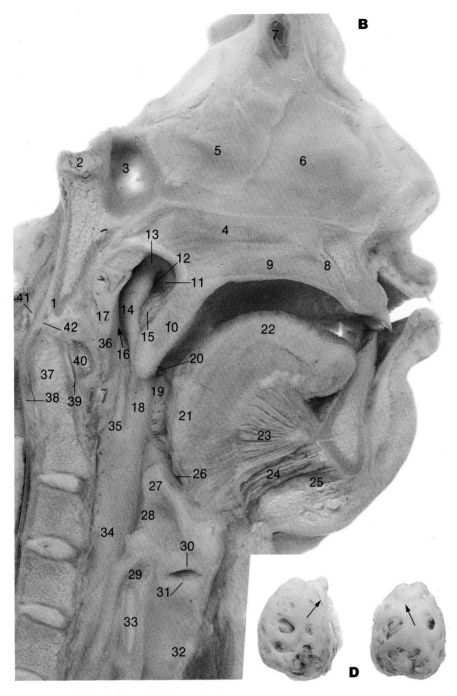

Nose, mouth, pharynx and larynx in sagittal section, from the right, B with the nasal septum intact, C with the nasal septum removed

Removal of the nasal septum (B4 to 6) reveals the superior, middle and inferior nasal conchae (C47, 49 and 51) on the lateral wall of the left half of the nasal cavity. The auditory tube (B12) opens into the upper part of the nasal part of the pharynx (B36). The palatoglossal folds (B20) form the boundary between the mouth (beneath the palate, B9 and 10) and the oral part of the pharynx (B35). The palatine tonsils lie between the palatoglossal and palatopharyngeal folds (B20 and 18)

1	Anterior margin of foramen magnum	27	Epiglottis
2	Pituitary gland	28	Aryepiglottic fold
3	Left sphenoidal sinus	29	Arytenoid cartilage
4	Vomer	30	Vestibular fold
5	Perpendicular plate of ethmoid } nasal septum	31	Vocal fold
6	Septal cartilage }	32	Arch } of cricoid
7	Frontal sinus	33	Lamina } cartilage
8	Incisive canal	34	Laryngeal } part
9	Hard palate	35	Oral } of
10	Soft palate	36	Nasal } pharynx
11	Salpingopalatal fold	37	Dens of axis
12	Opening of auditory tube	38	Transverse ligament of atlas
13	Tubal elevation	39	Median atlanto-axial joint
14	Salpingopharyngeal fold	40	Anterior arch of atlas
15	Levator elevation	41	Tectorial membrane
16	Pharyngeal recess	42	Apical ligament of dens
17	Pharyngeal tonsil	43	Intercavernous venous sinus
18	Palatopharyngeal fold	44	Optic nerve
19	Palatine tonsil	45	Right sphenoidal sinus
20	Palatoglossal fold	46	Spheno-ethmoidal recess
21	Pharyngeal } part of dorsum	47	Superior nasal concha
22	Oral } of tongue	48	Superior meatus
23	Genioglossus	49	Middle nasal concha
24	Geniohyoid	50	Middle meatus
25	Mylohyoid	51	Inferior nasal concha
26	Vallecula	52	Inferior meatus
		53	Atrium
		54	Vestibule

● The palatoglossal folds (20) form the boundary between the mouth and the oral part of the pharynx (35). The (palatine) tonsils (19) which lie between the palatoglossal (20) and palatopharyngeal folds (18) are therefore in the oral part of the pharynx, not in the mouth.
● In B the cricoid cartilage (32, 33) is lying at a higher level than normal (opposite the fourth and fifth cervical vertebrae, instead of the sixth).
● In C, the sphenoidal air sinuses (3, 45) are large, and both have extended across the midline.
● The sphenopalatine artery (the termination of the maxillary artery), supplying much of the lateral wall of the nose and nasal septum, enters the nasal cavity through the sphenopalatine foramen (page 18, B19) which lies immediately behind the posterior end of the middle nasal concha.

D Palatine tonsils

The pits on the medial surfaces of these operation specimens from a child aged 14 years are the openings of the tonsillar crypts. The arrows indicate the intratonsillar clefts (the remains of the embryonic second pharyngeal pouch)

● The palatine tonsils (commonly called simply 'the tonsils', B19) are masses of lymphoid tissue that are frequently enlarged in childhood but become much reduced in size in later life. Together with the lymphoid tissue in the posterior part of the tongue (lingual tonsil, B21) and in the posterior wall of the nasopharynx (pharyngeal tonsil, B17), they form a protective 'ring' of lymphoid tissue at the upper end of the respiratory and alimentary tracts.

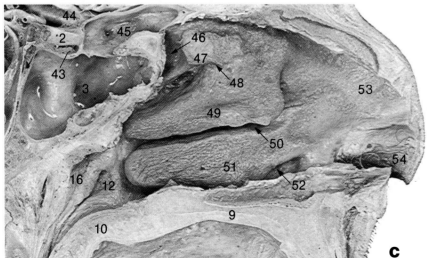

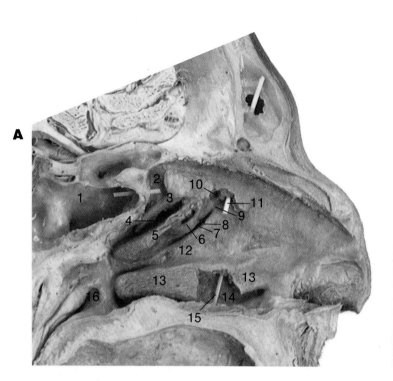

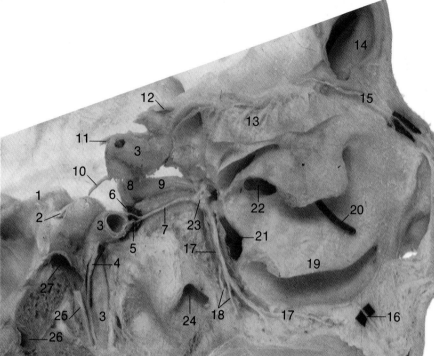

A Lateral wall of the left nasal cavity

The middle nasal concha (5) and part of the inferior concha (13) have been removed, and markers have been placed in the openings of the sphenoidal sinus (1), frontal sinus (11) and nasolacrimal duct (15)

1	Left sphenoidal sinus (marker in opening)
2	Spheno-ethmoidal recess
3	Superior nasal concha
4	Superior meatus
5	Cut edge of middle nasal concha
6	Ethmoidal bulla and opening of middle ethmoidal air cells
7	Semilunar hiatus
8	Marker in opening of maxillary sinus
9	Ethmoidal infundibulum
10	Opening of anterior ethmoidal air cells
11	Marker in frontonasal duct (opening of frontal sinus)
12	Middle meatus
13	Inferior nasal concha
14	Inferior meatus
15	Marker in opening of nasolacrimal duct
16	Opening of auditory tube

● The sites of the various openings into the different parts of the nasal cavity (referred to in the five notes below) can be summarized as follows:

Into the spheno-ethmoidal recess: the sphenoidal sinus
Into the superior meatus: the posterior ethmoidal air cells.
Into the middle meatus: the middle and anterior ethmoidal air cells and the maxillary sinus.
Into the inferior meatus: the nasolacrimal duct.

B Left nasal cavity and pterygopalatine ganglion, from the right

Behind the nasal cavity the perpendicular plate of the palatine bone (page 18, B22) has been removed to open up the greater palatine canal containing the greater palatine nerve and vessels (17). The left sphenoidal sinus has been dissected away to show the nerve of the pterygoid canal (7); the canal is below the floor of the sinus in the body of the sphenoid bone (page 30, 9)

● The olfactory area of the nasal mucosa occupies the mucosa overlying the superior nasal concha (A3), the corresponding part of the septum and the adjacent part of the roof of the nose.
● The nerve of the pterygoid canal (B7) is formed by the union of the greater petrosal nerve (B6, from the facial) and the deep petrosal nerve (B5, from the sympathetic plexus round the internal carotid artery—the internal carotid nerve, B4).

1	Arcuate eminence
2	Internal acoustic meatus and facial nerve
3	Internal carotid artery
4	Internal carotid (sympathetic) nerve
5	Deep petrosal nerve
6	Greater petrosal nerve
7	Nerve of pterygoid canal
8	Trigeminal ganglion
9	Maxillary nerve
10	Abducent nerve
11	Oculomotor nerve
12	Optic nerve
13	Olfactory nerve filaments
14	Frontal sinus and marker
15	Anterior ethmoidal nerve
16	Left nasopalatine nerve
17	Greater palatine nerve and vessels
18	Lesser palatine nerves
19	Inferior nasal concha
20	Marker emerging from frontonasal duct in middle meatus
21	Artificial opening into maxillary sinus and marker
22	Opening of maxillary sinus and marker
23	Pterygopalatine ganglion
24	Opening of auditory tube and marker
25	Inferior ganglion of vagus nerve
26	Vertebral artery
27	Internal jugular vein

● The sphenoidal sinus (A1) opens into the spheno-ethmoidal recess (A2).
● The posterior ethmoidal air cells open into the superior meatus (A4), the middle cells on or above the ethmoidal bulla (A6), in the middle meatus (A12), and the anterior cells into the infundibulum (A9) or frontonasal duct (A11), also in the middle meatus (A12).
● The frontal sinus opens into the middle meatus by the frontonasal duct (A11) or via the infundibulum (A9), which is the upward and anterior continuation of the semilunar hiatus (A7).
● The maxillary sinus opens into the semilunar hiatus (A7) of the middle meatus; occasionally there are two openings, one of which may be below the hiatus (as in the specimen on the page opposite, C14).
● The nasolacrimal duct (A15) opens into the inferior meatus (A14).

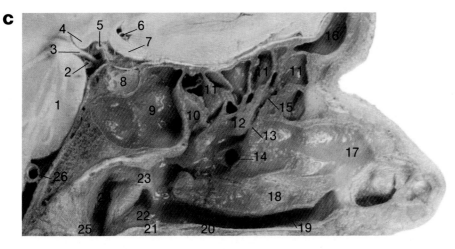

C

D

C Lateral wall of the left nasal cavity

In this sagittal section through the nose the superior and middle nasal conchae have been removed and the ethmoidal air cells (11) opened up

1	Pons	15	Ethmoidal infundibulum
2	Superior cerebellar artery	16	Frontal sinus
3	Oculomotor nerve	17	Atrium
4	Mamillary body	18	Inferior nasal concha
5	Posterior cerebral artery	19	Inferior meatus
6	Anterior cerebral artery	20	Hard palate
7	Optic nerve	21	Soft palate
8	Pituitary gland	22	Opening of auditory tube
9	Sphenoidal sinus	23	Tubal elevation
10	Spheno-ethmoidal recess	24	Pharyngeal recess
11	Ethmoidal air cells	25	Pharyngeal tonsil
12	Ethmoidal bulla	26	Basilar artery (tortuous)
13	Semilunar hiatus		
14	Opening of maxillary sinus		
	(unusually low)		

- When enlarged the lymphoid tissue of the pharyngeal tonsil constitutes the adenoids.

- The opening of the auditory tube lies over 1 cm behind the posterior end of the inferior nasal concha.

D Right trigeminal nerve, petrosal nerves and associated ganglia

Viewed from the right, much of the right side of the skull has been removed, leaving the medial sides of the right orbit (13) and maxillary sinus (22). Behind the sinus are seen the three branches of the trigeminal nerve: ophthalmic (7), maxillary (6) and mandibular (5)

1	Genicular ganglion of facial nerve	22	Medial wall of maxillary sinus and opening
2	Greater } petrosal nerve	23	Muscular branches of mandibular nerve
3	Lesser		
4	Trigeminal ganglion	24	Lower head of lateral pterygoid and lateral pterygoid plate
5	Mandibular nerve		
6	Maxillary nerve		
7	Ophthalmic nerve	25	Lingual nerve
8	Free margin of tentorium cerebelli	26	Medial pterygoid
		27	Tensor veli palatini
9	Oculomotor nerve	28	Chorda tympani
10	Frontal nerve	29	Otic ganglion
11	Nasociliary nerve	30	Facial nerve
12	Bristle in lacrimal canaliculus	31	Position of tympanic membrane
13	Medial wall of orbit		
14	Medial rectus	32	Glossopharyngeal nerve
15	Optic nerve	33	Internal carotid artery
16	Inferior rectus	34	Occipital artery
17	Ciliary ganglion	35	External carotid artery
18	Lacrimal nerve	36	Hypoglossal nerve
19	Pterygopalatine ganglion	37	Internal jugular vein and accessory nerve
20	Nerve of pterygoid canal		
21	Greater and lesser palatine nerves	38	Transverse process of atlas
		39	Rectus capitis lateralis

- The greater petrosal nerve (2) is a branch of the facial (1) and can be remembered as the nerve of tear secretion (though it also supplies nasal glands). It carries preganglionic fibres from the superior salivary nucleus (in the pons), and runs in the groove on the floor of the middle cranial fossa (page 17, 44) to enter the foramen lacerum and become the nerve of the pterygoid canal (20) which joins the pterygopalatine ganglion (19). Postganglionic fibres leave the ganglion to join the maxillary nerve and enter the orbit by the zygomatic branch which communicates with the lacrimal nerve, supplying the gland (page 56, D2).

- The lesser petrosal nerve (3), although having a communication with the facial nerve, is a branch of the glossopharyngeal nerve, being derived from the tympanic branch which supplies the mucous membrane of the middle ear by the tympanic plexus (page 58, B21). Its fibres are derived from the inferior salivary nucleus in the pons, and after leaving the middle ear and running in its groove on the floor of the middle cranial fossa (3, and page 17, 45), the nerve reaches the otic ganglion (29) via

the foramen ovale. From the ganglion secretomotor fibres join the mandibular nerve (5) to be distributed to the parotid gland by filaments from the auriculotemporal nerve.

- The chorda tympani (28) arises from the facial nerve before the latter leaves the stylomastoid foramen (30, upper leader line). It crosses the upper part of the tympanic membrane (31) underneath its mucosal covering and runs through the temporal bone to emerge from the petrotympanic fissure (page 15, 19) and join the lingual nerve (25). It carries preganglionic fibres to the submandibular ganglion (page 44, A20) for the submandibular and sublingual salivary glands, and also taste fibres for the anterior part of the tongue.

- The otic ganglion (29), which normally adheres to the deep surface of the mandibular nerve (5), has been teased off from the nerve and a black marker has been placed behind it.

A Pharynx, from behind

The back of the pharynx has been exposed by removing the vertebral column and prevertebral muscles. On the left only the uppermost parts of the main vessels and nerves have been preserved; the glossopharyngeal nerve (5) is seen winding round stylopharyngeus (31). On the right the internal carotid artery (3) has been displaced slightly laterally to show the pharyngeal branches of the glossopharyngeal and vagus nerves (15 and 16) which form the pharyngeal nerve plexus on the surface of the middle constrictor (30). On the left the accessory nerve (8) passes behind the internal jugular vein (9)—its usual relationship; on the right it runs in front of the vein, a common variation. Both pairs of parathyroid glands (21 and 22) are seen behind the lateral lobes of the thyroid gland (20)

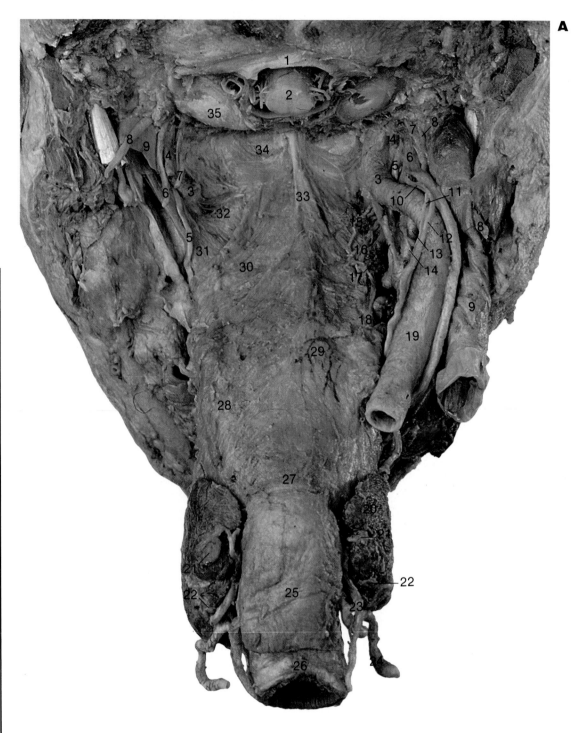

A

1	Margin of foramen magnum
2	Spinal cord
3	Internal carotid artery
4	Sympathetic trunk
5	Glossopharyngeal nerve
6	Vagus (inferior ganglion)
7	Hypoglossal nerve
8	Accessory nerve
9	Internal jugular vein
10	Superior laryngeal nerve
11	External laryngeal nerve
12	Internal laryngeal nerve
13	External carotid artery
14	Branches of glossopharyngeal and vagus nerves to carotid body and carotid sinus
15	Pharyngeal branch of glossopharyngeal nerve ⎫ pharyngeal
16	Pharyngeal branch of ⎬ plexus vagus nerve ⎭
17	Ascending pharyngeal artery
18	Tip of greater horn of hyoid bone
19	Common carotid artery
20	Lateral lobe of thyroid gland
21	Superior parathyroid gland
22	Inferior parathyroid gland
23	Recurrent laryngeal nerve
24	Inferior thyroid artery
25	Oesophagus
26	Trachea
27	Cricopharyngeal part ⎫ of inferior
28	Thyropharyngeal part ⎬ constrictor
29	Part of buccopharyngeal fascia and pharyngeal venous plexus
30	Middle constrictor
31	Stylopharyngeus
32	Superior constrictor
33	Pharyngeal raphe
34	Pharyngobasilar fascia
35	Occipital condyle

● The pharynx extends from the base of the skull to the level of the sixth cervical vertebra, and consists of nasal, oral and pharyngeal parts whose internal features (detailed below) are best seen in a sagittal section such as that on page 47, B.

● The nasal part (nasopharynx), as far down as the lower border of the soft palate, contains the openings of the auditory tubes, the pharyngeal tonsil and pharyngeal recesses, and opens anteriorly into the nasal cavity.

● The oral part, betwen the soft palate and the upper border of the epiglottis, contains the (palatine) tonsils and the palatopharyngeal arch and opens anteriorly into the mouth. The palatoglossal arch is the boundary between the mouth and the oral pharynx.

● The laryngeal part, below the upper border of the epiglottis, contains the piriform recess on either side of

the larynx, which bulges backwards into the pharynx with the laryngeal inlet below and behind the epiglottis.

● The lower end of the pharynx becomes continuous with the oesophagus, at the same level (opposite the sixth cervical vertebra) as the larynx continues as the trachea.

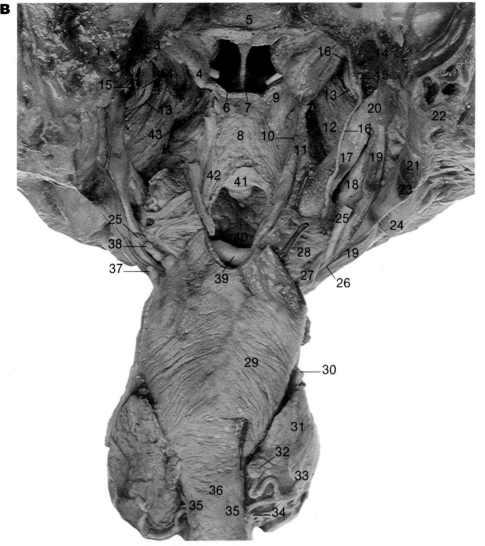

B Pharynx, from behind

By removing the upper part of the posterior pharyngeal wall, the posterior nasal apertures (6) can be seen above the back of the soft palate (8), while below it are the back of the tongue (40) and the tip of the epiglottis (39), seen through the arch formed by the two palatopharyngeus muscles (42) and the central uvula (41)

1	Sigmoid sinus	24	Angle of mandible
2	Jugular bulb	25	Hypoglossal nerve
3	Internal carotid artery	26	Nerve to thyrohyoid
4	Cartilaginous part of auditory tube (marker in opening)	27	Tip of greater horn of hyoid bone
5	Clivus	28	Middle constrictor (overlying red marker)
6	Posterior nasal aperture (choana)	29	Inferior constrictor (overlying blue marker)
7	Nasal septum (vomer)	30	Superior thyroid artery
8	Soft palate	31	Lateral lobe of thyroid gland
9	Levator veli palatini	32	Superior parathyroid gland
10	Salpingopharyngeus	33	Inferior thyroid artery
11	Superior constrictor (cut edge)	34	Recurrent laryngeal nerve
12	Medial pterygoid	35	Longitudinal ⎱ muscle of
13	Lingual nerve	36	Circular ⎰ oesophagus
14	Inferior alveolar nerve	37	Internal laryngeal nerve
15	Chorda tympani	38	Lingual artery
16	Glossopharyngeal nerve	39	Epiglottis
17	Stylopharyngeus	40	Foramen caecum in dorsum of tongue
18	Styloglossus	41	Uvula
19	Stylohyoid	42	Palatopharyngeus
20	Styloid process	43	Pterygoid hamulus
21	Posterior belly of digastric	44	Tensor veli palatini
22	Parotid gland		
23	Masseter		

• The palatopharyngeus (42) and salpingopharyngeus (10) pass downwards internal to the superior constrictor (11); the stylopharyngeus (17) passes downwards between the superior and middle constrictors (11 and 28).

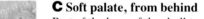

C Soft palate, from behind

Part of the base of the skull together with the pharynx and most other soft parts have been removed, leaving the central part of the soft palate (7)

1	Groove for sigmoid sinus	11	Tensor veli palatini (superficial to marker)
2	Tympanic membrane	12	Pterygoid hamulus
3	Apex of petrous part of temporal bone	13	Tendon of tensor veli palatini
4	Internal carotid artery	14	Styloid process
5	Clivus	15	Part of stylomandibular ligament
6	Vomer (nasal septum)	16	Sphenomandibular ligament
7	Soft palate	17	Angle of mandible
8	Uvula		
9	Marker in auditory tube		
10	Levator veli palatini		

• All the muscles of the pharynx and soft palate are supplied by the cranial part of the accessory nerve through the branches of the vagus that join the pharyngeal plexus, except for the stylopharyngeus which is supplied by the glossopharyngeal nerve and the tensor veli palatini by a branch from the nerve to the medial pterygoid muscle (mandibular nerve).
• Levator veli palatini (10), formerly called levator palati, is a short round muscle; tensor veli palatini (11), formerly called tensor palati, is a flat triangular muscle ending in a tendon (13) which hooks round the pterygoid hamulus (12) and then expands to become with its fellow of the opposite side the palatine aponeurosis.

51

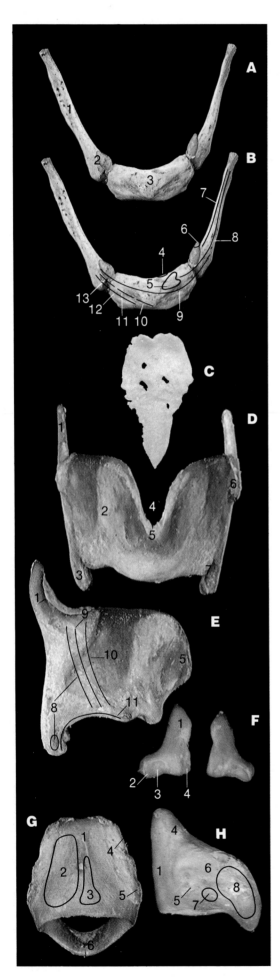

Hyoid bone, **A** from above and in front, **B** with muscle attachments

1 Greater horn
2 Lesser horn
3 Body
4 Genioglossus
5 Geniohyoid
6 Stylohyoid ligament
7 Middle constrictor
8 Hyoglossus
9 Mylohyoid
10 Sternohyoid
11 Omohyoid
12 Thyrohyoid
13 Stylohyoid

C Cartilage of the epiglottis, from the front. **D** Thyroid cartilage from the front, **E** from the right with attachments

1 Superior horn
2 Lamina
3 Inferior horn
4 Thyroid notch
5 Laryngeal prominence (Adam's apple)
6 Superior ⎱ tubercle
7 Inferior ⎰
8 Inferior constrictor
9 Sternothyroid
10 Thyrohyoid
11 Cricothyroid

F Arytenoid cartilages, from behind

1 Apex
2 Muscular process
3 Articular surface for cricoid cartilage
4 Vocal process

Cricoid cartilage and muscle attachments, **G** from behind and below, **H** from the right

1 Lamina
2 Posterior crico-arytenoid
3 Tendon of oesophagus
4 Articular surface for arytenoid cartilage
5 Articular surface for inferior horn of thyroid cartilage
6 Arch
7 Inferior constrictor
8 Cricothyroid

J Larynx, from behind

The left lamina of the thyroid cartilage has been reflected forwards and a glass rod (seen below the label 1 on the epiglottis) holds the pharynx open. Black markers underlie filaments from the recurrent and internal laryngeal nerves (7 and 10)

1 Epiglottis
2 Posterior pharyngeal wall
3 Cuneiform cartilage ⎱ in aryepi-
4 Corniculate cartilage ⎰ glottic fold
5 Transverse arytenoid muscle
6 Branch of internal laryngeal nerve
7 Branches of recurrent laryngeal nerve
8 Tendon of oesophagus
9 Circular fibres of oesophagus
10 Anastomosis between internal and recurrent laryngeal nerves
11 Cricothyroid muscle (reflected forwards with lamina of thyroid cartilage)

K Tongue and the inlet of the larynx, from above

1 Posterior wall of pharynx
2 Corniculate cartilage ⎱ in
3 Cuneiform cartilage ⎰ aryepi-glottic fold
4 Epiglottis
5 Median glosso-epiglottic fold
6 Vallecula
7 Lateral glosso-epiglottic fold
8 Pharyngeal part of dorsum of tongue
9 Foramen caecum
10 Sulcus terminalis
11 Vallate papilla
12 Fungiform papilla
13 Vestibular fold
14 Vocal fold

● The V-shaped sulcus terminalis (10), behind the row of vallate papillae (11), is not well marked in this tongue.

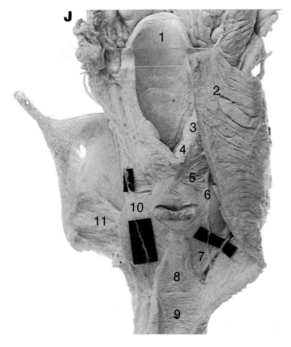

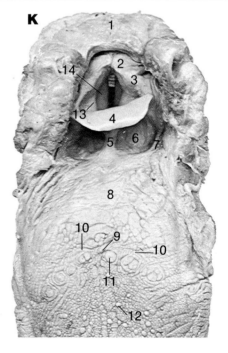

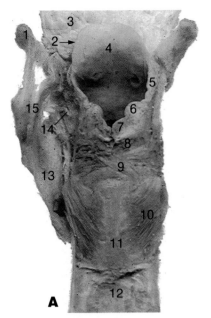

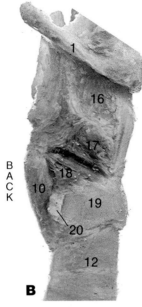

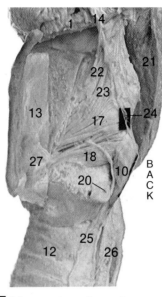

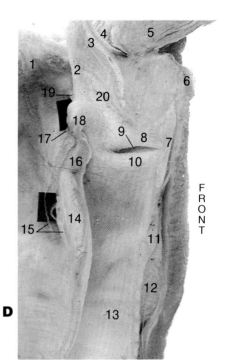

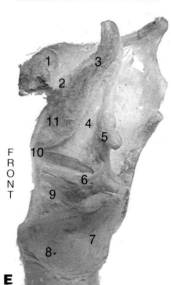

Intrinsic muscles of the larynx, A from behind, B from the right, C from the left

In B the right lamina of the thyroid cartilage has been removed, and in C part of the thyroid lamina has been turned forwards

1	Greater horn of hyoid bone
2	Vallecula
3	Dorsum of tongue
4	Epiglottis
5	Aryepiglottic fold
6	Cuneiform ⎫ cartilage
7	Corniculate ⎭
8	Transverse ⎫ arytenoid
9	Oblique ⎭ muscle
10	Posterior crico-arytenoid muscle
11	Area on lamina of cricoid cartilage for tendon of oesophagus
12	Trachea
13	Lamina of thyroid cartilage
14	Internal laryngeal nerve
15	Thyrohyoid membrane
16	Quadrangular membrane
17	Thyro-arytenoid muscle
18	Lateral crico-arytenoid muscle
19	Arch of cricoid cartilage
20	Cricothyroid joint
21	Posterior wall of pharynx
22	Aryepiglottic ⎫ muscle
23	Thyro-epiglottic ⎭
24	Anastomosis of internal and recurrent laryngeal nerves
25	Recurrent laryngeal nerve
26	Oesophagus
27	Cricothyroid muscle (reflected from cricoid attachment)

● The space between the vestibular and vocal folds is the sinus of the larynx (D9), and this is continuous with the saccule, a small pouch that extends upwards for a few millimetres between the vestibular fold and the inner surface of the thyro-arytenoid muscle (B17).

D Larynx, in sagittal section, from the right

The vocal fold (vocal cord, 10) lies below the vestibular fold (false vocal cord, 8)

1	Pharyngeal wall
2	Aryepiglottic fold and inlet of larynx
3	Epiglottis
4	Vallecula
5	Tongue
6	Body of hyoid bone
7	Lamina of thyroid cartilage
8	Vestibular fold
9	Sinus of larynx
10	Vocal fold
11	Arch of cricoid cartilage
12	Isthmus of thyroid gland
13	Trachea
14	Lamina of cricoid cartilage
15	Branches of recurrent laryngeal nerve
16	Transverse arytenoid muscle
17	Branches of internal laryngeal nerve anastomosing with recurrent laryngeal nerve
18	Corniculate cartilage and apex of arytenoid cartilage
19	Internal laryngeal nerve entering piriform recess
20	Vestibule of larynx

● The fissure between the two vestibular folds (D8) is the rima of the vestibule. The fissure between the vocal folds (vocal cords, D10) is the rima of the glottis.
● The vestibular folds are sometimes called the false vocal cords.

E Ligaments and membranes of the right side of the larynx, from the left

Most of the left side of the larynx has been removed but the whole of the cricoid cartilage remains intact

1	Hyoid bone
2	Hyo-epiglottic ligament
3	Epiglottis
4	Quadrangular membrane
5	Apex ⎫ of arytenoid
6	Vocal process ⎭ cartilage
7	Lamina ⎫ of cricoid
8	Arch ⎭ cartilage
9	Cricovocal membrane
10	Lamina of thyroid cartilage
11	Thyro-epiglottic ligament

● The intrinsic muscles of the larynx are supplied by the recurrent laryngeal nerve (C25), except the cricothyroid (page 39, B12) which is supplied by the external laryngeal nerve (page 39, B25).
● The mucous membrane of the larynx above the level of the vocal folds is supplied by the internal laryngeal nerve, and below the vocal folds by the recurrent laryngeal nerve (D17 and 15).
● The recurrent laryngeal nerve (C25) enters the larynx by passing beneath the lower border of the inferior constrictor of the pharynx, and here it lies immediately behind the cricothyroid joint (C20).
● The anterior part of the vocal fold (D10) is formed by the upper margin of the cricovocal membrane (E9), and the posterior part by the vocal process of the arytenoid cartilage (E6).
● The vestibular fold (false vocal cord, D8) is formed by the lower margin of the quadrangular membrane (E4), whose upper margin forms the aryepiglottic fold (D2, A5).
● The central (anterior) part of the cricothyroid membrane is usually known as the conus elasticus but sometimes this term is used for the cricovocal membrane.

A Cerebral dura mater, outer surface

The right half of the cranial vault has been removed to show branches of the middle meningeal vessels on the outer surface of the dura, i.e. in the extradural space. These vessels do not supply the brain

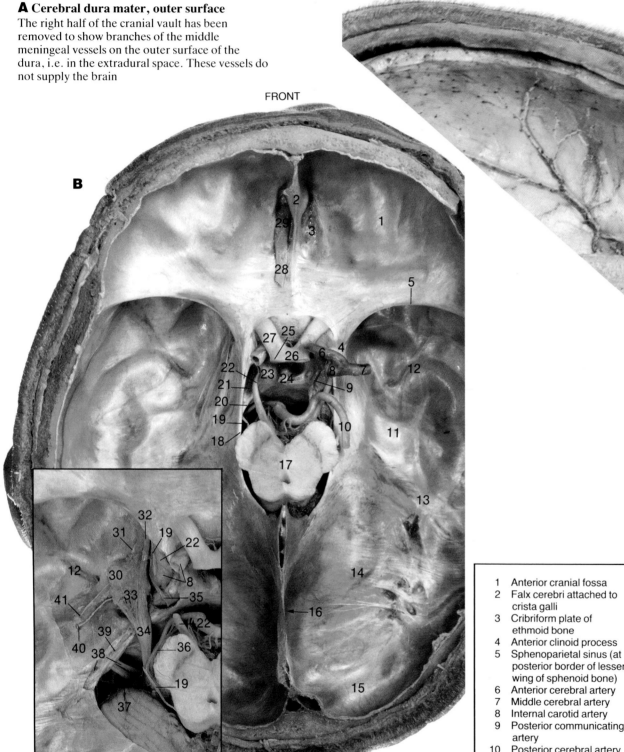

FRONT

Cranial fossae, B with dura mater intact, C with some dura removed

On the right the anterior, middle and posterior cerebral arteries (6, 7 and 10) and the posterior communicating artery (9) have been preserved, but on the left they have been removed to give a clearer view of the trochlear nerve (19) piercing the dura mater at the junction of the free (18) and attached (20) margins of the tentorium cerebelli, and the oculomotor nerve (22) piercing the roof of the cavernous sinus (21). In C some dura on the left side has been removed, including the roof of the cavernous sinus (B21) and segments of the oculomotor (22) and trochlear (19) nerves. The trigeminal nerve and its branches (30 to 34) are exposed, together with the petrosal nerves (40 and 41). With part of the tentorium missing the vestibulocochlear and facial nerves (37 and 38) are on view in the posterior cranial fossa

1	Anterior cranial fossa	18	Free margin of tentorium cerebelli
2	Falx cerebri attached to crista galli	19	Trochlear nerve
3	Cribriform plate of ethmoid bone	20	Attached margin of tentorium cerebelli
4	Anterior clinoid process	21	Roof of cavernous sinus
5	Sphenoparietal sinus (at posterior border of lesser wing of sphenoid bone)	22	Oculomotor nerve
		23	Posterior clinoid process
		24	Pituitary stalk
6	Anterior cerebral artery	25	Optic tract
7	Middle cerebral artery	26	Optic chiasma
8	Internal carotid artery	27	Optic nerve
9	Posterior communicating artery	28	Olfactory tract
		29	Olfactory bulb
10	Posterior cerebral artery	30	Mandibular nerve
11	Lateral part of middle cranial fossa	31	Maxillary nerve
		32	Ophthalmic nerve
12	Middle meningeal vessels	33	Trigeminal ganglion
13	Superior petrosal sinus (at attached margin of tentorium cerebelli)	34	Trigeminal nerve
		35	Abducent nerve
		36	Superior cerebellar artery
14	Tentorium cerebelli	37	Vestibulocochlear nerve
15	Transverse sinus (at attached margin of tentorium cerebelli)	38	Facial nerve
		39	Superior petrosal sinus
		40	Hiatus for greater petrosal nerve
16	Straight sinus (at junction of falx cerebri and tentorium cerebelli)	41	Hiatus for lesser petrosal nerve
17	Midbrain (superior colliculus level)		

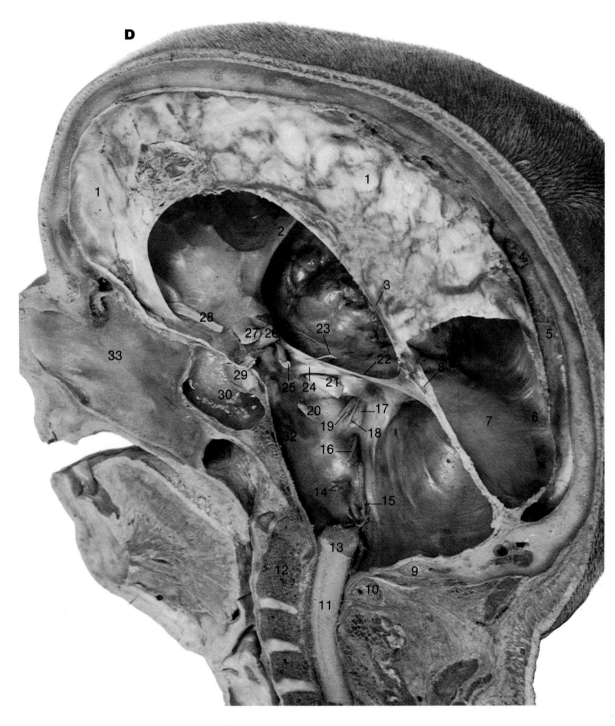

D

In this oblique view from the left and behind, the brain has been removed and a window has been cut in the posterior part of the falx cerebri (1) to show the upper surface of the tentorium cerebelli (7)

1	Falx cerebri
2	Sphenoparietal sinus
3	Inferior sagittal sinus
4	Arachnoid granulations
5	Superior sagittal sinus
6	Transverse sinus
7	Tentorium cerebelli
8	Straight sinus
9	Margin of foramen magnum
10	Posterior arch of atlas
11	Spinal cord
12	Dens of axis
13	Medulla oblongata
14	Rootlets of hypoglossal nerve
15	Spinal part of accessory nerve
16	Glossopharyngeal, vagus and accessory nerves
17	Vestibulocochlear nerve
18	Sensory root (nervus intermedius) ⎫ of facial nerve
19	Motor root ⎭
20	Abducent nerve
21	Trigeminal nerve
22	Free margin of tentorium cerebelli
23	Trochlear nerve
24	Attached margin of tentorium cerebelli
25	Oculomotor nerve
26	Internal carotid artery
27	Optic nerve
28	Olfactory tract
29	Pituitary gland
30	Sphenoidal sinus
31	Choana (posterior nasal aperture)
32	Clivus
33	Nasal septum

● The filaments of the olfactory (first cranial) nerve pierce the cribriform plate of the ethmoid to enter the olfactory bulb, at the front end of the olfactory tract (28) and just hidden by the curved edge of the falx cerebri (1).
● The optic (second cranial) nerve (27) emerges from the optic canal and passes medial to the internal carotid artery (26).
● The oculomotor (third cranial) nerve (25) pierces the dura mater of the roof of the cavernous sinus.
● The trochlear (fourth cranial) nerve (23) pierces the dura mater where the free margin of the tentorium cerebelli (22) crosses over the attached margin (24).
● The trigeminal (fifth cranial) nerve (21) crosses the apex of the petrous part of the temporal bone below the attached margin of the tentorium (24).
● The abducent (sixth cranial) nerve (20) pierces the dura mater on the clivus (32).
● The facial (seventh cranial) nerve (18 and 19) and the vestibulocochlear (eighth cranial) nerve (17) enter the internal acoustic meatus.
● The filaments of the glossopharyngeal, vagus and accessory nerves (ninth, tenth and eleventh cranial nerves respectively, 16), and including the spinal part of the accessory nerve (15) which has entered the skull through the foramen magnum (9), enter the jugular foramen.
● The rootlets of the hypoglossal (twelfth cranial) nerve (14) enter the hypoglossal canal as two separate bundles.

A

C

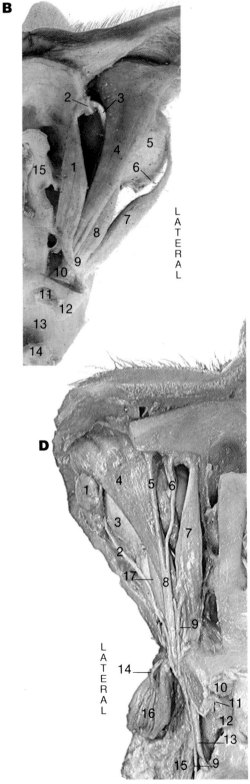

B

D

A Left eye. Surface features

With the eyelids in the normal open position, the lower margin of the upper lid (8) overlaps approximately the upper half of the iris (6); the margin of the lower lid (9) is level with the lower margin of the iris (6)

1	Lacrimal caruncle	6	Iris } behind
2	Lacrimal papilla	7	Pupil } cornea
3	Plica semilunaris	8	Upper eyelid
4	Sclera	9	Lower eyelid
5	Limbus (corneoscleral junction)		

- The cornea is the transparent anterior part of the outer coat of the eyeball and is continuous with the sclera (4) at the limbus (5).
- The pupil (7) is the central aperture of the iris (6), the circular pigmented diaphragm that lies in front of the lens.
- Each lacrimal papilla (2) contains the lacrimal punctum, the minute opening of the lacrimal canaliculus (H16, 6 and 7) which runs medially to open into the lacrimal sac, lying deep to the medial palpebral ligament (H3) and continuing downwards as the nasolacrimal duct (H4) within the nasolacrimal canal.

Right extra-ocular muscles, B from above, C from the right

The upper and lateral walls of the orbit have been removed, together with all fat, vessels and nerves, leaving only the muscles

1	Superior oblique
2	Trochlea
3	Tendon of superior oblique
4	Levator palpebrae superioris
5	Eyeball
6	Inferior oblique
7	Lateral rectus
8	Superior rectus
9	Tendinous ring
10	Optic nerve
11	Optic canal
12	Anterior clinoid process
13	Pituitary fossa (sella turcica)
14	Posterior clinoid process
15	Ethmoidal air cells
16	Inferior rectus

Left orbit, D from above, E from the left

The upper and lateral walls of the orbit have been removed, together with the blood vessels, leaving muscles and nerves. The lateral rectus (16) has been detached from the eyeball and turned backwards to show the abducent nerve (14) entering its deep (ocular) surface. In D the trochlear nerve (9) is seen entering the superficial (orbital) surface of the superior oblique (7). The frontal nerve (D8) divides on the upper surface of levator palpebrae superioris (4) into the supratrochlear (6) and supra-orbital (5) nerves. The levator muscle largely overlies the superior rectus (17), only a small part of which can be seen at the lateral border of the levator

1	Lacrimal gland
2	Lacrimal nerve
3	Eyeball
4	Levator palpebrae superioris
5	Supra-orbital nerve
6	Supratrochlear nerve
7	Superior oblique
8	Frontal nerve
9	Trochlear nerve
10	Optic nerve
11	Ophthalmic artery
12	Internal carotid artery
13	Oculomotor nerve
14	Abducent nerve
15	Trigeminal ganglion
16	Lateral rectus (reflected backwards)
17	Superior rectus
18	Ophthalmic nerve
19	Ciliary ganglion
20	Short ciliary nerves (superficial to marker)
21	Nerve to medial rectus
22	Inferior rectus
23	Nerve to inferior oblique
24	Inferior oblique
25	Lateral rectus

- The lateral rectus (E16) is supplied by the abducent nerve (E14).
- The superior oblique (D7) is supplied by the trochlear nerve (D9).
- All the other muscles that move the eyeball (medial, superior and inferior recti and the inferior oblique) are supplied by the oculomotor nerve. The branch to the inferior oblique (E23) is surprisingly large and runs above the floor of the orbit lateral to the inferior rectus (E22), to enter the posterior border of the oblique muscle (E24). All the other branches enter the deep (ocular) surfaces of the respective muscles.
- Levator palpebrae superioris (D4) is also supplied by the oculomotor nerve, but some of its fibres consist of visceral muscle which receives a sympathetic supply.

E

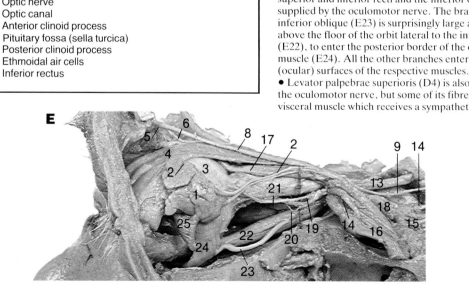

F Orbits, from above

Both orbits have been exposed from above, and most of levator palpebrae superioris (2) and the superior rectus (3) have been removed. On the right, as is usual, the ophthalmic artery (11) and nasociliary nerve (9) cross above the optic nerve (16) from lateral to medial; on the left the artery has crossed below the nerve, which is uncommon. The supra-orbital artery (4) is unusually small on the left and is absent on the right

```
 1  Lacrimal gland
 2  Levator palpebrae superioris
 3  Superior rectus
 4  Supra-orbital artery
 5  Supra-orbital nerve
 6  Supratrochlear nerve
 7  Eyeball
 8  Medial rectus
 9  Nasociliary nerve
10  Superior oblique
11  Ophthalmic artery
12  Trochlear nerve
13  Frontal nerve
14  Lacrimal nerve
15  Lateral rectus
16  Optic nerve (with overlying short ciliary
    nerves in left orbit)
17  Internal carotid artery
18  Middle cerebral artery
19  Anterior cerebral artery
20  Optic chiasma
21  Anterior communicating artery
22  Cribriform plate of ethmoid
23  Lacrimal artery
24  Posterior ciliary artery
25  Infratrochlear nerve and ophthalmic artery
26  Anterior ethmoidal artery and nerve
```

G Right orbit, from the front

The eye has been removed, leaving the cut end of the optic nerve (12) and the extra-ocular muscles

```
 1  Supra-orbital nerve
 2  Supratrochlear nerve
 3  Trochlea
 4  Tendon of superior oblique
 5  Superior oblique
 6  Anterior ethmoidal nerve
 7  Infratrochlear nerve
 8  Medial rectus
 9  Attachment of medial palpebral ligament
10  Inferior oblique
11  Inferior rectus
12  Optic nerve
13  Lateral rectus
14  Part of orbital septum
15  Lacrimal gland
16  Superior rectus
17  Levator palpebrae superioris
```

● The two oblique muscles (superior and inferior) both pass below the corresponding rectus muscles.
● The lateral palpebral ligament (connected to the tarsal plates of both eyelids) is attached to a small tubercle on the zygomatic bone (immediately in front of the part of the orbital septum seen in this specimen, 14). The medial palpebral ligament is attached to the anterior lacrimal crest of the frontal process of the maxilla, and therefore lies anterior to the lacrimal sac.
● The orbital septum is the continuation into the eyelids of the orbital periosteum (properly called the orbital fascia).

H Right nasolacrimal duct

Part of the maxilla has been dissected away to display the nasolacrimal duct (4). The upper end of the duct is continuous with the lacrimal sac (hidden behind the medial palpebral ligament, 3), into which the lacrimal canaliculi (1 and 6) open

```
 1  Superior canaliculus
 2  Dorsal nasal artery
 3  Medial palpebral ligament overlying
    lacrimal sac
 4  Nasolacrimal duct
 5  Infra-orbital nerve
 6  Inferior canaliculus
 7  Bristles in puncta of lacrimal canaliculi
```

● The most important branch of the ophthalmic artery—the central artery of the retina—is hidden below the optic nerve. It runs within the dural sheath of the nerve and pierces the inferomedial surface of the nerve 1.25 cm behind the eyeball, passing forwards in the centre of the nerve to reach the retina where its branches can be observed with the ophthalmoscope.

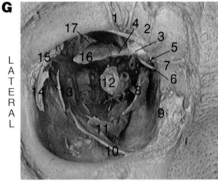

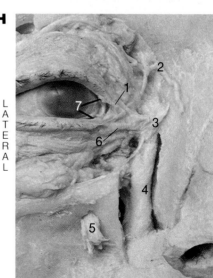

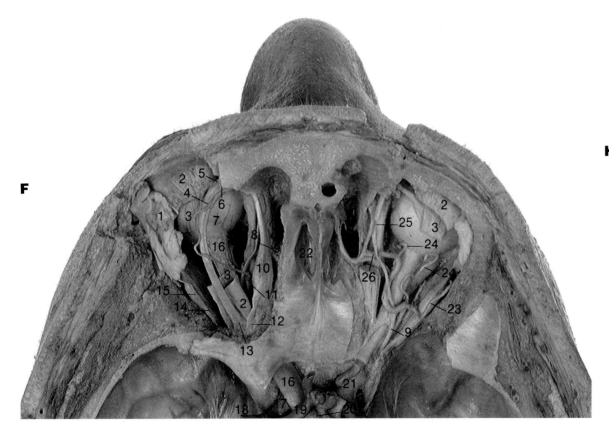

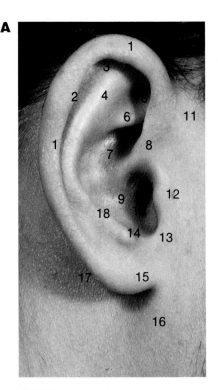

A Right external ear

1	Helix
2	Auricular tubercle
3	Scaphoid fossa
4	Upper crus of antihelix
5	Triangular fossa
6	Lower crus of antihelix
7	Upper part of concha
8	Crus of helix
9	Lower part of concha
10	External acoustic meatus
11	Superficial temporal vessels and auriculotemporal nerve
12	Tragus
13	Intertragic notch
14	Antitragus
15	Lobule
16	Transverse process of atlas
17	Mastoid process
18	Antihelix

● The external ear consists of the auricle (pinna) and external acoustic meatus (10)
● The concha (7 and 9) is the deepest part of the external ear. The lower part of the concha leads into the external acoustic meatus; the suprameatal triangle and mastoid antrum lie behind the upper part.

● For enlarged diagrams of the ear see page 61.
● The middle ear or tympanic cavity is an irregular space within the temporal bone, containing the auditory ossicles and filled with air that communicates with the nasopharynx through the auditory tube.

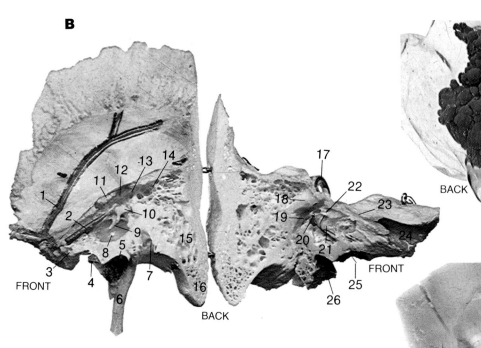

B Right temporal bone and ear

The bone has been bisected and opened out like opening a book, with some removal of the upper part of the petrous part. The section has opened up the tympanic (middle ear) cavity. On the left side of the figure the lateral wall of the middle ear, which includes the tympanic membrane (8), is seen from the medial side, while on the right the main features of the medial wall are in view

1	Groove for middle meningeal vessels
2	Tensor tympani muscle in its canal
3	Bony part of auditory tube
4	Part of carotid canal (red)
5	Part of jugular bulb (blue)
6	Styloid process
7	Stylomastoid foramen
8	Tympanic membrane
9	Malleus
10	Incus
11	Tegmen tympani
12	Epitympanic recess
13	Aditus to mastoid antrum
14	Mastoid antrum
15	Mastoid air cells
16	Mastoid process
17	Anterior ⎫
18	Lateral ⎬ semicircular canal
19	Canal for facial nerve (yellow)
20	Stapes in oval window and stapedius muscle
21	Promontory with overlying tympanic plexus
22	Lesser petrosal nerve
23	Groove for greater petrosal nerve (yellow)
24	Carotid canal (red)
25	Tympanic branch of glossopharyngeal nerve entering its canaliculus
26	Jugular bulb (blue)

● The epitympanic recess (12) is the part of the tympanic cavity that lies above the tympanic membrane (8), and lodges the head of the malleus (9) and the body of the incus (10). It leads backwards through the aditus (13) into the mastoid antrum (14), which is an enlarged mastoid air cell.
● The medial wall of the middle ear contains (from below upwards) the promontory (21, due to the first turn of the cochlea), the canal for the facial nerve (19) and the prominence due to the lateral semicircular canal (18). Below and behind the

C Cast of the right mastoid air cells, from the right

The air cells are seen within a transparent cast of the temporal bone. The styloid process projects downwards immediately below the external acoustic meatus, with the mastoid process behind

D Mastoid region of the right temporal bone, from the right

The mastoid air cells have been removed and the canal for the facial nerve (3) has been opened up to show the origin of the chorda tympani (5)

1	Sigmoid sinus
2	Dura mater of posterior cranial fossa
3	Facial nerve
4	Lateral semicircular canal
5	Chorda tympani
6	Tympanic membrane (upper part removed)

● The mastoid air cells are closely related to the sigmoid sinus (1) and posterior cranial fossa (2) posteromedially; above is the temporal lobe of the brain in the middle cranial fossa. The mastoid antrum and air cells can be approached surgically by opening up the bone through the suprameatal triangle (page 28, A13).

promontory (and just hidden by it in this view) is the round window (fenestra cochleae, closed by the secondary tympanic membrane), and above and behind it is the oval window (fenestra vestibuli, closed by the footplate of the stapes, 20).
● The roof of the middle ear is the tegmen tympani (11); the jugular bulb (5) lies below the floor, and the carotid canal (4) in the anterior wall.

Dissections of the middle and inner ear in the right temporal bone. E and F from the right and above. G and H from the left, above and in front. F and H are enlarged views of E and G respectively

Auditory ossicles: dark blue = malleus; red = incus; green = stapes. Margins of opened semicircular canals and cochlea: black.

E and F are viewed as when looking slightly downwards at the right side of the skull from the outside, through a window cut in the temporal bone, with the back of the skull (and mastoid process, 1) towards the left (see the adjacent diagram). G and H are of the same specimen, viewed as when looking at the inside of the skull from the left, above and in front, with the back of the skull towards the right (see the adjacent diagram). Note the depth of the middle ear in relation to the mastoid process

1	Mastoid process
2	Posterior
3	Anterior — semicircular canal
4	Lateral
5	Tympanic membrane and (dark blue) handle of malleus
6	Facial nerve (yellow)
7	Stapedius muscle
8	Chorda tympani (purple)
9	Margins of auditory tube (mauve)
10	Tensor tympani muscle
11	Cochleariform process
12	Tendon of tensor tympani
13	Cochlea
14	Cochlear part — of vestibulocochlear nerve
15	Vestibular part
16	Internal acoustic meatus
17	Genicular ganglion of facial nerve

E

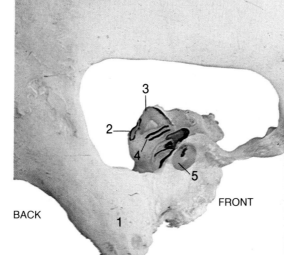

BACK

FRONT

F

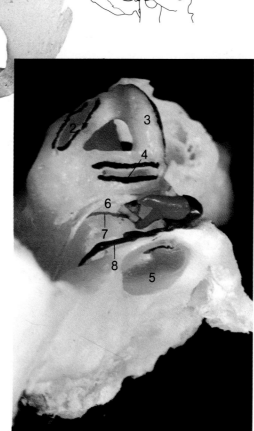

● The handle of the malleus is attached to the tympanic membrane (5).
● The chorda tympani (F8) passes between the fibrous and mucous layers of the tympanic membrane and crosses the handle of the malleus.
● From the genicular ganglion (H17) the facial nerve passes backwards in its canal (at label 6 in F) above the promontory (B21) and then downwards (B19) in the medial wall of the aditus to reach the stylomastoid foramen.
● Distinguish between semicircular and cochlear canals, and semicircular and cochlear ducts: the canals are the spaces within bone and contain perilymph, while the ducts (containing endolymph) are membranous structures inside the canals and therefore surrounded by perilymph.

G

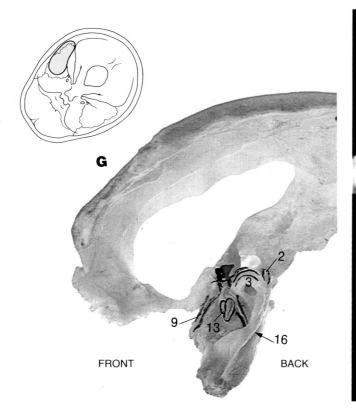

FRONT

BACK

H

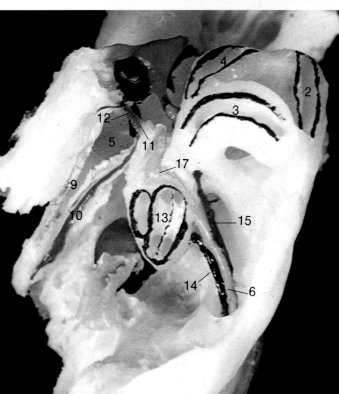

A

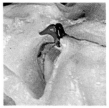 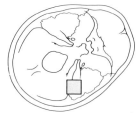

B

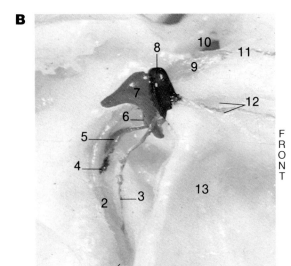

F
R
O
N
T

C

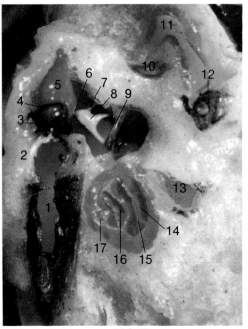

FRONT

D

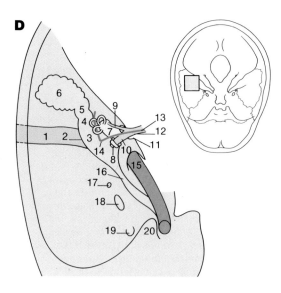

Right temporal bone. **A** Middle ear and the facial nerve and branches, **B** enlarged view of **A**

This dissection is seen from the right and above, looking forwards and medially. Bone has been removed to show the upper parts of the malleus (8) and incus (7) which normally project up into the epitympanic recess. The upper part of the facial canal (1) has been opened to show the facial nerve (2) giving off the chorda tympani (3) and the nerve to stapedius (4). The genicular ganglion of the facial nerve (9) is seen giving off the greater petrosal nerve (11)

1	Facial canal leading to stylomastoid foramen
2	Facial nerve
3	Chorda tympani
4	Nerve to stapedius
5	Stapedius
6	Stapes
7	Incus
8	Malleus
9	Genicular ganglion of facial nerve
10	Internal acoustic meatus
11	Greater petrosal nerve
12	Margin of auditory tube
13	Paraffin wax (for support) overlying tympanic membrane

● The stapedius (5) tendon emerges from a small conical projection on the posterior wall of the tympanic cavity, the pyramid (here dissected away).

C Right temporal bone. Middle ear and inner ear, enlarged

This dissection is viewed from above, looking slightly backwards and laterally. Within the cavity of the middle ear are the three auditory ossicles—malleus (3), incus (5) and stapes (8). The tympanic membrane and external acoustic meatus are not seen but lie below the label 4. The cochlea has been opened up to show its internal bony structure (14 to 17)

1	Auditory tube	
2	Chorda tympani	
3	Malleus	
4	Incudomallear joint	
5	Incus	
6	Incudostapedial joint	
7	Stapedius muscle	
8	Stapes	
9	Footplate of stapes in oval window of vestibule	
10	Lateral	
11	Posterior	semicircular canal
12	Anterior	
13	Internal acoustic meatus	
14	Bony canal	
15	Osseous spiral lamina	of
16	Modiolus	cochlea
17	Cupola	

● The spiral organ (the end organ of hearing) lies on the basilar membrane, which stretches between the free edge of the osseous spiral lamina (15) and the side of the bony cochlear canal.
● The modiolus (16) is the central axis of the cochlea, and the cupola (17) is its apex.

D Right ear, from above

This schematic diagram of part of the right side of the base of the skull indicates the position of the parts of the ear within the temporal bone. (The auditory ossicles have been omitted from the middle ear cavity, 3.) The external acoustic meatus (1) is at a right angle to the side of the skull, and the internal acoustic meatus (11) is level with it on the inner side of the temporal bone. The line (from front to back) of the auditory tube (16), middle ear cavity (3), mastoid antrum (4 and 5) and mastoid air cells (6) lies at about 60° to the line of the external meatus. The cochlear part of the inner ear (8) is in front of the vestibular part (7). The facial nerve (13) runs immediately above the vestibulocochlear nerve (12) and takes a right-angled turn backwards at the genicular ganglion (14) to pass below the lateral semicircular canal in the medial wall of the middle ear and then turns downwards in the medial wall of the aditus to the antrum (4) to reach the stylomastoid foramen

1	External acoustic meatus
2	Tympanic membrane
3	Middle ear
4	Aditus to mastoid antrum
5	Mastoid antrum
6	Mastoid air cells
7	Vestibular part of inner ear
8	Cochlear part of inner ear
9	Vestibular nerve
10	Cochlear nerve
11	Internal acoustic meatus
12	Vestibulocochlear nerve
13	Facial nerve
14	Genicular ganglion of facial nerve
15	Internal carotid artery emerging from foramen lacerum
16	Auditory tube
17	Foramen spinosum
18	Foramen ovale
19	Foramen rotundum
20	Anterior clinoid process

E Right ear, from the front

This schematic diagram shows a vertical section through the ear to indicate how the three auditory ossicles (malleus, incus and stapes—6, 7 and 8) bridge the tympanic cavity (4) so that vibrations of the tympanic membrane (2) are transmitted to the footplate of the stapes (9) in the oval window of the vestibule

1	External acoustic meatus
2	Tympanic membrane
3	Epitympanic recess
4	Middle ear cavity
5	Handle of malleus
6	Body of malleus
7	Incus
8	Stapes
9	Footplate of stapes in oval window
10	Round window
11	Auditory tube
12	Vestibule
13	Cochlea
14	Anterior
15	Posterior } semicircular canal
16	Lateral

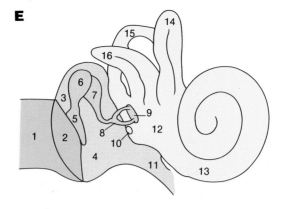

E

• The internal ear consists of the bony labyrinth and the membranous labyrinth.
• The bony labyrinth is a space within the temporal bone (61, F) and consists of the vestibule, semicircular canals and cochlea.
• The membranous labyrinth (61, G) is inside the bony labyrinth and consists of the utricle and saccule (within the vestibule), the semicircular ducts (within the semicircular canals) and the cochlear duct (within the cochlea).
• The membranous labyrinth contains endolymph and is separated from the walls of the bony labyrinth by perilymph. These two fluids do not communicate with one another, but the perilymph probably communicates with the subarachnoid space via the cochlear canaliculus (page 28, D23).

G

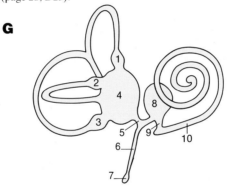

G Diagram of the membranous labyrinth

The utricle (4) and saccule (8) lie within the vestibule of the osseous labyrinth (F8), the cochlear duct (10) within the cochlea (F12), and the semicircular ducts (1, 2 and 3) within the semicircular canals (F2, 4 and 6). The endolymphatic duct (6) from the saccule (8) is joined by the utriculosaccular duct (5) from the utricle (4), and then runs in the aqueduct of the vestibule in the petrous part of the temporal bone (page 28, B21) to end under the dura mater there as the endolymphatic sac (7). The saccule (8) is connected to the cochlear duct (10) by the ductus reuniens (9)

1	Ampulla of anterior	
2	Ampulla of posterior	} semicircular duct
3	Ampulla of lateral	
4	Utricle	
5	Utriculosaccular duct	
6	Endolymphatic duct	
7	Endolymphatic sac	
8	Saccule	
9	Ductus reuniens	
10	Cochlear duct	

F

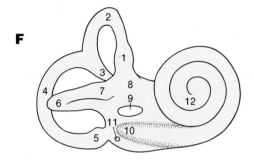

F Diagram of the osseous labyrinth

The drawing represents a cast of the space within the temporal bone. The central part is the vestibule (8) with the cochlea (12) at the front and the semicircular canals (2, 4 and 6) at the back. The beginning of the first turn of the cochlea (10) forms the promontory, between the oval window above and behind it (9) and the round window below and behind it (11). The promontory is one of the main features of the medial wall of the middle ear (see page 58, B21)

1	Ampulla of 2
2	Anterior semicircular canal
3	Common limb of 2 and 4
4	Posterior semicircular canal
5	Ampulla of 4
6	Lateral semicircular canal
7	Ampulla of 6
8	Vestibule
9	Oval window (fenestra vestibuli)
10	Promontory at base of first turn of cochlea
11	Round window (fenestra cochleae)
12	Cochlea

• The cochlear part of the ear is concerned with hearing.
• The vestibular part of the ear is concerned with balance (equilibrium).
• Vibrations of the footplate of the stapes in the oval window (E9, F9) cause vibrations in the perilymph of the cochlear canal (H1 and 2). This causes movement of the basilar membrane (H5) and stimulation of the hair cells on the surface of the spiral organ (H6), so causing impulses that proceed along the cochlear nerve (H9) to the brain for the sense of hearing.
• The round window (E10, F11) is closed by the secondary tympanic membrane, to prevent perilymph escaping from the cochlear canal. When the footplate of the stapes moves inwards, the secondary tympanic membrane moves outwards (to compensate for the increase of pressure in the perilymph) because the scala vestibuli and scala tympani parts of the cochlear canal (H1 and 2) are in continuity with one another at the apex of the cochlea.
• In the ampullae of the semicircular ducts (G1, 2 and 3) and in specialized areas (maculae) of the utricle and saccule (G4 and 8) there are receptors innervated by the vestibular nerve which respond to the movement of endolymph, so providing the basis for the sense of balance.

H

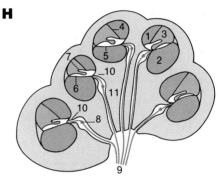

H Diagram of the cochlea

The basilar membrane (5) supports the spiral organ (6) which is supplied by fibres of the cochlear nerve (9) whose ganglion cells (8) lie within the petrous bone adjacent to the osseous spiral lamina (10)—the part of the cochlea that looks like the thread of a short fat screw (C15). For diagrammatic purposes only one nerve fibre and ganglion cell is shown in each of the representative canals passing through the central part (modiolus, 11) of the osseous labyrinth. The basilar membrane (5) and the vestibular membrane (4) are part of the cochlear duct (3) of the membranous labyrinth, and the roughly triangular space between those two membranes is filled with endolymph. The outer wall of the cochlear duct (the third side of the triangle) lies against the wall of the osseous labyrinth without an intervening space, but there are spaces above and below the cochlear duct; these are the parts of the cochlear canal called the scala vestibuli (1) and scala tympani, and are filled with perilymph

1	Scala vestibuli	} of cochlear canal,
2	Scala tympani	} containing perilymph
3	Cochlear duct, containing endolymph	
4	Vestibular membrane	
5	Basilar membrane	
6	Spiral organ	
7	Tectorial membrane	
8	Spiral (cochlear) ganglion	
9	Filaments of cochlear nerve	
10	Osseous spiral lamina	
11	Modiolus	

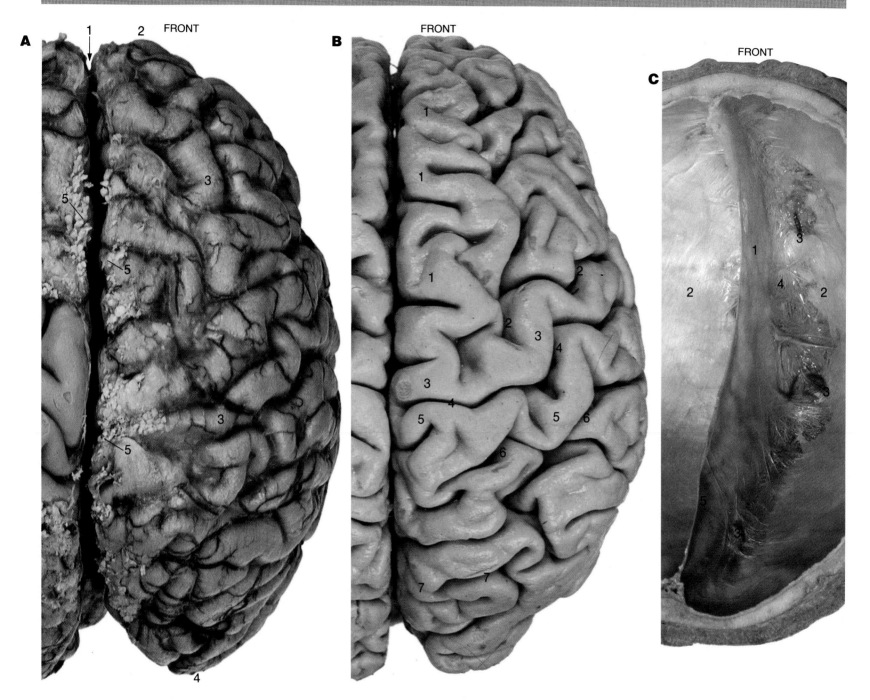

A Brain, from above

The right cerebral hemisphere is seen with the overlying arachnoid mater and arachnoid granulations (5) adjacent to the longitudinal fissure (1). Over the small part of the left hemisphere shown, a window has been cut in the arachnoid

1	Longitudinal fissure
2	Frontal pole
3	Superolateral surface
4	Occipital pole
5	Arachnoid granulations

● When removed from the cranial cavity the brain remains covered by the arachnoid mater which collapses on to most of the brain surface. In life the arachnoid is slightly separated from the brain surface by the cerebrospinal fluid in the subarachnoid space. In some areas the gap is larger, forming the cerebrospinal cisterns, e.g. the cerebellomedullary cistern (cisterna

magna) between the cerebellum and medulla oblongata (as shown on page 46, A18).
● The cerebral arteries and veins that appear to be on the brain surface are within the subarachnoid space, i.e. between the arachnoid and the pia mater which adheres intimately to the brain surface.

B Right cerebral hemisphere, from above

Removal of the arachnoid and the underlying vessels displays the gyri and sulci. Only a small number are named here; the most important are the central sulcus (4) and the precentral and postcentral gyri (3 and 5)

1	Superior frontal gyrus
2	Precentral sulcus
3	Precentral gyrus
4	Central sulcus
5	Postcentral gyrus
6	Postcentral sulcus
7	Parieto-occipital sulcus

C Cranial vault and falx, from below

Looking up into the cranial vault from below, the falx cerebri (1) is seen to be continuous with the dura over the vault (2), and has been cut off at the back (5) from the tentorium cerebelli. With the brain in place, the falx lies in the longitudinal fissure (A1) between the cerebral hemispheres (page 46), and the superior sagittal sinus (4) is within the dura at the top of the falx. The sinus receives superior cerebral veins (3 and D3) and is penetrated by the arachnoid granulations (A5) which make impressions on the bone (page 14, B2)

1	Falx cerebri
2	Dura mater over cranial vault
3	Superior cerebral veins
4	Superior sagittal sinus
5	Cut edge of falx cerebri

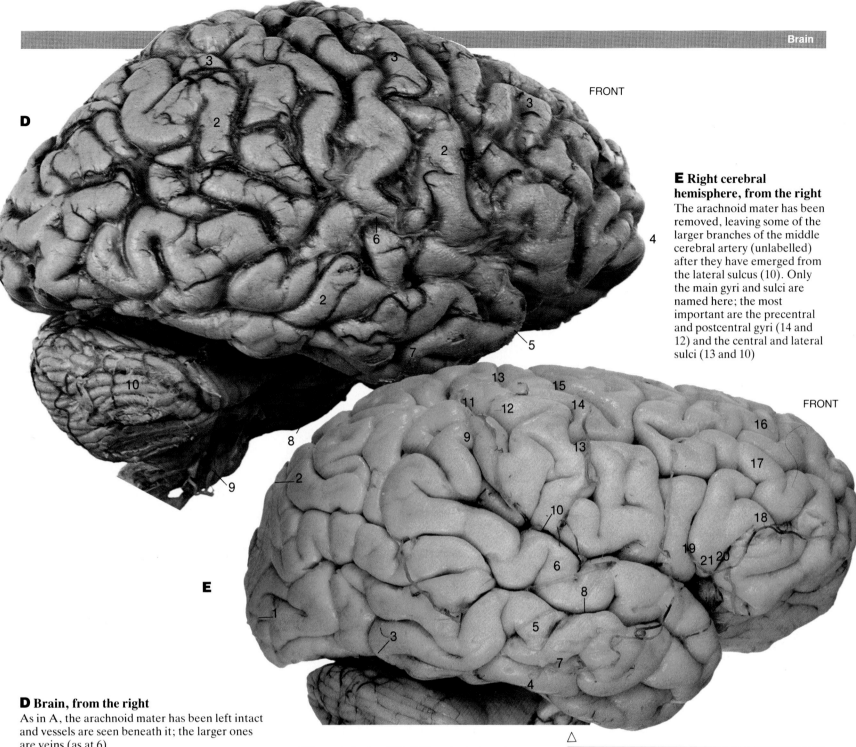

E Right cerebral hemisphere, from the right
The arachnoid mater has been removed, leaving some of the larger branches of the middle cerebral artery (unlabelled) after they have emerged from the lateral sulcus (10). Only the main gyri and sulci are named here; the most important are the precentral and postcentral gyri (14 and 12) and the central and lateral sulci (13 and 10)

D Brain, from the right
As in A, the arachnoid mater has been left intact and vessels are seen beneath it; the larger ones are veins (as at 6)

1	Occipital pole
2	Superolateral surface of right cerebral hemisphere
3	Superior cerebral veins
4	Frontal pole
5	Temporal pole
6	Superficial middle cerebral vein overlying lateral sulcus
7	Inferior cerebral veins
8	Pons and basilar artery
9	Medulla oblongata and vertebral artery
10	Right cerebellar hemisphere

● The brain consists of the forebrain (cerebrum, comprising the two cerebral hemispheres), the midbrain, and the hindbrain (comprising the pons, medulla oblongata and cerebellum).
● The midbrain, pons and medulla oblongata constitute the brainstem.

● The central sulcus (B4, E13) marks the boundary between the frontal and parietal lobes.
● An arbitrary line from the pre-occipital notch (E3) to the parieto-occipital sulcus (E2) marks the boundary between the parietal and occipital lobes, and the part of the hemisphere in front of this line and below the lateral sulcus (strictly, the posterior ramus of the lateral sulcus, E10) forms the temporal lobe.
● The precentral and postcentral gyri (B3 and 5, E14 and 12) contain the classically described 'motor' and 'sensory' areas of the cortex.
● The motor speech areas are in the region of the ascending and anterior rami of the lateral sulcus and the pars triangularis (E19 to 21).
● The auditory areas of the cortex probably comprise parts of the superior temporal gyrus (E6), especially the upper surface of it within the lateral sulcus (E10).

1	Lunate sulcus	
2	Parieto-occipital sulcus	
3	Pre-occipital notch	
4	Inferior	} temporal gyrus
5	Middle	
6	Superior	
7	Inferior	} temporal sulcus
8	Superior	
9	Supramarginal gyrus	
10	Lateral sulcus (posterior ramus)	
11	Postcentral sulcus	
12	Postcentral gyrus	
13	Central sulcus	
14	Precentral gyrus	
15	Precentral sulcus	
16	Superior	} frontal gyrus
17	Middle	
18	Inferior	
19	Ascending	} ramus of lateral sulcus
20	Anterior	
21	Pars triangularis	

A Brain, from below

This is the view of the under-surface of the brain as typically seen when first removed from the skull, without any dissection. Arachnoid mater, torn in places and with blood vessels beneath it, remains on the outer surface

1	Inferior surface of frontal lobe
2	Frontal pole
3	Longitudinal fissure
4	Gyrus rectus
5	Olfactory bulb
6	Olfactory tract
7	Anterior perforated substance
8	Optic nerve
9	Optic chiasma
10	Pituitary stalk (infundibulum)
11	Internal carotid artery
12	Posterior communicating artery
13	Oculomotor nerve
14	Crus of cerebral peduncle (midbrain)
15	Basilar artery
16	Pons
17	Trigeminal nerve
18	Abducent nerve
19	Facial nerve
20	Vestibulocochlear nerve
21	Vertebral artery
22	Medulla oblongata
23	Spinal part of accessory nerve
24	Cerebellar hemisphere
25	Inferior surface of temporal lobe
26	Uncus
27	Arachnoid mater overlying mamillary bodies
28	Temporal pole

FRONT

A

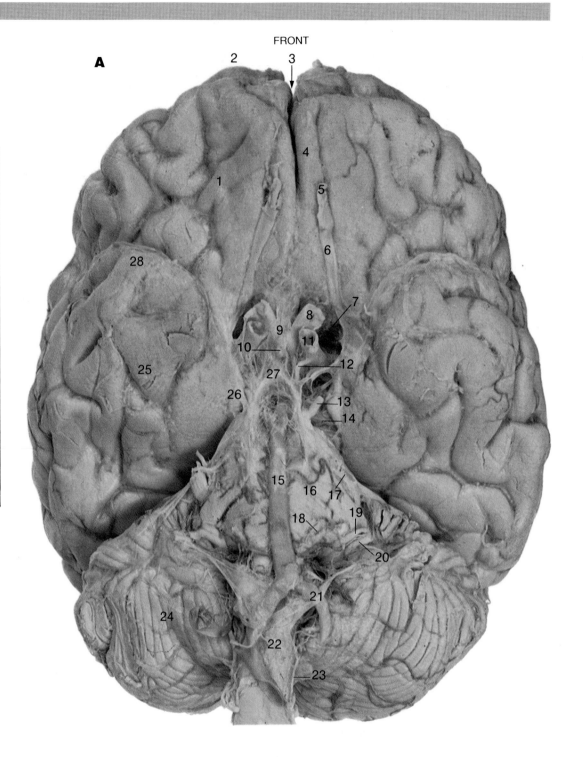

B Optic tract and geniculate bodies, from below

The brainstem has been mostly removed, leaving only the upper part of the midbrain. The most medial parts of each cerebral hemisphere have also been dissected away. To find the geniculate bodies (15 and 16), which are on the under-surface of the posterior part (pulvinar, 17) of the thalamus, identify the optic chiasma (4) and then follow the optic tract (9) backwards round the side of the midbrain (10)

● The lateral geniculate body is part of the visual pathway.
● The medial geniculate body is part of the acoustic pathway.

1	Olfactory tract	
2	Anterior perforated substance	
3	Optic nerve	
4	Optic chiasma	
5	Pituitary stalk (infundibulum)	
6	Tuber cinereum	
7	Mamillary body	
8	Posterior perforated substance	
9	Optic tract	
10	Crus	
11	Substantia nigra	
12	Tegmentum	of midbrain
13	Tectum	
14	Aqueduct	
15	Lateral	geniculate body
16	Medial	
17	Pulvinar of thalamus	
18	Splenium of corpus callosum	

FRONT

c

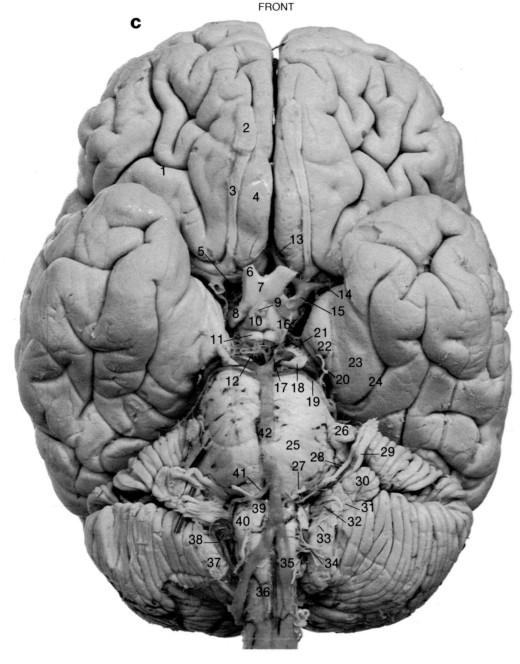

FRONT

B

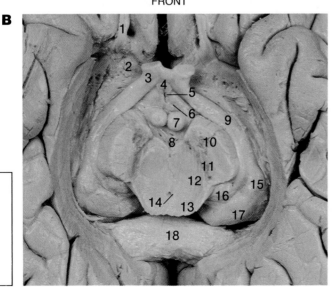

C Brain, from below.

After removal of the arachnoid mater the cranial nerves and the major blood vessels can be identified. The basilar artery (42) overlies the pons (25), and its terminal branches (the posterior cerebral arteries, 17) take part in the formation of the arterial circle (see page 68, B), whose other components are derived from the internal carotid arteries (15). The olfactory bulb (2) leads backwards into the olfactory tract (3), behind which is the anterior perforated substance (5). The pituitary stalk (9) is behind the optic chiasma (7), and the posterior perforated substance (12) is behind the mamillary bodies (11). For further details of the cranial nerves see page 67, C, and the notes on page 55

1	Orbital sulcus
2	Olfactory bulb
3	Olfactory tract
4	Gyrus rectus
5	Anterior perforated substance
6	Optic nerve
7	Optic chiasma
8	Optic tract
9	Pituitary stalk (infundibulum)
10	Tuber cinereum and median eminence
11	Mamillary body
12	Posterior perforated substance
13	Anterior cerebral artery
14	Middle cerebral artery
15	Internal carotid artery
16	Posterior communicating artery
17	Posterior cerebral artery
18	Oculomotor nerve
19	Superior cerebellar artery
20	Trochlear nerve
21	Crus of cerebral peduncle
22	Uncus
23	Parahippocampal gyrus
24	Collateral sulcus
25	Pons
26	Trigeminal nerve
27	Abducent nerve
28	Facial nerve
29	Vestibulocochlear nerve
30	Flocculus of cerebellum
31	Choroid plexus from lateral recess of fourth ventricle
32	Roots of glossopharyngeal, vagus and accessory nerves
33	Spinal part of accessory nerve
34	Rootlets of hypoglossal nerve (superficial to marker)
35	Vertebral artery
36	Medulla oblongata
37	Tonsil of cerebellum
38	Posterior inferior cerebellar artery
39	Pyramid } of medulla
40	Olive } oblongata
41	Anterior inferior cerebellar artery
42	Basilar artery

● A blue marker has been placed behind the right flocculus and the overlying facial and vestibulocochlear nerves (labelled 30, 28 and 29 on the left side).
● A red marker has been placed behind the roots of the right glossopharyngeal, vagus and accessory nerves (labelled 32 on the left side).

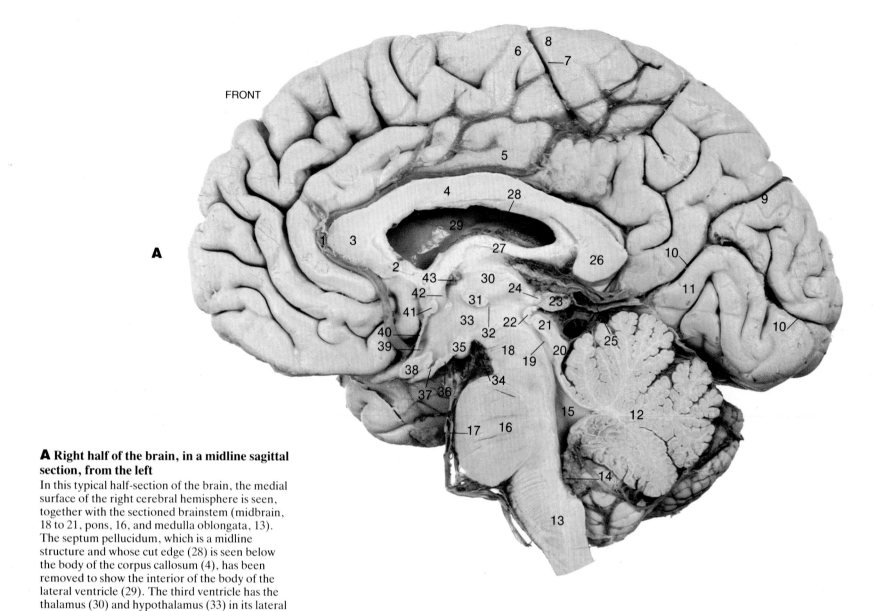

FRONT

A

A Right half of the brain, in a midline sagittal section, from the left

In this typical half-section of the brain, the medial surface of the right cerebral hemisphere is seen, together with the sectioned brainstem (midbrain, 18 to 21, pons, 16, and medulla oblongata, 13). The septum pellucidum, which is a midline structure and whose cut edge (28) is seen below the body of the corpus callosum (4), has been removed to show the interior of the body of the lateral ventricle (29). The third ventricle has the thalamus (30) and hypothalamus (33) in its lateral wall, while in its floor from front to back are the optic chiasma (38), the base of the pituitary stalk (37), the median eminence (36) and the posterior perforated substance (34)

1	Anterior cerebral artery	23	Pineal body
2	Rostrum	24	Suprapineal recess
3	Genu } of corpus callosum	25	Great cerebral vein
4	Body	26	Splenium of corpus callosum
5	Cingulate gyrus	27	Fornix
6	Precentral gyrus	28	Cut edge of septum pellucidum
7	Central sulcus	29	Body of lateral ventricle
8	Postcentral gyrus	30	Thalamus
9	Parieto-occipital sulcus	31	Interthalamic connexion
10	Calcarine sulcus	32	Hypothalamic sulcus
11	Lingual gyrus	33	Hypothalamus
12	Cerebellum	34	Posterior perforated substance
13	Medulla oblongata	35	Mamillary body
14	Median aperture of fourth ventricle	36	Tuber cinereum and median eminence
15	Fourth ventricle	37	Infundibular recess (base of pituitary stalk)
16	Pons	38	Optic chiasma
17	Basilar artery	39	Supra-optic recess
18	Tegmentum	40	Lamina terminalis
19	Aqueduct } of midbrain	41	Anterior commissure
20	Inferior colliculus	42	Anterior column of fornix
21	Superior colliculus	43	Interventricular foramen and choroid plexus
22	Posterior commissure		

● The third ventricle is the cavity which has in its lateral wall the thalamus (A30) and hypothalamus (A33).
● The fourth ventricle (A15) is largely between the pons (A16) and cerebellum (A12), although its lower end is behind the upper part of the medulla oblongata (A13) (see page 69, D).
●The aqueduct of the midbrain (A19) connects the third and fourth ventricles; cerebrospinal fluid normally flows through it from the third to the fourth ventricle.
● The interventricular foramen (A43) connects the third to the lateral ventricle, and is bounded in front by the anterior column of the fornix (A42) and behind by the thalamus (A30).
● The median eminence (A36) in the floor of the third ventricle is of great importance as the site of the neurosecretory cells whose products are released into the portal system of pituitary blood vessels (hypophysial portal system) and which control the secretion of anterior pituitary hormones.
● Posterior pituitary hormones are manufactured by cells of the supra-optic and paraventricular nuclei in the lateral wall of the hypothalamus (A33). The axons of these cells pass down the whole length of the pituitary stalk into the posterior part of the gland; the hormones are stored within the axons.

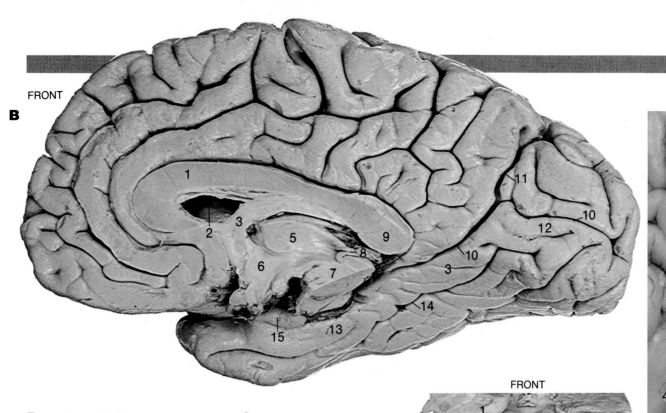

FRONT

B

FRONT

C

FRONT

D

B Medial surface of the right cerebral hemisphere

The brainstem has been removed through the midbrain (7) so that the lower part of the hemisphere can be seen; in A, opposite, the brainstem hides this part

1	Corpus callosum
2	Anterior horn of lateral ventricle
3	Anterior column of fornix
4	Interventricular foramen
5	Thalamus } in lateral wall
6	Hypothalamus } of third ventricle
7	Midbrain
8	Pineal body
9	Splenium of corpus callosum
10	Calcarine sulcus
11	Parieto-occipital sulcus
12	Lingual gyrus
13	Parahippocampal gyrus
14	Collateral sulcus
15	Uncus

● The parahippocampal gyrus (B13) is continuous anteriorly with the hook-like uncus (B15) and posteriorly with the lingual gyrus (B12).
● The visual area of the cerebral cortex occupies the upper and lower lips of the posterior part of the calcarine sulcus (B10, behind the parieto-occipital sulcus, B11), and part of the lower lip of the calcarine sulcus anterior to its junction with the parieto-occipital sulcus.

C Cranial nerves

In this ventral view of the central part of the brain, the right vertebral artery (on the left of the picture) has been removed almost at the junction with its fellow (21). The twelve cranial nerves on the right side are identified by their official numbers, although of course the filaments of the first nerve (olfactory) are not seen entering the olfactory bulb (1) as they are torn off when removing the brain. The roots forming the glossopharyngeal, vagus and accessory nerves (9, 10 and 11) cannot be clearly identified from one another, but the spinal part of the accessory nerve (11) is seen running up beside the medulla to join the cranial part (see the note on page 40)

1	Olfactory bulb	13	Pituitary stalk
2	Optic nerve	14	Internal carotid artery
3	Oculomotor nerve	15	Posterior communicating artery
4	Trochlear nerve	16	Posterior cerebral artery
5	Trigeminal nerve	17	Crus of cerebral peduncle
6	Abducent nerve	18	Superior cerebellar artery
7	Facial nerve	19	Basilar artery
8	Vestibulocochlear nerve	20	Pons
9	Glossopharyngeal nerve	21	Vertebral artery
10	Vagus nerve	22	Pyramid } of medulla
11	Accessory nerve	23	Olive } oblongata
12	Hypoglossal nerve		

D Roof of the fourth ventricle

In this dorsal view of the brainstem, the cerebellum has been removed by cutting through the cerebellar peduncles (6 to 8), but the pia mater and ependyma (10) forming the posterior part of the roof of the fourth ventricle have been preserved. The anterior part of the roof is the superior medullary velum (5)

1	Pulvinar of thalamus
2	Superior colliculus
3	Inferior colliculus
4	Trochlear nerve
5	Superior medullary velum and lingula of cerebellum
6	Superior }
7	Middle } cerebellar peduncle
8	Inferior }
9	Nodule of cerebellum
10	Pia mater and ependyma of roof of fourth ventricle
11	Median aperture
12	Lateral recess

● The median aperture (D11) in the posterior part of the roof of the fourth ventricle and the two lateral apertures (in the lateral recess of each side, D12) are the only sites of communication between the ventricular system and the subarachnoid space.

● The oculomotor nerve (C3) emerges on the *medial* side of the crus of the cerebral peduncle (C17), and the trochlear nerve (C4) winds round the *lateral* side of the peduncle. Both nerves pass between the posterior cerebral and superior cerebellar arteries (C16 and 18).
● The trochlear nerve (D4) is the only cranial nerve to emerge from the *dorsal* surface of the brainstem (from the midbrain, behind the inferior colliculus, D3).
● The trigeminal nerve (C5) emerges from the lateral side of the pons (C20).
● The abducent nerve (C6) emerges between the pons and the pyramid (C20 and 22).
● The facial and vestibulocochlear nerves (C7 and 8) emerge from the lateral pontomedullary angle.
● The glossopharyngeal and vagus nerves and the cranial root of the accessory nerve (C9, 10, 11) emerge from the medulla oblongata lateral to the olive (C23).
● The hypoglossal nerve (C12) emerges as two series of rootlets from the medulla oblongata between the pyramid (C22) and the olive (C23).
● The spinal part of the accessory nerve emerges from the lateral surface of the upper five or six cervical segments of the spinal cord, dorsal to the denticulate ligament.

A Injected arteries of the base of the brain

Part of the right cerebral hemisphere (on the left of the picture) has been removed to show the right middle cerebral artery (2)

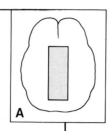

1	Anterior choroidal
2	Middle cerebral
3	Internal carotid
4	Anterior cerebral
5	Anterior communicating
6	Optic nerve
7	Olfactory tract
8	Posterior communicating
9	Posterior cerebral
10	Oculomotor nerve
11	Superior cerebellar
12	Basilar with pontine branches
13	Pons
14	Trigeminal nerve
15	Anterior inferior cerebellar
16	Abducent nerve
17	Pyramid
18	Olive
19	Unusually large branch of 15 overlying facial and vestibulocochlear nerves
20	Filaments of glossopharyngeal, vagus and accessory nerves
21	Vertebral
22	Posterior inferior cerebellar
23	Spinal cord
24	Spinal part of accessory nerve
25	Rootlets of first cervical nerve
26	Anterior spinal
27	Medulla oblongata

A FRONT

B FRONT

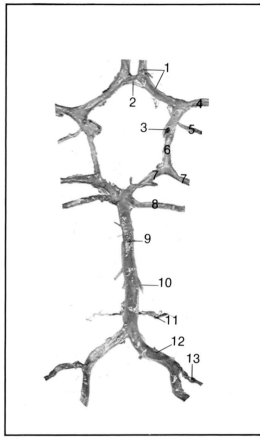

C

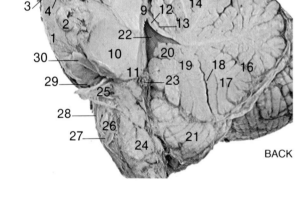

BACK

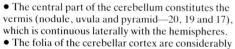

C Brainstem and cerebellum in sagittal section, from the left

The left half of the cerebellum has been removed by sagittal section in the midline and by transecting the left cerebellar peduncles (9 to 11)

1	Pons
2	Trigeminal nerve
3	Superior cerebellar artery
4	Trochlear nerve
5	Basal cerebral vein
6	Crus of cerebral peduncle
7	Posterior cerebral artery
8	Inferior colliculus
9	Superior
10	Middle } cerebellar peduncle
11	Inferior
12	Superior medullary velum
13	Lingula
14	Anterior lobe
15	Primary fissure
16	Prepyramidal fissure
17	Pyramid of vermis
18	Postpyramidal fissure
19	Uvula
20	Nodule
21	Tonsil
22	Fourth ventricle
23	Choroid plexus in lateral recess
24	Medulla oblongata
25	Roots of glossopharyngeal, vagus and accessory nerves
26	Olive
27	Rootlets of hypoglossal nerve
28	Pyramid of medulla oblongata
29	Abducent nerve
30	Facial and vestibulocochlear nerves

• The central part of the cerebellum constitutes the vermis (nodule, uvula and pyramid—20, 19 and 17), which is continuous laterally with the hemispheres.
• The folia of the cerebellar cortex are considerably narrower than the gyri of the cerebral cortex.
• The largest of the subcortical nuclei of the cerebellar hemisphere is the dentate nucleus, whose axons constitute the main efferent pathway from the cerebellum and leave in the superior peduncle.

B Arterial circle and basilar artery

The anastomosing vessels have been removed from the base of the brain and spread out in their relative positions

1	Anterior cerebral
2	Anterior communicating
3	Internal carotid
4	Middle cerebral
5	Anterior choroidal
6	Posterior communicating
7	Posterior cerebral
8	Superior cerebellar
9	Basilar
10	Labyrinthine
11	Anterior inferior cerebellar
12	Vertebral
13	Posterior inferior cerebellar

• The internal carotid artery (3) gives off the anterior cerebral (1) which passes forwards and medially to join its fellow by the anterior communicating artery. The middle cerebral (4) passes laterally from the carotid and the posterior communicating (6) passes backwards to join the posterior cerebral (7) which is the terminal branch of the basilar artery (9).
• The basilar artery (9) is formed by the union of the two vertebrals (12).

D

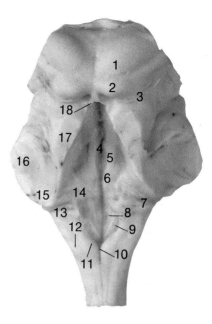

D Brainstem and floor of the fourth ventricle

In this view of the dorsal surface of the brainstem, it has been cut off from the rest of the brain at the top of the midbrain, just above the superior colliculi (1). The cerebellum has been removed by transecting the superior (17), middle (16) and inferior (15) cerebellar peduncles

1	Superior colliculus	10	Obex
2	Inferior colliculus	11	Gracile tubercle
3	Trochlear nerve	12	Cuneate tubercle
4	Median sulcus	13	Lateral recess
5	Medial eminence	14	Vestibular area
6	Facial colliculus	15	Inferior
7	Medullary striae	16	Middle } cerebellar peduncle
8	Hypoglossal triangle	17	Superior
9	Vagal triangle	18	Cut edge of superior medullary velum

E

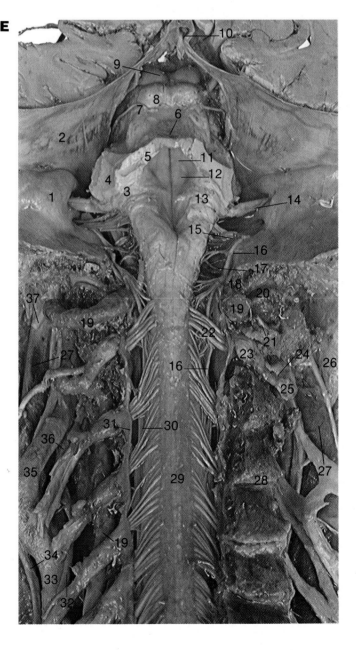

E Brainstem and upper part of the spinal cord, from behind

The posterior part of the skull, the cerebellum and vertebral arches have been removed, and the meninges have been dissected away to show the medulla oblongata passing through the foramen magnum (18) to become continuous with the spinal cord

1	Petrous part of temporal bone	18	Margin of foramen magnum
2	Tentorium cerebelli	19	Vertebral artery
3	Inferior	20	Lateral mass of atlas
4	Middle } cerebellar peduncle	21	Ventral ramus of first cervical nerve
5	Superior	22	Dorsal rootlets } of
6	Superior medullary velum	23	Dorsal root ganglion } second
7	Trochlear nerve	24	Ventral ramus } cervical
8	Inferior } colliculus	25	Dorsal ramus } nerve
9	Superior	26	Posterior belly of digastric
10	Straight sinus	27	Internal jugular vein
11	Medial eminence	28	Zygapophysial joint
12	Facial colliculus	29	Spinal cord
13	Medullary striae	30	Denticulate ligament
14	Facial and vestibulocochlear nerves and internal acoustic meatus	31	Dura mater
		32	Sympathetic trunk
15	Glossopharyngeal, vagus and accessory nerves and jugular foramen	33	Common carotid artery
		34	Vagus nerve
16	Spinal part of accessory nerve	35	Internal carotid artery
17	Rootlets of hypoglossal nerve and hypoglossal canal	36	Superior cervical sympathetic ganglion
		37	Hypoglossal nerve

● The medulla oblongata passes through the foramen magnum of the skull (E18); the spinal cord begins at the level of the atlas vertebra (E20), i.e. where the first cervical nerve rootlets emerge from the side of the cord (E29).
● The lower part of the diamond-shaped floor of the fourth ventricle containing the hypoglossal and vagal triangles (D8 and 9) is part of the medulla oblongata; the rest of the floor is part of the pons.
● The gracile and cuneate tubercles (D11 and 12) are caused by the underlying gracile and cuneate nuclei, where the fibres of the gracile and cuneate tracts (posterior white columns) end by synapsing with the cells of the nuclei. The fibres from these cells form the medial lemniscus which runs through the brainstem to the thalamus.
● The facial colliculus (D6), at the lower end of the medial eminence (D5) in the floor of the fourth ventricle, is caused by fibres of the facial nerve overlying the abducent nerve nucleus; it is not produced by the facial nerve nucleus, which lies at a deeper level in the pons.
● Occasionally (as in E) the dorsal root of the first cervical nerve is absent. The dorsal ramus of this nerve has been removed; the ventral ramus (E21) lies between the vertebral artery and the posterior arch of the atlas.
● After emerging from the foramen in the transverse process of the atlas the vertebral artery (E19) winds backwards round the lateral mass of the atlas (E20) before passing under the posterior atlanto-occipital membrane and piercing the dura and arachnoid mater to enter the skull.

A Cerebral hemispheres, sectioned horizontally

Viewed from above, the left cerebral hemisphere has been sectioned on a level with the interventricular foramen (11), and that on the right about 1.5 cm higher. The most important feature seen in the left hemisphere is the internal capsule (6 to 8), situated between the caudate (5) and lentiform (3 and 4) nuclei and the thalamus (9). On the right side a large part of the corpus callosum (17) has been removed, so opening up the lateral ventricle (19) from above and showing the caudate nucleus (5 and 18) arching backwards over the thalamus (9) with the thalamostriate vein (15) and choroid plexus (16) in the shallow groove between them

1	Insula	
2	Claustrum	
3	Putamen	} forming
4	Globus pallidus	} lentiform nucleus
5	Head of caudate nucleus	
6	Anterior limb	}
7	Genu	} of internal capsule
8	Posterior limb	}
9	Thalamus	
10	Third ventricle	
11	Interventricular foramen	
12	Anterior column of fornix	
13	Anterior horn of lateral ventricle	
14	Forceps minor (corpus callosum)	
15	Thalamostriate vein	
16	Choroid plexus	
17	Corpus callosum	
18	Body of caudate nucleus	
19	Body	}
20	Inferior horn	} of lateral ventricle
21	Posterior horn	}
22	Body of fornix	
23	Lunate sulcus	
24	Visual area of cortex	
25	Optic radiation	
26	Calcar avis	
27	Bulb	

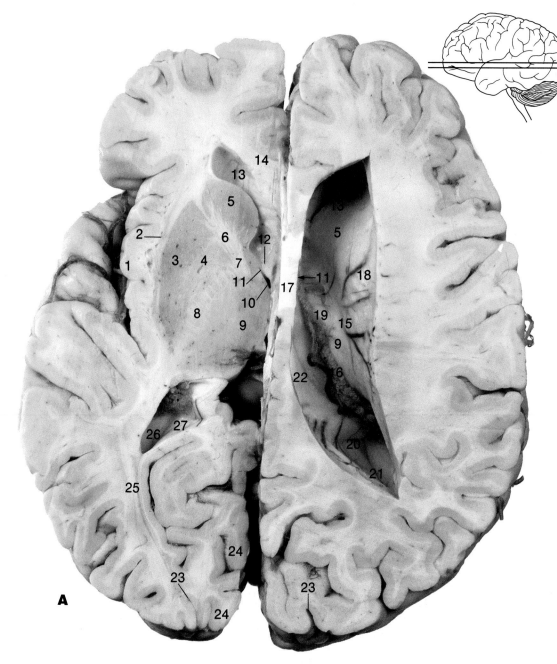

FRONT

● The anterior limb of the internal capsule (6) is bounded medially by the head of the caudate nucleus (5) and laterally by the lentiform nucleus (putamen and globus pallidus, 3 and 4).
● The genu of the internal capsule (7) lies at the most medial edge of the globus pallidus (4).
● The posterior limb of the internal capsule (8) is bounded medially by thalamus (9) and laterally by the lentiform nucleus (3 and 4).
● Corticonuclear fibres (motor fibres from the cerebral cortex to the motor nuclei of cranial nerves) pass through the genu of the internal capsule (7).
● Corticospinal fibres (motor fibres from the cerebral cortex to anterior horn cells of the spinal cord) pass through the anterior two-thirds of the posterior limb of the internal capsule (8).
● The genu and the posterior limb of the internal capsule, supplied by the striate branches of the anterior and middle cerebral arteries, are of the greatest clinical importance as they are the common sites for cerebral haemorrhage or thrombosis ('stroke').
● The choroid plexus of the third ventricle passes through the interventricular foramen into the body of the lateral ventricle and then into the inferior horn; there is no choroid plexus in the anterior or posterior horns.
● The optic radiation is alternatively known as the geniculocalcarine tract, and passes from the lateral geniculate body to the calcarine area of the cortex.

B Coronal section of the brain, from the front

This coronal section is not quite vertical but passes slightly backwards, through the third ventricle (14) and bodies of the lateral ventricles (7) from a level about 0.5 cm behind the interventricular foramina, and down through the pons (22) and the pyramid of the medulla (23). It has been cut in this way to show the path of the important corticospinal (motor) fibres passing down through the internal capsule (4) and pons (22) to form the pyramid of the medulla (23)

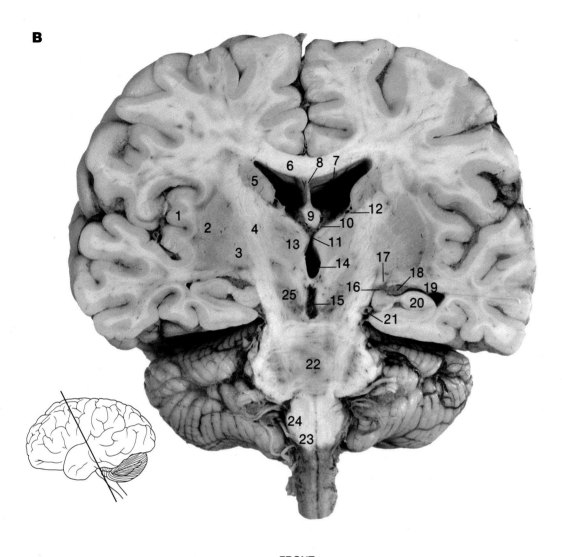

1	Insula
2	Putamen } lentiform
3	Globus pallidus } nucleus
4	Internal capsule
5	Body of caudate nucleus
6	Corpus callosum
7	Body of lateral ventricle
8	Septum pellucidum
9	Body of fornix
10	Choroid plexus of lateral ventricle
11	Choroid plexus of third ventricle
12	Thalamostriate vein
13	Thalamus
14	Third ventricle
15	Interpeduncular cistern
16	Choroidal fissure
17	Optic tract
18	Choroid plexus of inferior horn of lateral ventricle
19	Tail of caudate nucleus
20	Hippocampus
21	Posterior cerebral artery
22	Pons
23	Pyramid } of medulla
24	Olive } oblongata
25	Substantia nigra

FRONT

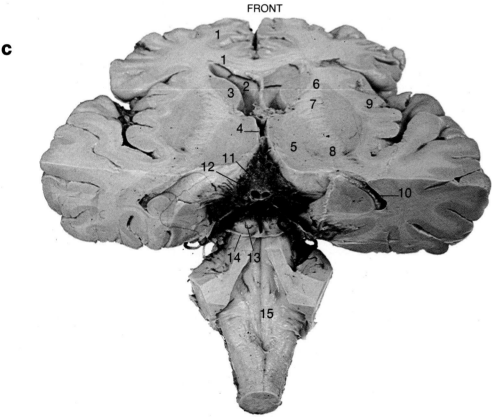

C Sectioned cerebral hemispheres and the brainstem, from above and behind

The cerebral hemispheres have been sectioned horizontally just above the level of the interventricular foramina, and the posterior parts of the hemispheres have been removed, together with the whole of the cerebellum, to show the tela choroidea (11) of the posterior part of the roof of the third ventricle and the underlying internal cerebral veins (12)

1	Forceps minor
2	Anterior horn of lateral ventricle
3	Head of caudate nucleus
4	Third ventricle
5	Thalamus
6	Anterior limb
7	Genu } of internal capsule
8	Posterior limb
9	Insula
10	Choroid plexus and junction of inferior and posterior horn
11	Tela choroidea of roof of third ventricle
12	Internal cerebral vein
13	Inferior colliculus
14	Trochlear nerve
15	Floor of fourth ventricle

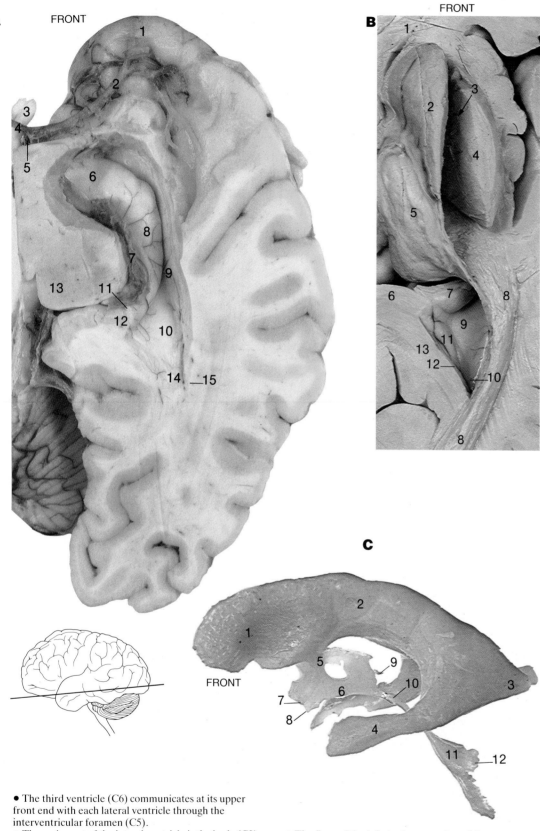

A FRONT

B FRONT

C FRONT

Compare this three-dimensional view of these structures with the brain sections on page 70

A Inferior horn of right lateral ventricle

Brain substance above the front part of the lateral sulcus has been removed, displaying the middle cerebral artery (2) running laterally over the upper surface of the front of the temporal lobe (1). Part of the temporal lobe has been opened up from above to show the hippocampus (6 and 8) in the floor of the inferior horn

1	Temporal pole
2	Middle cerebral artery
3	Optic nerve
4	Anterior cerebral artery
5	Anterior choroidal artery
6	Pes hippocampi
7	Choroid plexus
8	Hippocampus
9	Collateral eminence
10	Collateral trigone
11	Fimbria
12	Fornix
13	Thalamus
14	Posterior horn
15	Tapetum

B Dissection of the right cerebral hemisphere, from above

Much of the cerebral substance has been dissected away to show the caudate nucleus (2), thalamus (5) and lentiform nucleus (4). The intervening gap (3) is occupied by the internal capsule. The optic radiation (8) has also been dissected out; it runs backwards lateral to the posterior horn of the lateral ventricle. Compare this three-dimensional view of these structures with the brain sections on page 70

1	Forceps minor
2	Caudate nucleus
3	Internal capsule
4	Lentiform nucleus
5	Thalamus
6	Splenium of corpus callosum
7	Fornix
8	Optic radiation
9	Collateral trigone
10	Posterior horn of lateral ventricle
11	Calcar avis
12	Bulb
13	Forceps major

C Cast of the cerebral ventricles, from the left

In this side view the left lateral ventricle largely overlaps the right one

1	Anterior horn	
2	Body	of lateral
3	Posterior horn	ventricle
4	Inferior horn	
5	Interventricular foramen	
6	Third ventricle (with gap for interthalamic connexion)	
7	Supra-optic	
8	Infundibular	recess of third ventricle
9	Suprapineal	
10	Aqueduct of midbrain	
11	Fourth ventricle	
12	Lateral recess	

● The third ventricle (C6) communicates at its upper front end with each lateral ventricle through the interventricular foramen (C5).
● The main part of the lateral ventricle is the body (C2). The part in front of the interventricular foramen (C5) is the anterior horn (C1) which extends into the frontal lobe of the brain. At its posterior end the body divides into the posterior horn (C3, A14, B10) which extends backwards into the occipital lobe, and the inferior horn (C4, A) which passes downwards and forwards into the temporal lobe.
● The lower posterior part of the third ventricle (C6) communicates with the fourth ventricle (C11) through the aqueduct of the midbrain (C10).

● The floor of the inferior horn consists of the hippocampus (A6 and 8) medially and the collateral eminence (A9) laterally. At its junction with the posterior horn (A14, B10) the eminence broadens into the collateral trigone (A10, B9).
● The collateral eminence (A9) is produced by the inward projection of the collateral sulcus (page 67, B14).
● In the medial wall of the posterior horn, the bulb (B12) is produced by fibres of the corpus callosum, and the calcar avis (B11) by the inward projection of the calcarine sulcus (page 67, B10).

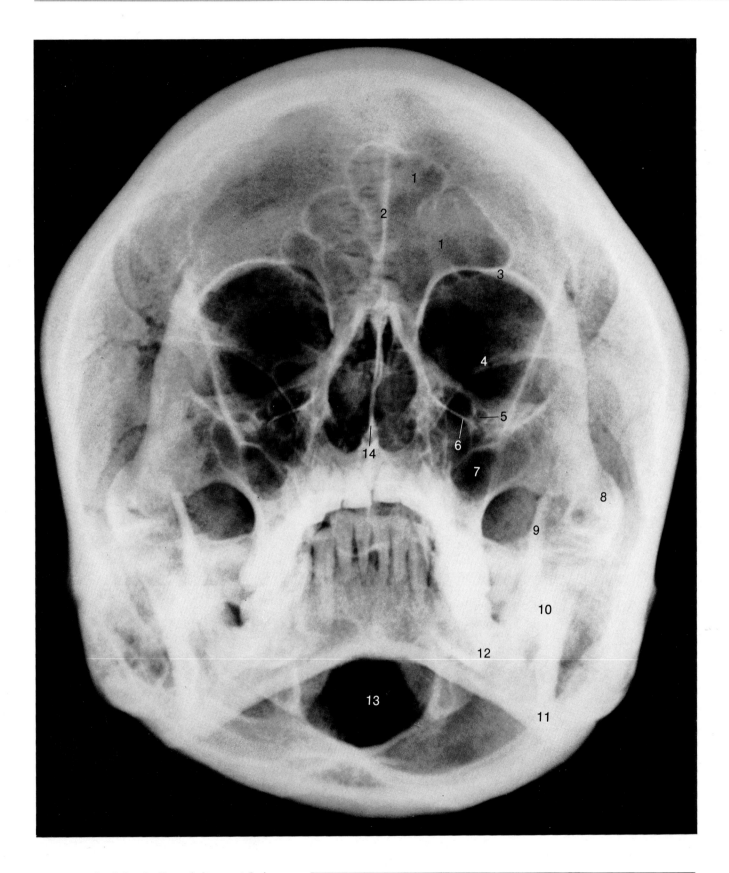

Radiograph of the skull, occipitomental view

This view of a dried skull is taken with the chin tilted upwards, a position used in the living to emphasise the frontal sinuses

1	Frontal sinus	8	Zygomatic arch	
2	Septum of frontal sinuses	9	Coronoid process	
3	Supra-orbital margin	10	Ramus	
4	Lesser wing of sphenoid	11	Angle	of mandible
5	Infra-orbital canal	12	Body	
6	Infra-orbital margin	13	Foramen magnum	
7	Maxillary sinus	14	Nasal septum	

73

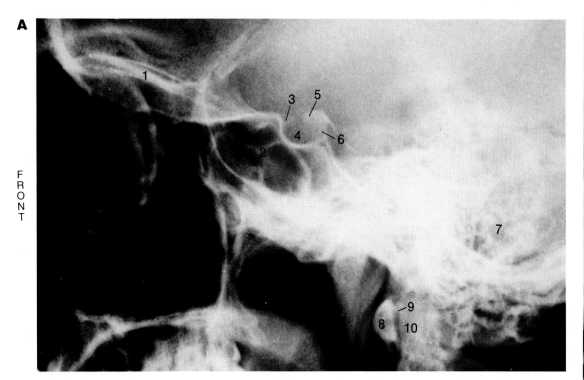

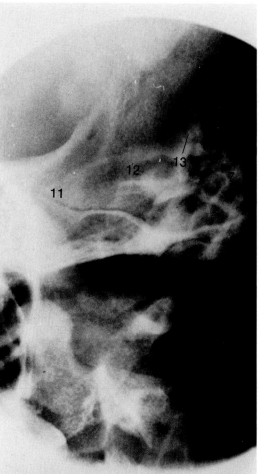

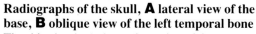

Radiographs of the skull, A lateral view of the base, B oblique view of the left temporal bone

The side view in A shows the region of the pituitary fossa (4), while B is a specialised view of the temporal bone with translucent areas indicating the internal acoustic meatus (12) and the anterior semicircular canal (13; compare with page 58, B17)

1	Floor of anterior cranial fossa
2	Sphenoidal sinus
3	Anterior clinoid process
4	Pituitary fossa (sella turcica)
5	Posterior clinoid process
6	Dorsum sellae
7	Mastoid air cells
8	Anterior arch of atlas
9	Median atlanto-axial joint
10	Dens of axis
11	Apex of petrous temporal
12	Internal acoustic meatus
13	Anterior semicircular canal

FRONT

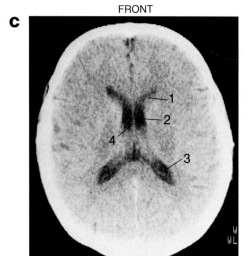

CT scans of the brain, C through the body of the lateral ventricle, D at the level of the pineal body

Scans of the head are viewed from above. The level of C is similar to the right side of the brain section A on page 70, and that of D is just above the midbrain, similar to C on page 71

1	Anterior horn	
2	Body	of lateral ventricle
3	Posterior horn	
4	Septum pellucidum	
5	Head of caudate nucleus	
6	Thalamus	
7	Calcified choroid plexus	
8	Subarachnoid space above colliculi (cisterna venae magnae cerebri)	
9	Calcified pineal body	

FRONT

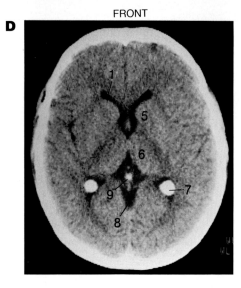

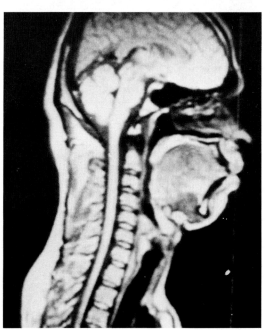

E MRI scan of head and neck

This MRI scan (magnetic resonance imaging) should be compared with the section of the head on page 46. Vertebral bodies and intervertebral discs are shown in front of the spinal cord, which is continuous with the brainstem. The tongue lies against the roof of the mouth, and the nasal cavity is on approximately the same level as the cerebellum behind the brainstem

Vertebral column and spinal cord

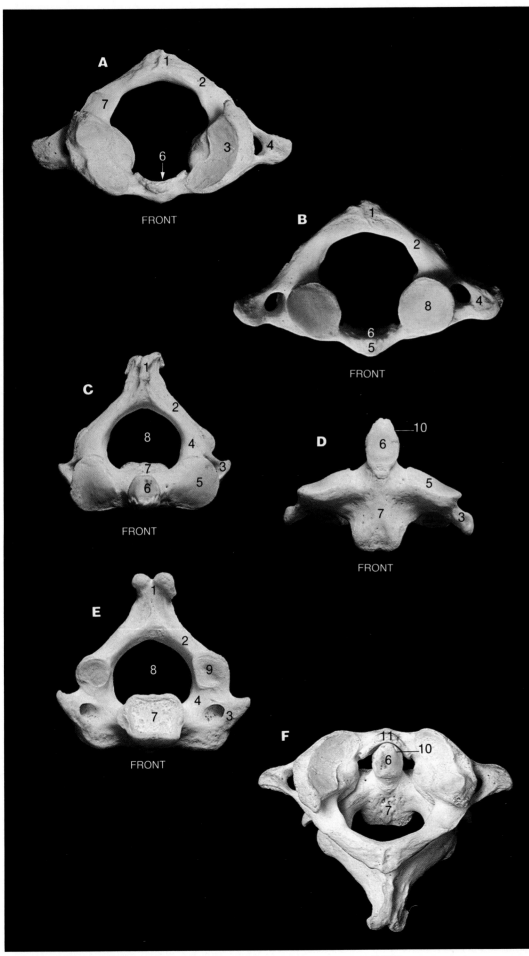

A — FRONT

B — FRONT

C — FRONT

D — FRONT

E — FRONT

F — BACK

Atlas (first cervical vertebra), **A** from above, **B** from below

1 Posterior tubercle
2 Posterior arch
3 Lateral mass with superior articular facet
4 Transverse process and foramen
5 Anterior arch and tubercle
6 Facet for dens of axis
7 Groove for vertebral artery
8 Lateral mass with inferior articular facet

● The superior articular facets (3) are concave and kidney-shaped.
● The inferior articular facets (8) are round and almost flat.
● The anterior arch (5) is straighter and shorter then the posterior arch (2), and contains on its posterior surface the facet for the dens of the axis (6).
● The atlas is the only vertebra that has no body.

Axis (second cervical vertebra), **C** from above, **D** from below, **E** from the front, **F** articulated with the atlas, from above and behind

1 Bifid spinous process
2 Lamina
3 Transverse process and foramen
4 Pedicle
5 Superior articular surface
6 Dens
7 Body
8 Vertebral foramen
9 Inferior articular process
10 Impression for alar ligament
11 Anterior arch of atlas

● The axis is unique in having the dens (6) which projects upwards from the body, and represents the body of the atlas.

Fifth cervical vertebra (a typical cervical vertebra), A from above, B from the front, C from the left

1	Bifid spinous process
2	Lamina
3	Superior articular process
4	Posterior tubercle
5	Intertubercular lamella } of transverse
6	Anterior tubercle } process
7	Foramen
8	Body
9	Posterolateral lip (uncus)
10	Pedicle
11	Vertebral foramen
12	Inferior articular process

D Seventh cervical vertebra (vertebra prominens), from above

1	Spinous process with tubercle
2	Lamina
3	Superior articular process
4	Posterior tubercle
5	Intertubercular lamella } of transverse
6	Anterior tubercle } process
7	Foramen
8	Posterolateral lip (uncus)
9	Body
10	Pedicle
11	Vertebral foramen

● All cervical vertebrae (1 to 7) have a foramen in each transverse process (as A7).
● Typical cervical vertebrae (3 to 6) have superior articular processes that face backwards and upwards (A3, C3), posterolateral lips on the upper surface of the body (A9), a triangular vertebral foramen (A11) and a bifid spinous process (A1).
● The anterior tubercle of the transverse process of the sixth cervical vertebra is large and known as the carotid tubercle.
● The seventh cervical vertebra (vertebra prominens) has a spinous process that ends in a single tubercle (D1).
● The rib element of a cervical vertebra is represented by the anterior root of the transverse process, the anterior tubercle, the intertubercular lamella (with groove for the ventral ramus of a spinal nerve), and the anterior part of the posterior tubercle (as at D6, 5 and 4).

Seventh thoracic vertebra (typical), E from above, F from the left, G from behind

1	Spinous process
2	Lamina
3	Superior articular process
4	Transverse process
5	Pedicle
6	Body
7	Vertebral foramen
8	Superior costal facet
9	Superior vertebral notch
10	Costal facet of transverse process
11	Inferior articular process
12	Inferior vertebral notch
13	Inferior costal facet

● Typical thoracic vertebrae (2 to 9) are characterised by costal facets on the bodies (F8, 13), costal facets on the transverse processes (F10), a round vertebral foramen (E7), a spinous process that points downwards as well as backwards (F1, G1), and superior articular processes that are vertical, flat and face backwards and laterally (E3, F3, G3).

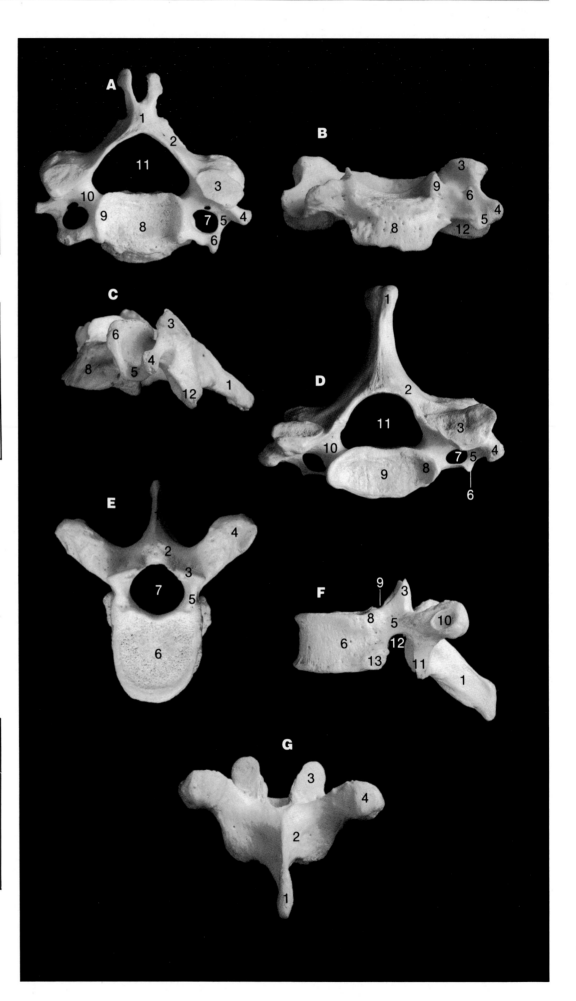

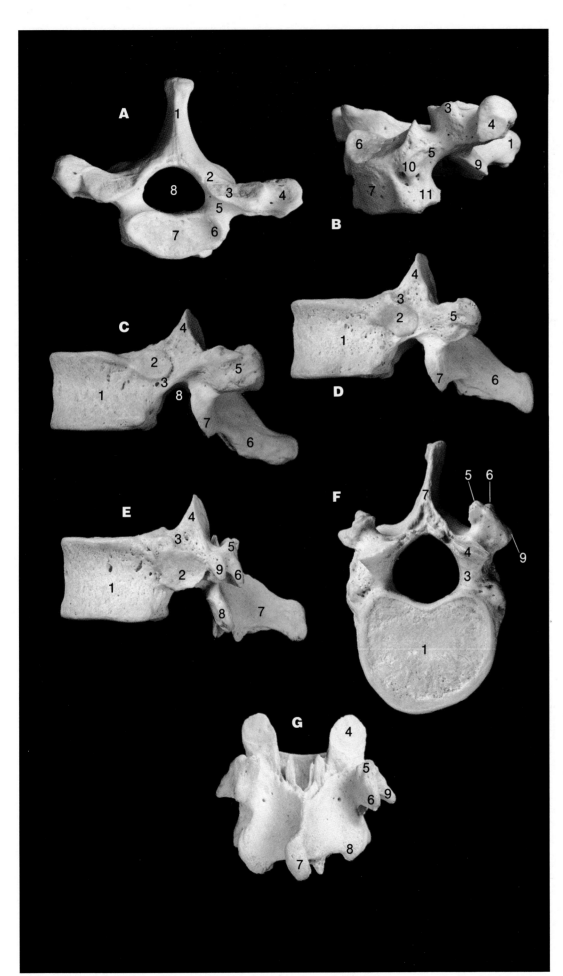

First thoracic vertebra, **A** from above, **B** from the front and the left

1	Spinous process
2	Lamina
3	Superior articular process
4	Transverse process with costal facet
5	Pedicle
6	Posterolateral lip (uncus)
7	Body
8	Vertebral foramen
9	Inferior articular process
10	Superior costal facet
11	Inferior costal facet

Tenth thoracic vertebra, **C** and eleventh thoracic vertebra, **D**, from the left

1	Body
2	Costal facet
3	Pedicle
4	Superior articular process
5	Transverse process
6	Spinous process
7	Inferior articular process
8	Inferior vertebral notch

Twelfth thoracic vertebra, **E** from the left, **F** from above, **G** from behind

1	Body
2	Costal facet
3	Pedicle
4	Superior articular process
5	Superior tubercle
6	Inferior tubercle
7	Spinous process
8	Inferior articular process
9	Lateral tubercle

● The atypical thoracic vertebrae are the first, tenth, eleventh and twelfth.

● The first thoracic vertebra has a posterolateral lip (A6, B6) on each side of the upper surface of the body and a triangular vertebral foramen (features like typical cervical vertebrae), and complete (round) superior costal facets (B10) on the sides of the body.

● The tenth, eleventh and twelfth thoracic vertebrae are characterised by a single complete costal facet on each side of the body that in the successive vertebrae comes to lie increasingly far from the upper surface of the body and encroaches increasingly on to the pedicle (C2, D2 and E2). There is also no articular facet on the transverse process.

● The transverse process of the twelfth thoracic vertebra is replaced by three tubercles—superior (E5, G5, corresponding to the mamillary process of a lumbar vertebra), lateral (F9, corresponding to a true transverse process) and inferior (E6, G6, corresponding to the accessory process of a lumbar vertebra).

●The inferior articular processes of the twelfth thoracic vertebra (E8) are curved to articulate with the curved superior processes of the first lumbar vertebra.

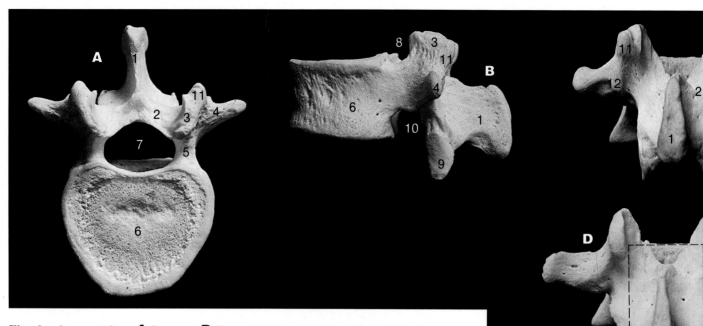

First lumbar vertebra, **A** from above, **B** from the left, **C** from behind

1	Spinous process
2	Lamina
3	Superior articular process
4	Transverse process
5	Pedicle
6	Body
7	Vertebral foramen
8	Superior vertebral notch
9	Inferior articular process
10	Inferior vertebral notch
11	Mamillary process
12	Accessory process

● Lumbar vertebrae are characterised by the large size of the bodies, the absence of costal facets on the bodies and the transverse processes, a triangular vertebral foramen (A7), a spinous process that points backwards and is quadrangular or hatchet-shaped (B1), and superior articular processes that are vertical, curved, face backwards and medially (A3) and possess a mamillary process at their posterior rim (A11).
● The rib element of a lumbar vertebra is represented by the transverse process (A4).

D Second lumbar vertebra, from behind, **E** third lumbar vertebra, from behind, **F** fourth lumbar vertebra, from behind, **G** fifth lumbar vertebra, from behind

● Viewed from behind, the four articular processes of the first and second lumbar vertebrae make a pattern (indicated by the interrupted line) of a vertical rectangle; those of the third or fourth vertebra make a square, and those of the fifth lumbar vertebra make a horizontal rectangle.

H Fifth lumbar vertebra, from above

1	Spinous process
2	Lamina
3	Superior articular process
4	Transverse process fusing with pedicle and body
5	Body
6	Vertebral foramen
7	Pedicle

● The fifth lumbar vertebra is unique in that the transverse process (H4) unites directly with the side of the body (H5) as well as with the pedicle (H7).

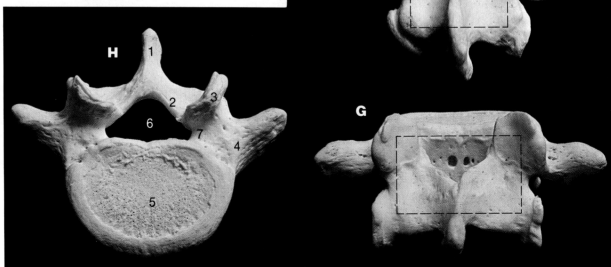

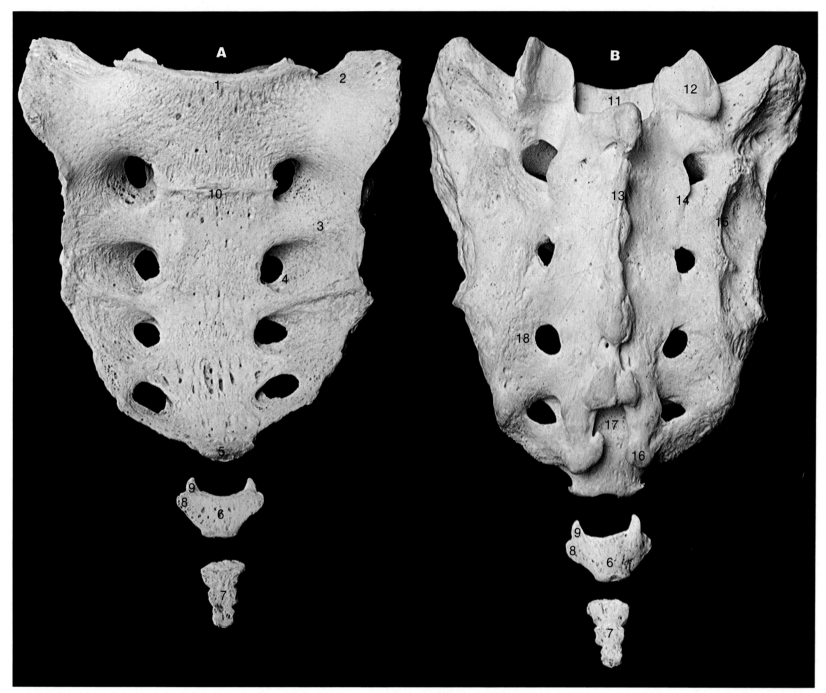

Sacrum and coccyx, A pelvic surface, B dorsal surface

1	Promontory	11	Sacral canal
2	Upper surface of lateral part (ala)	12	Superior articular process
3	Lateral part	13	Median sacral crest
4	Second pelvic sacral foramen	14	Intermediate sacral crest
5	Facet for coccyx	15	Lateral sacral crest
6	First coccygeal vertebra	16	Sacral cornu
7	Fused second to fourth vertebrae	17	Sacral hiatus
8	Transverse process	18	Third dorsal sacral foramen
9	Coccygeal cornu		
10	Site of fusion of first and second sacral vertebrae		

● The sacrum is formed by the fusion of the five sacral vertebrae. The median sacral crest (B13) represents the fused spinous processes, the intermediate crest (B14) the fused articular processes, and the lateral crest (B15) the fused transverse processes.
● The sacral hiatus (B17) is the lower opening of the sacral canal (B11).
● The coccyx is usually formed by the fusion of four rudimentary vertebrae but the number varies from three to five. In this specimen the first piece of the coccyx (6) is not fused with the remainder (7).

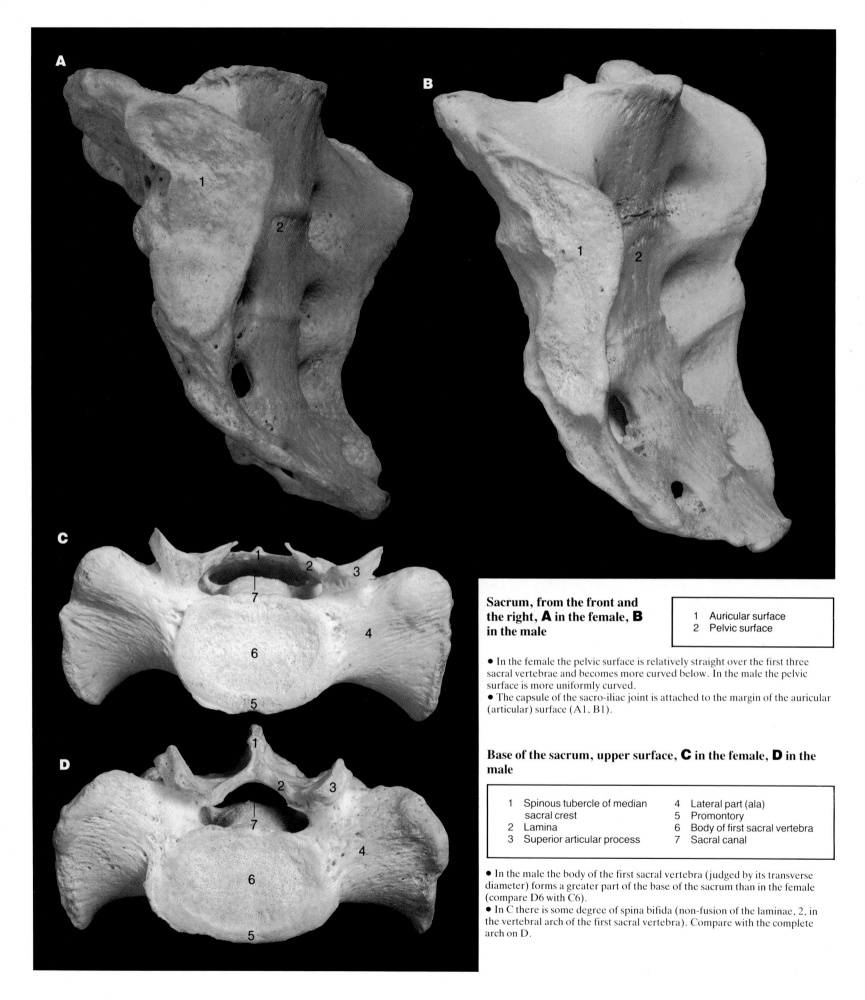

Sacrum, from the front and the right, A in the female, B in the male

1	Auricular surface
2	Pelvic surface

● In the female the pelvic surface is relatively straight over the first three sacral vertebrae and becomes more curved below. In the male the pelvic surface is more uniformly curved.
● The capsule of the sacro-iliac joint is attached to the margin of the auricular (articular) surface (A1, B1).

Base of the sacrum, upper surface, C in the female, D in the male

1	Spinous tubercle of median sacral crest	4	Lateral part (ala)
2	Lamina	5	Promontory
3	Superior articular process	6	Body of first sacral vertebra
		7	Sacral canal

● In the male the body of the first sacral vertebra (judged by its transverse diameter) forms a greater part of the base of the sacrum than in the female (compare D6 with C6).
● In C there is some degree of spina bifida (non-fusion of the laminae, 2, in the vertebral arch of the first sacral vertebra). Compare with the complete arch on D.

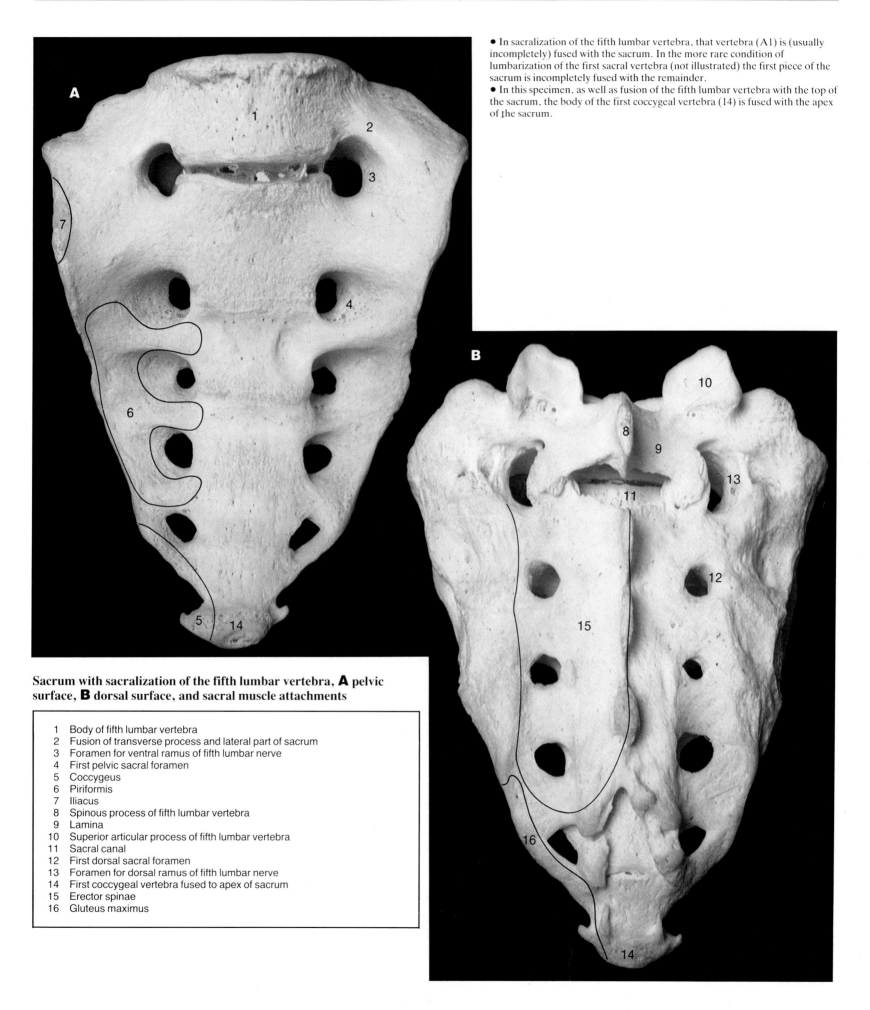

● In sacralization of the fifth lumbar vertebra, that vertebra (A1) is (usually incompletely) fused with the sacrum. In the more rare condition of lumbarization of the first sacral vertebra (not illustrated) the first piece of the sacrum is incompletely fused with the remainder.

● In this specimen, as well as fusion of the fifth lumbar vertebra with the top of the sacrum, the body of the first coccygeal vertebra (14) is fused with the apex of the sacrum.

Sacrum with sacralization of the fifth lumbar vertebra, A pelvic surface, B dorsal surface, and sacral muscle attachments

1	Body of fifth lumbar vertebra
2	Fusion of transverse process and lateral part of sacrum
3	Foramen for ventral ramus of fifth lumbar nerve
4	First pelvic sacral foramen
5	Coccygeus
6	Piriformis
7	Iliacus
8	Spinous process of fifth lumbar vertebra
9	Lamina
10	Superior articular process of fifth lumbar vertebra
11	Sacral canal
12	First dorsal sacral foramen
13	Foramen for dorsal ramus of fifth lumbar nerve
14	First coccygeal vertebra fused to apex of sacrum
15	Erector spinae
16	Gluteus maximus

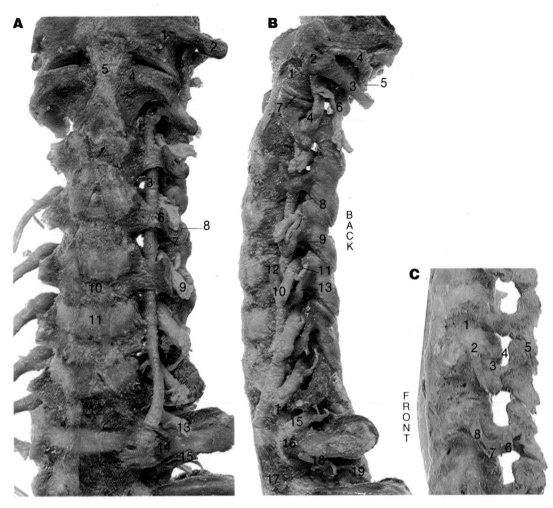

A Vertebral column, cervical region, from the front

The left vertebral artery (3) is seen within foramina of cervical transverse processes, which are partly removed from the sixth and seventh (12) cervical vertebrae. On the right side (left of the picture, unlabelled) all transverse processes have been removed and some dorsal root ganglia and nerve rami are displayed

1	Lateral mass } of atlas
2	Transverse process
3	Vertebral artery
4	Axis
5	Anterior longitudinal ligament
6	Anterior tubercle } of transverse process
7	Intertubercular lamella
8	Posterior tubercle
9	Ventral ramus of fifth cervical nerve
10	Body of fifth cervical vertebra
11	Intervertebral disc
12	Body of seventh cervical vertebra
13	Ventral ramus of eighth cervical nerve
14	Joint of head of first rib
15	Ventral ramus of first thoracic nerve

B Vertebral column, cervical and upper thoracic regions, from the left

Ventral and dorsal rami of spinal nerves (as at 10 and 11) are seen emerging from intervertebral foramina (as at 9)

1	Lateral mass } of atlas
2	Transverse process
3	Posterior arch
4	Vertebral artery
5	First cervical nerve
6	Dorsal root ganglion and rami of second cervical nerve
7	Atlanto-axial joint
8	Zygapophysial joint
9	Intervertebral foramen
10	Ventral } ramus of fifth cervical nerve
11	Dorsal
12	Anterior tubercle } of transverse process
13	Posterior tubercle } of fifth cervical vertebra
14	Body of seventh cervical vertebra
15	Ventral ramus of eighth cervical nerve
16	Head of first rib
17	Body of first thoracic vertebra
18	Ventral } ramus of first thoracic nerve
19	Dorsal

● The first and second cervical nerves pass respectively above and below the posterior arch of the atlas.
● On its upward course from the subclavian artery the vertebral artery enters the foramen of the transverse process of the sixth cervical vertebra.
● For the joints of the ribs with thoracic vertebrae see page 196.

C Vertebral column, cervical region, from the left

Soft tissue has been removed to show the boundaries of intervertebral foramina (as at 4). Compare with the cleared specimens of thoracic and lumbar vertebrae on page 85, C and D

1	Body of third cervical vertebra
2	Intervertebral disc
3	Pedicle
4	Intervertebral foramen
5	Zygapophysial joint
6	Posterior tubercle } of transverse
7	Intertubercular lamella } process of fifth
8	Anterior tubercle } cervical vertebra

● Each intervertebral foramen (as at C4) is bounded in front by a vertebral body and intervertebral disc (C1 and 2), above and below by pedicles (C3), and behind by a zygapophysial joint (C5).
● In the thoracic and lumbar regions there are the same number of pairs of spinal nerves as there are vertebrae (twelve thoracic and five lumbar), and spinal nerves are numbered from the vertebra beneath whose pedicles they emerge. In the cervical region there are seven cervical vertebrae and eight cervical nerves. The first nerve emerges between the occipital bone of the skull and the atlas, and the eighth (A13) below the pedicle of the seventh cervical vertebra (A12).
● The zygapophysial joints between the articular processes of adjacent vertebrae are commonly called facet joints (between the articular facets of those processes).
● For further details of spinal nerves see the notes on the opposite page.

D Vertebral column and spinal cord, lower cervical and upper thoracic regions, from behind

The vertebral arches and most of the dura mater and arachnoid have been removed, to show dorsal nerve rootlets (2) emerging from the spinal cord (1) to unite as a dorsal nerve root and enter the dural sheath (as at 6). Ventral nerve roots do the same from the ventral aspect of the cord but are not seen in this view as they are obscured by the dorsal roots

1	Spinal cord and posterior spinal vessels
2	Dorsal rootlets } of eighth
3	Dorsal root ganglion } cervical nerve
4	Pedicle of first thoracic vertebra
5	Dura mater
6	Dural sheath } of second
7	Dorsal root ganglion } thoracic nerve
8	Ventral } ramus of fifth
9	Dorsal } thoracic nerve
10	Angulation of nerve roots entering dural sheath

- The spinal cord is properly called the spinal medulla (not to be confused with the medulla oblongata, the lowest part of the brainstem, which continues as the spinal medulla).
- Each spinal nerve is formed by the union of ventral and dorsal nerve roots.
- Each nerve root is formed by the union of several rootlets (as at D2).
- The union of ventral and dorsal nerve roots to form a spinal nerve occurs immediately distal to the ganglion on the dorsal root (as at D3), within the intervertebral foramen, and the nerve at once divides into a ventral and a dorsal ramus (formerly called ventral and dorsal primary rami) (as at D8 and 9). The spinal nerve proper is thus only a millimetre or two in length, but is often so short that the rami appear to be branches of the ganglion itself.
- The lowest cervical and upper thoracic nerve roots become acutely angled in order to enter their dural sheaths (as at D10).

E Vertebral column and spinal cord, cervical and upper thoracic regions, from the left

Parts of the vertebral arches and meninges have been removed, to show the denticulate ligament (9). Dorsal nerve rootlets lie behind it (as at 11) and ventral nerve roots in front of it (as at 10 but largely hidden in this view)

1	Spinal part of accessory nerve
2	Medulla oblongata
3	Foramen magnum
4	Occipital bone
5	Posterior arch of atlas
6	Spinous process of axis (abnormally large)
7	Spinal cord
8	Dura mater
9	Denticulate ligament
10	Ventral rootlets
11	Dorsal rootlets — of fifth
12	Dorsal root ganglion — cervical
13	Dorsal ramus — nerve
14	Ventral ramus
15	Spinous process of seventh cervical vertebra
16	Dorsal root ganglion of eighth cervical nerve
17	Body of first thoracic vertebra
18	Arachnoid mater
19	Sympathetic trunk

F Cervical region of the spinal cord, from the front

For this ventral view of the upper part of the spinal cord (1), the dura and arachnoid mater have been incised longitudinally and turned aside (3) to show the ventral nerve rootlets and roots (as at 4) passing laterally in front of the denticulate ligament (2) to enter meningeal nerve sheaths with dorsal roots (as at 5) and form a spinal nerve. On some roots branches of radicular vessels (as at 6) are seen anastomosing with anterior spinal vessels (7)

1	Spinal cord
2	Denticulate ligament
3	Arachnoid and dura mater
4	Ventral root of fifth cervical nerve entering dural sheath
5	Dorsal root of sixth cervical nerve
6	Radicular vessels
7	Anterior spinal vessels

- The denticulate ligament (F2) is composed of pia mater. The ventral and dorsal nerve roots pass respectively ventral and dorsal to the ligament, which extends laterally from the side of the cord and is attached by its spiky denticulations (as at F2) to the arachnoid and dura mater in the intervals between dural nerve sheaths. The highest denticulation is above the first cervical nerve and the lowest below the twelfth thoracic nerve.
- For the continuity of the spinal cord with the brainstem see page 69, E.

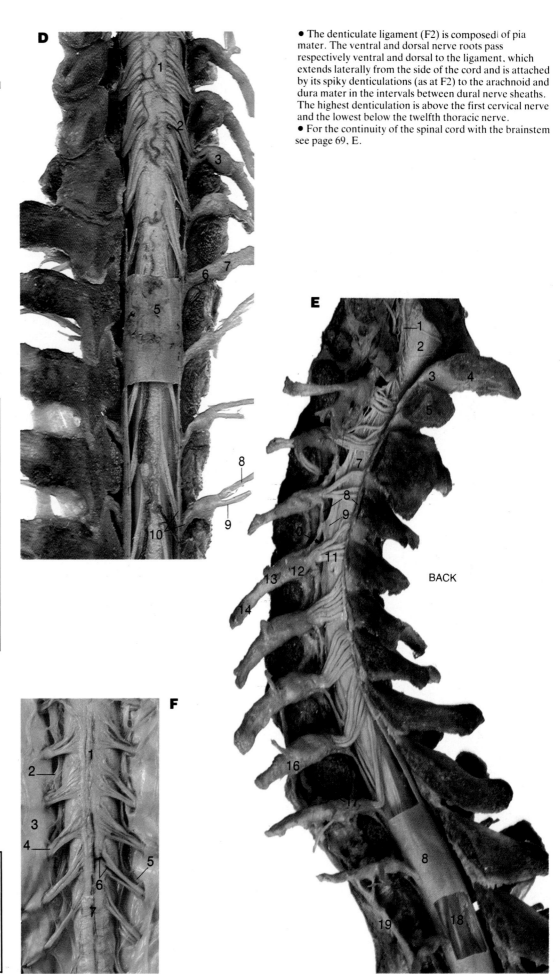

A

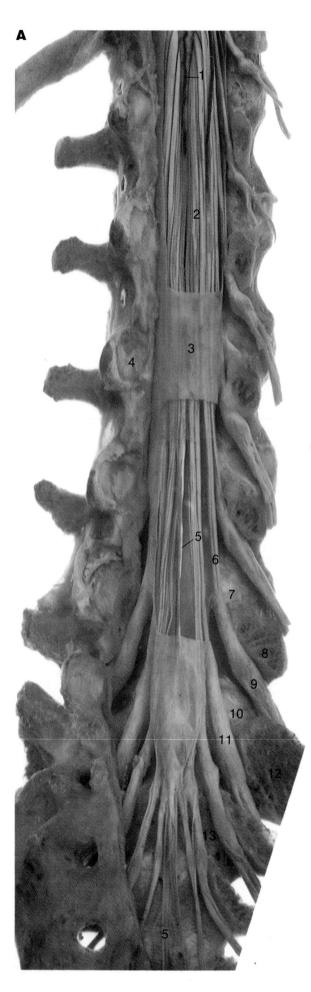

B

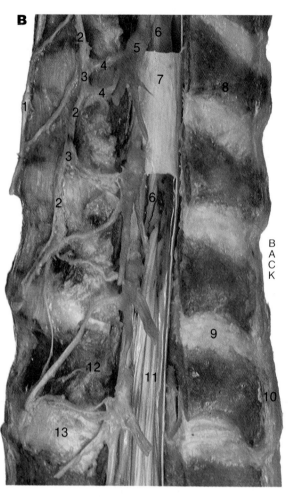

BACK

B Vertebral column and spinal cord, lower thoracic and upper lumbar regions

The specimen is seen from the left with parts of the vertebral arches and meninges removed, to show (at the front) part of the sympathetic trunk (2) on the vertebral bodies and (at the back) the spinous ligaments (9 and 10)

1	Greater splanchnic nerve
2	Sympathetic trunk
3	Sympathetic ganglion
4	Rami communicantes
5	Dorsal root ganglion of tenth thoracic nerve
6	Spinal cord
7	Dura mater
8	Spinous process of tenth thoracic vertebra
9	Interspinous ligament
10	Supraspinous ligament
11	Cauda equina
12	Body of first lumbar vertebra
13	First lumbar intervertebral disc

A Vertebral column, lumbar and sacral regions, from behind

Parts of the vertebral arches and meninges have been removed, to show the cauda equina (2) and nerve roots entering their meningeal sheaths (as at 6)

1	Conus medullaris of spinal cord
2	Cauda equina
3	Dura mater
4	Superior articular process of third lumbar vertebra
5	Filum terminale
6	Roots of fifth lumbar nerve
7	Fourth lumbar invertebral disc
8	Pedicle of fifth lumbar vertebra
9	Dorsal root ganglion of fifth lumbar nerve
10	Fifth lumbar (lumbosacral) intervertebral disc
11	Dural sheath of first sacral nerve roots
12	Lateral part of sacrum
13	Second sacral vertebra

• The spinal cord ends at the level of the first lumbar vertebra.
• The subarachnoid space ends at the level of the second sacral vertebra.
• The conus medullaris (1) is the lower, pointed end of the spinal cord.

• The cauda equina (2) consists of the dorsal and ventral roots of the lumbar, sacral and coccygeal nerves. Note that it is nerve roots which form the cauda, not the spinal nerves themselves; these are not formed until ventral and dorsal roots unite at the level of an intervertebral foramen, immediately distal to the dorsal root ganglion (as at A9).
• If the fifth lumbar intervertebral disc protrudes backwards (the commonest 'slipped disc') it may irritate the roots of the first sacral nerve (A11). This is the general rule for any part of the vertebral column—a protruded disc may irritate the roots of the nerve numbered one below the disc. Note for example that the fifth lumbar nerve roots (A6) within their dural sheath pass laterally immediately below the pedicle of the fifth lumbar vertebra (A8) and so do not come to lie immediately behind the fifth lumbar disc (A10); it is the first sacral roots (A11) which lie in this position. The fifth nerve roots (A6) lie behind the fourth disc (A7).

C

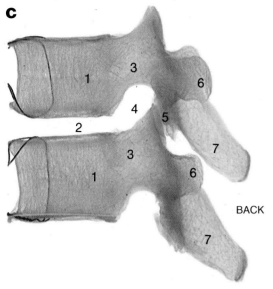

Cleared specimens, **C** thoracic vertebrae, **D** lumbar vertebrae

The pairs of vertebrae are seen from the side and articulated to show the boundaries of an intervertebral foramen (4)

1	Body
2	Space for intervertebral disc
3	Pedicle
4	Intervertebral foramen
5	Zygapophysial joint
6	Transverse process
7	Spinous process

BACK

• The intervertebral foramen (4) is bounded in front by the lower part of the vertebral body (1) and the intervertebral disc (2), above and below by the pedicles (3), and behind by the zygapophysial joint (5).

D

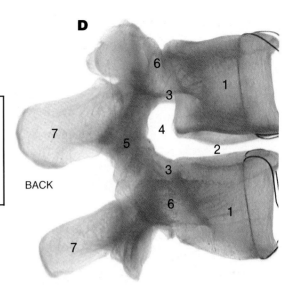

BACK

E Vertebral column, lumbar region. Posterior longitudinal ligament

The vertebral arches of the three upper lumbar vertebrae have been cut away through their pedicles (as at 1) and the meninges have been removed to show the posterior longitudinal ligament. Part of the internal vertebral venous plexus has been preserved

1	Pedicle of first lumbar vertebra
2	Posterior longitudinal ligament
3	Intervertebral disc
4	Intervertebral foramen
5	Internal vertebral venous plexus

• The posterior longitudinal ligament (E2) is broad where it is firmly attached to the intervertebral discs (E3), but narrow and less firmly attached to the vertebral bodies, leaving vascular foramina patent and allowing the basivertebral veins which emerge from them to enter the internal vertebral venous plexus (E5).
• The anterior longitudinal ligament (F1) is uniformly broad and firmly attached to discs and vertebral bodies.

F Vertebral column, lower lumbar region, from the front

At the top the anterior longitudinal ligament (1) has a marker behind it, and lower down part of it has been reflected off an intervertebral disc (3) and vertebral bodies (2 and 4)

1	Anterior longitudinal ligament
2	Body of fourth lumbar vertebra
3	Fourth lumbar intervertebral disc
4	Body of fifth lumbar vertebra
5	Ventral ramus of fifth lumbar nerve
6	Lateral part of sacrum

G Vertebral column, upper lumbar region, from the right

This side view shows lumbar nerves emerging from intervertebral foramina (as at 6)

1	Twelfth rib
2	Sympathetic trunk ganglion
3	Anterior longitudinal ligament
4	First lumbar vertebra
5	Rami communicantes
6	First lumbar nerve emerging from intervertebral foramen
7	Ventral } ramus of first lumbar nerve
8	Dorsal } ramus of first lumbar nerve
9	First lumbar intervertebral disc
10	Ventral } ramus of second lumbar nerve
11	Dorsal } ramus of second lumbar nerve
12	Zygapophysial joint
13	Spinous process of second lumbar vertebra
14	Interspinous ligament
15	Supraspinous ligament

F

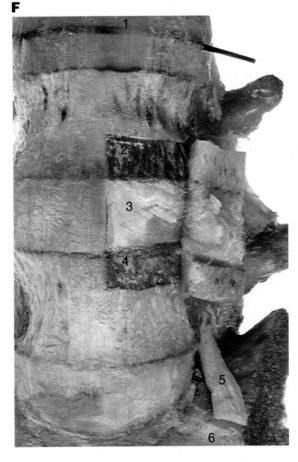

E

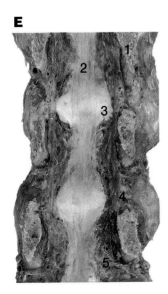

G

BACK

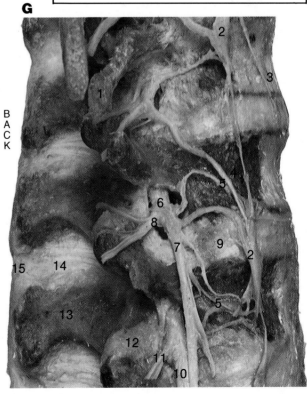

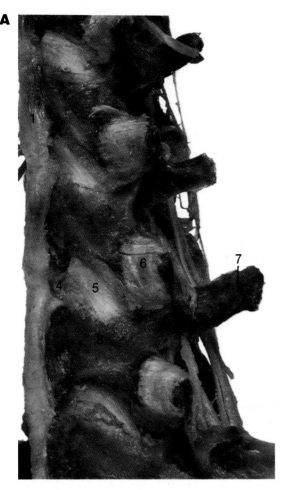

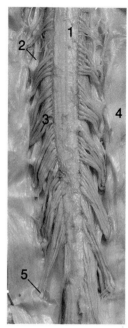

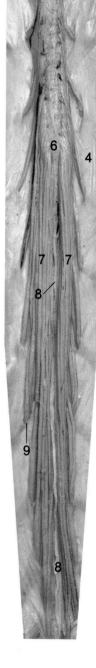

Dorsal surface of the spinal cord, **B** upper end, **C** lower end and cauda equina

The dura and arachnoid mater have been incised longitudinally and turned outwards (B4 and C4) to show the nerve roots entering their dural sheaths (as at B5 and C9). Below the level of the conus medullaris (the lower end of the spinal cord, C6) the nerve roots constitute the cauda equina (C7). Compare B with the ventral surface of the cervical part of the cord (page 83, F)

1	Spinal cord
2	Denticulate ligament
3	Dorsal rootlets of fifth cervical nerve
4	Arachnoid overlying dura mater
5	Eighth cervical nerve roots entering dural sheath
6	Conus medullaris
7	Cauda equina
8	Filum terminale
9	Fifth lumbar nerve roots entering dural sheath

● The filum terminale (C8), which consists of connective tissue, not neural elements, extends from the tip of the conus medullaris (C6) through the subarachnoid space to the level of the second sacral vertebra where it fuses with the dura mater and continues downwards to become attached to the first piece of the coccyx.

A Vertebral column, lumbar region, from the right and behind

This posterior view of the right side of some lumbar vertebrae shows ligamenta flava (as at 5), which pass between the laminae of adjacent vertebrae (as at 3 and 8)

1	Supraspinous ligament	
2	Spinous process	of second
3	Lamina	lumbar vertebra
4	Interspinous ligament	
5	Ligamentum flavum	
6	Zygapophysial joint	
7	Transverse process	of third
8	Lamina	lumbar vertebra

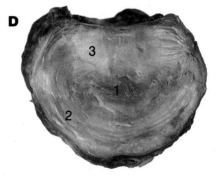

FRONT

D Intervertebral disc

This disc, on the upper surface of the body of a lumbar vertebra, has been cut horizontally to show the central nucleus pulposus (1) and the concentric fibrocartilaginous laminae of the surrounding annulus fibrosus (2). At the back the annulus has been shaved off to reveal part of the plate of hyaline cartilage (3) on the surface of the vertebra

1	Nucleus pulposus
2	Annulus fibrosus
3	Plate of hyaline cartilage

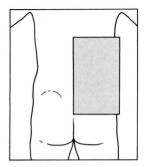

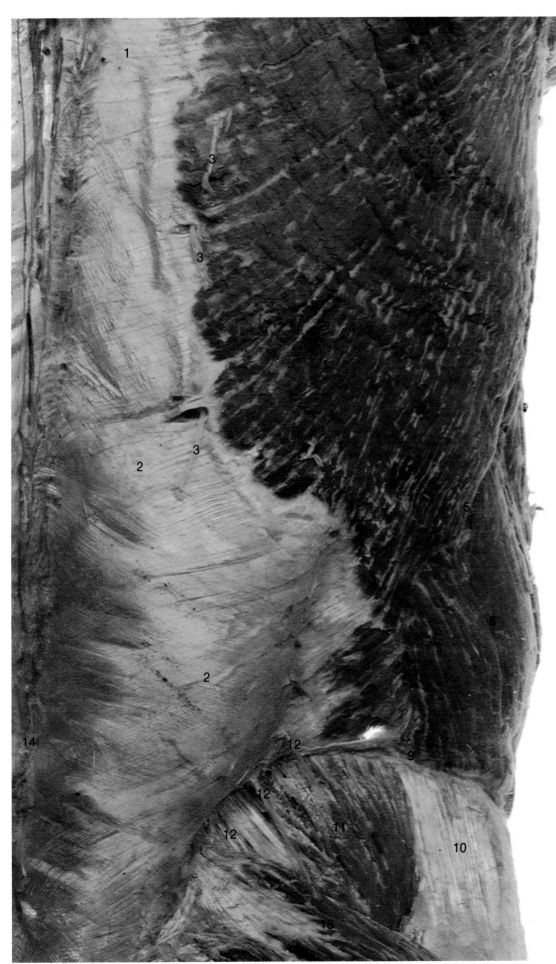

Muscles of the vertebral column. Right erector spinae and thoracolumbar fascia

The thoracolumbar fascia (1 and 2) covers erector spinae and laterally gives origin to latissimus dorsi (4, a muscle of the upper limb) and internal oblique (8, a muscle of the anterolateral abdominal wall)

1	Thoracic part of thoracolumbar fascia overlying erector spinae
2	Posterior layer of lumbar part of thoracolumbar fascia overlying erector spinae
3	Branches of dorsal rami of thoracic nerves
4	Latissimus dorsi
5	Free lateral border of 4
6	External oblique
7	Free posterior border of 6
8	Internal oblique
9	Iliac crest
10	Gluteal fascia
11	Gluteus medius
12	Cutaneous branches of dorsal rami of first three lumbar nerves
13	Gluteus maximus
14	Level of fourth lumbar spinous process

● The thoracolumbar fascia consists of a thoracic part, single-layered, covering the thoracic part of the erector spinae (1), and a lumbar part (where there are no ribs) which is commonly called simply the lumbar fascia and which consists of three layers.

● The posterior layer (2) is continuous with the thoracic part (1). The middle and anterior layers are usually studied with the posterior abdominal wall; the quadratus lumborum muscle lies between them, and psoas major is in front of the anterior layer (page 240). The lumbar part of erector spinae is between the posterior and middle layers. The three layers come together approximately at the lateral border of erector spinae (see the transverse section on page 240, B).

● For other parts of erector spinae see pages 88 and 157.

A

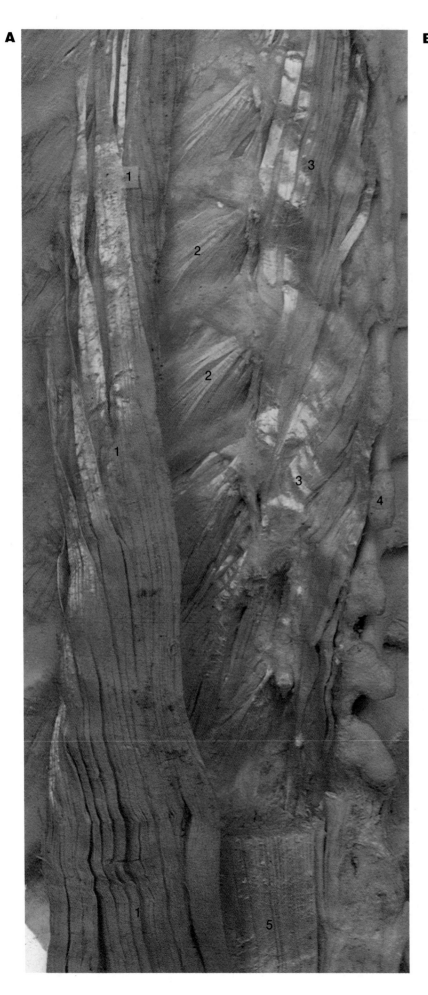

B

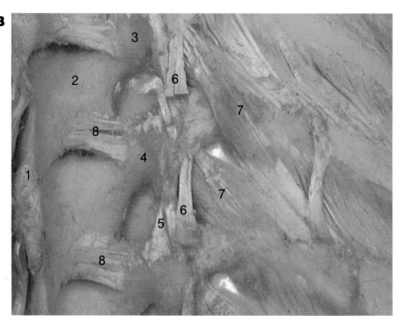

B Muscles of the vertebral column, right midthoracic region

All parts of erector spinae have been removed to show some rotator muscles (8) and intertransverse muscles and ligaments (5)

1	Spinous process
2	Lamina } of fourth thoracic vertebra
3	Transverse process
4	Transverse process of fifth thoracic vertebra
5	Intertransverse muscle and ligament
6	Tendons of longissimus
7	Levator costae
8	Rotator muscle

• The rotator muscles (8) pass from the transverse process of one vertebra (4) to the lamina of the vertebra above (2). They are only prominent in the thoracic region.
• The intertransverse muscles and ligaments (5 and 6) pass between adjacent transverse processes. The muscles are best developed in the cervical region and are usually absent over most of the thorax.

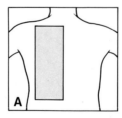

A Muscles of the vertebral column, left thoracolumbar region

Some of the iliocostalis (1), longissimus (5) and spinalis (3) parts of erector spinae are shown, together with levator costae muscles (2)

1	Iliocostalis
2	Levator costae
3	Parts of spinalis
4	Spine of eighth thoracic vertebra
5	Lower part of longissimus

• In the upper lumbar region, erector spinae divides into three muscle masses: iliocostalis (1) laterally, an intermediate longissimus (5, mostly removed in this specimen), and spinalis (3) medially.
• The levator costae muscles (2) are classified as muscles of the thorax, not of the vertebral column. They are revealed here because much of the longissimus part of the erector spinae (5) has been removed.

A

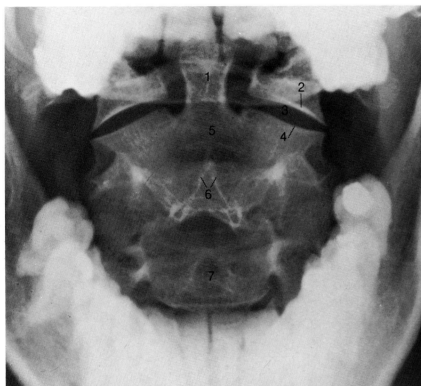

A Radiograph of upper cervical vertebrae

This is a standard radiographic view of the axis and its dens (1). The correct angle must be chosen with the mouth open to avoid overlying shadows of the teeth and jaws. The surfaces of the lateral atlanto-axial joints (2 and 3) do not appear congruent because the hyaline cartilage which covers the bony surfaces is not radio-opaque (this applies to any synovial joint). The outlines of the arches of the atlas are seen faintly between the sides of the shadow of the dens (1) and the lateral masses of the atlas (2)

1	Dens of axis	4	Superior articular surface of axis
2	Inferior articular surface of lateral mass of atlas	5	Body of axis
3	Lateral atlanto-axial joint	6	Bifid spinous process of axis
		7	Body of third cervical vertebra

B Radiograph of lower cervical and upper thoracic vertebrae, from the front

Note the tracheal shadow produced by the translucency of its contained air

1	Body of sixth cervical vertebra	9	Head	
2	Margin of tracheal shadow	10	Neck	of second rib
3	Body } of first	11	Tubercle	
4	Transverse process } thoracic vertebra			
5	Head			
6	Neck } of first rib			
7	Tubercle			
8	Shaft			

B

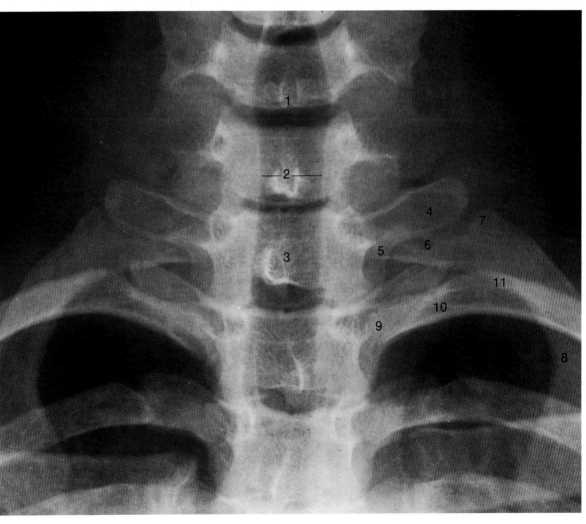

A

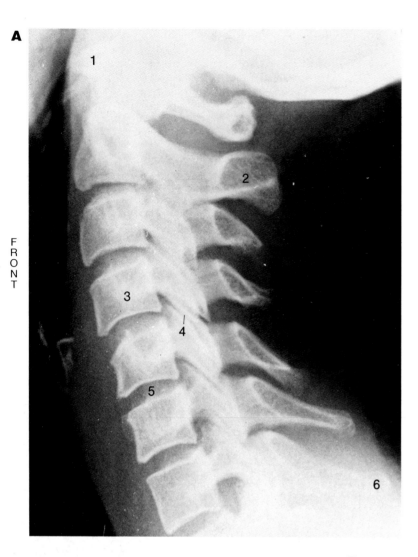

FRONT

B

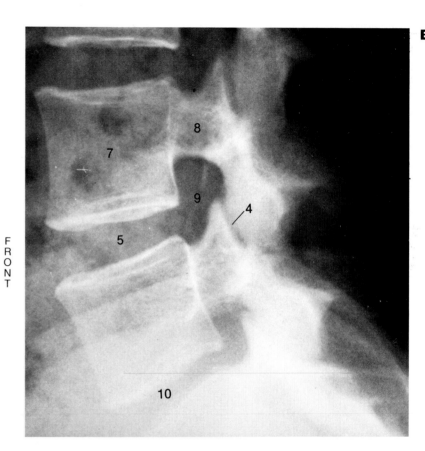

FRONT

C

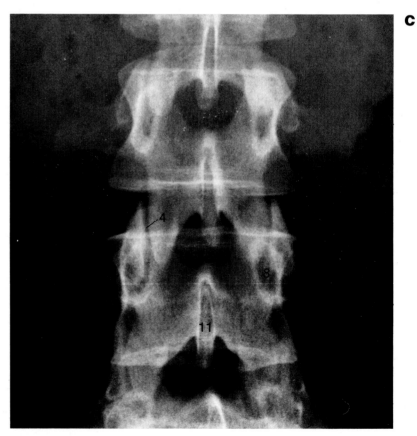

Radiographs of vertebrae, **A** cervical region, lateral view, **B** lumbar region, lateral view, **C** lumbar region, posterior view

In A note the (normal) large size of the spine of the axis (2), and the facet joints (4) between the articular processes of adjacent vertebrae. The intervertebral disc spaces and intervertebral foramina are largest in the lumbar region (B5, 9 and 10); compare with the cleared specimens on page 85, D. In the posterior view of the lumbar vertebrae, the pedicles appear as oval outlines over the lateral third of the vertebral bodies (C8)

1	Anterior arch of atlas	7	Body ⎫ of fourth
2	Spinous process of axis	8	Pedicle ⎰ lumbar vertebra
3	Body of fourth cervical vertebra	9	Intervertebral foramen
4	Zygapophysial (facet) joint	10	Lumbosacral disc space
5	Intervertebral disc space	11	Spinous process of fourth
6	Spinous process of seventh cervical vertebra		lumbar vertebra

Upper limb

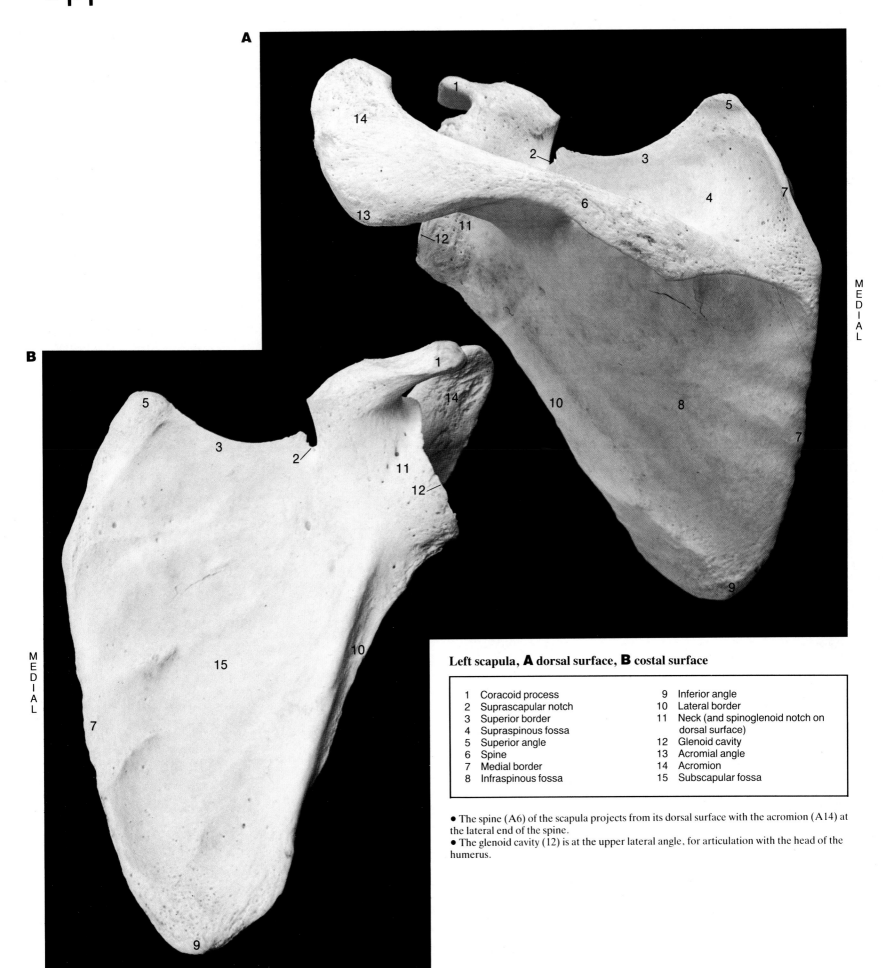

Left scapula, A dorsal surface, B costal surface

1	Coracoid process	9	Inferior angle
2	Suprascapular notch	10	Lateral border
3	Superior border	11	Neck (and spinoglenoid notch on dorsal surface)
4	Supraspinous fossa	12	Glenoid cavity
5	Superior angle	13	Acromial angle
6	Spine	14	Acromion
7	Medial border	15	Subscapular fossa
8	Infraspinous fossa		

- The spine (A6) of the scapula projects from its dorsal surface with the acromion (A14) at the lateral end of the spine.
- The glenoid cavity (12) is at the upper lateral angle, for articulation with the head of the humerus.

91

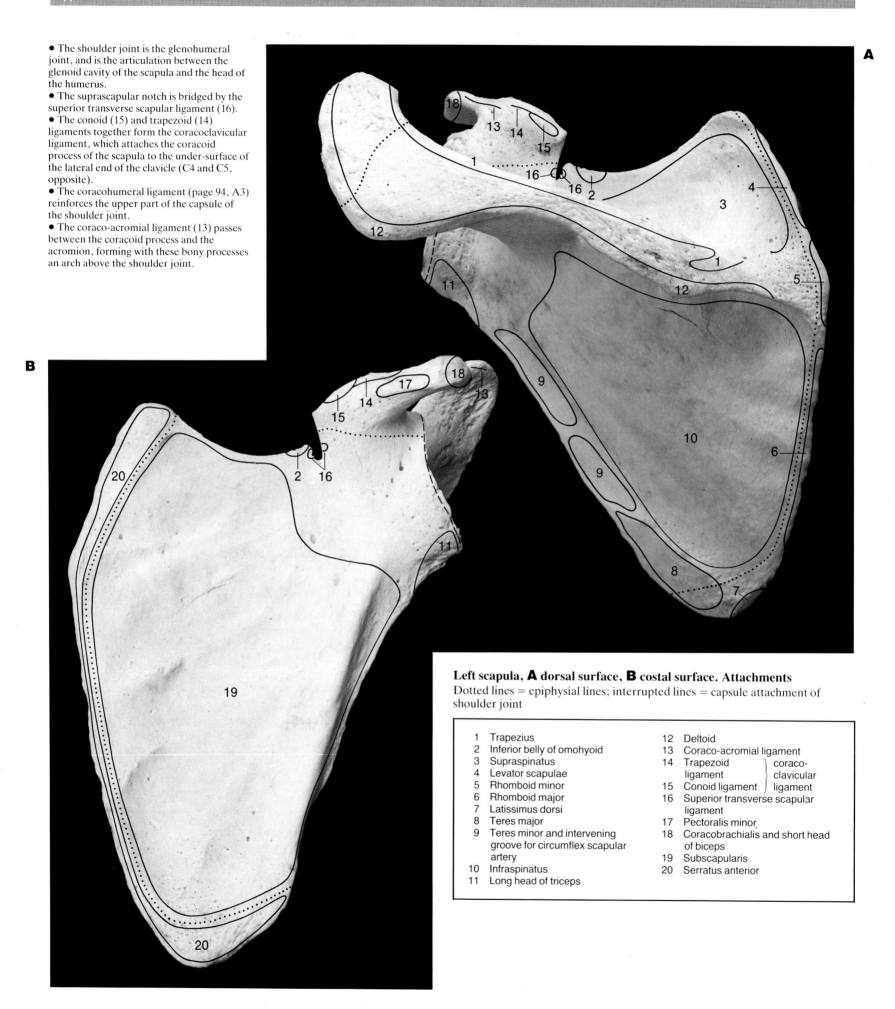

● The shoulder joint is the glenohumeral joint, and is the articulation between the glenoid cavity of the scapula and the head of the humerus.

● The suprascapular notch is bridged by the superior transverse scapular ligament (16).

● The conoid (15) and trapezoid (14) ligaments together form the coracoclavicular ligament, which attaches the coracoid process of the scapula to the under-surface of the lateral end of the clavicle (C4 and C5, opposite).

● The coracohumeral ligament (page 94, A3) reinforces the upper part of the capsule of the shoulder joint.

● The coraco-acromial ligament (13) passes between the coracoid process and the acromion, forming with these bony processes an arch above the shoulder joint.

Left scapula, A dorsal surface, B costal surface. Attachments
Dotted lines = epiphysial lines; interrupted lines = capsule attachment of shoulder joint

1	Trapezius	12	Deltoid
2	Inferior belly of omohyoid	13	Coraco-acromial ligament
3	Supraspinatus	14	Trapezoid ligament } coraco-
4	Levator scapulae		clavicular
5	Rhomboid minor	15	Conoid ligament } ligament
6	Rhomboid major	16	Superior transverse scapular
7	Latissimus dorsi		ligament
8	Teres major	17	Pectoralis minor
9	Teres minor and intervening	18	Coracobrachialis and short head
	groove for circumflex scapular		of biceps
	artery	19	Subscapularis
10	Infraspinatus	20	Serratus anterior
11	Long head of triceps		

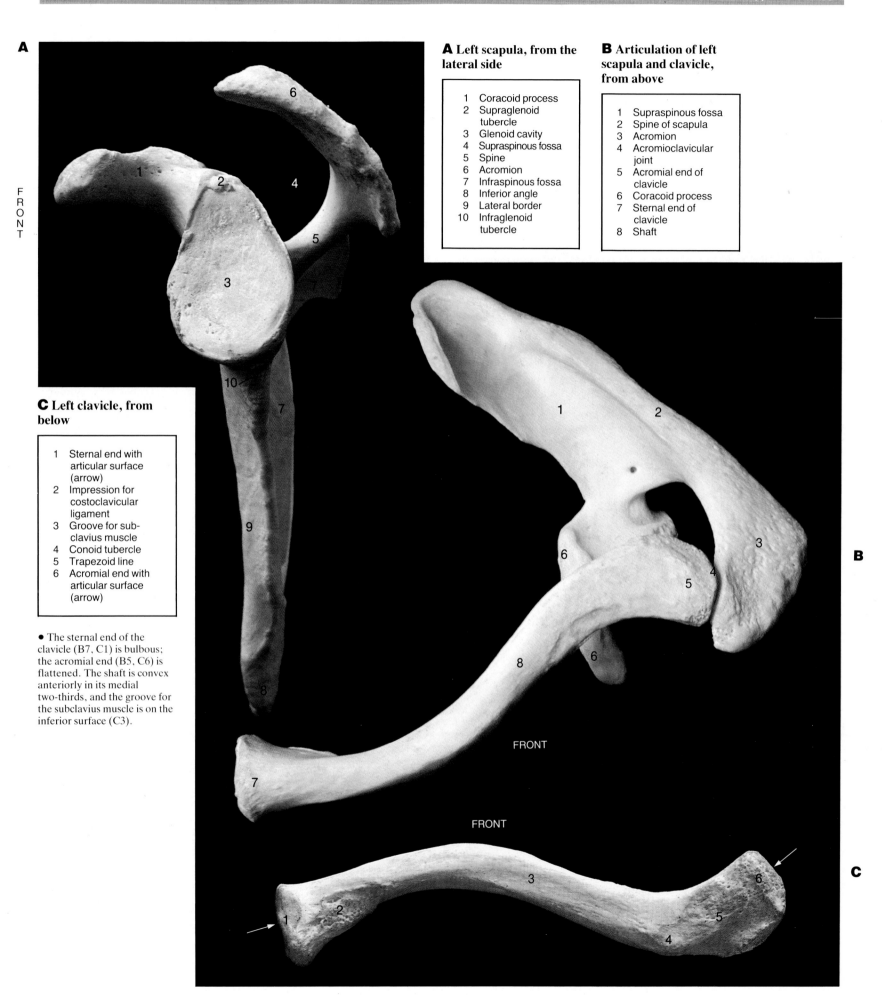

A

F
R
O
N
T

A Left scapula, from the lateral side

1	Coracoid process
2	Supraglenoid tubercle
3	Glenoid cavity
4	Supraspinous fossa
5	Spine
6	Acromion
7	Infraspinous fossa
8	Inferior angle
9	Lateral border
10	Infraglenoid tubercle

B Articulation of left scapula and clavicle, from above

1	Supraspinous fossa
2	Spine of scapula
3	Acromion
4	Acromioclavicular joint
5	Acromial end of clavicle
6	Coracoid process
7	Sternal end of clavicle
8	Shaft

C Left clavicle, from below

1	Sternal end with articular surface (arrow)
2	Impression for costoclavicular ligament
3	Groove for sub-clavius muscle
4	Conoid tubercle
5	Trapezoid line
6	Acromial end with articular surface (arrow)

● The sternal end of the clavicle (B7, C1) is bulbous; the acromial end (B5, C6) is flattened. The shaft is convex anteriorly in its medial two-thirds, and the groove for the subclavius muscle is on the inferior surface (C3).

FRONT

FRONT

B

C

93

A

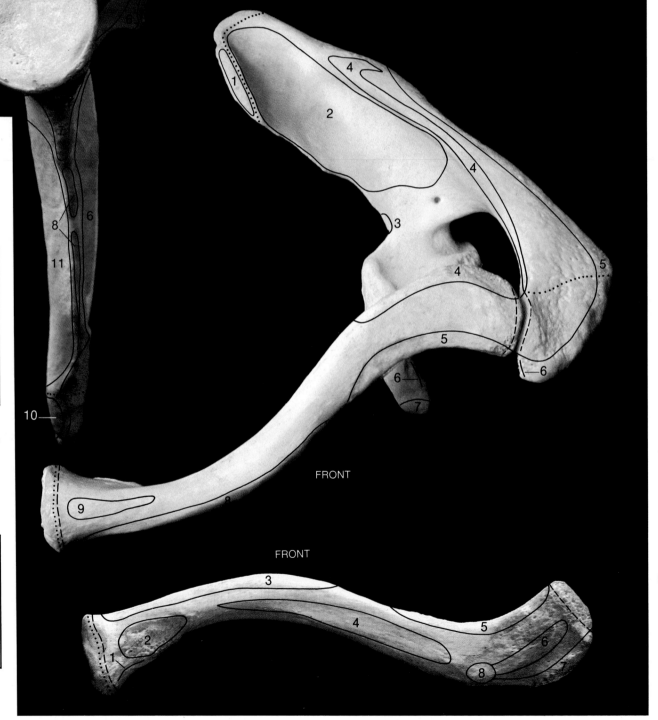

A Left scapula, from the lateral side. Attachments

Dotted lines = epiphysial lines; interrupted line = capsule attachment of shoulder joint

1	Coracobrachialis and short head of biceps	7	Long head of triceps
2	Coraco-acromial ligament	8	Teres minor (with intervening groove for circumflex scapular artery)
3	Coracohumeral ligament		
4	Long head of biceps	9	Teres major
5	Deltoid	10	Serratus anterior
6	Infraspinatus	11	Subscapularis

B Articulation of left scapula and clavicle, from above

Dotted lines = epiphysial lines; interrupted lines = capsule attachments of sternoclavicular and acromioclavicular joints

1	Levator scapulae
2	Supraspinatus
3	Inferior belly of omohyoid
4	Trapezius
5	Deltoid
6	Coraco-acromial ligament
7	Coracobrachialis and short head of biceps
8	Pectoralis major
9	Sternocleidomastoid

C Left clavicle, from below. Attachments

Dotted lines = epiphysial lines; interrupted lines = capsule attachments of sternoclavicular and acromioclavicular joints

1	Sternohyoid
2	Costoclavicular ligament
3	Pectoralis major
4	Subclavius and clavipectoral fascia
5	Deltoid
6	Trapezoid ligament
7	Trapezius
8	Conoid ligament

FRONT

FRONT

B

C

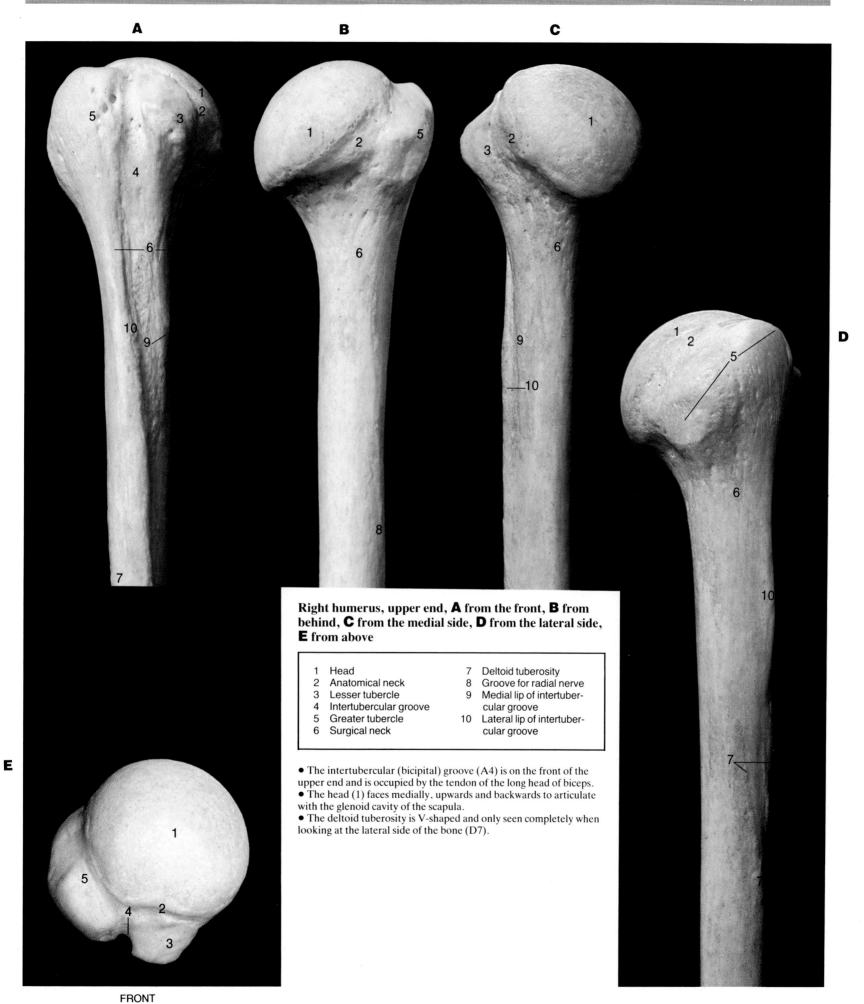

A

B

C

D

E

FRONT

Right humerus, upper end, A from the front, B from behind, C from the medial side, D from the lateral side, E from above

1	Head	7	Deltoid tuberosity
2	Anatomical neck	8	Groove for radial nerve
3	Lesser tubercle	9	Medial lip of intertuber-
4	Intertubercular groove		cular groove
5	Greater tubercle	10	Lateral lip of intertuber-
6	Surgical neck		cular groove

● The intertubercular (bicipital) groove (A4) is on the front of the upper end and is occupied by the tendon of the long head of biceps.
● The head (1) faces medially, upwards and backwards to articulate with the glenoid cavity of the scapula.
● The deltoid tuberosity is V-shaped and only seen completely when looking at the lateral side of the bone (D7).

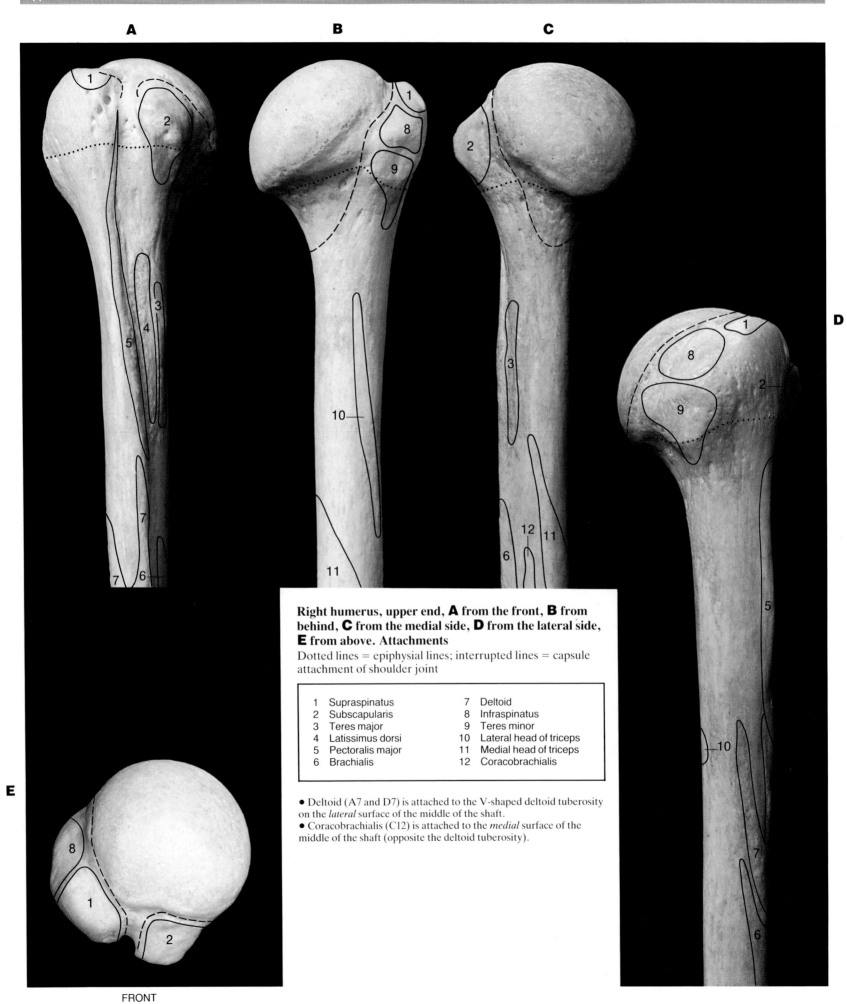

Right humerus, upper end, A from the front, B from behind, C from the medial side, D from the lateral side, E from above. Attachments

Dotted lines = epiphysial lines; interrupted lines = capsule attachment of shoulder joint

1	Supraspinatus	7	Deltoid
2	Subscapularis	8	Infraspinatus
3	Teres major	9	Teres minor
4	Latissimus dorsi	10	Lateral head of triceps
5	Pectoralis major	11	Medial head of triceps
6	Brachialis	12	Coracobrachialis

● Deltoid (A7 and D7) is attached to the V-shaped deltoid tuberosity on the *lateral* surface of the middle of the shaft.
● Coracobrachialis (C12) is attached to the *medial* surface of the middle of the shaft (opposite the deltoid tuberosity).

FRONT

96

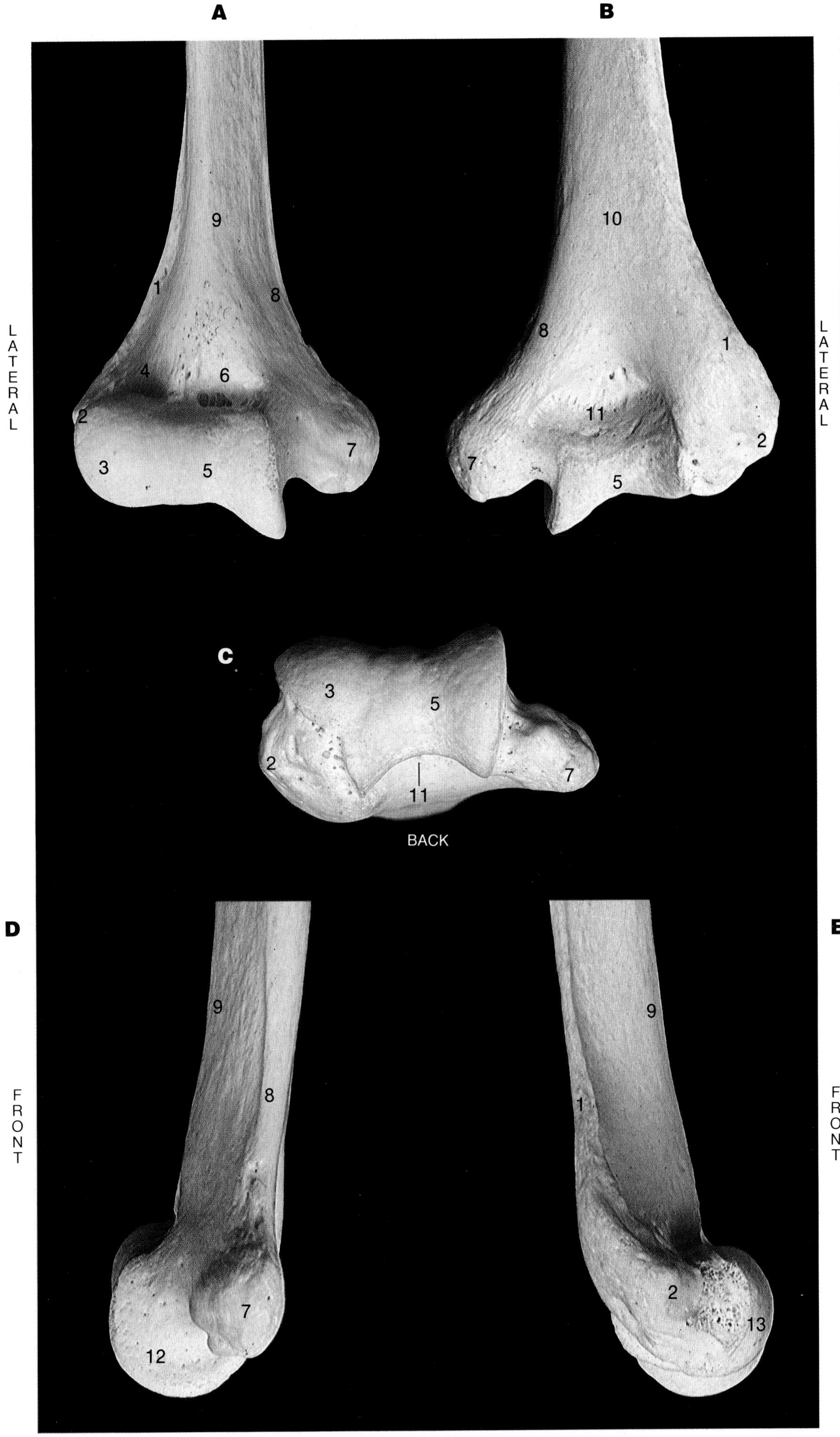

A

B

**Right humerus, lower end, A from the front,
B from behind, C from below, D from the
medial side, E from the lateral side**

1 Lateral supracondylar ridge
2 Lateral epicondyle
3 Capitulum
4 Radial fossa
5 Trochlea
6 Coronoid fossa
7 Medial epicondyle
8 Medial supracondylar ridge
9 Anterior surface
10 Posterior surface
11 Olecranon fossa
12 Medial surface of trochlea
13 Lateral edge of capitulum

● The medial epicondyle (7) is more prominent than the
lateral (2).
● The medial part of the trochlea (5) is more prominent
than the lateral part.
● The olecranon fossa (11) on the posterior surface is
deeper than the radial and coronoid fossae on the
anterior surface (4 and 6).

LATERAL

LATERAL

C

BACK

D

E

FRONT

FRONT

Right humerus, lower end, A from the front, B from behind, C from below, D from the medial side, E from the lateral side.
Attachments
Dotted lines = epiphysial lines; interrupted lines = capsule attachment of elbow joint

1 Brachialis
2 Pronator teres
3 Common flexor origin
4 Common extensor origin
5 Extensor carpi radialis longus
6 Brachioradialis
7 Anconeus
8 Medial head of triceps

● The ulnar and radial collateral ligaments of the elbow joint are attached to the medial and lateral epicondyles respectively (beneath the common flexor and extensor origins, 3 and 4).

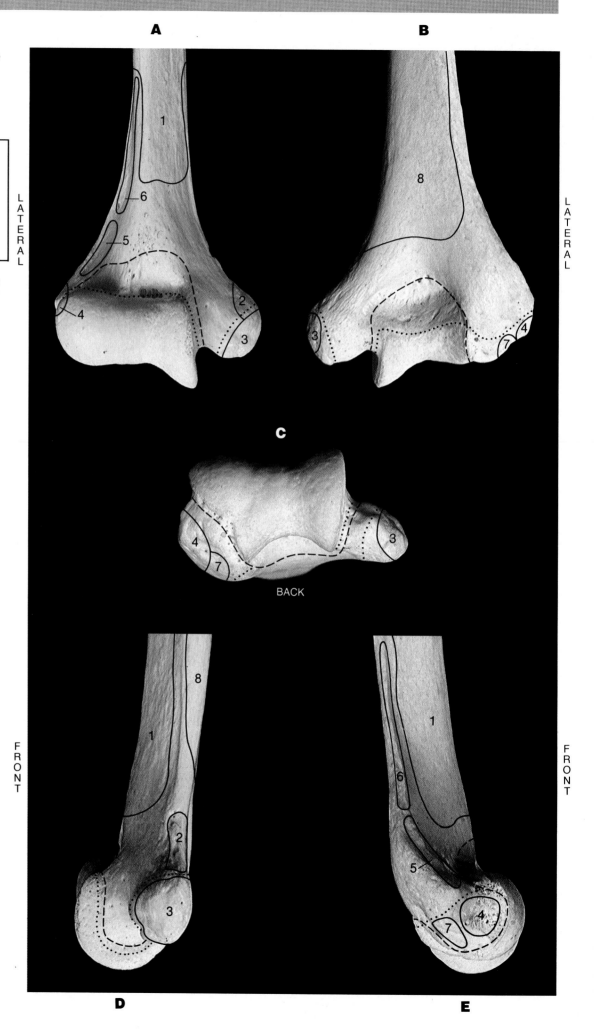

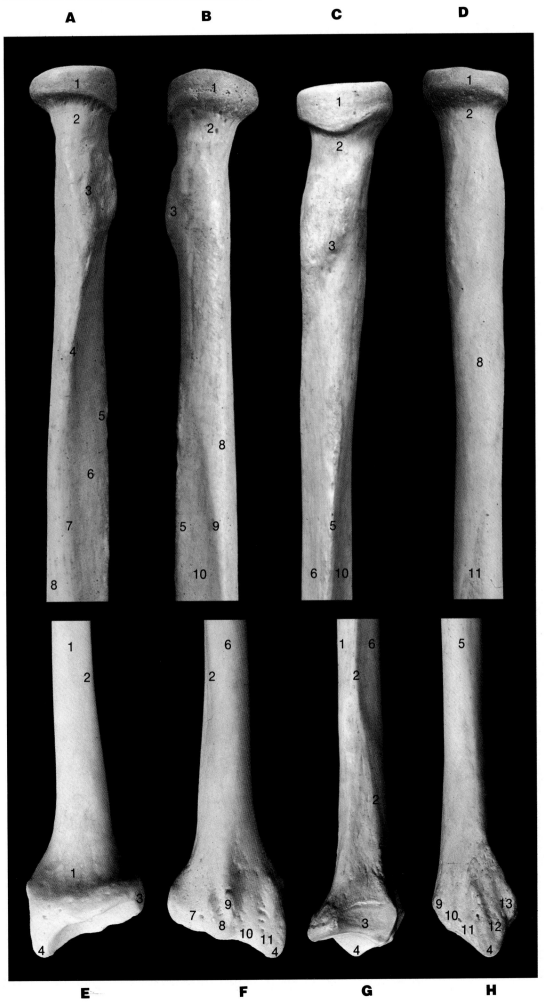

A   **B**   **C**   **D**

E   **F**   **G**   **H**

Right radius, upper end, A from the front, B from behind, C from the medial side, D from the lateral side

1	Head
2	Neck
3	Tuberosity
4	Anterior oblique line
5	Interosseous border
6	Anterior surface
7	Anterior border
8	Lateral surface
9	Posterior border
10	Posterior surface
11	Rough area for pronator teres

● The head of the radius (1) is at its upper end; the head of the ulna is at its lower end (page 100, E3).
● The tuberosity (3) is rough posteriorly for the attachment of the biceps tendon, and smooth anteriorly where it is covered by the intervening bursa.
● The shaft is triangular in cross section, and its surfaces are anterior (6), posterior (10) and lateral (8); its borders are interosseous (5), anterior (7) and posterior (9) (compare with the ulna, page 100).

Right radius, lower end, E from the front, F from behind, G from the medial side, H from the lateral side

1	Anterior surface
2	Interosseous border
3	Ulnar notch
4	Styloid process
5	Lateral surface
6	Posterior surface
7	Groove for extensor digitorum and extensor indicis
8	Groove for extensor pollicis longus
9	Dorsal tubercle
10	Groove for extensor carpi radialis brevis
11	Groove for extensor carpi radialis longus
12	Groove for extensor pollicis brevis
13	Groove for abductor pollicis longus

● The lower end of the radius is concave anteriorly (at the lower label 1 in E), with the ulnar notch medially (G3) and the dorsal tubercle on the posterior surface (F9).

Right ulna, upper end, A from the front, **B** from behind, **C** from the medial side, **D** from the lateral side

1	Olecranon
2	Trochlear notch
3	Coronoid process
4	Tuberosity
5	Radial notch
6	Supinator crest
7	Interosseous border
8	Anterior surface
9	Anterior border
10	Posterior surface
11	Posterior border
12	Medial surface

● The trochlear notch (2) faces forwards, with the radial notch (5) on the lateral side.
● The upper part of the shaft is triangular in cross section but the lower quarter is almost cylindrical. The surfaces of the shaft are anterior (8), posterior (10) and medial (12); the borders are interosseous (7), anterior (9) and posterior (11) (compare with the radius, page 99).

Right ulna, lower end, E from the front, **F** from behind, **G** from the medial side, **H** from the lateral side

1	Interosseous border
2	Anterior surface
3	Head
4	Posterior surface
5	Groove for extensor carpi ulnaris
6	Styloid process
7	Medial surface

● The head of the ulna (3) is at its lower end, with the styloid process (6) situated posteromedially. The head of the radius is at its upper end (page 99).

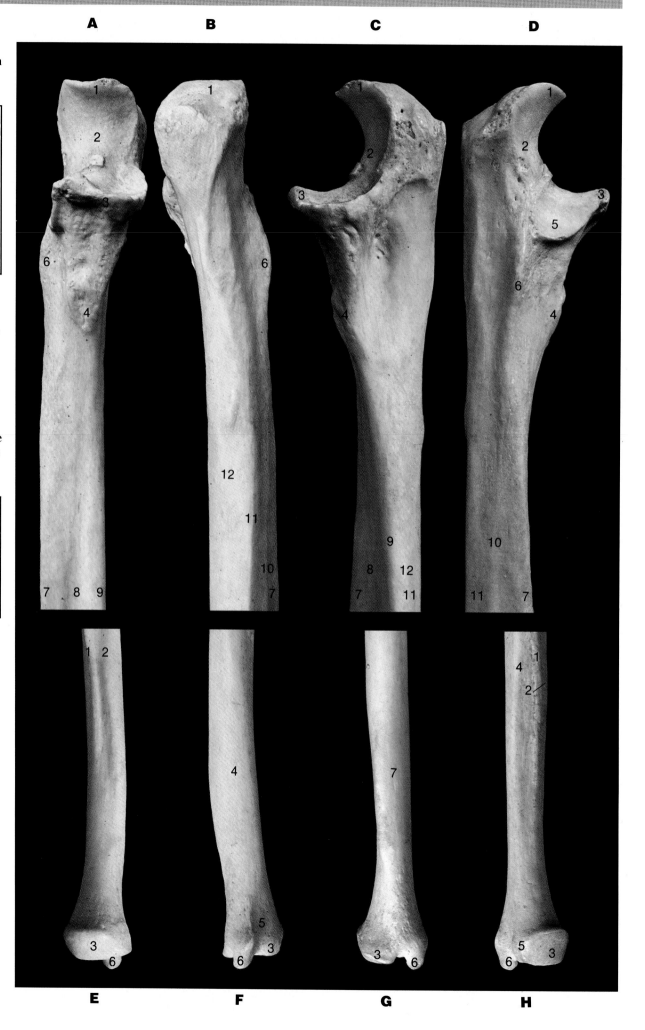

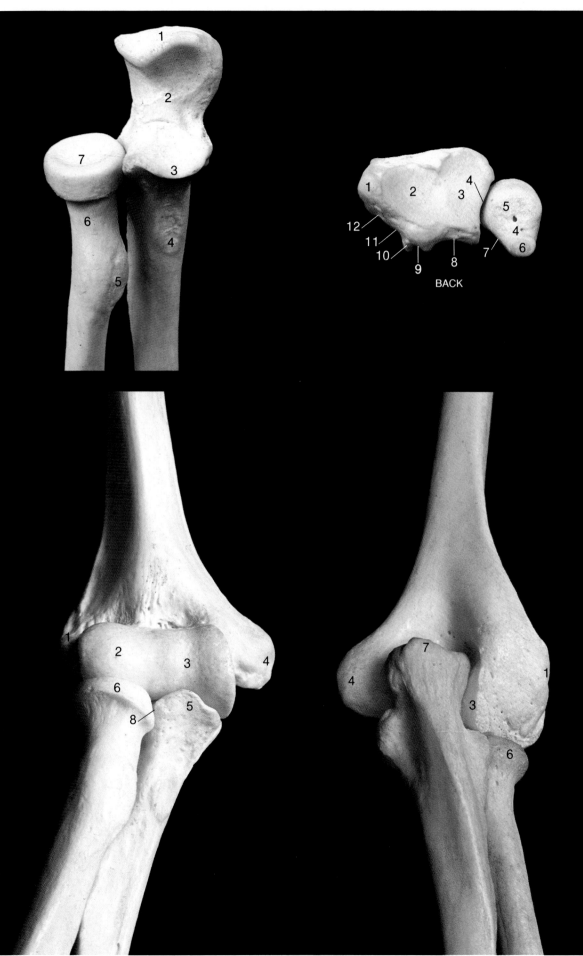

A Right radius and ulna, upper ends, from above and in front

1 Olecranon
2 Trochlear notch
3 Coronoid process
4 Tuberosity of ulna
5 Tuberosity of radius
6 Neck
7 Head

B Right radius and ulna, lower ends, from below

1 Styloid process of radius
2 Surface for scaphoid
3 Surface for lunate
4 Attachment of articular disc
5 Surface for disc
6 Styloid process of ulna
7 Groove for extensor carpi ulnaris
8 Groove for extensor digitorum and extensor indicis
9 Groove for extensor pollicis longus
10 Dorsal tubercle
11 Groove for extensor carpi radialis brevis
12 Groove for extensor carpi radialis longus

Articulation of right humerus, radius and ulna, **C** from the front, **D** from behind

1 Lateral epicondyle ⎫
2 Capitulum   ⎬ of
3 Trochlea   ⎬ humerus
4 Medial epicondyle ⎭
5 Coronoid process of ulna
6 Head of radius
7 Olecranon ⎫ of ulna
8 Radial notch ⎭

● The elbow joint is the articulation of the humerus with the radius and ulna—the capitulum of the humerus (2) with the head of the radius (6), and the trochlea of the humerus (3) with the trochlear notch of the ulna.
● The head of the radius (6) also articulates with the radial notch of the ulna (8), forming the proximal radio-ulnar joint.
● The elbow joint and the proximal radio-ulnar joint share a common synovial cavity.

Right radius and ulna, **A** from the front, **B** from behind. Attachments

Dotted lines = epiphysial lines; interrupted lines = capsule attachments of elbow and wrist joints

1	Flexor digitorum superficialis, ulnar head
2	Pronator teres
3	Brachialis
4	Flexor digitorum profundus
5	Pronator quadratus
6	Brachioradialis
7	Flexor pollicis longus
8	Flexor digitorum superficialis, radial head
9	Pronator teres
10	Supinator
11	Biceps
12	Triceps
13	Anconeus
14	Abductor pollicis longus
15	Extensor pollicis brevis
16	Extensor indicis
17	Extensor pollicis longus
18	Aponeurotic attachment of flexor digitorum profundus, flexor carpi ulnaris and extensor carpi ulnaris

• Abductor pollicis longus (14) and extensor pollicis brevis (15) are the only two muscles to have an origin from the posterior surface of the radius (although both extend on to the interosseous membrane and the abductor also has an origin from the posterior surface of the ulna). These muscles remain companions as they wind round the lateral side of the radius (page 127, C4 and 5) and form the radial boundary of the anatomical snuffbox (page 139, C6 and 7).

• Flexor pollicis longus has an occasional small additional origin from the lateral (or rarely the medial) side of the coronoid process of the ulna (beside the lower part of the brachialis attachment).

A   **B**

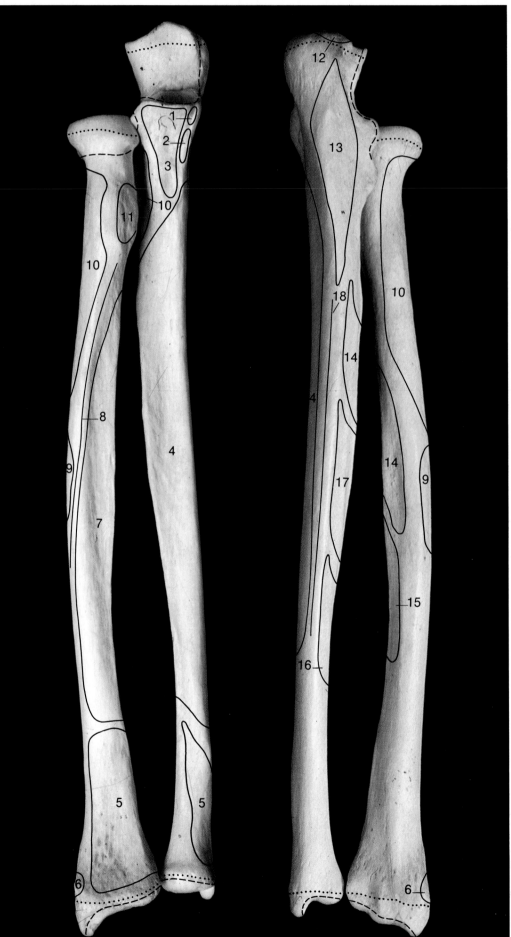

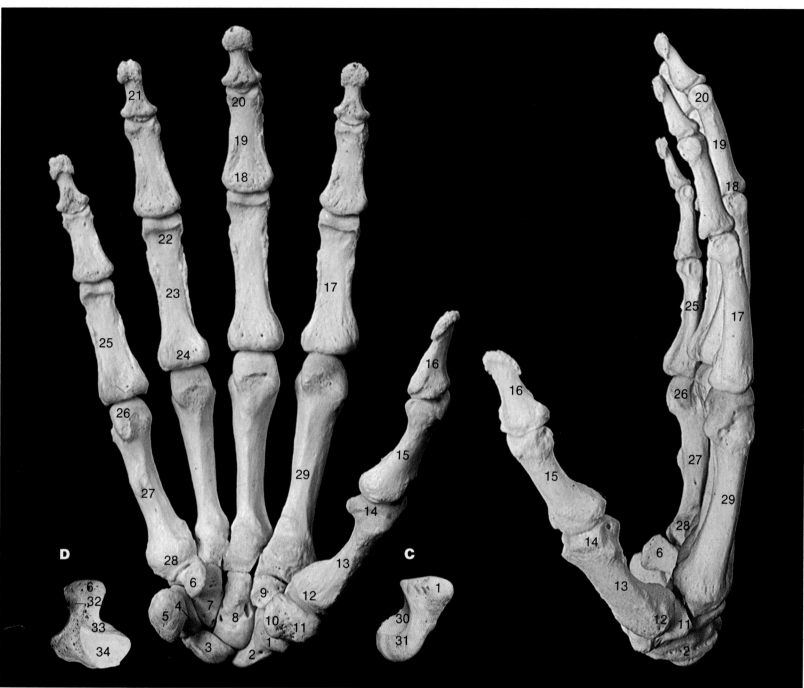

A

B

C

D

Bones of the right hand, A palmar surface, B from the lateral side, C scaphoid, palmar surface, D hamate from the medial side

● The scaphoid, lunate, triquetral and pisiform bones form the proximal row of carpal bones.
● The trapezium, trapezoid, capitate and hamate bones form the distal row of carpal bones.

1	Tubercle of scaphoid	
2	Scaphoid	
3	Lunate	
4	Triquetral	
5	Pisiform	
6	Hook of hamate	
7	Hamate	
8	Capitate	
9	Trapezoid	
10	Tubercle of trapezium	
11	Trapezium	
12	Base	} of first metacarpal
13	Shaft	
14	Head	
15	Proximal	} phalanx of thumb
16	Distal	
17	Proximal phalanx of index finger	

18	Base	} of middle phalanx of middle finger
19	Shaft	
20	Head	
21	Distal phalanx of ring finger	
22	Head	} of proximal phalanx of ring finger
23	Shaft	
24	Base	
25	Proximal phalanx of little finger	
26	Head	} of fifth metacarpal
27	Shaft	
28	Base	
29	Second metacarpal	
30	Surface for capitate	
31	Surface for lunate	
32	Groove for deep branch of ulnar nerve	
33	Palmar surface	
34	Surface for triquetral	

Bones of the right hand, **A** dorsal surface

1	Styloid process of radius	13	Proximal } phalanx of
2	Scaphoid	14	Distal } thumb
3	Lunate	15	Third metacarpal
4	Triquetral	16	Proximal } phalanx
5	Styloid process of ulna	17	Middle } of middle
6	Hamate	18	Distal } finger
7	Capitate	19	Fifth metacarpal
8	Trapezoid		
9	Trapezium		
10	Base }		
11	Shaft } of first metacarpal		
12	Head }		

Bones of the right hand, **B** palmar surface, **C** dorsal surface. Attachments

1 Flexor carpi ulnaris
2 Abductor digiti minimi
3 Pisohamate ligament
4 Pisometacarpal ligament
5 Flexor digiti minimi brevis
6 Opponens digiti minimi
7 Fourth ⎫
8 Third ⎬ palmar interosseous
9 Second ⎪
10 First ⎭
11 First ⎫
12 Second ⎬ dorsal interosseous
13 Third ⎪
14 Fourth ⎭
15 Transverse ⎫ head of adductor pollicis
16 Oblique ⎭
17 Flexor carpi radialis
18 Flexor pollicis brevis
19 Opponens pollicis
20 Abductor pollicis brevis
21 Abductor pollicis longus
22 Extensor pollicis brevis
23 Extensor pollicis longus
24 Flexor digitorum superficialis
25 Flexor digitorum profundus
26 Flexor pollicis longus
27 Extensor expansion
28 Extensor carpi ulnaris
29 Extensor carpi radialis brevis
30 Extensor carpi radialis longus

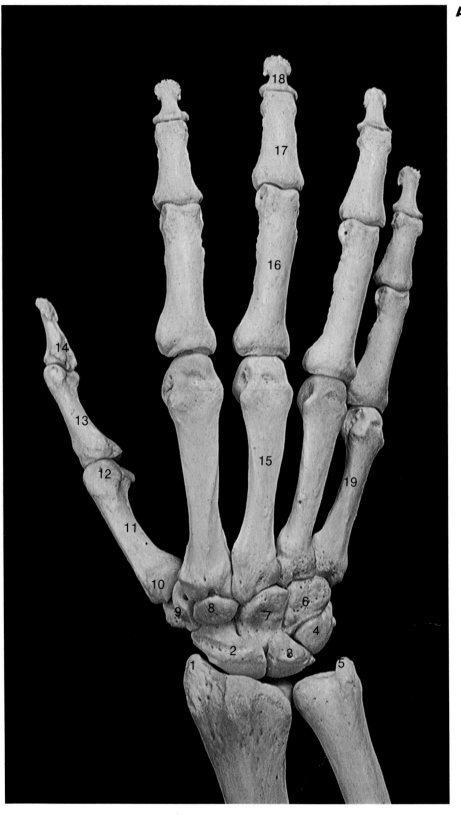

A

- The wrist joint (properly called the radiocarpal joint) is the joint between (proximally) the lower end of the radius and the interarticular disc which holds the lower ends of the radius and ulna together, and (distally) the scaphoid, lunate and triquetral bones.
- The midcarpal joint is the joint between the proximal and distal rows of carpal bones (see the note on page 103).
- The carpometacarpal joint of the thumb is the joint between the trapezium and the base of the first metacarpal.

B

C

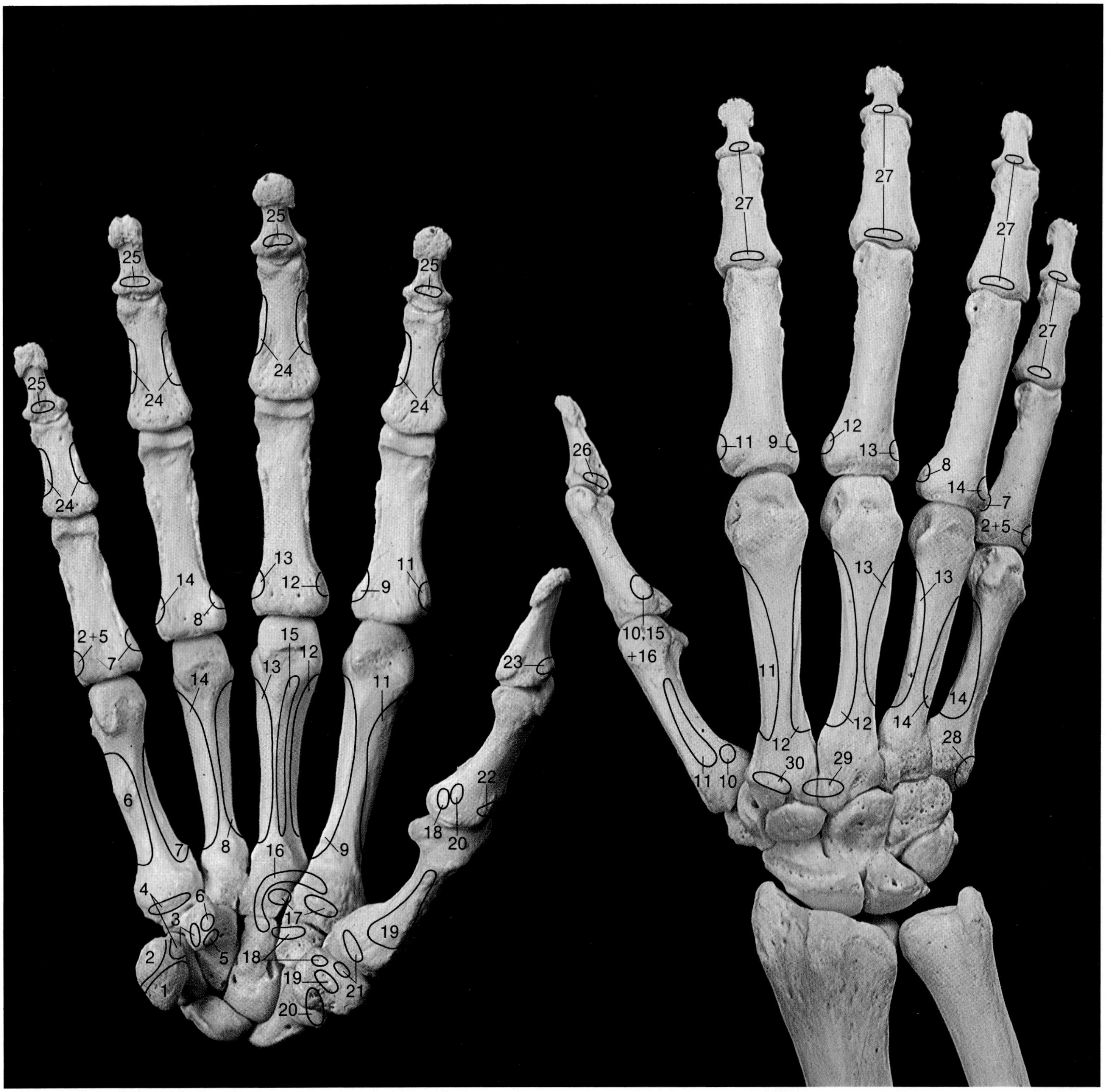

• The metacarpophalangeal joints are the joints between the heads of the metacarpals and the bases of the proximal phalanges.
• The interphalangeal joints are the joints between the head of one phalanx and the base of the adjoining phalanx.
• The pisiform is a sesamoid bone in the tendon of flexor carpi ulnaris and is anchored by the pisohamate and pisometacarpal ligaments.
• In official anatomical terminology, the origin of flexor pollicis brevis from the trapezium (and flexor

retinaculum) is referred to as the superficial head, and that from the trapezoid and capitate as the deep head (often small or even absent, and to be distinguished from the first palmar interosseous which is sometimes considered to be synonymous with the deep head).
• Dorsal interossei arise from the sides of two adjacent metacarpal bones (as at C12, from the sides of the second and third metacarpals); palmar interossei arise only from the metacarpal of their own finger (as at B9 from the second metacarpal). Compare with the dissection on page 137 and note that when looking at the palm, parts of

the dorsal interossei can be seen as well as the palmar interossei, but when looking at the dorsum of the hand (as on page 143, C) only dorsal interossei are seen.

105

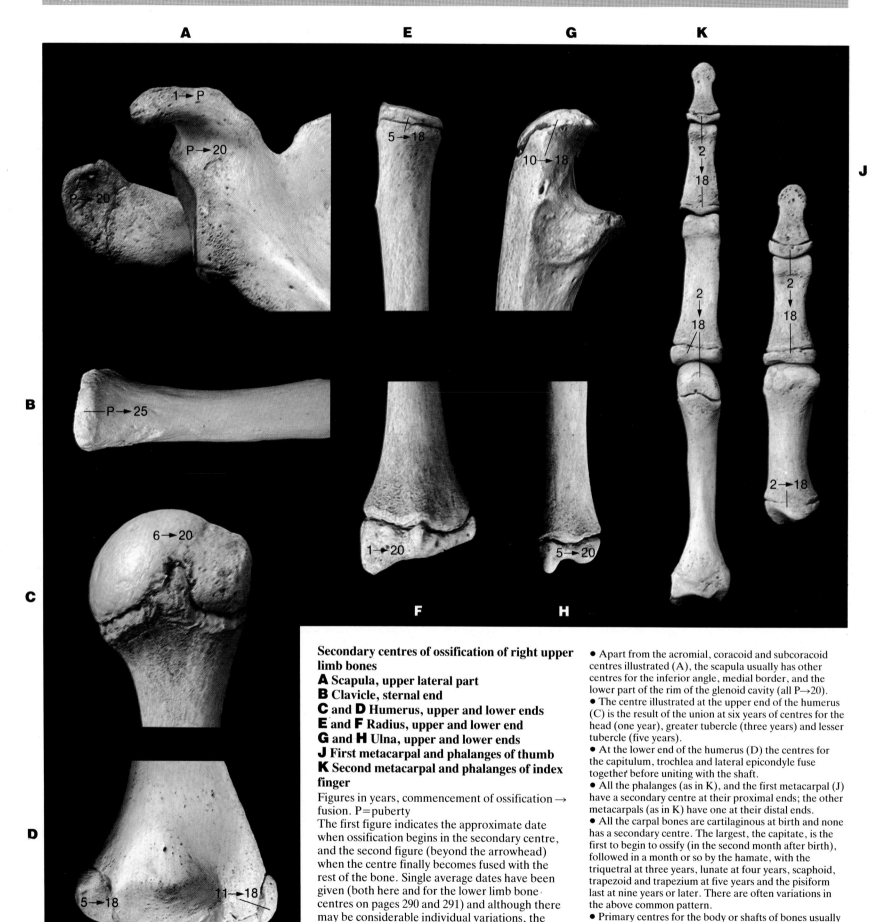

Secondary centres of ossification of right upper limb bones

A Scapula, upper lateral part

B Clavicle, sternal end

C and D Humerus, upper and lower ends

E and F Radius, upper and lower end

G and H Ulna, upper and lower ends

J First metacarpal and phalanges of thumb

K Second metacarpal and phalanges of index finger

Figures in years, commencement of ossification → fusion. P=puberty

The first figure indicates the approximate date when ossification begins in the secondary centre, and the second figure (beyond the arrowhead) when the centre finally becomes fused with the rest of the bone. Single average dates have been given (both here and for the lower limb bone centres on pages 290 and 291) and although there may be considerable individual variations, the 'growing end' of the bone (where fusion occurs last) is constant. The dates in females are often a year or more earlier than in males.

● Apart from the acromial, coracoid and subcoracoid centres illustrated (A), the scapula usually has other centres for the inferior angle, medial border, and the lower part of the rim of the glenoid cavity (all P→20).

● The centre illustrated at the upper end of the humerus (C) is the result of the union at six years of centres for the head (one year), greater tubercle (three years) and lesser tubercle (five years).

● At the lower end of the humerus (D) the centres for the capitulum, trochlea and lateral epicondyle fuse together before uniting with the shaft.

● All the phalanges (as in K), and the first metacarpal (J) have a secondary centre at their proximal ends; the other metacarpals (as in K) have one at their distal ends.

● All the carpal bones are cartilaginous at birth and none has a secondary centre. The largest, the capitate, is the first to begin to ossify (in the second month after birth), followed in a month or so by the hamate, with the triquetral at three years, lunate at four years, scaphoid, trapezoid and trapezium at five years and the pisiform last at nine years or later. There are often variations in the above common pattern.

● Primary centres for the body or shafts of bones usually begin to ossify about the eighth week of fetal life, but the clavicle is the first bone to commence ossification, between the fifth and sixth week.

Right shoulder, from the front

The arm is slightly abducted. Compare the positions of the features noted here with the dissection on the next page

1	Deltoid overlying greater tubercle of humerus
2	Acromion
3	Acromioclavicular joint
4	Acromial end of clavicle
5	Trapezius
6	Supraclavicular fossa
7	Infraclavicular fossa
8	Upper margin of pectoralis major
9	Anterior margin of deltoid
10	Deltopectoral groove and cephalic vein
11	Lower margin of pectoralis major
12	Serratus anterior
13	Biceps
14	Areola
15	Nipple

● The nipple in the male (15) normally lies at the level of the fourth intercostal space.
● The deltopectoral groove containing the cephalic vein (10) is formed by the adjacent borders of deltoid (9) and pectoralis major (8).
● The lower border of pectoralis major (11) forms the anterior axillary fold.

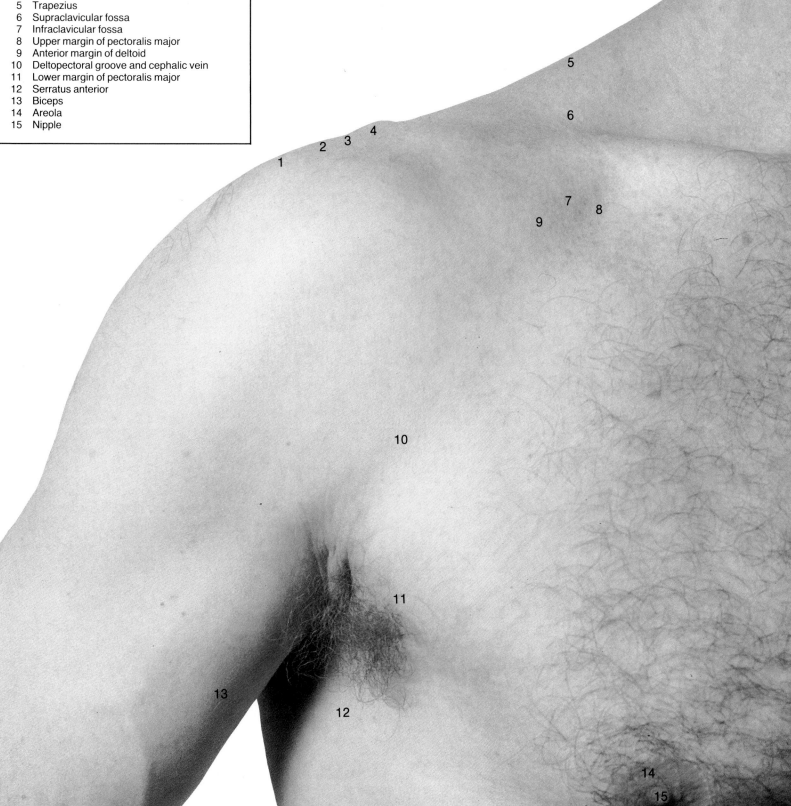

A Right shoulder, from the front. Superficial dissection

Removal of skin and fascia displays branches of the supraclavicular nerve (9) crossing the clavicle (10), and the cephalic vein (17) lying in the deltopectoral groove between deltoid (2) and pectoralis major (15)

1 Tip of shoulder
2 Deltoid
3 Acromion of scapula
4 Acromioclavicular joint
5 Acromial end of clavicle
6 Trapezius
7 Accessory nerve
8 Cervical nerve to trapezius
9 Branches of supraclavicular nerve
10 Clavicle
11 A superficial venous plexus
12 Clavicular head ⎫ of sterno-
13 Sternal head ⎭ cleidomastoid
14 Sternocostal part ⎫ of pectoralis
15 Clavicular part ⎭ major
16 Clavipectoral fascia
17 Cephalic vein

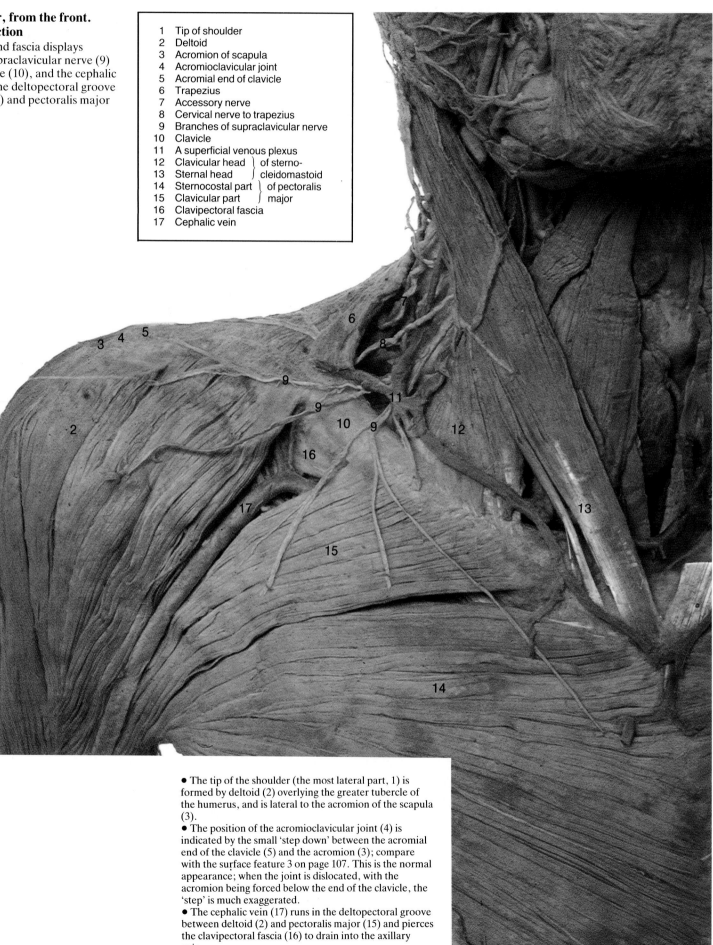

A

● The tip of the shoulder (the most lateral part, 1) is formed by deltoid (2) overlying the greater tubercle of the humerus, and is lateral to the acromion of the scapula (3).
● The position of the acromioclavicular joint (4) is indicated by the small 'step down' between the acromial end of the clavicle (5) and the acromion (3); compare with the surface feature 3 on page 107. This is the normal appearance; when the joint is dislocated, with the acromion being forced below the end of the clavicle, the 'step' is much exaggerated.
● The cephalic vein (17) runs in the deltopectoral groove between deltoid (2) and pectoralis major (15) and pierces the clavipectoral fascia (16) to drain into the axillary vein.

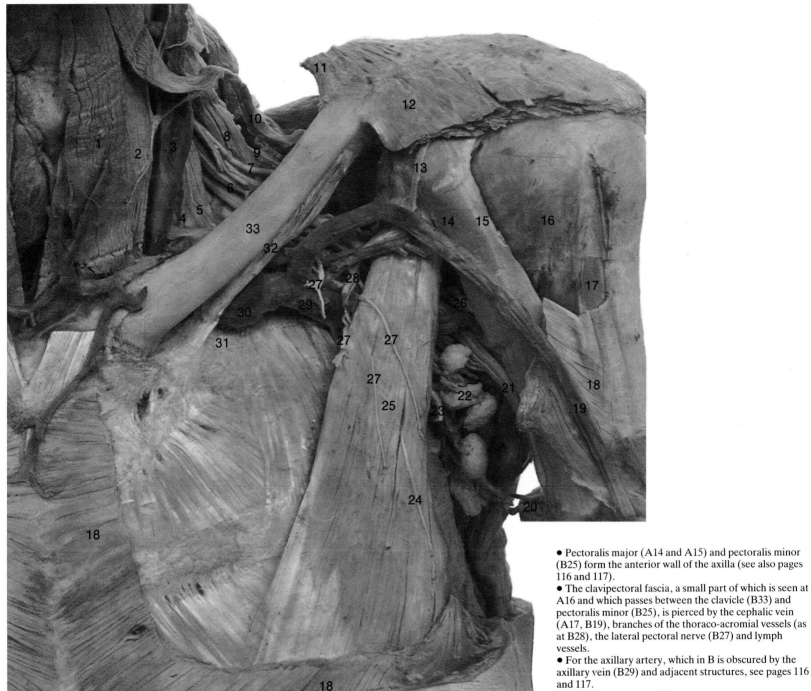

● Pectoralis major (A14 and A15) and pectoralis minor (B25) form the anterior wall of the axilla (see also pages 116 and 117).

● The clavipectoral fascia, a small part of which is seen at A16 and which passes between the clavicle (B33) and pectoralis minor (B25), is pierced by the cephalic vein (A17, B19), branches of the thoraco-acromial vessels (as at B28), the lateral pectoral nerve (B27) and lymph vessels.

● For the axillary artery, which in B is obscured by the axillary vein (B29) and adjacent structures, see pages 116 and 117.

B Left shoulder, from the front. Deeper dissection

Most of deltoid (12) and pectoralis major (18) have been removed to show the underlying pectoralis minor (25) and its associated vessels and nerves. The clavipectoral fascia which passed between the clavicle (33) and the upper (medial) border of the pectoralis minor (25) has also been removed to show the axillary vein (29) receiving the cephalic vein (19) and continuing as the subclavian vein (30) as it crosses the first rib (31). Above the clavicle, the inferior belly of omohyoid (10) has been displaced upwards to give a clear view of some brachial plexus branches (4 to 7, 9)

1	Sternohyoid	18	Pectoralis major
2	Sternothyroid	19	Cephalic vein
3	Internal jugular vein	20	Intercostobrachial nerve
4	Phrenic nerve overlying scalenus anterior	21	Median nerve
5	Nerve to subclavius	22	Axillary lymph nodes
6	Trunks of brachial plexus	23	Lateral thoracic artery
7	Suprascapular nerve	24	Branch of medial pectoral nerve
8	Scalenus medius	25	Pectoralis minor
9	Long thoracic nerve (to serratus anterior)	26	Anterior circumflex humeral artery and
10	Inferior belly of omohyoid (displaced upwards)		musculocutaneous nerve
11	Trapezius	27	Branches of lateral pectoral nerve
12	Deltoid	28	Pectoral branch of thoraco-acromial artery
13	Coracoid process and acromial branch of	29	Axillary vein
	thoraco-acromial artery	30	Subclavian vein
14	Coracobrachialis	31	First rib
15	Short head of biceps	32	Subclavius
16	Subscapularis	33	Clavicle
17	Tendon of long head of biceps		

A

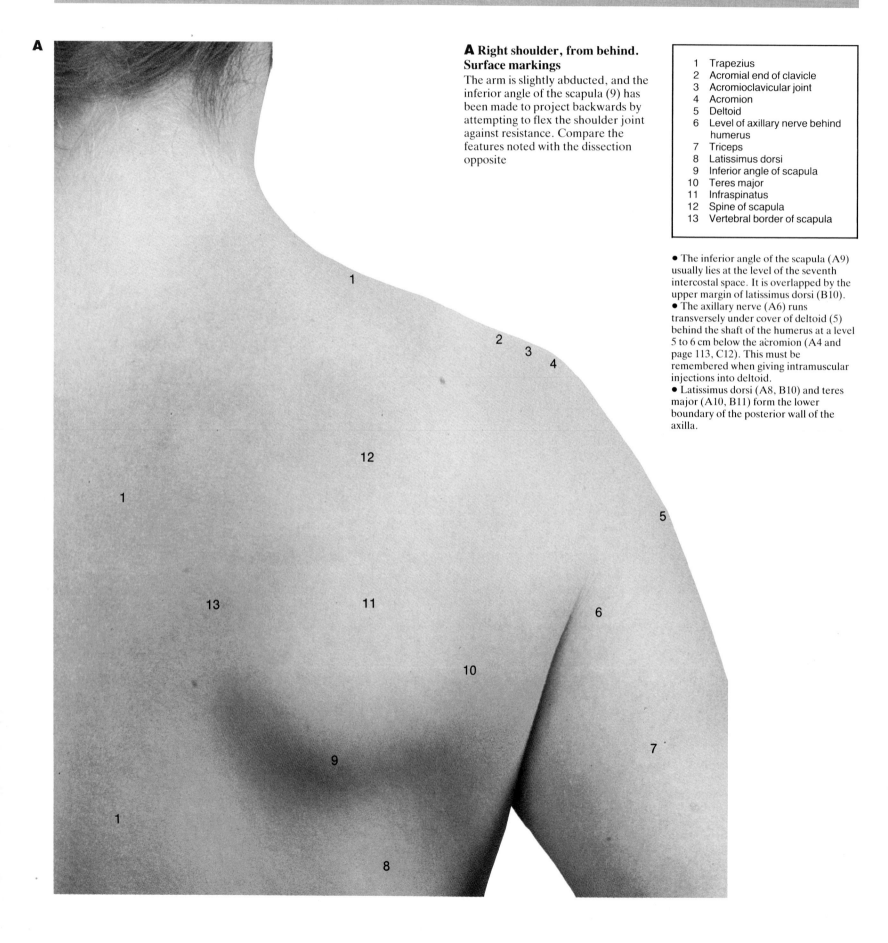

A Right shoulder, from behind. Surface markings

The arm is slightly abducted, and the inferior angle of the scapula (9) has been made to project backwards by attempting to flex the shoulder joint against resistance. Compare the features noted with the dissection opposite

1 Trapezius
2 Acromial end of clavicle
3 Acromioclavicular joint
4 Acromion
5 Deltoid
6 Level of axillary nerve behind humerus
7 Triceps
8 Latissimus dorsi
9 Inferior angle of scapula
10 Teres major
11 Infraspinatus
12 Spine of scapula
13 Vertebral border of scapula

● The inferior angle of the scapula (A9) usually lies at the level of the seventh intercostal space. It is overlapped by the upper margin of latissimus dorsi (B10).
● The axillary nerve (A6) runs transversely under cover of deltoid (5) behind the shaft of the humerus at a level 5 to 6 cm below the acromion (A4 and page 113, C12). This must be remembered when giving intramuscular injections into deltoid.
● Latissimus dorsi (A8, B10) and teres major (A10, B11) form the lower boundary of the posterior wall of the axilla.

B

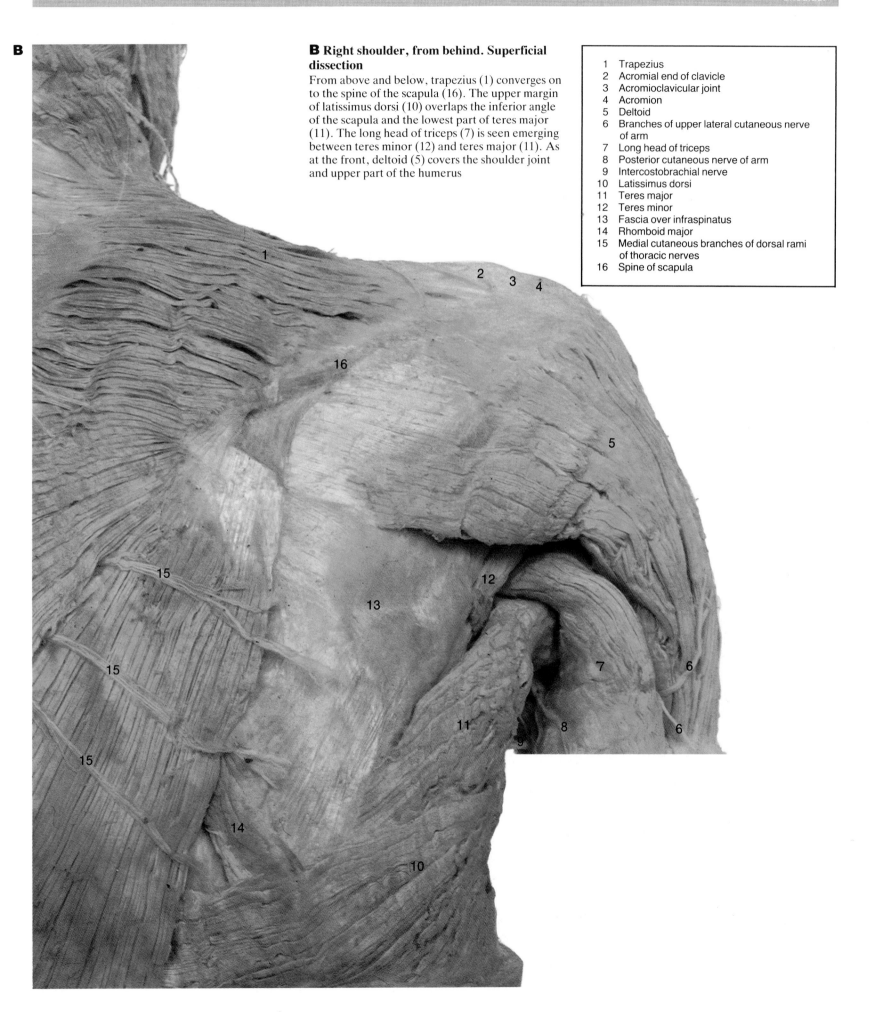

B Right shoulder, from behind. Superficial dissection

From above and below, trapezius (1) converges on to the spine of the scapula (16). The upper margin of latissimus dorsi (10) overlaps the inferior angle of the scapula and the lowest part of teres major (11). The long head of triceps (7) is seen emerging between teres minor (12) and teres major (11). As at the front, deltoid (5) covers the shoulder joint and upper part of the humerus

1	Trapezius
2	Acromial end of clavicle
3	Acromioclavicular joint
4	Acromion
5	Deltoid
6	Branches of upper lateral cutaneous nerve of arm
7	Long head of triceps
8	Posterior cutaneous nerve of arm
9	Intercostobrachial nerve
10	Latissimus dorsi
11	Teres major
12	Teres minor
13	Fascia over infraspinatus
14	Rhomboid major
15	Medial cutaneous branches of dorsal rami of thoracic nerves
16	Spine of scapula

A Left shoulder, from behind

Most of trapezius (5) and deltoid (1) have been removed to show the underlying muscles. The medial cut edge of trapezius remains near the line of the thoracic spines (11). Levator scapulae (7), rhomboid minor (8) and rhomboid major (9) are seen converging on to the vertebral border of the scapula, and supraspinatus (6) lies above the spine of the scapula (20)

1 Deltoid	12 Erector spinae
2 Acromion	13 Thoracic part of thoracolumbar fascia
3 Acromioclavicular joint	14 Latissimus dorsi
4 Acromial end of clavicle	15 Teres major
5 Trapezius	16 Long head of triceps
6 Supraspinatus	17 Posterior circumflex humeral vessels and
7 Levator scapulae	axillary nerve
8 Rhomboid minor	18 Teres minor
9 Rhomboid major	19 Infraspinatus
10 Branch of dorsal ramus of a thoracic nerve	20 Spine of scapula
11 Third thoracic spinous process	

● Muscles producing movements at the shoulder joint:

Abduction: supraspinatus and deltoid (middle fibres) for about 120°; further abduction requires scapular rotation produced by serratus anterior and trapezius.
Adduction: pectoralis major, latissimus dorsi, teres major, teres minor.

Flexion: deltoid (anterior fibres), pectoralis major, biceps, coracobrachialis.
Extension: deltoid (posterior fibres), latissimus dorsi, teres major.

Lateral rotation: infraspinatus, teres minor.
Medial rotation: pectoralis major, subscapularis, latissimus dorsi, teres major.

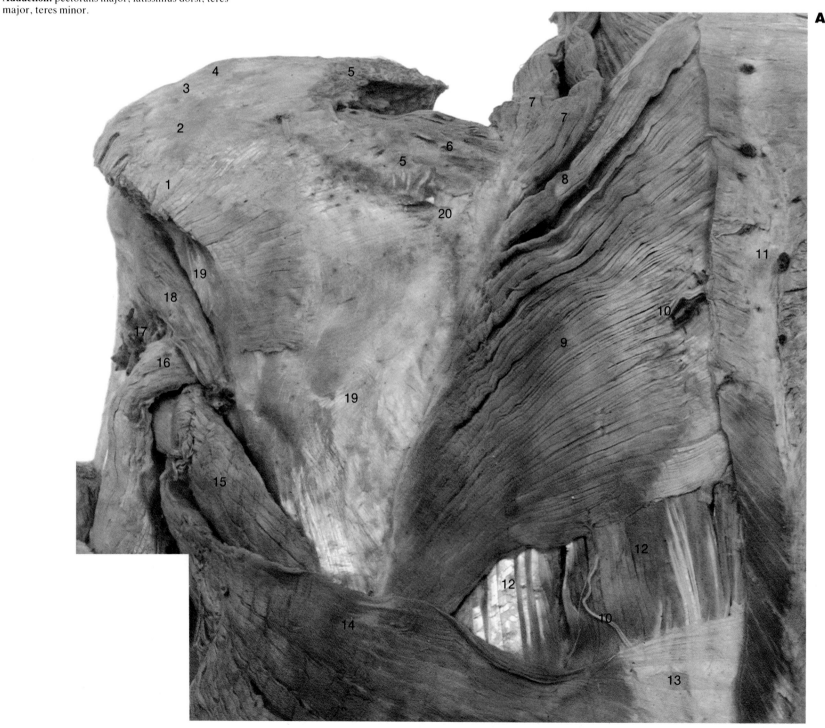

A

B

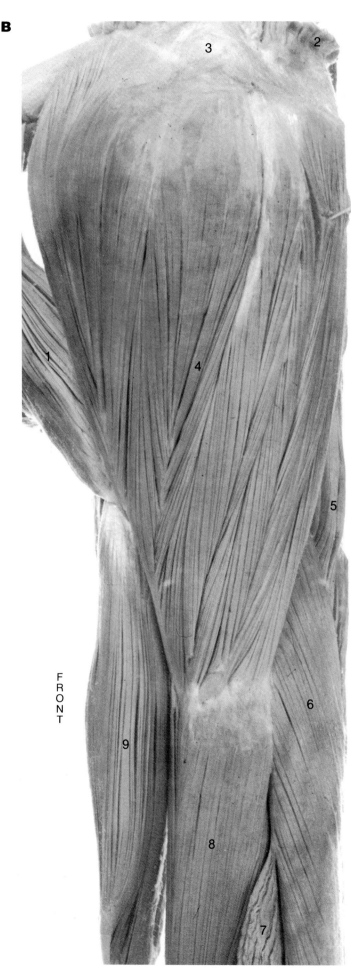

FRONT

C

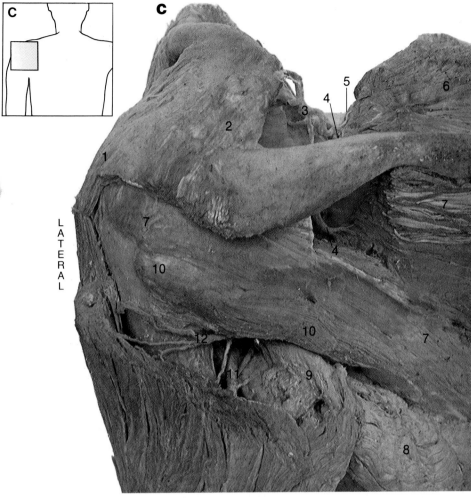

LATERAL

B Left shoulder and upper arm, from the left

Deltoid (4) extends over the tip of the shoulder to its attachment half way down the lateral side of the shaft of the humerus. Biceps (9) is on the front of the arm below pectoralis major (1) and triceps (5 and 6) is at the back

1	Pectoralis major
2	Trapezius
3	Acromion
4	Deltoid
5	Long head of triceps
6	Lateral head of triceps
7	Brachioradialis
8	Brachialis
9	Biceps

C Left shoulder, from the left and behind

The central part of supraspinatus (6) and part of infraspinatus (7) have been removed to show the suprascapular nerve (4) which supplies both muscles. Part of deltoid (1) has also been removed to show the axillary nerve (12) which supplies the muscle passing backwards through the quadrilateral space (see note below)

1	Deltoid
2	Acromioclavicular joint
3	Suprascapular artery
4	Suprascapular nerve
5	Superior transverse scapular (suprascapular) ligament
6	Supraspinatus
7	Infraspinatus
8	Teres major
9	Long head of triceps
10	Teres minor
11	Posterior circumflex humeral artery
12	Axillary nerve

● As it lies just beneath the capsule of the shoulder joint, the axillary nerve may be injured by dislocation of the joint.
● The suprascapular artery (C3) passes into the supraspinous fossa superficial to the superior transverse scapular ligament (C5); the suprascapular nerve (C4) passes deep to the ligament.

● The axillary nerve (C12) and posterior circumflex humeral vessels (C11) pass backwards through the quadrilateral space which (viewed from behind) is bounded above by teres minor (C10), below by teres major (C8), medially by the long head of triceps (C9) and laterally by the humerus. (Viewed from the front, the upper boundary of the space is subscapularis—see page 118, A17)

113

A

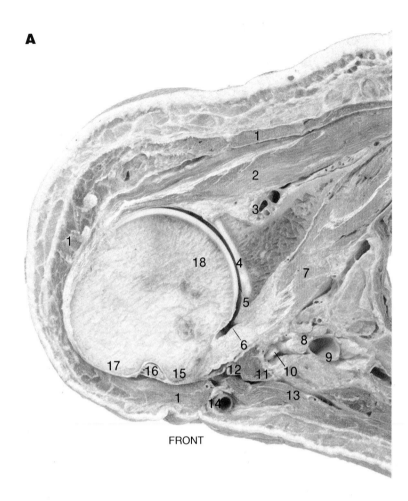

FRONT

B

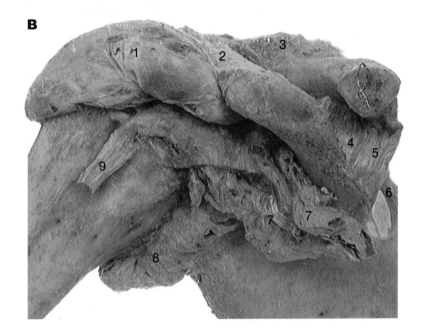

C

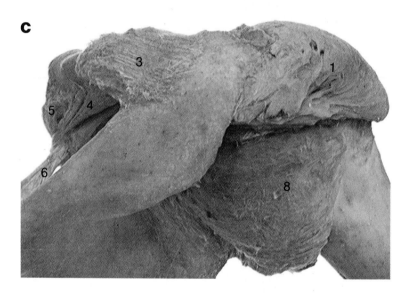

D

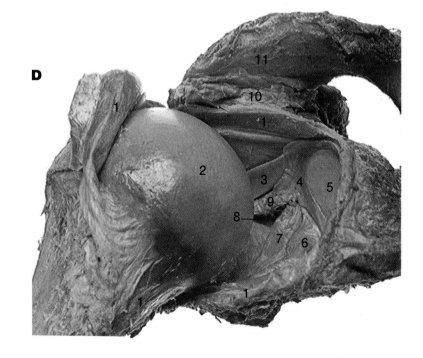

A Right shoulder joint, horizontal section

Viewed from above, this section shows the articulation of the head of the humerus (18) with the glenoid cavity of the scapula (4). The tendon of the long head of biceps (16) lies in the groove between the greater and lesser tubercles of the humerus (17 and 15). Subscapularis (7) passes immediately in front of the joint, and infraspinatus (2) behind it

1	Deltoid
2	Infraspinatus
3	Suprascapular nerve and vessels
4	Glenoid cavity
5	Glenoid labrum
6	Capsule
7	Subscapularis
8	Cords of brachial plexus
9	Axillary artery
10	Musculocutaneous nerve
11	Coracobrachialis
12	Short head of biceps
13	Pectoralis major
14	Cephalic vein
15	Lesser tubercle
16	Tendon of long head of biceps in intertubercular groove
17	Greater tubercle
18	Head of humerus

Right shoulder joint, **B** from the front, **C** from behind

The synovial joint cavity inside the capsule (8) and the subacromial bursa (1) have been injected separately with green resin

1	Subacromial bursa
2	Coraco-acromial ligament
3	Acromioclavicular joint
4	Trapezoid ligament
5	Conoid ligament
6	Superior transverse scapular (suprascapular) ligament
7	Subscapularis bursa
8	Capsule of shoulder joint
9	Tendon of long head of biceps

● The subscapularis bursa (B7) normally communicates with the synovial cavity of the shoulder joint.
● The subacromial bursa (B and C1) does *not* normally communicate with the shoulder joint; it is separated from the joint by the supraspinatus tendon. Only if the tendon is ruptured can the two cavities become continuous with one another.

D Left shoulder joint, opened from behind

In this view, after removing all the posterior part of the capsule, the inner surface of the front of the capsule (1) is seen, with its reinforcing glenohumeral ligaments (6, 7 and 9)

1	Capsule
2	Head of humerus
3	Long head of biceps
4	Glenoid labrum
5	Glenoid cavity
6	Inferior glenohumeral ligament
7	Middle glenohumeral ligament
8	Opening into subscapularis bursa
9	Superior glenohumeral ligament
10	Supraspinatus
11	Acromion

● The joint cavity communicates with the subscapularis bursa through an opening (8) between the superior (9) and middle (7) glenohumeral ligaments.
● The tendon of the long head of biceps (3) is continuous with the glenoid labrum (4).

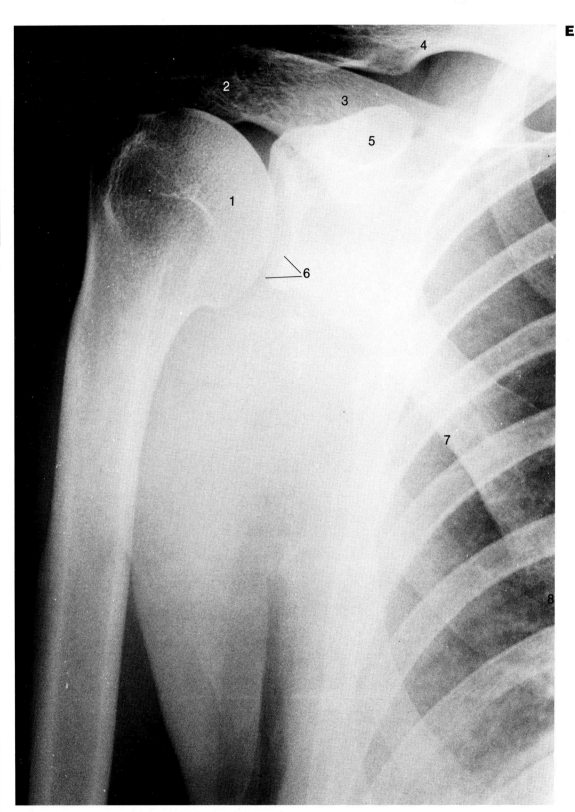

E

E Radiograph of the right shoulder, from the front

The head of the humerus (1) lies against the glenoid cavity of the scapula (6), whose coracoid process (5) is seen end-on

1	Head of humerus	
2	Acromion	
3	Spine of scapula	
4	Clavicle.	
5	Coracoid process	
6	Rim of glenoid cavity	
7	Lateral border	} of scapula
8	Inferior angle	

115

A Left axilla, anterior wall

Pectoralis major (1) has been reflected upwards and laterally, and the clavipectoral fascia which passes from subclavius (3) to pectoralis minor (7) has been removed

1	Pectoralis major
2	Clavicle
3	Subclavius
4	Cephalic vein
5	Thoraco-acromial vessels
6	Lateral pectoral nerve
7	Pectoralis minor
8	Axillary sheath surrounding axillary vessels and brachial plexus
9	Branches of medial pectoral nerve
10	First rib
11	Subclavian vein

• The clavipectoral fascia (here removed, between subclavius, 3, and pectoralis minor, 7) is pierced by the cephalic vein (4), thoraco-acromial vessels (5), lateral pectoral nerve (6) and lymphatics.
• The axillary sheath (8) is the downward continuation of the prevertebral fascia of the neck and forms a dense covering for the axillary vessels and the surrounding parts of the brachial plexus.
• The *lateral* pectoral nerve (6) is related to the *medial* (upper) border of pectoralis minor (7). The *medial* pectoral nerve (9) is related to the *lateral* (lower) border of pectoralis minor.

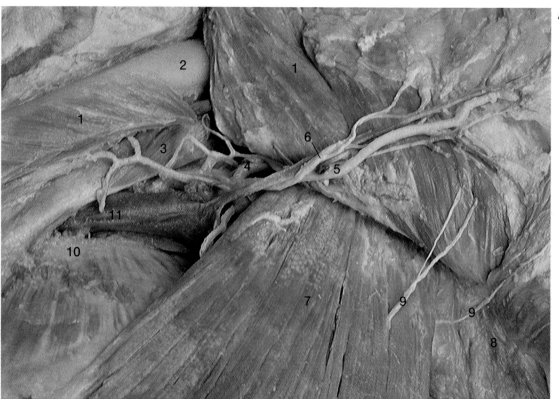

B Left axilla and brachial plexus, from the front

Pectoralis major (1) has been reflected and the clavipectoral fascia removed, together with the axillary sheath (A8) which surrounded the axillary vessels and brachial plexus

1	Pectoralis major
2	Clavicle
3	Deltoid
4	Thoraco-acromial vessels and lateral pectoral nerve
5	Lateral cord of brachial plexus
6	Axillary artery
7	Pectoralis minor
8	Musculocutaneous nerve
9	Coracobrachialis
10	Lateral root ⎫ of median nerve
11	Medial root ⎬
12	Median nerve
13	Ulnar nerve
14	Medial cutaneous nerve of forearm
15	Axillary vein
16	Medial cutaneous nerve of arm
17	Latissimus dorsi
18	Teres major
19	Circumflex scapular artery
20	Thoracodorsal artery
21	Thoracodorsal nerve
22	Subscapularis
23	Serratus anterior
24	Entry of cephalic vein
25	Subclavian vein
26	First rib
27	Subclavius

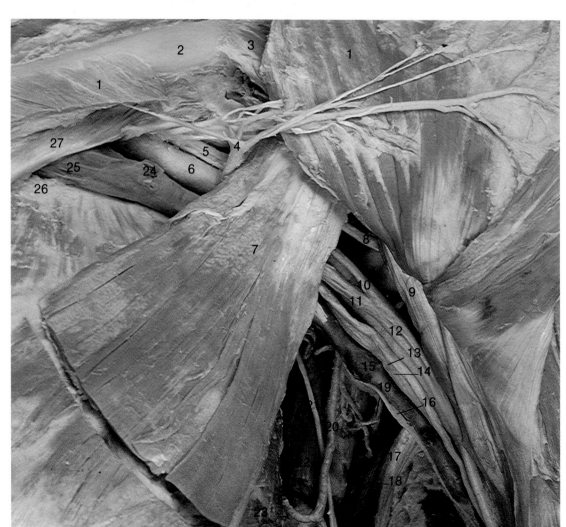

c

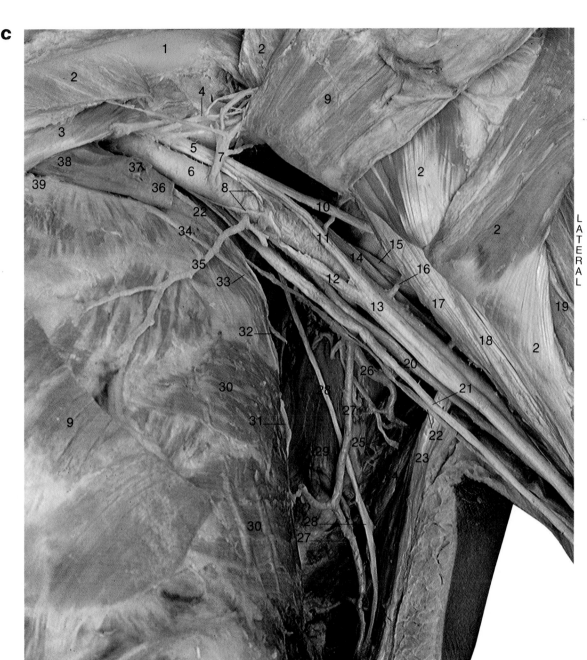

C Left brachial plexus, from the front

Pectoralis major and minor (2 and 9) have been reflected and the axillary sheath (A8) removed, together with most of the axillary vein (36) and its tributaries

```
 1  Clavicle
 2  Pectoralis major
 3  Subclavius
 4  Lateral pectoral nerve
 5  Lateral cord
 6  Axillary artery
 7  Thoraco-acromial artery
 8  Loop between medial and lateral pectoral
    nerves
 9  Pectoralis minor
10  Musculocutaneous nerve
11  Lateral root  ⎫
12  Medial root   ⎬ of median nerve
13  Median nerve
14  Radial nerve
15  Axillary nerve
16  Anterior circumflex humeral artery
17  Coracobrachialis and short head of biceps
18  Long head of biceps
19  Deltoid
20  Ulnar nerve
21  Medial cutaneous nerve of forearm
22  Medial cutaneous nerve of arm
23  Latissimus dorsi
24  Teres major
25  Lower subscapular nerve
26  Circumflex scapular artery
27  Thoracodorsal artery
28  Thoracodorsal nerve
29  Subscapularis
30  Serratus anterior
31  Long thoracic nerve
32  Intercostobrachial nerve (cut end)
33  Communication between 22 and 32
34  Branch from first thoracic nerve to
    intercostobrachial nerve
35  Lateral thoracic artery
36  Axillary vein
37  Entry of cephalic vein
38  Subclavian vein
39  First rib
```

• The thoracodorsal artery (27) is the name given to the continuation of the subscapular artery distal to the origin of the circumflex scapular branch (26).
• To sort out the major branches of the medial and lateral cords, note that the largest branches form the shape of a capital M. Identify the median nerve (13, the middle stem of the M) in front of the axillary artery. Follow its lateral root (11) upwards to the lateral cord (5), from which the musculocutaneous nerve arises (10, as the lateral stem of the M) to run into the coracobrachialis muscle (17). Follow the medial root of the median nerve (12) upwards to the medial cord (obscured by the axillary artery below the label 6), whose largest branch is the ulnar nerve (20, the medial stem of the M).
• The radial nerve (14, one of the two terminal branches of the posterior cord and the largest of all the branches of the plexus) is most easily identified as it lies behind the axillary artery and in front of the latissimus dorsi tendon. Follow the nerve upwards to find the axillary nerve (15, the other terminal branch of the posterior cord) passing laterally and backwards through the quadrilateral space (see page 113).

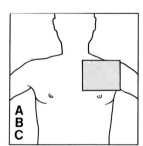

• Boundaries of the axilla:
Anterior wall: pectoralis major and minor (B1 and 7) and the clavipectoral fascia.
Posterior wall: subscapularis (C29), teres major (C24) and latissimus dorsi (C23).
Medial wall: serratus anterior (C30) overlying the first four ribs and intercostal muscles.
Lateral wall: the intertubercular groove of the humerus, coracobrachialis and biceps (C17).
Apex: the space between the clavicle (C1), first rib (C39) and upper border of the scapula.
Base: the concavity of skin and axillary fascia between the lower borders of pectoralis major and latissimus dorsi.

A Right brachial plexus and branches

In this front view of the plexus, all the blood vessels have been removed to show the cords of the plexus and their branches more clearly. Note the 'capital M' pattern (referred to in the notes on page 117) formed by the musculocutaneous nerve (5), the lateral root of the median nerve (7), the median nerve itself (24), the medial root of the median nerve (9) and the ulnar nerve (14). In this specimen the tendon of latissimus dorsi (19) is unusually broad and has become blended with the long head of triceps (20)

A

1	Lateral cord
2	Posterior cord
3	Medial cord
4	Pectoralis minor and lateral pectoral nerve
5	Musculocutaneous nerve
6	Axillary nerve
7	Lateral root of median nerve
8	Radial nerve
9	Medial root of median nerve
10	Upper subscapular nerves
11	Thoracodorsal nerve
12	Lower subscapular nerve
13	Medial cutaneous nerve of arm
14	Ulnar nerve
15	Medial cutaneous nerve of forearm
16	Intercostobrachial nerve
17	Subscapularis
18	Teres major
19	Latissimus dorsi
20	Long head of triceps
21	Lateral head of triceps
22	Medial head of triceps
23	Radial nerve branches to triceps
24	Median nerve
25	Coracobrachialis
26	Biceps
27	Deltoid

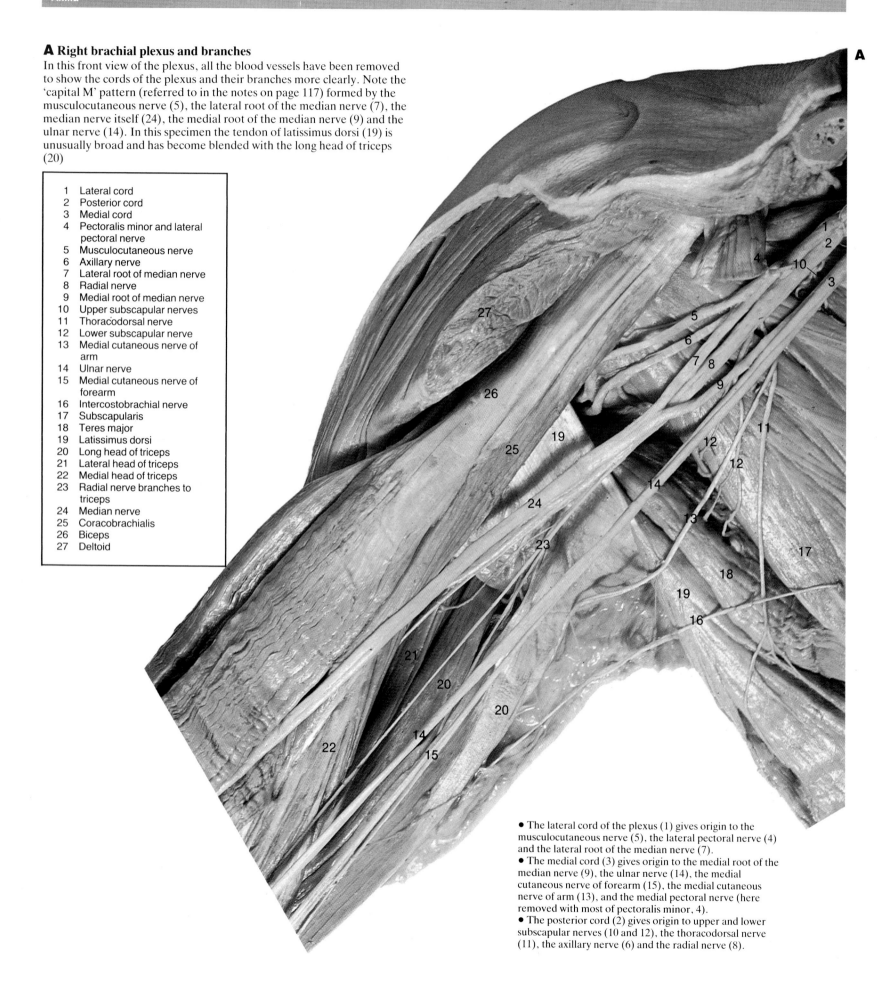

- The lateral cord of the plexus (1) gives origin to the musculocutaneous nerve (5), the lateral pectoral nerve (4) and the lateral root of the median nerve (7).
- The medial cord (3) gives origin to the medial root of the median nerve (9), the ulnar nerve (14), the medial cutaneous nerve of forearm (15), the medial cutaneous nerve of arm (13), and the medial pectoral nerve (here removed with most of pectoralis minor, 4).
- The posterior cord (2) gives origin to upper and lower subscapular nerves (10 and 12), the thoracodorsal nerve (11), the axillary nerve (6) and the radial nerve (8).

FRONT

B

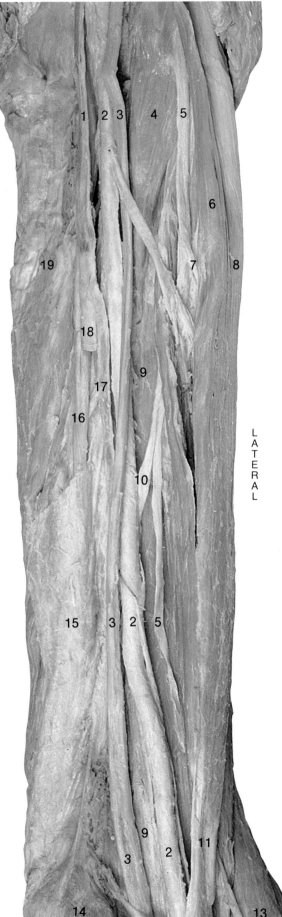

LATERAL

C

LATERAL

B Left arm. Vessels and nerves, from the front

Biceps (6 and 8) has been turned laterally to show the musculocutaneous nerve (5) emerging from coracobrachialis (4), giving branches to biceps and brachialis (7 and 10) and becoming the lateral cutaneous nerve of the forearm (12) on the lateral side of the biceps tendon (11). The median nerve (3) gradually crosses over in front of the brachial artery (2) from the lateral to the medial side. The ulnar nerve (16) passes behind the medial intermuscular septum (15), and the end of the basilic vein (18) is seen joining a vena comitans (17) of the brachial artery to form the brachial vein (1)

1	Brachial vein
2	Brachial artery
3	Median nerve
4	Coracobrachialis
5	Musculocutaneous nerve
6	Short head of biceps
7	Nerve to short head of biceps
8	Long head of biceps
9	Brachialis
10	Nerve to brachialis
11	Tendon of biceps
12	Lateral cutaneous nerve of forearm
13	Brachioradialis
14	Pronator teres
15	Medial intermuscular septum
16	Ulnar nerve
17	Vena comitans of brachial artery
18	Basilic vein (cut end)
19	Long head of triceps

● The musculocutaneous nerve (B5) supplies coracobrachialis (B4), biceps (B6 and 8) and brachialis (B9), and at the level where the muscle fibres of biceps become tendinous (B11) it pierces the deep fascia to become the lateral cutaneous nerve of the forearm (B12).
● The median nerve does not give off any muscular branches in the arm (unless the nerve to pronator teres has a high origin—page 124, C).

C Cross section of the left arm, from below

Looking from the elbow towards the shoulder, the section is taken through the middle of the arm. The musculocutaneous nerve (13) lies between brachialis (3) and biceps (2), and the median nerve (11) is on the medial side of the brachial artery (12) which has several venae comitantes adjacent (unlabelled). The ulnar nerve (7), with the superior ulnar collateral artery (8) beside it, is behind the median nerve (11) and the basilic vein (9). The radial nerve and the profunda brachii vessels (4) are in the posterior compartment at the lateral side of the humerus (5)

1	Cephalic vein
2	Biceps
3	Brachialis
4	Radial nerve and profunda brachii vessels
5	Humerus
6	Triceps
7	Ulnar nerve
8	Superior ulnar collateral artery
9	Basilic vein
10	Medial cutaneous nerve of forearm
11	Median nerve
12	Brachial artery
13	Musculocutaneous nerve

● The ulnar nerve (B16) leaves the anterior compartment of the arm by piercing the medial intermuscular septum (B15), and does not give off any muscular branches in the arm.

119

A Left arm, from behind. **A** triceps, **B** and **C**, radial nerve

In their normal position in A, the long and lateral heads of triceps (A3 and 10) cover the medial head except low down on the medial side, where it can be seen (A4) below the long head (A3). In B deltoid (1) has been displaced laterally and the long and lateral heads (B3 and 10) have been separated by a vertical incision to show the radial nerve (11) giving off its branches to triceps (see notes) as it lies medial to the humerus. Lower down in C with the long and lateral heads further separated (C3 and 10), the radial nerve (C11) crosses the medial head (C4) obliquely before lying against the radial groove (C18) at the lateral side of the humerus

1	Deltoid
2	Teres major
3	Long head of triceps
4	Medial head of triceps
5	Medial intermuscular septum
6	Medial epicondyle
7	Tendon of triceps
8	Extensor carpi radialis longus
9	Brachioradialis
10	Lateral head of triceps
11	Radial nerve
12	Nerve to long head
13	Nerve to medial head
14	Ulnar nerve
15	Profunda brachii artery
16	Nerve to medial head
17	Nerve to lateral head
18	Radial nerve at radial groove

● Triceps has three heads but four nerves—the medial head receives two branches. All the muscular branches (B12, 13, 16 and 17) arise from the radial nerve (B11) high up, well before the nerve has reached the radial groove (C18) at the lateral side of the humerus (page 95, B8). The usual order of origin of the branches from above downwards is: nerve to the long head (B12), medial head (B13), lateral head (B17). and medial head (B16). The first branch to the medial head (B13) runs for part of its course close to the ulnar nerve (B14), and is therefore sometimes called the ulnar collateral nerve.
● The medial head (4) of triceps would be better known as the deep head, since most of it is under cover of the long and lateral heads (3 and 10 in A and B), but on the lower medial side of the arm part of the medial head (A4) does project below the long head (A3).

A

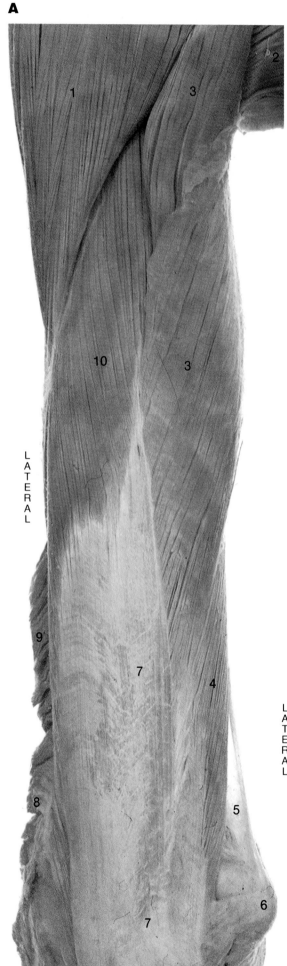

B

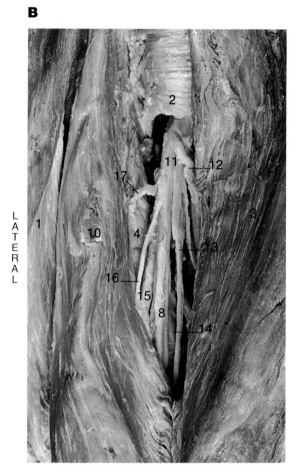

C

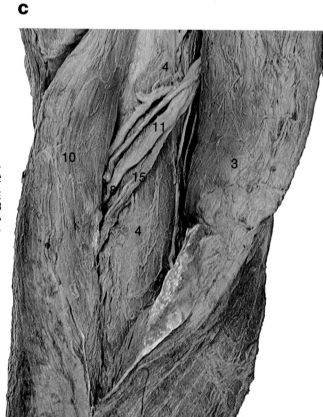

D

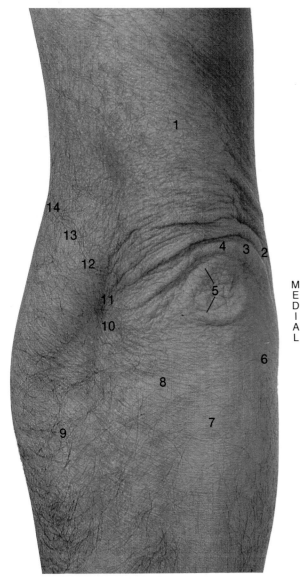

E

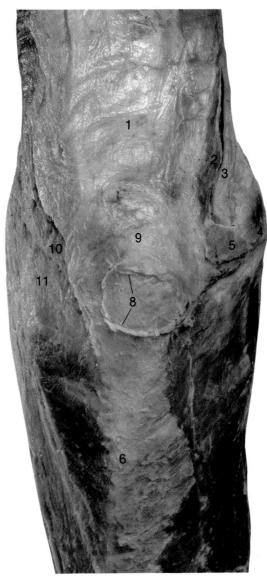

M
E
D
I
A
L

L
A
T
E
R
A
L

D Left elbow, from behind. Surface markings

With the elbow fully extended, the extensor muscles (9, 13) form a bulge on the lateral side. In the adjacent hollow can be felt the head of the radius (10) and the capitulum of the humerus (11) which indicate the line of the humeroradial part of the elbow joint. The lateral and medial epicondyles of the humerus (12 and 2) are palpable on each side. Wrinkled skin lies at the back of the prominent olecranon of the ulna (4), and in this arm the margin of the olecranon bursa (5) is outlined. The most important structure in this region is the ulnar nerve (3) which is palpable as it lies in contact with the humerus behind the medial epicondyle (2). The posterior border of the ulna (7) is subcutaneous throughout its whole length

1	Triceps
2	Medial epicondyle of humerus
3	Ulnar nerve
4	Olecranon of ulna
5	Margin of olecranon bursa
6	Flexor carpi ulnaris
7	Posterior border of ulna
8	Anconeus
9	Extensor muscles
10	Head of radius
11	Capitulum of humerus
12	Lateral epicondyle of humerus
13	Extensor carpi radialis longus
14	Brachioradialis

● With the elbow extended (straight) the medial and lateral epicondyles of the humerus (D2 and 12; E4 and 10) and the olecranon of the ulna (D4 and E9) are on the same level, but with flexion of the elbow the olecranon moves to a lower level.
● The subcutaneous position of the ulnar nerve (D3, E3) behind the medial epicondyle of the humerus (D2, E4) makes it easily palpable; here it can be rolled against the bone or injured, with paraesthesia (tingling sensation) in the distribution of the nerve on the ulnar side of the hand.
● The region of the medial epicondyle of the humerus is colloquially called the 'funny bone'.

E Left elbow, from behind. Superficial dissection

Skin and subcutaneous tissue and some deep fascia have been removed, but the margin of the olecranon bursa (8) has been preserved. The ulnar nerve (3) is behind the medial epicondyle (4) and passes downwards under cover of flexor carpi ulnaris (5)

1	Triceps tendon
2	Medial head of triceps
3	Ulnar nerve
4	Medial epicondyle of humerus
5	Flexor carpi ulnaris
6	Posterior border of ulna
7	Anconeus
8	Margin of olecranon bursa
9	Olecranon of ulna
10	Lateral epicondyle of humerus
11	Common extensor origin

A

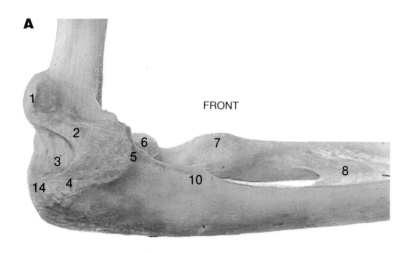

FRONT

B

FRONT

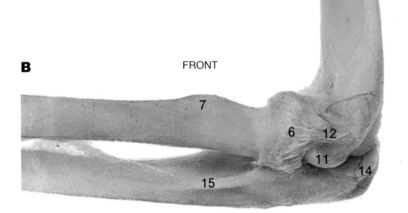

C

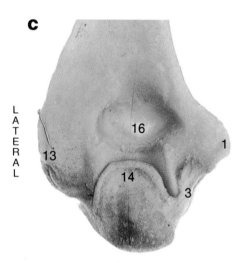

D

FRONT

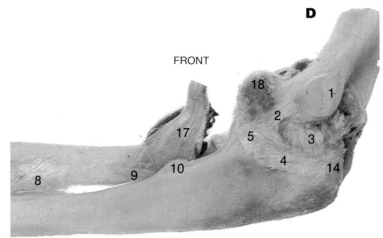

E

FRONT

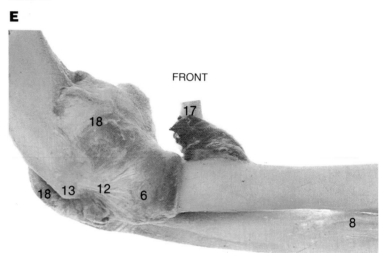

F

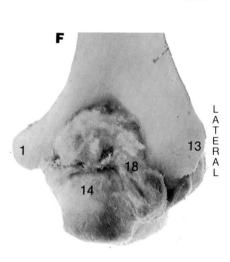

Left elbow joint and proximal radio-ulnar joint, A from the medial side, B from the lateral side, C from behind
Right elbow joint and proximal radio-ulnar joint, D from the medial side, E from the lateral side, F from behind

In A, B and C the forearm is flexed to a right angle. In D, E and F the forearm is partially flexed, and the synovial cavity within the capsule (18) and the bursa beneath the biceps tendon (17) have been injected with green resin

1	Medial epicondyle
2	Upper band ⎫
3	Posterior band ⎬ of ulnar collateral ligament
4	Oblique band ⎭
5	Coronoid process of ulna
6	Head of radius covered by annular ligament
7	Tuberosity of radius
8	Interosseous membrane
9	Oblique cord
10	Tuberosity of ulna
11	Capitulum
12	Radial collateral ligament
13	Lateral epicondyle
14	Olecranon of ulna
15	Supinator crest of ulna
16	Olecranon fossa
17	Biceps tendon and underlying bursa
18	Capsule (distended)

• The synovial cavity of the proximal radio-ulnar joint is continuous with that of the elbow joint (the synovial cavity of the distal radio-ulnar joint is *not* continuous with that of the wrist joint).
• Posteriorly and above, the capsule of the elbow joint is attached to the upper part of the *floor* of the olecranon fossa, not to the upper margin of the fossa (page 98, B).
• The main ligaments of the elbow and proximal radio-ulnar joints are the capsule (18), the ulnar and radial collateral ligaments (2 to 4 and 12) and the annular ligament (6).

• Muscles producing movements at the elbow joint:
Flexion: brachialis, biceps, brachioradialis.
Extension: triceps, anconeus.
• Muscles producing movements at the proximal and distal radio-ulnar joints:
Pronation: pronator quadratus, pronator teres.
Supination: supinator, biceps.

A

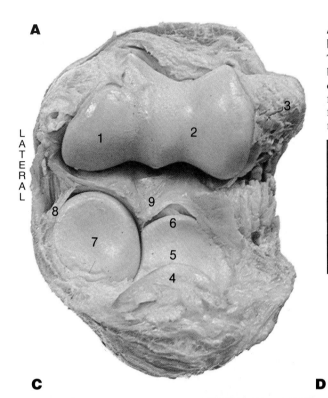

LATERAL

A Left elbow joint, opened from behind

The joint has been 'forced open' from behind: the capitulum (1) and trochlea (2) of the lower end of the humerus are seen from below with the forearm in forced flexion to show the upper ends of the radius and ulna (7 and 5) from above

1	Capitulum	⎫
2	Trochlea	⎬ of humerus
3	Medial epicondyle	⎭
4	Olecranon	⎫
5	Trochlear notch	⎬ of ulna
6	Coronoid process	⎭
7	Head of radius	
8	Annular ligament	
9	Anterior part of capsule	

B

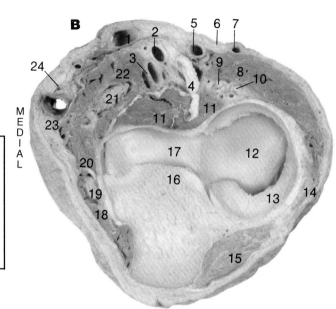

MEDIAL

B Cross section of the left elbow

The section is viewed from below, looking towards the shoulder, and is just below the point where the brachial artery has divided into radial and ulnar arteries (2 and 3). The cut has passed immediately below the trochlea (17) and capitulum (12) of the humerus, and has gone through the coronoid process of the ulna (16). The radial nerve (9) and its posterior interosseous branch (10) lie between brachioradialis (8) and brachialis (11). The median nerve (21) is under the main part of pronator teres (22), and the ulnar nerve (19) is passing under flexor carpi ulnaris (18)

1	Median basilic vein	14	Extensor carpi radialis longus and brevis
2	Radial artery	15	Anconeus
3	Ulnar artery	16	Coronoid process of ulna
4	Tendon of biceps	17	Trochlea of humerus
5	Median cephalic vein	18	Flexor carpi ulnaris
6	Lateral cutaneous nerve of forearm	19	Ulnar nerve
7	Cephalic vein	20	Common flexor origin
8	Brachioradialis	21	Median nerve
9	Radial nerve	22	Pronator teres
10	Posterior interosseous nerve	23	Basilic vein
11	Brachialis	24	Medial cutaneous nerve of forearm
12	Capitulum of humerus		
13	Fringe of synovial membrane		

C   **D**

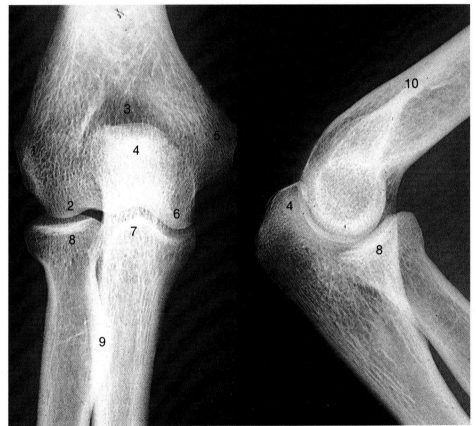

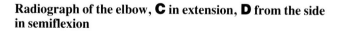

Radiograph of the elbow, **C** in extension, **D** from the side in semiflexion

1	Lateral epicondyle of humerus	7	Coronoid process of ulna
2	Capitulum	8	Head of radius (in D superimposed on coronoid process of ulna)
3	Olecranon fossa		
4	Olecranon of ulna	9	Tuberosity of radius
5	Medial epicondyle	10	Medial supracondylar ridge
6	Medial margin of trochlea		

123

Left cubital fossa, A surface markings, B superficial veins, C after removal of the deep fascia

In A there is an M-shaped pattern of superficial veins (see notes). In B the cephalic (1) and basilic (11) veins are joined by a median cubital vein (15) into which drain two small median forearm veins (8). In C the deep fascia has been removed but the bicipital aponeurosis (18) is preserved; it runs downwards and medially from the biceps tendon (5), crossing the brachial artery (6) and the median nerve (7). The musculocutaneous nerve becomes the lateral cutaneous nerve of the forearm (13) at the lateral border of biceps where the muscle becomes tendinous. Brachioradialis (3) forms the lateral boundary and pronator teres (9) the medial boundary of the cubital fossa

1	Cephalic vein
2	Lateral epicondyle
3	Brachioradialis
4	Median cephalic vein
5	Biceps tendon
6	Brachial artery
7	Median nerve
8	Median forearm vein
9	Pronator teres
10	Median basilic vein
11	Basilic vein
12	Medial epicondyle
13	Lateral cutaneous nerve of forearm
14	Medial cutaneous nerve of forearm
15	Median cubital vein
16	Brachialis
17	Radial artery
18	Bicipital aponeurosis
19	Nerve to pronator teres
20	A muscular artery
21	Medial intermuscular septum
22	Medial head of triceps

● The superficial veins on the front of the elbow such as the cephalic (1) and basilic (11) and their intercommunicating tributaries are those most commonly used for intravenous injections and obtaining specimens of venous blood. The pattern of veins is typically M-shaped (as in A) or H-shaped (as in B), but there is much variation and it is not always possible or necessary to name every vessel.
● The order of the structures in the cubital fossa from lateral to medial is: biceps tendon (5), brachial artery (6) and median nerve (7).

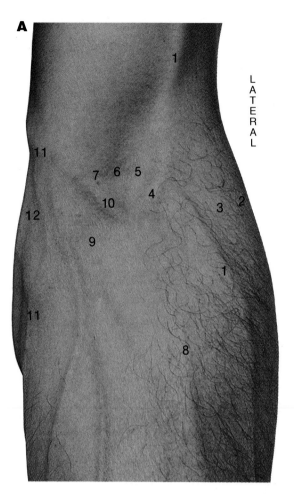

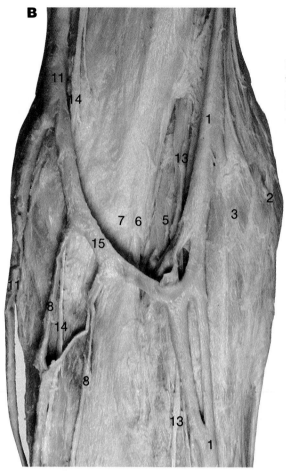

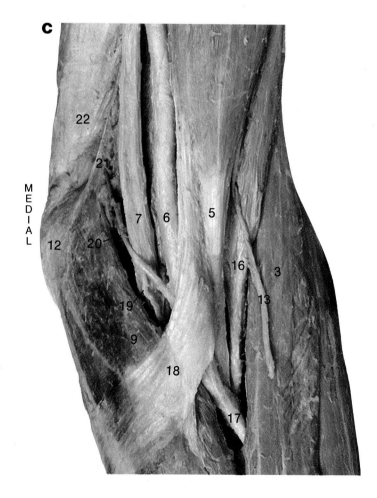

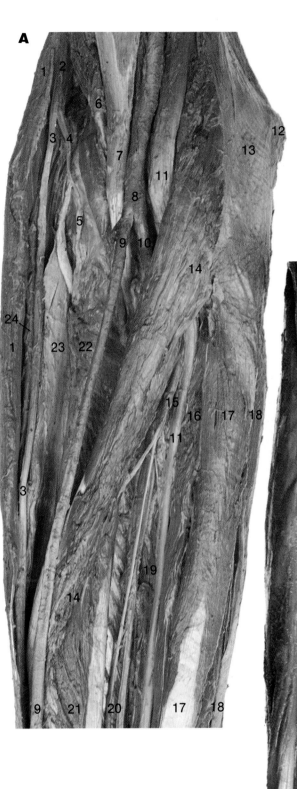

• The median nerve (B5) passes between the humeral (superficial) and ulnar (deep) heads of pronator teres; the ulnar artery (B16) passes deep to the ulnar head. In B most of the humeral head (B6) has been removed to show the ulnar head (B15) lying between the median nerve (B5) and the ulnar artery (B16).

• In the lower part of B flexor carpi ulnaris (B9) has been displaced medially to show the underlying ulnar nerve and artery (B10).

• At the level of the lateral epicondyle and under cover of brachioradialis (A1) the radial nerve (A2) divides into its superficial (A3) and deep (A4) terminal branches. The deep terminal branch is commonly called the posterior interosseous nerve.

A Right cubital fossa and forearm. Arteries and nerves

Pronator teres (14) and flexor carpi radialis (17) have been separated below the level of the cubital fossa and palmaris longus and the radial head of flexor digitorum superficialis removed, to show the median nerve (11) and its anterior interosseous branch (15)

1	Brachioradialis (displaced laterally)
2	Radial nerve
3	Superficial terminal branch of radial nerve
4	Posterior interosseous nerve (deep terminal branch of radial nerve)
5	Nerve to supinator
6	Brachialis
7	Biceps
8	Brachial artery
9	Radial artery
10	Ulnar artery
11	Median nerve
12	Medial epicondyle
13	Common flexor origin
14	Pronator teres
15	Anterior interosseous nerve
16	Humero-ulnar head of flexor digitorum superficialis
17	Flexor carpi radialis (displaced medially)
18	Flexor carpi ulnaris
19	Flexor digitorum profundus
20	Anterior interosseous nerve and artery overlying interosseous membrane
21	Flexor pollicis longus
22	Supinator
23	Extensor carpi radialis brevis
24	Extensor carpi radialis longus

B Right cubital fossa and forearm. Arteries and nerves

Most of the humeral origins of pronator teres and flexor carpi radialis (from the common flexor origin, 6 and 7) and palmaris longus have been removed to show the median nerve (5) passing superficial to the deep head of pronator teres (15) and then deep to the upper border of the radial head of flexor digitorum superficialis (13)

1	Lateral cutaneous nerve of forearm
2	Brachialis
3	Biceps
4	Brachial artery
5	Median nerve
6	Humeral head of pronator teres
7	Common flexor origin
8	Humero-ulnar head of flexor digitorum superficialis
9	Flexor carpi ulnaris (displaced medially)
10	Ulnar nerve and artery
11	Radial artery
12	Superficial terminal branch of radial nerve overlying extensor carpi radialis longus
13	Radial head of flexor digitorum superficialis
14	Anterior interosseous nerve
15	Ulnar head of pronator teres
16	Ulnar artery
17	A muscular branch of median nerve
18	Radial recurrent artery
19	Brachioradialis (displaced laterally)

125

A

B

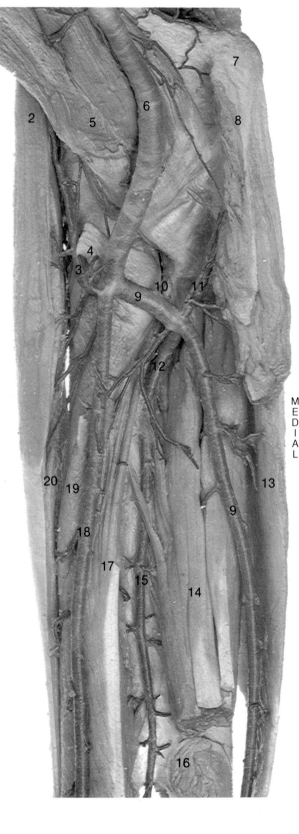

A Left forearm, from the front. Deep muscles

All vessels and nerves have been removed, together with the superficial muscles, to show the deep flexor group—flexor digitorum profundus (15), flexor pollicis longus (6) and pronator quadratus (11)

1	Common flexor origin
2	Brachialis
3	Biceps
4	Supinator
5	Pronator teres
6	Flexor pollicis longus
7	Extensor carpi radialis brevis
8	Extensor carpi radialis longus
9	Brachioradialis
10	Abductor pollicis longus
11	Pronator quadratus
12	Flexor carpi radialis
13	Flexor retinaculum
14	Flexor carpi ulnaris
15	Flexor digitorum profundus

B Right cubital fossa and forearm. Arteries

The arteries have been injected, and after removal of most of the superficial muscles the brachial artery (6) is seen dividing into the radial artery (18) and the ulnar artery (9). The radial artery gives off the radial recurrent (3) which runs upwards in front of supinator, giving branches to the carpal extensor muscles (2 and 20). The ulnar artery gives off the anterior and posterior ulnar recurrent vessels (11 and 10), and its common interosseous branch (12) is seen giving off the anterior interosseous (15) which passes down in front of the interosseous membrane between flexor pollicis longus (17) and flexor digitorum profundus (14)

1	Brachioradialis
2	Extensor carpi radialis longus
3	Radial recurrent artery overlying supinator
4	Biceps tendon
5	Brachialis
6	Brachial artery
7	Medial epicondyle of humerus
8	Common flexor origin
9	Ulnar artery
10	Posterior ulnar recurrent artery
11	Anterior ulnar recurrent artery
12	Common interosseous artery
13	Flexor carpi ulnaris
14	Flexor digitorum profundus
15	Anterior interosseous artery overlying interosseous membrane
16	Pronator quadratus
17	Flexor pollicis longus
18	Radial artery
19	Pronator teres
20	Extensor carpi radialis brevis

● The radial artery (18) usually appears to be the direct continuation of the brachial, as here, and the ulnar artery (9) branches off from the parent trunk almost at a right angle.

● The unnamed vessels are muscular branches.

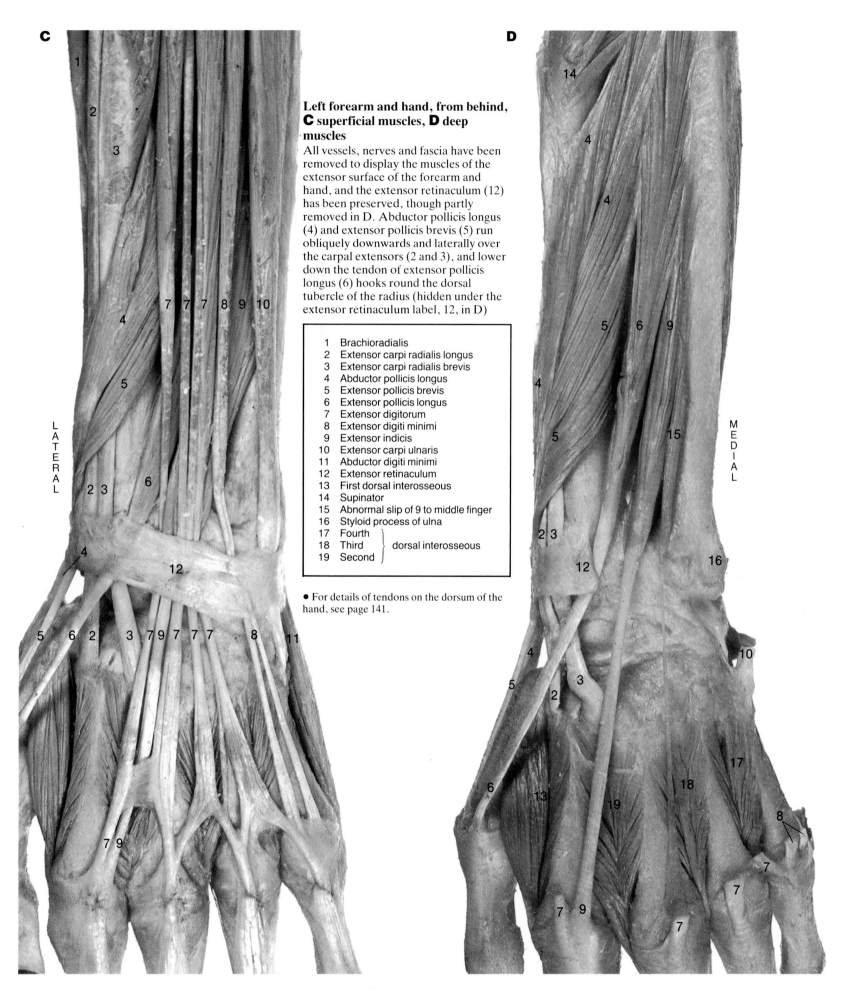

C

D

Left forearm and hand, from behind, C superficial muscles, D deep muscles

All vessels, nerves and fascia have been removed to display the muscles of the extensor surface of the forearm and hand, and the extensor retinaculum (12) has been preserved, though partly removed in D. Abductor pollicis longus (4) and extensor pollicis brevis (5) run obliquely downwards and laterally over the carpal extensors (2 and 3), and lower down the tendon of extensor pollicis longus (6) hooks round the dorsal tubercle of the radius (hidden under the extensor retinaculum label, 12, in D)

1	Brachioradialis
2	Extensor carpi radialis longus
3	Extensor carpi radialis brevis
4	Abductor pollicis longus
5	Extensor pollicis brevis
6	Extensor pollicis longus
7	Extensor digitorum
8	Extensor digiti minimi
9	Extensor indicis
10	Extensor carpi ulnaris
11	Abductor digiti minimi
12	Extensor retinaculum
13	First dorsal interosseous
14	Supinator
15	Abnormal slip of 9 to middle finger
16	Styloid process of ulna
17	Fourth
18	Third dorsal interosseous
19	Second

● For details of tendons on the dorsum of the hand, see page 141.

LATERAL

MEDIAL

A Left forearm, from the lateral side. Deep muscles

All vessels, nerves and fascia and the superficial group of flexor muscles have been removed, but the attachment of pronator teres (3) halfway down the lateral side of the radius remains. Above it the radius is covered by supinator (2), and below it abductor pollicis longus (4) and extensor pollicis brevis (5) curl obliquely round the lower part of the radius. The three most radial compartments of the extensor retinaculum (8) have been preserved, containing the tendons of abductor pollicis longus and extensor pollicis brevis (4 and 5), extensor carpi radialis longus and brevis (10 and 9) and extensor pollicis longus (6)

1	Biceps
2	Supinator
3	Pronator teres
4	Abductor pollicis longus
5	Extensor pollicis brevis
6	Extensor pollicis longus
7	Extensor indicis
8	Extensor retinaculum
9	Extensor carpi radialis brevis
10	Extensor carpi radialis longus (double)
11	Flexor pollicis longus

● Distal to the extensor retinaculum (8) the tendons of extensor carpi radialis longus and brevis (10 and 9) pass deep to the tendon of extensor pollicis longus (6).

B Left forearm, from behind. Posterior interosseous nerve

The forearm is in the mid-prone position. Most of the deep fascia has been removed and the extensor group of muscles has been split between extensor digitorum (5, which has been displaced medially) and extensor carpi radialis brevis (2). The posterior interosseous nerve (4) emerges from supinator (3) and gives off branches to the adjacent muscles

1	Extensor carpi radialis longus
2	Extensor carpi radialis brevis
3	Supinator
4	Posterior interosseous nerve
5	Extensor digitorum
6	Extensor carpi ulnaris
7	Extensor retinaculum
8	Extensor indicis
9	Extensor pollicis longus
10	Extensor pollicis brevis
11	Abductor pollicis longus
12	Branch of posterior interosseous artery

● Abductor pollicis longus (11) and extensor pollicis brevis (10) are the only muscles attached to the posterior surface of the radius. The abductor also has an attachment to the posterior surface of the ulna (as well as the intervening interosseous membrane), and below it on this bone extensor pollicis longus (9) and extensor indicis (8) have an origin (see page 102, B).
● For details of supinator, see the opposite page.

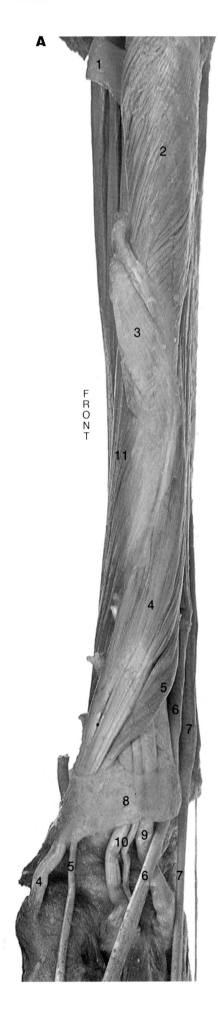

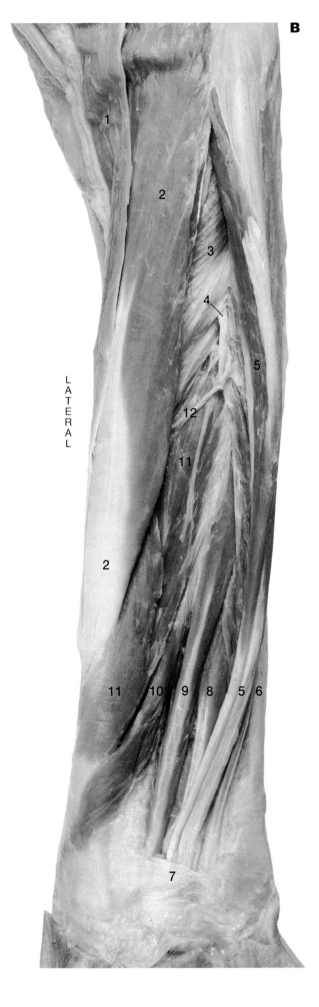

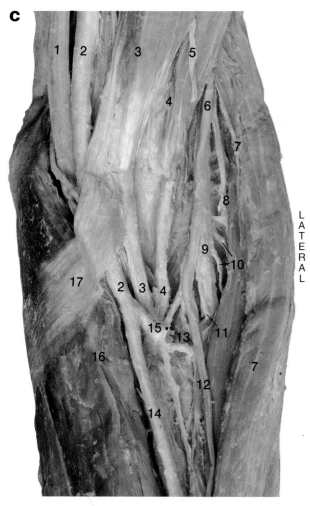

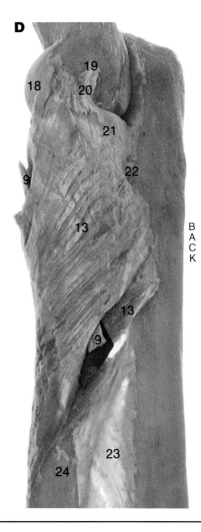

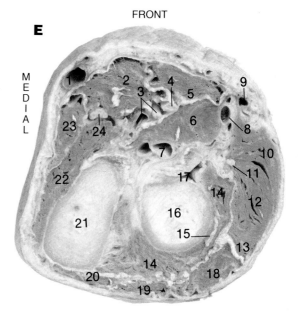

FRONT

Left elbow and upper forearm, **C** from the front, **D** in the midprone position from the lateral side

In C brachioradialis (7) and extensor carpi radialis longus (8) have been displaced laterally to show the radial nerve (6) giving off branches to those muscles and then dividing into the superficial (cutaneous) branch (12) and the deep (posterior interosseous) branch (9) which enters supinator. In D, with the forearm in midpronation and seen from the lateral side so that the radius (24) lies in front of the ulna, all muscles have been removed except supinator (13) to show its humeral and ulnar origins (see notes)

- The fibres of the interosseous membrane (23) pass obliquely downwards from the radius (24) to the ulna, so transmitting weight from the hand and radius to the ulna.
- The supinator muscle (13) arises from the lateral epicondyle of the humerus (19), radial collateral ligament (20), annular ligament (21), supinator crest of the ulna (22) and bone in front of the crest (page 100, D6), and an aponeurosis overlying the muscle. From these origins the fibres wrap themselves round the upper end of the radius above the pronator teres attachment, to be attached to the lateral surface of the radius and extending anteriorly and posteriorly as far as the tuberosity of the radius.
- The posterior interosseous nerve (9) passes through the muscle, dividing it into superficial and deep layers. In D there is a black marker behind the nerve as it emerges from between the two layers.

1	Median nerve
2	Brachial artery
3	Biceps
4	Brachialis
5	Lateral cutaneous nerve of forearm
6	Radial nerve
7	Brachioradialis and nerve
8	Extensor carpi radialis longus and nerve
9	Posterior interosseous nerve
10	Branches to extensor carpi radialis brevis
11	Nerve to supinator
12	Superficial branch of radial nerve
13	Supinator
14	Radial artery
15	Radial recurrent artery
16	Pronator teres
17	Bicipital aponeurosis
18	Capitulum of humerus
19	Lateral epicondyle
20	Radial collateral ligament
21	Annular ligament
22	Supinator crest of ulna
23	Interosseous membrane
24	Radius

E Cross section of the left upper forearm, from below

The section, seen from below looking towards the elbow, shows the posterior interosseous nerve (15) within the supinator muscle (14) which curls round the radius (16)

1	Basilic vein
2	Flexor digitorum superficialis
3	Anterior interosseous nerve and vessels
4	Median nerve
5	Flexor carpi radialis and palmaris longus
6	Pronator teres
7	Ulnar artery
8	Radial artery
9	Cephalic vein
10	Brachioradialis
11	Superficial branch of radial nerve
12	Extensor carpi radialis longus
13	Extensor carpi radialis brevis
14	Supinator
15	Posterior interosseous nerve
16	Radius
17	Tendon of biceps and bursa
18	Extensor digitorum
19	Extensor carpi ulnaris
20	Anconeus
21	Ulna
22	Flexor digitorum profundus
23	Flexor carpi ulnaris
24	Ulnar nerve

A Palm of the left hand

The surface markings of various structures within the wrist and hand are indicated; not all of them are palpable, e.g. the superficial and deep palmar arches (5 and 6), but their relative positions are important

1	Head of metacarpal	13	Distal ⎫
2	Longitudinal crease	14	Middle ⎬ wrist crease
3	Proximal ⎫ transverse	15	Proximal ⎭
4	Distal ⎬ crease	16	Flexor carpi ulnaris
5	Level of superficial palmar arch	17	Palmaris longus
6	Level of deep palmar arch	18	Median nerve
7	Abductor digiti minimi	19	Flexor carpi radialis
8	Flexor digiti minimi brevis	20	Radial artery
9	Palmaris brevis	21	Abductor pollicis brevis
10	Hook of hamate	22	Flexor pollicis brevis
11	Pisiform	23	Thenar eminence
12	Ulnar artery and nerve	24	Adductor pollicis

B Left wrist, from the front. Cutaneous nerves

The hand is in ulnar deviation at the wrist joint, so the radial border (with the base of the thumb and thenar muscles, 1) is in line with the radial border of the forearm. The palmar cutaneous branch of the median nerve (2) pierces the fascia between flexor carpi radialis (9) and palmaris longus (8). The palmar cutaneous branch of the ulnar nerve (6) in this specimen is on the ulnar side of flexor carpi ulnaris (5); it is usually on the radial side

1	Lateral part of palmar aponeurosis overlying thenar muscles
2	Palmar cutaneous branch of median nerve overlying palmaris longus attachment to flexor retinaculum
3	Medial part of palmar aponeurosis overlying hypothenar muscles
4	Branches of dorsal branch of ulnar nerve
5	Flexor carpi ulnaris
6	Palmar cutaneous branch of ulnar nerve
7	Medial cutaneous nerve of forearm and fascia overlying flexor digitorum superficialis
8	Palmaris longus
9	Flexor carpi radialis
10	Lateral cutaneous nerve of forearm
11	Superficial terminal branch of radial nerve

● The curved lines (1) proximal to the bases of the fingers indicate the ends of the heads of the metacarpals and the level of the metacarpophalangeal joints.
● The creases on the fingers indicate the level of the interphalangeal joints.
● The middle crease at the wrist indicates the level of the wrist joint.
● The radial artery at the wrist (20) is the commonest site for feeling the pulse. The vessel is on the radial side of the tendon of flexor carpi radialis (19) and can be compressed against the lower end of the radius.
● The median nerve at the wrist (18) lies on the ulnar side of the tendon of flexor carpi radialis (19) and is slightly overlapped from the ulnar side by the tendon of palmaris longus (17) (although this muscle is absent in 13 per cent of limbs).

● The ulnar nerve and artery at the wrist (12) are on the radial side of the tendon of flexor carpi ulnaris (16) and the pisiform bone (11). The artery is on the radial side of the nerve and its pulsation can be felt, though less easily than that of the radial artery (20).
● Abductor pollicis brevis (21) and flexor pollicis brevis (22), together with the underlying opponens pollicis, are the muscles which form the thenar eminence, the 'bulge' at the base of the thumb. Abductor digiti minimi (7) and flexor digiti minimi brevis (8), together with the underlying opponens digiti minimi, form the muscles of the hypothenar eminence, the less prominent bulge on the ulnar side of the palm where palmaris brevis (9) lies subcutaneously.

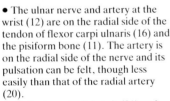

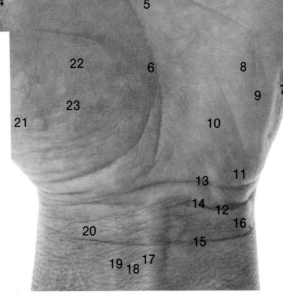

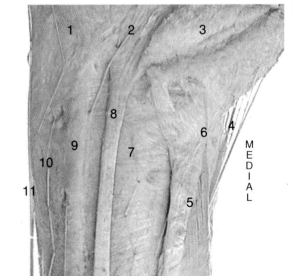

C Palm of the left hand. Palmar aponeurosis

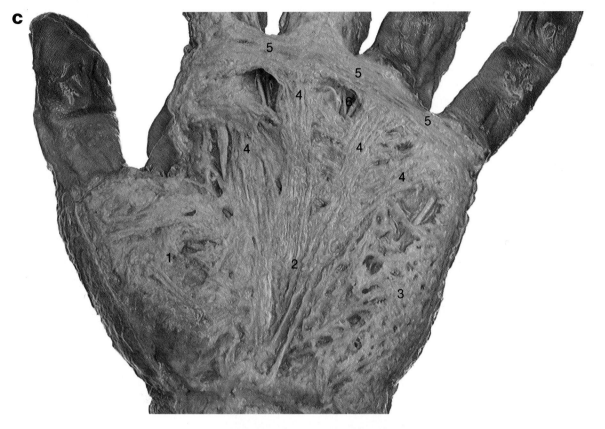

Removal of skin reveals the palmar aponeurosis with its thick central part (2) and the thin lateral and medial parts (1 and 3) which overlie the thenar and hypothenar muscles respectively. The central part divides into slips (4) for each finger; in the intervals between adjacent slips (as at 6) digital vessels and nerves are seen

1 Lateral part of aponeurosis overlying thenar muscles
2 Central part of aponeurosis
3 Medial part of aponeurosis overlying hypothenar muscles
4 Digital slips of aponeurosis
5 Superficial transverse metacarpal ligaments
6 Palmar digital vessels and nerves in interval between slips

● The palmar aponeurosis is continuous with the distal edge of the flexor retinaculum; the palmaris longus tendon is attached to the aponeurosis and the distal part of the retinaculum.

D Palm of the left hand. Superficial dissection

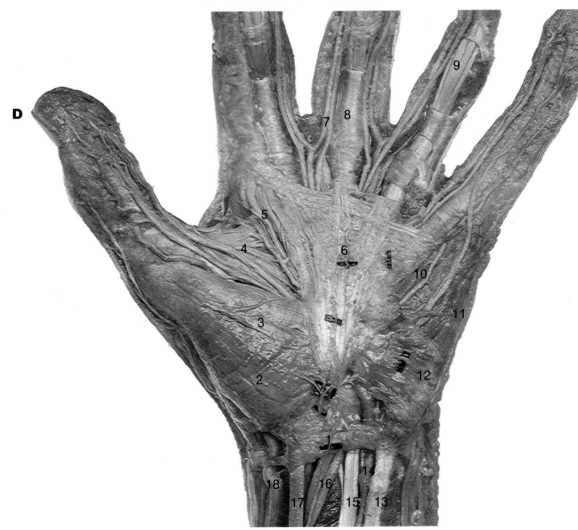

The central part of the aponeurosis remains (6) but the medial and lateral parts have been removed to show the underlying muscles. At the base of the thumb, abductor pollicis brevis (2) lies lateral to flexor pollicis brevis (3). On the ulnar side, palmaris brevis (12) overlies the proximal part of abductor digiti minimi (11) and flexor digiti minimi brevis (10). At the wrist the median nerve (16) is on the ulnar side of the tendon of flexor carpi radialis (17)

1 Flexor retinaculum and palmar branch of median nerve
2 Abductor pollicis brevis
3 Flexor pollicis brevis and muscular branch of median nerve
4 Adductor pollicis and digital branches of median nerve
5 First lumbrical
6 Central part of palmar aponeurosis and filaments of palmar branch of median nerve
7 Palmar digital vessels and nerves
8 Fibrous sheath (partly removed)
9 Flexor digitorum profundus tendon overlying superficialis tendon
10 Flexor digiti minimi brevis
11 Abductor digiti minimi
12 Palmaris brevis and filament of palmar branch of ulnar nerve
13 Flexor carpi ulnaris
14 Ulnar nerve and artery passing beneath superficial part of flexor retinaculum
15 Flexor digitorum superficialis
16 Median nerve and overlying palmar branch
17 Flexor carpi radialis
18 Radial artery

131

A Left wrist and hand. Muscles and tendons of the palmar surface

All vessels, nerves and fascia have been removed, and parts of the fibrous flexor sheaths of the fingers (9) have also been excised to show the contained tendons of flexor digitorum superficialis (8) and flexor digitorum profundus (7). In the palm the lumbrical muscles (6, 10, 11 and 12) are seen arising from the profundus tendons. At the wrist, palmaris longus (16) becomes attached to the flexor retinaculum (17) and flexor carpi ulnaris to the pisiform bone (15)

1	Abductor pollicis longus overlying extensor pollicis brevis
2	Abductor pollicis brevis
3	Flexor pollicis brevis
4	Adductor pollicis
5	First dorsal interosseous
6	First lumbrical
7	Flexor digitorum profundus
8	Flexor digitorum superficialis
9	Remaining parts of fibrous flexor sheath
10	Second lumbrical
11	Third lumbrical
12	Fourth lumbrical
13	Flexor digiti minimi brevis
14	Abductor digiti minimi
15	Flexor carpi ulnaris and pisiform
16	Palmaris longus
17	Flexor retinaculum
18	Flexor pollicis longus
19	Flexor carpi radialis
20	Pronator quadratus
21	Brachioradialis

● Near the base of the proximal phalanges each flexor digitorum superficialis tendon divides (as at the two adjacent 8 labels on the middle finger) to allow the profundus tendon (as at 7 on the middle finger) to pass through to its attachment to the base of the distal phalanx. The divided superficialis slips reunite and partially decussate (cross over) before becoming attached to the sides of the shaft of the middle phalanx.

B Left wrist and hand, from the lateral side

This side view of the specimen seen in A shows the two most lateral compartments of the extensor retinaculum (11), one containing the tendons of abductor pollicis longus (7) and extensor pollicis brevis (6), and the other containing the two extensor carpi radialis tendons, longus (5) and brevis (4)

1	Extensor digitorum
2	First dorsal interosseous
3	Extensor pollicis longus
4	Extensor carpi radialis brevis
5	Extensor carpi radialis longus
6	Extensor pollicis brevis
7	Abductor pollicis longus (giving slip to brevis)
8	Abductor pollicis brevis
9	Flexor carpi radialis
10	Flexor pollicis longus
11	Extensor retinaculum

● Three tendons pass to different levels of the thumb: abductor pollicis longus (7) to the base of the first metacarpal, extensor pollicis brevis (6) to the base of the proximal phalanx, and extensor pollicis longus (3) to the base of the distal phalanx.

● The lumbrical muscles have no bony attachments. They arise from the tendons of flexor digitorum profundus (A7)—the first and second (A6 and A10) from the tendons of the index and middle fingers respectively, and the third and fourth (A11 and A12) from adjacent sides of the middle and ring, and ring and little fingers respectively. Each is attached distally to the radial side of the dorsal digital expansion of each finger (page 137).

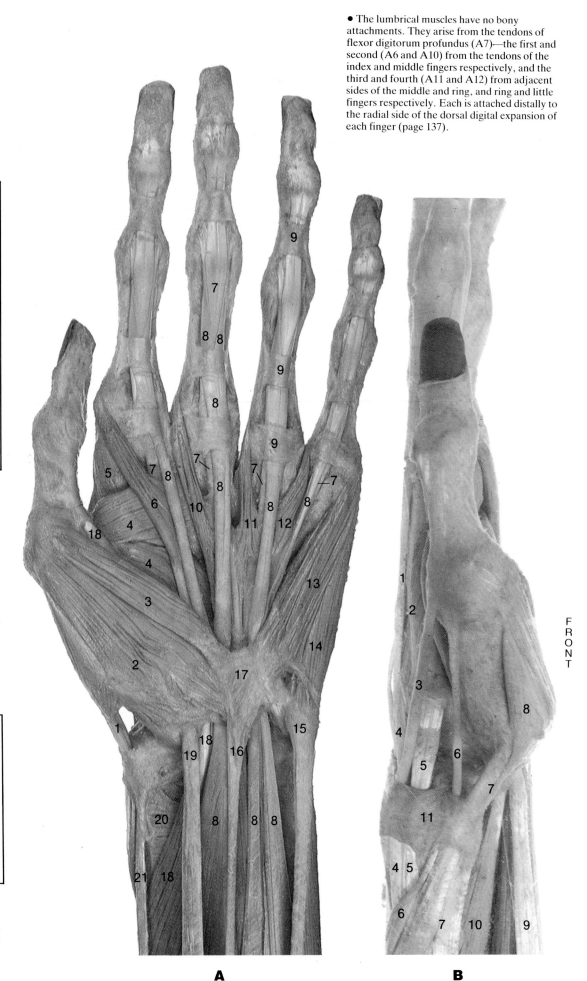

A

B

A

Superficial palmar arch, A incomplete in the left hand, B complete in the right hand

The superficial palmar (arterial) arch (6) and its branches (as at 7) in the palm are superficial to branches of the median and ulnar nerves (4 and 13). The arch, the continuation of the ulnar artery (21) in the palm, is usually incomplete as in A (see notes), but in B is completed by the superficial palmar branch (32) of the radial artery (26). In B the thenar muscles and long flexor tendons have been removed, and in both hands flexor digiti minimi brevis has been excised to show the deep branches of the ulnar nerve and artery (18 and 17) passing through opponens digiti minimi (14)

1	Abductor pollicis brevis	16	Palmaris brevis
2	Flexor pollicis brevis	17	Deep branch of ulnar artery
3	Muscular (recurrent) branch of median nerve	18	Deep branch of ulnar nerve
4	Median nerve dividing into common palmar digital branches	19	Flexor carpi ulnaris and pisiform
		20	Ulnar nerve
5	First lumbrical	21	Ulnar artery
6	Superficial palmar arch	22	Flexor retinaculum
7	A common palmar digital artery	23	Median nerve
8	A palmar digital nerve	24	Flexor pollicis longus
9	A palmar digital artery	25	Flexor carpi radialis
10	Flexor digitorum superficialis	26	Radial artery
11	Flexor digitorum profundus	27	Abductor pollicis longus
12	Fourth lumbrical	28	Deep palmar arch
13	Common palmar digital branch of ulnar nerve	29	Common stem of 30 and 31
		30	Radialis indicis artery
14	Opponens digiti minimi	31	Princeps pollicis artery
15	Abductor digiti minimi	32	Superficial branch of radial artery

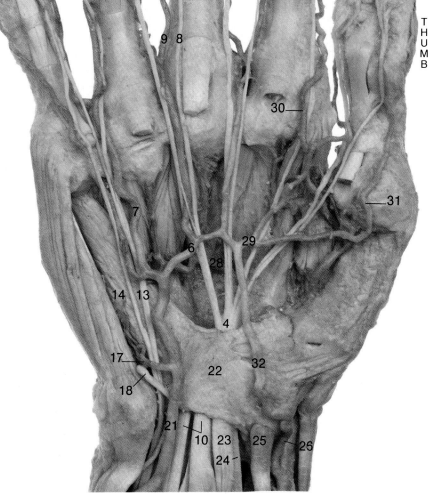

B

● In two-thirds of hands the superficial palmar arch is not complete (as in A, 6). In the other third it is usually completed by the superficial palmar branch of the radial artery (B32).
● In the palm the superficial arterial arch (6) and its branches (as at 7) lie superficial to the common palmar digital nerves (4 and 13), but on the fingers the palmar digital nerves (as at 8) lie superficial (anterior) to the palmar digital arteries (as at 9).
● The ulnar nerve (20) supplies the skin of the ulnar side of the palm and of the ulnar one-and-a-half or two fingers; the rest of the palm and the palmar surfaces of the remaining fingers and thumb are supplied by the median nerve (23).
● In B the radial side of the superficial arch gives off a common stem (B29) which divides into the radialis indicis and princeps pollicis arteries (B30 and 31); these vessels usually arise from the radial artery.

133

A

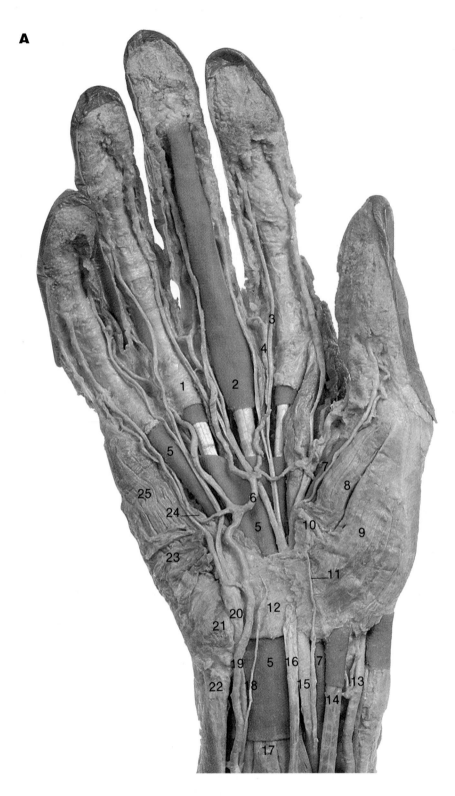

A Palm of the right hand, with synovial sheaths

The synovial sheaths of the wrist and fingers have been emphasized by blue tissue. On the middle finger the fibrous flexor sheath has been removed (but retained on the other fingers, as at 1) to show the whole length of the synovial sheath (2). On the index and ring fingers the synovial sheath projects slightly proximal to the fibrous sheath. The synovial sheath of the little finger is continuous with the sheath surrounding the finger flexor tendons under the flexor retinaculum (the ulnar bursa, 5), and the sheath of flexor pollicis longus is the radial bursa (7) which also continues under the retinaculum (12)

1	Fibrous flexor sheath
2	Synovial sheath
3	Palmar digital nerve
4	Palmar digital artery
5	Ulnar bursa
6	Superficial palmar arch
7	Radial bursa and flexor pollicis longus
8	Flexor pollicis brevis
9	Abductor pollicis brevis
10	Muscular branch of median nerve
11	Palmar branch of median nerve
12	Flexor retinaculum
13	Radial artery
14	Flexor carpi radialis
15	Median nerve
16	Palmaris longus
17	Flexor digitorum superficialis
18	Palmar branch of ulnar nerve
19	Ulnar artery
20	Ulnar nerve
21	Pisiform bone
22	Flexor carpi ulnaris
23	Palmaris brevis
24	Flexor digiti minimi brevis
25	Abductor digiti minimi

● In the carpal tunnel (beneath the flexor retinaculum), one synovial sheath envelops the eight tendons of flexor digitorum superficialis and profundus (A5), another envelops the flexor pollicis longus tendon (A7), and the flexor carpi radialis (in its own compartment of the flexor retinaculum) has its own sheath also (A14). The synovial sheaths for flexor carpi radialis and flexor pollicis longus extend as far as the tendon insertions.
● The sheath of the long finger flexors is continuous with the digital synovial sheath of the little finger, but is *not* continuous with the digital synovial sheaths of the ring, middle or index fingers; these fingers have their own synovial sheaths whose proximal ends project slightly beyond the *fibrous* sheaths within which the digital *synovial* sheaths lie.
● The muscular (recurrent) branch (A10) of the median nerve usually supplies abductor pollicis brevis, flexor pollicis brevis and opponens pollicis, but of all the muscles in the body flexor pollicis brevis (A8) is the one most likely to have an anomalous supply: in about one-third of hands by the median nerve, in another third by the ulnar nerve, and in the rest by both the median and ulnar nerves.

B Long flexor tendons and vincula of the right middle finger, from the front and the right

The fibrous and synovial sheaths have been removed, and the flexor tendons (1 and 2) have been pulled anteriorly to show the vincula (3 to 6), which are small fibrous bands carrying blood vessels from the sheaths to the tendons

1	Flexor digitorum superficialis
2	Flexor digitorum profundus
3	Short vinculum of profundus tendon
4	Long vinculum of profundus tendon
5	Position of short vinculum of superficialis tendon
6	Long vincula of superficialis tendon

B

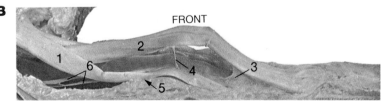

FRONT

A

B

C

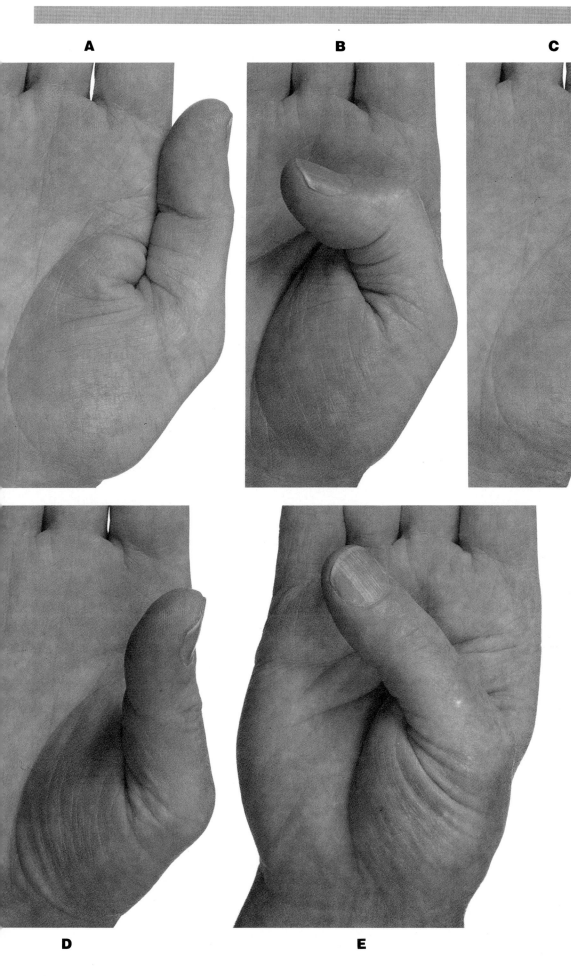

D

E

Movements of the thumb. A, in the anatomical position, B in flexion, C in extension, D in abduction, E in opposition

With the thumb in the anatomical position (A), the thumb nail is at right angles to the fingers, because the first metacarpal is at right angles to the others (page 103). This is a rather artificial position; in the normal position of rest the thumb makes an angle of about 60° with the plane of the palm (i.e. it is partially abducted). Flexion (B) means bending the thumb across the palm, keeping the phalanges at right angles to the palm. Extension (C) is the opposite movement, away from the palm. In abduction (D) the thumb is lifted forwards from the plane of the palm, and continuation of this movement inevitably leads to opposition (E), with rotation of the first metacarpal, twisting the whole digit so that the pulp of the thumb can be brought towards the palm at the base of the little finger (or more commonly in everyday use, to contact or overlap any of the flexed fingers). Opposition is a combination of abduction with flexion and medial rotation at the carpometacarpal joint; it is not necessarily accompanied by flexion at the other thumb joints

● Muscles producing movements at the carpometacarpal joint of the thumb:

Flexion: flexor pollicis brevis, opponens pollicis, and (when the other thumb joints are flexed) flexor pollicis longus.
Extension: abductor pollicis longus, extensor pollicis longus, extensor pollicis brevis.
Abduction: abductor pollicis brevis, abductor pollicis longus.
Adduction: adductor pollicis.
Opposition: opponens pollicis, flexor pollicis brevis, reinforced by adductor pollicis and flexor pollicis longus.

A

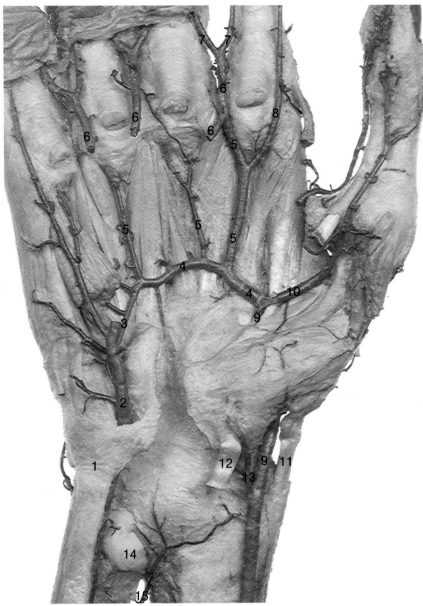

B

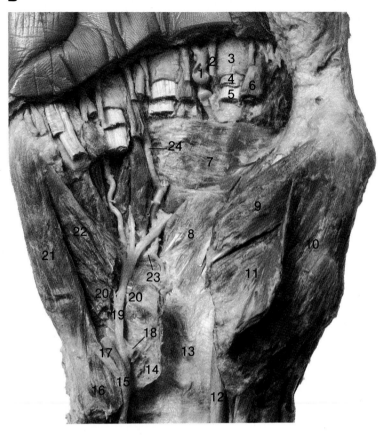

B Palm of the right hand. Deep branch of the ulnar nerve

The long flexor tendons (4 and 5) and lumbricals (6) have been cut off near the heads of the metacarpals and parts of the hypothenar muscles removed to show the deep branches of the ulnar nerve and artery (19 and 18) running into the palm and curling laterally to pass between the transverse and oblique heads of adductor pollicis (7 and 8)

A Palm of the right hand. Deep palmar arch

Most muscles and tendons have been removed and the arteries have been distended by injection. The deep palmar arch (4) is seen giving off the palmar metacarpal arteries (5) which join the common palmar digital arteries (6) from the superficial arch

1	Flexor carpi ulnaris and pisiform
2	Ulnar artery
3	Deep branch of ulnar artery
4	Deep palmar arch
5	Palmar metacarpal arteries
6	Common palmar digital arteries (from superficial arch)
7	Palmar digital arteries
8	Radialis indicis artery (anomalous origin)
9	Radial artery
10	Princeps pollicis artery
11	Abductor pollicis longus
12	Flexor carpi radialis
13	Superficial palmar branch of radial artery
14	Head of ulna
15	Branch of anterior interosseous artery to anterior carpal arch

- Unlike the superficial arch (page 133), the deep palmar arch (A4) is usually complete, being formed by the terminal part of the radial artery (A9) anastomosing with the deep branch of the ulnar artery (A3).
- The most distal part of the deep arch lies about 1 cm proximal to the superficial arch. For the surface markings, see page 130.
- The radialis indicis artery (A8) is usually a branch of the deep arch (A4), but in A it has arisen from the first palmar metacarpal artery (A5).
- The deep branch of the ulnar nerve (B19) normally supplies all the interossei, the hypothenar muscles (B10, B11 and B12), adductor pollicis (B7 and B8), and the two medial (third and fourth) lumbricals (not labelled in B but their cut ends are seen adjacent to the cut flexor tendons of the ring and little fingers). This branch may thus be said to supply all the small muscles of the hand except those supplied by the median nerve (the three thenar muscles—flexor and abductor pollicis brevis and opponens pollicis—and the two lateral lumbricals; but see the note on page 134 for the nerve supply of flexor pollicis brevis).
- For identification of the interossei see opposite page.

1	A common palmar digital artery
2	A palmar digital nerve
3	Fibrous flexor sheath
4	Flexor digitorum superficialis
5	Flexor digitorum profundus
6	First lumbrical
7	Transverse head ⎱ of adductor pollicis
8	Oblique head ⎰
9	Flexor pollicis brevis
10	Abductor pollicis brevis
11	Opponens pollicis
12	Flexor pollicis longus
13	Carpal tunnel
14	Flexor retinaculum (cut edge)
15	Ulnar nerve
16	Pisiform
17	Digital branches of ulnar nerve
18	Deep branch of ulnar artery
19	Deep branch of ulnar nerve
20	Opponens digiti minimi
21	Abductor digiti minimi
22	Flexor digiti minimi brevis
23	Deep palmar arch
24	A palmar metacarpal artery

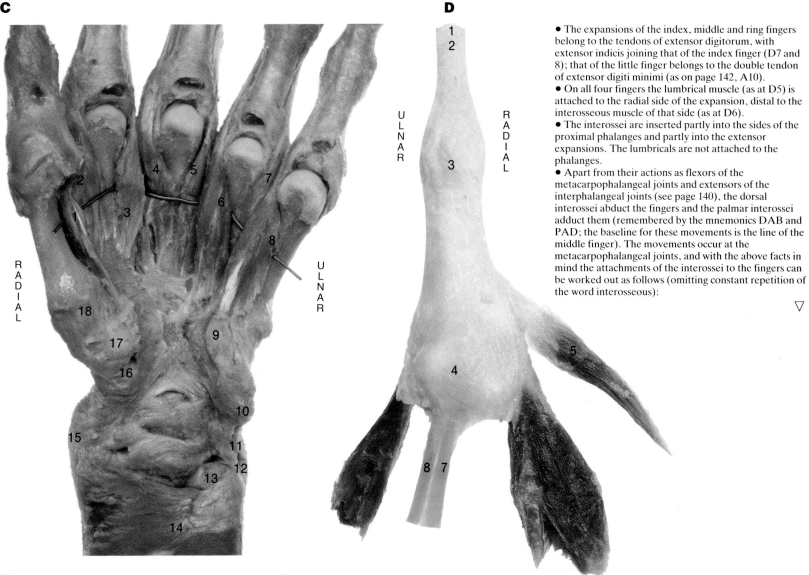

C

D

- The expansions of the index, middle and ring fingers belong to the tendons of extensor digitorum, with extensor indicis joining that of the index finger (D7 and 8); that of the little finger belongs to the double tendon of extensor digiti minimi (as on page 142, A10).
- On all four fingers the lumbrical muscle (as at D5) is attached to the radial side of the expansion, distal to the interosseous muscle of that side (as at D6).
- The interossei are inserted partly into the sides of the proximal phalanges and partly into the extensor expansions. The lumbricals are not attached to the phalanges.
- Apart from their actions as flexors of the metacarpophalangeal joints and extensors of the interphalangeal joints (see page 140), the dorsal interossei abduct the fingers and the palmar interossei adduct them (remembered by the mnemonics DAB and PAD; the baseline for these movements is the line of the middle finger). The movements occur at the metacarpophalangeal joints, and with the above facts in mind the attachments of the interossei to the fingers can be worked out as follows (omitting constant repetition of the word interosseous):

▽

C Left wrist and palm. Interosseous muscles

In this deep dissection with most other muscles removed, the palmar interossei (1, 3, 6 and 8) are shown superficial to the blue marker and the dorsal interossei (2, 4, 5 and 7) deep to it. The capsule of the distal radio-ulnar joint has been opened up to show the head of the ulna (13)

1	First palmar
2	First dorsal
3	Second palmar
4	Second dorsal
5	Third dorsal
6	Third palmar
7	Fourth dorsal
8	Fourth palmar
9	Hook of hamate
10	Pisiform
11	Ulnar collateral ligament
12	Styloid process of ulna
13	Head of ulna
14	Pronator quadratus
15	Styloid process of radius
16	Scaphoid
17	Trapezium
18	Capsule of carpometacarpal joint of thumb

D Extensor expansion of the left index finger

The extensor expansion (often called the dorsal digital expansion) of the left index finger has been removed from the finger with its attached lumbrical (5) and interosseous muscles (6 and 9) and extensor tendons (7 and 8), and is seen from the dorsal surface (as in the right hand on page 142) but with the lower 'angles' somewhat spread out

1	End attached to distal phalanx
2	Part overlying distal interphalangeal joint
3	Part overlying proximal interphalangeal joint
4	Part overlying metacarpophalangeal joint
5	First lumbrical
6	First dorsal interosseous (two heads)
7	Extensor digitorum tendon
8	Extensor indicis tendon
9	Second palmar interosseous

- The expansion of the index finger (shown in D) has the first dorsal on its radial side (D6), and the second palmar on its ulnar side (D9).
- The expansion of the middle finger has the second dorsal on its radial side and the third dorsal on its ulnar side (to abduct the finger to either side of its own baseline).
- The expansion of the ring finger has the third palmar on its radial side and the fourth dorsal on its ulnar side.
- The expansion of the little finger has the fourth palmar on its radial side and part of abductor digiti minimi on its ulnar side.
- The first palmar (C1) belongs to the thumb, not to a finger.
- The above attachments reflect the order of the interossei as seen in the palm dissection C.
- For the bony attachments of the interossei, see page 105. Note that the dorsal interossei have two heads of origin, from adjacent metacarpals, but the palmar interossei have only one, arising from the metacarpal of the digit which they are inserted.
- When viewing a palmar dissection, as in C, all the interossei (palmar and dorsal) can be seen, but on the dorsum of the hand, as on page 141, only the dorsal interossei are visible.

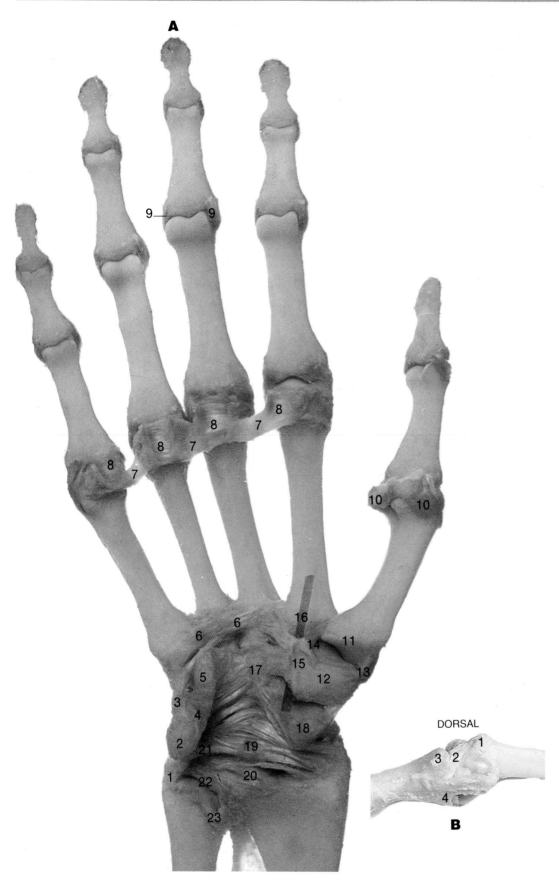

A Palm of the right hand. Ligaments and joints

The capsule of the carpometacarpal joint of the thumb (between the base of the first metacarpal and the trapezium) has been removed, to show the saddle-shaped joint surfaces which allow the unique movement of opposition of the thumb to occur. The palmar and lateral ligaments (14 and 13) of the joint remain intact. The capsule of the distal radio-ulnar joint has also been removed to show the articular disc, but the wrist joint, the ulnar part of which lies distal to the disc, has not been opened

1	Ulnar collateral ligament of wrist joint
2	Pisiform
3	Pisometacarpal ligament
4	Pisohamate ligament
5	Hook of hamate
6	Interosseous metacarpal ligament
7	Deep transverse metacarpal ligament
8	Palmar ligament of metacarpophalangeal joint with groove for flexor tendon
9	Collateral ligament of interphalangeal joint
10	Sesamoid bones of flexor pollicis brevis tendons (with adductor pollicis on ulnar side)
11	Base of first metacarpal
12	Trapezium
13	Lateral ligament of carpometacarpal joint of thumb
14	Palmar ligament of carpometacarpal joint
15	Tubercle of trapezium
16	Marker in groove on trapezium for flexor carpi radialis tendon
17	Head of capitate
18	Tubercle of scaphoid
19	Lunate
20	Palmar radiocarpal ligament
21	Palmar ulnocarpal ligament
22	Articular disc of distal radio-ulnar joint
23	Sacciform recess of capsule of distal radio-ulnar joint

● The collateral ligaments of the metacarpophalangeal and interphalangeal joints (A9, B2) pass obliquely forwards from the posterior part of the side of the head of the proximal bone to the anterior part of the side of the base of the distal bone. They become tightest in flexion.

● Opposition of the thumb is a combination of flexion and abduction with medial rotation of the first metacarpal (page 135). The saddle-shape of the joint between the base of the first metacarpal and the trapezium, together with the way that the capsule and its reinforcing ligaments are attached to the bones, ensures that when flexor pollicis brevis and opponens pollicis contract they produce the necessary metacarpal rotation.

● The articular disc (22) holds the lower ends of the radius and ulna together, and separates the distal radio-ulnar joint from the wrist joint, so that the cavities of these joints are not continuous (unlike those of the elbow and proximal radio-ulnar joints, which have one continuous cavity—page 122).

B Metacarpophalangeal joint of the right index finger, from the radial side

Part of the capsule has been removed to define the collateral ligament (2)

1	Head of second metacarpal
2	Collateral ligament
3	Base of proximal phalanx
4	Fibrous flexor sheath

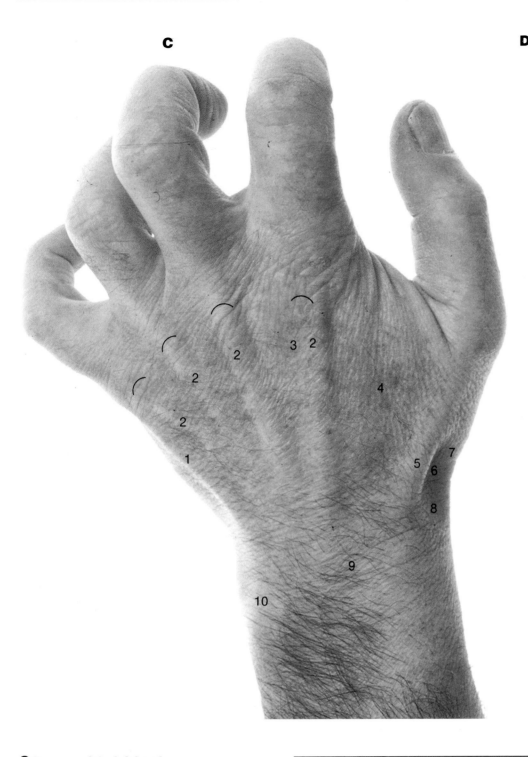

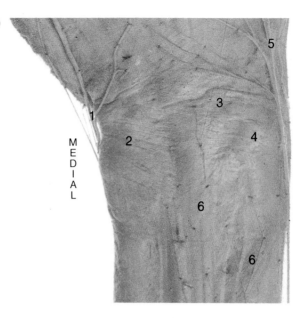

D Dorsum of the left wrist. Cutaneous nerves

Cutaneous nerves have been dissected out from the subcutaneous tissues. Branches of the radial nerve (5) overlie the region of the anatomical snuffbox (C6), while on the ulnar side are filaments from the dorsal branch of the ulnar nerve (1)

1	Branches of dorsal branch of ulnar nerve
2	Head of ulna
3	Extensor retinaculum
4	Lower end of radius
5	Superficial terminal branches of radial nerve
6	Branches of lateral cutaneous nerve of forearm

C Dorsum of the left hand

The fingers are extended at the metacarpophalangeal joints, causing the extensor tendons of the fingers (1, 2 and 3) to stand out, and partially flexed at the interphalangeal joints. The thumb is extended at the carpometacarpal joint and partially flexed at the metacarpophalangeal and interphalangeal joints. The lines proximal to the bases of the fingers indicate the ends of the heads of the metacarpals and the level of the metacarpophalangeal joints. The anatomical snuffbox (6) is the hollow between the tendons of abductor pollicis longus and extensor pollicis brevis laterally (7) and extensor pollicis longus medially (5)

1	Extensor digiti minimi
2	Extensor digitorum
3	Extensor indicis
4	First dorsal interosseous
5	Extensor pollicis longus
6	Anatomical snuffbox
7	Extensor pollicis brevis and abductor pollicis longus
8	Styloid process of radius
9	Extensor retinaculum
10	Head of ulna

Movements of the fingers. A flexion of the metacarpophalangeal joints and flexion of the interphalangeal joints, **B** extension of the metacarpophalangeal joints and flexion of the interphalangeal joints, **C** extension of the metacarpophalangeal and interphalangeal joints

When 'making a fist' with all finger joints flexed (A), the heads of the metacarpals (2) form the knuckles. To extend the metacarpophalangeal joints (B3) requires the activity of the long extensor tendons of the fingers, but to extend the interphalangeal joints (C6 and 9) as well requires the activity of the interossei and lumbricals, pulling on the dorsal extensor expansions (page 137). Only if the metacarpophalangeal joints remain flexed can the long extensors extend the interphalangeal joints

1	Base ⎫ of metacarpal
2	Head ⎭
3	Metacarpophalangeal joint
4	Base ⎫ of proximal phalanx
5	Head ⎭
6	Proximal interphalangeal joint
7	Base ⎫ of middle phalanx
8	Head ⎭
9	Distal interphalangeal joint
10	Base of distal phalanx

• Muscles producing movements at the metacarpophalangeal joints:

Flexion: flexor digitorum profundus, flexor digitorum superficialis, lumbricals, interossei, with flexor digiti minimi brevis for the little finger and flexor pollicis longus, flexor pollicis brevis and the first palmar interosseous for the thumb.

Extension: extensor digitorum, extensor indicis (index finger) and extensor digiti minimi (little finger), with extensor pollicis longus and extensor pollicis brevis for the thumb.

Adduction: palmar interossei; when flexed, the long flexors assist.

Abduction: dorsal interossei and the long extensors, with abductor digiti minimi for the little finger.

• Muscles producing movements at the interphalangeal joints:

Flexion: at the proximal joints, flexor digitorum superficialis and flexor digitorum profundus; at the distal joints, flexor digitorum profundus. For the thumb, flexor pollicis longus.

Extension: with the metacarpophalangeal joints flexed, extensor digitorum, extensor indicis and extensor digiti minimi; with the metacarpophalangeal joints extended, interossei and lumbricals. For the thumb, extensor pollicis longus.

• Muscles producing movements at the wrist joint:

Flexion: flexor carpi radialis, flexor carpi ulnaris, palmaris longus, with assistance from flexor digitorum superficialis, flexor digitorum profundus, flexor pollicis longus and abductor pollicis longus.

Extension: extensor carpi radialis longus and brevis, extensor carpi ulnaris, assisted by extensor digitorum, extensor indicis, extensor digiti minimi and extensor pollicis longus.

Abduction: flexor carpi radialis, extensor carpi radialis longus and brevis, abductor pollicis longus and extensor pollicis brevis.

Adduction: flexor carpi ulnaris, extensor carpi ulnaris.

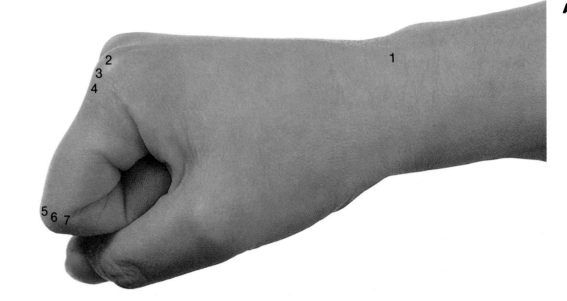

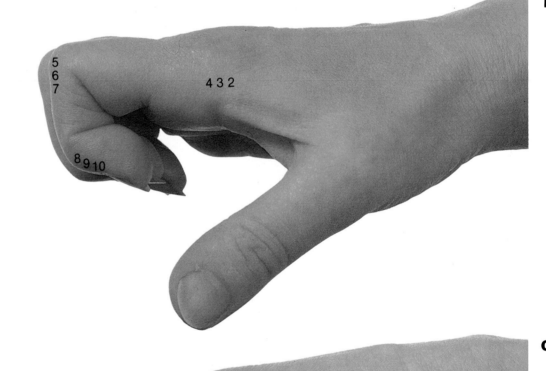

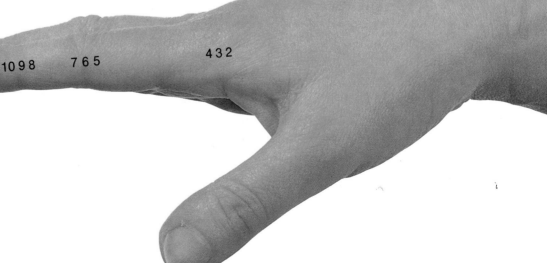

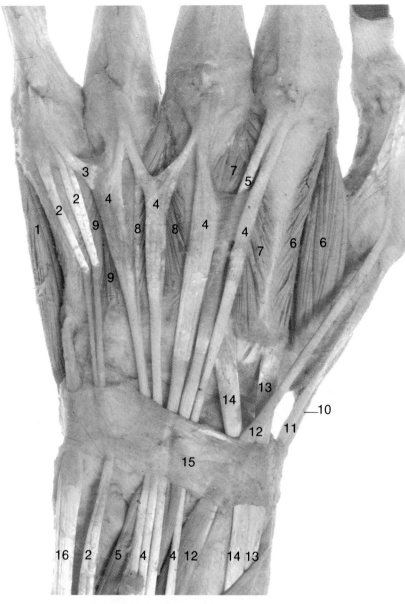

D Dorsum of the left hand. Muscles and tendons

All vessels, nerves and fascia have been removed to show the long tendons passing under the extensor retinaculum (15). See the notes below for the identification of finger tendons

1	Abductor digiti minimi
2	Extensor digiti minimi
3	Slip from extensor digitorum to little finger
4	Extensor digitorum
5	Extensor indicis
6	First
7	Second
8	Third } dorsal interosseous
9	Fourth
10	Abductor pollicis longus
11	Extensor pollicis brevis
12	Extensor pollicis longus
13	Extensor carpi radialis longus
14	Extensor carpi radialis brevis
15	Extensor retinaculum
16	Extensor carpi ulnaris

● On the dorsum of the hand the tendon of extensor indicis (D5) lies on the ulnar side of the extensor digitorum tendon to the index finger (D4).
● It is normal for the tendon of extensor digiti minimi (D2) to be double. In this specimen the extensor digitorum tendon (D4) to the ring finger is also double.
● The 'tendon' of extensor digitorum to the little finger (D3) normally consists, as here, of a slip from the digitorum tendon to the ring finger (D4), joining the digiti minimi tendon (D2) just proximal to the metacarpophalangeal joint. Similar slips may join adjacent digitorum tendons on other fingers, as here between the ring and middle fingers.

E Dorsum of the right wrist and hand. Synovial sheaths

Fascia and cutaneous branches of the ulnar nerve have been removed; the extensor retinaculum (10) and the radial nerve (2) have been preserved and the synovial sheaths have been emphasized by blue tissue. From the radial to the ulnar side, the six compartments of the extensor retinaculum contain the tendons of: a, abductor pollicis longus and extensor pollicis brevis (13 and 12); b, extensor carpi radialis longus and brevis (4 and 5); c, extensor pollicis longus (3); d, extensor digitorum and extensor indicis (7 and 8); e, extensor digiti minimi (9); f, extensor carpi ulnaris (11)

1	Cephalic vein
2	Branches of radial nerve
3	Extensor pollicis longus
4	Extensor carpi radialis longus
5	Extensor carpi radialis brevis
6	Common sheath for 4 and 5
7	Extensor digitorum
8	Extensor indicis
9	Extensor digiti minimi
10	Extensor retinaculum
11	Extensor carpi ulnaris
12	Extensor pollicis brevis
13	Abductor pollicis longus

A Dorsum of the right hand. Muscles and tendons

All vessels and nerves (except the radial artery, 3) have been removed; the extensor retinaculum (13) is preserved, together with some fascia distal to it to give some support to synovial sheaths which have been partially injected with green resin (compare with page 141, E). The margins of the distal parts of the extensor digital expansions (as at 5 and 6) have been emphasized by removal of the intervening connective tissue

1	Extensor pollicis brevis	8	Extensor digitorum
2	Extensor pollicis longus	9	Extensor indicis
3	Radial artery	10	Extensor digiti minimi
4	First dorsal interosseous	11	Extensor carpi ulnaris
5	Extensor expansion	12	Head of ulna
6	Collateral slip of expansion to distal phalanx	13	Extensor retinaculum
7	Intermediate part of expansion to middle phalanx	14	Extensor carpi radialis brevis
		15	Extensor carpi radialis longus

B Right hand. Muscles and tendons, from the radial side

This is the specimen seen in A, now rotated to show muscles and tendons on the radial (lateral) side. The synovial sheaths of extensor pollicis brevis (4) and extensor pollicis longus (6) show some injected resin. Between the thumb and index finger the first dorsal interosseous (10) passes to the expansion (11), with the first lumbrical (9) running into the expansion just beyond the interosseous. Adductor pollicis (8) passes to the proximal phalanx of the thumb

1	Abductor pollicis brevis	8	Adductor pollicis
2	Opponens pollicis	9	First lumbrical
3	Abductor pollicis longus	10	First dorsal interosseous
4	Extensor pollicis brevis	11	Extensor expansion
5	Radial artery	12	Extensor carpi radialis brevis
6	Extensor pollicis longus	13	Extensor carpi radialis longus
7	Princeps pollicis artery (unusual origin)	14	Extensor retinaculum

C Dorsum of the right hand. Arteries

The arteries have been injected and the long finger tendons removed to display the dorsal carpal arch (6) and dorsal metacarpal arteries (as at 2 and 3). Above the wrist pronator quadratus has been removed to show the branch (9) of the anterior interosseous artery (7) which continues towards the palm; the anterior interosseous itself passes to the dorsal surface to join the posterior interosseous artery (8)

1	Adductor pollicis and branch of princeps pollicis artery	8	Posterior interosseous artery
2	First dorsal interosseous and first dorsal metacarpal artery	9	Branch of anterior interosseous artery to anterior carpal arch
3	Second dorsal interosseous and second dorsal metacarpal artery	10	Extensor pollicis brevis
		11	Abductor pollicis longus
4	Abductor digiti minimi	12	Brachioradialis
5	Extensor carpi ulnaris	13	Extensor carpi radialis brevis
6	Dorsal carpal arch	14	Extensor carpi radialis longus
7	Anterior interosseous artery	15	Radial artery
		16	Extensor pollicis longus

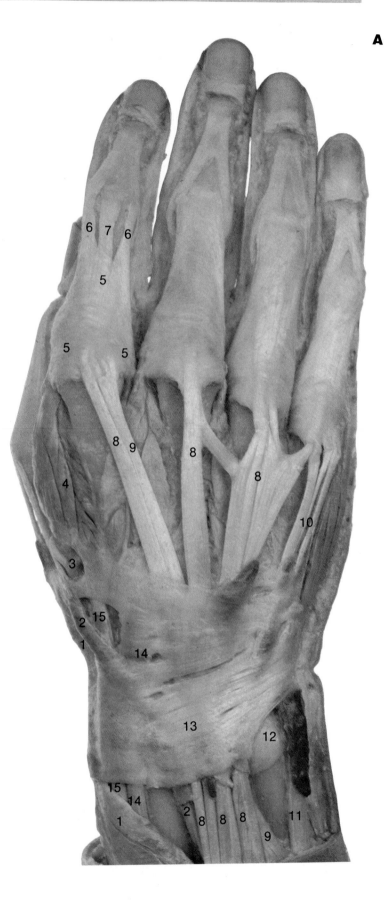

A

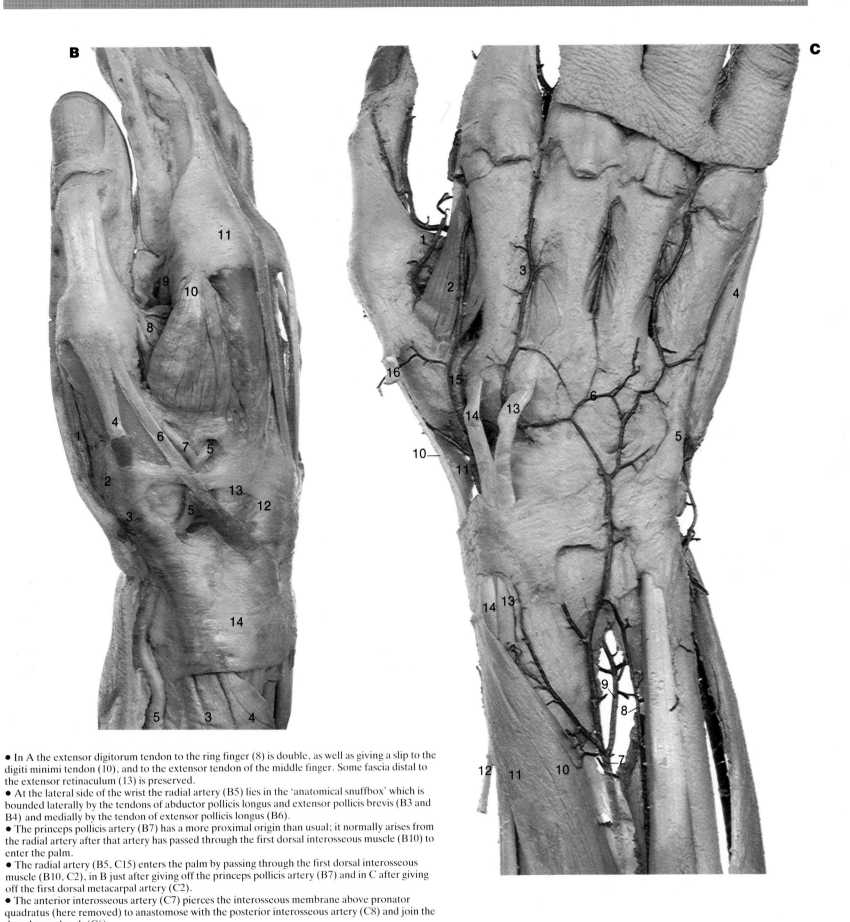

B **C**

- In A the extensor digitorum tendon to the ring finger (8) is double, as well as giving a slip to the digiti minimi tendon (10), and to the extensor tendon of the middle finger. Some fascia distal to the extensor retinaculum (13) is preserved.
- At the lateral side of the wrist the radial artery (B5) lies in the 'anatomical snuffbox' which is bounded laterally by the tendons of abductor pollicis longus and extensor pollicis brevis (B3 and B4) and medially by the tendon of extensor pollicis longus (B6).
- The princeps pollicis artery (B7) has a more proximal origin than usual; it normally arises from the radial artery after that artery has passed through the first dorsal interosseous muscle (B10) to enter the palm.
- The radial artery (B5, C15) enters the palm by passing through the first dorsal interosseous muscle (B10, C2), in B just after giving off the princeps pollicis artery (B7) and in C after giving off the first dorsal metacarpal artery (C2).
- The anterior interosseous artery (C7) pierces the interosseous membrane above pronator quadratus (here removed) to anastomose with the posterior interosseous artery (C8) and join the dorsal carpal arch (C6).

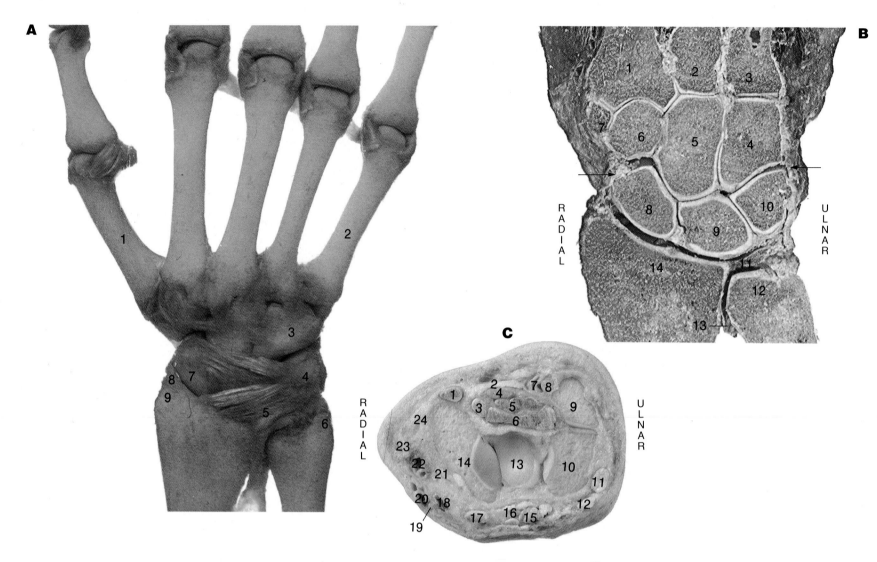

A

B

C

A Dorsum of the right hand. Ligaments and joints

Most joint capsules have been removed, including the radial part of the wrist joint capsule, so showing the articulation between the scaphoid (7) and the lower end of the radius (9)

1	First metacarpal
2	Fifth metacarpal
3	Hamate
4	Triquetral
5	Dorsal radiocarpal ligament
6	Styloid process of ulna
7	Scaphoid
8	Radial collateral ligament of wrist joint
9	Styloid process of radius

• The wrist (radiocarpal) joint is the joint between the lower end of the radius and the articular disc of the distal radio-ulnar joint proximally, and the scaphoid, lunate and triquetral bones distally.
• The midcarpal joint is the joint between the scaphoid, lunate and triquetral proximally, and the trapezium, trapezoid, capitate and hamate distally.
• Extension of the wrist occurs at the wrist and midcarpal joints, but most of the movement takes place at the wrist joint.
• Flexion of the wrist occurs at the wrist and midcarpal joints, but most of the movement takes place at the midcarpal joint.

B Coronal section of the right hand

Viewed from the dorsal surface, the section has passed through the wrist near this surface, and the first and fifth metacarpals have not been included in the cut. The arrows between the two rows of carpal bones indicate the line of the midcarpal joint

1	Base of second metacarpal
2	Base of third metacarpal
3	Base of fourth metacarpal
4	Hamate
5	Capitate
6	Trapezoid
7	Trapezium
8	Scaphoid
9	Lunate
10	Triquetral
11	Articular disc
12	Head of ulna
13	Sacciform recess of distal radio-ulnar joint
14	Lower end of radius

C Cross section of the right wrist joint, from below

The section, seen as when looking towards the elbow, is at the level of the scaphoid (14) and pisiform (9), and shows the flexor retinaculum (2) and the structures deep to it (in the carpal tunnel), in particular the median nerve (4)

1	Flexor carpi radialis
2	Flexor retinaculum
3	Flexor pollicis longus
4	Median nerve
5	Flexor digitorum superficialis
6	Flexor digitorum profundus
7	Ulnar artery
8	Ulnar nerve
9	Pisiform
10	Triquetral
11	Extensor carpi ulnaris
12	Extensor digiti minimi
13	Lunate with surface for capitate
14	Scaphoid with surface for capitate
15	Extensor digitorum
16	Extensor indicis
17	Extensor carpi radialis brevis
18	Extensor pollicis longus
19	Radial nerve
20	Cephalic vein
21	Extensor carpi radialis longus
22	Radial artery
23	Extensor pollicis brevis
24	Abductor pollicis longus

D

PALMAR

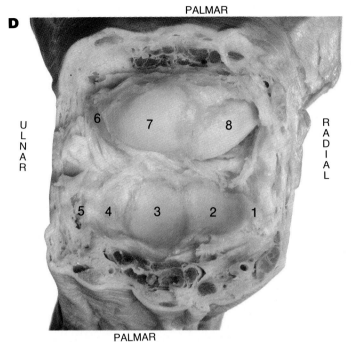

PALMAR

E

DORSAL

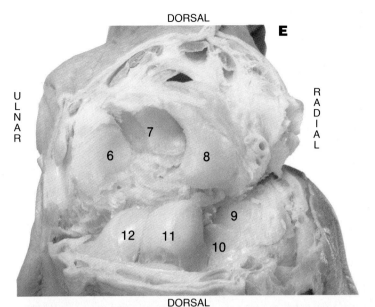

DORSAL

F

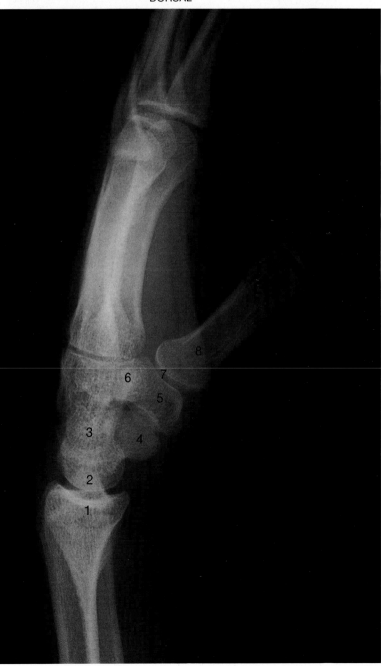

Right wrist and midcarpal joints, D wrist joint, opened up in forced extension, E midcarpal joint, opened up in forced flexion

Both joints have been opened up (far beyond the normal range of movement) in order to demonstrate the bones of the joint surfaces. The wrist joint in A has been forced open in extension, since extension takes place mostly at this joint, and the midcarpal joint in B has been forced open in flexion, since flexion takes place mostly at this joint. The proximal (wrist joint) surfaces of the scaphoid (8), lunate (7) and triquetral (6) are seen in D, and their distal (midcarpal joint) surfaces in E

1	Styloid process of radius
2	Surface on radius for scaphoid
3	Surface on radius for lunate
4	Articular disc
5	Styloid process of ulna
6	Triquetral
7	Lunate
8	Scaphoid
9	Trapezium
10	Trapezoid
11	Capitate
12	Hamate

F Radiograph of the wrist and hand, lateral view

In this side view there is much superimposition of bones, but the carpometacarpal joint of the thumb (7) between the base of the first metacarpal (8) and the trapezium (5) is clearly defined, and so is the proximal end of the lunate (2) at its articulation with the lower end of the radius (1)

1	Lower end of radius
2	Lunate
3	Capitate
4	Pisiform
5	Trapezium
6	Hook of hamate
7	Carpometacarpal joint of thumb
8	First metacarpal

A

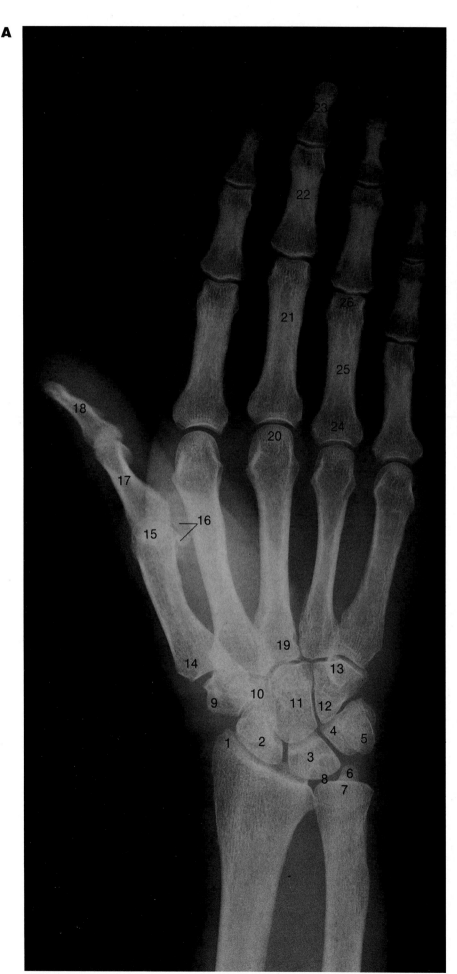

B

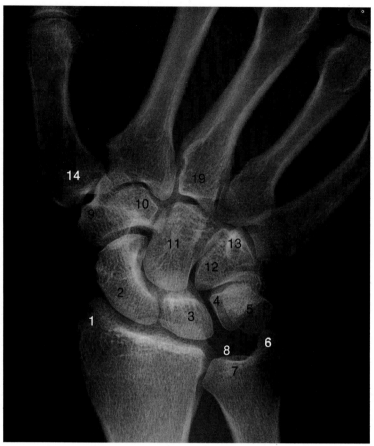

Radiographs of the left wrist and hand, **A** in the anatomical position, **B** in adduction (ulnar deviation)

Compare the position of the scaphoid (2), lunate (3) and the triquetral (4) in relation to the lower end of the radius (1) in A and B

1	Styloid process at lower end of radius
2	Scaphoid
3	Lunate
4	Triquetral
5	Pisiform
6	Styloid process of ulna
7	Head of ulna
8	Position of articular disc of distal radio-ulnar joint
9	Trapezium
10	Trapezoid
11	Capitate
12	Hamate
13	Hook of hamate
14	Base ⎫
15	Head ⎬ of first metacarpal
16	Sesamoid bones in flexor pollicis brevis and adductor pollicis tendons
17	Proximal phalanx ⎫
18	Distal phalanx ⎬ of thumb
19	Base ⎫
20	Head ⎬ of third metacarpal
21	Proximal ⎫
22	Middle ⎬ phalanx of middle finger
23	Distal ⎭
24	Base ⎫
25	Shaft ⎬ of phalanx
26	Head ⎭

● The wrist (radiocarpal) joint is the joint between the lower end of the radius (1) and articular disc (8) of the distal radio-ulnar joint proximally, and the scaphoid (2), lunate (3) and triquetral (4) distally.

● In the normal position the lunate (A3) articulates with the radius and the articular disc, but in adduction (B) it moves completely on to the radius. In extreme adduction part of the triquetral may also make contact with the radius.

Thorax

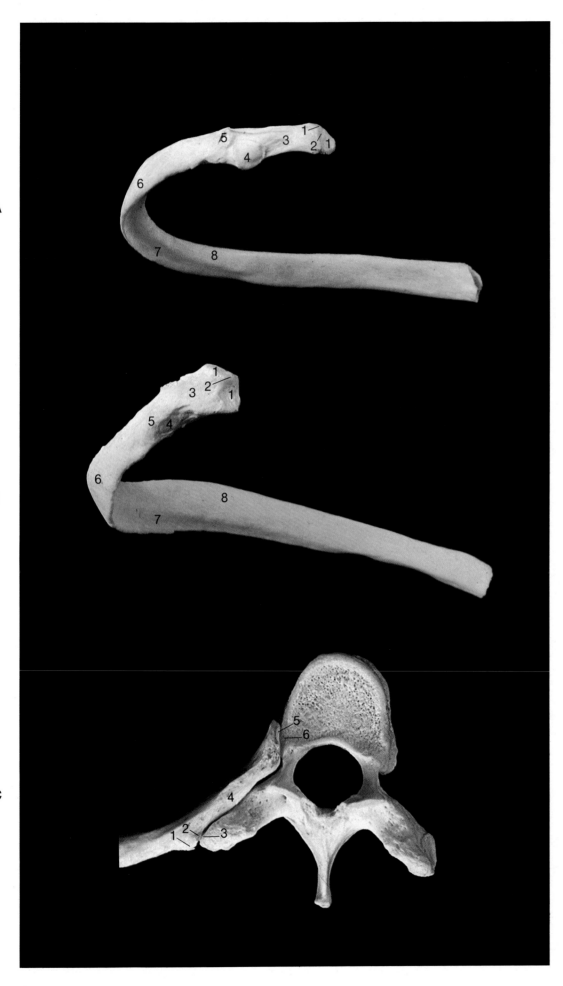

Typical ribs, from behind, A the left fifth rib (a typical upper rib), B the left seventh rib (a typical lower rib)

1	Articular facets of head
2	Crest of head
3	Neck
4	Articular facet of tubercle
5	Non-articular part of tubercle
6	Angle
7	Costal groove
8	Shaft

● The typical ribs are the third to the ninth.
● Typical ribs have a head with two facets (1), and a tubercle with articular and non-articular parts (4 and 5) at the junction of the neck (3) and shaft. The shaft has external and internal surfaces, an angle (6) and a costal groove (7).
● In typical upper ribs the articular facet of the tubercle is curved (A4) but becomes increasingly flattened in lower ribs (B4).

C Typical rib and vertebra articulated, from above

1	Non-articular ⎫ part of tubercle
2	Articular ⎭
3	Articular facet of transverse process
4	Neck of rib
5	Upper costal facet of head of rib
6	Upper costal facet of vertebral body

● The lower of the two facets on the head of a typical rib articulates with the upper costal facet (6) on the vertebral body having the same number as the rib. The upper facet on the head of the rib (5) articulates with the vertebral body above. These form the joints of the heads of the ribs.
● The articular facet of the tubercle of a rib (C2) articulates with the costal facet of the transverse process of a vertebra. These are the costotransverse joints.
● The joints of the heads of the ribs and the costotransverse joints collectively form the costovertebral joints.

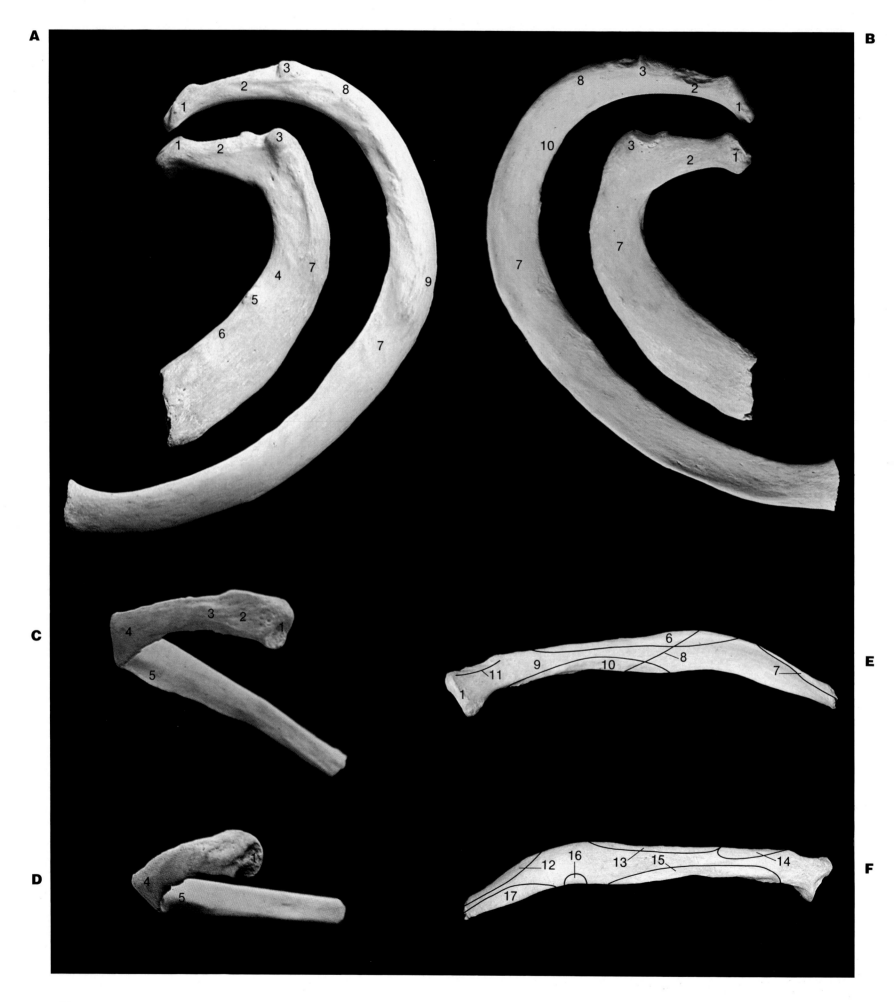

G   **H**

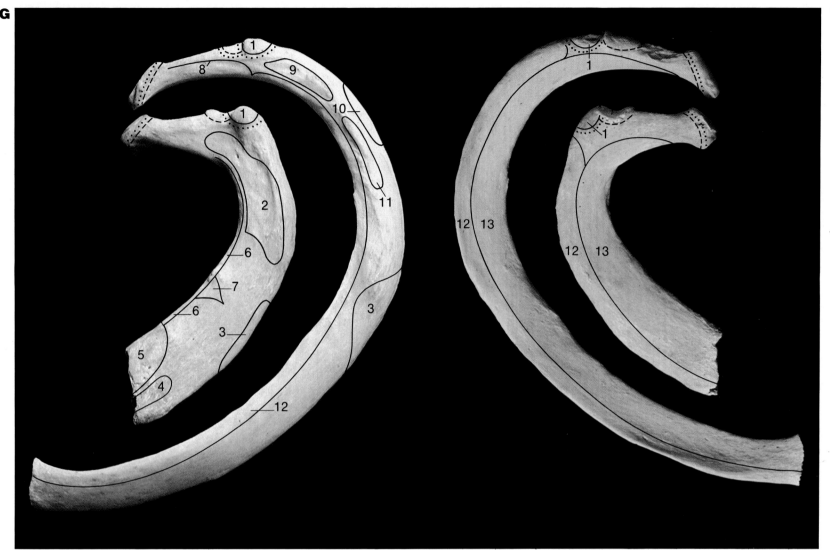

Left first rib (inner) and second rib (outer), A from above, B from below

1	Head
2	Neck
3	Tubercle
4	Groove for subclavian artery and first thoracic nerve
5	Scalene tubercle
6	Groove for subclavian vein
7	Shaft
8	Angle
9	Serratus anterior tuberosity
10	Costal groove

● The second rib gives origin to part of the first, and the whole of the second, digitation of serratus anterior.
● The atypical ribs are the first, second, tenth, eleventh and twelfth.
● The first rib has a head with one facet (A1), a prominent tubercle (A3), no angle and no costal groove. The shaft has superior and inferior surfaces.
● The second rib has a head with two facets (B1), an angle (B8) near the tubercle (B3), a broad costal groove (B10) posteriorly, and an external surface facing upwards and outwards with the inner surface facing correspondingly downwards and inwards.
● The tenth rib has a head with one or two facets (C1), a tubercle with or without an articular facet (C3), and a costal groove (C5).

Atypical left lower ribs, C tenth rib from behind, D eleventh rib from behind, E twelfth rib from the front, with attachments, F twelfth rib from behind, with attachments

1	Head
2	Neck
3	Tubercle
4	Angle
5	Costal groove
6	Internal intercostal
7	Diaphragm
8	Line of pleural reflexion
9	Area covered by pleura
10	Quadratus lumborum
11	Costotransverse ligament
12	Latissimus dorsi
13	External intercostal
14	Levator costae
15	Erector spinae
16	Serratus posterior inferior
17	External oblique

● The eleventh rib has a head with one facet (D1), no tubercle but there is an angle (D4) and a slight costal groove (D5).
● The twelfth rib has a head with one facet (E1) but there is no tubercle, no angle and no costal groove. The shaft tapers at its end (the ends of all other ribs widen slightly).

Left first rib (inner) and second rib (outer), G from above, H from below. Attachments

Dotted lines = epiphysial lines; interrupted lines = capsule attachments of costovertebral joints

1	Lateral costotransverse ligament
2	Scalenus medius
3	Serratus anterior
4	Subclavius
5	Costoclavicular ligament
6	Suprapleural membrane
7	Scalenus anterior
8	Superior costotransverse ligament
9	Levator costae
10	Serratus posterior superior
11	Scalenus posterior
12	Intercostal muscles and membranes
13	Area covered by pleura

149

A **B** **C** **D**

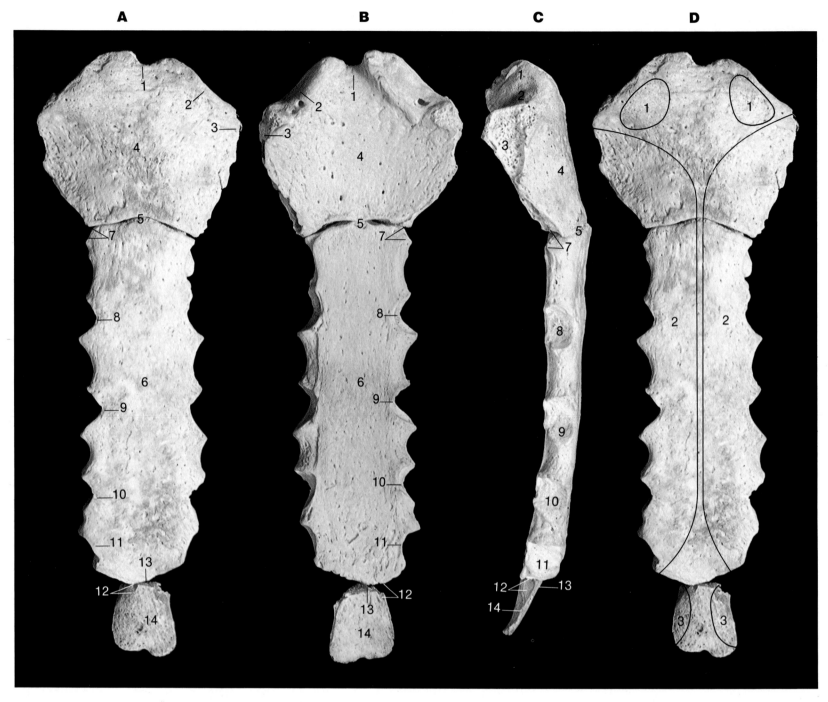

The sternum, A from the front, B from behind, C from the right

1	Jugular notch
2	Clavicular notch
3	Notch for first costal cartilage
4	Manubrium
5	Sternal angle and manubriosternal joint
6	Body
7	Notches for second
8	Notch for third
9	Notch for fourth
10	Notch for fifth	costal cartilage
11	Notch for sixth
12	Notches for seventh
13	Xiphisternal joint
14	Xiphoid process

• The sternum consists of the manubrium (4), body (6) and xiphoid process (14).

• The body of the sternum (6) is formed by the fusion of four sternebrae, the sites of the fusion sometimes being indicated by three slight transverse ridges.

• The manubrium (4) and body (6) are bony but the xiphoid process (14), which varies considerably in size and shape, is cartilaginous although it frequently shows some degree of ossification.

• The manubriosternal and xiphisternal joints (5 and 13) are both symphyses, the surfaces being covered by hyaline cartilage and united by a fibrocartilaginous disc.

The sternum, D from the front, E from behind. Attachments

1	Sternocleidomastoid
2	Pectoralis major
3	Rectus abdominis
4	Sternohyoid
5	Sternothyroid
6	Area covered by right pleura
7	Area covered by left pleura
8	Area in contact with pericardium
9	Transverse thoracic
10	Diaphragm

• The two pleural sacs are in contact from the levels of the second to fourth costal cartilages.

E

F

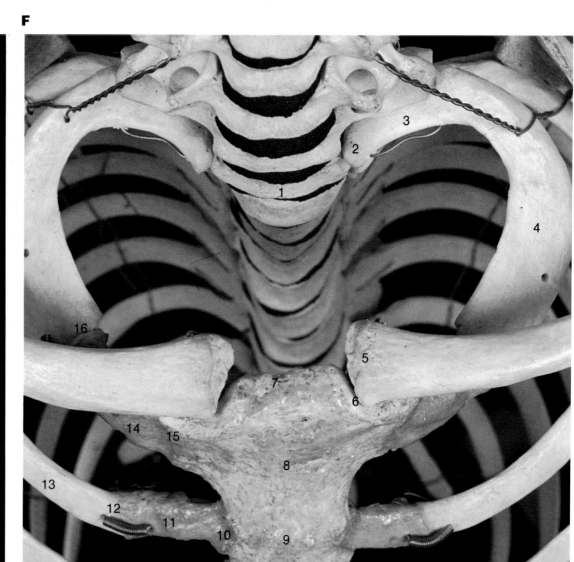

F Thoracic inlet, from above and in front, in an articulated skeleton

- The thoracic inlet (upper aperture of the thorax) is approximately the same size and shape as the outline of the kidney, and is bounded by the first thoracic vertebra (1), first ribs (4), and costal cartilages (14), and the upper border of the manubrium of the sternum (jugular notch, 7). It does not lie in a horizontal plane but slopes downwards and forwards.
- The second costal cartilage (11) joins the manubrium and body of the sternum (10) at the level of the manubriosternal joint (9). This is an important landmark, since the joint line is palpable as a ridge at the slight angle between the manubrium and body, and the second costal cartilage and rib can be identified lateral to it. Other ribs can be identified by counting down from the second; the first costal cartilage and the end of the first rib are under cover of the clavicle and not easily felt.

1	First thoracic vertebra
2	Head ⎫
3	Neck ⎬ of first rib
4	Shaft ⎭
5	Sternal end of clavicle
6	Sternoclavicular joint
7	Jugular notch
8	Manubrium of sternum
9	Manubriosternal joint (angle of Louis)
10	Second sternocostal joint
11	Second costal cartilage
12	Costochondral joint
13	Second rib
14	First costal cartilage
15	First sternocostal joint
16	First costochondral joint

A Surface markings of the heart, left pleura and lung, in the female

Interrupted line = heart; dotted line = pleura

The positions of the four heart valves are indicated by ellipses, and the sites where the sounds of the corresponding valves are best heard with the stethoscope are indicated by the circles

1	Jugular notch
2	Sternocleidomastoid
3	Sternoclavicular joint
4	Midpoint of clavicle
5	Acromioclavicular joint
6	Axillary tail
7	Areola
8	Nipple
9	Areolar gland
10	Costal margin (at eighth costal cartilage)
11	Apex of heart
12	Xiphisternal joint
13	Sixth
14	Fourth
15	Third
16	Second
17	Manubriosternal joint
18	Pulmonary
19	Aortic
20	Mitral
21	Tricuspid

(6–9) of breast
(13–16) costal cartilage
(18–21) valve

● The manubriosternal joint (17) is palpable and a guide to identifying the second costal cartilage (16) which joins the sternum at this level (see page 151, 9 to 11).

● The pleura and lung extend into the neck for 2.5 cm above the medial third of the clavicle.

● In the midclavicular line the lower limit of the *pleura* reaches the eighth costal cartilage, in the midaxillary line it reaches the tenth rib, and at the lateral border of the erector spinae muscle it crosses the twelfth rib. The lower border of the *lung* is about two ribs higher than the pleural reflexion.

● Behind the sternum the pleural sacs are adjacent to one another in the midline from the level of the second to fourth costal cartilages, but then diverge due to the mass of the heart on the left.

● The four heart valves are approximately in or just to the left of the midline—pulmonary, aortic, mitral, tricuspid in that order from above downwards (18 to 21).

● Because of the overlying bone and cartilage and the direction of blood flow, the sites where the sounds of the valves closing are best heard are not usually over the valves themselves, except for the tricuspid valve (21). For pulmonary valve (18) sounds, the stethoscope is placed over the second left intercostal space at the costal margin (below 16), for the aortic valve (19) over the second right interspace (above 15), and for the mitral valve (20) near the apex of the heart (11).

● For a radiograph of the chest and heart see pages 198 to 199.

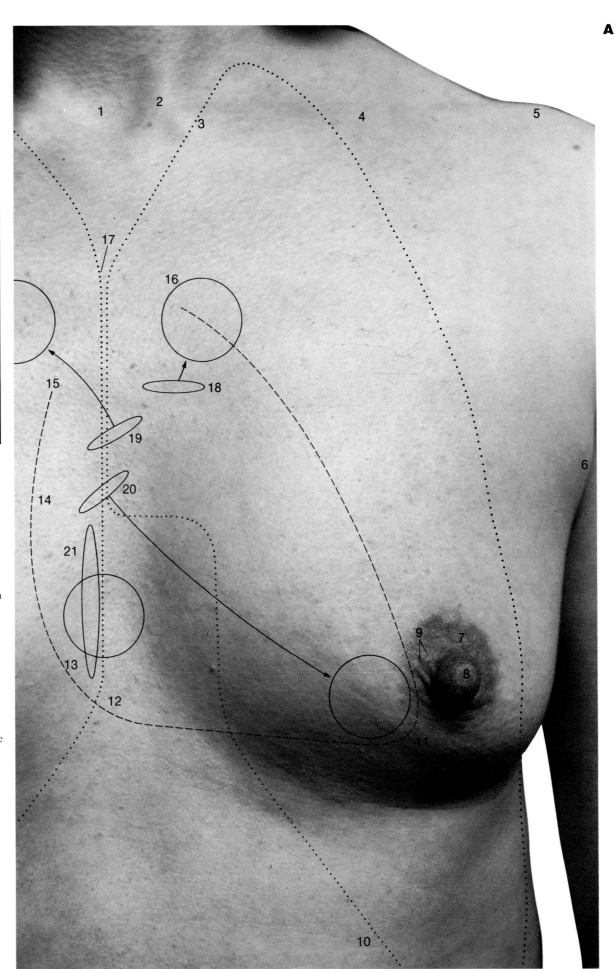

A

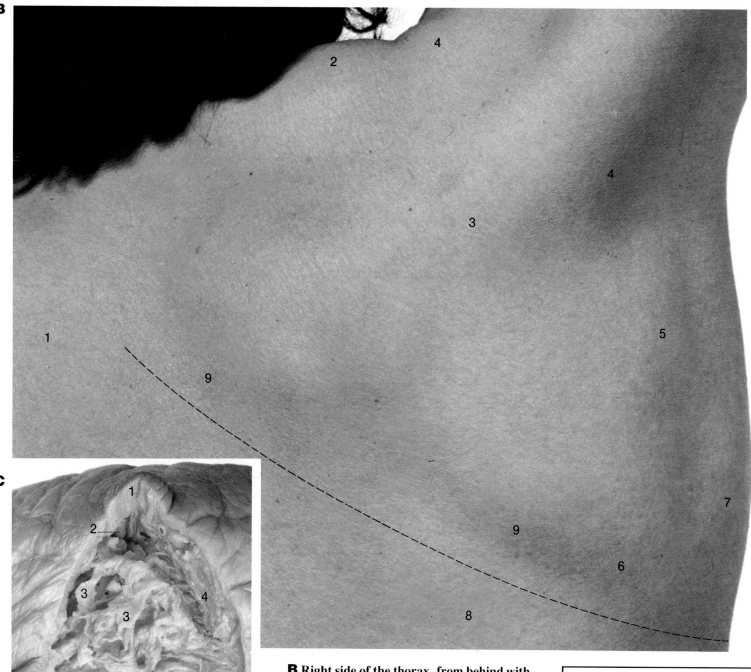

B

C

C Female breast (mammary gland)

Fat has been dissected away to show the irregular fibrous tissue septa which pass from the overlying skin to the underlying fascia over pectoralis major. The glandular elements lie among the fat and end in lactiferous ducts which have a dilated ampulla (2) before opening on to the surface of the nipple

1	Nipple
2	Ampulla of lactiferous duct
3	Fibrous septum
4	Fat
5	Fascia over pectoralis major

B Right side of the thorax, from behind with the arm abducted

With the arm fully abducted, the medial (vertebral) border of the scapula (9) comes to lie at an angle of about 60° to the vertical, and indicates approximately the line of the oblique fissure of the lung (interrupted line)

• Lymph from the lateral part of the breast drains mainly to axillary lymph nodes, and that from the medial part to internal thoracic nodes, but there is no rigid division between these patterns of lymph flow, especially when channels become affected by disease, and lymph from any part may reach either group of nodes, as well as crossing to the opposite breast and passing down to the abdominal wall.

1	Spinous process of third thoracic vertebra
2	Trapezius
3	Spine of scapula
4	Deltoid
5	Teres major
6	Inferior angle of scapula
7	Latissimus dorsi
8	Fifth intercostal space
9	Medial border of scapula

• The line of the oblique fissure of the lung runs from the level of the spine of the third thoracic vertebra (1) to the sixth costal cartilage at the lateral border of the sternum (see page 154). With the arm fully abducted the vertebral border of the scapula (9) is a good guide to the direction of this fissure.

A

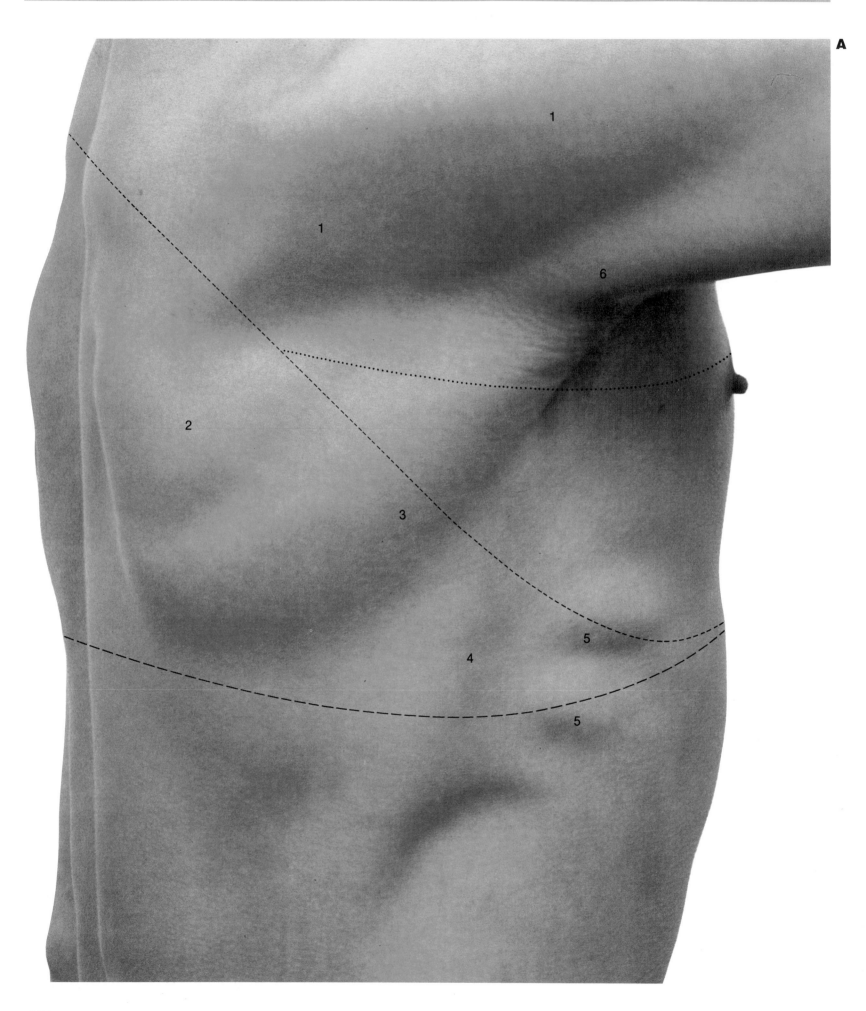

A Right side of the thorax, from the right

The arm is flexed at the shoulder joint. The transverse fissure of the right lung is indicated by the dotted line, the oblique fissure by the short interrupted line, and the lower border by the long interrupted line. Some digitations of serratus anterior are prominent (as at 5) on the chest wall, and there are also contours produced by the lower part of latissimus dorsi (4), by teres major (3), and infraspinatus (2). On the arm, deltoid (1) envelops the shoulder region, and the long head of triceps (6) forms the posterior margin of the arm

1	Deltoid
2	Infraspinatus
3	Teres major
4	Latissimus dorsi
5	Serratus anterior
6	Long head of triceps

• The transverse fissure of the right lung is represented by a line drawn horizontally backwards from the fourth costal cartilage until it meets the line of the oblique fissure (described on page 153) running forwards to the sixth costal cartilage. The triangle so outlined indicates the middle lobe of the lung, with the superior lobe above it and the inferior lobe below and behind it.
• On the left side where the lung has only two lobes, superior and inferior, there is no transverse fissure; the surface marking for the oblique fissure is similar to that on the right.

B Muscles of the thorax. Left external and internal intercostal muscles, from the front

Pectoral and abdominal muscles have been removed, together with all vessels and nerves and the anterior intercostal membranes, to show the external and internal intercostal muscles (as at 4 and 5)

1	Sternal angle
2	Second costal cartilage
3	Second rib
4	External intercostal
5	Internal intercostal
6	Xiphoid process
7	Seventh ⎫
8	Eighth ⎬ costal cartilage
9	Ninth ⎪
10	Tenth ⎭

• The fibres of the external intercostal muscles (4) run downwards and medially, and near the costochondral junctions (as between 2 and 3) give place to the anterior intercostal membrane (here removed); these are thin sheets of connective tissue through which the underlying internal intercostal muscles (5) can be seen.
• The fibres of the internal intercostal muscles (5) run downwards and laterally. At the front they are covered by the anterior intercostal membranes, and at the back of the thorax they give place to the posterior intercostal membranes. The different directions of the muscle fibres enable the two muscle groups to be distinguished—down and medially for the externals (4), down and laterally for the internals (5).
• The seventh costal cartilage (7) is the lowest to join the sternum and together with the eighth, ninth and tenth cartilages (8 to 10) forms the costal margin.

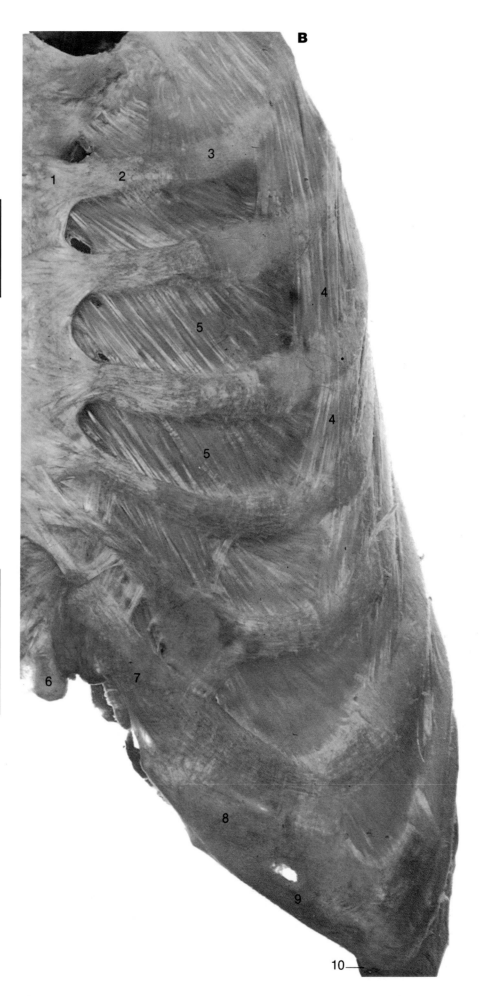

Muscles of the thorax. Right intercostal muscles, A from the outside, B from the inside

In A each intercostal space has been dissected to a different depth, showing from above downwards an external intercostal muscle (2), internal intercostal (4), innermost intercostal (7) and pleura (9). The main intercostal vessels and nerve lie between the internal and innermost muscles; the nerve (6) is seen in the sixth interspace immediately below the sixth rib (5) and lying on the outer surface of the innermost intercostal (7), but the artery and vein are under cover of the costal groove. The vessels as well as the nerve are seen in the fifth intercostal space when this is dissected from the inside of the thorax, as in B; here the pleura and innermost intercostal muscle have been removed, and the vessels (11 and 12) and fifth intercostal nerve (13) lie against the inner surface of the internal intercostal (4)

1	Fourth rib
2	External intercostal
3	Fifth rib
4	Internal intercostal
5	Sixth rib
6	Sixth intercostal nerve
7	Innermost intercostal
8	Seventh rib
9	Pleura
10	Eighth rib
11	Fifth posterior intercostal vein
12	Fifth posterior intercostal artery
13	Fifth intercostal nerve

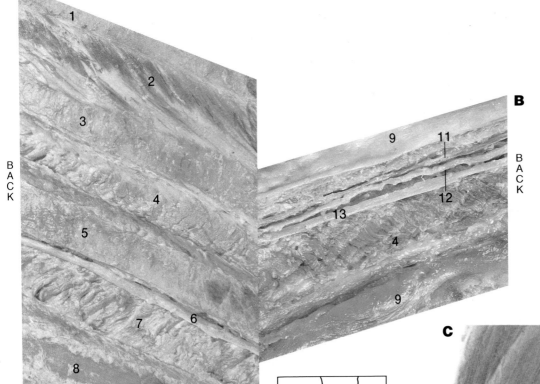

C Muscles of the thorax. Levator costae muscles, left side, from behind

The left erector spinae and latissimus dorsi have been removed from the left side of the vertebral column and adjacent ribs to show the levator costae muscles (as at 3) and the medial ends of the external intercostals (as at 2)

1	Seventh rib
2	External intercostal
3	Levator costae
4	Lateral costotransverse ligament
5	Transverse process of eighth thoracic vertebra
6	Lamina of eighth thoracic vertebra
7	Tubercle of ninth rib
8	Angle of ninth rib

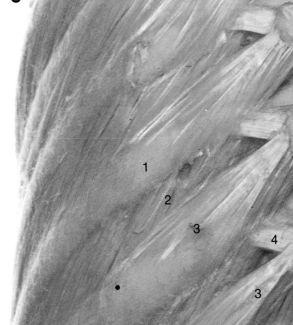

● Each levator costae muscle (as at C3) passes from the tip of the transverse process of one vertebra (as at C5) to the rib below between the tubercle (C7) and angle (C8).
● The internal intercostal muscles are continuous posteriorly with the posterior intercostal membranes which are covered up by the medial ends of the external intercostals (as at C2).

D

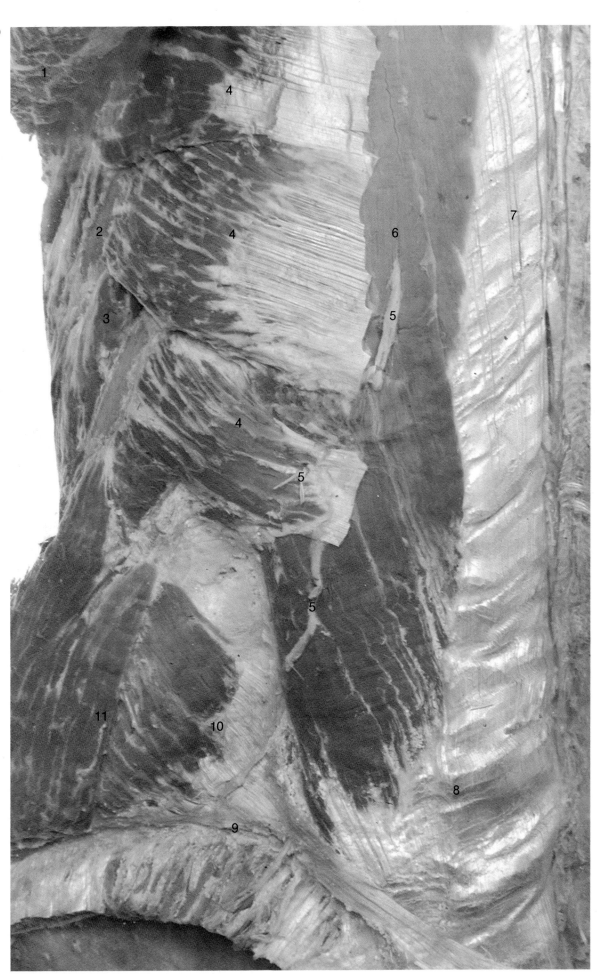

In this view of the lower left thorax and
lumbar region from behind, latissimus
dorsi has been removed to display
serratus posterior inferior (4), part of
whose aponeurotic origin from vertebral
spines has also been removed to uncover
part of erector spinae (6, 7 and 8) (which
belongs to the vertebral column group of
muscles—pages 87 and 88)

1	Latissimus dorsi
2	Tenth rib
3	External intercostal
4	Serratus posterior inferior
5	Dorsal rami of lower thoracic and
	upper lumbar nerves
6	Longissimus part of erector spinae
7	Spinalis part of erector spinae
8	Erector spinae
9	Iliac crest
10	Internal oblique
11	Posterior (free) border of external
	oblique

● The medial part of serratus posterior *inferior*
(4) (arising from the last two thoracic and
upper two lumbar spinous processes and the
supraspinous ligament, and blending with the
underlying lumbar part of the thoracolumbar
fascia) has been removed, so displaying the
medial and intermediate parts of erector
spinae (6 and 7) which belongs to the muscles
of the vertebral column (page 88). The lateral
(iliocostalis) part of erector spinae is under
cover of the lateral part of the serratus muscle,
which becomes attached to the lower four ribs
lateral to their angles.

● The serratus posterior *superior* muscle (not
illustrated) passes to the second to fifth ribs
lateral to their angles, under cover of the
rhomboid muscles (page 112), having arisen
from the lower part of the ligamentum nuchae
and the spinous processes of the seventh
cervical and upper two or three thoracic
vertebrae and the supraspinous ligament.

● On each side there is one serratus *anterior*
muscle (belonging to the group connecting the
upper limb to the trunk) and two serratus
posterior muscles (belonging to the muscles of
the thorax).

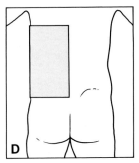

A

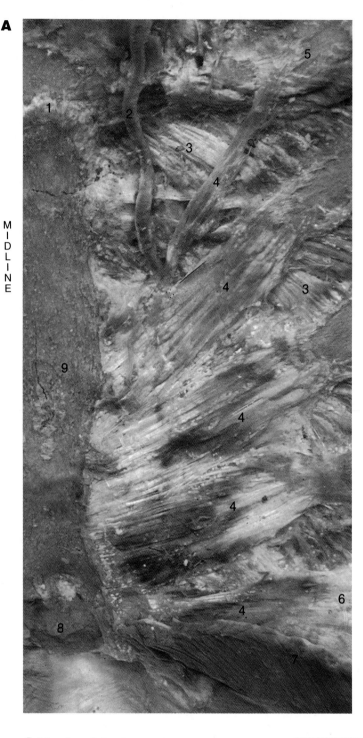

B

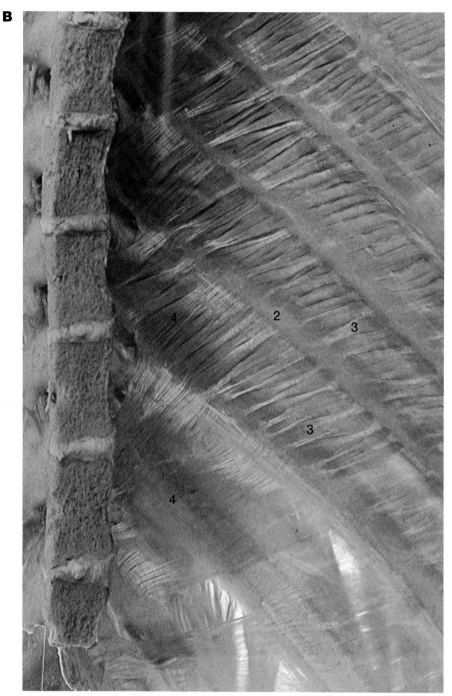

A Muscles of the thorax. Right transversus thoracis, from behind

This view of the internal surface of the thoracic wall shows the posterior surface of the right half of the sternum and adjacent wall, with the pleura removed. The internal thoracic artery (2) is seen passing deep to the slips of transversus thoracis (4, previously called sternocostalis)

● Transversus thoracis (A4) is in the same plane as the innermost intercostal muscles at the lateral side of the thoracic wall (B3) and the subcostal muscles on the posterior part (B4).

● The subcostal muscles (B4) span more than one rib. They and the innermost intercostals (B3, intercostales intimi) are often poorly developed or absent in the upper part of the thorax.

1	Sternal angle
2	Internal thoracic artery
3	Internal intercostal
4	Slips of transversus thoracis muscle
5	Second rib
6	Sixth rib
7	Diaphragm
8	Xiphoid process
9	Body of sternum

B Muscles of the thorax. Left lower subcostal and innermost intercostal muscles

This view of the lower left hemithorax is seen from the right and in front, with vertebral bodies (as at 1) sectioned and the pleura, vessels and nerves removed, and shows part of the innermost layer of thoracic wall muscles (3 and 4)

1	Eighth thoracic vertebra
2	Eighth rib
3	Innermost intercostal
4	Subcostal

RIGHT

LEFT

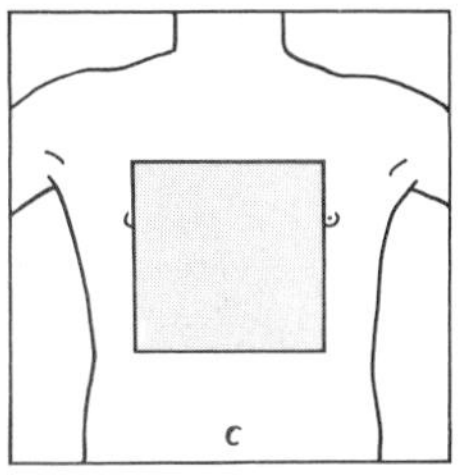

Lungs and pericardium, from the front

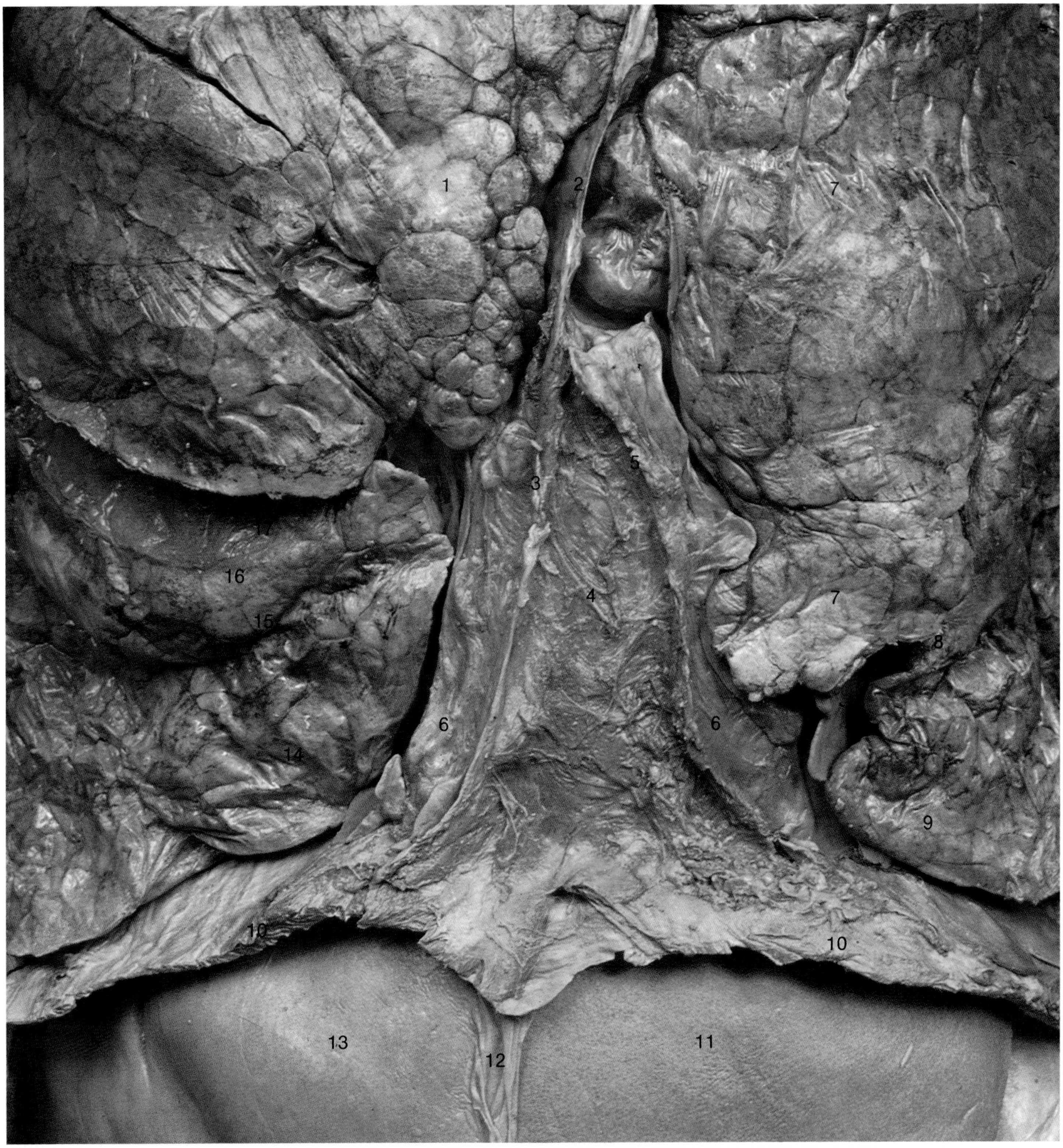

The anterior thoracic and abdominal walls have been removed. The cut edges of the two pleural sacs are seen lying adjacent to one another (2), but lower down over the front of the pericardium (4) they become separated (3 and 5)

• The pleurae become separated at the level of the fourth costal cartilage (junction of 2, 3 and 5) due to the leftward bulge of the heart, and the central part of the fibrous pericardium (4) is not covered by pleura.

1 Superior lobe of right lung	10 Diaphragm
2 Right and left parietal pleurae in contact	11 Left lobe of liver
3 Line of reflexion of right pleura	12 Falciform ligament
4 Fibrous pericardium	13 Right lobe of liver
5 Line of reflexion of left pleura	14 Inferior lobe } of right lung
6 Pleura overlying pericardium	15 Oblique fissure } of right lung
7 Superior lobe of left lung	16 Middle lobe } of right lung
8 Oblique fissure	17 Transverse fissure } of right lung
9 Inferior lobe of left lung	

A

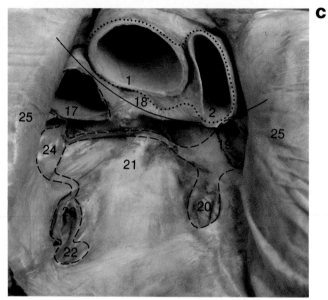

B

C

Heart and pericardium, **A** from the front, **B** with marker in the transverse sinus, **C** oblique sinus after removal of the heart

In A the pericardium has been incised and turned back (3) to display the anterior surface of the heart. The pulmonary trunk (2) leaves the right ventricle (9) in front and to the left of the ascending aorta (1) which is overlapped by the auricle (16) of the right atrium (15). The superior vena cava (17) is to the right of the aorta and still largely covered by pericardium. The anterior interventricular branch (6) of the left coronary artery and the great cardiac vein (7) lie in the interventricular groove between the right and left ventricles (9 and 5), and the right coronary artery (13) is in the atrioventricular groove between the right ventricle (9) and right atrium (15). In B only the upper part of another heart is shown, with a marker in the transverse sinus, the space behind the aorta (1) and pulmonary trunk (2). In C the heart has been removed from the pericardium, leaving the orifices of the great vessels. The dotted line indicates the attachment of the single sleeve of serous pericardium surrounding the aorta (1) and pulmonary trunk (2). The interrupted line indicates the attachment of another more complicated but still single sleeve of serous pericardium surrounding all the other six great vessels (the four pulmonary veins, 19, 20, 23 and 24, and the superior and inferior venae cavae, 17 and 22). The narrow interval between the two sleeves is the transverse sinus; the solid line in C indicates the path of the marker in B. The area of the pericardium (21) between the pulmonary veins

and limited above by the reflexion of the serous pericardium on to the back of the heart is the oblique sinus

1	Ascending aorta
2	Pulmonary trunk
3	Serous pericardium overlying fibrous pericardium (turned laterally)
4	Auricle of left atrium
5	Left ventricle
6	Anterior interventricular branch of left coronary artery
7	Great cardiac vein
8	Diaphragm
9	Right ventricle
10	Marginal branch of right coronary artery
11	Small cardiac vein
12	Pericardium fused with tendon of diaphragm
13	Right coronary artery
14	Anterior cardiac vein
15	Right atrium
16	Auricle of right atrium
17	Superior vena cava
18	Marker in transverse sinus
19	Left superior pulmonary vein
20	Left inferior pulmonary vein
21	Posterior wall of pericardial cavity and oblique sinus
22	Inferior vena cava
23	Right inferior pulmonary vein
24	Right superior pulmonary vein
25	Pericardium turned laterally over lung

● The right border of the heart is formed by the right atrium (A15).
● The left border is formed mostly by the left ventricle (A5) with at the top the uppermost part (infundibulum) of the right ventricle (A9) and the tip of the left auricle (A4).
● The inferior border is formed by the right ventricle (A9) with a small part of the left ventricle at the apex (D9).

D

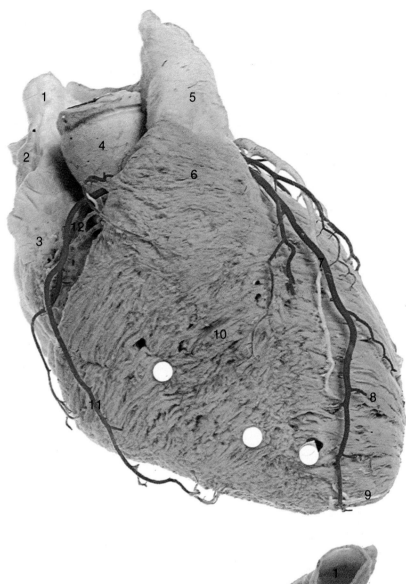

D Heart, from the front, with blood vessels injected

The coronary arteries have been injected with red latex and the cardiac veins with gray latex. The pulmonary trunk (5) passes upwards from the infundibulum (6) of the right ventricle (10), and at its commencement it is just in front and to the left of the ascending aorta (4)

1	Superior vena cava
2	Right atrium
3	Auricle of right atrium (displaced laterally)
4	Ascending aorta
5	Pulmonary trunk
6	Infundibulum of right ventricle
7	Anterior interventricular branch of left coronary artery and great cardiac vein in interventricular groove
8	Left ventricle
9	Apex
10	Right ventricle
11	Marginal branch of right coronary artery
12	Right coronary artery in anterior atrioventricular groove

● The *sternocostal* surface of the heart is the *anterior* surface (as seen in A and D) formed mainly by the right ventricle (A9, D10), with parts of the left ventricle (A5, D8) and right atrium (A15 and D2).
● The *apex* of the heart (D9) is formed by the left ventricle.
● The infundibulum (D6) is the part of the right ventricle (D10) from which the pulmonary trunk arises (D5).
● In D the anterior atrioventricular groove has been opened up by displacing the auricle (D3) of the right atrium to show the right coronary artery (D12) more clearly. The marginal branch (11) of this vessel has an unusually high origin.
● The *base* of the heart is the *posterior* surface, formed mainly by the left atrium (E5) with a small part of the right atrium (E7).
● The *inferior* surface is the *diaphragmatic* surface, formed by the two ventricles (mainly the left) (E15 and 14).
● In E there is a large ventricular branch of the left coronary artery passing superficial to the great cardiac vein (E17).

E

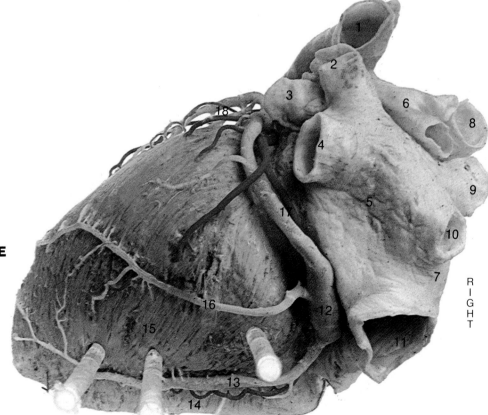

E Heart, from behind, with blood vessels injected

This posterior view of the same specimen as in D shows the coronary sinus (12) in the posterior atrioventricular groove and three large tributaries entering it—the great cardiac vein (17), the posterior vein of the left ventricle (16) and the middle cardiac vein (13). The four pulmonary veins (2, 4, 9 and 10) enter the left atrium (5)

1	Left pulmonary artery
2	Superior left pulmonary vein
3	Auricle of left atrium
4	Inferior left pulmonary vein
5	Left atrium
6	Right pulmonary artery
7	Right atrium
8	Superior vena cava
9	Superior right pulmonary vein
10	Inferior right pulmonary vein
11	Inferior vena cava
12	Coronary sinus in posterior atrioventricular groove
13	Middle cardiac vein and posterior interventricular branch of right coronary artery in posterior interventricular groove
14	Right ventricle
15	Left ventricle
16	Posterior vein of left ventricle
17	Great cardiac vein and circumflex branch of left coronary artery
18	Great cardiac vein and anterior interventricular branch of left coronary artery

161

A **Right atrium, from the front and right**

The anterior wall has been incised near its left margin and reflected to the right, showing on its internal surface the vertical crista terminalis (2) and horizontal pectinate muscles (1). The fossa ovalis (11) is on the interatrial septum, and the opening of the coronary sinus (7) is to the left of the inferior vena caval opening (10)

1	Pectinate muscles	8	Valve of coronary sinus
2	Crista terminalis	9	Valve of inferior vena cava
3	Superior vena cava		cava
4	Auricle	10	Inferior vena cava
5	Tricuspid valve	11	Fossa ovalis
6	Position of	12	Limbus
	atrioventricular node	13	Position of intervenous
7	Coronary sinus		tubercle

● The intervenous tubercle, which is rarely detectable in the human heart(13), may have served in the embryo to direct blood from the superior vena cava towards the tricuspid orifice.
● The fossa ovalis (11) forms part of the interatrial septum, and is part of the embryonic primary septum.
● The limbus (12), which forms the margin of the fossa ovalis (11), represents the lower margin of the embryonic secondary septum. Before the primary and secondary septa fuse (at birth), the gap between them forms the foramen ovale.
● The sinuatrial node (SA node, not illustrated) is embedded in the anterior wall of the atrium at the upper end of the crista terminalis, just below the opening of the superior vena cava.
● The atrioventricular node (AV node, 6) is embedded in the interatrial septum, just above and to the left of the opening of the coronary sinus (7).

B **Right ventricle, from the front**

Most of the anterior wall has been removed, but the part to which the anterior papillary muscle (5) is attached remains. The septomarginal trabecula (4) joins the anterior papillary muscle (5), and the anterior cusp of the tricuspid valve (7) largely obscures the other cusps (they are shown in A on page 164)

1	Pulmonary trunk	7	Anterior cusp of
2	Infundibulum of right		tricuspid valve
	ventricle	8	Chordae tendineae
3	Trabeculae on	9	Ascending aorta
	interventricular septum	10	Auricle of right atrium
4	Septomarginal	11	Right atrium
	trabecula	12	Inferior vena cava
5	Anterior ⎫ papillary	13	Superior vena cava
6	Posterior ⎭ muscle		

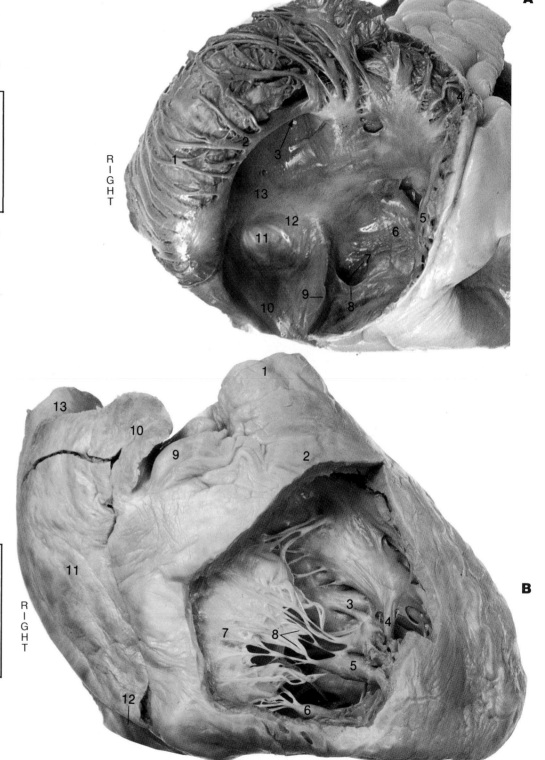

● The septomarginal trabecula (4), which conducts the right limb of the atrioventricular bundle from the interventricular septum (3) to the anterior papillary muscle (5), was formerly known as the moderator band.
● The chordae tendineae (8) connect the cusps of the tricuspid valve to the papillary muscles. The usual arrangement of the connexions is given in the following notes.
● The anterior papillary muscle (5) is large and connected to the anterior (7) and posterior cusps.
● The posterior papillary muscle (6) is small and connected to the posterior and septal cusps.
● Several small septal papillary muscles are connected to the septal and anterior cusps.
● The posterior papillary muscle (6) is so called because it is *behind* the anterior cusp (7), but it might be better named *inferior* because it is on the *floor* of the ventricle.

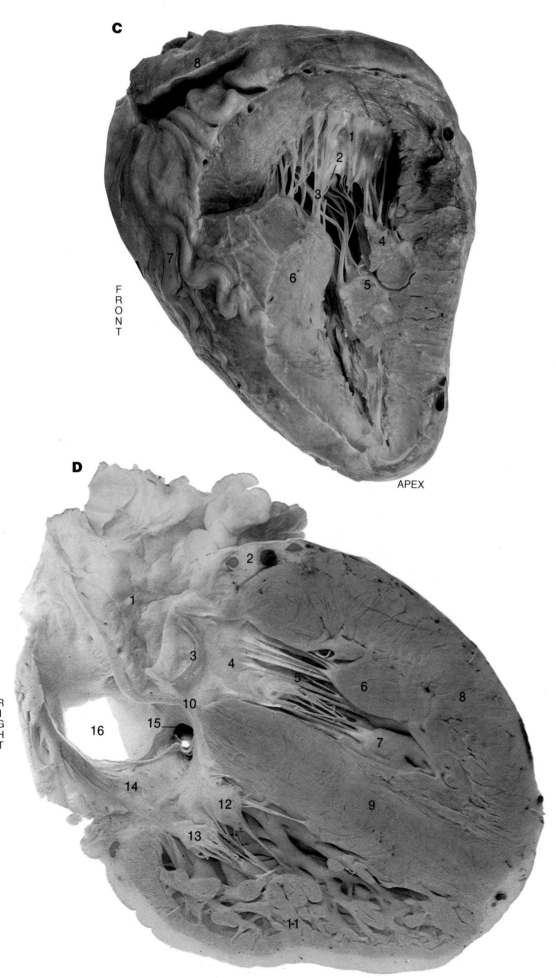

C

FRONT

APEX

D

RIGHT

C Left ventricle, from the left and below

The ventricle has been opened by removing much of the left, anterior and posterior walls, and is viewed from below, looking upwards to the under-surface of the cusps of the mitral valve (1 and 2) which are anchored to the anterior and posterior papillary muscles (4 and 5) by chordae tendineae (3). The posterior cusp (2) is largely hidden by the anterior cusp (1) in this view

1	Anterior ⎫ cusp of mitral valve
2	Posterior ⎭
3	Chordae tendineae
4	Anterior ⎫ papillary muscle
5	Posterior ⎭
6	Anterior ventricular wall
7	Anterior interventricular branch of left coronary artery
8	Auricle of left atrium

• The anterior and posterior papillary muscles (4 and 5) are both connected by chordae tendineae (3) to both valve cusps (1 and 2).

D Coronal section of the ventricles

The heart has been cut in two in the coronal plane, and this is the posterior section seen from the front, looking towards the back of both ventricles. The section has passed immediately in front of the anterior cusp of the mitral valve (4) and the posterior cusp of the aortic valve (3)

1	Ascending aorta
2	Left coronary artery branches and great cardiac vein
3	Posterior cusp of aortic valve
4	Anterior cusp of mitral valve
5	Chordae tendineae
6	Anterior papillary muscle
7	Posterior papillary muscle
8	Left ventricular wall
9	Muscular ⎫ part of interventricular septum
10	Membranous ⎭
11	Right ventricular wall
12	Septal ⎫ cusp of tricuspid valve
13	Posterior ⎭
14	Right atrium
15	Coronary sinus
16	Inferior vena cava

• The wall of the left ventricle (8) is normally three times as thick as the wall of the right ventricle (11).
• The mitral orifice (which is immediately behind the anterior cusp of the mitral valve, 4) and aortic orifice (whose posterior cusp is at 3) are adjacent to one another and separated from each other only by the anterior cusp of the mitral valve (4).

• The cusps of the aortic and pulmonary valves are here given their official names but some English texts use slightly different alternatives, as follows:

	Official	English
Aortic	Right	Anterior
	Left	Left posterior
	Posterior	Right posterior
Pulmonary	Left	Posterior
	Anterior	Left anterior
	Right	Right anterior

163

A Tricuspid valve, from the right atrium

The right atrium has been opened by incising the anterior wall (3) and turning the flap outwards so that the atrial surface of the atrioventricular orifice is seen, guarded by the three cusps of the tricuspid valve—anterior (4), posterior (5) and septal (6)

1	Superior vena cava
2	Auricle of right atrium
3	Anterior wall of right atrium
4	Anterior ⎫
5	Posterior ⎬ cusp of tricuspid valve
6	Septal ⎭
7	Interatrial septum
8	Crista terminalis
9	Pectinate muscles

● The posterior cusp (5) of the tricuspid valve is the smallest.

B Pulmonary, aortic and mitral valves, from above

The pulmonary trunk (1) and ascending aorta (5) have been cut off immediately above the three cusps of the pulmonary and aortic valves (2 to 4, 7 to 9). The upper part of the left atrium (14) has been removed to show the upper surface of the mitral valve cusps (15 and 16)

1	Pulmonary trunk
2	Left ⎫
3	Anterior ⎬ cusp of pulmonary valve
4	Right ⎭
5	Ascending aorta
6	Marker in ostium of right coronary artery
7	Right ⎫
8	Posterior ⎬ cusp of aortic valve
9	Left ⎭
10	Ostium of left coronary artery
11	Auricle of right atrium
12	Right atrium
13	Superior vena cava
14	Left atrium
15	Posterior ⎫ cusp of mitral valve
16	Anterior ⎭

C Fibrous framework of the heart

The heart is seen from the right and behind after removing both atria, looking down on to the fibrous rings (11) that surround the mitral and tricuspid orifices and form the attachments for the bases of the valve cusps. The cusps of the pulmonary valve are seen at the top of the infundibulum of the right ventricle, and the aortic valve cusps have been dissected out from the beginning of the ascending aorta

1	Left ⎫	11	Fibrous ring
2	Anterior ⎬ cusps of pulmonary valve	12	Right fibrous trigone
3	Right ⎭	13	Posterior ⎫ cusps of mitral valve
4	Infundibulum of right ventricle	14	Anterior ⎭
5	Right ⎫	15	Left fibrous trigone
6	Posterior ⎬ cusps of aortic valve		
7	Left ⎭		
8	Anterior ⎫		
9	Posterior ⎬ cusps of tricuspid valve		
10	Septal ⎭		

● The fibrous framework of the heart consists of the fibrous rings which form a figure-of-eight round the atrioventricular orifices, and which extend round the pulmonary and aortic orifices.
● The red marker is in the right fibrous trigone (12) at the junction of the mitral, tricuspid and aortic orifices; it is continuous below with the membranous part of the interventricular septum, through which the atrioventricular bundle passes.

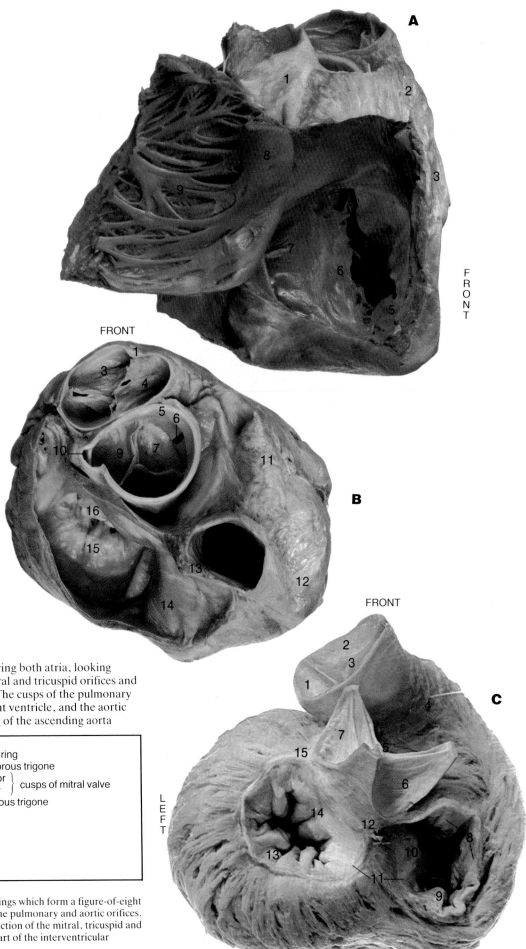

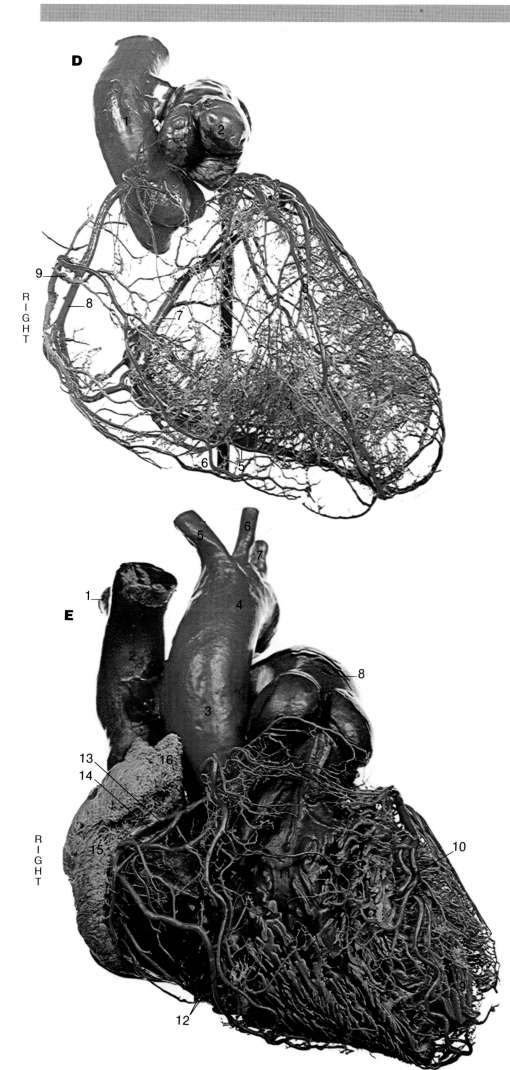

D Cast of the cardiac vessels, from the front

The aorta and coronary vessels have been injected with red resin, and the cardiac veins with blue resin. The pulmonary trunk has also been separately injected with blue resin. At the lower end of the aorta (1) and pulmonary trunk (2) note the three 'bulges' indicating the aortic and pulmonary sinuses above the aortic and pulmonary valves. The interventricular septum (4) is outlined by the many deeply penetrating branches of the anterior and posterior interventricular arteries and their accompanying veins (3 and 5)

1	Ascending aorta
2	Pulmonary trunk and sinuses above pulmonary valve cusps
3	Anterior interventricular branch of left coronary artery and great cardiac vein
4	Vessels of interventricular septum
5	Middle cardiac vein and posterior interventricular branch of right coronary artery
6	Marginal branch of right coronary artery and small cardiac vein
7	Coronary sinus
8	Right coronary artery
9	Anterior cardiac vein

E Cast of the heart and great vessels, from the front

The left ventricle (9) and the aorta (3 and 4) and its branches including the coronary vessels have been injected with red resin. The superior vena cava (2), right atrium (15), right ventricle (11) and the pulmonary trunk (8) have been injected with blue resin. In the lower part of the right ventricle (11) note the rough pattern produced by the muscular trabeculae, but the upper part of the ventricular wall (the 'outflow' part, leading to the pulmonary trunk) is smooth

1	Azygos vein
2	Superior vena cava
3	Ascending aorta
4	Arch of aorta
5	Brachiocephalic trunk
6	Left common carotid artery
7	Left subclavian artery
8	Pulmonary trunk
9	Left ventricle
10	Anterior interventricular branch of left coronary artery and great cardiac vein
11	Right ventricle
12	Marginal branch of right coronary artery and small cardiac vein
13	Right coronary artery
14	Anterior cardiac vein
15	Right atrium
16	Auricle of right atrium

● For a view of this specimen from behind see page 169, D.
● Like the veins of the brain, the veins of the heart do not usually have the same names as those of the arteries.
● The great cardiac vein accompanies the anterior interventricular (D3, E10) and circumflex branches of the left coronary artery.
● The middle cardiac vein accompanies the posterior interventricular branch of the right coronary artery (D5).
● The small cardiac vein accompanies the marginal branch of the right coronary artery (D6, E12).
● The above veins normally all drain into the coronary sinus (page 169) but the small cardiac vein, as in D, often enters the right atrium directly.

165

A Cast of the coronary arteries, from the front

Compare this cast with the dissection A on page 160 and the combined dissection and cast D on page 161

1	Ascending aorta
2	Left coronary artery
3	Circumflex
4	Anterior interventricular } branch of left coronary artery
5	Right coronary artery
6	Marginal } branch of right coronary
7	Posterior interventricular } artery
8	Atrioventricular nodal artery

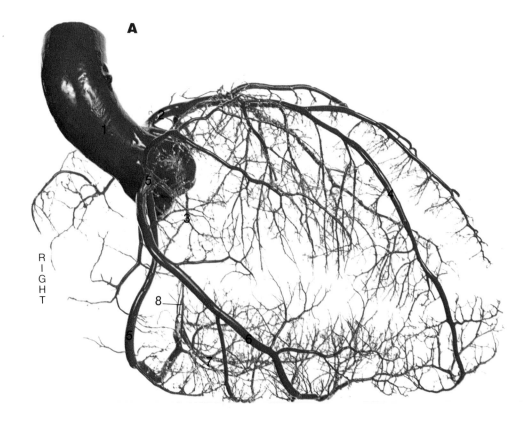

• The left coronary artery (A2, B5) gives off two main branches—the circumflex (A3, B7) which is really the continuation of the main vessel into the posterior atrioventricular groove, and the anterior interventricular (A4, B8) which runs down the front of the heart in the interventricular groove. Many other atrial and ventricular vessels are given off from these branches, including septal branches to the interventricular septum, which are the only branches to penetrate deeply into the myocardium, and frequently the sinuatrial nodal artery (see the page opposite).

• The right coronary artery (A5, B13) gives off two main branches—the marginal (A6) which runs along the lower border of the heart but which frequently has a high origin (as on page 165, E12), and the posterior interventricular (A7) which runs in the interventricular groove on the under-surface of the heart. Many other atrial and ventricular vessels are given off from these branches, including the sinuatrial nodal artery (see the page opposite) and septal branches to the interventricular septum, which like their fellows from the anterior interventricular artery penetrate deeply into the septum. One of them is the atrioventricular nodal artery (A8).

• The interventricular branches are often called by clinicians the descending branches.

B Cast of the heart and vessels, from the front and above

The pulmonary trunk has been removed from the top of the right ventricle (11) so that the origin of the left coronary artery (5) can be seen clearly

1	Superior vena cava
2	Left atrium
3	Left pulmonary veins
4	Auricle of left atrium
5	Left coronary artery
6	Left aortic sinus
7	Circumflex branch
8	Anterior interventricular branch
9	Great cardiac vein
10	Left ventricle
11	Right ventricle
12	Marginal branch of right coronary artery and small cardiac vein
13	Right coronary artery
14	Right aortic sinus
15	Ascending aorta
16	Auricle of right atrium

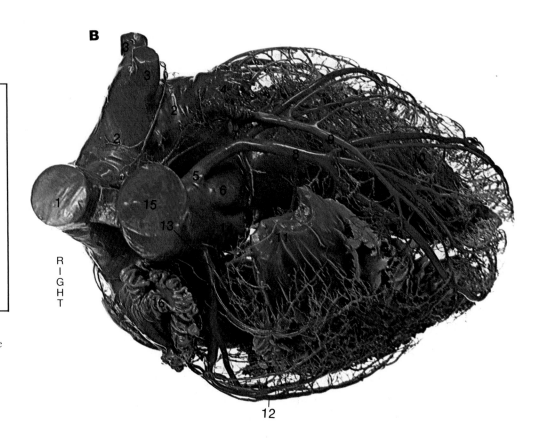

• The origin of the right coronary artery (B13, from the right aortic sinus) is easily seen when dissecting the heart from the front, but the origin of the left coronary artery (B5, from the left aortic sinus) is hidden behind the pulmonary trunk (page 168, A).

C

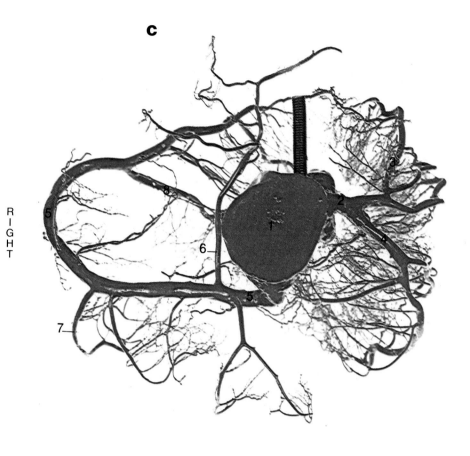

RIGHT

C Cast of the coronary arteries, from above

The largest atrial branch of the right coronary artery (5) is the sinuatrial nodal artery (6)

1	Ascending aorta	5	Right coronary artery
2	Left coronary artery	6	Sinuatrial nodal artery
3	Circumflex branch	7	Marginal branch
4	Anterior interventricular branch	8	Posterior interventricular branch

D

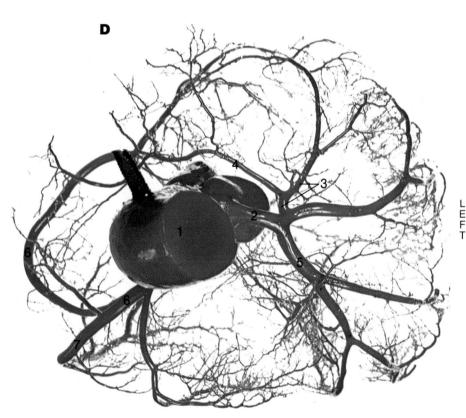

LEFT

D Cast of the coronary arteries, from above

This cast illustrates the origin of the sinuatrial nodal artery (4) from the circumflex branch of the left coronary (3); it passes behind the ascending aorta (1)

1	Ascending aorta	5	Anterior interventricular branch
2	Left coronary artery		
3	Circumflex branch	6	Right coronary artery
4	Sinuatrial nodal artery	7	Marginal branch

● In about 55 per cent of hearts the sinuatrial nodal artery arises from the right coronary; in 45 per cent it comes from the circumflex branch of the left coronary.

● From either origin the artery penetrates the wall of the right atrium and makes an arterial ring within the atrial wall just below the entry of the superior vena cava. The node is in the front of the atrial wall at the top of the crista terminalis (page 162, A2).

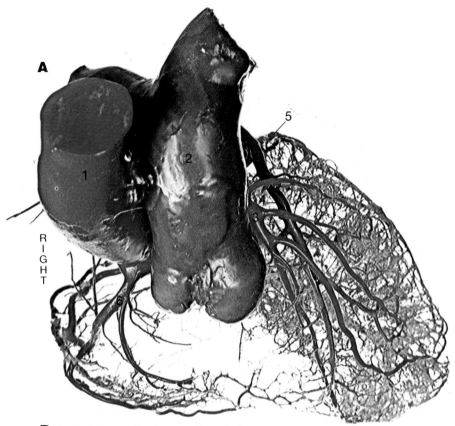

A

R
I
G
H
T

2

1

5

3

6

A Cast of the cardiac and great vessels, from above

With the pulmonary trunk (2) in its normal position, the origin of the left coronary artery is obscured but that of the right coronary (6) is seen easily

1	Ascending aorta
2	Pulmonary trunk
3	Anterior interventricular branch of left coronary artery
4	Great cardiac vein
5	Circumflex branch of left coronary artery
6	Right coronary artery

B Cast of the aortic sinuses, from below

The ascending aorta has been filled with resin, so outlining the aortic sinuses (the dilatations above the cusps of the aortic valve), which are seen here as when looking upwards through the aortic valve

1	Right	}
2	Left	} aortic sinus
3	Posterior	}
4	Right coronary artery	
5	Left coronary artery	

• Strictly speaking, there is only one aortic sinus, with right, left and posterior parts, but the parts are commonly called the right, left and posterior sinuses.
• The aortic and pulmonary valve cusps (and sinuses) are named from their approximate positions in the adult heart (see the last note on page 163).
• The right coronary artery (B4, A6) arises from the right aortic sinus (B1).
• The left coronary artery (B5) arises from the left aortic sinus.

C Cast of the pulmonary trunk and arteries, from the front

As with the aorta shown in B, the filling of the pulmonary trunk (4) with resin has outlined the position of the cusps of the pulmonary valve and sinuses

1	Right	}
2	Anterior	} pulmonary sinus
3	Left	}
4	Pulmonary trunk	
5	Left pulmonary artery	
6	Right pulmonary artery and branch to superior lobe of right lung	

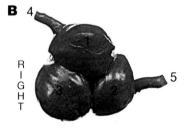

B 4

R
I
G
H
T

1

3   2

5

D Cast of the heart and great vessels, from behind

This view from behind shows the base or posterior surface of the heart which is formed by the left atrium (15), with a small part of the right atrium (10) on the right. The two pairs of pulmonary veins (16 and 9) are seen entering the left atrium, while below it the coronary sinus (13) lies in the atrioventricular groove

1	Left pulmonary artery
2	Arch of aorta
3	Left subclavian artery
4	Left common carotid artery
5	Brachiocephalic trunk
6	Azygos vein
7	Superior vena cava
8	Right pulmonary artery
9	Right pulmonary veins
10	Right atrium
11	Inferior vena cava
12	Middle cardiac vein
13	Coronary sinus
14	Posterior vein of left ventricle
15	Left atrium
16	Left pulmonary veins
17	Pulmonary trunk

E Cast of the heart and great vessels, from the left, below and behind

This specimen, similar to that in D, has been tilted downwards to show the coronary sinus (10) in the atrioventricular groove

1	Pulmonary trunk
2	Left coronary artery
3	Ascending aorta
4	Superior vena cava
5	Right pulmonary veins
6	Right atrium
7	Inferior vena cava
8	Posterior interventricular branch of right coronary artery
9	Middle cardiac vein
10	Coronary sinus
11	Left ventricle
12	Posterior vein of left ventricle
13	Great cardiac vein
14	Circumflex branch of left coronary artery
15	Oblique vein of left coronary artery
16	Left atrium
17	Left pulmonary veins
18	Auricle of left atrium

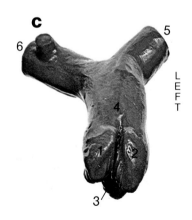

C

6

5

L
E
F
T

4

1   2

3

• There is no such thing as *the* pulmonary artery; the pulmonary *trunk* divides into *right* and *left* pulmonary arteries.

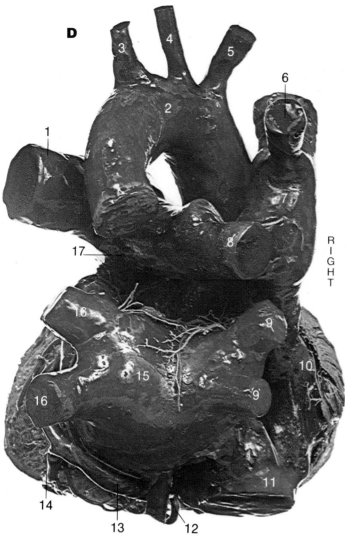

F Cast of the heart and great vessels, from the vessels, below and behind

In contrast to D and E, only the vessels and not the chambers of the heart have been filled with resin, giving a clearer view of the coronary sinus (7). Compare with E on page 161

1	Left pulmonary artery
2	Right pulmonary artery
3	Ascending aorta
4	Right coronary artery
5	Marginal branch of 4 and small cardiac vein
6	Posterior interventricular branch of 4 and middle cardiac vein
7	Coronary sinus
8	Posterior vein of left ventricle
9	Great cardiac vein
10	Circumflex branch of left coronary artery

● The base of the heart (like the base of the prostate) is its posterior surface, formed largely by the left atrium (D15, E16). Note that the base is not the part of the heart which joins the superior vena cava, aorta and pulmonary trunk; this part has no special name.

● The very small oblique vein of the left atrium (E5) marks the point where the great cardiac vein (E13) becomes the coronary sinus (E10), but in E the junction is unusually far to the right so that the posterior vein of the left ventricle (E12) joins the great cardiac vein (E13) instead of the coronary sinus itself.

● The coronary sinus (D13, E10, F7), which receives most of the venous blood from the heart, lies in the posterior part of the atrioventricular groove between the left atrium and left ventricle (page 161, E12), and opens into the right atrium (page 162).

● The coronary sinus normally receives as tributaries the great cardiac vein (E13, F9), middle cardiac vein (E9, F6), and the small cardiac vein (F5), the posterior vein of the left ventricle (E12, F8) and the oblique vein of the left atrium (E15).

● The small cardiac vein (F5) frequently drains directly into the right atrium and not into the coronary sinus.

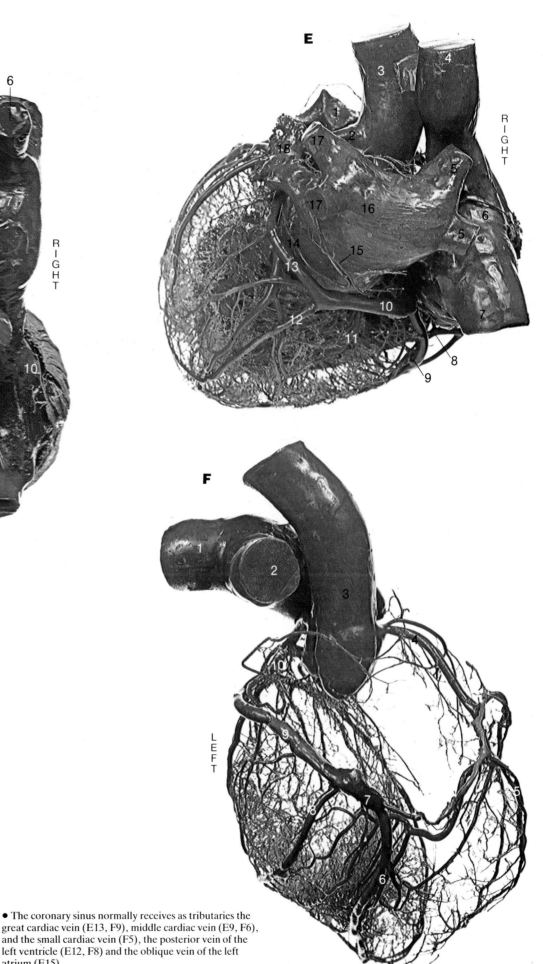

A Cast of the cardiac vessels, from the right and behind

This view looks at the interventricular septum (6) end-on, between the left and right ventricles (11 and 5)

1	Ascending aorta
2	Right coronary artery
3	Anterior cardiac vein
4	Small cardiac vein entering right atrium
5	Right ventricle
6	Vessels of interventricular septum
7	Posterior interventricular branch of right coronary artery
8	Middle cardiac vein
9	Coronary sinus
10	Posterior vein of left ventricle
11	Left ventricle
12	Great cardiac vein
13	Circumflex branch of left coronary artery
14	Left coronary artery

● The position of the muscular interventricular septum is indicated by the deeply penetrating branches of the anterior and posterior interventricular arteries and their accompanying veins.

B Cast of the heart and vessels, from the right and behind

The left atrium (2), left ventricle and ascending aorta (4) have been filled with red resin, and the four pulmonary veins (1) are shown entering the left atrium. The vessels outlining the interventricular septum (8) overlie the resin in the left ventricle

1	Pulmonary veins
2	Left atrium
3	Auricle of left atrium
4	Ascending aorta
5	Right coronary artery
6	Marginal branch and small cardiac vein
7	A large atrial branch
8	Vessels of interventricular septum
9	Posterior interventricular branch and middle cardiac vein
10	Coronary sinus

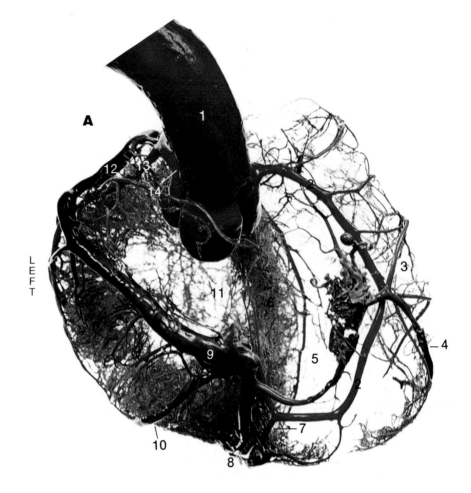

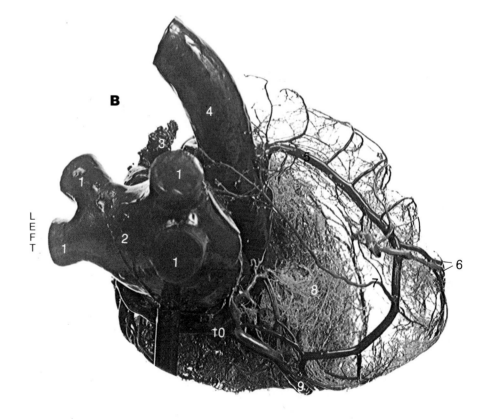

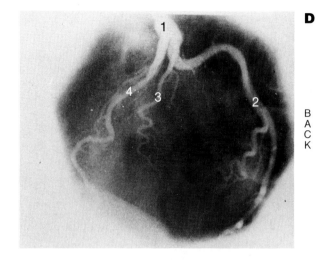

D

BACK

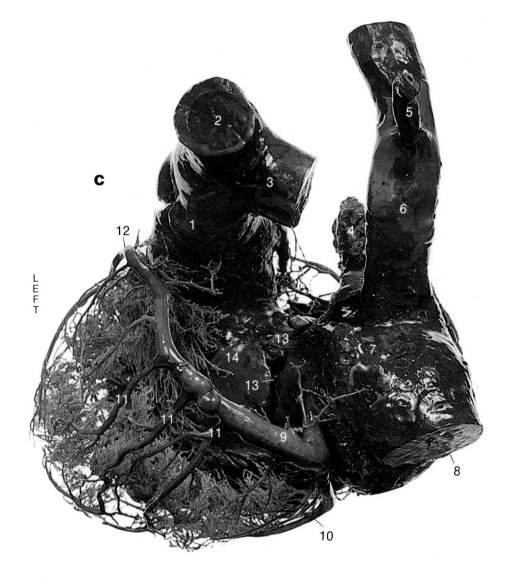

C

LEFT

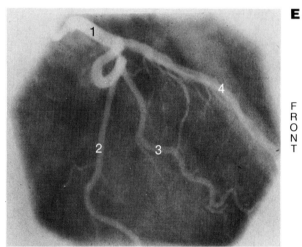

E

FRONT

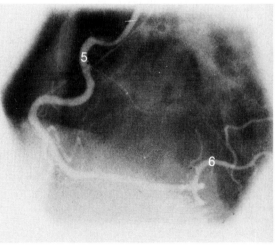

F

FRONT

C Cast of the cardiac veins, from behind

The pulmonary trunk (1) passes upwards to divide into the two pulmonary arteries (2 and 3). The azygos vein (5) is seen running into the back of the superior vena cava (6) which enters the right atrium (7), with the inferior vena cava (8) entering the atrium from below. Numerous large veins from the left ventricle (11) join the coronary sinus (9) as well as the great (12) and middle (10) cardiac veins seen here

1 Pulmonary trunk
2 Left pulmonary artery
3 Right pulmonary artery
4 Auricle of right atrium
5 Azygos vein
6 Superior vena cava
7 Right atrium
8 Inferior vena cava
9 Coronary sinus
10 Middle cardiac vein
11 Various veins of left ventricle
12 Great cardiac vein
13 Position of right atrioventricular (tricuspid) valve
14 Right ventricle

Coronary arteriograms, D left, coronary artery, from the left, E left coronary artery, from the right and in front, F right coronary artery, from the right and in front

These arteriograms illustrate how the pattern of coronary vessels can be visualised in the living, by injecting contrast medium into the openings of the coronary arteries via a catheter threaded through the femoral (or brachial) arteries into the ascending aorta. There are standard views for examining the branching of the arteries; only the major vessels are identified here. Compare with the casts on page 166

1 Left coronary artery
2 Circumflex branch
3 Marginal branch
4 Anterior interventricular branch
5 Right coronary artery
6 Posterior interventricular branch

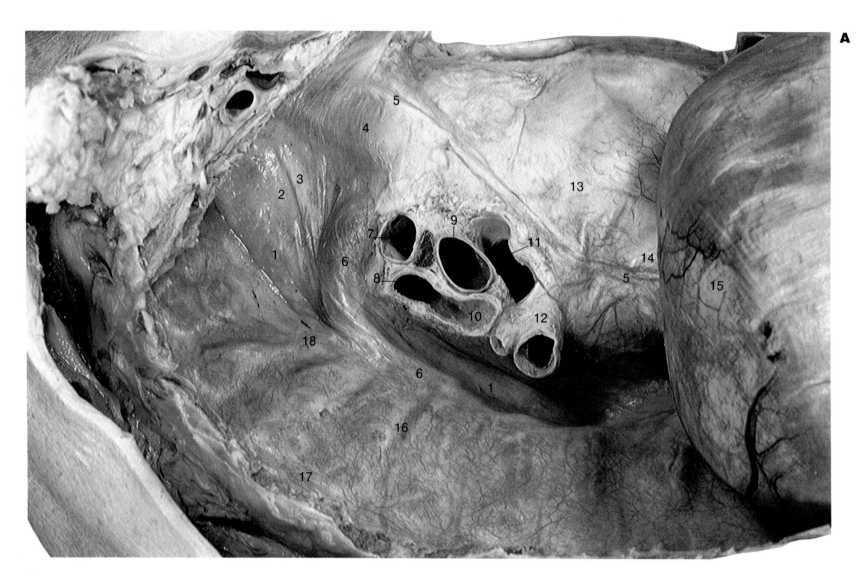

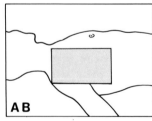

A

A Right lung root and mediastinal pleura

This is the view of the right side of the mediastinum after removing the lung but with the pleura still intact (with the body lying on its back, head towards the left). Compare the features seen here with those in the dissection opposite (a different specimen), from which the pleura has been removed

1	Oesophagus
2	Trachea
3	Right vagus nerve
4	Superior vena cava
5	Right phrenic nerve and pericardiacophrenic vessels
6	Azygos vein
7	Branch of right pulmonary artery to superior lobe
8	Superior lobe bronchus
9	Right pulmonary artery
10	Right principal bronchus
11	Right superior pulmonary vein
12	Right inferior pulmonary vein
13	Mediastinal pleura and pericardium overlying right atrium
14	Inferior vena cava
15	Diaphragm
16	Posterior intercostal vessels under parietal pleura
17	Sympathetic trunk
18	Right superior intercostal vein

AB

● The right vagus nerve (A3, B10) passes obliquely downwards and backwards under the mediastinal pleura across the side of the trachea (A2, B11).

● The right phrenic nerve (A5, B7) passes downwards under the mediastinal pleura on the side of the superior vena cava (A4, B8), the pericardium over the right atrium (A13, B25) and the inferior vena cava (A14, B26).

● The pleura on the right is in close contact with the side of the trachea (A2) above the arch of the azygos vein (A6), but on the left above the arch of the aorta (page 174) the left common carotid and subclavian arteries intervene between the trachea and pleura.

● The order of the main structures in the right lung root from before backwards is: vein, artery, bronchus (A11, 9 and 10, and B19, 18 and 17). The lowest structure is the inferior pulmonary vein (A12, B20). The highest structures are the branches of the artery and bronchus to the superior lobe (A7 and 8, B15 and 16).

B

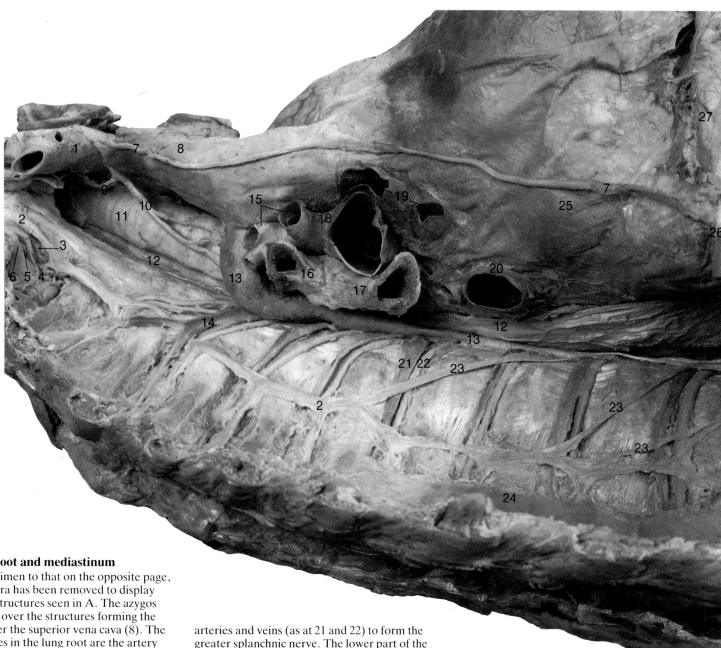

B Right lung root and mediastinum

In a similar specimen to that on the opposite page, most of the pleura has been removed to display the underlying structures seen in A. The azygos vein (13) arches over the structures forming the lung root to enter the superior vena cava (8). The highest structures in the lung root are the artery (15) and bronchus (16) to the superior lobe of the lung. The right superior pulmonary vein (19) is in front of the right pulmonary artery, with the right inferior pulmonary vein (20) the lowest structure in the root. Above the arch of the azygos vein the trachea (11), with the right vagus nerve (10) in contact with it, lies in front of the oesophagus (12). Part of the first rib has been cut away to show the structures lying in front of its neck (5)—the sympathetic trunk (2), supreme intercostal vein (3), superior intercostal artery (4) and the ventral ramus of the first thoracic nerve (6). The right recurrent laryngeal nerve (9) hooks underneath the subclavian artery (1). The right phrenic nerve (7) runs down over the superior vena cava (8) and the pericardium overlying the right atrium (25), and pierces the diaphragm (27) beside the inferior vena cava (26). Contributions from the sympathetic trunk (23) pass over the sides of vertebral bodies superficial to posterior intercostal

arteries and veins (as at 21 and 22) to form the greater splanchnic nerve. The lower part of the oesophagus (12) behind the lung root and heart has the azygos vein (13) on its right side

1	Right subclavian artery	16	Superior lobe bronchus
2	Sympathetic trunk and ganglion	17	Right principal bronchus
3	Supreme intercostal vein	18	Right pulmonary artery
4	Superior intercostal artery	19	Right superior pulmonary vein
5	Neck of first rib	20	Right inferior pulmonary vein
6	Ventral ramus of first thoracic nerve	21	Sixth right posterior intercostal vein
7	Right phrenic nerve	22	Sixth right posterior intercostal artery
8	Superior vena cava	23	Branches of sympathetic trunk to greater
9	Right recurrent laryngeal nerve		splanchnic nerve
10	Right vagus nerve	24	Pleura (cut edge)
11	Trachea	25	Pericardium over right atrium
12	Oesophagus	26	Inferior vena cava
13	Azygos vein	27	Diaphragm
14	Superior intercostal vein		
15	Branch of right pulmonary artery to superior lobe		

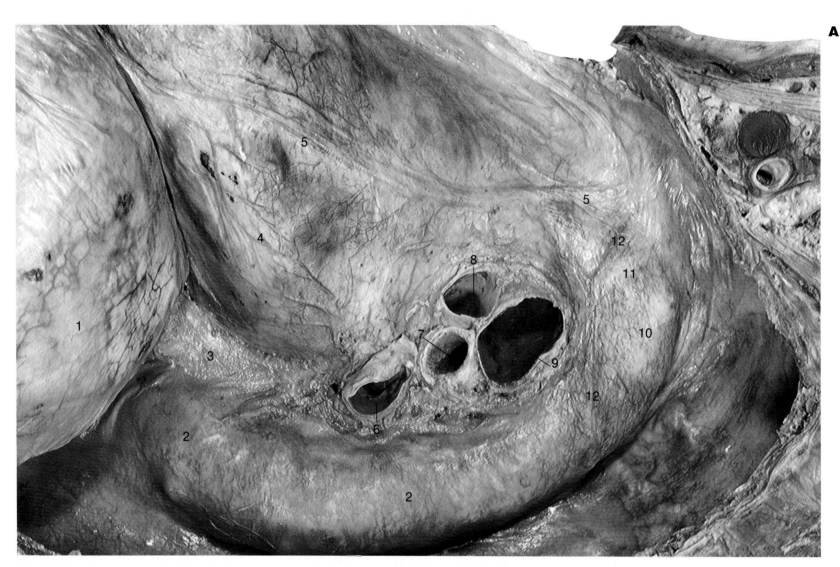

A Left lung root and mediastinal pleura

This is the view of the left side of the mediastinum after removing the lung but with the pleura still intact (with the body lying on its back, head towards the right). Compare the features seen here with those in the dissection opposite (a different specimen), from which the pleura has been removed

1	Diaphragm
2	Thoracic aorta
3	Oesophagus
4	Mediastinal pleura and pericardium overlying left ventricle
5	Left phrenic nerve and pericardiacophrenic vessels
6	Left inferior pulmonary vein
7	Left principal bronchus
8	Left superior pulmonary vein
9	Left pulmonary artery
10	Arch of aorta
11	Left vagus nerve
12	Left superior intercostal vein

● The left vagus nerve (A11, B9) and the left phrenic nerve (A5, B2) pass downwards over the arch of the aorta (A10, B10), the phrenic in front of the vagus.
● The left superior intercostal vein (A12, B11) crosses the upper part of the arch of the aorta transversely, passing over the vagus (B9) and under the phrenic (B2).
● The order of the main structures in the left lung root from before backwards is: vein, artery, bronchus (A8, 9 and 7, B4, 6 and 5). The lowest structure is the inferior pulmonary vein (A6, B3), and the highest structure the pulmonary artery (A9, B6).
● On the left side above the diaphragm the lower end of the oesophagus lies in a triangle bounded by the diaphragm below (A1), the heart in front (A4, B1) and the descending aorta behind (A2, B26).

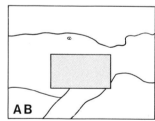

B

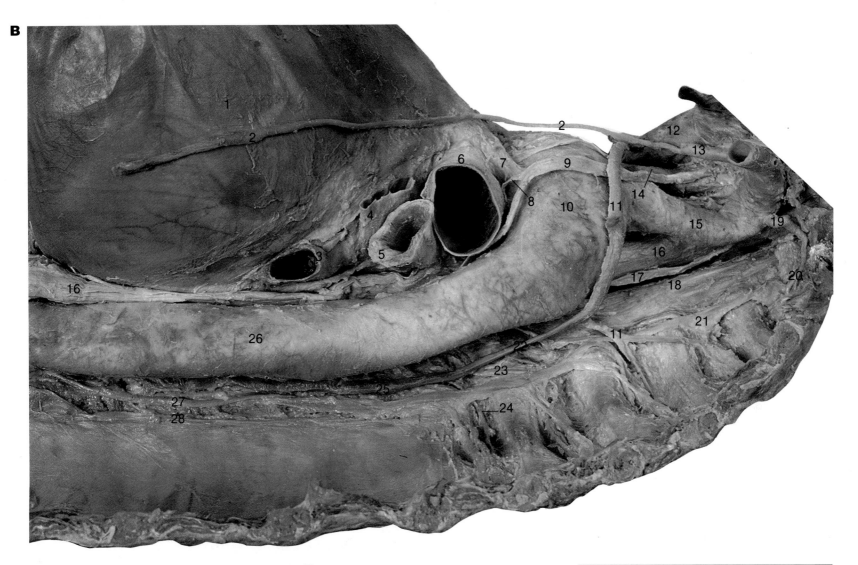

B Left lung root and mediastinum

In a similar specimen to that on the opposite page, most of the pleura has been removed to show the underlying structures seen in A. The left vagus nerve (9) crosses the arch of the aorta (10) with the left phrenic nerve (2) anterior to it; the superior intercostal vein (11) runs over the vagus and under the phrenic. The left recurrent laryngeal nerve (8) hooks round the ligamentum arteriosum (7) while the vagus nerve continues behind the structures forming the lung root. The left pulmonary artery (6) is the highest structure in the root, and the inferior pulmonary vein (3) the lowest. The left superior pulmonary vein (4) is in front of the principal bronchus. The thoracic duct (17) is seen behind the left edge of the oesophagus and the origin of the left superior intercostal artery (20) from the costocervical trunk (19) of the subclavian artery (15) is shown. In this specimen there is an uncommon communication (22) between the left superior intercostal vein (11) and the accessory hemi-azygos vein (25). Above the diaphragm (not shown, having been pushed beyond the edge of the picture with the lower end of the phrenic nerve, 2) the oesophagus (16) bulges towards the left between the heart and pericardium (1) in front and the descending aorta (26) behind

1	Pericardium overlying left ventricle
2	Left phrenic nerve
3	Left inferior pulmonary vein
4	Left superior pulmonary vein
5	Left principal bronchus
6	Left pulmonary artery
7	Ligamentum arteriosum
8	Left recurrent laryngeal nerve
9	Left vagus nerve
10	Arch of aorta
11	Left superior intercostal vein
12	Left brachiocephalic vein
13	Left internal thoracic artery
14	Left common carotid artery
15	Left subclavian artery
16	Oesophagus
17	Thoracic duct
18	Anterior longitudinal ligament
19	Costocervical trunk
20	Left superior intercostal artery
21	Sympathetic trunk and ganglion
22	Communication between 11 and 25
23	Fourth left posterior intercostal artery
24	Fifth left posterior intercostal vein
25	Accessory hemi-azygos vein
26	Thoracic aorta
27	Hemi-azygos vein
28	Pleura (cut edge)

Cast of the bronchial tree

The bronchi of the bronchopulmonary segments have been coloured and labelled with their conventional numbers

● For notes on the lobar and segmental bronchi see page 187

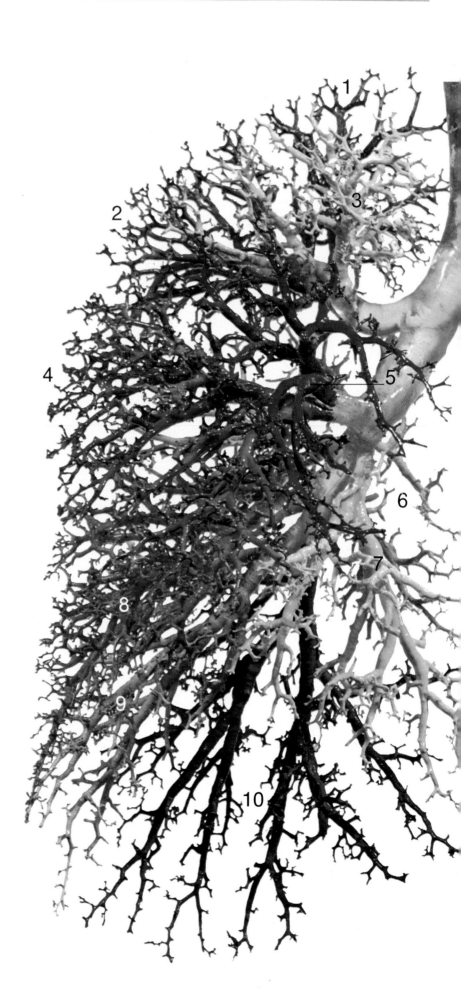

RIGHT LUNG

Superior lobe
1 Apical
2 Posterior
3 Anterior

Middle lobe
4 Lateral
5 Medial

Inferior lobe
6 Apical (superior)
7 Medial basal
8 Anterior basal
9 Lateral basal
10 Posterior basal

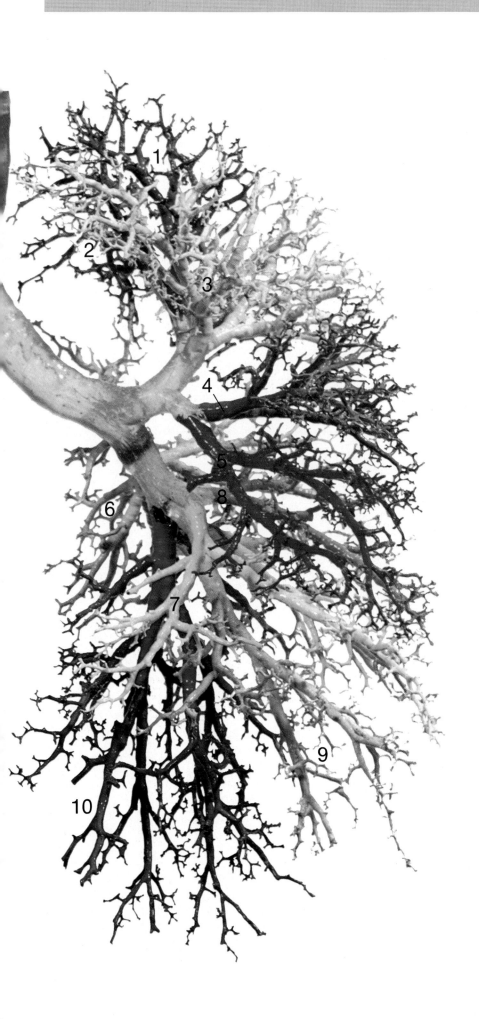

LEFT LUNG

Superior lobe
1 Apical
2 Posterior
3 Anterior
4 Superior lingular
5 Inferior lingular

Inferior lobe
6 Apical (superior)
7 Medial basal (cardiac)
8 Anterior basal
9 Lateral basal
10 Posterior basal

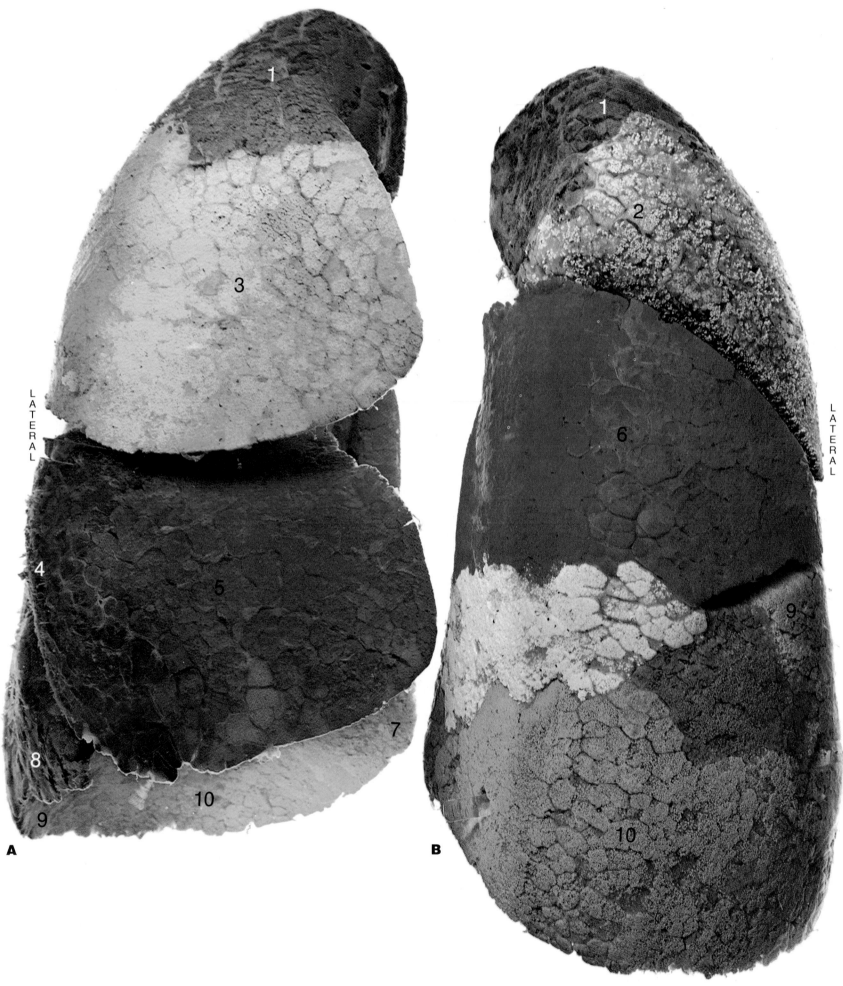

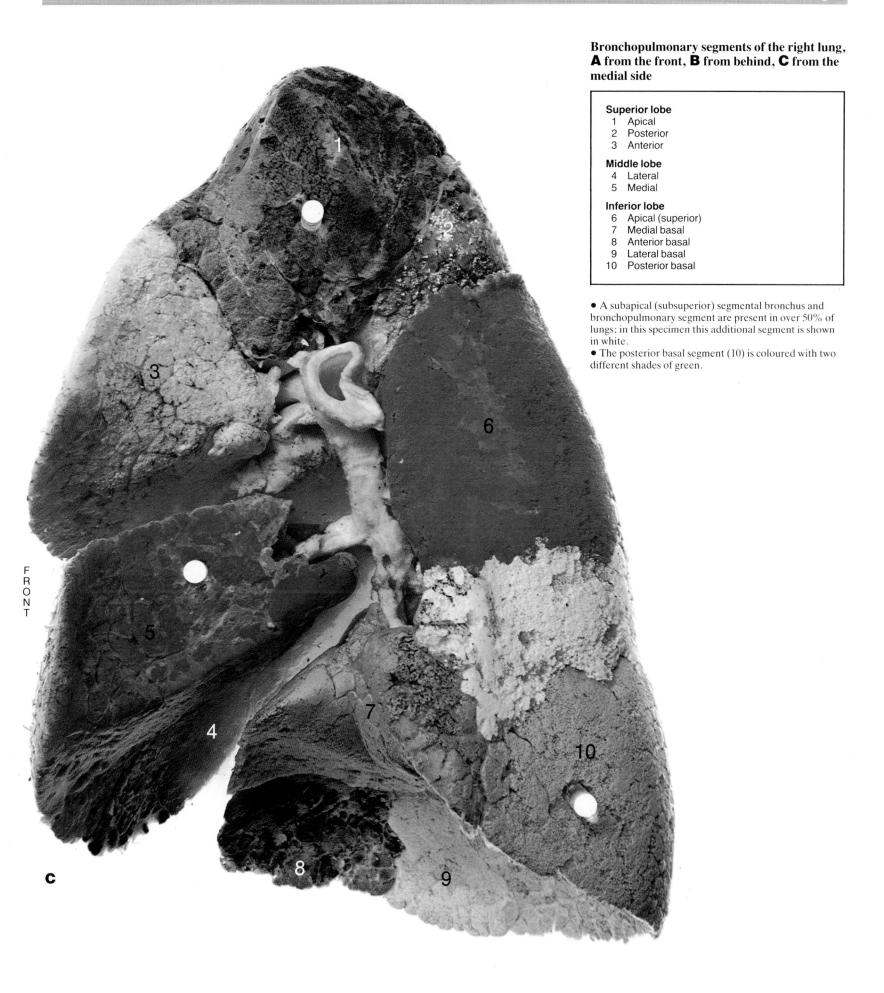

Bronchopulmonary segments of the right lung, A from the front, B from behind, C from the medial side

Superior lobe
1 Apical
2 Posterior
3 Anterior

Middle lobe
4 Lateral
5 Medial

Inferior lobe
6 Apical (superior)
7 Medial basal
8 Anterior basal
9 Lateral basal
10 Posterior basal

● A subapical (subsuperior) segmental bronchus and bronchopulmonary segment are present in over 50% of lungs; in this specimen this additional segment is shown in white.
● The posterior basal segment (10) is coloured with two different shades of green.

FRONT

c

Bronchopulmonary segments of the right lung, from the lateral side

Superior lobe
1 Apical
2 Posterior
3 Anterior

Middle lobe
4 Lateral
5 Medial

Inferior lobe
6 Apical (superior)
7 Medial basal
8 Anterior basal
9 Lateral basal
10 Posterior basal

● The medial basal segment (7) is not seen in this view.
● The posterior basal segment (10) is coloured with two different shades of green.

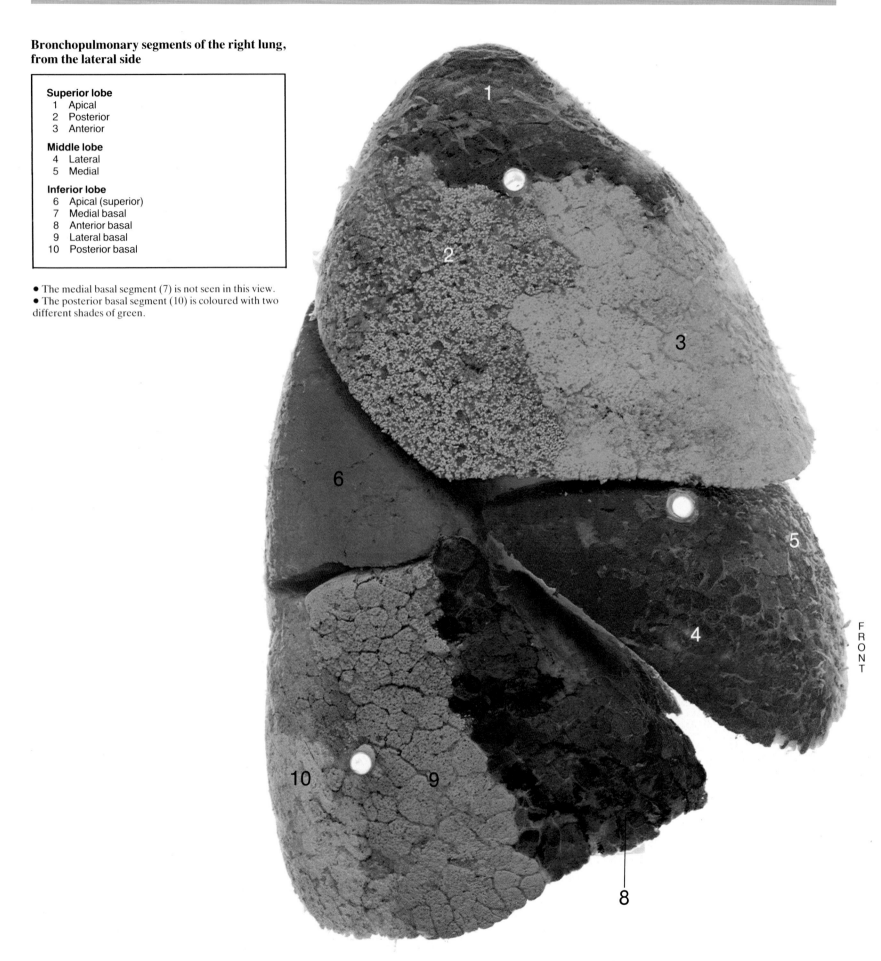

FRONT

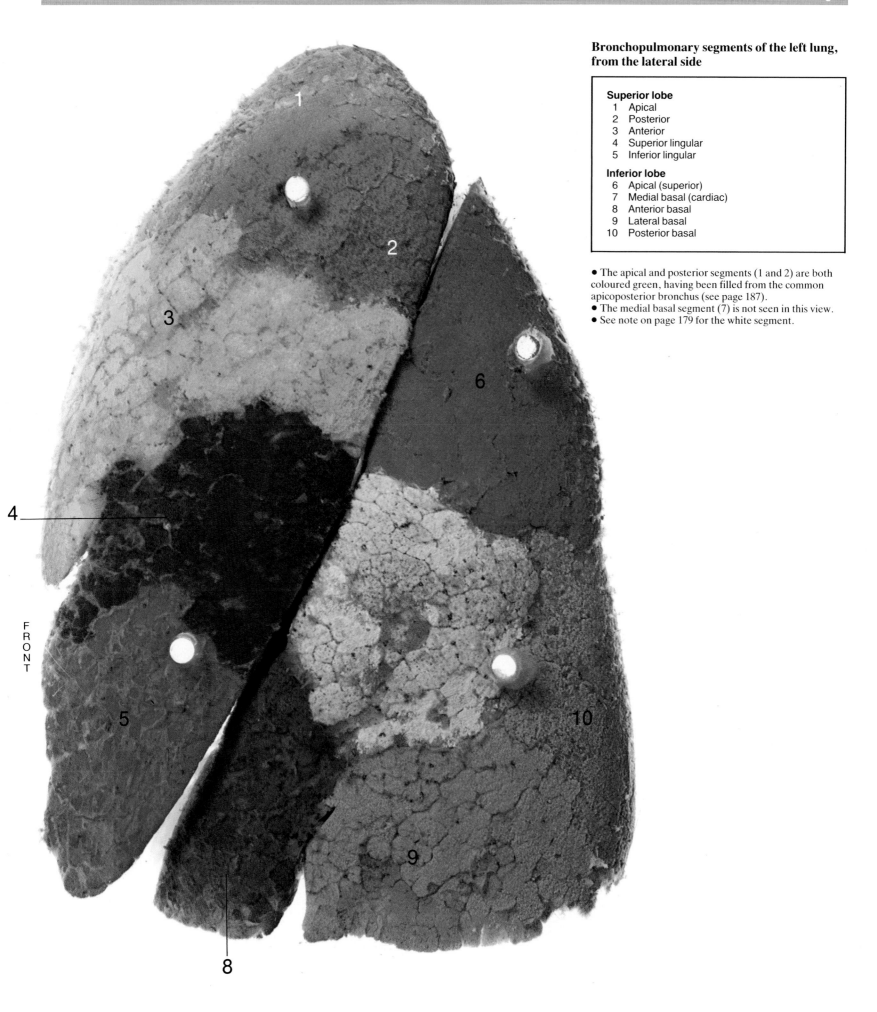

Bronchopulmonary segments of the left lung, from the lateral side

Superior lobe
1 Apical
2 Posterior
3 Anterior
4 Superior lingular
5 Inferior lingular

Inferior lobe
6 Apical (superior)
7 Medial basal (cardiac)
8 Anterior basal
9 Lateral basal
10 Posterior basal

● The apical and posterior segments (1 and 2) are both coloured green, having been filled from the common apicoposterior bronchus (see page 187).
● The medial basal segment (7) is not seen in this view.
● See note on page 179 for the white segment.

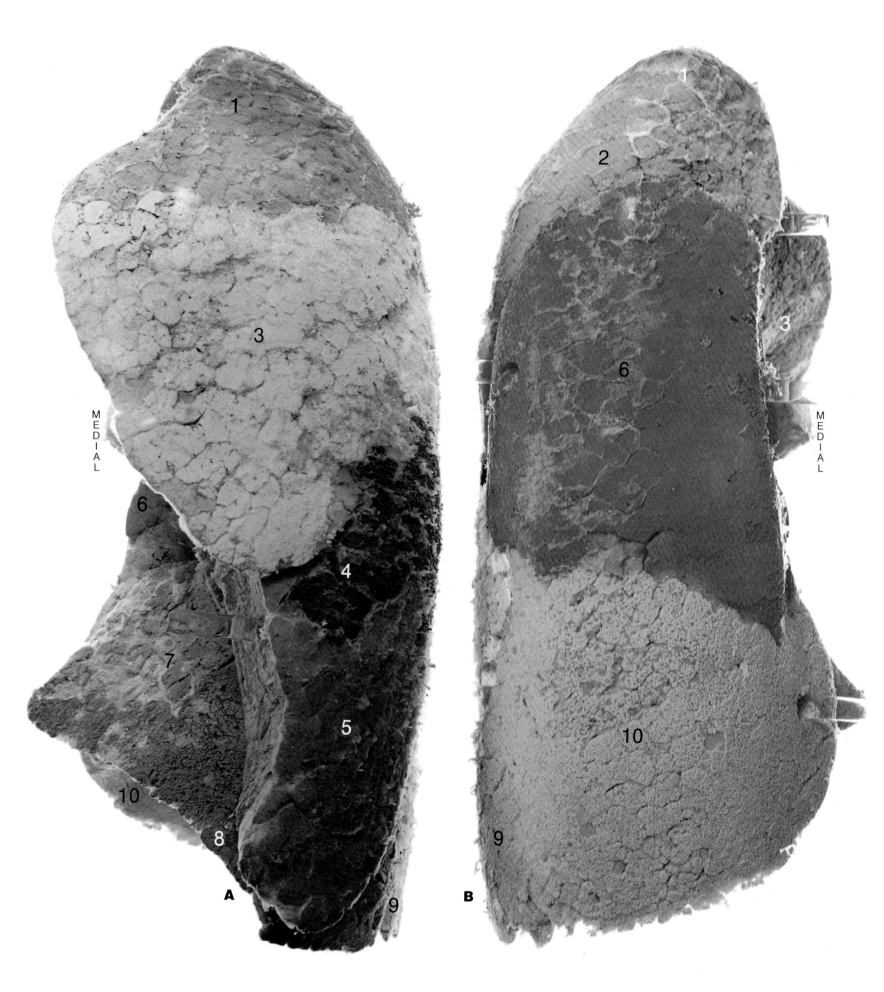

Bronchopulmonary segments of the left lung, A from the front, B from behind, C from the medial side

Superior lobe
1 Apical
2 Posterior
3 Anterior
4 Superior lingular
5 Inferior lingular

Inferior lobe
6 Apical (superior)
7 Medial basal (cardiac)
8 Anterior basal
9 Lateral basal
10 Posterior basal

● The apical and posterior segments (1 and 2) are both coloured green, having been filled from the common apicoposterior bronchus (see page 187).
● See note on page 179 for the white segment in B.

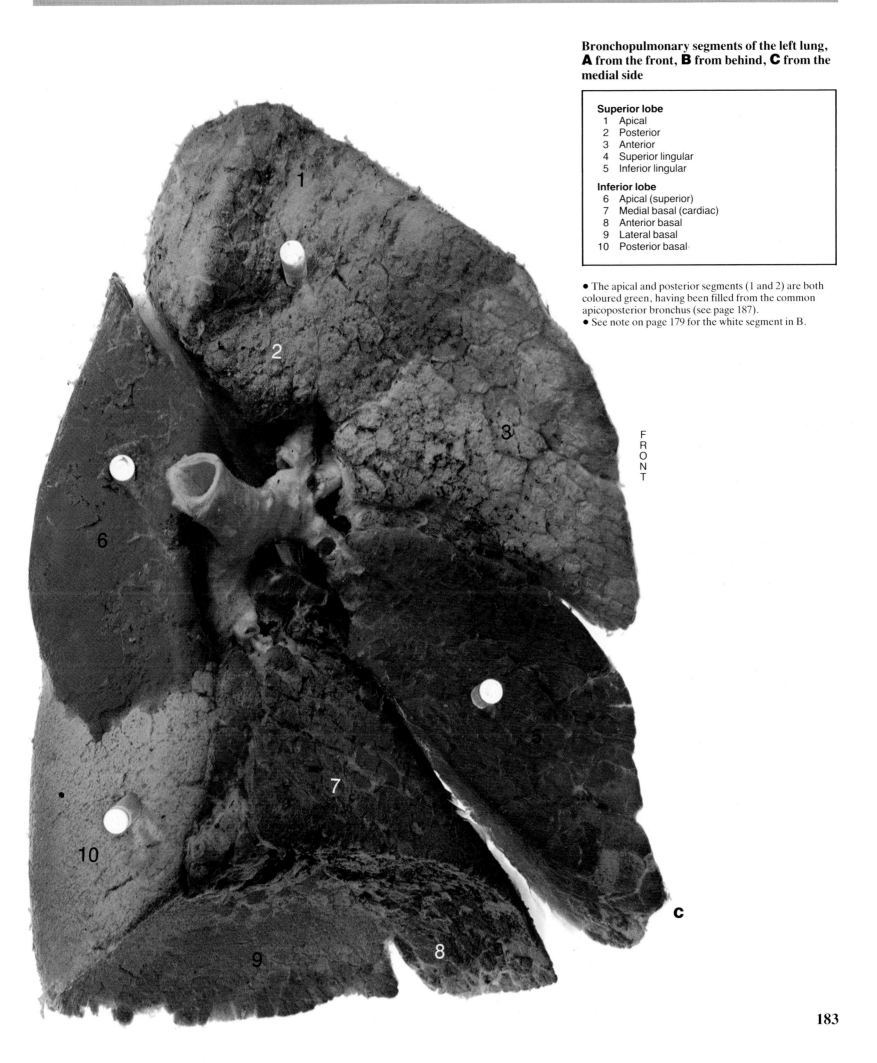

FRONT

C

A

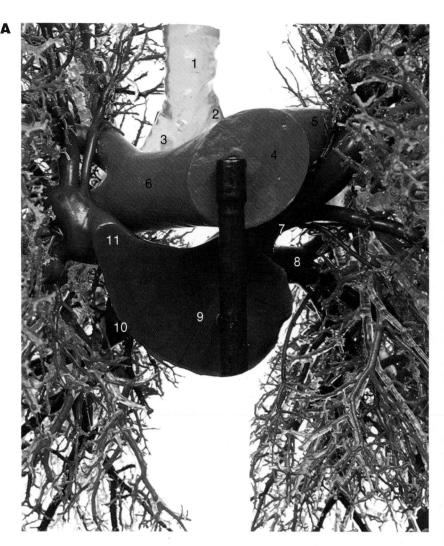

B

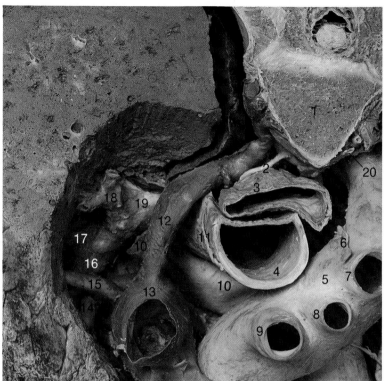

C

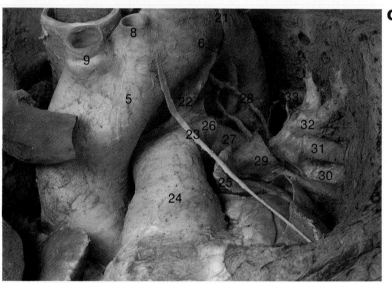

A Cast of the bronchial tree and pulmonary vessels, from the front

The pulmonary trunk (4) divides into the left and right pulmonary arteries (5 and 6), and these vessels have been injected with red resin. The four pulmonary veins (7, 8, 10 and 11) which drain into the left atrium (9) have been filled with blue resin. Note that in the living body the pulmonary veins are filled with oxygenated blood from the lungs and would normally be represented by a red colour; similarly the pulmonary arteries contain deoxygenated blood and should be represented by a blue colour (as in the casts of the heart on pages 165 to 171)

1	Trachea		7	Superior	left pulmonary
2	Left	principal	8	Inferior	vein
3	Right	bronchus	9	Left atrium	
4	Pulmonary trunk		10	Inferior	right pulmonary
5	Left	pulmonary	11	Superior	vein
6	Right	artery			

Lung roots and bronchial arteries, B right side from above, C left side from the front

In B the thorax has been sectioned transversely at the level of the third thoracic vertebra (1), just above the arch of the aorta (5) whose three large branches have been removed (7, 8 and 9), and lung tissue at the hilum has been dissected away from above. The oesophagus (3) and trachea (4) have been tilted forwards to show one of the bronchial arteries (2). In C lung tissue has been removed from the region of the left hilum and the lung root structures are seen from the front, including the left bronchial artery (28) which ran behind the principal bronchus (27) with a branch passing on to the front of the bronchus

1	Third thoracic vertebra	17	Middle lobe bronchus
2	Right bronchial artery	18	Superior lobe bronchus
3	Oesophagus	19	Right principal bronchus
4	Trachea	20	Thoracic duct
5	Arch of aorta	21	Left vagus nerve
6	Left recurrent laryngeal nerve	22	Ligamentum arteriosum
7	Left subclavian artery	23	Left phrenic nerve
8	Left common carotid artery	24	Pulmonary trunk
9	Brachiocephalic trunk	25	Auricle of left atrium
10	Right pulmonary artery	26	Left pulmonary artery
11	Right vagus nerve	27	Left principal bronchus
12	Azygos vein	28	A left bronchial artery
13	Superior vena cava	29	Inferior pulmonary vein
14	Inferior lobe artery	30	Inferior lobe bronchus
15	Tributary of inferior pulmonary vein	31	Inferior lobe artery
16	Inferior lobe bronchus	32	Superior lobe bronchus
		33	Superior lobe artery

● For notes on the position of the main structures in the lung roots see pages 172 and 174.

D

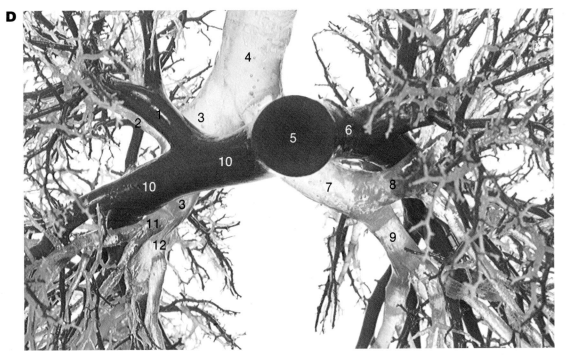

D Cast of the pulmonary arteries and bronchi, from the front

The upper part of the pulmonary trunk (5) is seen end-on after cutting off the lower part, and the bifurcation of the trunk into the left (6) and right (10) pulmonary arteries is in front of the beginning of the left main bronchus (7). In the living body these pulmonary vessels contain deoxygenated blood and would normally be represented by a blue colour (as in the casts of the heart on pages 165 to 170), but here they have been filled with red resin

1	Branch of right pulmonary artery to superior lobe
2	Superior lobe bronchus
3	Right principal bronchus
4	Trachea
5	Pulmonary trunk
6	Left pulmonary artery
7	Left principal bronchus
8	Superior lobe bronchus
9	Inferior lobe bronchus
10	Right pulmonary artery
11	Middle lobe bronchus
12	Inferior lobe bronchus

E

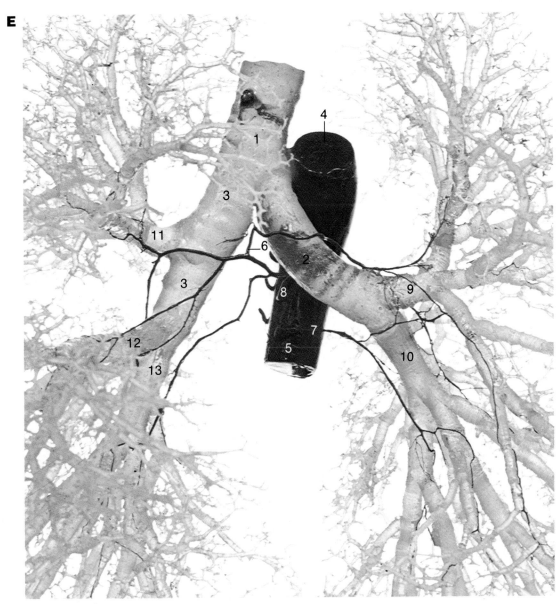

E Cast of the bronchi and bronchial arteries, from the front

Part of the aorta (4 and 5) has been injected with red resin to fill the bronchial arteries. These vessels normally run behind the bronchi and their branches but in this specimen they are in front

1	Trachea
2	Left principal bronchus
3	Right principal bronchus
4	Arch of aorta
5	Thoracic aorta
6	Origin of upper left bronchial artery
7	Origin of lower left bronchial artery
8	Origin of right bronchial artery
9	Superior lobe bronchus
10	Inferior lobe bronchus
11	Superior lobe bronchus
12	Middle lobe bronchus
13	Inferior lobe bronchus

● Compare the order of the main structures in the lung roots and casts on these two pages with the mediastinal dissections on pages 172 and 174. Note for example the order vein, artery, bronchus from before backwards in the cast of the right lung root (A11, 6 and 3).
● The left pulmonary artery (D6) hooks over the left principal bronchus (D7) and descends behind the lobar bronchi.
● The right pulmonary artery (D10) passes below the bifurcation of the trachea (D4) and hooks over the right principal bronchus (D3), but its branch to the superior lobe (D1) remains in front of the superior lobe bronchus (D2).
● The pulmonary trunk (D5, C24) divides into the two pulmonary arteries in front of the left principal bronchus (D7, C27).
● There are usually two left bronchial arteries (from the aorta; one is seen at C28) and one right bronchial artery (from the third right posterior intercostal or upper left bronchial artery; B2). The cast E is unusual in that the vessels run in front of the bronchi rather than behind them, and the upper left artery (E6) arises from the right bronchial artery (E8).

185

A **Medial surface of the upper part of the right lung**

In the hardened dissecting room specimen, adjacent structures make impressions on the medial surface of the lung. The most prominent feature on the right side is the groove for the azygos vein (5), above and behind the structures of the lung root (7 to 9)

1	Groove for first rib
2	Groove for subclavian vein
3	Groove for subclavian artery
4	Oesophageal and tracheal area
5	Groove for azygos vein
6	Groove for superior vena cava
7	Right pulmonary veins
8	Branches of right pulmonary artery
9	Branches of right principal bronchus

B **Medial surface of the upper part of the left lung**

Compare with the right lung in A, and note the large size of the impression made by the aorta on the left lung (B1), in contrast to the smaller azygos groove on the right (A5)

1	Groove for aorta
2	Groove for left subclavian artery
3	Groove for left subclavian and brachiocephalic vein
4	Groove for first rib
5	Left pulmonary veins
6	Branches of left principal bronchus
7	Branches of left pulmonary artery

● The upper end of the medial surface of the right lung lies against the oesophagus and trachea (A4) with only the pleura intervening, but on the left the subclavian artery (B2) (and the left common carotid in front of it) keep the lung further away from these structures.

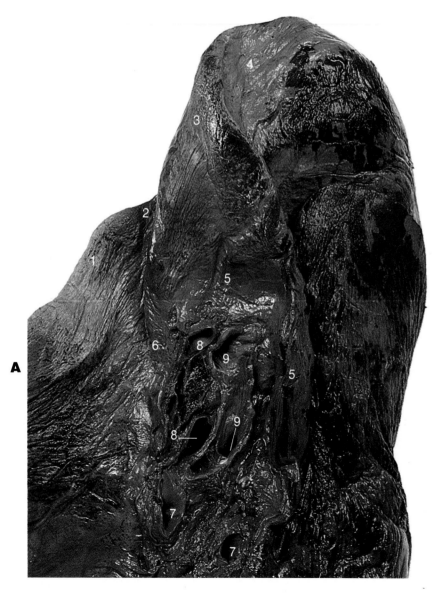

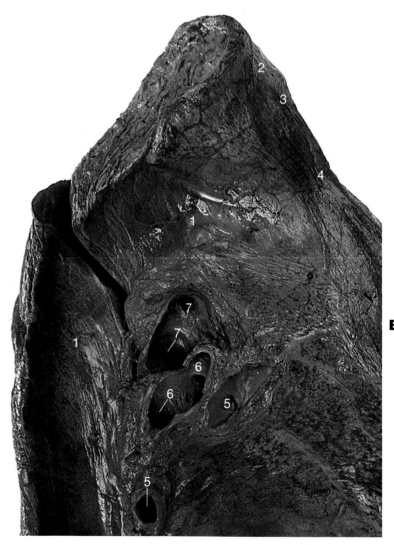

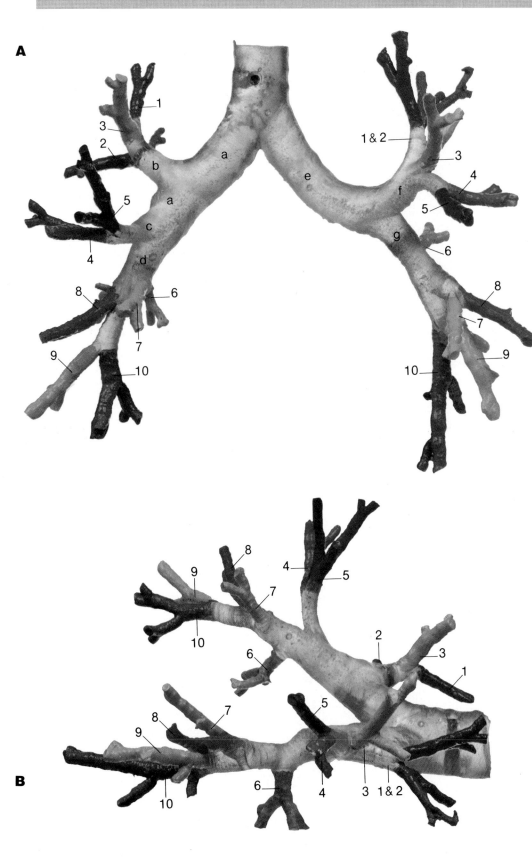

A

B

Cast of the lower trachea and bronchi, **A** vertical, from the front, **B** horizontal, from the left

The main bronchi and lobar bronchi are labelled with letters; the segmental bronchi are labelled with their conventional numbers. In the horizontal side view in B, the cast has been tilted to avoid overlap, and the right side is higher than the left.

● The trachea divides into right and left principal bronchi (a and e).
● The right principal bronchus (a) is shorter, wider and more vertical than the left (e).
● The left principal bronchus (e) is longer and narrower and lies more transversely than the right. Foreign bodies are therefore more likely to enter the right principal bronchus than the left.
● The right principal bronchus (a) gives off a superior lobe bronchus (b) and then enters the hilum of the right lung before dividing into middle and inferior lobe bronchi (c and d).
● The left principal bronchus (e) enters the hilum of the lung before dividing into superior and inferior lobe bronchi (f and g).
● The branches of the lobar bronchi are called segmental bronchi and each supplies a segment of lung tissue—bronchopulmonary segment. The segmental bronchi and the bronchopulmonary segments have similar names, and the ten segments of each lung are officially numbered (as on pages 176 to 183) as well as being named. The bronchi here have been numbered to conform with those of the segments.
● The segmental bronchi of the left and right lungs are essentially similar except that the apical and posterior bronchi of the superior lobe of the left lung arise from a common stem, thus called the apicoposterior bronchus and labelled here as 1 and 2; also there is no middle lobe in the left lung—the superior and inferior lingular bronchi (4 and 5) of its superior lobe correspond to the lateral and medial bronchi of the middle lobe of the right lung, and so the corresponding segments bear similar numbers; and the medial basal bronchus (7) of the left lung usually arises in common with the anterior basal (8).
● The apical (superior) bronchus of the inferior lobe (6) of both lungs is the first or highest bronchus to arise from the *posterior* surface of the bronchial tree. When lying on the back fluid may therefore gravitate into this bronchus; the side view in B has been orientated to illustrate this point.

RIGHT LUNG	LEFT LUNG
Lobar bronchi	
a Principal	e Principal
b Superior lobe	f Superior lobe
c Middle lobe	g Inferior lobe
d Inferior lobe	
Segmental bronchi	
Superior lobe	**Superior lobe**
1 Apical	1 & 2 Apicoposterior
2 Posterior	3 Anterior
3 Anterior	4 Superior lingular
	5 Inferior lingular
Middle lobe	
4 Lateral	**Inferior lobe**
5 Medial	6 Apical (superior)
	7 Medial basal (cardiac)
Inferior lobe	8 Anterior basal
6 Apical (superior)	9 Lateral basal
7 Medial basal	10 Posterior basal
8 Anterior basal	
9 Lateral basal	
10 Posterior basal	

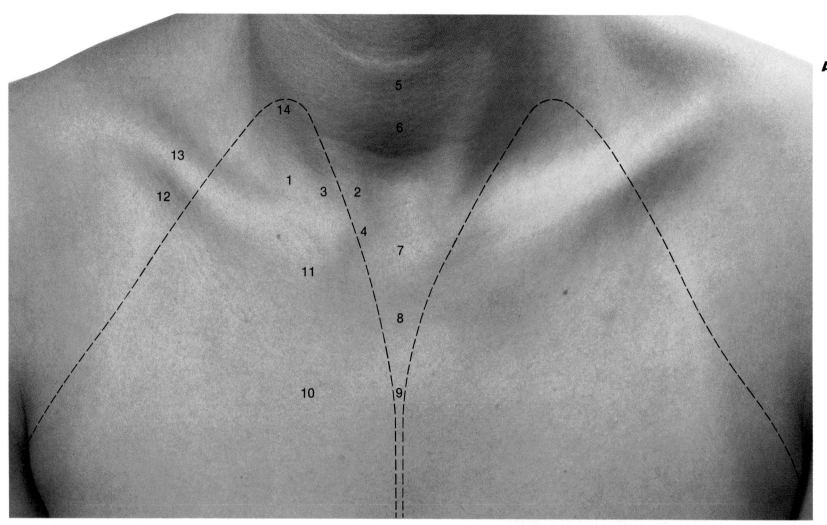

A Lower neck and upper thorax. Surface markings

The interrupted line indicates the extent of the pleura and lung on each side; the apices of the pleura and lung (14) rise into the neck for about 4 cm above the medial third of the clavicle. The lower end of the internal jugular vein (3) lies behind the interval between the sternal (2) and clavicular (1) heads of sternocleidomastoid. Behind the sternoclavicular joint (4) the internal jugular and subclavian veins unite to form the brachiocephalic vein. The trachea (6) is felt in the midline above the jugular notch (7), and the arch of the cricoid cartilage (5) is 4 to 5 cm above the notch, with the manubriosternal joint (sternal angle, 9) 4 to 5 cm below the notch. The joint is at the level of the second costal cartilage (10) and opposite the lower border of the body of the fourth thoracic vertebra, and the horizontal plane through these points indicates the junction between the superior and inferior parts of the mediastinum. The left brachiocephalic vein passes behind the upper half of the manubrium to unite with the right brachiocephalic at the lower border of the right first costal cartilage (11) to form the superior vena cava. The midpoint of the manubrium (8) marks the highest level of the arch of the aorta and the origin of the brachiocephalic trunk. Compare many of the features mentioned here with the structures in the dissections below and opposite

1	Clavicular head ⎫ of sterno-	8	Midpoint of manubrium of
2	Sternal head ⎭ cleidomastoid		sternum
3	Internal jugular vein	9	Manubriosternal joint
4	Sternoclavicular joint	10	Second costal cartilage
5	Cricoid cartilage	11	First costal cartilage
6	Trachea and isthmus of thyroid	12	Infraclavicular fossa
	gland	13	Clavicle
7	Jugular notch	14	Apex of pleura and lung

A

B

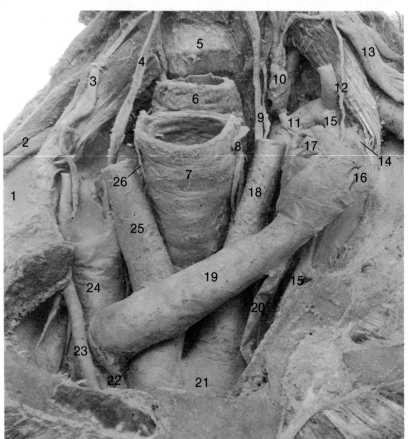

B Thoracic inlet, from the front

The manubrium and the first right costal cartilage have been removed to show the left brachiocephalic vein (19) crossing in front of the left common carotid artery (18) and the brachiocephalic trunk (25)

1	First rib
2	Lowest roots of brachial plexus
3	Right phrenic nerve and scalenus anterior
4	Right vagus nerve
5	Cervical vertebral column
6	Oesophagus
7	Trachea
8	Left recurrent laryngeal nerve
9	Left vagus nerve
10	Middle cervical sympathetic ganglion
11	Ansa subclavia and left subclavian artery
12	Left thyrocervical trunk, phrenic nerve and scalenus anterior
13	Upper trunk of brachial plexus
14	Apex of lung
15	Left internal thoracic artery
16	Left subclavian vein
17	Left internal jugular vein
18	Left common carotid artery
19	Left brachiocephalic vein
20	Left internal thoracic vein
21	Arch of aorta
22	Superior vena cava
23	Right internal thoracic artery
24	Right brachiocephalic vein
25	Brachiocephalic trunk
26	Right recurrent laryngeal nerve

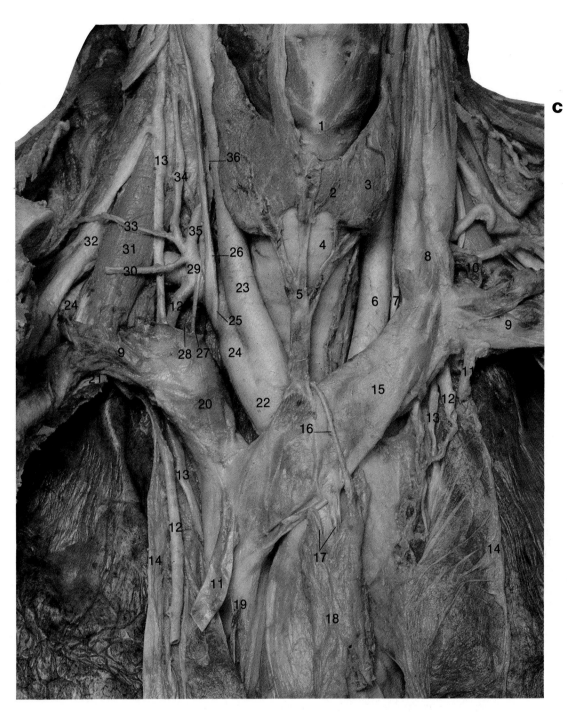

C

C Thoracic inlet and mediastinum, from the front

The anterior thoracic wall and the medial ends of the clavicles have been removed, but part of the parietal pleura (14) remains over the medial part of each lung. The right internal jugular vein has also been removed, displaying the thyrocervical trunk (29) and the origin of the internal thoracic artery (12). Inferior thyroid veins (5) run down over the trachea (4) to enter the left brachiocephalic vein (15). The thymus (18) has been dissected out from mediastinal fat; thymic veins (17) enter the left brachiocephalic vein, and an unusual thymic artery (16) arises from the brachiocephalic trunk (22)

1	Arch of cricoid cartilage	19	Superior vena cava
2	Isthmus ⎫ of thyroid	20	Right brachiocephalic vein
3	Lateral lobe ⎭ gland	21	First rib
4	Trachea	22	Brachiocephalic trunk
5	Inferior thyroid veins	23	Right common carotid artery
6	Left common carotid artery	24	Right subclavian artery
7	Left vagus nerve	25	Right recurrent laryngeal nerve
8	Internal jugular vein	26	Right vagus nerve
9	Subclavian vein	27	Unusual cervical tributary of 20
10	Thoracic duct	28	Vertebral vein
11	Internal thoracic vein	29	Thyrocervical trunk
12	Internal thoracic artery	30	Suprascapular artery
13	Phrenic nerve	31	Scalenus anterior
14	Parietal pleura (cut edge) over lung	32	Upper trunk of brachial plexus
15	Left brachiocephalic vein	33	Superficial cervical artery
16	A thymic artery	34	Ascending cervical artery
17	Thymic veins	35	Inferior thyroid artery
18	Thymus	36	Sympathetic trunk

● The internal jugular (8) and subclavian (9) veins unite behind the sternoclavicular joint to form the brachiocephalic vein (left, 15, and right, 20).
● The left and right brachiocephalic veins (15 and 20) unite at the lower border of the right first costal cartilage to form the superior vena cava (19).
● The brachiocephalic trunk (22) divides into the right subclavian and common carotid arteries (24 and 23). (The left subclavian and common carotid arteries, like the brachiocephalic trunk, are direct branches from the arch of the aorta.)
● At its attachment to the first rib (21), scalenus anterior (31) has the subclavian vein (9) in front and the subclavian artery (24) behind but at a higher level, due to the obliquity of the rib.
● The remains of the thymus (18) are in front of the pericardium, but in the child, where the thymus is much larger, it may extend upwards in front of the great vessels as high as the lower part of the thyroid gland (3).

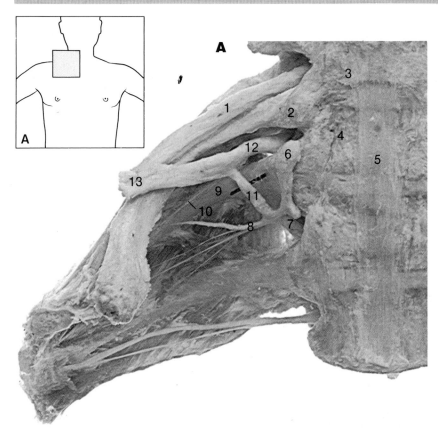

A Thoracic inlet. Right upper ribs, from the front

This dissection shows the nerves related to the first and second ribs. The ventral ramus of the first thoracic nerve (12) is joined by the ventral ramus of the eighth cervical nerve (1) to form the lower trunk of the brachial plexus (13). In this specimen there is a large communication (11) between the second and first nerves

1	Ventral ramus of eighth cervical nerve
2	Head of first rib
3	Seventh cervical vertebra
4	First thoracic vertebra
5	Anterior longitudinal ligament
6	Sympathetic trunk and ganglion
7	Ventral ramus of second thoracic nerve
8	Second intercostal nerve
9	Second rib
10	First intercostal nerve
11	Communication with first thoracic nerve
12	Ventral ramus of first thoracic nerve
13	Lower trunk of brachial plexus

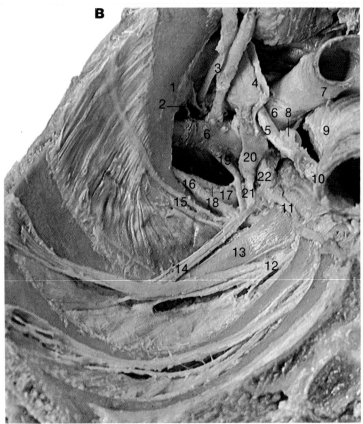

• The neck of the first rib (17) is crossed in order from medial to lateral by the sympathetic trunk (11), supreme intercostal vein (21), superior intercostal artery (19) and the ventral ramus of the first thoracic nerve (16).

B Thoracic inlet. Right upper ribs, from below

This is the view looking upwards into the right side of the thoracic inlet—the region occupied by the cervical pleura, here removed. The under-surface of most of the first rib (1) is seen from below, with the subclavian artery (6) passing over the top of it after giving off the internal thoracic branch (3) which runs towards the top of the picture (to the anterior thoracic wall), and the costocervical trunk whose superior intercostal branch (19) runs down over the neck of the first rib (17). The vertebral vein (20) has come down from the neck and is labelled on its posterior surface before entering the brachiocephalic vein (4, labelled at its opened cut edge). The vertebral vein receives an unusually large supreme intercostal vein (21). On its medial side is the sympathetic trunk (11) with the cervicothoracic ganglion (22). The neck of the first rib (17) has the ventral ramus of the eighth cervical nerve (18) above it and the ventral ramus of the first thoracic nerve (16) below it

1	First rib
2	Subclavian vein
3	Internal thoracic vessels
4	Brachiocephalic vein
5	Vagus nerve
6	Subclavian artery
7	Brachiocephalic trunk
8	Recurrent laryngeal nerve
9	Trachea
10	Right principal bronchus
11	Sympathetic trunk
12	Second intercostal nerve
13	Second rib
14	Superior intercostal vein
15	First intercostal nerve
16	Ventral ramus of first thoracic nerve
17	Neck of first rib
18	Ventral ramus of eighth cervical nerve
19	Superior intercostal artery
20	Vertebral vein
21	Supreme intercostal vein (unusually large)
22	Cervicothoracic (stellate) ganglion

C

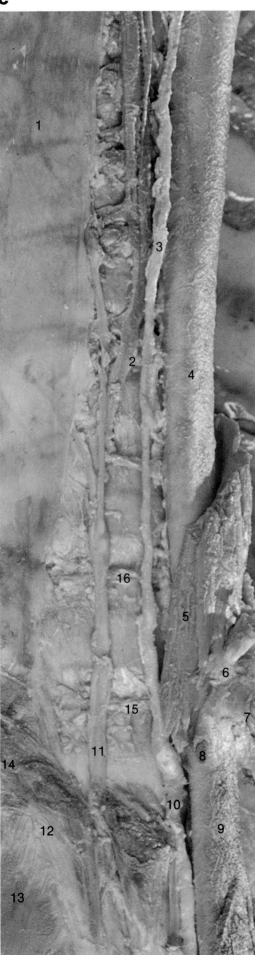

D

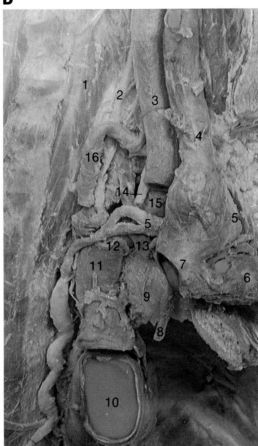

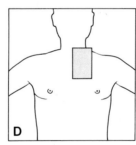

C Thoracic duct, thoracic part

All viscera and part of the pleura have been removed to show the aorta (4 and 9) in front of the vertebral column and viewed from the right, with the thoracic duct (3) lying between the aorta (4) and azygos vein (2); the lower part of the vein was overlying the duct and has been removed. The cisterna chyli (10), where the thoracic duct begins, is in the abdomen under cover of the right crus of the diaphragm (5)

1	Sympathetic trunk underlying pleura
2	Azygos vein
3	Thoracic duct
4	Thoracic aorta
5	Right crus of diaphragm
6	Coeliac trunk
7	Superior mesenteric artery
8	Right renal artery
9	Abdominal aorta
10	Cisterna chyli
11	Greater splanchnic nerve
12	Medial arcuate ligament
13	Psoas major
14	Diaphragm
15	First lumbar artery and first lumbar vertebra
16	Twelfth thoracic vertebra and subcostal artery

D Thoracic duct, cervical part

In this deep dissection of the left side of the root of the neck and upper thorax, the internal jugular vein (4) joins the subclavian vein (6) to form the left brachiocephalic vein (7). The thoracic duct (5) is double for a short distance just before passing in front of the vertebral artery (15) and behind the common carotid artery (3, whose lower end has been cut away to show the duct). The duct then runs behind the internal jugular vein (4) before draining into the junction of that vein with the subclavian vein (6)

1	Longus colli
2	Sympathetic trunk
3	Common carotid artery
4	Internal jugular vein
5	Thoracic duct
6	Subclavian vein
7	Brachiocephalic vein
8	Phrenic nerve
9	Pleura
10	Arch of aorta
11	Subclavian artery
12	Ansa subclavia
13	Internal thoracic artery
14	Vagus nerve
15	Origin of vertebral artery
16	Inferior thyroid artery

● From the cisterna chyli (C10), situated under cover of the left margin of the right crus of the diaphragm (C5) at the level of the first and second lumbar vertebrae, the thoracic duct passes upwards (through the aortic opening in the diaphragm) on the right side of the front of the thoracic vertebral column between the aorta (C4) and azygos vein (C2), crossing to the left at the level of the fifth thoracic vertebra and ending by opening into the left side of the union of the left internal jugular (D4) and subclavian (D6) veins after passing between the common carotid artery (in front, D3) and the vertebral artery (behind, D15).

191

A

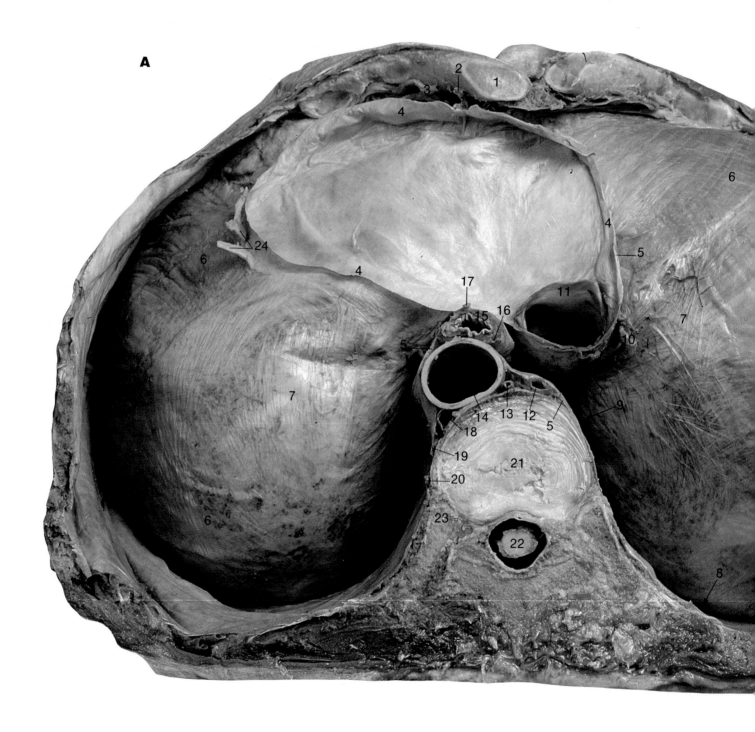

A Diaphragm, from above

The thorax has been transected at the level of the disc between the ninth and tenth thoracic vertebrae. The diaphragm is seen from above after removing the lungs and heart, but the lowest part of the fibrous pericardium (4) has been retained. The aorta (14) has the oesophagus (15) in front of it and the inferior vena cava (11) on its right. The right phrenic nerve (10) goes through the foramen for the inferior vena cava (11) in the tendinous part of the diaphragm (7, right label), while the left phrenic nerve (24) pierces the muscular part (6, left label) in front of the left part of the tendon (7, left label)

1	Seventh left costal cartilage
2	Left internal thoracic artery
3	Left musculophrenic artery
4	Fibrous pericardium (cut edge)
5	Pleura (cut edge)
6	Muscle of diaphragm
7	Tendon of diaphragm
8	Costodiaphragmatic recess
9	Costomediastinal recess
10	Right phrenic nerve
11	Inferior vena cava
12	Azygos vein
13	Thoracic duct
14	Thoracic aorta
15	Oesophagus
16	Posterior vagal trunk
17	Anterior vagal trunk
18	Hemi-azygos vein
19	Left greater splanchnic nerve
20	Left sympathetic trunk
21	Intervertebral disc
22	Spinal cord
23	Head of left ninth rib
24	Left phrenic nerve

● After forming the oesophageal plexus behind the lower part of the oesophagus, the two vagus nerves become reconstituted as the anterior and posterior vagal trunks (17 and 16) which enter the abdomen with the oesophagus (15; see also page 224).
● According to the standard textbook description, the foramen for the vena cava is at the level of the disc between the eighth and ninth thoracic vertebrae, the oesophageal opening at the level of the tenth thoracic vertebra and the aortic opening opposite the twelfth thoracic vertebra. However, it is common for the oesophageal opening to be nearer the midline, as in this specimen (15), and the vena caval foramen (11) is lower than usual.
● The vena caval foramen is in the tendinous part of the diaphragm and the oesophageal opening in the muscular part. The so-called aortic opening is not in the diaphragm but behind it (page 241).
● The central tendon of the diaphragm has the shape of a trefoil leaf and has no bony attachment.
● The right phrenic nerve (10) passes through the vena caval opening, i.e. through the tendinous part, but the left phrenic nerve (24) pierces the muscular part in front of the central tendon just lateral to the overlying pericardium.
● The phrenic nerves are the *only motor* nerves to the diaphragm, including the crura. The supply from lower thoracic (intercostal and subcostal) nerves is purely afferent. Damage to one phrenic nerve completely paralyses its own half of the diaphragm.

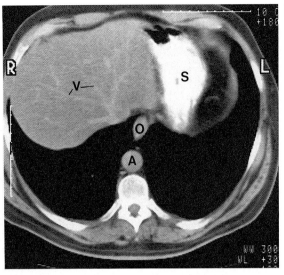

B

B CT scan of the lower thorax

Looking towards the domes of the diaphragm from below, the liver is on the right and shows some hepatic vein tributaries (V), with the stomach (S) on the left. The apparently empty black space on each side is occupied by the translucent lungs. The thoracic aorta (A) is in front of the vertebral column, and in front of the aorta lies the oesophagus (O)

A Oesophagus, lower thoracic part, from the front

The heart has been removed from the pericardial cavity by transecting the great vessels, the pulmonary trunk being cut at the point where it divides into the two pulmonary arteries (3 and 4). Part of the pericardium (9) at the back has been removed to reveal the oesophagus (5). It is seen below the left principal bronchus (6) and is being crossed by the beginning of the right pulmonary artery (3)

1　Ascending aorta
2　Superior vena cava
3　Right pulmonary artery
4　Left pulmonary artery
5　Oesophagus
6　Left principal bronchus
7　Left superior pulmonary vein
8　Left inferior pulmonary vein
9　Pericardium (cut edge)
10　Anterior vagal trunk
11　Inferior vena cava
12　Right inferior pulmonary vein
13　Right superior pulmonary vein

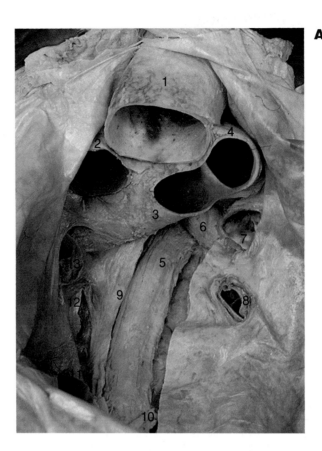

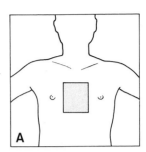

B Intercostal spaces

This dissection shows the medial ends of some intercostal spaces of the right side, viewed from the front and slightly from the right. The pleura has been removed, revealing subcostal muscles (1) laterally, the nerves and vessels (3, 4 and 5) in the intercostal spaces, and the sympathetic trunk (6) and greater splanchnic nerve (8) on the sides of the vertebral bodies (as at 7)

1　Subcostal muscle
2　Eighth rib
3　Eighth posterior intercostal vein
4　Eighth posterior intercostal artery
5　Eighth intercostal nerve
6　Sympathetic trunk and ganglia
7　Body of ninth thoracic vertebra
8　Greater splanchnic nerve

● In the medial part of an intercostal space near the vertebral column, the neurovascular structures lie in the middle of the space; only farther laterally do they take up their positions in the upper part of the space below the costal groove (as shown on page 156, A and B).

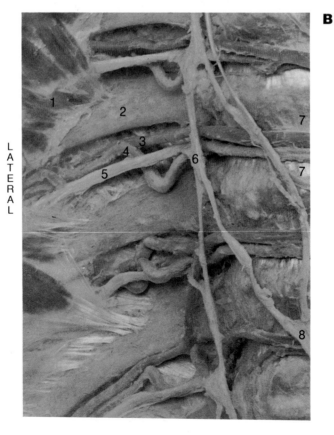

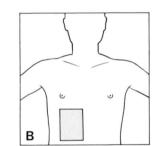

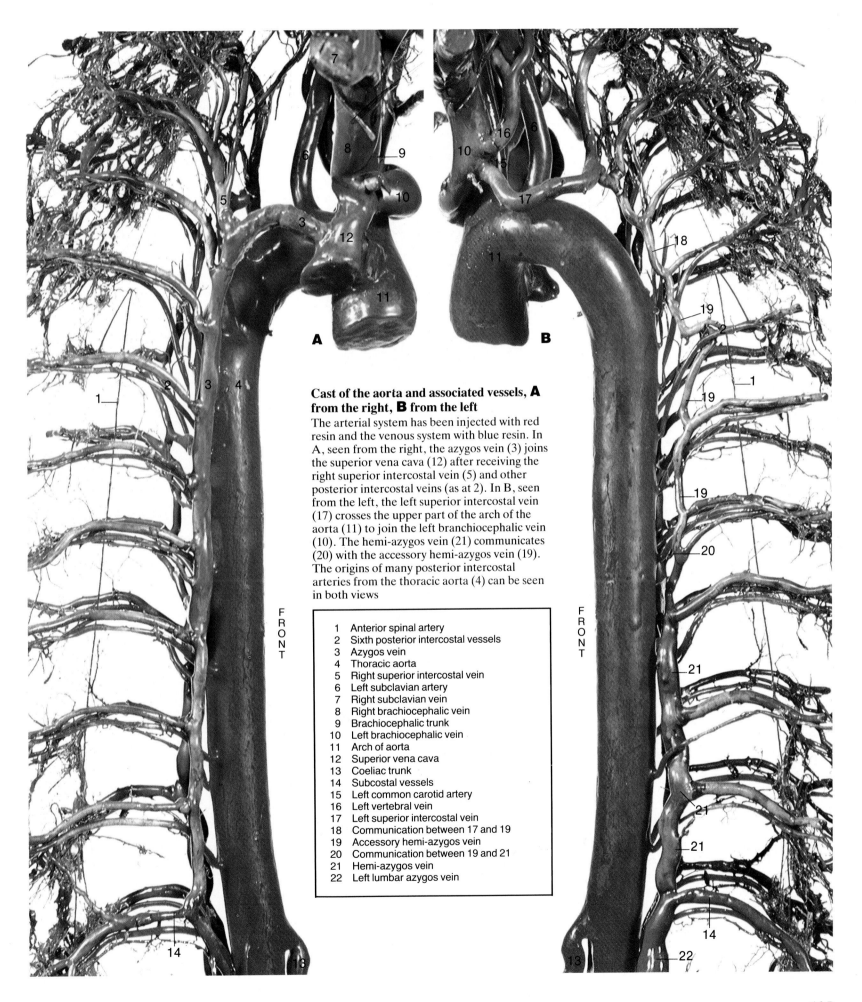

Cast of the aorta and associated vessels, A from the right, B from the left

The arterial system has been injected with red resin and the venous system with blue resin. In A, seen from the right, the azygos vein (3) joins the superior vena cava (12) after receiving the right superior intercostal vein (5) and other posterior intercostal veins (as at 2). In B, seen from the left, the left superior intercostal vein (17) crosses the upper part of the arch of the aorta (11) to join the left branchiocephalic vein (10). The hemi-azygos vein (21) communicates (20) with the accessory hemi-azygos vein (19). The origins of many posterior intercostal arteries from the thoracic aorta (4) can be seen in both views

1	Anterior spinal artery
2	Sixth posterior intercostal vessels
3	Azygos vein
4	Thoracic aorta
5	Right superior intercostal vein
6	Left subclavian artery
7	Right subclavian vein
8	Right brachiocephalic vein
9	Brachiocephalic trunk
10	Left brachiocephalic vein
11	Arch of aorta
12	Superior vena cava
13	Coeliac trunk
14	Subcostal vessels
15	Left common carotid artery
16	Left vertebral vein
17	Left superior intercostal vein
18	Communication between 17 and 19
19	Accessory hemi-azygos vein
20	Communication between 19 and 21
21	Hemi-azygos vein
22	Left lumbar azygos vein

A Joints of the heads of the ribs, from the right

In this part of the right mid-thoracic region, the ribs have been cut short beyond their tubercles, and the joints that the two facets of the head of a rib make with the facets on the sides of adjacent vertebral bodies and the intervening disc are shown, as at 6 to 8, where the radiate ligament (6) covers the capsule of these small synovial joints

1	Neck of rib
2	Superior costotransverse ligament
3	Ventral ramus of spinal nerve
4	Rami communicantes
5	Sympathetic trunk
6	Radiate ligament of joint of head of rib
7	Vertebral body
8	Intervertebral disc
9	Greater splanchnic nerve

B Costotransverse joints, from behind

In this view of the right half of the thoracic vertebral column from behind, costotransverse joints between the transverse processes of vertebrae and the tubercles of ribs are covered by the lateral costotransverse ligaments (as at 5). The dorsal rami of spinal nerves (8) pass medial to the superior costotransverse ligaments (4); ventral rami (7) run in front of these ligaments

1	Spinous process
2	Lamina
3	Transverse process
4	Superior ⎫ costotransverse
5	Lateral ⎭ ligament
6	Costotransverse ligament
7	Ventral ⎫ ramus of
8	Dorsal ⎭ spinal nerve

● There are two types of costovertebral joint—the joints of the heads of the ribs (A and C) with the facets on the vertebral bodies, and the costotransverse joints (B and C) between the articular facets on the tubercles of the ribs and the facets on the transverse processes.
● There are three kinds of costotransverse ligament: *the* costotransverse ligament (B6) between the back of the neck of a rib and the front of the corresponding transverse process; the *lateral* costotransverse ligament (B5), between the tip of a transverse process and the non-articular part of the tubercle of the corresponding rib; and the *superior* costotransverse ligament (B4, C7), having anterior and posterior layers and passing from the (upper) crest of the neck of a rib to the transverse process of the vertebra above.
● The dorsal rami of spinal nerves pass backwards *medial* to the superior costotransverse ligaments (B8), dividing into medial and lateral branches.
● The ventral rami of spinal nerves (B7) pass laterally *in front of* the superior costotransverse ligaments.

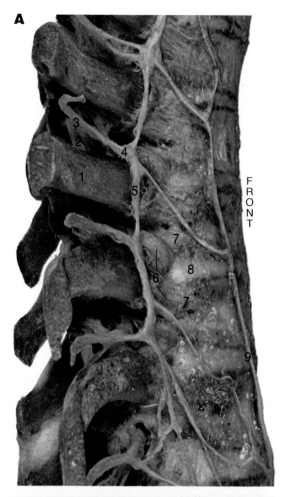

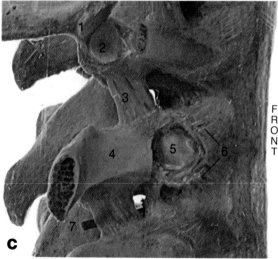

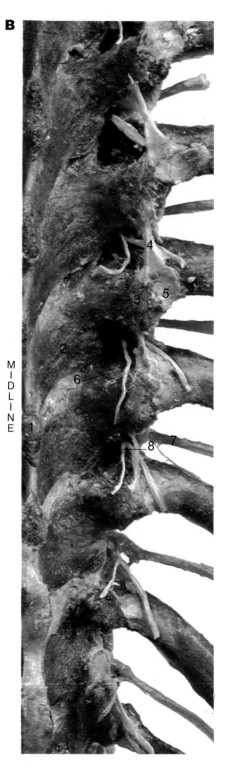

C Costovertebral joints, disarticulated, from the right

In the upper part of the figure, the upper rib has been severed through its neck (4) and the part with the tubercle attached has been turned upwards after cutting through the capsule of the costotransverse joint, to show the articular facet of the tubercle (1) and the transverse process (2). The head of the lower rib has been removed after transecting the radiate ligament (6) and underlying capsule of the joint of the head of the rib (5)

1	Articular facet of tubercle of rib
2	Articular facet of transverse process
3	Superior costotransverse ligament
4	Neck of rib
5	Cavity of joint of head of rib
6	Radiate ligament
7	Marker between anterior and posterior parts of superior costotransverse ligament

A

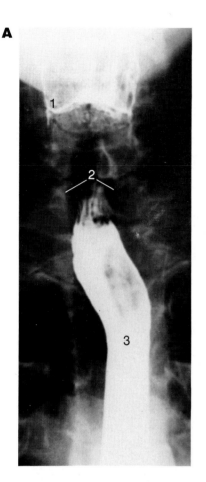

B

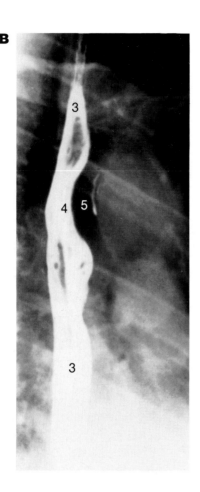

D

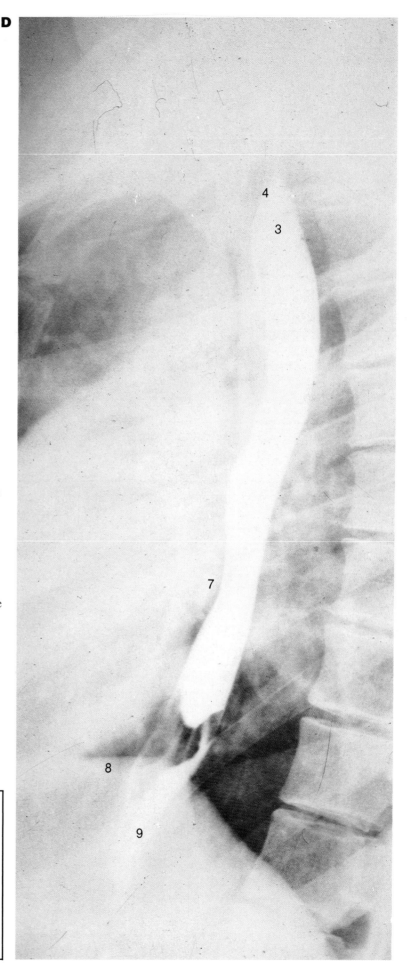

C

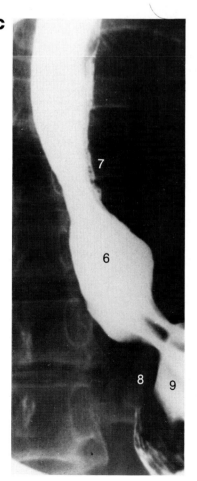

Radiographs of the oesophagus during a barium swallow. A Lower pharynx and upper oesophagus, B middle part, C lower end, D whole length

In A, viewed from the front, some of the barium paste adheres to the pharyngeal wall, outlining the piriform recesses (1), but most of it has passed into the oesophagus (3). In B, viewed obliquely from the left, the oesophagus is indented by the arch of the aorta (5) which shows some calcification in its wall—a useful aid to its identification. In C there is some dilatation at the lower end of the thoracic oesophagus (6) and it is constricted where it passes through the diaphragm (8) to join the stomach (9). The left atrium of the heart lies in front of the lower thoracic oesophagus (page 194, A5), but only when enlarged does the atrium cause an indentation in the oesophagus. In D, the whole length is seen in front of the vertebral column

1	Piriform recess in laryngeal part of pharynx
2	Margins of trachea (translucent with contained air)
3	Barium in oesophagus
4	Aortic impression in oesophagus
5	Arch of aorta with plaque of calcification
6	Lower thoracic oesophagus
7	Position of left atrium
8	Diaphragm
9	Stomach

A

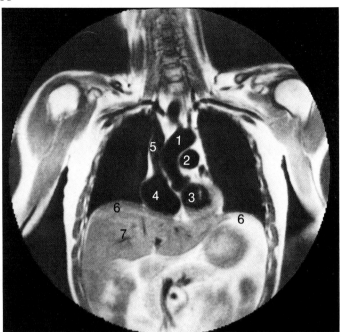

A MRI scan of the thorax (coronal section)

The section shows the heart and great vessels in the mediastinum, above the domes of the diaphragm (6) and liver (7). The plane of the image is through the left ventricle (3) and right atrium (4)

1	Arch of aorta	5	Superior vena cava
2	Pulmonary trunk	6	Dome of diaphragm
3	Left ventricle	7	Liver
4	Right atrium		

B

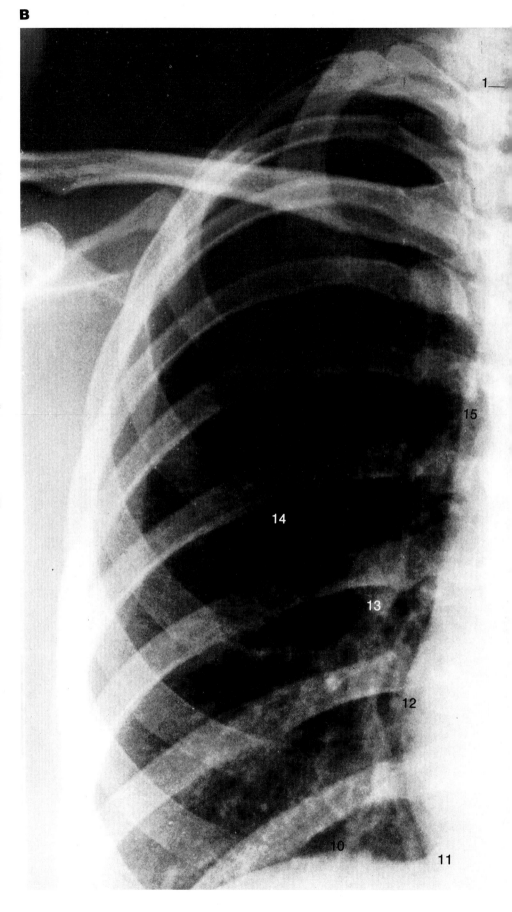

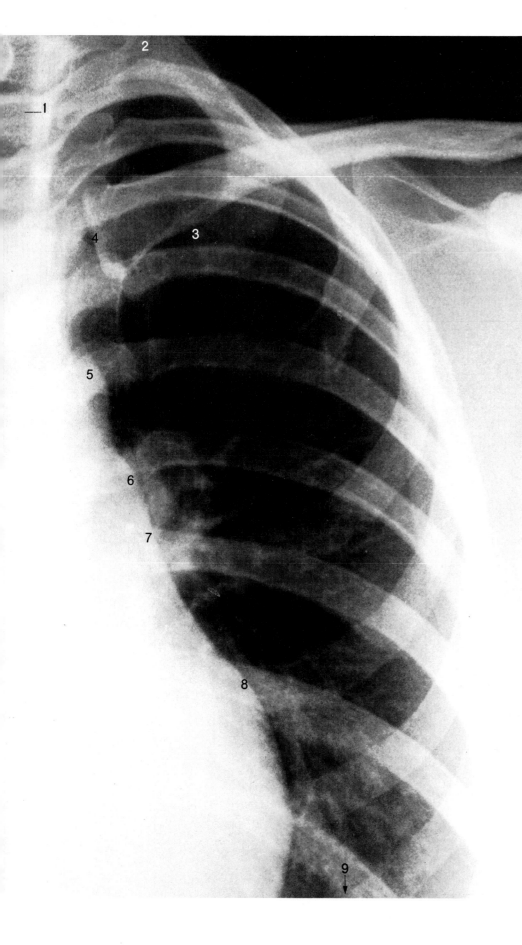

B Radiograph of the thorax

This standard postero-anterior view of the thorax is commonly called a 'straight x-ray of the chest' or 'plain film of the chest'—taken from behind with the film at the front of the thorax. It shows in particular (see notes) the outline of the heart, the hilar regions of the lungs and the more peripheral parts of the lungs (lung fields), and the domes of the diaphragm

1	Margin of trachea
2	Tubercle ⎫ of first rib
3	Anterior end ⎭
4	Sternal end of clavicle
5	Arch of aorta (aortic knuckle)
6	Infundibulum of right ventricle
7	Position of tip of auricle of left atrium
8	Left ventricle
9	Left ⎫ dome of diaphragm
10	Right ⎭
11	Position of inferior vena cava
12	Right atrium
13	Hilar shadows of right lung
14	Anterior end of third rib
15	Superior vena cava

● The shadow of the right border of the heart is formed by the right atrium (12).
● The arch of the aorta (5) produces a characteristic bulge, commonly known radiologically as the aortic knuckle.
● The shadow of the left border of the heart below the aortic knuckle is formed by the infundibulum (outflow tract) of the right ventricle (6) and the left ventricle (8). Contrary to most textbook statements, the auricle of the left atrium (7) does not normally form part of the left margin radiologically; only when enlarged does it do so. Compare this radiograph with the dissection A on page 160, and note how little of the left auricle can be seen there (A4) when looking at the heart from the front.
● The shadows in the hilar regions of the lungs (as at 13) are caused by the pulmonary vessels; when seen end-on they appear as round opacities. The bronchi being filled with air are not radio-opaque but when seen end-on may appear as round translucent areas. The more peripheral parts of the normal lung fields, where the vessels are much smaller, are relatively clear.
● Note the obliquity of the ribs, e.g. from the tubercle (2) to the anterior end (3) of the first rib, and identify the others by counting downwards from it. The normal cartilaginous costal cartilages are not radio-opaque, but their positions can be imagined beyond the anterior ends of the ribs. Thus the third right costal cartilage at the end of the third rib (14) indicates the level at which the superior vena cava (15) enters the right atrium (12).

A

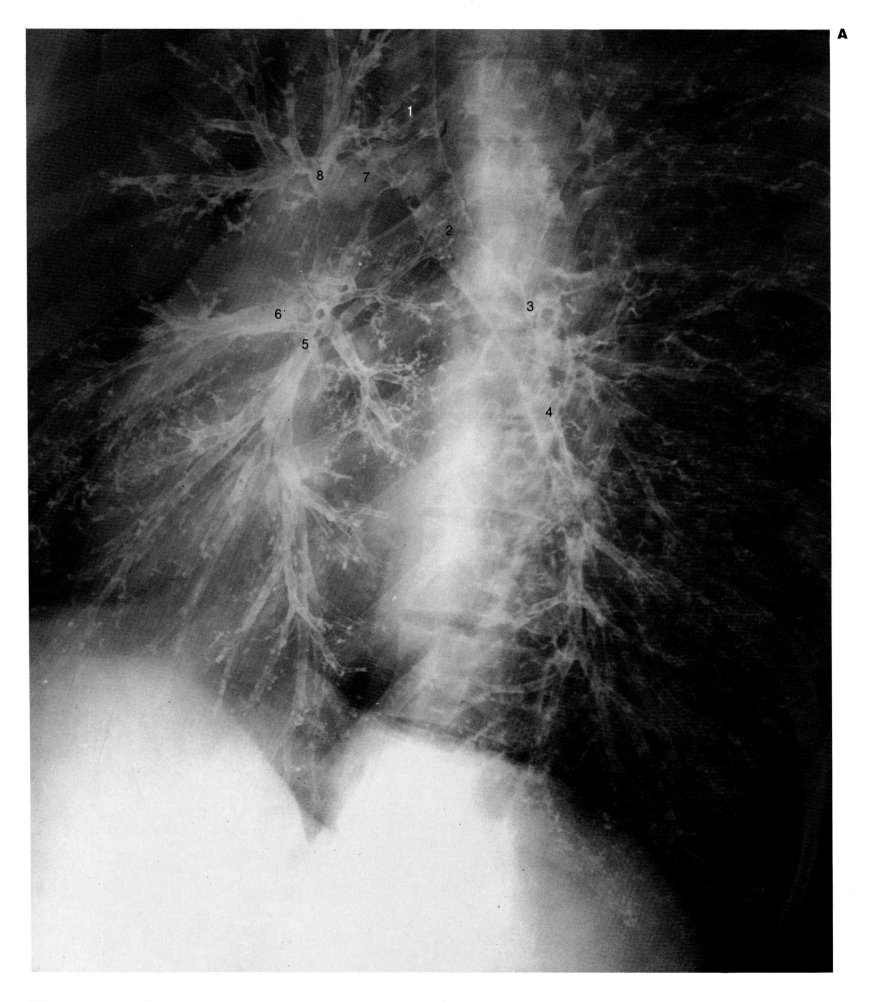

A Bronchogram, viewed obliquely from the front and the left

Bronchograms, which are radiographs taken after the instillation of contrast medium into the trachea and bronchi, are now not commonly performed but provide good demonstrations of the branching pattern of the bronchial tree. In this oblique view only the principal and lobar bronchi are identified. Compare with the cast B on page 187 which when held sideways shows the bronchi in positions very similar to those in which they are seen in this bronchogram

1	Trachea
2	Left principal bronchus
3	Left superior lobe bronchus
4	Left inferior lobe bronchus
5	Right inferior lobe bronchus
6	Right middle lobe bronchus
7	Right principal bronchus
8	Right superior lobe bronchus

B, C, D, E and F CT scans of the thorax

All scans are viewed from below, and are at four different levels: B shows the great arteries (2, 3 and 4) that have arisen from the arch of the aorta (7) seen in C. D is just below the point where the trachea has divided into the two principal bronchi (11 and 12), and in E a pulmonary vein (16) enters the left atrium (15). In F, which is at the same level as D, the image setting has been manipulated to show vessels within the lungs which are not visualized at the settings required for mediastinal structures

1	Superior vena cava
2	Brachiocephalic trunk
3	Left common carotid artery
4	Left subclavian artery
5	Oesophagus
6	Trachea
7	Arch of aorta
8	Azygos vein
9	Ascending aorta
10	Left pulmonary artery
11	Left principal bronchus
12	Right principal bronchus
13	Thoracic (descending) aorta
14	Pulmonary trunk
15	Left atrium
16	Left inferior pulmonary vein
17	Right auricle

B

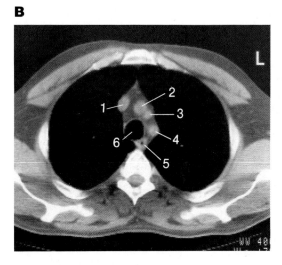

C

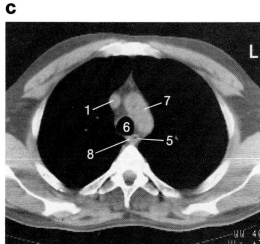

D

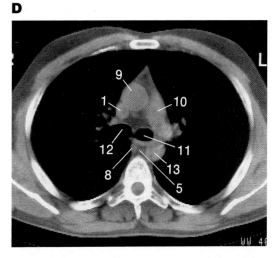

E

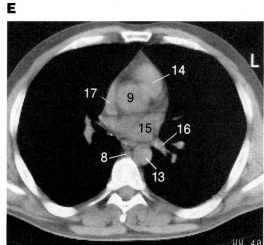

F

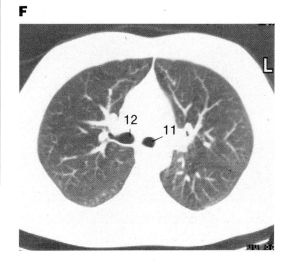

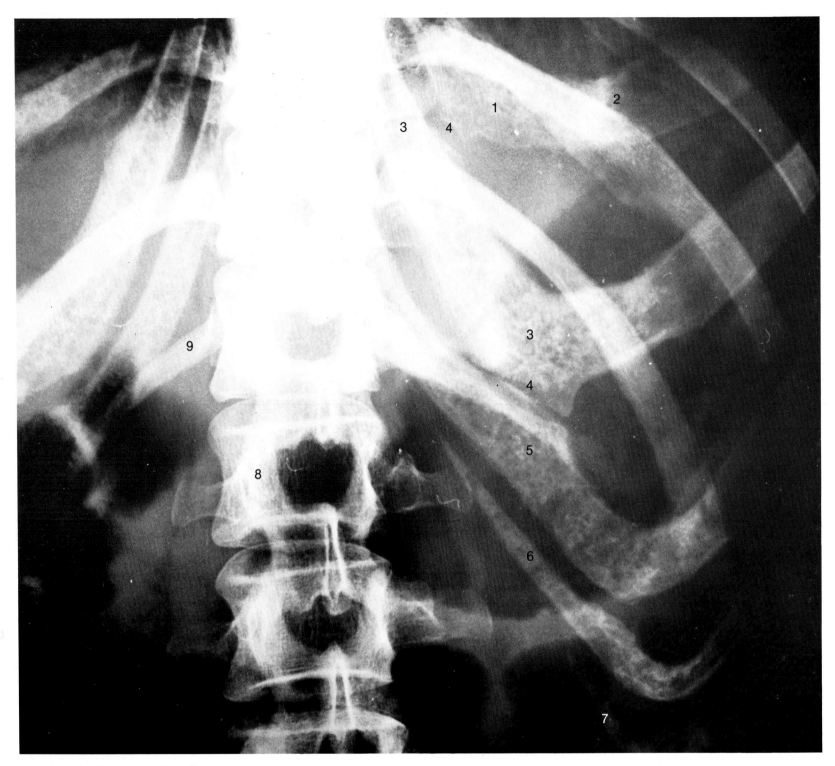

Radiograph of lower costal cartilages

In this radiograph of the lower thorax and costal margins there is some calcification of the costal cartilages which emphasises their outlines

1	Sixth costal cartilage
2	Anterior end of sixth rib
3	Seventh costal cartilage
4	Interchondral joint
5	Eighth ⎤
6	Ninth ⎬ costal cartilage
7	Tenth ⎦
8	First lumbar vertebra
9	Medial end of twelfth rib

● The costal margin on each side is formed by the seventh to tenth costal cartilages (3, 5, 6 and 7 on the left side).
● The seventh costal cartilage (3) is the lowest to join the sternum.
● The tenth costal cartilage (7) forms the lowest part of the margin.

Abdomen and pelvis

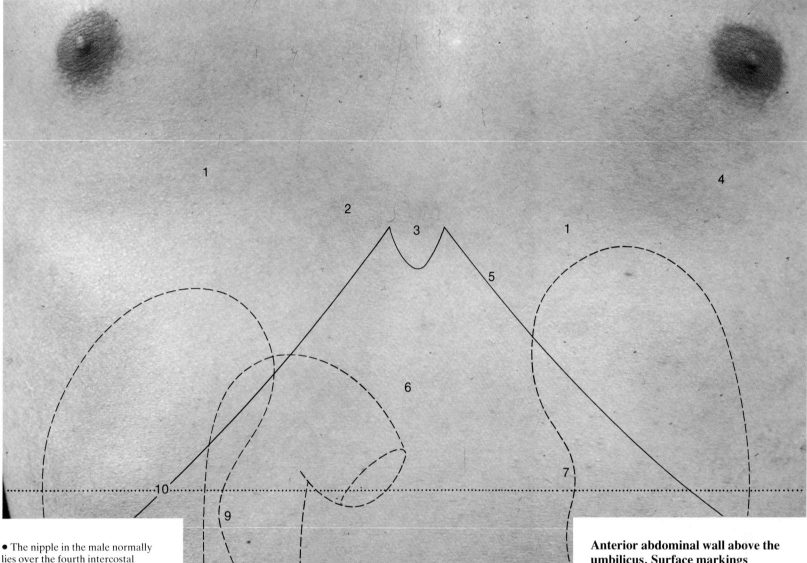

- The nipple in the male normally lies over the fourth intercostal space.
- The umbilicus normally lies at the level of the disc between the third and fourth lumbar vertebrae.
- The transpyloric plane lies midway between the jugular notch of the sternum and the upper border of the pubic symphysis, or approximately a hand's breadth below the xiphisternal joint (3), and level with the lower part of the body of the first lumbar vertebra.
- The foramen for the inferior vena cava in the diaphragm (2) is about 2.5 cm from the midline at the level of the disc between the eighth and ninth thoracic vertebrae.
- The oesophageal opening in the diaphragm (5) is at the level of the tenth thoracic vertebra about 2.5 cm from the midline (but is often near or in the midline).
- The aortic opening in the diaphragm (6) is in the midline at the level of the twelfth thoracic vertebra.
- The hilum of each kidney is about 5 cm from the midline, that of the left (7) being just above the transpyloric plane and that of the right (9) just below it.

- In life the duodenum and the head of the pancreas (8) may lie at one or more vertebral levels lower than in the standard textbook or cadaveric position, shown here.

- The fundus of the gall bladder (10) lies behind the point where the lateral border of the right rectus sheath meets the costal margin at the ninth costal cartilage.

Anterior abdominal wall above the umbilicus. Surface markings

The solid line indicates the costal margin. The transverse dotted line indicates the transpyloric plane. The C-shaped duodenum is outlined by the short interrupted lines, and the kidneys by the longer interrupted lines

1	Dome of diaphragm and upper margin of liver
2	Foramen for inferior vena cava in diaphragm
3	Xiphisternal joint
4	Apex of heart in fifth intercostal space
5	Oesophageal ⎱ opening in
6	Aortic ⎰ diaphragm
7	Hilum of left kidney
8	Head of pancreas and level of second lumbar vertebra
9	Hilum of right kidney
10	Fundus of gall bladder, and junction of ninth costal cartilage and lateral border of rectus sheath

A Anterior abdominal wall, right upper quadrant

In this right upper quadrant of the anterior abdominal wall, above the umbilicus (12), part of the rectus sheath (3) has been removed to show the upper part of rectus abdominis (4) and two of its tendinous intersections (5). The lateral cutaneous branches of intercostal nerves (as at 13, with their anterior ends removed with the overlying skin and fascia) run round on the muscle fibres of the external oblique, which becomes aponeurotic (2) before taking part in the formation of the anterior wall of the rectus sheath (3). The anterior cutaneous branches of intercostal nerves pierce the rectus muscle (as at 6) and then pierce the anterior wall of the sheath (as at 10 and 11)

1	External oblique muscle
2	External oblique aponeurosis
3	Rectus sheath
4	Rectus abdominis
5	Tendinous intersection
6	Anterior cutaneous nerve (eighth intercostal)
7	Linea alba
8	Posterior layer } of internal
9	Anterior layer } oblique aponeurosis
10	Anterior cutaneous nerve (ninth intercostal)
11	Anterior cutaneous nerve (tenth intercostal)
12	Umbilicus
13	Lateral cutaneous nerve (eighth intercostal)

● The rectus sheath (A3) is formed by the internal oblique aponeurosis (B16) which splits at the lateral border of the rectus muscle (B4) into two layers. The posterior (B12) passes behind the muscle to blend with the aponeurosis of transversus abdominis (B7) to form the posterior wall of the sheath (B6), and the anterior layer (B13) passes in front of the muscle to blend with the external oblique aponeurosis (A2) as the anterior wall (A3).
● The anterior and posterior walls of the sheath unite at the medial border of the rectus muscle to form the midline linea alba (A7, B2).
● The tendinous intersections of the rectus muscle (A5, B14) are irregular and usually incomplete fibrous bands which adhere to the anterior wall of the rectus sheath but not to the posterior wall. There are usually three—one below the xiphoid process, one at umbilical level and one between these two—but there may be others (as on page 207, B, unlabelled below the umbilicus).

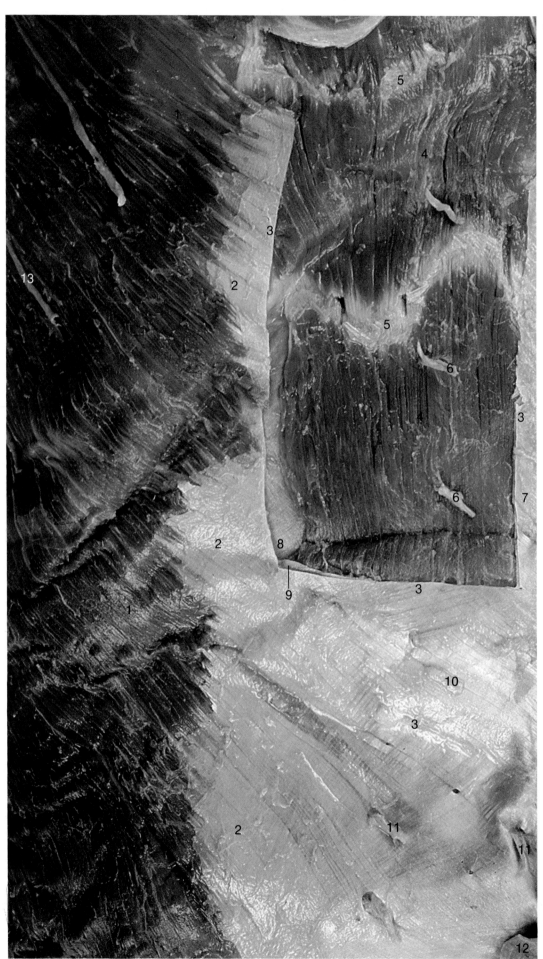

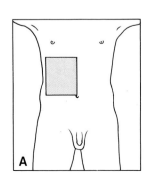

B

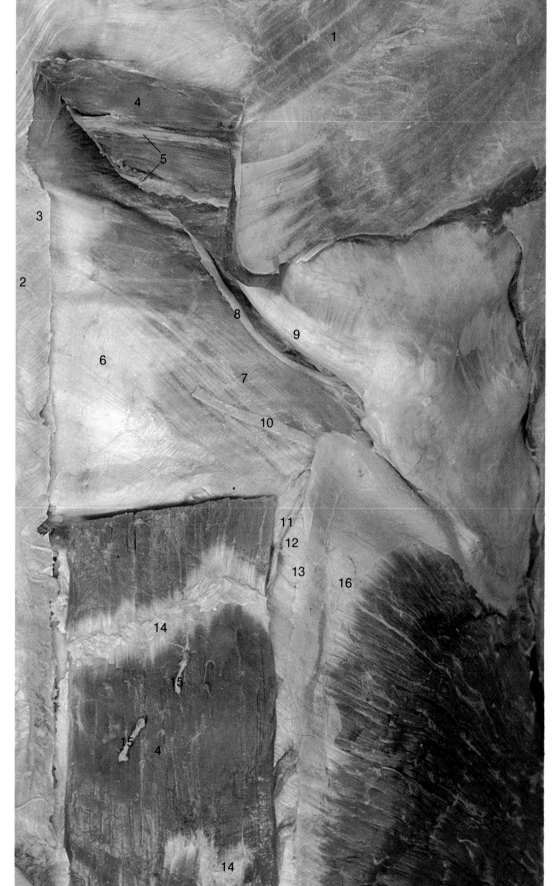

MIDLINE

B Anterior abdominal wall, left upper quadrant

The anterior wall of the rectus sheath and most of the external oblique muscle (1) and aponeurosis have been removed, together with a segment of the rectus muscle (4), whose upper end has been turned upwards to show branches of the superior epigastric vessels (5) on its deep surface. The aponeurosis (16) of the internal oblique muscle (17) splits at the lateral border of the rectus muscle into anterior (13) and posterior (12) layers which, when fused with the external oblique and transversus abdominis aponeuroses respectively, become the anterior (3) and posterior (6) walls of the rectus sheath. Below the costal margin (as at 9) the muscle fibres of transversus abdominis (7) run for some distance behind the rectus muscle before becoming aponeurotic. The seventh intercostal nerve (8) runs upwards parallel with the costal margin under the rectus muscle; other intercostal nerves (as at 11) are seen piercing the posterior layer (12) of the internal oblique aponeurosis before entering the rectus muscle (4)

1	External oblique
2	Linea alba
3	Anterior wall of rectus sheath
4	Rectus abdominis
5	Superior epigastric vessels
6	Posterior wall of rectus sheath
7	Transversus abdominis
8	Seventh intercostal nerve
9	Ninth costal cartilage
10	Eighth intercostal nerve
11	Ninth intercostal nerve
12	Posterior layer ⎫ of internal
13	Anterior layer ⎬ oblique aponeurosis
14	Tendinous intersection
15	Anterior cutaneous nerve (ninth intercostal)
16	Internal oblique aponeurosis
17	Internal oblique muscle
18	Umbilicus

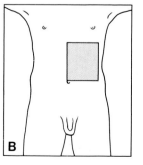

B

A Anterior abdominal wall, right lower quadrant

The external oblique muscle (1) and aponeurosis (2) and the rectus sheath (3) remain intact. Over the inguinal region parts of the fatty layer (7) and fibrous layer (8) of the superficial fascia have been preserved. As the fibrous layer passes down below the level of the upper margin of the pubic symphysis (14) it becomes the superficial perineal fascia (15)

1 External oblique muscle
2 External oblique aponeurosis
3 Anterior wall of rectus sheath
4 Anterior cutaneous nerve
  (eleventh intercostal)
5 Anterior superior iliac spine
6 Inguinal ligament
7 Fatty layer ⎫ of superficial
8 Fibrous layer ⎬ fascia
9 Superficial circumflex iliac artery
10 Superficial epigastric artery
11 A superficial inguinal lymph node
12 Position of saphenous opening
13 Suspensory ligament of penis
14 Level of pubic symphysis
15 Superficial perineal fascia
16 Umbilicus

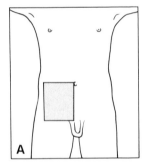

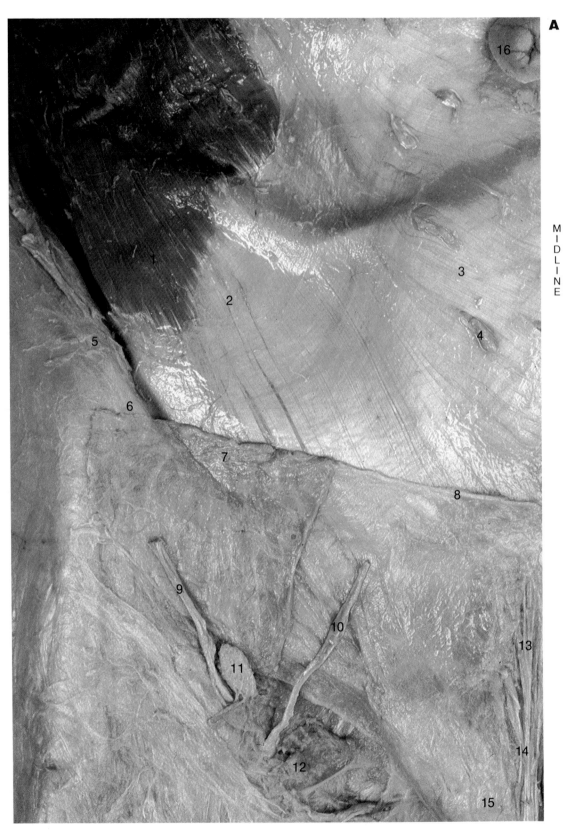

B

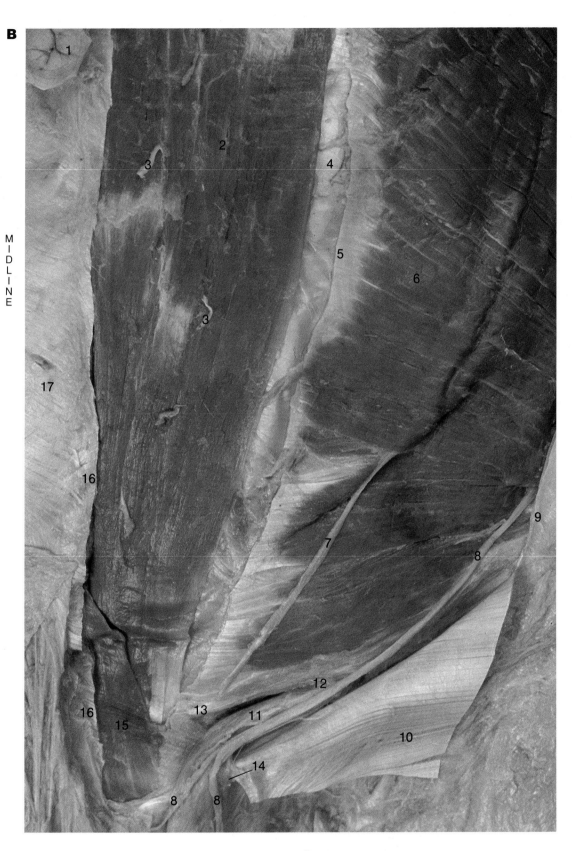

MIDLINE

• For further details of the inguinal canal in the male see pages 208 and 246, and in the female page 247.

B Anterior abdominal wall, left lower quadrant

The anterior wall of the rectus sheath and most of the external oblique have been removed but a small part of the external oblique aponeurosis has been turned down (10) to show the spermatic cord (11) and ilio-inguinal nerve (8) in the inguinal canal. The iliohypogastric nerve (7) is at a higher level and does not enter the inguinal canal

1	Umbilicus
2	Rectus abdominis
3	Anterior cutaneous nerve (eleventh intercostal)
4	Eleventh intercostal nerve
5	Lateral border of rectus sheath
6	Internal oblique
7	Iliohypogastric nerve
8	Ilio-inguinal nerve
9	Anterior superior iliac spine
10	External oblique aponeurosis
11	Spermatic cord
12	Margin of deep inguinal ring
13	Conjoint tendon
14	External spermatic fascia and margin of superficial inguinal ring
15	Pyramidalis
16	Medial border of rectus sheath
17	Linea alba

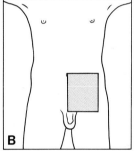

C CT scan of the lower abdomen

Viewed from below looking towards the thorax (as are all scans of the trunk), the rectus abdominis muscles (RA) are seen on either side of the midline of the anterior abdominal wall, and continuing backwards from them the three flat anterolateral muscles (external and internal obliques and transversus) can be distinguished as a 'sandwich' (M)

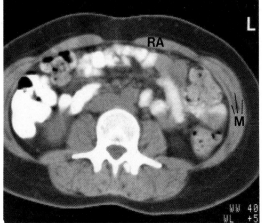

C

● McBurney's point (4) indicates the opening of the appendix into the caecum, and lies at the junction of the lateral and middle thirds of a line drawn from the anterior superior iliac spine (3) to the umbilicus.

● The superficial inguinal ring (9, at the medial end of the inguinal canal) lies 1 cm above the pubic tubercle (8).

● The deep inguinal ring (15, at the lateral end of the inguinal canal) lies 1 cm above the midpoint of the inguinal ligament.

● The femoral artery (12, whose pulsation should normally be palpable) enters the thigh midway between the pubic symphysis (7) and the anterior superior iliac spine (3).

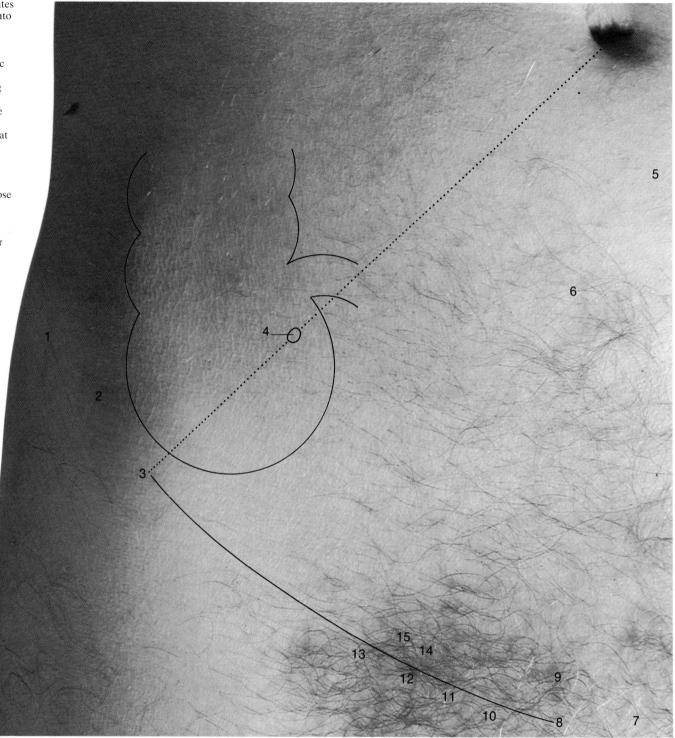

Anterior abdominal wall, right lower quadrant. Surface markings

The caecum with the ileum opening into it from the left and the ascending colon continuing upwards from it are indicated by the continuous line. McBurney's point (4; see notes) overlies the opening of the appendix into the caecum, and is on the line (here dotted) from the anterior superior iliac spine (3) to the umbilicus. The inguinal ligament, between the anterior superior iliac spine (3) and the pubic tubercle (8), is indicated by the interrupted line. The femoral artery (12) has the femoral vein (11) on its medial side and the femoral nerve (13) on its lateral side. The femoral canal (10) is on the medial side of the vein. The deep inguinal ring (15) and inferior epigastric vessels (14) are above the artery, while the superficial inguinal ring (9) is above the pubic tubercle (8)

1	Tubercle of iliac crest	8	Pubic tubercle
2	Iliac crest	9	Superficial inguinal ring
3	Anterior superior iliac spine	10	Femoral canal
4	McBurney's point	11	Femoral vein
5	Bifurcation of aorta (fourth lumbar vertebra)	12	Femoral artery
6	Lower end of inferior vena cava (fifth lumbar vertebra)	13	Femoral nerve
		14	Inferior epigastric vessels
7	Pubic symphysis	15	Deep inguinal ring

A

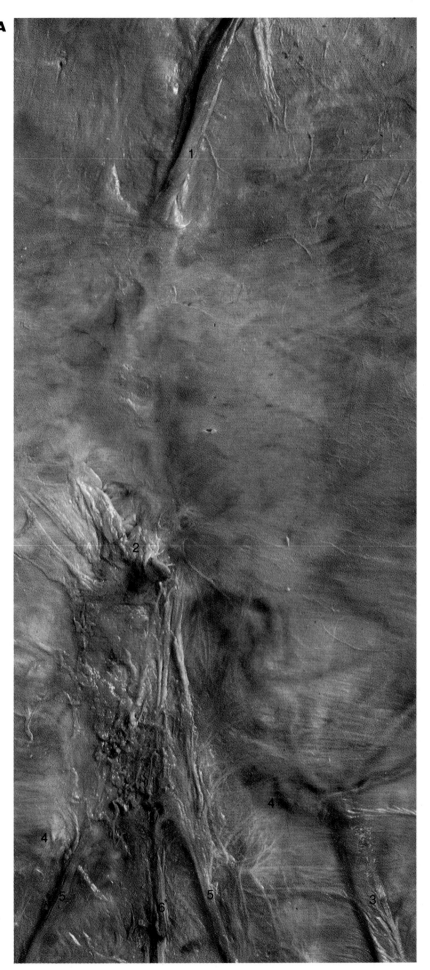

B

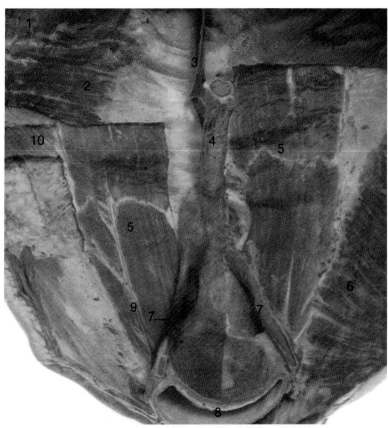

A Anterior abdominal wall, from behind. Umbilical folds

This view of the peritoneal surface of the central region of the anterior abdominal wall shows the peritoneal folds raised by underlying structures. There is one fold above the umbilicus—the falciform ligament (1)—and there are five below it: the median umbilical fold (6) in the midline, and a pair of medial and lateral umbilical folds on each side (5 and 3). See the notes for the contents of the folds

1	Falciform ligament	4	Arcuate line
2	Umbilicus	5	Medial umbilical fold
3	Lateral umbilical fold	6	Median umbilical fold

B Fetal anterior abdominal wall, from behind

In this full-term fetus the peritoneum and extraperitoneal tissues have been removed from the anterior abdominal wall to show the umbilical arteries (7) and left umbilical vein (4) converging at the back of the (unlabelled) umbilicus

1	Diaphragm	6	Internal oblique
2	Transversus abdominis	7	Umbilical artery
3	Falciform ligament	8	Urinary bladder
4	Left umbilical vein	9	Inferior epigastric vessels
5	Rectus abdominis	10	External oblique

● The falciform ligament (A1) contains the ligamentum teres, which is the obliterated remains of the left umbilical vein (B4). In A the ligamentum teres has not raised a fold until some distance above the umbilicus.

● The median umbilical fold (A6) contains the median umbilical ligament, which is the obliterated remains of the urachus (formed from the allantois, the embryonic connexion between the bladder and umbilicus).

● The medial umbilical fold (A5) contains the medial umbilical ligament, which is the obliterated remains of the umbilical artery (B7).

● The lateral umbilical fold (A3) contains the inferior epigastric vessels, conducting them from the external iliac vessels to the rectus sheath. Although called an umbilical fold, it does not extend as far as the umbilicus, since the vessels enter the rectus sheath by passing beneath the arcuate line (A4), which is the lower border of the posterior wall of the sheath. Below this level the three aponeuroses that form the sheath (page 204) all pass in front of the rectus muscle.

A

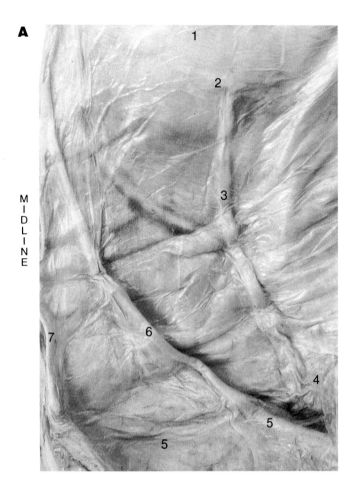

MIDLINE

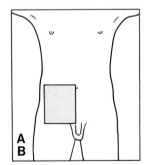

B

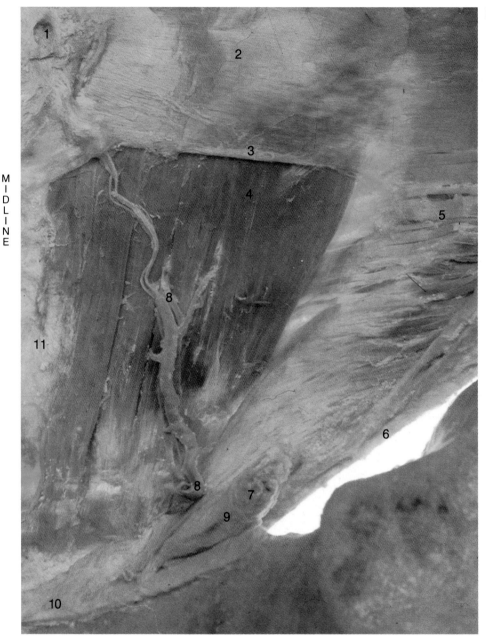

MIDLINE

A Anterior abdominal wall, right side, from behind

This view shows the posterior surface of the anterior abdominal wall to the right of the midline and above the pelvic brim (5), with the peritoneum intact. The medial umbilical fold (6) is prominent, and the inferior epigastric vessels (3) are seen passing deep to the arcuate line (2)

1	Posterior layer of rectus sheath
2	Arcuate line
3	Inferior epigastric vessels in lateral umbilical fold
4	Position of deep inguinal ring
5	Pelvic brim
6	Medial umbilical fold
7	Median umbilical fold

B Anterior abdominal wall, right side, from behind

In a similar specimen to that in A, the peritoneum and extraperitoneal tissues have been removed, leaving the inferior epigastric vessels (8) coursing over the back of the rectus muscle (4) to enter the rectus sheath (2) beneath the arcuate line (3)

1	Umbilicus
2	Posterior wall of rectus sheath
3	Arcuate line
4	Rectus abdominis
5	Transversus abdominis
6	Inguinal ligament
7	Spermatic cord
8	Inferior epigastric vessels
9	Position of deep inguinal ring
10	Pubic crest
11	Linea alba

● The arcuate line (A2, B3) is sometimes called the semicircular fold (not to be confused with the semilunar line, which is the name sometimes given to the lateral border of the rectus sheath, nor with the arcuate line of the ilium—page 267, 12).
● The umbilicus is a midline scar in the anterior abdominal wall at the level of the disc between the third and fourth lumbar vertebrae (page 203). It contains on its deep (posterior) surface the obliterated remains of the two umbilical arteries (page 209, B7), the left umbilical vein (page 209, B4), the urachus and perhaps the remains of the vitello-intestinal duct (which normally disappears completely; in early fetal life it connected the yolk sac to the intestine. If the intestinal end persists it forms the ileal or Meckel's diverticulum which when present is about 60 cm from the ileocaecal junction).
● The right umbilical vein disappears very early in development; it is the left one which persists and eventually becomes the ligamentum teres within the falciform ligament (page 209, A1).
●For notes on the peritoneal folds see previous page.

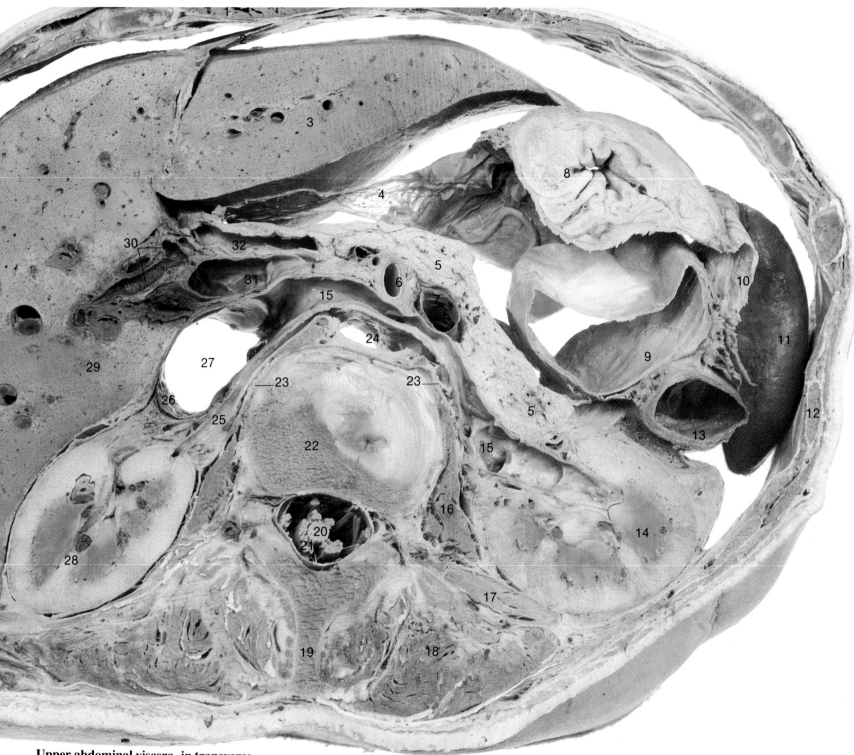

Upper abdominal viscera, in transverse section

This section through the upper abdomen at the level of the first lumbar vertebra, seen from below looking towards the thorax, shows the general disposition of some of the viscera. The vertebral column (22) bulges forwards into the abdominal cavity, with the kidneys (14 and 28) lying in the trough on either side. The bulk of the liver (29) is on the right side, extending towards the left (3) to overlap part of the stomach (8), and the pancreas (5) lies centrally, also extending towards the left (but on a deeper plane) to overlap part of the left kidney (14). Parts of the colon (9 and 13) are adjacent to the spleen (11) which lies against the part of the diaphragm attached to the thoracic wall in the region of the tenth rib (12)

1	Right rectus abdominis	17	Quadratus lumborum
2	Falciform ligament	18	Erector spinae
3	Left lobe of liver	19	Spine of first lumbar vertebra
4	Lesser omentum	20	Conus medullaris of spinal cord
5	Pancreas	21	Nerve roots of cauda equina
6	Superior mesenteric artery	22	Body of first lumbar vertebra
7	Splenic vein	23	Sympathetic trunk
8	Stomach	24	Abdominal aorta
9	Transverse colon	25	Right renal artery
10	Greater omentum	26	Right renal vein
11	Spleen	27	Inferior vena cava
12	Tenth rib	28	Right kidney
13	Descending colon	29	Right lobe of liver
14	Left kidney	30	Hepatic ducts
15	Left renal vein	31	Portal vein
16	Psoas major	32	Hepatic artery

A Upper abdominal viscera, from the front

The thoracic and abdominal walls and the anterior part of the diaphragm have been removed to show the undisturbed viscera. The liver (5 and 6) and stomach (7) are immediately below the diaphragm (3). The greater omentum (9) hangs down from the greater curvature (lower margin) of the stomach (7), overlying much of the small and large intestine but leaving some of the transverse colon (11) and small intestine (10) uncovered. The fundus (tip) of the gall bladder (12) is seen between the right lobe of the liver (5) and transverse colon (11)

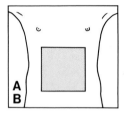

1	Inferior lobe of right lung
2	Pericardial fat
3	Diaphragm
4	Falciform ligament
5	Right lobe of liver
6	Left lobe of liver
7	Stomach
8	Inferior lobe of left lung
9	Greater omentum
10	Small intestine
11	Transverse colon
12	Gall bladder

● For an explanation of peritoneal structures see the diagrams on page 219.

B Upper abdominal viscera, from the front

In this view of the undisturbed abdomen the upper part of the greater omentum (as at 5) overlies much of the transverse colon and mesocolon (with the right part of the transverse colon seen at 11).

The lower part of the omentum (6) covers coils of small intestine, some of which (7) are visible beyond the right margin of the omentum. The caecum (8) is at the lower end of the ascending colon (9) which continues upwards into the right colic flexure (hepatic flexure, 10) and then becomes the transverse colon (11)

1	Right lobe of liver
2	Falciform ligament
3	Left lobe of liver
4	Stomach
5	Greater omentum overlying transverse colon and mesocolon
6	Greater omentum overlying coils of small intestine
7	Small intestine
8	Caecum
9	Ascending colon
10	Right colic flexure
11	Transverse colon
12	Fundus of gall bladder

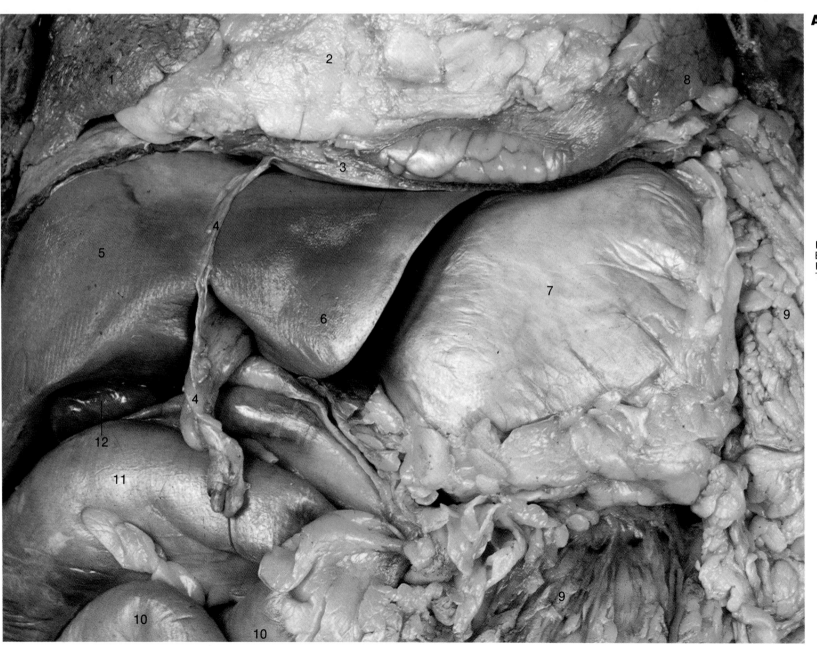

A

RIGHT

LEFT

B

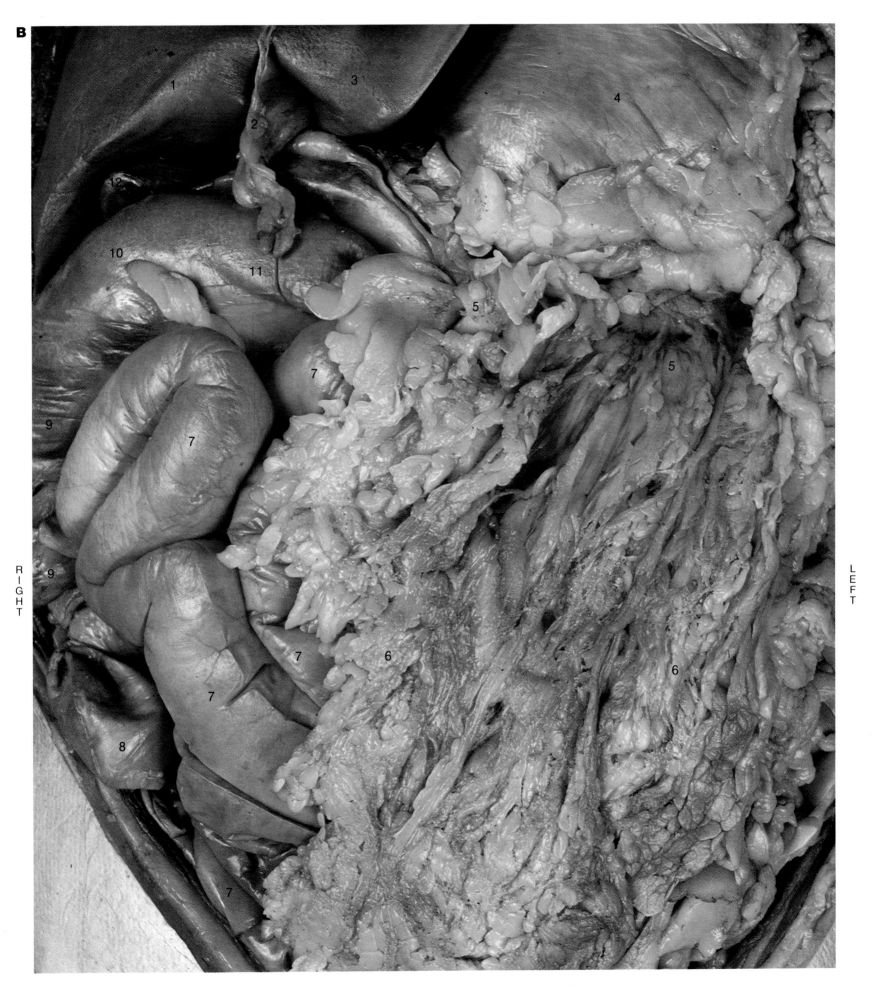

RIGHT

LEFT

A Upper abdominal viscera, from the front

In this view of the same specimen as on pages 212 and 213, the greater omentum (4) has been lifted upwards to show its adherence to the transverse colon (5) (see page 219)

1	Right lobe of liver
2	Falciform ligament
3	Left lobe of liver
4	Posterior surface of greater omentum
5	Transverse colon
6	Appendices epiploicae
7	Small intestine
8	Gall bladder

● For further details of the peritoneum and greater omentum in a less obese subject, see pages 216 to 218.
● The appendices epiploicae (A6) are fat-filled appendages of peritoneum on the various parts of the colon (ascending, transverse, descending and sigmoid). They are not present on the small intestine or the rectum, and may be rudimentary on the caecum and appendix. In abdominal operations they are one feature that helps to distinguish colon from other parts of the intestine.

● In strict anatomical nomenclature the term 'small intestine' includes the duodenum, jejunum and ileum, but clinically it is frequently used to mean jejunum and ileum, with the duodenum being referred to by its own name.
● The parts of the duodenum are properly called superior, descending, horizontal and ascending, but are more commonly known as the first, second, third and fourth parts respectively.

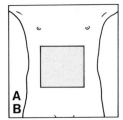

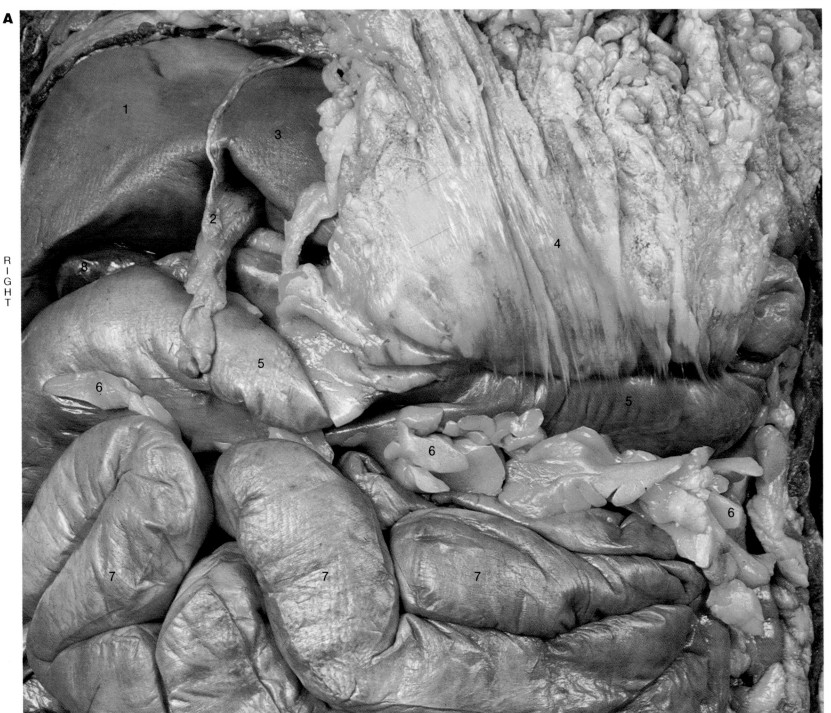

B

FRONT

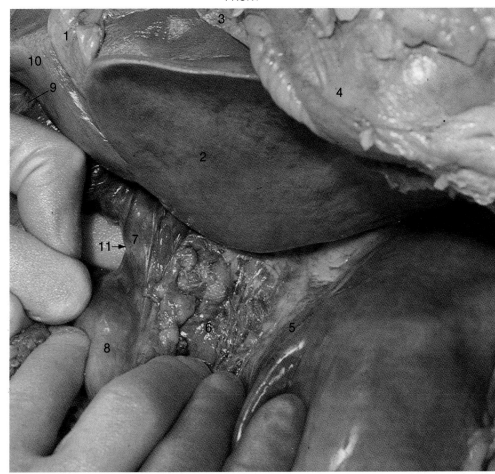

LEFT

C

HEAD

FRONT

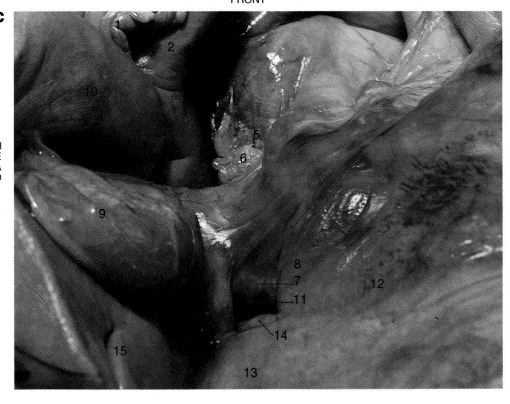

Lesser omentum and epiploic foramen, **B** from the front, **C** from the right

In B a finger has been placed in the epiploic foramen (11) behind the right free margin of the lesser omentum (7), and the tip can be seen in the lesser sac, through the transparent lesser omentum (6) which stretches between the liver (2) and the lesser curvature of the stomach (5). In the side view in C, seen from the right with the body lying on its back (with the head to the left), the foramen (11) is identified between the right free margin of the lesser omentum (7) in front and the inferior vena cava (14) behind, above the first part of the duodenum (8)

1	Falciform ligament
2	Left lobe of liver
3	Diaphragm
4	Pericardium
5	Lesser curvature of stomach
6	Lesser omentum
7	Right free margin of lesser omentum
8	Superior (first) part of duodenum
9	Gall bladder
10	Quadrate lobe of liver
11	Epiploic foramen
12	Descending (second) part of duodenum
13	Upper pole of right kidney
14	Inferior vena cava
15	Right lobe of liver

● The epiploic foramen (of Winslow, B11 and C11) is the communication between the general peritoneal cavity (sometimes called the greater sac) and the lesser sac (omental bursa), a space lined by peritoneum behind the stomach (5) and lesser omentum (B6 and B7) and in front of parts of the pancreas and left kidney.
● The epiploic foramen, the opening into the lesser sac (11), has the following boundaries:

Behind—the inferior vena cava (C14).
In front—the right free margin of the lesser omentum (B7) which contains the portal vein, hepatic artery and bile duct (page 220, A22, 21 and 18). The portal vein is the most posterior of these structures, so the foramen may be said to lie between the two great veins—inferior vena cava and portal vein.
Below—the first part of the duodenum (8 in B and C) which passes backwards as well as to the right.
Above—the caudate process of the liver (page 227, B18).

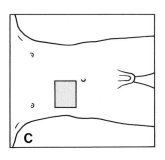

C

A Upper abdominal viscera, from the front

The stomach (4 and 7) is contracted and the lesser curvature (5) sufficiently low to allow the pancreas to be seen through the lesser omentum (3). The transverse colon (13) is very tortuous, and the greater omentum (9) is rather sparse and short, not covering much of the transverse colon and ending with its lower free border above the segments of small intestine labelled 11. For a dissection of this specimen see page 220

1	Gall bladder	9	Greater omentum overlying transverse mesocolon and transverse colon
2	Left lobe of liver	10	Descending colon
3	Lesser omentum overlying pancreas	11	Small intestine and mesentery
4	Body ⎫	12	Ascending colon
5	Lesser curvature ⎬ of stomach	13	Transverse colon
6	Greater curvature ⎪	14	Superior (first) part of duodenum
7	Pyloric part ⎭		
8	Position of pylorus		

● The pyloric part of the stomach (A7) consists of the pyloric antrum, pyloric canal and the pylorus.
● The distal end of the pyloric antrum narrows to become the pyloric canal, and the pylorus (A8) is a sphincter formed by a thickening of the circular layer of gastric muscle at the gastroduodenal junction.

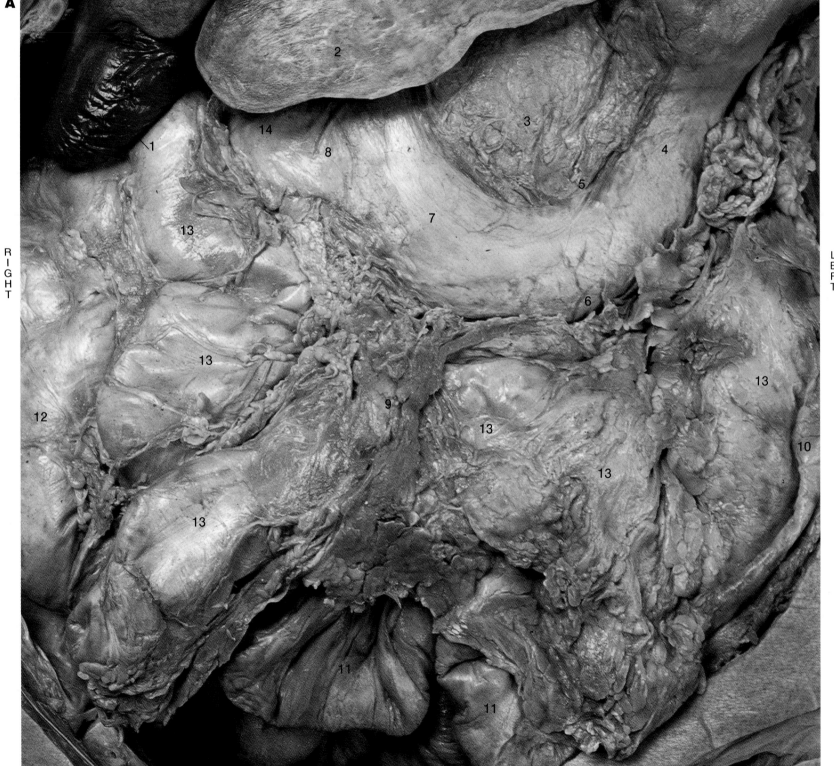

RIGHT

LEFT

FRONT

B

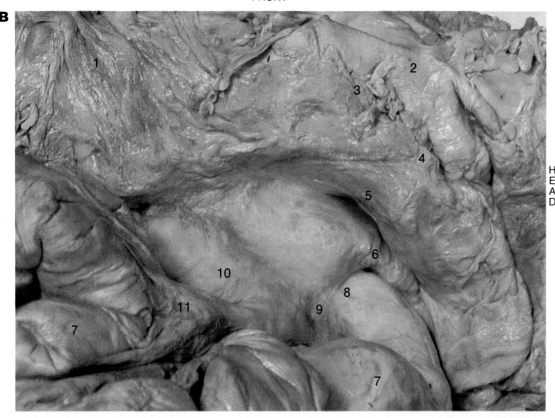

HEAD

B Upper abdominal viscera, from the left and below

In this view from the left with the body lying on its back (with the head to the right), the stomach (4 and 5), transverse colon (2) and greater omentum (1) have been lifted up to show the region of the duodenojejunal flexure (8). The left end of the horizontal part of the duodenum (10) turns upwards (to the right as seen here) as the ascending part (9) which is continuous with the jejunum at the duodenojejunal flexure (8) below the lower border of the pancreas (6)

1	Greater omentum (posterior surface)
2	Transverse colon (posterior surface)
3	Transverse mesocolon (posterior surface)
4	Greater ⎫
5	Lesser ⎬ curvature of stomach
6	Lower border of pancreas
7	Jejunum
8	Duodenojejunal flexure
9	Ascending (fourth) ⎫
10	Horizontal (third) ⎬ part of duodenum
11	Mesentery

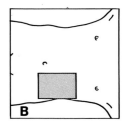
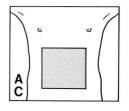

C

RIGHT

LEFT

C Lesser sac and transverse mesocolon, from the front

The greater omentum (1) hanging down from the greater curvature of the stomach (2) has been separated from the underlying transverse colon (7) and mesocolon (6) and lifted upwards, and an opening made into the lesser sac (as in E on page 219). This view therefore shows the posterior surface of the greater omentum (1), stomach and lesser omentum (4), and the anterior surface of the transverse mesocolon (6)

1	Greater omentum (posterior surface)
2	Greater ⎫
3	Lesser ⎬ curvature of stomach
4	Lesser omentum (posterior surface)
5	Peritoneum of lesser sac overlying pancreas
6	Transverse mesocolon
7	Transverse colon
8	Mesentery
9	Coils of jejunum and ileum

• The greater omentum (A9) hanging down from the greater curvature of the stomach (A6) overlies the transverse mesocolon and transverse colon (A13) and fuses with them (as in A), so that when the greater omentum is lifted up the transverse colon is lifted also (as in B1, 2 and 3). When the greater omentum (C1) is dissected off the transverse colon (C7) and mesocolon (C6) and lifted up (as in C), the transverse colon is left behind, suspended from the lower border of the pancreas (C5) by its mesocolon (C6).

217

A Mesentery and descending colon, from the left

With the body lying on its back and seen from the left (with the head to the right), the stomach (6) and transverse colon (7) have been displaced upwards to show the left end of the root of the mesentery (3) at the duodenojejunal flexure (5). The descending colon (9) which is retroperitoneal becomes the sigmoid colon (11) when it ceases to be retroperitoneal and acquires a mesocolon (12)

```
 1   Coils of jejunum and ileum
 2   Mesentery
 3   Root of mesentery
 4   Horizontal (third) part of duodenum
 5   Duodenojejunal flexure
 6   Greater curvature of stomach
 7   Transverse colon
 8   Left colic flexure
 9   Descending colon
10   Peritoneum overlying external iliac vessels
11   Sigmoid colon
12   Sigmoid mesocolon
```

• The root of the mesentery (A3) begins at the duodenojejunal flexure (A5) and passes downwards and to the right, crossing the horizontal part of the duodenum (A4); the superior mesenteric vessels enter the mesentery at this point (see page 221).

• The sigmoid colon (A11), like the transverse colon, has its own mesentery, the sigmoid mesocolon (A12).

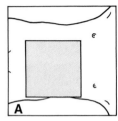

FRONT

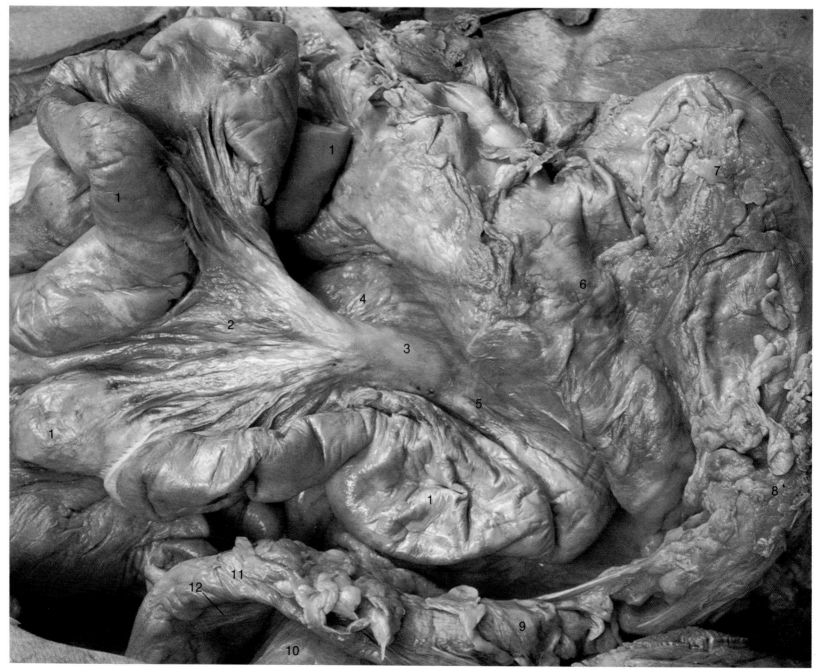

HEAD

FRONT

B

HEAD

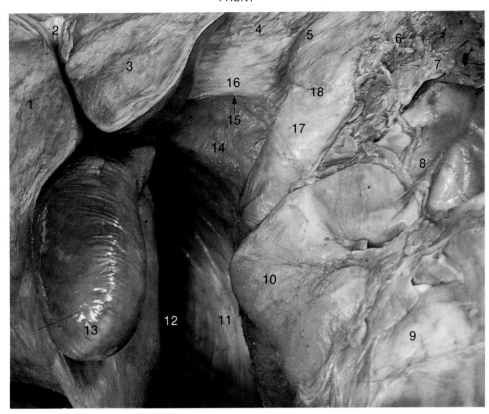

B Hepatorenal pouch of peritoneum, from the right and below

With the body lying on its back and seen from the right (with the head towards the left), the liver (1) has been turned upwards (towards the left) to open up the gap between the liver and the upper pole of the right kidney (11)—the hepatorenal pouch of peritoneum (12, Morison's pouch or the right subhepatic compartment of the peritoneal cavity)

1	Right lobe of liver
2	Falciform ligament
3	Left lobe of liver
4	Lesser omentum overlying pancreas
5	Lesser ⎫ curvature of stomach
6	Greater ⎭
7	Greater omentum
8	Transverse colon
9	Ascending colon
10	Right colic flexure
11	Upper pole of right kidney
12	Hepatorenal (Morison's) pouch
13	Gall bladder
14	Inferior vena cava
15	Epiploic foramen
16	Right free margin of lesser omentum
17	Superior (first) part of duodenum
18	Gastroduodenal junction

● The upper boundary of the hepatorenal pouch is the inferior layer of the coronary ligament, where the peritoneum is reflected from the lower margin of the bare area of the liver to the upper pole of the right kidney (see page 227).

B

Diagrams of peritoneum. C Normal position, D with the lower part of the greater omentum lifted up, E with the greater omentum lifted up and separated from the transverse mesocolon and colon, with an opening into the lesser sac, F with the greater omentum and transverse mesocolon and colon lifted up, with an opening into the lesser sac

These drawings of a sagittal section through the middle of the abdomen, viewed from the left, illustrate theoretically how the peritoneum forms the lesser omentum (L, passing down to the stomach, S), greater omentum (G), transverse mesocolon (TM) passing to the transverse colon, and the mesentery (M) of the small intestine (SI). The layer in blue represents the peritoneum of the lesser sac. The superior mesenteric artery passes between the head and uncinate process of the pancreas

(P and U), and continues across the duodenum (D) into the mesentery (M) to the small intestine (SI), giving off the middle colic artery which runs in the transverse mesocolon (TM) to the transverse colon (TC). The greater omentum (G) is formed by four layers fused together and also fused with the front of the transverse mesocolon (TM, two layers) and transverse colon. On dissection, no separation between any layers is possible except between the greater omentum and the transverse mesocolon. The six layers between the stomach and transverse colon are sometimes collectively known as the gastrocolic omentum. C corresponds to the dissections on pages 212 and 213, D to page 214, E to page 217C, and F to page 222. The arrows in E and F indicate the layers cut to make artificial openings into the lesser sac

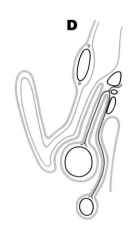
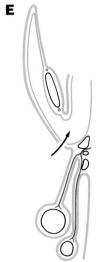
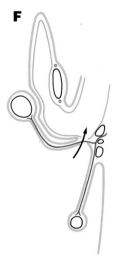
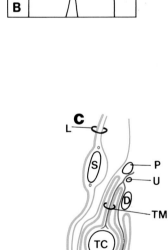
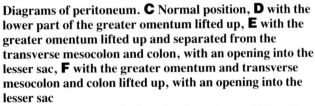

A

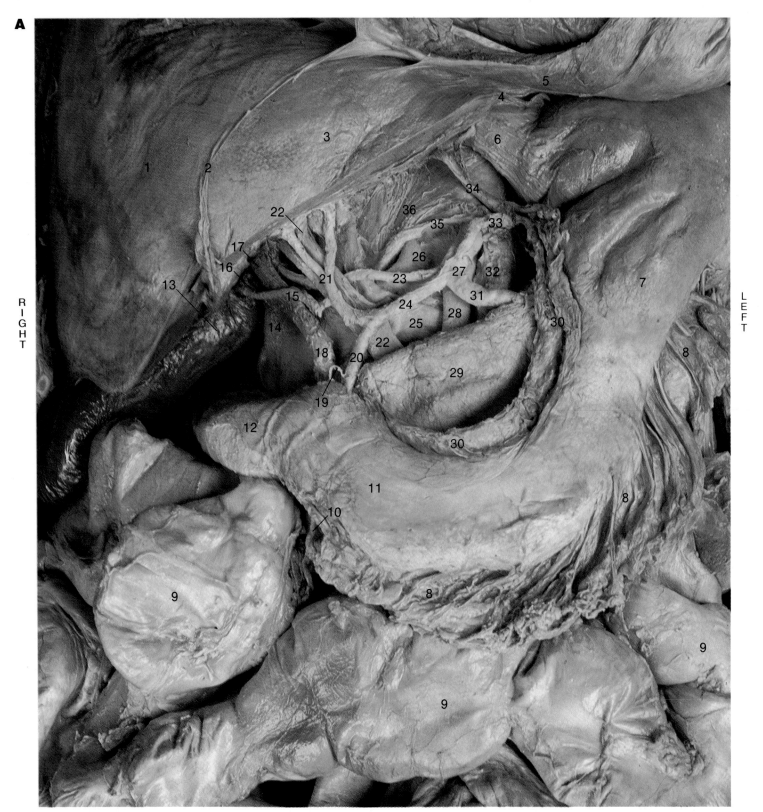

RIGHT

LEFT

- The portal vein (22), hepatic artery (21) and bile duct (18) are contained within the right free margin of the lesser omentum, the duct being the structure farthest to the right.
- The cystic artery (15) is normally derived from the right branch of the hepatic artery and passes behind the common hepatic and cystic ducts. Here it comes from the hepatic artery itself (21) and passes in front of the bile duct (18).
- If an accessory hepatic artery is present (as in this specimen, 23) it passes *behind* the portal vein (22), not in front like the normal artery.

- It is normal for the right gastric artery (19) to be much smaller than the left (33).
- The coeliac trunk (27) gives off three branches: the left gastric artery (33), the splenic artery (31) and the common hepatic artery (24).
- The left gastric artery (33) passes upwards and to the left and then turns down to run along the lesser curvature of the stomach between the two layers of peritoneum that form the lesser omentum (30). It gives off an oesophageal branch which passes up through the oesophageal opening in the diaphragm and supplies the lower part of the oesophagus (6). The accompanying

veins (not shown here) drain to the left gastric vein and thence to the portal vein, making the lower end of the oesophagus one of the most important sites of portal–systemic anastomosis (see page 224, A6).
- The splenic artery (31) passes to the left along the upper border of the pancreas (29).
- The common hepatic artery (24) passes to the right, to give off the gastroduodenal artery (20) and then turns upwards in the right free margin of the lesser omentum as the hepatic artery (21) which divides into right and left branches to enter the porta hepatis of the liver.

◁ **A Coeliac trunk and surrounding area**

Part of the left lobe of the liver (3), and most of the lesser and greater omentum (30 and 8) have been removed, together with peritoneum of the central part of the posterior abdominal wall (posterior wall of the lesser sac), to show some of the most important structures in the upper abdomen: the coeliac trunk (27) and its branches (33, 31 and 24), the portal vein (22), and the bile duct (18) formed by the union of the cystic duct (16) from the gall bladder (13) with the common hepatic duct (17) from the liver (1 and 3)

1	Right lobe of liver
2	Falciform ligament
3	Left lobe of liver
4	Left triangular ligament
5	Diaphragm
6	Abdominal part of oesophagus
7	Body of stomach
8	Branches of left and right gastro-epiploic arteries in greater omentum
9	Transverse colon
10	Right gastro-epiploic artery
11	Pyloric part of stomach
12	Superior (first) part of duodenum
13	Gall bladder
14	Inferior vena cava
15	Cystic artery
16	Cystic duct
17	Common hepatic duct
18	Bile duct
19	Right gastric artery
20	Gastroduodenal artery
21	Hepatic artery and right and left branches
22	Portal vein
23	Accessory hepatic artery
24	Common hepatic artery
25	Left renal vein
26	Abdominal aorta
27	Coeliac trunk
28	Superior mesenteric artery
29	Body of pancreas
30	Lesser omentum containing right and left gastric arteries
31	Splenic artery
32	Left crus of diaphragm
33	Left gastric artery
34	Oesophageal branch of left gastric artery
35	Median arcuate ligament
36	Right crus of diaphragm

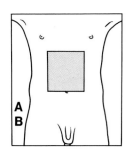

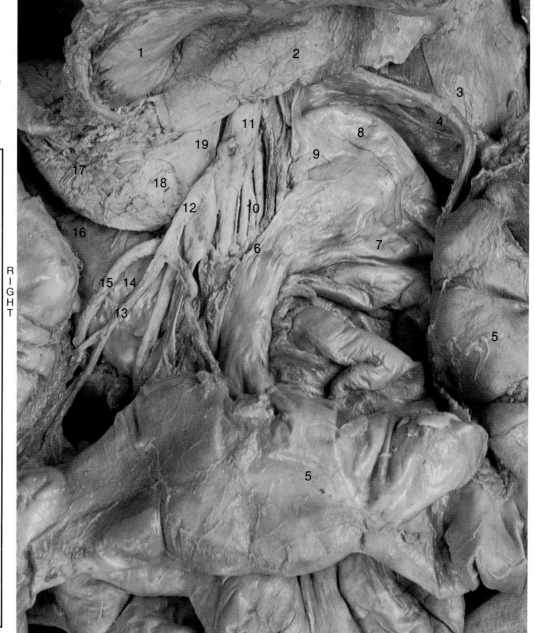

B

RIGHT

LEFT

B Superior mesenteric vessels

The stomach (1) has been lifted upwards and transverse mesocolon removed, leaving the transverse colon (5) in its normal position. Part of the peritoneum of the mesentery (6) has been dissected away to show branches of the superior mesenteric artery (11)

1	Posterior surface of pyloric part of stomach
2	Body of pancreas
3	Lower pole of left kidney
4	Branches of left colic vessels
5	Transverse colon
6	Cut edge of peritoneum at root of mesentery
7	Jejunum
8	Duodenojejunal flexure
9	Ascending (fourth) part of duodenum
10	Jejunal and ileal arteries
11	Superior mesenteric artery
12	Middle colic artery
13	Right colic artery
14	Horizontal (third) part of duodenum
15	Ileocolic artery
16	Descending (second) part of duodenum
17	Head of pancreas
18	Uncinate process of head of pancreas
19	Superior mesenteric vein

● The right colic artery (13) is normally a branch of the superior mesenteric artery (11) but often (as here) arises from its middle colic branch (12).
● The superior mesenteric vein (19) lies on the right side of its companion artery (11). They appear at the lower border of the pancreas (2), crossing the uncinate process (18) of the head of the pancreas (17) and lower down crossing the third part of the duodenum (14) which is where they enter or leave the root of the mesentery (6).

A Superior mesenteric vessels

This dissection is similar to that on page 221, B, but here the stomach (2) and transverse colon (1) have both been lifted upwards, so lifting the middle colic artery (13) upwards also. The root of the mesentery (10) begins at the duodenojejunal flexure (7) and passes obliquely downwards to the right over the horizontal (third) part of the duodenum (15), where the superior mesenteric vessels and their branches (14, 12 and 11) become enclosed between the two layers of the peritoneum that form the mesentery (see C on page 219)

1	Transverse colon
2	Posterior surface of body of stomach
3	Body of pancreas
4	Left kidney
5	Left colic vessels
6	Descending colon
7	Duodenojejunal flexure
8	Jejunum
9	Mesentery
10	Cut edge of peritoneum at root of mesentery
11	Jejunal and ileal arteries
12	Superior mesenteric artery
13	Middle colic artery
14	Superior mesenteric vein
15	Horizontal (third) part of duodenum
16	Ileocolic artery
17	Descending (second) part of duodenum
18	Uncinate process of head of pancreas
19	Head ⎫ of pancreas
20	Neck ⎭
21	Right branch of middle colic artery

• In its normal position the middle colic artery runs downwards from its superior mesenteric origin (page 221, B12), but obviously when the transverse colon is lifted upwards (as here, A1, and in F on page 219), the vessel (A13) passes upwards also. Textbook drawings of the arteries of the colon often illustrate it in this position, but it must be remembered that with the body in the normal anatomical position it runs downwards.

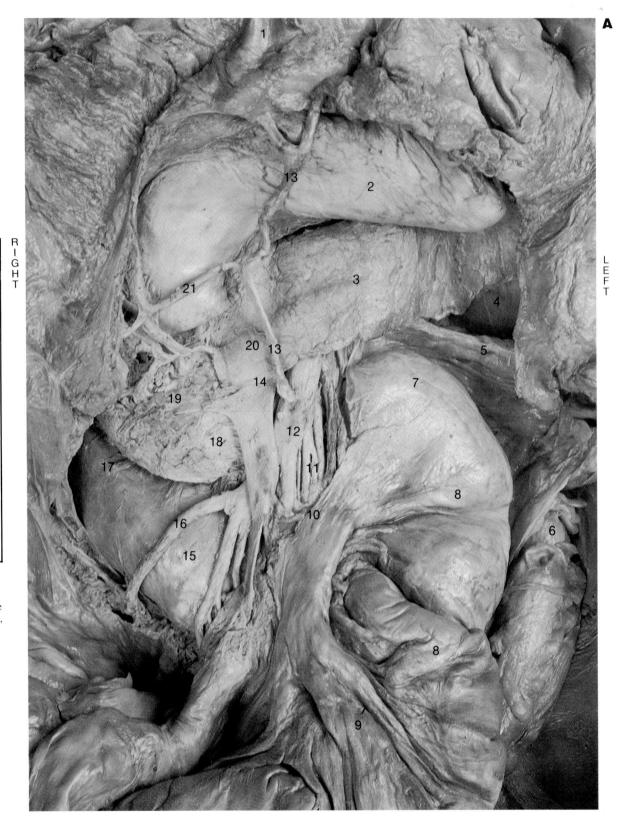

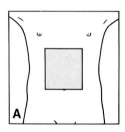

FRONT

B

HEAD

B Inferior mesenteric vessels, from the left

The body is lying on its back and viewed from the left (with the head to the right), with the stomach (13) and transverse colon (15) lifted upwards (to the right). The peritoneum of the posterior abdominal wall has been removed and the left-sided parts of the duodenum (3 and 4) reflected towards the right (i.e. towards the top of the picture), to show the origin of the inferior mesenteric artery (5) from the aorta (6). The lower border of the pancreas (11) has been lifted up, revealing the splenic vein (10) with the inferior mesenteric (24) running into it. The ureter (27) has the gonadal vessels (22 and 23) in front of it and the genitofemoral nerve (26) behind it, lying on psoas major (25)

● In this specimen (as in D on page 241) the gonadal (testicular) artery (22) arises from the renal artery (17) and not from the aorta (6).

1	Mesentery		16	Splenic artery
2	Horizontal (third)	part of duodenum	17	Left renal artery
3	Ascending (fourth)		18	Lower pole of left kidney
4	Duodenojejunal flexure		19	Branches of left colic vessels
5	Inferior mesenteric artery		20	Descending colon
6	Abdominal aorta		21	Pelvis of kidney
7	Suspensory muscle of duodenum (muscle of Treitz)		22	Gonadal artery
8	Superior mesenteric artery		23	Gonadal vein
9	Superior mesenteric vein		24	Inferior mesenteric vein
10	Splenic vein		25	Psoas major
11	Body of pancreas		26	Genitofemoral nerve
12	Middle colic artery		27	Ureter
13	Posterior surface of pyloric part of stomach		28	Left colic artery
14	Left renal vein		29	Cut edge of peritoneum
15	Transverse colon			

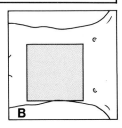

223

A

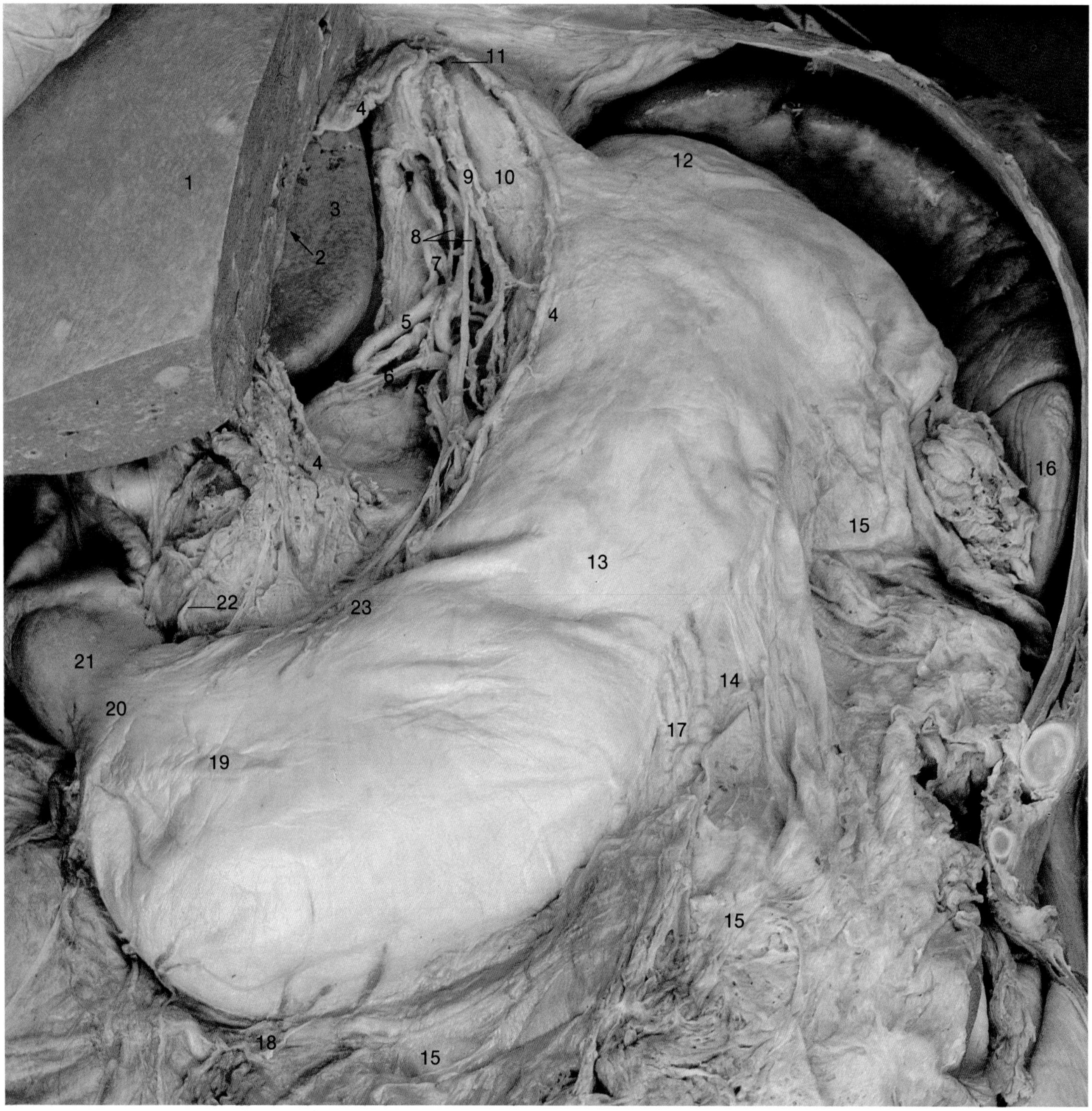

A Stomach, with vessels and vagus nerves, from the front

The anterior thoracic and abdominal walls and the left lobe of the liver have been removed, with part of the lesser omentum (4), to show the stomach (12, 13, 19 and 20) in its undisturbed position. The removal of the upper part of the lesser omentum between the liver (1) and the lesser curvature of the stomach (23) has displayed the left gastric vessels (5 and 6) and branches, with the anterior and posterior vagal trunks (9 and 7) which enter the abdomen with the lower end of the oesophagus (10) through the oesophageal opening in the diaphragm (11). The greater omentum (15) remains at the greater curvature, with the

gastro-epiploic vessels (17 and 18) between the layers of the omentum

● For a diagrammatic representation of the peritoneal layers forming the omenta see page 219.

1	Right lobe of liver	12	Fundus	⎫
2	Fissure for ligamentum venosum	13	Body	of stomach
3	Caudate lobe of liver	14	Greater curvature	⎬
4	Lesser omentum (cut edge)	15	Greater omentum	⎭
5	Left gastric artery	16	Lower end of spleen	
6	Left gastric vein	17	Branches of left gastro-epiploic vessels	
7	Posterior vagal trunk	18	Right gastro-epiploic vessels and branches	
8	Oesophageal branches of left gastric vessels	19	Pyloric part of stomach	
9	Anterior vagal trunk	20	Pylorus	
10	Oesophagus	21	Superior (first) part of duodenum	
11	Oesophageal opening in diaphragm	22	Right gastric artery	
		23	Lesser curvature	

B
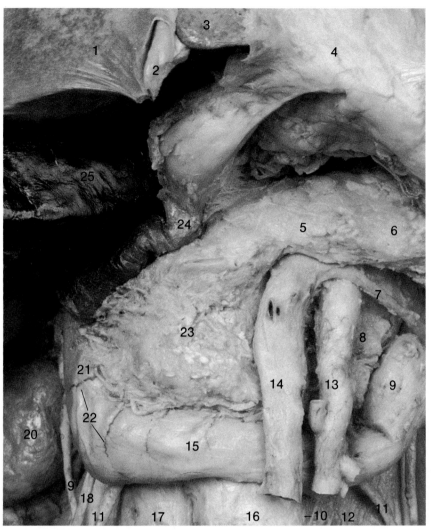

C
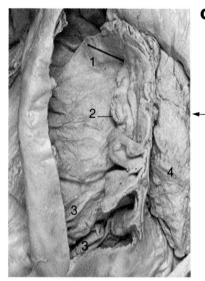

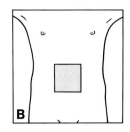

D
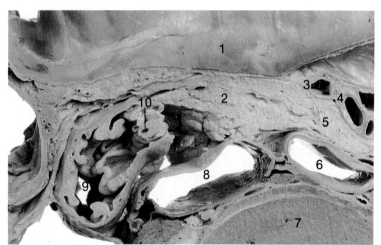

B Duodenum and pancreas

The stomach (4) has been lifted up, the colon and the peritoneum of the posterior abdominal wall removed and branches of the superior mesenteric vessels (13 and 14) cut off. The C-shaped duodenum (24, 21, 15 and 9) is seen embracing the head of the pancreas (23); the neck (5) and body (6) of the pancreas have been displaced slightly upwards to show the splenic vein (7) joining the superior mesenteric vein (14) (to form the portal vein behind the neck of the pancreas). The descending (second) part of the duodenum (21) overlaps the hilum of the right kidney (20). The superior mesenteric artery (13) and vein (14) cross the uncinate process (8) of the head of the pancreas and then the horizontal (third) part of the duodenum (15)

C Duodenal papillae

The anterior wall of the descending (second) part of the duodenum has been removed. A bristle has been placed in the opening of the minor duodenal papilla (1), which is about 1.5 cm above the major papilla (2). The arrow indicates the level of the section in D

1	Bristle in minor duodenal papilla
2	Major duodenal papilla
3	Circular folds of mucous membrane
4	Head of pancreas

D Transverse section of the abdomen, through the major duodenal papilla

The section shows the central part of the abdomen, with the aorta (6) and inferior vena cava (8) in front of the second lumbar vertebra (7) and the duodenum (9) transected through the major duodenal papilla (10), at the level of the arrow in C

1	Lumen of transverse colon
2	Head of pancreas
3	Superior mesenteric vein
4	Superior mesenteric artery
5	Uncinate process of head of pancreas
6	Abdominal aorta
7	Body of second lumbar vertebra
8	Inferior vena cava
9	Descending (second) part of duodenum
10	Major duodenal papilla

• The bile duct and the main pancreatic duct join within the wall of the descending (second) part of the duodenum to form the hepatopancreatic ampulla, which opens on the summit of the major duodenal papilla (C2, D10). This is on the posteromedial wall of the duodenum, about 8 to 10 cm beyond the pylorus. The visceral muscle that surrounds the ampulla and the ends of the ducts constitutes the ampullary sphincter (of Oddi).
• The accessory pancreatic duct opens on the summit of the minor duodenal papilla (C1).

1	Right lobe of liver	13	Superior mesenteric artery
2	Falciform ligament	14	Superior mesenteric vein
3	Left lobe of liver	15	Horizontal (third) part of duodenum
4	Posterior surface of greater omentum overlying stomach	16	Abdominal aorta
		17	Inferior vena cava
5	Neck ⎱ of pancreas	18	Gonadal vein
6	Body ⎰	19	Ureter
7	Splenic vein	20	Right kidney
8	Uncinate process of head of pancreas	21	Descending (second) part of duodenum
9	Ascending (fourth) part of duodenum	22	Branches of pancreaticoduodenal vessels
10	Sympathetic trunk	23	Head of pancreas
11	Gonadal artery	24	Superior (first) part of duodenum
12	Psoas major	25	Gall bladder

225

A Liver, from above and in front

Part of the diaphragm (2 and 6) remains attached, with a portion of fibrous pericardium (5)

1	Right triangular ligament
2	Diaphragm overlying bare area
3	Superior layer of coronary ligament
4	Inferior vena cava
5	Fibrous pericardium
6	Diaphragm overlying left triangular ligament
7	Superior ⎫ surface of left lobe
8	Anterior ⎭
9	Falciform ligament
10	Anterior ⎫ surface of right lobe
11	Superior ⎭
12	Right surface

- The caudate (B8) and quadrate (B24) lobes are classified *anatomically* as part of the right lobe (B14), but *functionally* they belong to the left lobe (B3), since they receive blood from the left branches of the hepatic artery and portal vein, and drain bile to the left hepatic duct.
- The caudate *process* (B18) joins the caudate lobe (B8) to the right lobe (B14). It is the caudate process (not the caudate lobe) that forms the upper boundary of the epiploic foramen (page 215).
- The surfaces of the liver are named as diaphragmatic and visceral (or inferior).
- The diaphragmatic surface can be subdivided into anterior (A8 and 10), superior (A7 and 11), right (A12), and posterior surfaces, but they merge into one another without distinct boundaries, as does the inferior or visceral surface with the posterior.
- The posterior surface contains the bare area (B10), the groove for the inferior vena cava (B7), the caudate lobe

(B8) and the fissure for the ligamentum venosum (B6), the suprarenal impression (B17) and most of the right renal impression (B13).
- The inferior (visceral) surface contains the porta hepatis where the hepatic artery (B21), portal vein (B20) and hepatic ducts (B22) enter or leave, enclosed within the peritoneum forming the right free margin of the lesser omentum (B19). It also contains the quadrate lobe (B24), the fossa for the gall bladder (B23), the fissure for the ligamentum teres (B25), and the gastric (B4), duodenal (B16) and colic (B15) impressions.

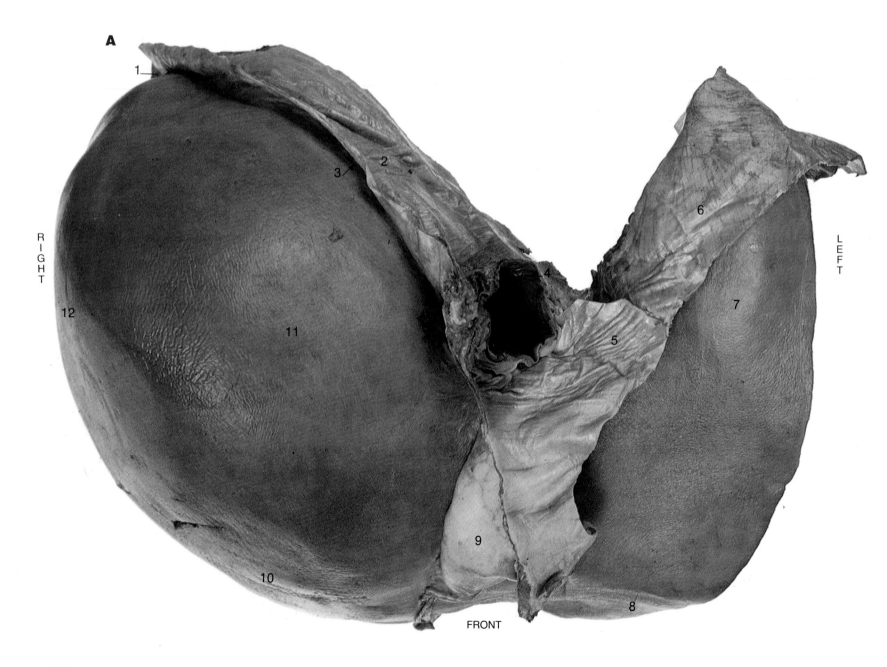

A

RIGHT

LEFT

FRONT

B Liver, from above and behind

Looking from above and behind, this view shows the posterior and inferior (visceral) surfaces, with no clear demarcation between them. As a general guide, note that the bare area (10) and groove for the inferior vena cava (7) are on the posterior surface, and the fossa for the gall bladder (23) and the structures of the porta hepatis (19 to 22) on the inferior surface

1 Left triangular ligament
2 Diaphragm
3 Left lobe
4 Gastric impression
5 Oesophageal groove
6 Lesser omentum in fissure for ligamentum venosum
7 Inferior vena cava
8 Caudate lobe
9 Diaphragm on part of bare area
10 Bare area
11 Inferior layer of coronary ligament
12 Right triangular ligament
13 Renal impression
14 Right lobe
15 Colic impression
16 Duodenal impression
17 Suprarenal impression
18 Caudate process
19 Right free margin of lesser omentum in porta hepatis
20 Portal vein
21 Hepatic artery
22 Common hepatic duct
23 Gall bladder
24 Quadrate lobe
25 Ligamentum teres and falciform ligament in fissure for ligamentum teres
26 Omental tuberosity

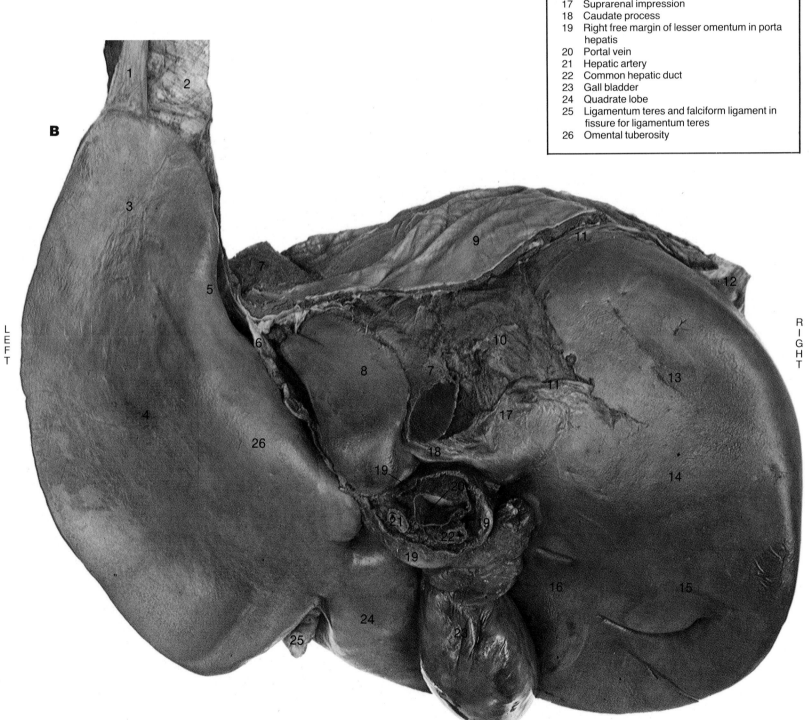

LEFT

RIGHT

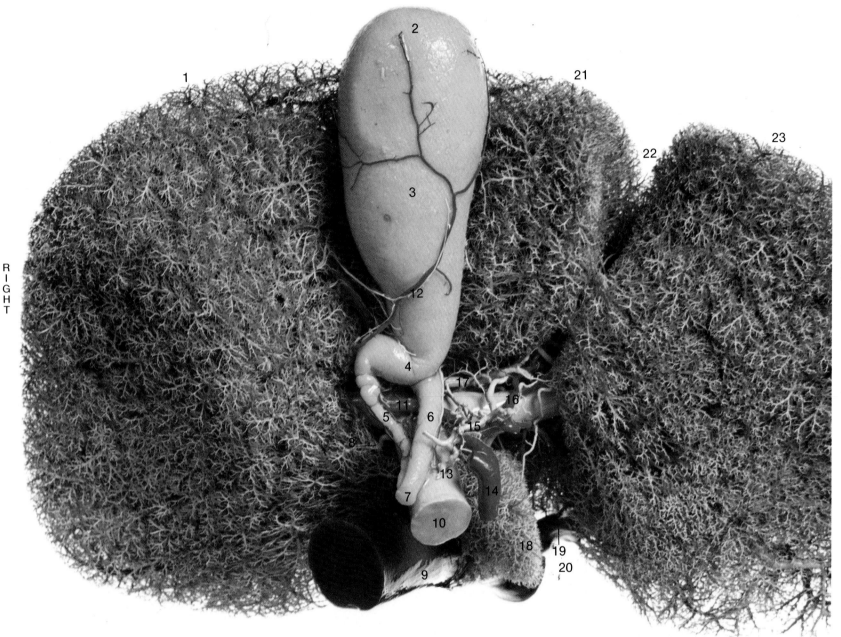

Cast of the liver, extrahepatic biliary tract and associated vessels, from behind

Yellow = gall bladder and biliary tract
Red = hepatic artery and branches
Light blue = portal vein and tributaries
Dark blue = inferior vena cava, hepatic veins and tributaries

This view shows the inferior and posterior surfaces, as when looking into the abdomen from below with the lower border of the liver pushed up towards the thorax

● The hepatic artery (14) divides like a Y into left (16) and right (11) branches.
● The portal vein (10) divides like a T into left (16) and right (11) branches.
● The common hepatic duct (6) is formed by the union of the left (17) and right (obscured) hepatic ducts, and is joined by the cystic duct (5) to form the bile duct (7).

1	Right lobe	
2	Fundus	} of gall bladder
3	Body	
4	Neck	
5	Cystic duct	
6	Common hepatic duct	
7	Bile duct	
8	Caudate process	
9	Inferior vena cava	
10	Portal vein	
11	Right branch of hepatic artery overlying right branch of portal vein	
12	Cystic artery and veins	
13	Right gastric vein	
14	Hepatic artery	
15	Left gastric vein	
16	Left branch of hepatic artery overlying left branch of portal vein	
17	Left hepatic duct	
18	Caudate lobe	
19	Left hepatic vein	
20	Fissure for ligamentum venosum	
21	Quadrate lobe	
22	Fissure for ligamentum teres	
23	Left lobe	

Cast of the duodenum, liver, biliary tract and associated vessels, from the front

Yellow = biliary tract, pancreatic duct and urinary tract
Red = arteries
Blue = portal venous system
Clear yellow = small intestine
In this combined cast there is inevitably overlap of structures. Identify first the C-shaped duodenum (22, 25 and 18) and the duodenojejunal flexure (15), then the gall bladder and bile duct (2 and 3) with the adjacent hepatic artery (4) and portal vein (5). The main pancreatic duct (14) is seen above the duodenojejunal flexure (15) and also where it enters the second part of the duodenum (25) just below the bile duct (3)

1 Right branch of portal vein and hepatic artery and right hepatic duct
2 Gall bladder
3 Bile duct
4 Hepatic artery
5 Portal vein
6 Left branch of portal vein and hepatic artery and left hepatic duct
7 Left gastric artery
8 Left gastric vein
9 Splenic artery
10 Splenic vein
11 Short gastric vessels
12 Left gastro-epiploic vessels
13 Vessels of left kidney
14 Pancreatic duct
15 Duodenojejunal flexure
16 Superior mesenteric artery
17 Superior mesenteric vein
18 Horizontal (third) part of duodenum
19 Right gastro-epiploic vessels
20 Pyloric canal
21 Pylorus
22 Superior (first) part of duodenum
23 Right gastric vessels
24 Branches of superior and inferior pancreaticoduodenal vessels
25 Descending (second) part of duodenum
26 Vessels of right kidney

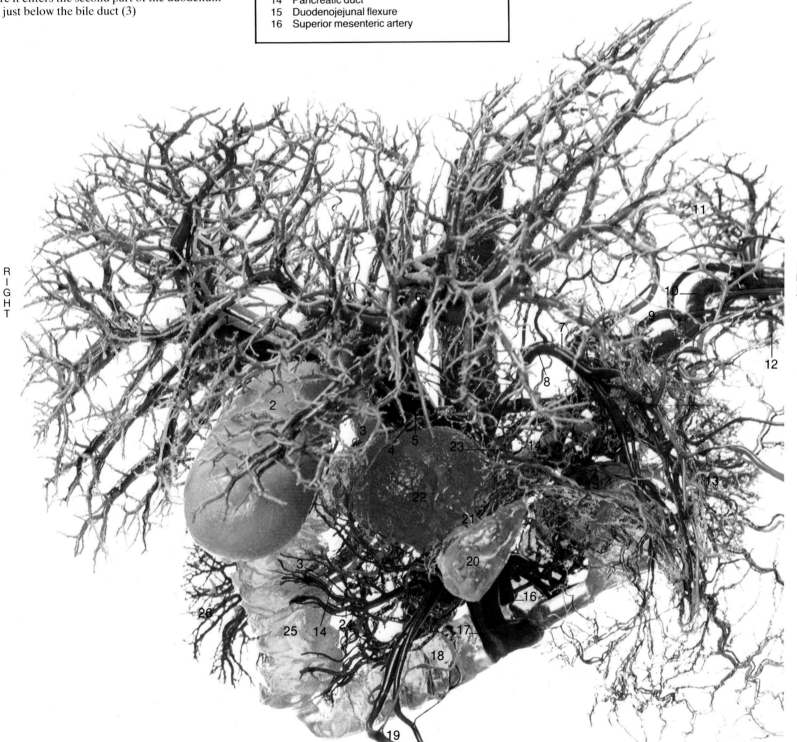

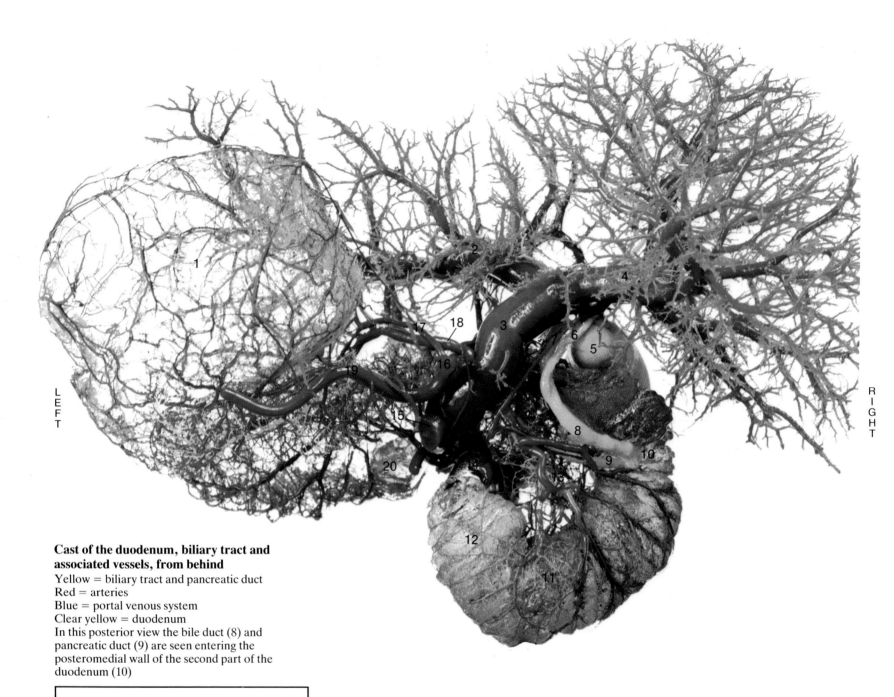

Cast of the duodenum, biliary tract and associated vessels, from behind

Yellow = biliary tract and pancreatic duct
Red = arteries
Blue = portal venous system
Clear yellow = duodenum
In this posterior view the bile duct (8) and pancreatic duct (9) are seen entering the posteromedial wall of the second part of the duodenum (10)

1	Stomach outlined by its vessels
2	Left branch of portal vein and hepatic artery and left hepatic duct
3	Portal vein
4	Right branch of portal vein and hepatic artery and right hepatic duct
5	Gall bladder
6	Cystic duct
7	Common hepatic duct
8	Bile duct
9	Pancreatic duct
10	Descending (second)
11	Horizontal (third) — part of duodenum
12	Ascending (fourth)
13	Branches of pancreaticoduodenal vessels
14	Superior mesenteric vein
15	Splenic vein
16	Coeliac trunk
17	Left gastric artery
18	Left gastric vein
19	Splenic artery
20	Pyloric canal

Cast of the hepatic vessels and associated structures, from above and behind

Green = biliary tract
Yellow = pancreatic duct
Red = arteries
Blue = portal venous system
Clear yellow = duodenum
The areas 1 to 4 demarcated by the interrupted lines indicate the four main segments of the liver. The specimen shows an accessory left hepatic artery (19) arising from the left gastric (18), a comon occurrence. The accessory pancreatic duct (7) is seen entering the duodenum (6) proximal to the entry of the bile duct (8) and main pancreatic duct (9)

1	Left lateral	segments
2	Left medial	
3	Right anterior	
4	Right posterior	
5	Gall bladder	
6	Descending (second) part of duodenum	
7	Accessory pancreatic duct	
8	Bile duct	
9	Pancreatic duct	
10	Inferior pancreaticoduodenal vessels	
11	Superior mesenteric vein	
12	Superior mesenteric artery	
13	Portal vein	
14	Left gastric vein	
15	Common hepatic artery	
16	Gastroduodenal artery	
17	Coeliac trunk	
18	Left gastric artery	
19	Accessory hepatic artery	
20	Splenic artery	
21	Splenic vein	

• The main liver segments are the left lateral and medial (1 and 2), and the right anterior and posterior (3 and 4). These are determined by the way the hepatic artery and portal vein branch within the liver.

• The left lateral segment (1) corresponds to the left lobe, and the left medial segment (2) to the caudate and quadrate lobes.
• The right lobe is divided into two segments, anterior (3) and posterior (4).

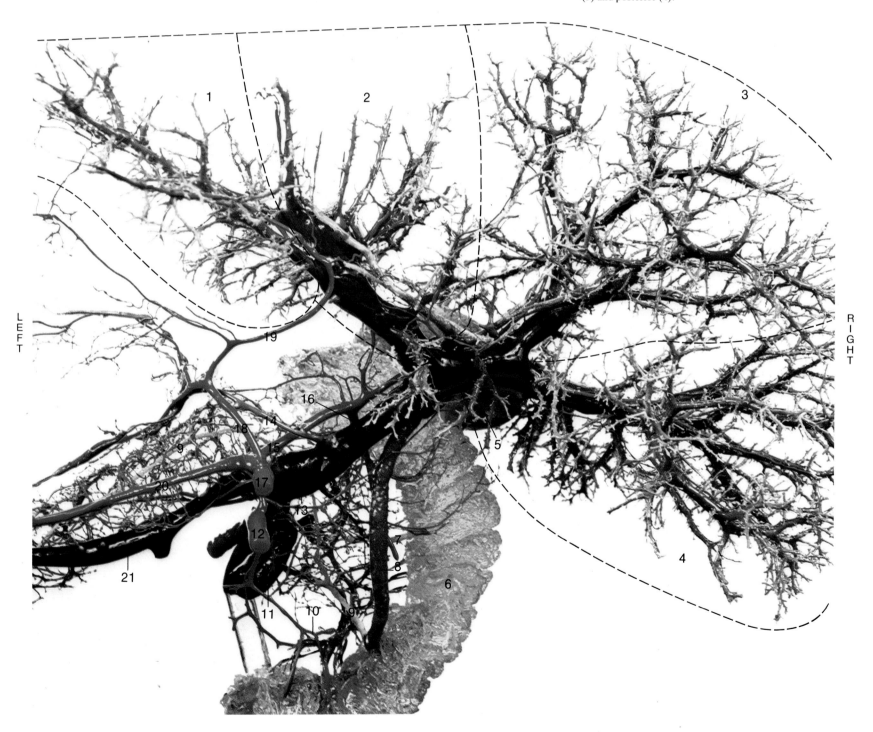

Cast of the portal vein and tributaries, and the mesenteric vessels, from behind

Yellow = biliary tract and pancreatic ducts
Red = arteries
Blue = portal venous system
In this posterior view (chosen in preference to the anterior view, where the many very small vessels to the intestines would have obscured the larger branches), the superior mesenteric vein (22) is seen continuing upwards to become the portal vein (8) after it has been joined by the splenic vein (2). In the porta hepatis the portal vein divides into its right and left branches (9 and 10). Due to removal of the aorta, the upper part of the inferior mesenteric artery (17) has become displaced slightly to the right and appears to have given origin to the ileocolic artery (16), but this is simply an overlap of the vessels; the origin of the ileocolic from the superior mesenteric is not seen in this view

1	Pancreatic duct
2	Splenic vein
3	Splenic artery
4	Coeliac trunk
5	Left gastric artery and vein
6	Left ⎫ branch of
7	Right ⎬ hepatic artery
8	Portal vein
9	Left ⎫
10	Right ⎬ branch of portal vein
11	Bile duct
12	Pancreaticoduodenal vessels
13	Pancreatic ducts in head of pancreas
14	Branches of middle colic vessels
15	Right colic vessels
16	Ileocolic vessels
17	Inferior mesenteric artery
18	Sigmoid vessels
19	Inferior mesenteric vein
20	Left colic vessels
21	Superior mesenteric artery
22	Superior mesenteric vein

● The inferior mesenteric vein (19) normally drains into the splenic vein (2) behind the body of the pancreas, but it may join the splenic vein nearer the union with the superior mesenteric vein or (as in this specimen) enter the superior mesenteric vein itself (22)
● The colic arteries (14, 15, 16, 20) anastomose with one another near the colonic wall forming what is often called the marginal artery (as at the arrows).

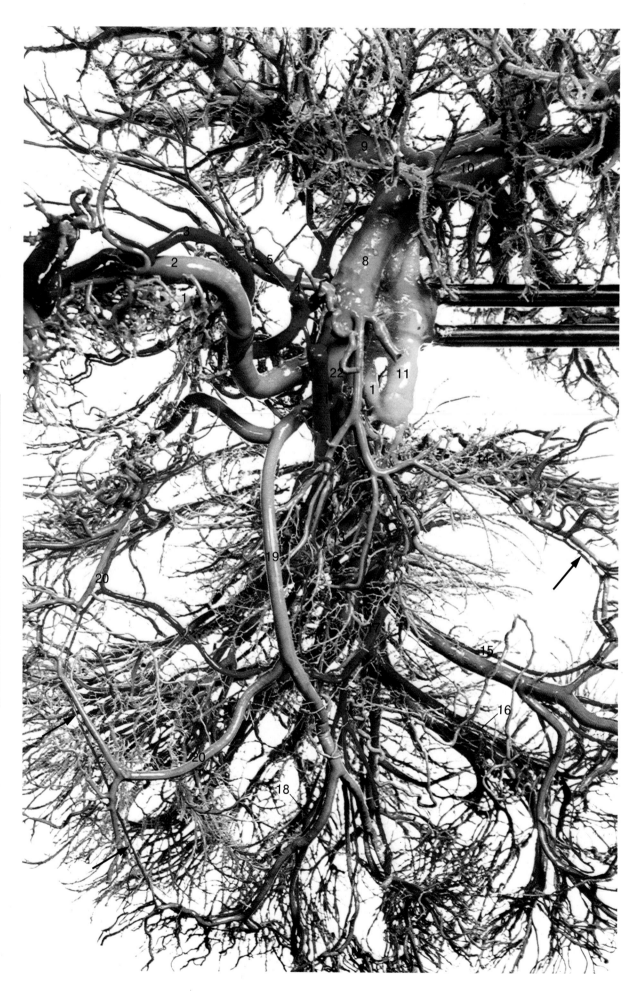

A **Spleen, from the front**

The left upper anterior abdominal and lower anterior thoracic walls have been removed and part of the diaphragm (1) turned upwards to show the spleen in its normal position, lying adjacent to the stomach (2) and colon (9), with the lower part against the kidney (shown in C)

1	Diaphragm
2	Stomach
3	Gastrosplenic ligament
4	Gastric impression
5	Superior border
6	Notch
7	Diaphragmatic surface
8	Inferior border
9	Left colic flexure
10	Costodiaphragmatic recess
11	Thoracic wall

- The gastrosplenic ligament contains the short gastric and left gastro-epiploic branches of the splenic vessels.
- The lienorenal ligament contains the tail of the pancreas and the splenic vessels.

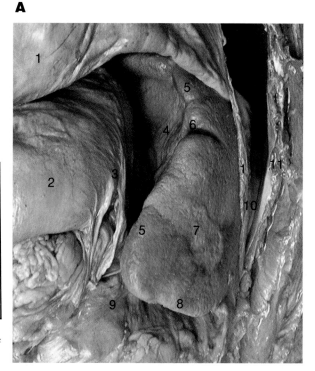

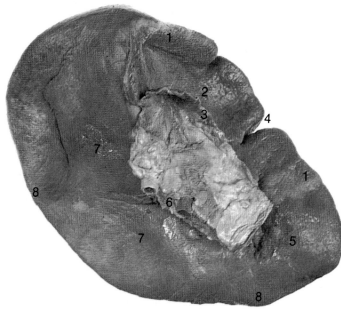

B **Spleen, visceral surface**

The spleen has been removed and its visceral or medial surface is shown, with a small part of the gastrosplenic (3) and lienorenal (6) ligaments remaining attached

1	Superior border
2	Gastric impression
3	Gastrosplenic ligament
4	Notch
5	Colic impression
6	Tail of pancreas and splenic vessels in lienorenal ligament
7	Renal impression
8	Inferior border

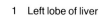

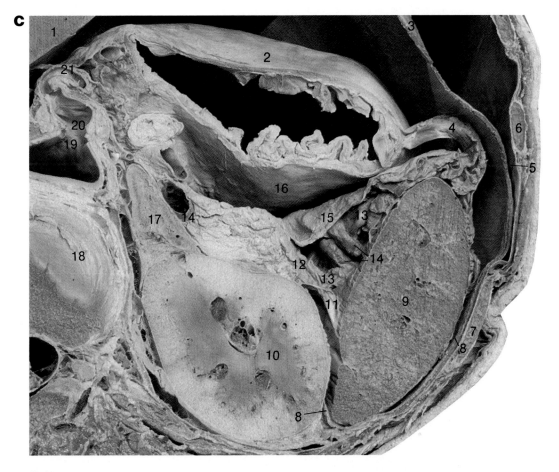

C **Spleen, in a transverse section of the left upper abdomen**

The section is at the level of the disc (18) between the twelfth thoracic and first lumbar vertebrae, and is viewed from below looking towards the thorax. The spleen (9) lies against the diaphragm (3) and left kidney (10) but separated from them by peritoneum of the greater sac (8). The peritoneum behind the stomach (2) forming part of the gastrosplenic (4) and lienorenal (15) ligaments belongs to the lesser sac (16)

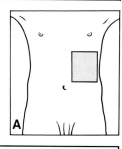

1	Left lobe of liver
2	Stomach
3	Diaphragm
4	Gastrosplenic ligament
5	Costodiaphragmatic recess of pleura
6	Ninth rib
7	Tenth rib
8	Peritoneum of greater sac
9	Spleen
10	Left kidney
11	Posterior layer of lienorenal ligament
12	Tail of pancreas
13	Splenic artery
14	Splenic vein
15	Anterior layer of lienorenal ligament
16	Lesser sac
17	Left suprarenal gland
18	Intervertebral disc
19	Abdominal aorta
20	Coeliac trunk
21	Left gastric artery

A Caecum and appendix, from the front

The terminal ileum (5) is seen joining the large intestine at the junction of the caecum (2) and ascending colon (1), and the appendix (7) joins the caecum just below the ileocaecal junction

1	Ascending colon
2	Caecum
3	Anterior taenia coli
4	Superior ileocaecal recess
5	Terminal ileum
6	Inferior ileocaecal recess
7	Base ⎫
8	Tip ⎭ of appendix
9	Peritoneum overlying external iliac vessels
10	Retrocaecal recess

B Interior of the caecum

The anterior wall has been cut open and reflected to show the lips of the ileocaecal valve (2) and the opening of the appendix (3)

1	Ascending colon
2	Lips of ileocaecal valve
3	Opening of appendix

● The position of the *base* (A7) of the appendix (properly called the vermiform appendix) is constant, opening (B3) just below and behind the ileocaecal valve (B2), but the *tip* may lie in a variety of positions—over the pelvic brim, behind the caecum or ascending colon, below the caecum, or behind the terminal part of the ileum.
● The three taeniae coli of the ascending colon and caecum converge on the base of the appendix (A3 and A7), and serve as useful guides to the base.

C Appendix, ileocolic artery and related structures, from the front

Most of the peritoneum of the mesentery and posterior abdominal wall have been removed, and coils of small intestine (3) have been displaced to the right, to show the ileocolic artery (2), terminal ileum (4) and appendix (6) with its appendicular artery (7)

1	Descending (second) part of duodenum
2	Ileocolic artery
3	Mesentery and coils of jejunum and ileum
4	Terminal part of ileum
5	Mesoappendix
6	Appendix
7	Appendicular artery in mesoappendix
8	Caecum
9	Ascending colon
10	Ileal and caecal vessels
11	Psoas major
12	Right colic artery
13	Lower pole of kidney
14	Ureter
15	Testicular vein
16	Genitofemoral nerve
17	Inferior vena cava˙
18	Testicular artery

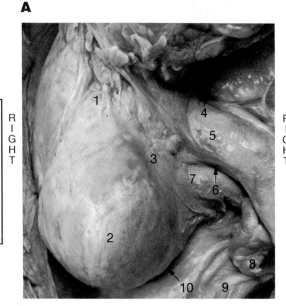

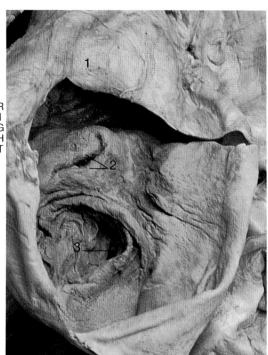

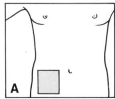

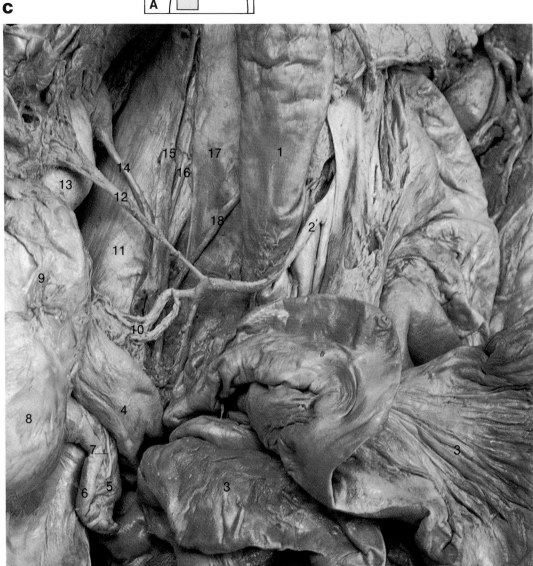

D

E

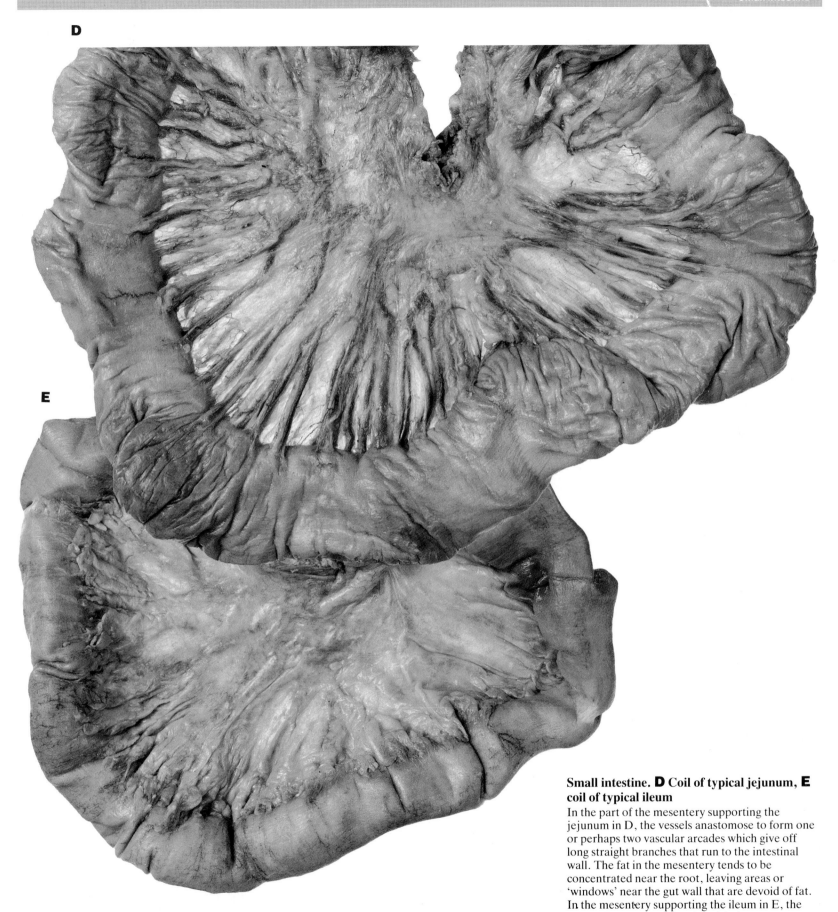

Small intestine. D Coil of typical jejunum, E coil of typical ileum

In the part of the mesentery supporting the jejunum in D, the vessels anastomose to form one or perhaps two vascular arcades which give off long straight branches that run to the intestinal wall. The fat in the mesentery tends to be concentrated near the root, leaving areas or 'windows' near the gut wall that are devoid of fat. In the mesentery supporting the ileum in E, the vessels form several arcades with shorter branches, and there are no fat-free areas. The jejunal wall (D) is thicker than that of the ileum (E) and has a larger lumen. The jejunum also feels thicker, because the folds of its mucous membrane are more numerous than in the ileum

• The appendix gets its blood supply from the appendicular artery (C7), normally a branch of one of the caecal arteries (C10), usually the posterior caecal. The vessel is not at first closely applied to the appendix but approaches it through the mesoappendix (C5), the peritoneal fold continuous with the lower part of the mesentery of the terminal ileum (C4). If this arterial supply becomes obstructed, the appendix becomes necrotic, as there is no collateral circulation.

A Kidneys and suprarenal glands

The kidneys (13 and 30) and suprarenal glands (11 and 33) are displayed on the posterior abdominal wall after the removal of all other viscera. The left renal vein (15) receives the left suprarenal (12) and gonadal veins (17) (and in this specimen an unusually large tributary from lumbar veins, 16) and then passes over the aorta (22) and deep to the superior mesenteric artery (10) to reach the inferior vena cava (24). In the hilum of the right kidney (30) a large branch of the renal artery (31) passes in front of the renal vein (32). The origins of the renal arteries from the aorta are not seen because they underlie the left renal vein (15) and inferior vena cava (24)

1	Right crus of diaphragm	19	Left psoas major
2	Common hepatic artery	20	Left gonadal artery
3	Left gastric artery	21	Left sympathetic trunk
4	Splenic artery	22	Abdominal aorta and aortic plexus
5	Left crus of diaphragm	23	Inferior mesenteric artery
6	Left inferior phrenic artery	24	Inferior vena cava
7	Left inferior phrenic vein	25	Right gonadal artery
8	Coeliac trunk	26	Right gonadal vein
9	Left coeliac ganglion	27	Right ureter
10	Superior mesenteric artery	28	Right ilio-inguinal nerve
11	Left suprarenal gland	29	Right iliohypogastric nerve
12	Left suprarenal vein	30	Right kidney
13	Left kidney	31	Right renal artery
14	Left renal artery	32	Right renal vein
15	Left renal vein	33	Right suprarenal gland
16	Lumbar tributary of renal vein	34	Right inferior phrenic artery
17	Left gonadal vein	35	Right coeliac ganglion
18	Left ureter	36	A hepatic vein

● Because of the forward bulge of the lumbar part of the vertebral column on the posterior abdominal wall, the kidneys do not lie flat but are tilted at an angle, each hanging down into the 'gutter' at the side of the lumbar vertebrae and the psoas major muscle (A19), as though suspended there by the renal vessels (A14 and 15) extending into the hilum from the aorta and inferior vena cava (A22 and 24).

● The hilum of the kidney (see the notes opposite) is the region at the medial border occupied by the renal vessels (as at A31 and 32) and by the renal pelvis (hidden behind the vessels) which becomes the ureter (as at A27).

● Because of the bulk of the liver on the right side, the right kidney lies at a slightly lower level than the left (see the surface markings on page 203).

● The right suprarenal gland (A33) overlaps the top of the upper pole of the right kidney (A30).

● The left suprarenal gland (A11) lies along the medial border of the upper pole of the left kidney (A13).

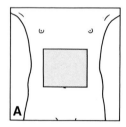

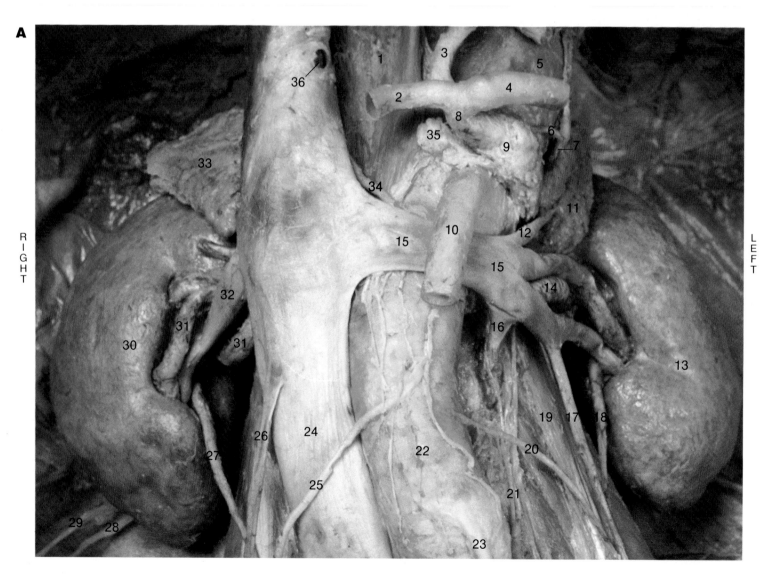

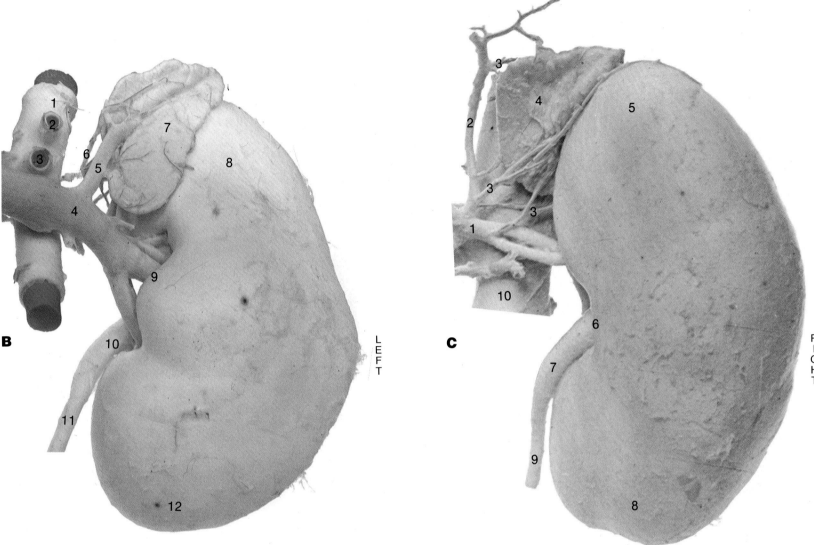

B Left kidney, suprarenal gland and related vessels, from the front

The vessels have been distended by injection of resin, and all fascia has been removed, but the suprarenal gland (7) has been retained in its normal position, lying against the medial side of the upper pole of the kidney (8)

1	Abdominal aorta
2	Coeliac trunk
3	Superior mesenteric artery
4	Left renal vein overlying renal artery
5	Left suprarenal gland
6	Suprarenal arteries
7	Suprarenal gland
8	Upper pole of kidney
9	Hilum of kidney
10	Pelvis of kidney
11	Ureter
12	Lower pole of kidney

● The ureter (B11, C9) is the constricted downward continuation of the pelvis of the kidney (B10, C7). Note that the correct term is pelvis of the kidney or renal pelvis, not pelvis of the ureter.
● In the hilum of the kidney, the order of the principal structures from front to back is usually remembered as vein, artery, ureter (strictly speaking, pelvis—see note above), although small branches of the vessels may sometimes get out of order. Compare with vein, artery, bronchus in the hilum of the lung (page 174).

C Right kidney, suprarenal gland and related vessels, from behind

Similar to B, but note that this is the right kidney from behind, not the left; the hilum of each kidney faces medially

1	Right renal artery
2	Right inferior phrenic artery
3	Suprarenal arteries
4	Suprarenal gland
5	Upper pole of kidney
6	Hilum of kidney
7	Pelvis of kidney
8	Lower pole of kidney
9	Ureter
10	Inferior vena cava

● Each suprarenal gland receives arteries from three sources—the inferior phrenic artery, the aorta and the renal artery—but there are not just three arteries; there are several from each source, perhaps up to a total of 20, and only some of the larger ones are shown (as at C3).
● There is usually only one suprarenal vein on each side. On the left (B5) it drains into the renal vein (B4); on the right it is very short and runs directly into the inferior vena cava (in C it is hidden by the gland itself, but is shown in the cast on page 239, D2).
● For details of the renal arteries see pages 238 and 239.

D CT scan of the kidneys

In the right kidney the white opacity in the hilum is the renal pelvis (P), and the left ureter (U) lies on the medial side of the left kidney

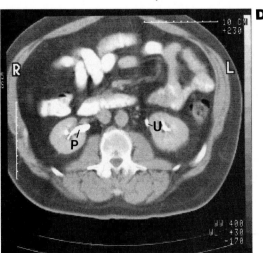

A

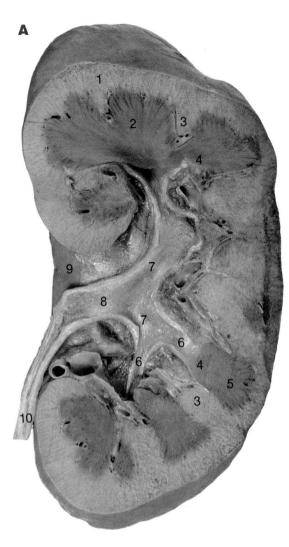

A Kidney. Internal structure in longitudinal section

The section is through the centre of the kidney and has included the renal pelvis (8) and beginning of the ureter (10). The major vessels in the hilum (9) have been removed

1	Cortex
2	Medulla
3	Renal column
4	Renal papilla
5	Medullary pyramid
6	Minor calyx
7	Major calyx
8	Renal pelvis
9	Hilum
10	Ureter

- The renal medulla (2) is made up of the medullary pyramids (5), whose apices form the renal papillae (4) which project into the minor calyces (6).
- The renal columns (3) are the parts of the cortex that intervene between pyramids (5).
- Several minor calyces (6), which receive urine discharged into them from the collecting ducts that open on the renal papillae (4), unite to form a major calyx (7).
- The two or three major calyces (7) unite to form the renal pelvis (8) which passes out through the hilum (9) to become the ureter (10), often with a slight constriction at the junction.
- The hilum is the slit-like space on the medial surface of the kidney where the vessels and renal pelvis enter or leave.

C Cast of the aorta and kidneys, from the front

Red = arteries
Yellow = urinary tracts
On the right side the ureters (unlabelled) are double, each arising from a separate set of calyces. On the left the arteries are double (4 and 5)

1	Early branching of right renal artery
2	Coeliac trunk
3	Superior mesenteric artery
4	Accessory left renal artery
5	Left renal artery

D Cast of the kidneys and great vessels, from the front

Red = arteries
Blue = veins
Yellow = urinary tracts
Here both kidneys show double ureters (unlabelled), and there are accessory renal arteries (10) to the lower poles of both kidneys. The suprarenal glands (also unlabelled) are outlined by their venous patterns, and the short right suprarenal vein (2) is shown draining directly to the inferior vena cava (3). On the left there are two suprarenal veins (8), both draining to the left renal vein (7)

1	Right renal vein
2	Right suprarenal vein
3	Inferior vena cava
4	Aorta
5	Coeliac trunk
6	Superior mesenteric artery
7	Left renal vein
8	Left suprarenal veins
9	Left renal artery
10	Accessory renal arteries
11	Right renal artery

B Cast of the right kidney, from the front

Red = renal artery
Yellow = urinary tract
The posterior division (2) of the renal artery (1) here passes behind the pelvis (10) and upper calyx (upper 8), but all other vessels are in front of the urinary tract; hence this is a right kidney seen from the front (vein, artery, ureter from front to back, and the hilum on the medial side—see page 237), not a left kidney from behind

1	Renal artery
2	Posterior division (forming posterior segment artery)
3	Anterior division
4	Superior segment artery
5	Anterior superior segment artery (double)
6	Anterior inferior segment artery
7	Inferior segment artery
8	Major calyx
9	Minor calyx
10	Pelvis of kidney
11	Ureter

- The kidney has five arterial segments, named posterior, superior, anterior superior, anterior inferior and inferior. Typically the renal artery (1) divides into anterior (3) and posterior (2) divisions; the posterior supplies the posterior segment and the anterior supplies the remainder. However, the pattern of branching displays many variations.
- This specimen shows a fairly typical pattern, although the superior segment (4) obtains a small additional branch from the posterior division (2), and the anterior superior segment receives two major branches (5).

B

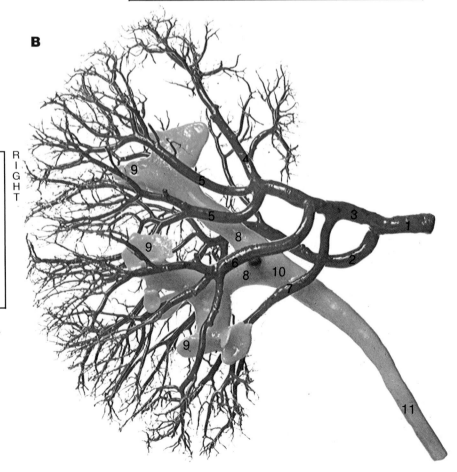

RIGHT

238

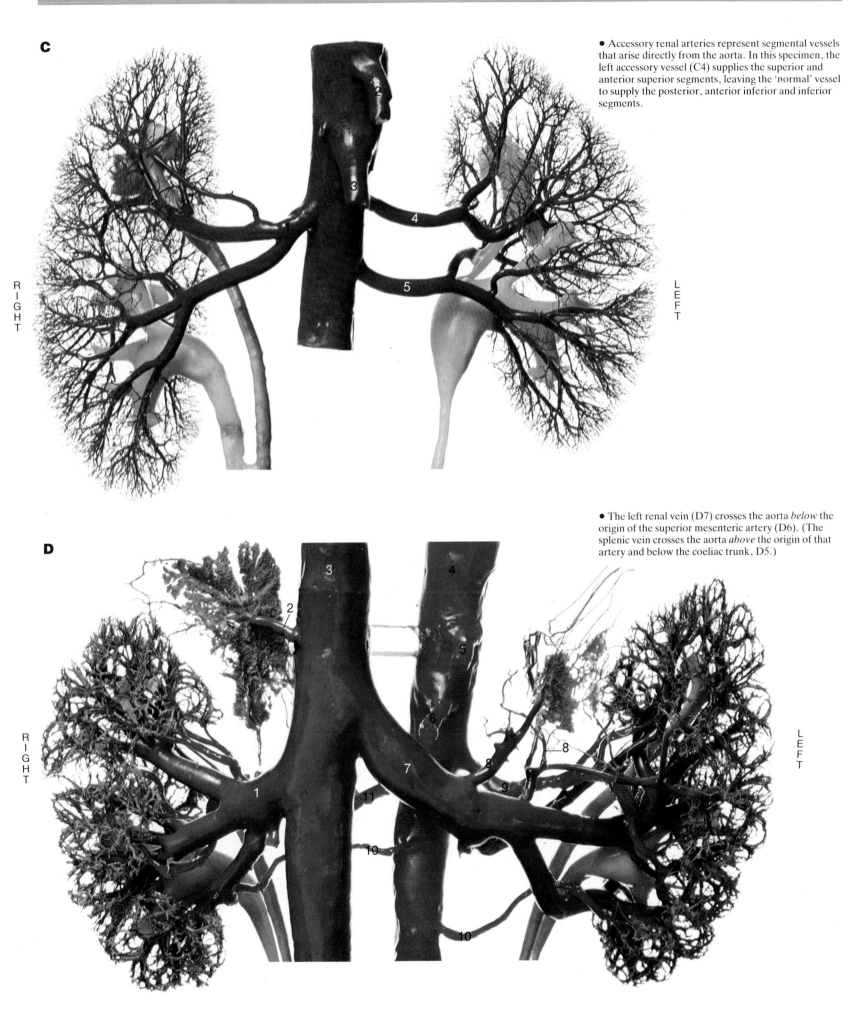

C

• Accessory renal arteries represent segmental vessels that arise directly from the aorta. In this specimen, the left accessory vessel (C4) supplies the superior and anterior superior segments, leaving the 'normal' vessel to supply the posterior, anterior inferior and inferior segments.

D

• The left renal vein (D7) crosses the aorta *below* the origin of the superior mesenteric artery (D6). (The splenic vein crosses the aorta *above* the origin of that artery and below the coeliac trunk, D5.)

RIGHT

LEFT

239

A Left kidney and suprarenal gland, from the left

With the body lying on its back (with the head to the right), the left kidney (20) and suprarenal gland (17) are seen on the posterior abdominal wall. Much of the diaphragm has been removed but the oesophageal opening remains, with the end of the oesophagus (12) opening out into the cardiac part of the stomach and a (double) anterior vagal trunk (11) overlying the red marker. The posterior vagal trunk (10) is behind and to the right of the oesophagus. Part of the pleura has been cut away (16) to show the sympathetic trunk (15) on the side of the lower thoracic vertebrae. The left coeliac ganglion and the coeliac plexus (5) are at the root of the coeliac trunk (6)

1	Abdominal aorta
2	Superior mesenteric artery
3	Left renal vein
4	Left crus of diaphragm
5	Left coeliac ganglion and coeliac plexus
6	Coeliac trunk
7	Common hepatic artery
8	Splenic artery
9	Left gastric artery
10	Posterior vagal trunk
11	Anterior vagal trunk (double, over marker)
12	Lower end of oesophagus
13	Inferior phrenic vessels
14	Thoracic aorta
15	Sympathetic trunk
16	Pleura (cut edge)
17	Left suprarenal gland
18	Left suprarenal vein
19	Left renal artery
20	Left kidney
21	Left ureter
22	Left gonadal vein
23	Psoas major

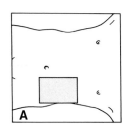

B Right kidney and renal fascia, in transverse section from below

In this transverse section of the lower part of the right kidney, seen from below looking towards the thorax, the renal fascia (3) has been dissected out from the perirenal fat (4) and the kidney's own capsule (5). (There was a small cyst on the surface of this kidney.) The section also displays the three layers (8, 9 and 10) of the lumbar fascia (12; see the notes on page 87)

1	Psoas major
2	Psoas sheath
3	Renal fascia
4	Perirenal fat
5	Renal capsule
6	Right kidney
7	Erector spinae
8	Posterior layer ⎫
9	Middle layer ⎬ of lumbar fascia
10	Anterior layer ⎭
11	Quadratus lumborum
12	Lumbar fascia
13	External oblique
14	Internal oblique
15	Transversus abdominis
16	Peritoneum
17	Right lobe of liver
18	Coil of small intestine

• Outside the kidney's own capsule (renal capsule, 5), there is a variable amount of fat (perirenal fat, 4) and outside this is a condensation of connective tissue forming the renal fascia (3). Peritoneum (16) and retroperitoneal fat lie outside this fascia, which forms a separate compartment for the suprarenal gland (too high to be seen in this section).

FRONT

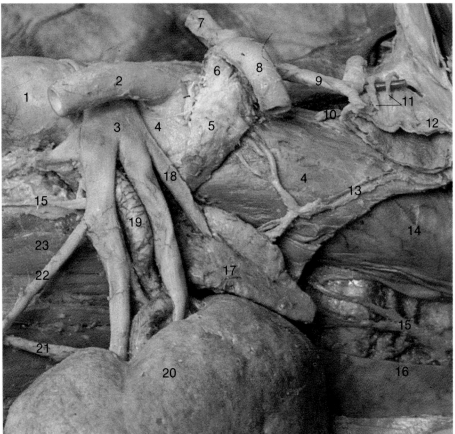

A

FRONT

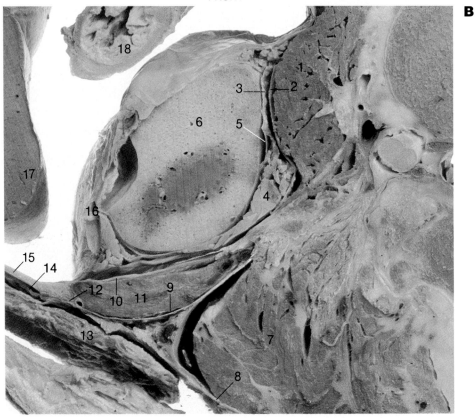

B

C Posterior abdominal wall. **Crura of the diaphragm**

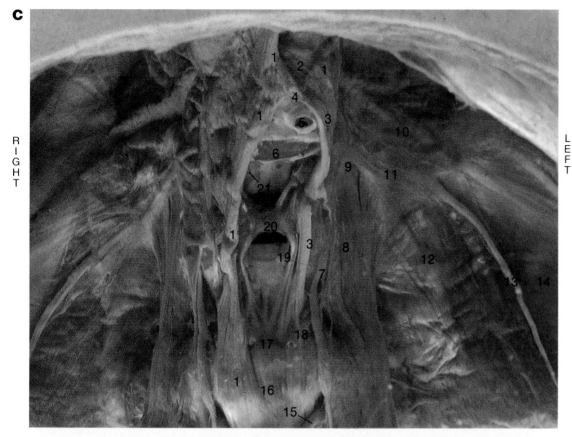

Abdominal contents have been removed and the aorta (6) has been transected immediately below the origin of the coeliac trunk (5), which is just below the median arcuate ligament (4) where the two crura (1 and 3) unite.

1	Right crus
2	Oesophageal opening
3	Left crus
4	Median arcuate ligament
5	Coeliac trunk
6	Aorta
7	Sympathetic trunk
8	Psoas major
9	Medial arcuate ligament
10	Diaphragm
11	Lateral arcuate ligament
12	Quadratus lumborum
13	Subcostal nerve
14	Lumbar part of thoracolumbar fascia
15	Third lumbar artery
16	Second lumbar intervertebral disc
17	Second lumbar vertebra
18	Second lumbar artery
19	First lumbar artery
20	Abnormal communication between crura (superficial to marker)
21	Subcostal artery

● The right crus of the diaphragm (C1) has a more extensive origin (from the upper three lumbar vertebrae) than the left (C3) (from the upper two) because of the greater bulk of the liver on the right; the crura help to pull the liver downwards when the diaphragm contracts.
● Fibres of the *right* crus (C1) form the *right and left* boundaries of the oesophageal opening (C2).

D Posterior abdominal wall, **left side**

The ureter (5) passes down on psoas major (17) deep to the testicular artery (16) and vein (15); in this specimen the artery has arisen from the renal artery under cover of the renal vein (3) and not from the aorta (20) which is its normal origin. The subcostal, iliohypogastric and ilio-inguinal nerves (11, 9 and 7) emerge from behind the kidney (6). The fourth lumbar artery (14) runs laterally superficial to the lower part of quadratus lumborum (8) above the iliolumbar ligament (13)

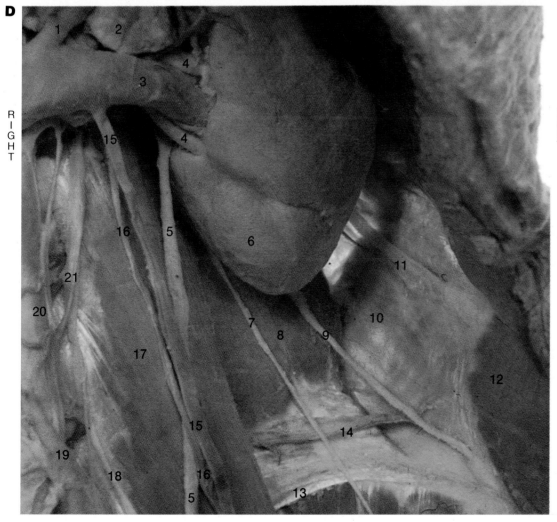

1	Suprarenal vein
2	Suprarenal gland
3	Renal vein
4	Renal artery
5	Ureter
6	Lower pole of kidney
7	Ilio-inguinal nerve
8	Quadratus lumborum
9	Iliohypogastric nerve
10	Lumbar part of thoracolumbar fascia
11	Subcostal nerve
12	Transversus abdominis
13	Iliac crest and iliolumbar ligament
14	Fourth lumbar artery
15	Testicular vein
16	Testicular artery
17	Psoas major
18	Genitofemoral nerve
19	Inferior mesenteric artery
20	Aorta and aortic plexus
21	Sympathetic trunk and ganglion

241

A Posterior abdominal and pelvic walls

All peritoneum and viscera (except for the bladder, 40, ureter, 3, and ductus deferens or vas deferens, 31) have been removed, to display vessels and nerves

1	Psoas major
2	Testicular vessels
3	Ureter
4	Genitofemoral nerve
5	Inferior vena cava
6	Aorta and aortic plexus
7	Inferior mesenteric artery and plexus
8	Sympathetic trunk and ganglia

9	Femoral } branch of genitofemoral
10	Genital } nerve
11	Quadratus lumborum
12	Fourth lumbar artery
13	Ilio-inguinal nerve
14	Iliohypogastric nerve
15	Lumbar part of thoracolumbar fascia
16	Iliolumbar ligament

17	Iliacus and branches from femoral nerve and iliolumbar artery
18	Lateral femoral cutaneous nerve arising from femoral nerve
19	Deep circumflex iliac artery
20	Femoral nerve
21	External iliac artery
22	External iliac vein
23	Inguinal ligament
24	Femoral artery
25	Femoral vein
26	Position of femoral canal
27	Spermatic cord
28	Rectus abdominis
29	Lacunar ligament
30	Pectineal ligament
31	Ductus deferens
32	Inferior hypogastric (pelvic) plexus and pelvic splanchnic nerves
33	Hypogastric nerve
34	Internal iliac artery
35	Common iliac artery
36	Common iliac vein
37	Superior hypogastric plexus
38	Obturator nerve and vessels
39	Rectum (cut edge)
40	Bladder

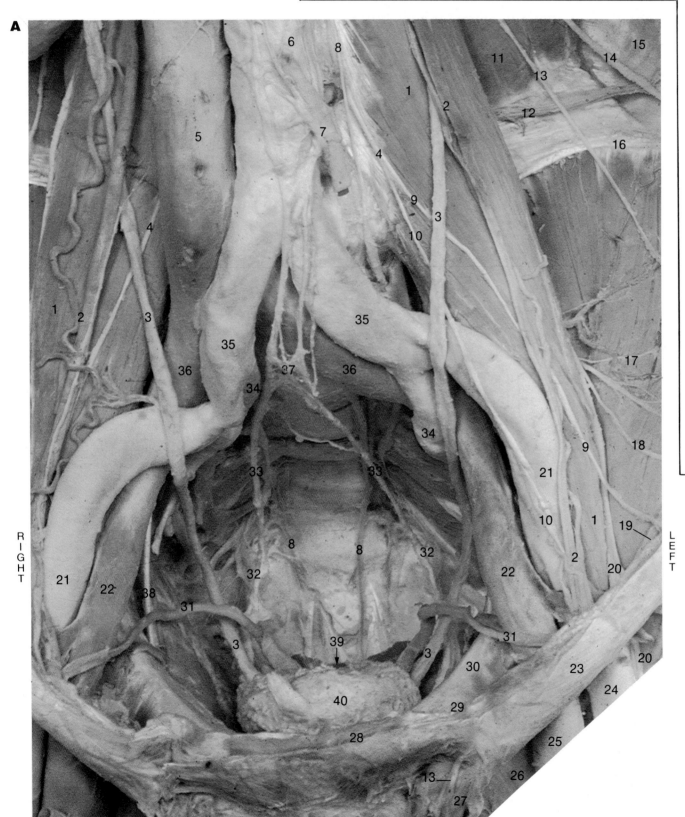

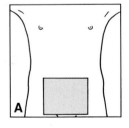

• The aorta (A6) bifurcates into the common iliac arteries (A35) at the level of the fourth lumbar vertebra.
• The common iliac veins (A36) unite at the level of the fifth lumbar vertebra to form the inferior vena cava (A5), which lies on the right of the aorta (A6).
• On psoas major (A1) the ureter (A3) lies with the genitofemoral nerve (A4) behind it and the testicular vessels (A2) in front of it. A normal genitofemoral nerve is seen on the right side of this specimen, but on the left it has divided unusually early (above the level of the aortic bifurcation) into its genital and femoral branches (A9 and 10).
• The ureter (A3) enters the pelvis at the bifurcation of the common iliac artery (A35) crossing the external iliac artery (A21) and running down in front of the internal iliac artery (A34).
• In the pelvis the ureter (A3) is crossed superficially by the ductus deferens (A31).
• The single midline superior hypogastric plexus (A37) divides to form the right and left hypogastric nerves (A33) which enter the pelvis to contribute to the right and left inferior hypogastric plexuses (A32), collectively known as the pelvic plexus.
• The external iliac vessels (A21 and 22) pass beneath the inguinal ligament (A23) to become the femoral vessels, the vein (A25) lying medial to the artery (A24). The femoral nerve (A20) is lateral to the artery.

B Left lumbar plexus, from the front

Psoas major has been removed to show the constituent nerves of the plexus which are embedded within the muscle. Because of the removal of most of the anterolateral abdominal wall (except for the lowest parts of the external oblique, 11, internal oblique, 10, and transversus, 15), the iliohypogastric (8) and ilio-inguinal (7) nerves have fallen too far medially; they should not overlie iliacus (9)

1	Third lumbar vertebra and anterior longitudinal ligament
2	Sympathetic trunk and ganglia
3	Rami communicantes
4	Ventral ramus of fourth lumbar nerve
5	Iliolumbar ligament
6	Quadratus lumborum
7	Ilio-inguinal nerve
8	Iliohypogastric nerve
9	Iliacus
10	Internal oblique
11	External oblique
12	External oblique aponeurosis
13	Upper surface of inguinal ring
14	Superficial inguinal ring
15	Transversus abdominis
16	Obturator nerve
17	Femoral nerve
18	Genitofemoral nerve
19	Lateral femoral cutaneous nerve
20	Ventral ramus of fifth lumbar nerve
21	Lumbosacral trunk
22	Ventral ramus of first sacral nerve

• The lumbosacral trunk (21), formed by part of the ventral ramus of the fourth lumbar nerve (4) and the whole of the ventral ramus of the fifth lumbar nerve (20) is the contribution which the lumbar plexus makes to the sacral plexus.

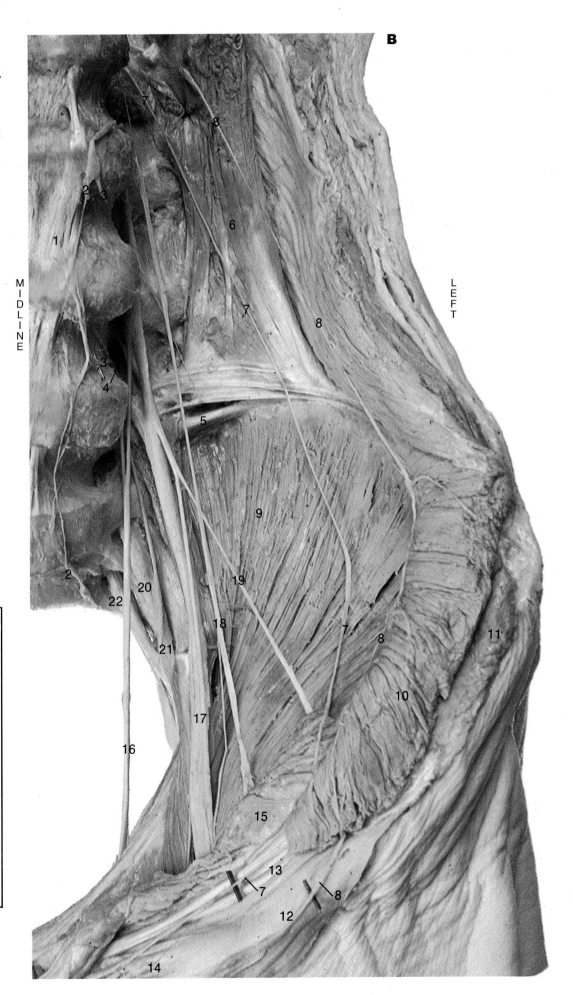

A Muscles of the left half of the pelvis and upper thigh, from the front

All fasciae have been removed but the inguinal ligament (16), formed from part of the external oblique aponeurosis, has been preserved. Psoas major (3) and iliacus (4) are seen entering the thigh deep to the inguinal ligament. On the front of the thigh there is an unusually large gap between the adjacent borders of pectineus (14) and adductor longus (11), revealing part of the adductor brevis (13)

1	Promontory of sacrum
2	Fifth lumbar intervertebral disc
3	Psoas major
4	Iliacus
5	Iliac crest
6	Anterior superior iliac spine
7	Tensor fasciae latae
8	Vastus lateralis
9	Rectus femoris
10	Sartorius
11	Adductor longus
12	Gracilis
13	Adductor brevis
14	Pectineus
15	Pubic tubercle
16	Inguinal ligament
17	Coccygeus
18	Obturator internus
19	Piriformis

● The medial border of psoas major (A3) overlaps the side of the pelvic brim.
● Above the inguinal ligament (A16) iliacus (A4) forms the floor of the iliac fossa. On the right side, this is where the caecum and appendix lie (page 234, A).
● Piriformis (A19) and obturator internus (A18) are muscles of the posterior and lateral walls of the pelvis; they are also classified as muscles of the lower limb.
● Coccygeus (A17, B and C2) and levator ani (C18 and 21) are the muscles of the pelvic floor, otherwise known as the pelvic diaphragm.
● Below the inguinal ligament (A16), iliacus (A4), psoas major (A3), pectineus (A14), adductor brevis (A13) and adductor longus (A11) form the floor of the femoral triangle (page 296), whose lateral boundary is the medial border of sartorius (A10) and medial boundary the medial border of adductor longus (A11). Adductor longus is usually adjacent to pectineus (A14), so excluding adductor brevis (A13) from the floor of the triangle.
● Gracilis (A12, B13) is the most medial muscle of the thigh.
● The anterior superior iliac spine (A6) and the pubic tubercle (A15), which give attachment to the ends of the inguinal ligament (A16), are important palpable landmarks in the inguinal region (see page 208).

A

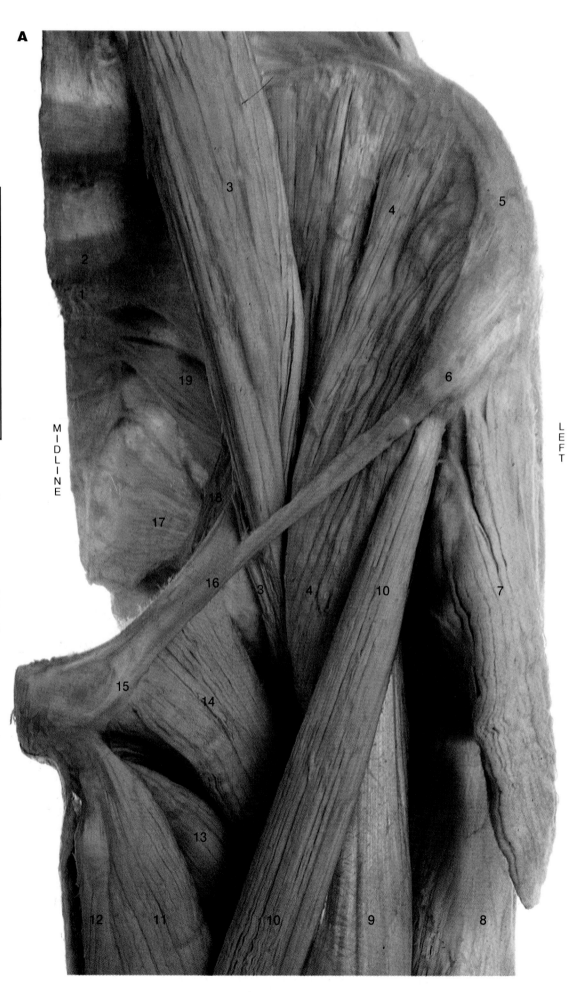

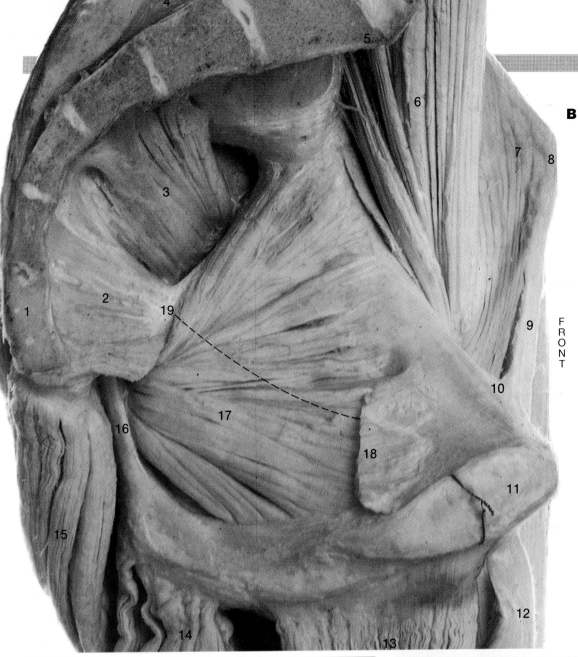

B **Muscles of the left half of the pelvis, from the right, B with most of levator ani removed, C with levator ani intact in the female**

Piriformis (3) is on the posterior pelvic wall, and obturator internus (17) on the lateral wall. Coccygeus (2) forms the posterior part of the pelvic floor (pelvic diaphragm), with levator ani (18 and 21) at the side and in front; in B most of levator ani has been removed (from the attachment indicated by the interrupted line) to show more of obturator internus (17), from whose overlying fascia (20) much of the levator ani arises. Here the iliococcygeus part of the levator ani (21) is more fibrous than usual. In C the lower ends of the urethra (23), vagina (24) and rectum (25) have been preserved

● The part of obturator internus (17) *above* the attachment of levator ani (interrupted line in B) is part of the lateral wall of the pelvic cavity, while the part *below* the attachment is in the perineum and forms part of the lateral wall of the ischiorectal fossa (page 256).
● Piriformis (3) passes out of the pelvis into the gluteal region through the *greater* sciatic foramen *above* the ischial spine (19), while obturator internus (17) passes out through the *lesser* sciatic foramen *below* the ischial spine (19).
● The posterior part of the *ilio*coccygeus part of the levator ani (C21) arises from the *ischial* spine (19), not from any part of the ilium; the name is derived from animals in which the muscle has a higher origin.

F
R
O
N
T

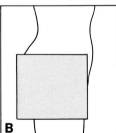

1 Coccyx
2 Coccygeus
3 Piriformis
4 Sacral canal
5 Promotory of sacrum
6 Psoas major
7 Iliacus
8 Anterior superior iliac spine
9 Inguinal ligament
10 Lacunar ligament
11 Pubic symphysis
12 Adductor longus
13 Gracilis
14 Adductor magnus
15 Gluteus maximus
16 Sacrotuberous ligament
17 Obturator internus
18 Pubococcyeus part of levator ani
19 Ischial spine
20 Fascia over obturator internus
21 Iliococcygeus part of levator ani
22 Branch of fourth sacral nerve
23 Urethra
24 Vagina
25 Rectum

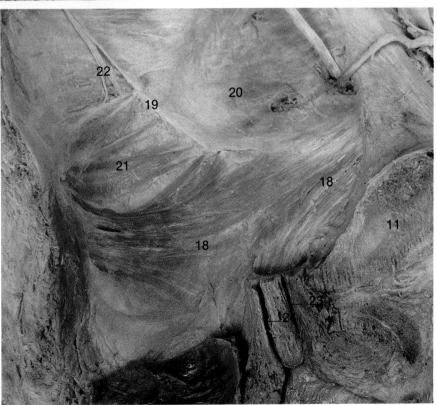

C

A

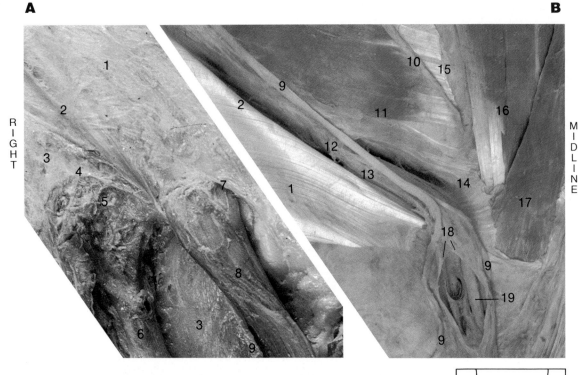

RIGHT

MIDLINE

B

Right inguinal region in the male, A superficial dissection, B with the external oblique aponeurosis and spermatic cord incised

In A the spermatic cord (8) is seen emerging from the superficial inguinal ring (7) and covered by the external spermatic fascia. In B, with the external oblique aponeurosis reflected and the anterior wall of the rectus sheath removed, the cord is emerging from the deep inguinal ring (12) with the cremasteric fascia (13) now the most superficial covering. All three coverings of the cord have been incised (18) to show the ductus deferens (19)

1	External oblique aponeurosis
2	Inguinal ligament
3	Fascia lata
4	Upper margin of saphenous opening
5	Cribriform fascia
6	Great saphenous vein
7	Upper margin of superficial inguinal ring
8	Spermatic cord
9	Ilio-inguinal nerve
10	Iliohypogastric nerve
11	Internal oblique
12	Deep inguinal ring
13	Cremasteric fascia over spermatic cord
14	Conjoint tendon
15	Edge of rectus sheath
16	Rectus abdominis
17	Pyramidalis
18	Incised margin of coverings of cord
19	Ductus deferens

● The spermatic cord (8) consists of the ductus deferens, the obliterated remains of the processus vaginalis of peritoneum, three arteries (testicular, cremasteric and deferential), the pampiniform plexus of veins, the genital branch of the genitofemoral nerve, sympathetic nerve fibres (accompanying the arteries) from the testicular and pelvic plexuses, and lymph vessels from the testis.
● The *coverings* of the cord consist of the internal spermatic fascia (derived from the transversalis fascia at the deep inguinal ring), the cremasteric fascia (B13, from the transversus and internal oblique muscles), and the external spermatic fascia (from the external oblique aponeurosis at the superficial inguinal ring, A7).
● The external oblique aponeurosis (A1) and the external spermatic fascia (which is the outermost covering of the spermatic cord, as at A8) are in continuity at the superficial inguinal ring (A7). The 'ring' only becomes a gap with a free margin if the fascia is cut away from the aponeurosis—as has been done for a short distance exactly at the label A7 on the medial side of the cord.
● The lowest fibres of the internal oblique (11), together with the underlying transversus fibres, arch over the cord (as at B11) to form the conjoint tendon (B14).
● The inguinal canal is the oblique gap in the anterior abdominal wall above the inguinal ligament and between the deep inguinal ring (B12) laterally and the superficial inguinal ring (A7) medially.
● In the male the inguinal canal contains the spermatic cord and the ilio-inguinal nerve; the cord enters the canal through the deep inguinal ring (B12), but the ilio-inguinal nerve (B9) enters from the side by running deep to the external oblique aponeurosis (in A it can be seen shining through the aponeurosis just below and to the right of the label 2). Both the cord and the nerve leave the canal through the superficial inguinal ring (7).

C

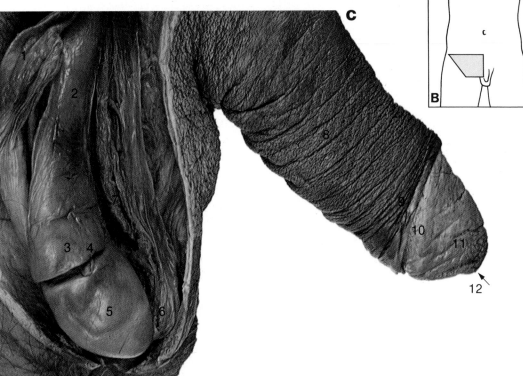

C Right testis and epididymis, and the penis, from the right

The scrotum, spermatic cord (2) and the tunica vaginalis (1) of the testis (5) have been opened up. The testis has been rotated to show that the ductus deferens (7) is the upward continuation of the tail of the epididymis (6); in its normal position the testis (5) hangs with the epididymis (3 and 6) on its posterolateral side, not anteromedial as here

1	Tunica vaginalis
2	Spermatic cord
3	Head of epididymis
4	Appendix of testis
5	Testis
6	Tail of epididymis
7	Ductus deferens
8	Body of penis
9	Foreskin (retracted)
10	Corona of glans
11	Glans penis
12	External urethral orifice

D Right inguinal region, in the female

The external oblique aponeurosis (1) has been incised and reflected to show the position of the deep inguinal ring (5) which marks the lateral end of the inguinal canal. The round ligament of the uterus (8) emerges from the superficial inguinal ring (7), which marks the medial end of the canal, and becomes lost in the fat of the labium majus (9). The ilio-inguinal nerve (2) also passes through the canal and out of the superficial ring

1	External oblique aponeurosis
2	Ilio-inguinal nerve
3	Upper surface of inguinal ligament
4	Internal oblique
5	Position of deep inguinal ring
6	Conjoint tendon
7	Position of superficial inguinal ring
8	Round ligament of uterus
9	Fat of labium majus
10	Great saphenous vein

• In the female the inguinal canal contains the round ligament of the uterus and the ilio-inguinal nerve.
• The processus vaginalis is normally obliterated, but if it remains patent within the female inguinal canal it is sometimes known as the canal of Nuck.

E Right inguinal and femoral regions, in the female

Part of the fascia lata of the thigh has been removed to show the femoral nerve (21), artery (20) and vein (18) beneath the inguinal ligament (19), and also the position of the femoral canal (17), medial to the vein (18). The femoral structures have been included here because of the importance of the femoral canal as a site for hernia in the female (see page 249)

1	Anterior superior iliac spine
2	External oblique aponeurosis
3	Cut edge of rectus sheath
4	Rectus abdominis
5	Superficial epigastric vein
6	Superficial inguinal ring
7	Round ligament of uterus
8	Mons pubis
9	Gracilis
10	Adductor longus
11	Pectineus
12	Great saphenous vein
13	Superficial external pudendal vessels
14	Fascia lata
15	Accessory saphenous vein
16	Lower edge of saphenous opening
17	Position of femoral canal
18	Femoral vein
19	Inguinal ligament
20	Femoral artery
21	Femoral nerve
22	Medial ⎱ femoral cutaneous nerve
23	Intermediate ⎰
24	Sartorius
25	Superficial circumflex iliac vessels
26	Fascia lata overlying tensor fasciae latae

• The round ligament of the uterus (D8, E7) is a very much smaller structure than the spermatic cord of the male but it pursues a similar course through the inguinal canal. Theoretically it has similar coverings to those of the cord but they are usually too small to be defined. The round ligament disappears into the labium majus (D9).

• The round ligament of the uterus (D8, E7) is a very much smaller structure than the spermatic cord of the male but it pursues a similar course through the inguinal canal. Theoretically it has similar coverings to those of the cord but they are usually too small to be defined. The round ligament disappears into the labium majus (D9).

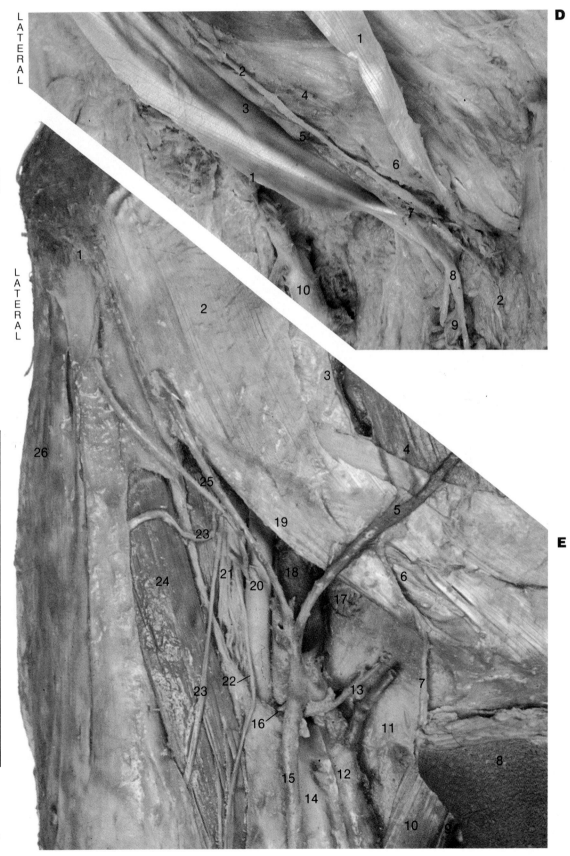

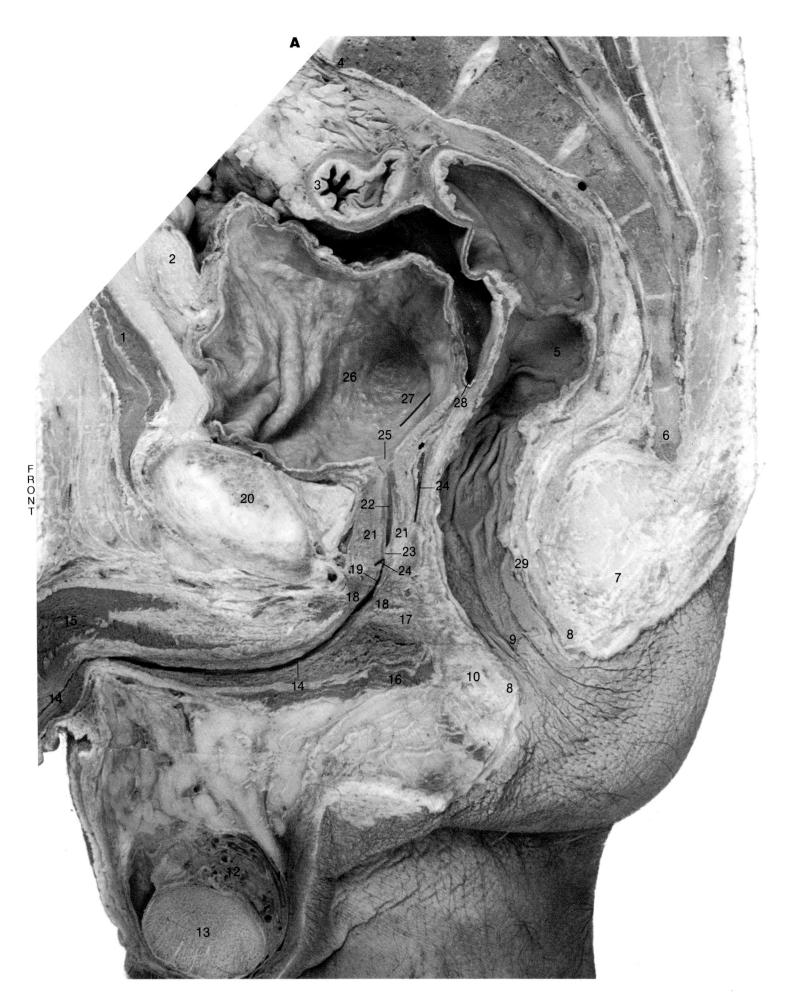

A

FRONT

A Right half of a midline sagittal section of the male pelvis

The section has passed exactly through the midline of the anal canal (9) and the prostatic, membranous and spongy parts of the urethra (22, 19 and 14) but has transected the left side of the scrotum and the left testis (13) and epididymis (12). The prostate (21) and bladder (26) are somewhat higher than usual; the empty bladder should not extend above the pubic symphysis (20)

1	Rectus abdominis
2	Extraperitoneal fat
3	Sigmoid colon
4	Promontory of sacrum
5	Rectum
6	Coccyx
7	Anococcygeal body
8	External anal sphincter
9	Anal canal with anal columns of mucous membrane
10	Perineal body
11	Ductus deferens
12	Epididymis
13	Testis
14	Spongy part of urethra and corpus spongiosum
15	Corpus cavernosum
16	Bulbospongiosus
17	Perineal membrane
18	Sphincter urethrae
19	Membranous part of urethra
20	Pubic symphysis
21	Prostate
22	Prostatic part of urethra
23	Seminal colliculus
24	Bristle in ejaculatory duct
25	Internal urethral orifice
26	Bladder
27	Bristle passing up into right ureteral orifice
28	Rectovesical pouch
29	Puborectalis fibres of levator ani

• The lowest part of the peritoneal cavity is the rectovesical pouch (A28), between the front of the rectum (A5) and the posterior surface (base) of the bladder (A26).

• The lower end of the rectum (A5) and the anal canal (A9) are maintained at right angles to one another by a sling formed by the puborectalis fibres of both levator ani muscles (A29), which become continuous with the upper end of the external anal sphincter (A8).

• The various constituents of the spermatic cord come together at the deep inguinal ring (B5), which is in the transversalis fascia (B4) *lateral* to the inferior epigastric vessels (B3). The ductus deferens (B9) therefore appears to emerge from the ring by hooking round the lateral side of the vessels.

• The inguinal triangle is the area bounded laterally by the inferior epigastric vessels (B3), medially by the lateral border of rectus abdominis (B1) and below by the inguinal ligament (B19). A *direct* inguinal hernia passes forwards through this triangle, *medial* to the inferior epigastric vessels.

• An *indirect* inguinal hernia passes through the deep inguinal ring (B5) *lateral* to the inferior epigastric vessels (B3).

• A femoral hernia passes into the femoral canal through the femoral ring (B18), bounded medially by the lacunar ligament (B16) and laterally by the femoral vein (the external iliac vein, B8, becomes the femoral vein as it passes beneath the inguinal ligament).

B

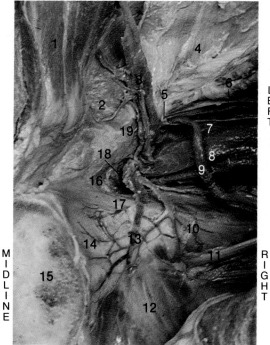

B Right deep inguinal ring and inguinal triangle, in the male

This is a view looking into the right half of the pelvis from the left, showing the posterior surface of the lower part of the anterior abdominal wall, above the pubic symphysis. The femoral ring (18), the entrance to the femoral canal, is below the medial end of the inguinal ligament (19). The inferior epigastric vessels (3) lie medial to the deep inguinal ring (5)

1	Rectus abdominis
2	Conjoint tendon
3	Inferior epigastric vessels
4	Transversalis fascia overlying transversus abdominis
5	Deep inguinal ring
6	Testicular vessels
7	External iliac artery
8	External iliac vein
9	Ductus deferens
10	Superior ramus of pubis
11	Obturator nerve
12	Origin of levator ani from fascia overlying obturator internus
13	Pubic branches of inferior epigastric vessels
14	Body of pubis
15	Pubic symphysis
16	Lacunar ligament
17	Pectineal ligament
18	Femoral ring
19	Inguinal ligament

C

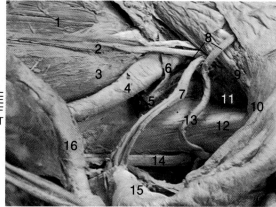

C Left accessory obturator artery in the male, from the right

This is a similar view to that in B but on the left side, showing an accessory obturator artery (13) passing from the inferior epigastric (8) over the superior pubic ramus (12) to enter the obturator foramen with the obturator nerve (14)

1	Iliacus
2	Testicular vessels
3	Psoas major
4	External iliac artery
5	External iliac vein (cut end)
6	Deep circumflex iliac vein
7	Ductus deferens
8	Inferior epigastric artery
9	Inguinal ligament
10	Lacunar ligament
11	Femoral ring
12	Superior ramus of pubis and pectineal ligament
13	Accessory obturator artery
14	Obturator nerve
15	Bladder
16	Right common iliac artery and vein

• The anastomosis between the pubic branches of the inferior epigastric and obturator arteries may be unusually large, forming the vessel known as the accessory or abnormal obturator artery (C13), in which case the normal obturator branch from the internal iliac may be absent.

• The accessory obturator artery *usually* lies at the *lateral* margin of the femoral ring (C11) but rarely it lies at the medial edge of the ring, i.e. at the lateral margin of the lacunar ligament (C10), where it may be at risk if the ligament has to be incised to enlarge the femoral ring in operations to reduce a femoral hernia.

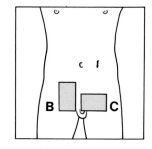

A Pelvis, right inguinal region and penis, from above

In the pelvis, most of the bladder (18) has been removed to show part of the base (upper surface) of the prostate (17), and the left seminal vesicle (16) lying lateral to the ductus deferens (15). The ductus in the pelvis crosses superficial to the ureter (9). The external iliac artery (8) passes under the inguinal ligament (1) to become the femoral artery (36). On the dorsum of the penis the fascia has been removed, showing the single midline deep dorsal vein (27) with a dorsal artery (28) and dorsal nerve (29) on each side

1	External oblique aponeurosis and inguinal ligament
2	Internal oblique
3	Iliacus
4	Femoral nerve
5	Psoas major
6	Femoral ⎞ branch of genitofemoral
7	Genital ⎠ nerve
8	External iliac artery
9	Ureter
10	Common iliac artery
11	Internal iliac artery
12	Fifth lumbar intervertebral disc
13	Sigmoid colon (cut lower end)
14	Rectum
15	Ductus deferens
16	Seminal vesicle
17	Base of prostate
18	Trigone of bladder
19	Internal urethral orifice
20	Ureteral orifice
21	Superior vesical artery
22	Inferior vesical artery
23	Obturator artery
24	Obturator nerve
25	Spermatic cord
26	Inferior epigastric artery
27	Deep dorsal vein ⎞
28	Dorsal artery ⎟ of penis
29	Dorsal nerve ⎠
30	Adductor longus
31	Pectineus
32	Deep external pudendal artery
33	Femoral vein
34	Great saphenous vein
35	Superficial circumflex iliac vein
36	Femoral artery

● The trigone of the bladder (A18, C38), at the lower part of the base or posterior surface, is the relatively fixed area with smooth mucous membrane between the internal urethral orifice (A19, C37) and the two ureteral openings (A20 on the right side, C39 on the left).

● In the male pelvis the ureter (A9, C11) is crossed superficially by the ductus deferens (A15, C6). (In the female pelvis it is crossed superficially by the uterine artery—page 255.)

● The ureter (A9, C11) enters the pelvis at the bifurcation of the common iliac artery (A10), crossing the external iliac artery and vein (C4 and 5) and running down the side wall of the pelvis in front of the internal iliac artery (A11, C12) and being crossed superficially by the ductus deferens (A15, C6).

● The obturator artery (A23, C19) runs below the obturator nerve (A24, C10), with the vein below the artery, but in C there is an accessory obturator vein (C8) draining to the inferior epigastric vein (C40).

● Each ductus deferens (A15, B3, C6) lies on the medial side of its own seminal vesicle (A16, B2), and crosses superficial to the ureter (A9, C11).

● The neck of the bladder is the part containing the internal urethral orifice (A19, C37), at the lower angle of the trigone (A18, C38).

● The base of the bladder is its posterior surface (B5).

● The base of the prostate is not its posterior surface (B6) but its upper surface (A17), in contact with the neck of the bladder and pierced by the urethra (A19, C37).

B

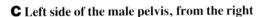

B Bladder and prostate, from behind
The bladder (5) has been distended and the left half of the prostate removed to show the ductus deferens (3) and the seminal vesicle (2) uniting to form the ejaculatory duct (4)

1	Ureter
2	Seminal vesicle
3	Ductus deferens
4	Left ejaculatory duct
5	Base of bladder
6	Posterior surface of prostate

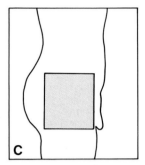

C

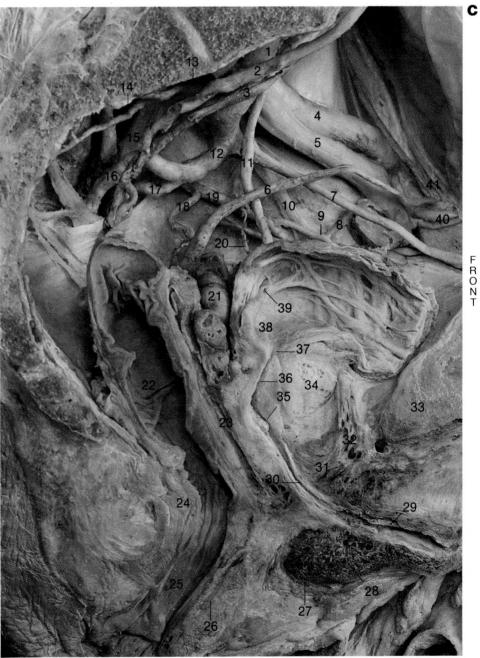

FRONT

C Left side of the male pelvis, from the right
In this midline sagittal section, the prostate (34) is enlarged, lengthening the prostatic urethra (36). The mucous membrane of the bladder (whose trigone is labelled at 38) has been removed to show muscular trabeculae in the wall. Variations in the branches of the internal iliac artery (12) are common, and here the obturator artery (19) gives origin to the superior vesical (9) and inferior vesical (20) as well as the middle rectal (18). The largest branch of the internal iliac, the superior gluteal (13) is largely hidden behind the superior rectal vessels (2 and 3). The ureter (11) is crossed superficially by the ductus deferens (6)

1	Common iliac artery	24	Puborectalis part of levator ani
2	Superior rectal artery		
3	Superior rectal vein	25	Anal canal
4	External iliac artery	26	External anal sphincter
5	External iliac vein	27	Bulbospongiosus
6	Ductus deferens	28	Bulb of penis
7	Obliterated umbilical artery	29	Bulbar part of spongy urethra
8	Accessory obturator vein		
9	Superior vesical artery	30	Membranous part of urethra
10	Obturator nerve		
11	Ureter	31	Urogenital diaphragm
12	Internal iliac artery	32	Vesicoprostatic venous plexus
13	Superior gluteal artery		
14	Lateral sacral artery	33	Pubic symphysis
15	Ventral ramus of second sacral nerve	34	Prostate (enlarged)
		35	Seminal colliculus
16	Inferior gluteal artery	36	Prostatic part of urethra
17	Internal pudendal artery	37	Internal urethral orifice
18	Middle rectal artery	38	Trigone of bladder
19	Obturator artery	39	Ureteral orifice
20	Inferior vesical artery	40	Inferior epigastric vessels
21	Seminal vesical	41	Testicular vessels and deep inguinal ring
22	Lower end of rectum		
23	Rectovesical fascia		

251

A Arteries and nerves of the pelvis, left side

In this left half section of the pelvis, all peritoneum, fascia, veins and visceral arteries have been removed together with the left levator ani, so displaying the whole of the internal surface of obturator internus (20). On the posterior pelvic wall the vessels in general lie superficial to the nerves. In this specimen the external iliac artery (15) is unusually tortuous, and the anterior trunk of the internal iliac artery (12) has divided unusually high up into its terminal branches, the internal pudendal (13) and the inferior gluteal (5). The superior gluteal artery (8) has perforated the lumbosacral trunk

1	Sacrococcygeal joint
2	Coccygeus and sacrospinous ligament
3	Union of ventral rami of second and third sacral nerves
4	Piriformis
5	Inferior gluteal artery
6	Ventral ramus of first sacral nerve
7	Lateral sacral artery
8	Superior gluteal artery piercing lumbosacral trunk
9	Posterior trunk of internal iliac artery
10	Sacral promontory
11	Internal iliac artery
12	Anterior trunk of internal iliac artery
13	Internal pudendal artery
14	Obturator nerve and artery
15	External iliac artery
16	Inferior epigastric artery
17	Inguinal ligament
18	Lacunar ligament
19	Pubic symphysis
20	Obturator internus
21	Ischial tuberosity

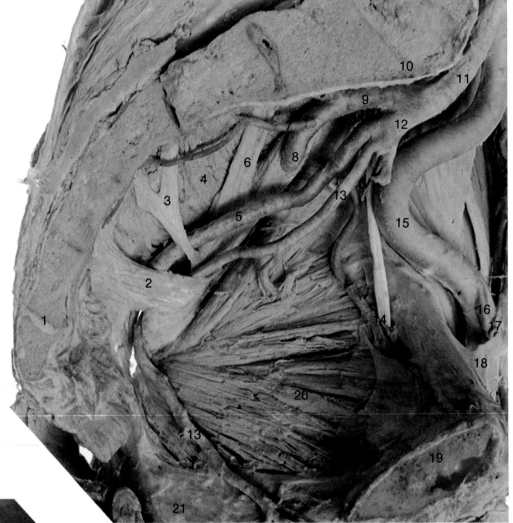

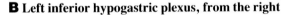

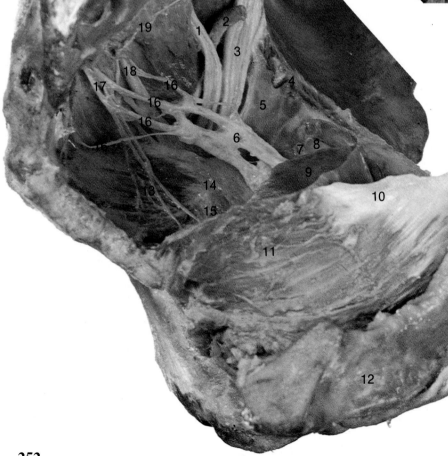

B Left inferior hypogastric plexus, from the right

In this view of the left side of the pelvis from the right, the right pelvic wall has been removed but the right levator ani (11) forming part of the pelvic floor (pelvic diaphragm) has been preserved and is seen from its right (perineal) side. Pelvic splanchnic nerves (16) arise from the ventral rami of the second and third sacral nerves (18 and 17) and contribute to the inferior hypogastric plexus (6)

1	Ventral ramus of first sacral nerve
2	Superior gluteal artery
3	Lumbosacral trunk
4	Arcuate line of ilium
5	Fascia overlying obturator internus
6	Left inferior hypogastric plexus
7	Left seminal vesicle
8	Left ductus deferens
9	Rectum
10	Lateral surface of fascia overlying right obturator internus
11	Right levator ani and ischiorectal fossa
12	Right ischiopubic ramus
13	Left coccygeus and nerves to levator ani
14	Ischial spine
15	Left levator ani
16	Pelvic splanchnic nerves (nervi erigentes)
17	Ventral ramus of third sacral nerve
18	Ventral ramus of second sacral nerve
19	Part of left sympathetic trunk

● Before they leave the pelvis, the internal pudendal artery (A13) lies in front of the inferior gluteal (A5). The perineal part of the internal pudendal is seen here overlying the lower part of the obturator internus (A20) because the fascia forming the pudendal canal (in which it lies, page 257, F13) has been removed.

● The superior gluteal artery (A8) usually passes backwards above piriformis (A4) between the lumbosacral trunk and the ventral ramus of the first sacral nerve (A6) (but sometimes between the first and second ventral rami). Here it has passed between fibres of the lumbosacral trunk.

● The inferior gluteal artery (A5) passes backwards below piriformis (A4) between the ventral rami of the first (A6) and second (A3) (or second and third) sacral nerves.

● The left and right inferior hypogastric plexuses (B6) together form the pelvic plexus. Their parasympathetic fibres are from the pelvic splanchnic nerves (B16), and the sympathetic contributions are from the hypogastric nerves (page 242, A33) and ganglia of the sacral part of the sympathetic trunk (B19).

C Pelvic ligaments, left side, from the right

In this median sagittal section of the pelvis all soft tissues have been removed except the ligaments

1	Sacral promontory
2	Iliac fossa
3	Anterior superior iliac spine
4	Anterior inferior iliac spine and origin of straight head of rectus femoris
5	Inguinal ligament
6	Lacunar ligament
7	Pectineal ligament
8	Pubic symphysis
9	Obturator foramen
10	Obturator membrane
11	Falciform process of sacrotuberous ligament
12	Ischial tuberosity
13	Sacrotuberous ligament
14	Lesser sciatic foramen
15	Ischial spine
16	Sacrospinous ligament
17	Greater sciatic foramen
18	Ventral sacro-iliac ligament

● The ligaments classified as 'the ligaments of the pelvis' (vertebropelvic ligaments) are the sacrotuberous (13), sacrospinous (16) and iliolumbar (seen in the posterior view on page 301, B2).

● The sacrotuberous and sacrospinous ligaments convert the greater and lesser sciatic *notches* of the hip bone (page 265, 18 and 15) into *foramina* (C17 and C14).

● The lacunar ligament (C6) passes backwards from the medial end of the inguinal ligament (C5) to the medial end of the pectineal line of the pubis, to which the pectineal ligament (C7) is attached.

● The lower attachment of the sacrotuberous ligament is to the medial side of the ischial tuberosity, but it gives off two slips. One is the falciform process (C11), which passes towards the ischial ramus to form the lower boundary of the pudendal canal (page 257, F13). The other runs into the ischial attachment of the long head of biceps (page 295, B5).

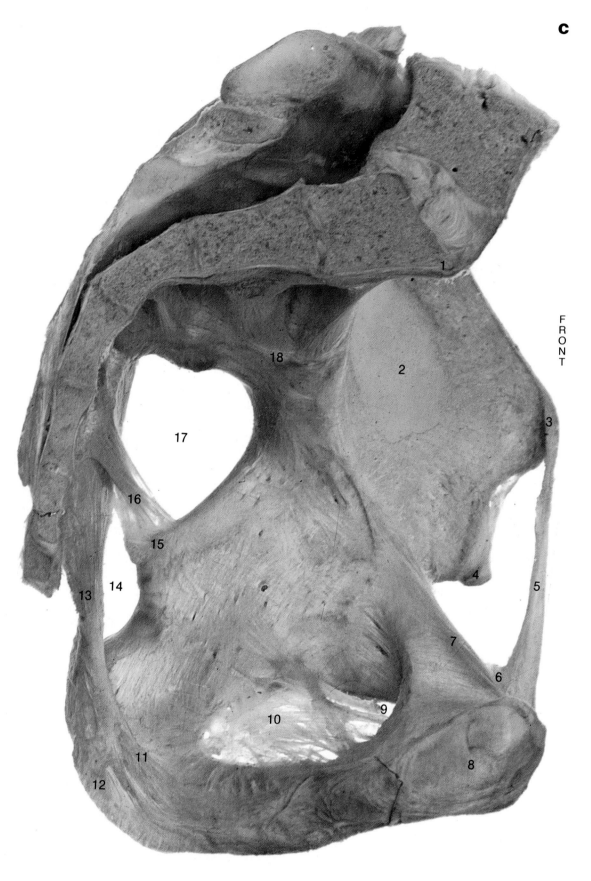

C

FRONT

A Left half of a midline sagittal section of the female pelvis

The lower end of the rectum (32) is dilated, and the bladder (16), uterus (11) and vagina (27 and 28) are contracted. The section has opened up the whole length of the urethra (19), but the cervix of the uterus (12) is rarely exactly in the midline and the line of the cervical canal is indicated by the marker in the internal and external os (13 and 14)

1	Line of attachent of right limb of sigmoid mesocolon
2	Fifth lumbar intervertebral disc
3	Apex of sigmoid mesocolon
4	Ureter underlying peritoneum
5	Ovary
6	Uterine tube
7	Suspensory ligament of ovary containing ovarian vessels
8	Left limb of sigmoid mesocolon overlying external iliac vessels
9	Sigmoid colon (reflected to left and upwards)
10	Fundus ⎫
11	Body ⎬ of uterus
12	Cervix ⎭
13	Marker in internal os
14	Marker in external os
15	Vesico-uterine pouch
16	Bladder
17	Marker in left ureteral orifice
18	Internal urethral orifice
19	Urethra
20	External urethral orifice
21	Pubic symphysis
22	Rectus abdominis (turned forwards)
23	Fat of mons pubis
24	Labium minus
25	Labium majus
26	Vestibule ⎫
27	Anterior wall ⎮
28	Posterior wall ⎬ of vagina
29	Anterior fornix ⎮
30	Posterior fornix ⎭
31	Recto-uterine pouch
32	Rectum
33	Perineal body
34	Anal canal
35	External anal sphincter

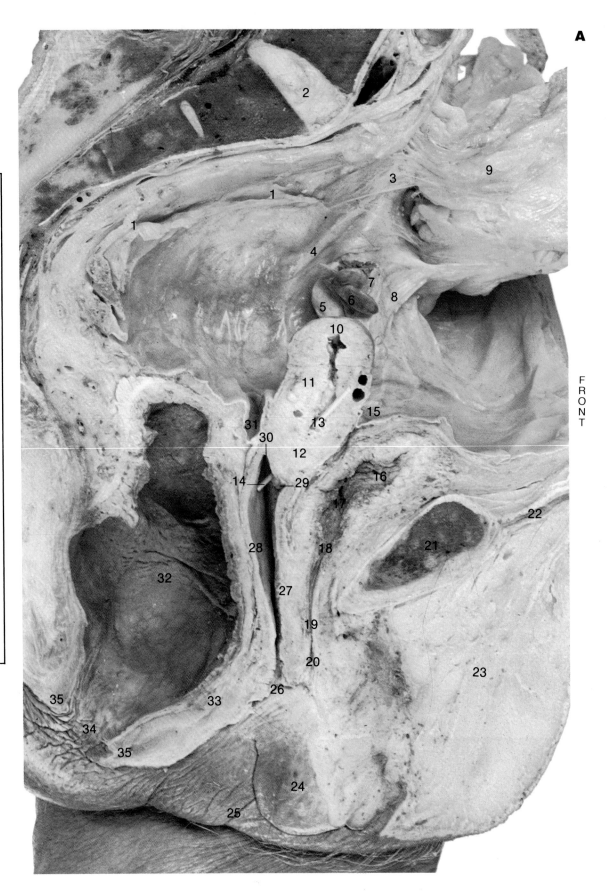

FRONT

B

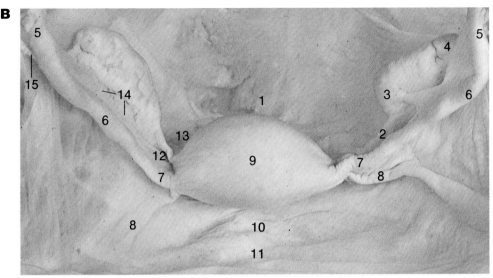

FRONT

C

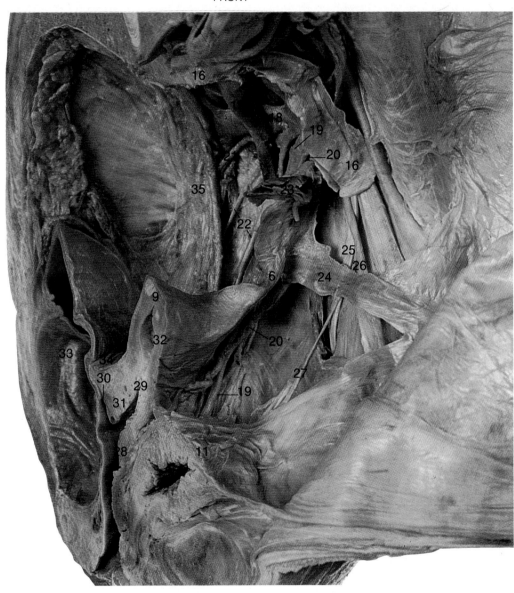

F
R
O
N
T

Female pelvis. **B** Uterus and ovaries, from above and in front. **C** Left half, obliquely from above and in front

In B, looking down into the pelvis from the front, the fundus of the uterus (9) overlies the bladder (11) with the peritoneum of the vesico-uterine pouch (10) intervening. In C, looking obliquely into the left half of the pelvis from the front, with the anterior abdominal wall turned forwards, the peritoneum of the vesico-uterine pouch has been incised and the uterus (32) displaced backwards to show the ureter (19) running towards the bladder and being crossed by the uterine artery (20)

1	Recto-uterine pouch
2	Ligament of ovary
3	Uterine ⎫
4	Tubal ⎭ extremity of ovary
5	Infundibulum ⎫
6	Ampulla ⎬ of uterine tube
7	Isthmus ⎭
8	Round ligament of uterus
9	Fundus of uterus
10	Vesico-uterine pouch
11	Peritoneum overlying bladder
12	Mesosalpinx
13	Posterior surface of broad ligament
14	Mesovarium
15	Suspensory ligament of ovary with ovarian vessels
16	Sigmoid mesocolon
17	Internal iliac vein
18	Internal iliac artery
19	Ureter
20	Uterine artery
21	Middle rectal artery
22	Vaginal artery (double)
23	Fimbriated end of uterine tube
24	Round ligament of uterus
25	Obturator nerve
26	Obliterated umbilical artery
27	Superior vesical artery
28	Cavity ⎫
29	Anterior fornix ⎬ of vagina
30	Posterior fornix ⎭
31	Cervix ⎫ of uterus
32	Body ⎭
33	Rectum
34	Recto-uterine pouch
35	Uterosacral ligament

● The apex of the sigmoid mesocolon (A3, C16) is a guide to the left ureter (A4, C19) which enters the pelvis under the peritoneum at this point (in both sexes).
● Farther forward in the pelvis the ureter (C19) is crossed superficially by the uterine artery (C20). In the male pelvis it is crossed by the ductus deferens (pages 250 and 251).
● The recto-uterine pouch (A31, C34, pouch of Douglas) overlies the posterior fornix of the vagina (A30, C30), but the vesico-uterine pouch (A15) does not reach the anterior fornix (A29).
● The uterosacral ligaments (C35), passing backwards on either side of the rectum to the sacrum and internal iliac vessels, and the lateral cervical ligaments (tissue underlying the ureter and uterine artery, C19 and 20, often called the cardinal or Mackenrodt's ligaments and passing to the lateral pelvic wall) are condensations of retroperitoneal tissue of great importance in supporting the uterine cervix (A12, C31) in its normal position.

A Male perineum

The central area is shown, with the scrotum (1) pulled upwards and forwards

1	Scrotum overlying left testis
2	Raphe overlying bulb of penis
3	Perineal body
4	Margin of anus
5	Anococcygeal body

● In both sexes the ischiorectal fossa has the pudendal canal (E11, F13) in its lateral wall. In B the canal has been opened up to display its contents: the internal pudendal artery (B18) and the terminal branches of the pudendal nerve—the perineal nerve (B17) and the dorsal nerve of the penis (B21) or clitoris.

A FRONT

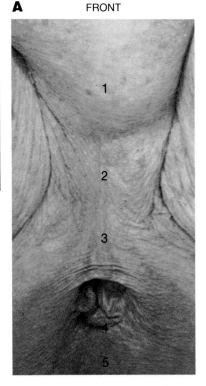

C Root of penis, from in front and below

The front part of the penis has been removed to show the root, formed by the two corpora cavernosa dorsally (8) and the single corpus spongiosum ventrally (9) containing the urethra (10)

1	Pubic tubercle	8	Corpus cavernosum
2	Pubic crest	9	Corpus spongiosum
3	Pubic symphysis	10	Urethra
4	Suspensory ligament	11	Perineal membrane
5	Deep dorsal vein	12	Ischiopubic ramus
6	Dorsal artery	13	Obturator membrane
7	Dorsal nerve		

C

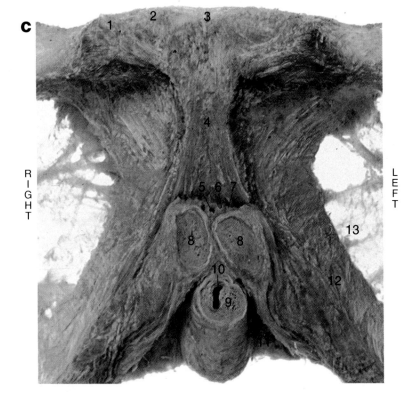

B

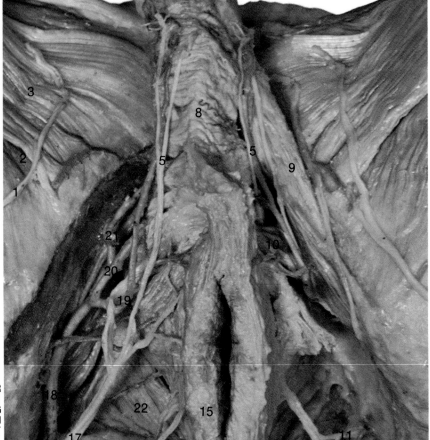

B Male perineum and ischiorectal fossae

All the fat has been removed from the ischiorectal fossae so that a clear view is obtained of the perineal surface of levator ani (22) and of the vessels and nerves within the fossae. On the left side (right of the picture) the perineal membrane (10) is intact but on the right side it and the underlying muscle (urogenital diaphragm) have been removed

1	Perineal branch of posterior femoral cutaneous nerve	11	Inferior rectal vessels and nerve in ischiorectal fossa
2	Adductor magnus	12	Perforating cutaneous nerve
3	Gracilis	13	Gluteus maximus
4	Adductor longus	14	Anococcygeal body
5	Posterior scrotal vessels and nerves	15	Margin of anus
6	Corpus cavernosum of penis	16	Sacrotuberous ligament
7	Corpus spongiosum of penis	17	Perineal nerve
8	Bulbospongiosus overlying bulb of penis	18	Internal pudendal artery
9	Ischiocavernosus overlying crus of penis	19	Perineal artery
10	Superficial transverse perineal muscle overlying posterior border of perineal membrane	20	Artery to bulb
		21	Dorsal nerve and artery of penis
		22	Levator ani

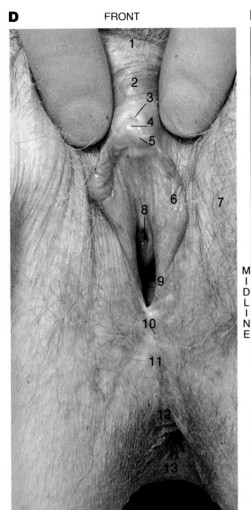

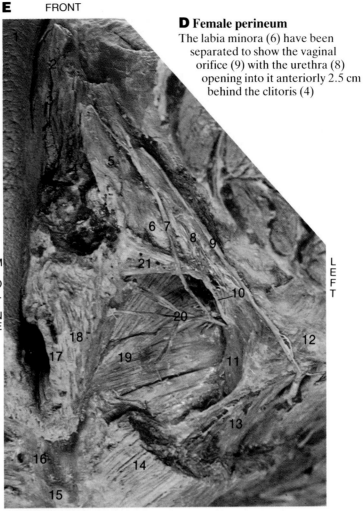

D Female perineum
The labia minora (6) have been separated to show the vaginal orifice (9) with the urethra (8) opening into it anteriorly 2.5 cm behind the clitoris (4)

1	Mons pubis
2	Anterior commissure
3	Prepuce of clitoris
4	Clitoris
5	Frenulum of clitoris
6	Labium minus
7	Labium majus
8	External urethral orifice
9	Vaginal orifice
10	Posterior commissure
11	Perineal body
12	Margin of anus
13	Anococcygeal body

E Left ischiorectal fossa and perineum in the female, from below
The nerves are preserved but the accompanying vessels have been removed

1	Labium majus
2	Labium minus
3	External urethral orifice
4	Vagina
5	Bulbospongiosus overlying bulb of vestibule
6	Perineal membrane
7	Posterior labial nerve
8	Ischiocavernosus overlying crus of clitoris
9	Perineal branch of posterior femoral cutaneous nerve
10	Pudendal nerve
11	Pudendal canal
12	Ischial tuberosity
13	Sacrotuberous ligament
14	Gluteus maximus
15	Coccyx
16	Anococcygeal body
17	Anal margin
18	External anal sphincter
19	Levator ani
20	Inferior rectal nerve
21	Superficial transverse perineal muscle overlying posterior border of perineal membrane

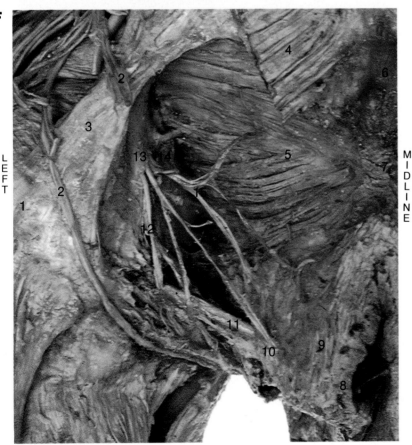

F Left ischiorectal fossa and perineum in the female, from behind
This view shows obturator internus with its overlying fascia (14) forming the lateral wall of the fossa, with levator ani (5) sloping downwards and medially as the roof

1	Ischial tuberosity
2	Perineal branch of posterior femoral cutaneous nerve
3	Sacrotuberous ligament
4	Gluteus maximus
5	Levator ani
6	Coccyx
7	Anococcygeal body
8	Anal margin
9	External anal sphincter
10	Posterior labial nerve
11	Posterior border of perineal membrane
12	Pudendal nerve
13	Pudendal canal
14	Obturator internus and fascia
15	Inferior rectal nerve

● The ischiorectal fossa is now properly and more correctly called the ischio-anal fossa; the anal canal (E17 and 18, F8 and 9), not the rectum, is its lower medial boundary. The walls and contents are similar in both sexes.

● The vulva is the anterior part of the female perineum containing the external genitalia.

● The external genitalia consist of the mons pubis (D1), labia majora (D7), labia minora (D6), clitoris (D4), vestibule of the vagina (the lower end with the vaginal orifice, D9), the bulb of the vestibule (E5), the greater vestibular (Bartholin's) glands (under the posterior end of the bulb of the vestibule), and the lesser vestibular glands (small mucous glands in the labia minora).

● The vestibule of the vagina is bounded by the labia minora (D6), and contains the external urethral orifice (D8), the vaginal orifice (D9, with the hymen at its margin in the virgin) and the ducts of the greater and lesser vestibular glands.

● The pudendal cleft is the region between the two labia majora (D7).

A

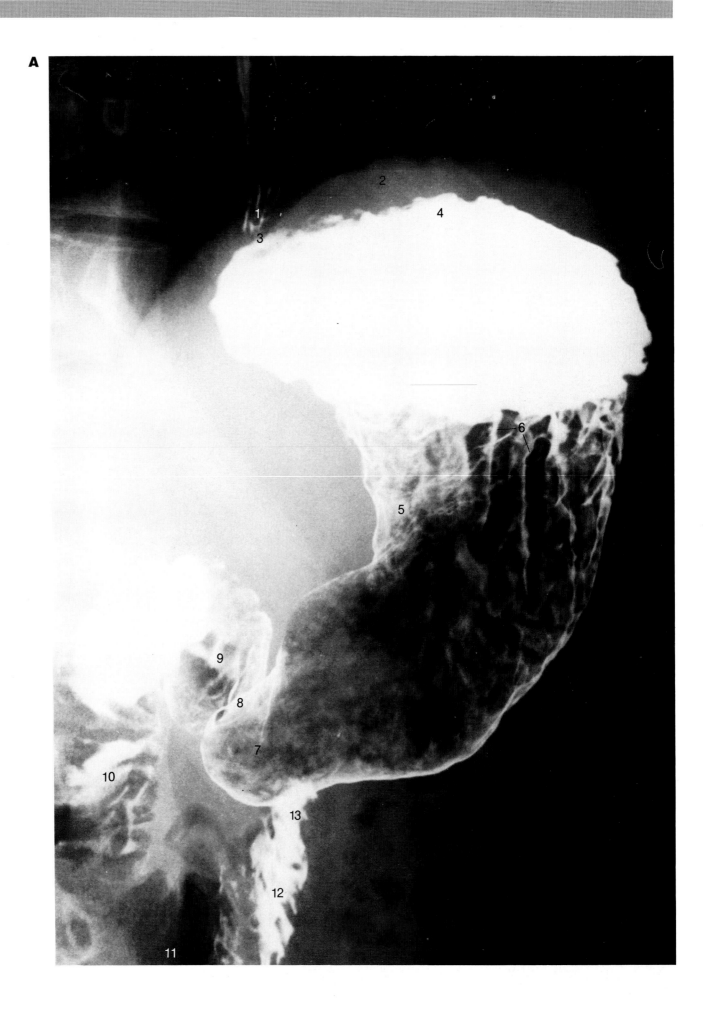

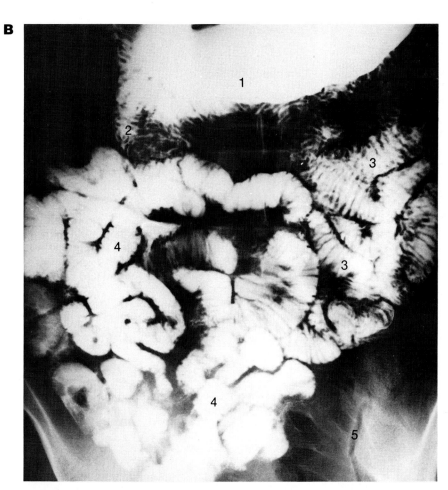

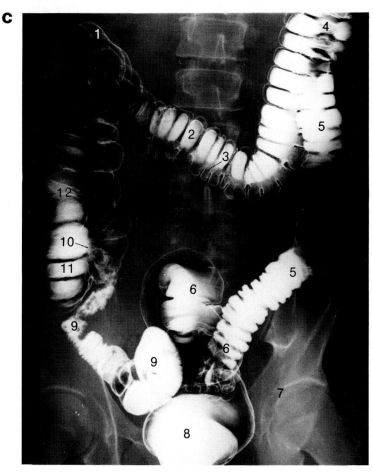

A Radiograph of the stomach, after a barium meal

In this double-contrast barium meal (barium and air, with the patient lying supine), the contrast medium is concentrated in the fundus and upper part of the body of the stomach (4 and 5) and at the junction of the superior (first) and descending (second) parts of the duodenum (9 and 10). The sparse barium in the rest of the stomach outlines some of the rugae (folds, 6) of the mucous membrane, and the constricted area (8) indicates the pylorus and gastroduodenal junction. Some barium has passed through into the ascending (fourth) part of the duodenum (12) and the region of the duodenojejunal flexure (13). Some barium also adheres to the oesophageal wall (1)

1	Oesophagus	8	Pylorus and gastroduodenal junction	
2	Diaphragm			
3	Cardia (gastro-oesophageal junction)	9	Superior (first)	part
		10	Descending (second)	of
4	Fundus	11	Horizontal (third)	duo-
5	Body of	12	Ascending (fourth)	denum
6	Rugae stomach	13	Duodenojejunal flexure	
7	Pyloric part			

● The C-shaped curve of the duodenum (9 to 12) is often known radiologically as the duodenal loop.

B Radiograph of the jejunum and ileum

In this 'follow through' after a barium meal, the contrast medium has filled the coils of small intestine, and although much remains in the stomach the duodenum is largely empty. The radiograph shows the typical 'feathery' pattern of the jejunum (3), mainly on the left side of the abdomen, and the non-feathery ileum (4); the difference in appearance results from the greater number of mucosal folds in the jejunum

1	Stomach	3	Coils of jejunum
2	Descending (second) part of duodenum	4	Coils of ileum
		5	Left sacro-iliac joint

C Radiograph of the large intestine

In this double-contrast barium enema (barium and air), the sacculations (haustrations, 3) of the various parts of the colon allow it to be distinguished from the narrower terminal ileum (9), which has become partly filled by barium flowing into it through the ileocaecal junction (10)

1	Right colic (hepatic) flexure	7	Hip joint
2	Transverse colon	8	Rectum
3	Sacculations	9	Terminal ileum
4	Left colic (splenic) flexure	10	Ileocaecal junction
5	Descending colon	11	Caecum
6	Sigmoid colon	12	Ascending colon

● For the appendix, which has not become filled with contrast medium here, see the next page.

A

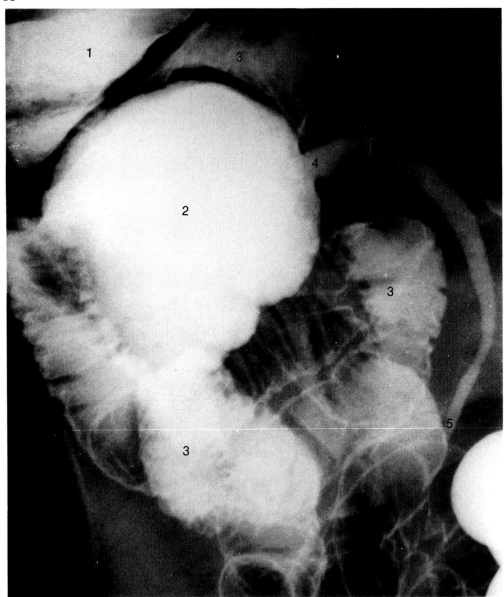

A Radiograph of the caecum and appendix

In this barium enema, the contrast medium has not only passed into the terminal ileum (3) from the caecum but has also filled the appendix (4) whose tip (5) lies in the pelvis

1	Ascending colon	4	Base of appendix
2	Caecum	5	Tip of appendix
3	Terminal ileum	6	Iliac crest

CT scans of the upper abdomen, B at the level of the coeliac trunk, C at the level of the left renal vein

All CT (computerised tomography) scans of the trunk are, by convention, viewed from below (as with the body lying on the back and the viewer looking towards the head). In B both oral and intravenous contrast media have been used (to emphasise the outlines of the gut and vascular system); in C there is no intravenous contrast. To avoid too many labels, only some key features have been numbered, and the various parts of the alimentary tract are unlabelled. The coeliac trunk arising from the aorta (9) is seen to divide as a Y into the splenic artery running towards the left behind the pancreas (5) and the common hepatic artery passing to the right near the portal vein (3). On the left side the spleen (6) and the upper pole of the kidney (7) are shown, but on the right the plane of the scan is too high to show the right kidney. In C, at a lower level, both kidneys are seen (7 and 11) with the left renal vein (12) crossing in front of the aorta (9) to enter the inferior vena cava (4)

1	Gall bladder	8	Twelfth thoracic
2	Liver		vertebra
3	Portal vein	9	Abdominal aorta
4	Inferior vena cava	10	Right crus of diaphragm
5	Pancreas	11	Right kidney
6	Spleen	12	Left renal vein
7	Left kidney	13	First lumbar vertebra

B FRONT

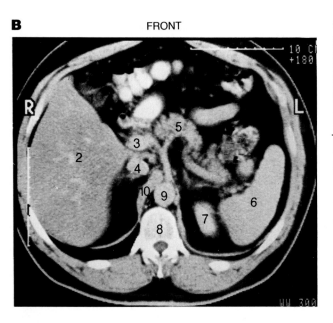

C FRONT

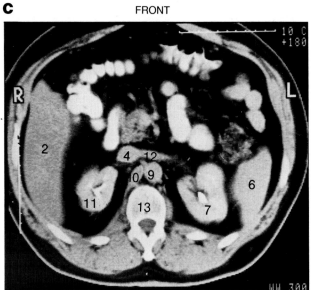

**D Radiography of the gall bladder.
Endoscopic retrograde
cholecystopancreatography (ERCP)**

In ERCP an endoscope is passed through the
mouth, pharynx, oesophagus and stomach into
the duodenum, and through it a cannula is
introduced into the major duodenal papilla
(page 225, C2) and bile duct so that contrast
medium can be injected up the biliary tract.
(The pancreatic duct can also be cannulated in
this way)

1	Liver shadow and tributaries of hepatic ducts
2	Right hepatic duct
3	Left hepatic duct
4	Common hepatic duct
5	Cystic duct
6	Gall bladder
7	Bile duct

D

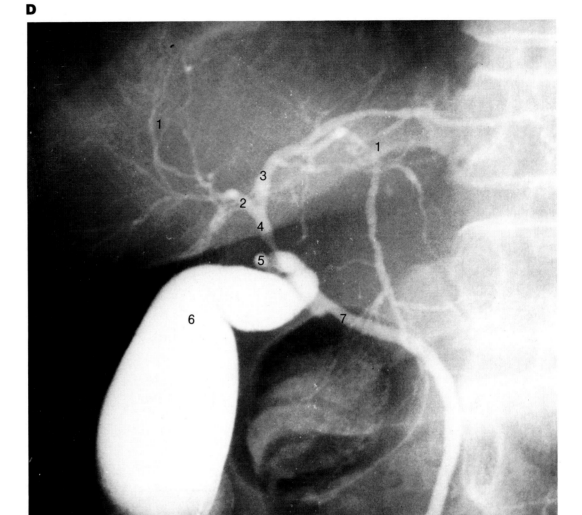

**E Radiography of the gall bladder.
Ultrasound scan**

To an untrained observer, ultrasound scans are
difficult to interpret but here the gall bladder
can be distinguished as a sausage-shaped cavity
(2)

1	Liver
2	Gall bladder
3	Diaphragm

E

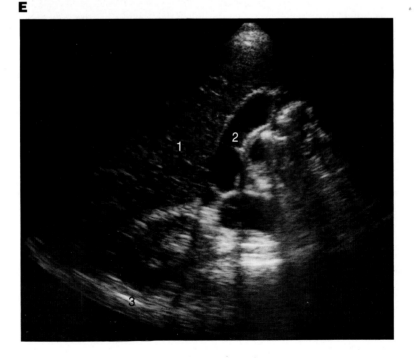

A

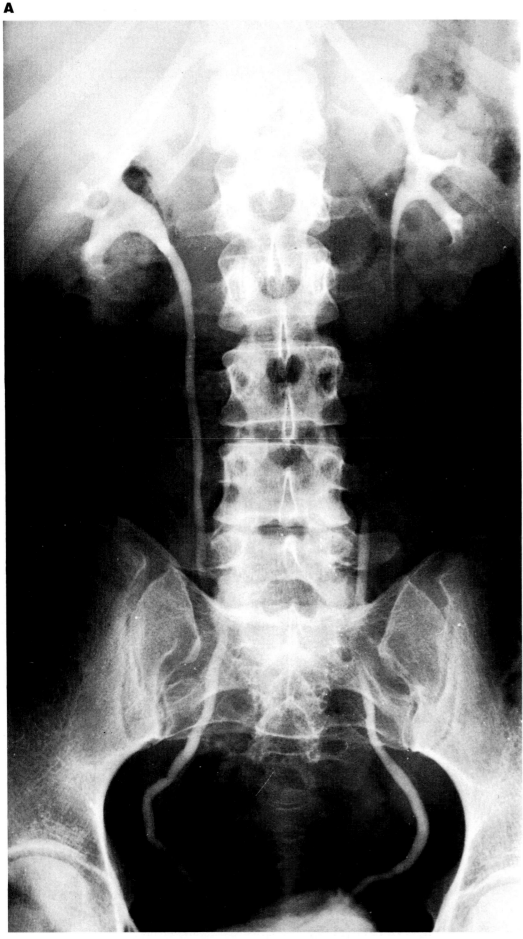

● Radiologically the ureters normally lie near the tips of the transverse processes of the lumbar vertebrae.

B   FRONT

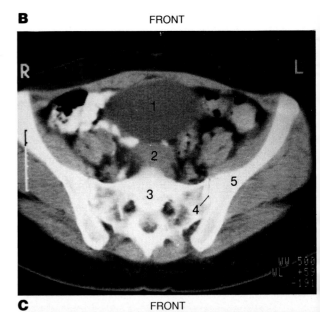

C   FRONT

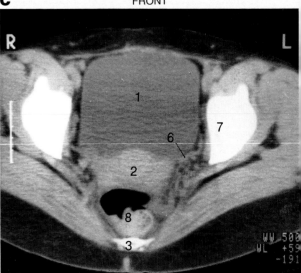

A Radiography of the urinary tract. Intravenous urogram (IVU)

Contrast medium injected intravenously is excreted by the kidneys to outline the calyces (page 238, A), renal pelvis and the ureters which enter the bladder in the pelvis

CT scans of the female pelvis, B at the level of the sacro-iliac joints, C at the level of the lower part of the sacrum

As in the abdomen (page 260, B and C), the scans are viewed from below as if looking up towards the thorax. The uterus (2) is behind the distended bladder (1). Coils of the gut are not labelled

1	Bladder (distended)
2	Uterus
3	Sacrum
4	Sacro-iliac joint
5	Hip bone
6	Uterine tube
7	Hip joint region
8	Rectum (gas black)

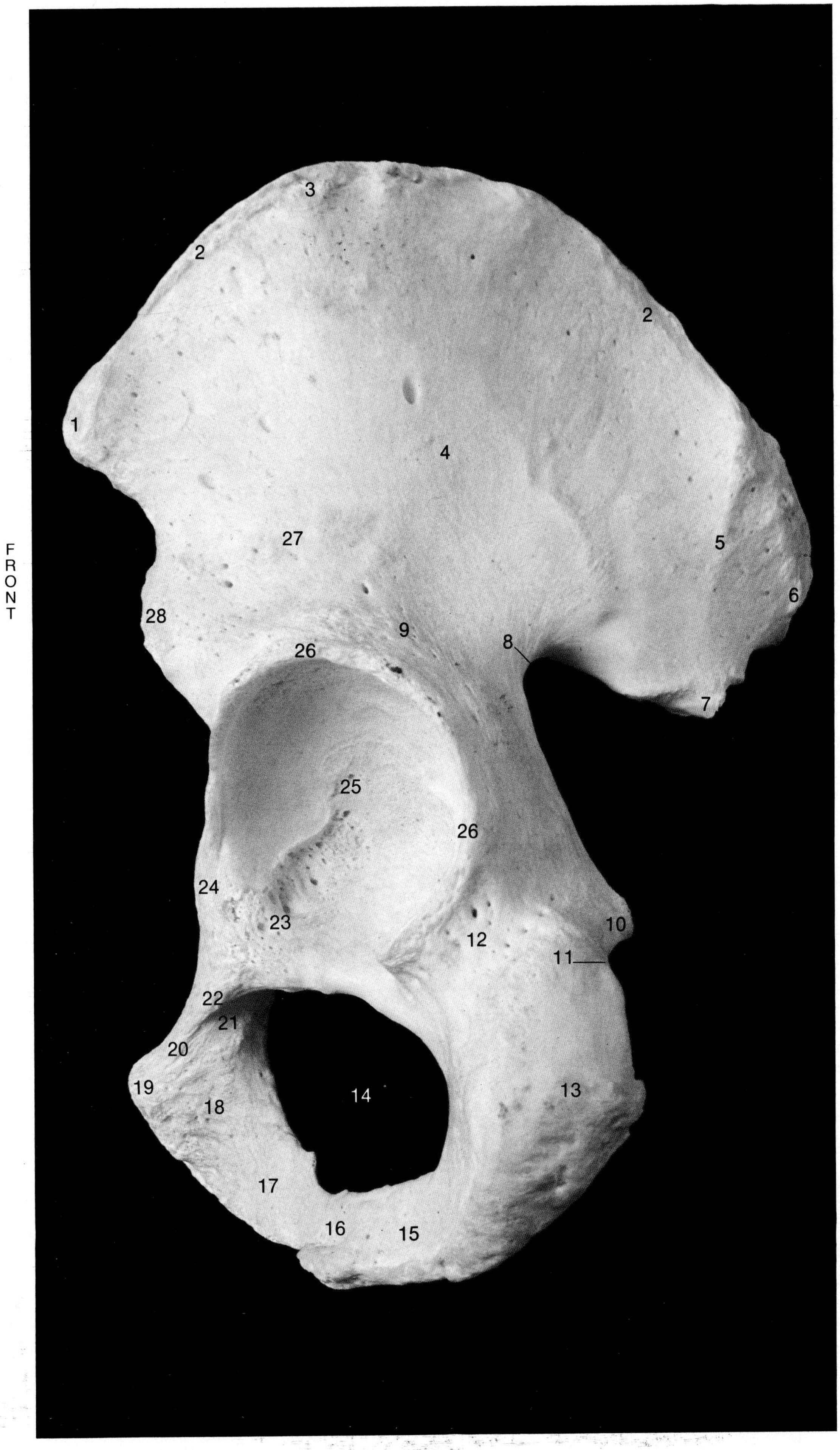

Left hip bone, lateral surface

1	Anterior superior iliac spine
2	Iliac crest
3	Tubercle of iliac crest
4	Anterior gluteal line
5	Posterior gluteal line
6	Posterior superior iliac spine
7	Posterior inferior iliac spine
8	Greater sciatic notch
9	Body of ilium
10	Ischial spine
11	Lesser sciatic notch
12	Body of ischium
13	Ischial tuberosity
14	Obturator foramen
15	Ramus of ischium
16	Junction of 15 and 17
17	Inferior ramus of pubis
18	Body of pubis
19	Pubic tubercle
20	Superior ramus of pubis
21	Obturator groove
22	Obturator crest
23	Acetabular notch
24	Iliopubic eminence
25	Acetabulum
26	Rim of acetabulum
27	Inferior gluteal line
28	Anterior inferior iliac spine

● The hip (innominate) bone is formed by the union of the ilium (9), ischium (12) and pubis (18).
● It bears on its lateral surface the cup-shaped acetabulum (25), to which the ilium, ischium and pubis each contribute a part (see page 290).
● The two hip bones articulate in the midline anteriorly at the pubic symphysis; posteriorly they are separated by the sacrum, forming the sacro-iliac joints. The two hip bones with the sacrum and coccyx constitute the pelvis.
● The ischiopubic ramus is formed by the union (16) of the ramus of the ischium (15) with the inferior ramus of the pubis (17).

263

**Left hip bone, lateral surface.
Attachments**

Dotted lines = epiphysial lines;
interrupted line = capsule attachment of
hip joint

1 External oblique
2 Tensor fasciae latae
3 Gluteus minimus
4 Gluteus medius
5 Gluteus maximus
6 Piriformis
7 Ischiofemoral ligament
8 Superior gemellus
9 Semimembranosus
10 Semitendinosus and long head
    of biceps
11 Quadratus femoris
12 Adductor magnus
13 Obturator externus
14 Gracilis
15 Adductor brevis
16 Adductor longus
17 Transverse ligament
18 Reflected head of rectus femoris
19 Iliofemoral ligament
20 Straight head of rectus femoris
21 Sartorius
22 Inguinal ligament

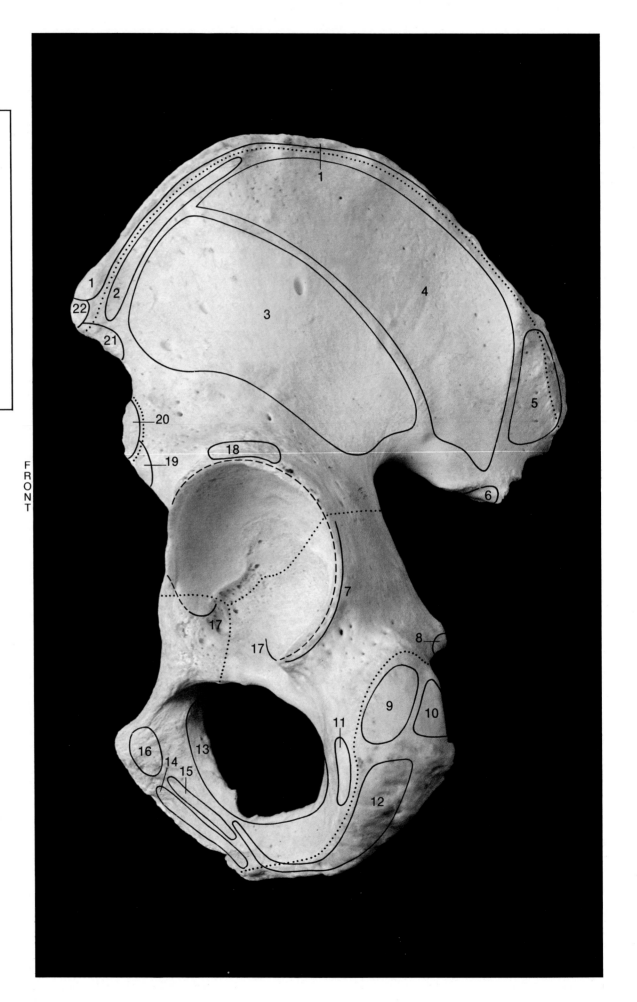

FRONT

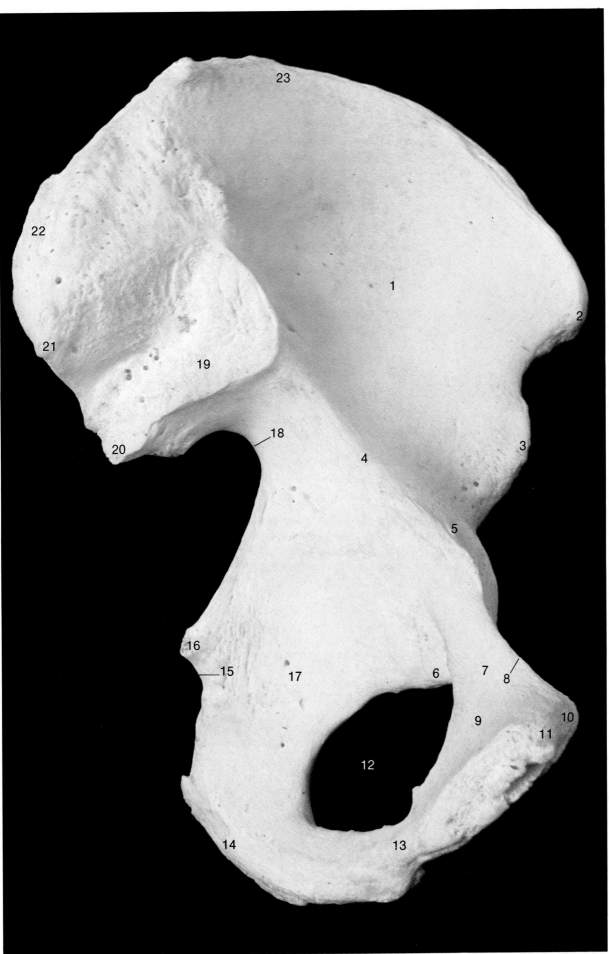

Left hip bone, medial surface

1	Iliac fossa
2	Anterior superior iliac spine
3	Anterior inferior iliac spine
4	Arcuate line
5	Iliopubic eminence
6	Obturator groove
7	Superior ramus of pubis
8	Pecten of pubis (pectineal line)
9	Body of pubis
10	Pubic tubercle
11	Pubic crest
12	Obturator foramen
13	Ischiopubic ramus
14	Ischial tuberosity
15	Lesser sciatic notch
16	Ischial spine
17	Body of ischium
18	Greater sciatic notch
19	Auricular surface
20	Posterior inferior iliac spine
21	Posterior superior iliac spine
22	Iliac tuberosity
23	Iliac crest

● The auricular surface of the ilium (19) is the articular surface for the sacro-iliac joint.

FRONT

**Left hip bone, medial surface.
Attachments**

Dotted lines = epiphysial lines;
interrupted line = capsule
attachment of sacro-iliac joint

1 Erector spinae
2 Interosseous ligament
3 Iliolumbar ligament
4 Quadratus lumborum
5 Transversus abdominis
6 Iliacus
7 Inguinal ligament
8 Sartorius
9 Straight head of rectus
 femoris
10 Psoas minor
11 Levator ani
12 Pubic symphysis
13 Obturator internus
14 Sphincter urethrae
15 Superficial transverse
 perineal and
 ischiocavernosus
16 Falciform process of sacrotuberous ligament
17 Sacrotuberous ligament
18 Inferior gemellus
19 Coccygeus and
 sacrospinous ligament

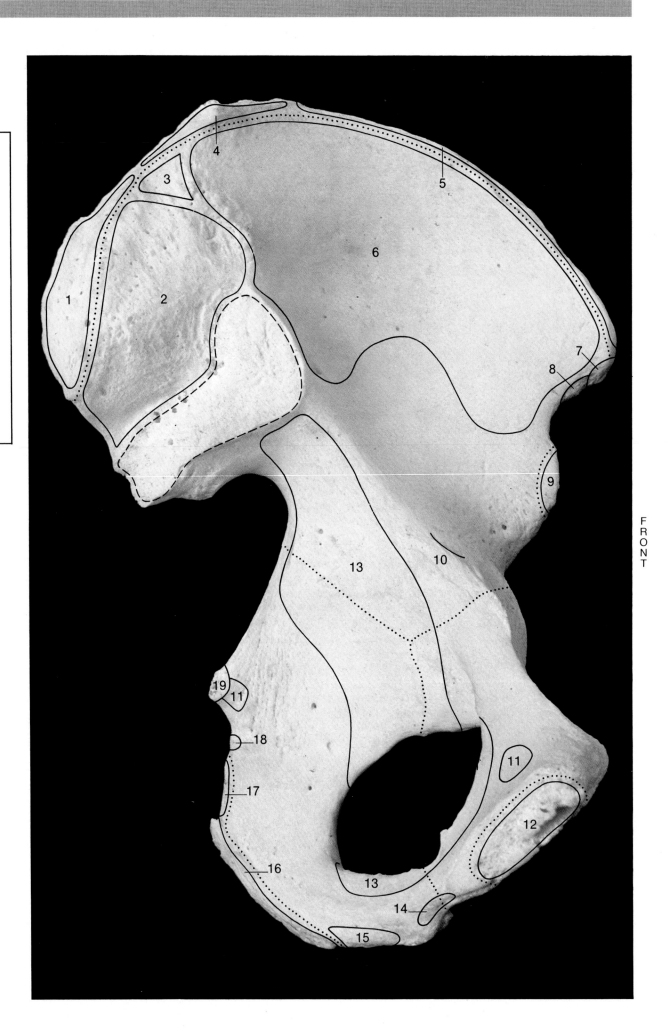

FRONT

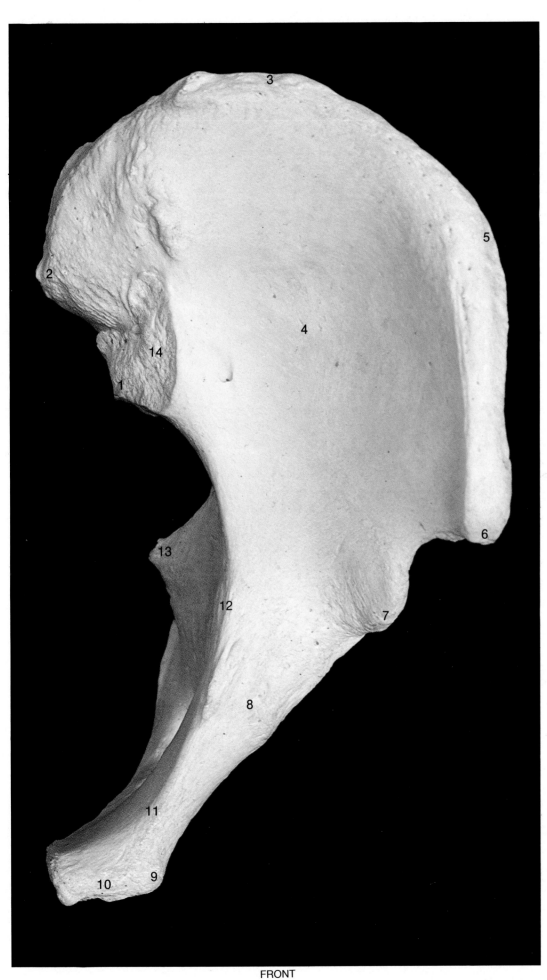

FRONT

Left hip bone, from above

1	Posterior inferior iliac spine
2	Posterior superior iliac spine
3	Iliac crest
4	Iliac fossa
5	Tubercle of iliac crest
6	Anterior superior iliac spine
7	Anterior inferior iliac spine
8	Iliopubic eminence
9	Pubic tubercle
10	Pubic crest
11	Pecten of pubis (pectineal line)
12	Arcuate line
13	Ischial spine
14	Auricular surface

● The arcuate line on the ilium (12) and the pecten and crest of the pubis (11 and 10) form part of the brim of the pelvis (the rest of the brim being formed by the promontory and upper surface of the lateral part of the sacrum—see page 79).
● The pecten of the pubis (11) is more commonly called the pectineal line.

L
E
F
T

Left hip bone from above. Attachments

Dotted lines = epiphysial lines; interrupted line = capsule attachment of sacro-iliac joint

1	Interosseous sacro-iliac ligament
2	Iliolumbar ligament
3	Quadratus lumborum
4	Iliacus
5	Transversus abdominis
6	Internal oblique
7	External oblique
8	Inguinal ligament
9	Straight head of rectus femoris
10	Iliofemoral ligament
11	Psoas minor
12	Pectineal ligament
13	Pectineus
14	Lacunar ligament
15	Anterior wall of rectus sheath
16	Pyramidalis
17	Lateral head of rectus abdominis
18	Conjoint tendon
19	Medial head of rectus abdominis

● The inguinal ligament (8) is formed by the lower border of the aponeurosis of the external oblique muscle, and extends from the anterior superior iliac spine to the pubic tubercle.

● The lacunar ligament (14, sometimes called the pectineal part of the inguinal ligament) is the part of the inguinal ligament that extends backwards from the medial end of the inguinal ligament to the pecten of the pubis.

● The pectineal ligament (12) is the lateral extension of the lacunar ligament along the pecten. It is not classified as a part of the inguinal ligament, and must not be confused with the alternative name for the lacunar ligament, i.e. with the pectineal part of the inguinal ligament.

● The conjoint tendon (18) is formed by the aponeuroses of the internal oblique and transversus muscles, and is attached to the pubic crest and the adjoining part of the pecten, blending medially with the anterior wall of the rectus sheath.

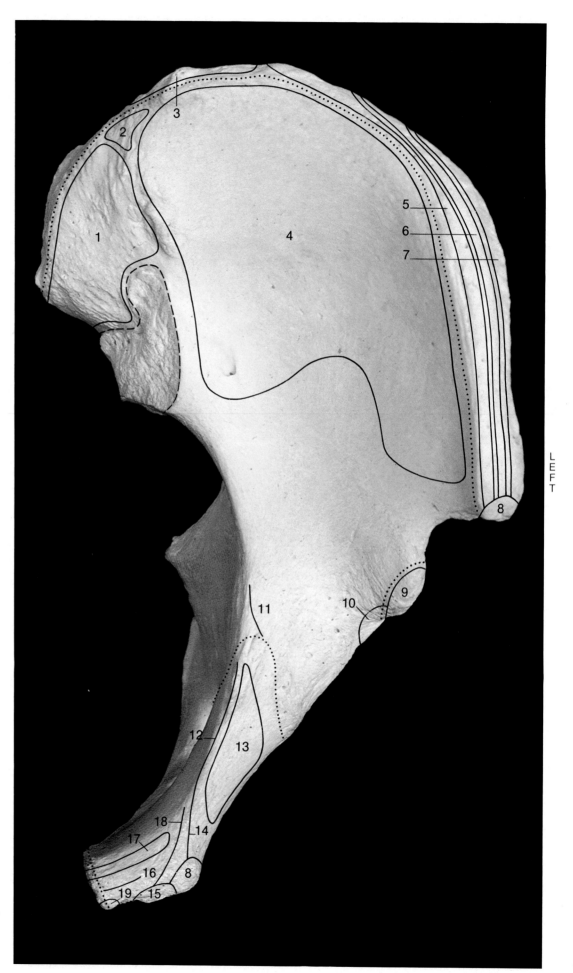

LEFT

FRONT

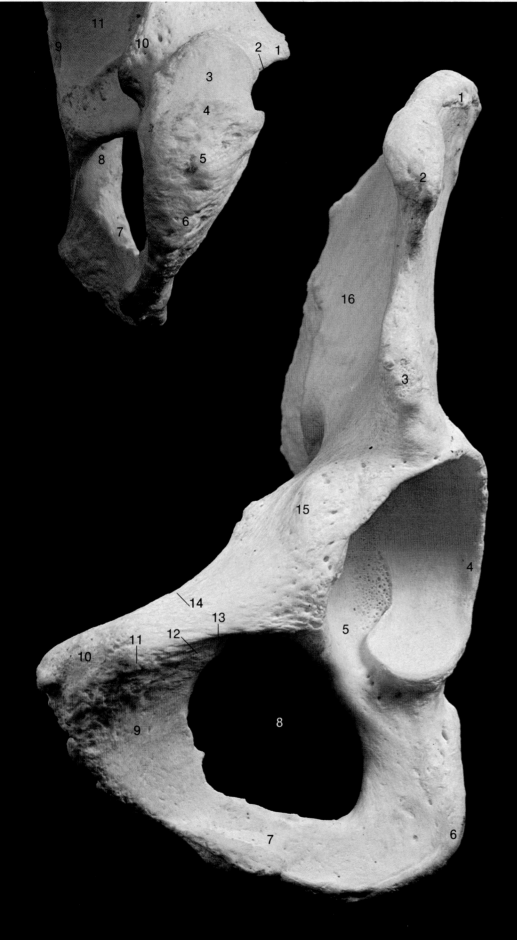

A LATERAL

B LATERAL

LATERAL

A Left hip bone. Ischial tuberosity, from behind and below

1	Ischial spine
2	Lesser sciatic notch
3	Upper part of tuberosity
4	Transverse ridge
5	Lower part of tuberosity
6	Longitudinal ridge
7	Ischiopubic ramus
8	Obturator groove
9	Acetabular notch
10	Rim of acetabulum
11	Acetabulum

B Left hip bone, from the front

1	Tubercle of iliac crest
2	Anterior superior iliac spine
3	Anterior inferior iliac spine
4	Rim of acetabulum
5	Acetabular notch
6	Ischial tuberosity
7	Ischiopubic ramus
8	Obturator foramen
9	Body of pubis
10	Pubic crest
11	Pubic tubercle
12	Obturator groove
13	Obturator crest
14	Pecten of pubis (pectineal line)
15	Iliopubic eminence
16	Iliac fossa

269

A Left hip bone. Ischial tuberosity, from behind and below. Attachments

Dotted lines = epiphysial lines; interrupted line = capsule attachment of hip joint

1	Superior gemellus
2	Inferior gemellus
3	Semitendinosus and long head of biceps
4	Semimembranosus
5	Adductor magnus
6	Ischiofemoral ligament

● The area on the ischial tuberosity medial to the adductor magnus attachment (5) is covered by fibrofatty tissue and the ischial bursa underlying gluteus maximus.

B Left hip bone, from the front. Attachments

Dotted lines = epiphysial lines; interrupted line = capsule attachment of hip joint

1	Transversus abdominis
2	Internal oblique
3	External oblique and inguinal ligament
4	Sartorius
5	Straight head of rectus femoris
6	Iliofemoral ligament
7	Reflected head of rectus femoris
8	Psoas minor
9	Pubofemoral ligament
10	Transverse ligament
11	Semimembranosus
12	Quadratus femoris
13	Adductor magnus
14	Obturator externus
15	Gracilis
16	Adductor brevis
17	Adductor longus
18	Medial head of rectus abdominis
19	Rectus sheath
20	Inguinal ligament
21	Pyramidalis
22	Lateral head of rectus abdominis
23	Conjoint tendon
24	Lacunar ligament
25	Pectineus
26	Pectineal ligament

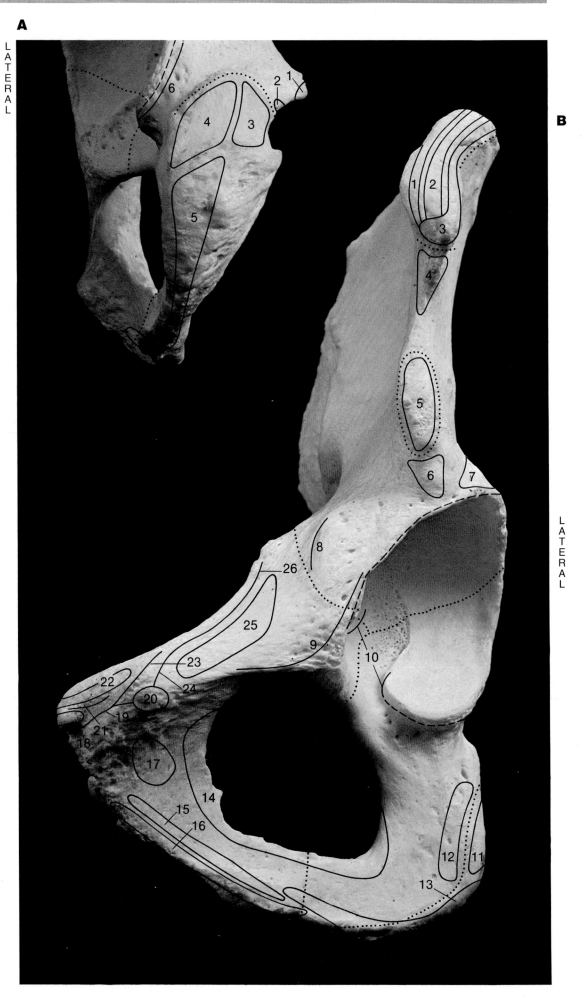

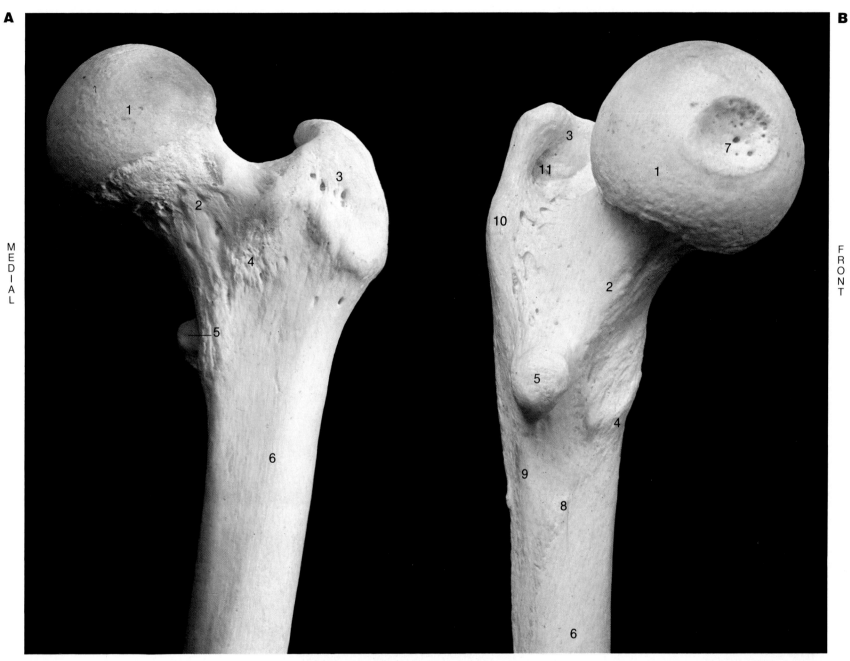

Left femur, upper end, A from the front, B from the medial side

1	Head
2	Neck
3	Greater trochanter
4	Intertrochanteric line
5	Lesser trochanter
6	Shaft
7	Facet of head
8	Spiral line
9	Pectineal line
10	Quadrate tubercle on intertrochanteric crest
11	Trochanteric fossa

● The intertrochanteric *line* (4) is at the junction of the neck (2) and shaft (6) on the anterior surface; the intertrochanteric *crest* is in a similar position on the posterior surface (10, and page 272, A9).
● The neck makes an angle with the shaft of about 125°.
● The pectineal line of the femur (9) must not be confused with the pectineal line (pecten) of the pubis (page 267), nor with the spiral line of the femur (8) which is usually more prominent than the pectineal line.

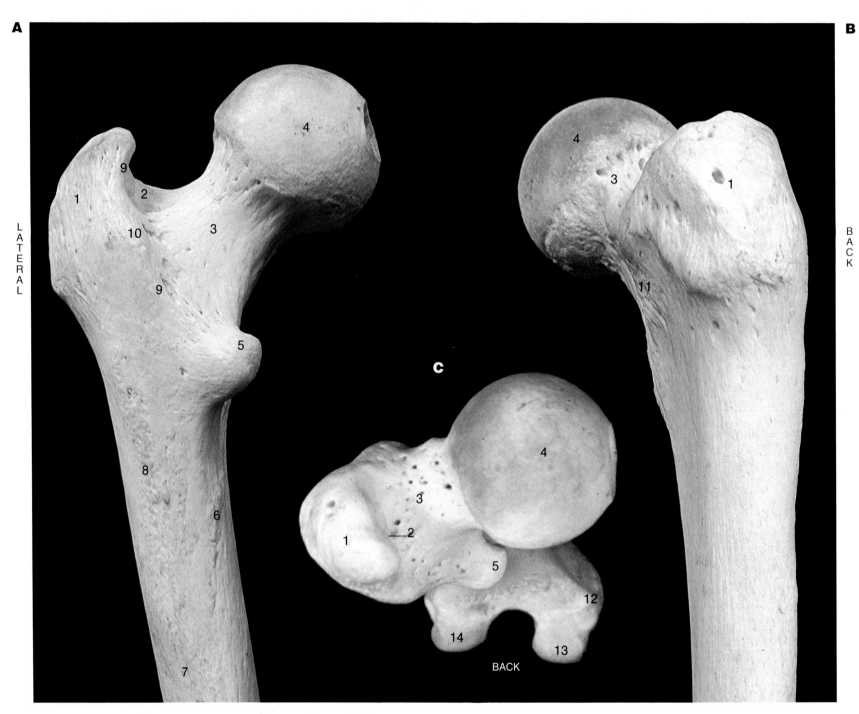

Left femur, upper end, A from behind, B from the lateral side, C from above

● The neck of the femur passes forwards as well as upwards and medially (C3), making an angle of about 15° with the transverse axis of the lower end (the angle of femoral torsion).

● The lesser trochanter (5) projects backwards and medially.

1	Greater trochanter
2	Trochanteric fossa
3	Neck
4	Head
5	Lesser trochanter
6	Spiral line
7	Linea aspera
8	Gluteal tuberosity
9	Intertrochanteric crest
10	Quadrate tubercle
11	Intertrochanteric line
12	Adductor tubercle ⎫
13	Medial condyle ⎬ at lower end
14	Lateral condyle ⎭

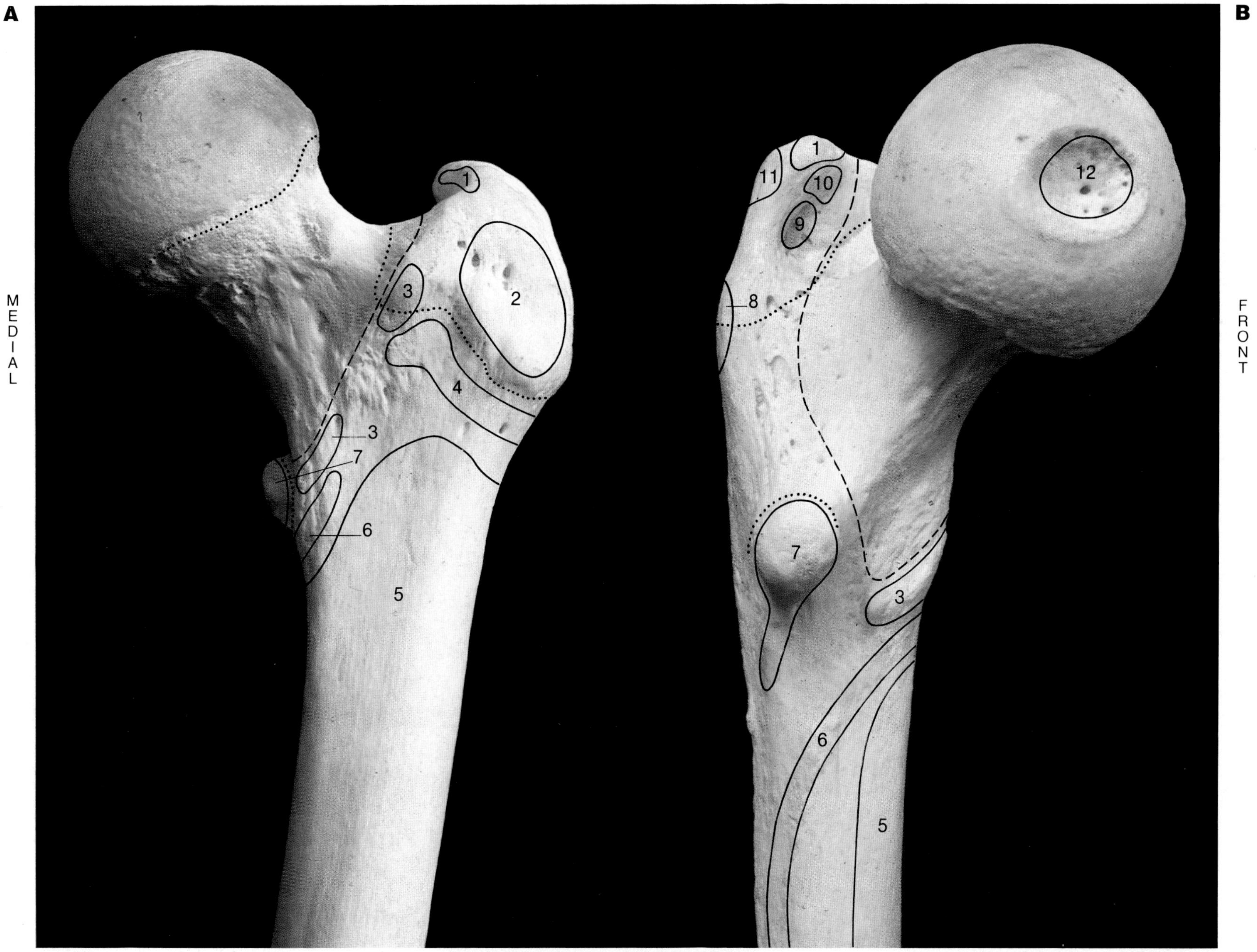

A

B

M
E
D
I
A
L

F
R
O
N
T

Left femur, upper end, **A** from the front, **B** from the medial side. Attachments

Dotted lines = epiphysial lines; interrupted line = capsule attachment of hip joint

1	Piriformis
2	Gluteus minimus
3	Iliofemoral ligament
4	Vastus lateralis
5	Vastus intermedius
6	Vastus medialis
7	Psoas major and iliacus
8	Quadratus femoris
9	Obturator externus
10	Obturator internus
11	Gluteus medius
12	Ligament of head of femur

● The iliofemoral ligament has the shape of an inverted Y, with the stem attached to the anterior inferior iliac spine of the hip bone (page 270, 6), and the limbs attached to the upper (lateral) and lower (medial) ends of the intertrochanteric line (3), blending with the capsule of the hip joint.

● The tendon of psoas major is attached to the lesser trochanter (7); many of the muscle fibres of iliacus are inserted into the psoas tendon but some reach the femur below the trochanter.

273

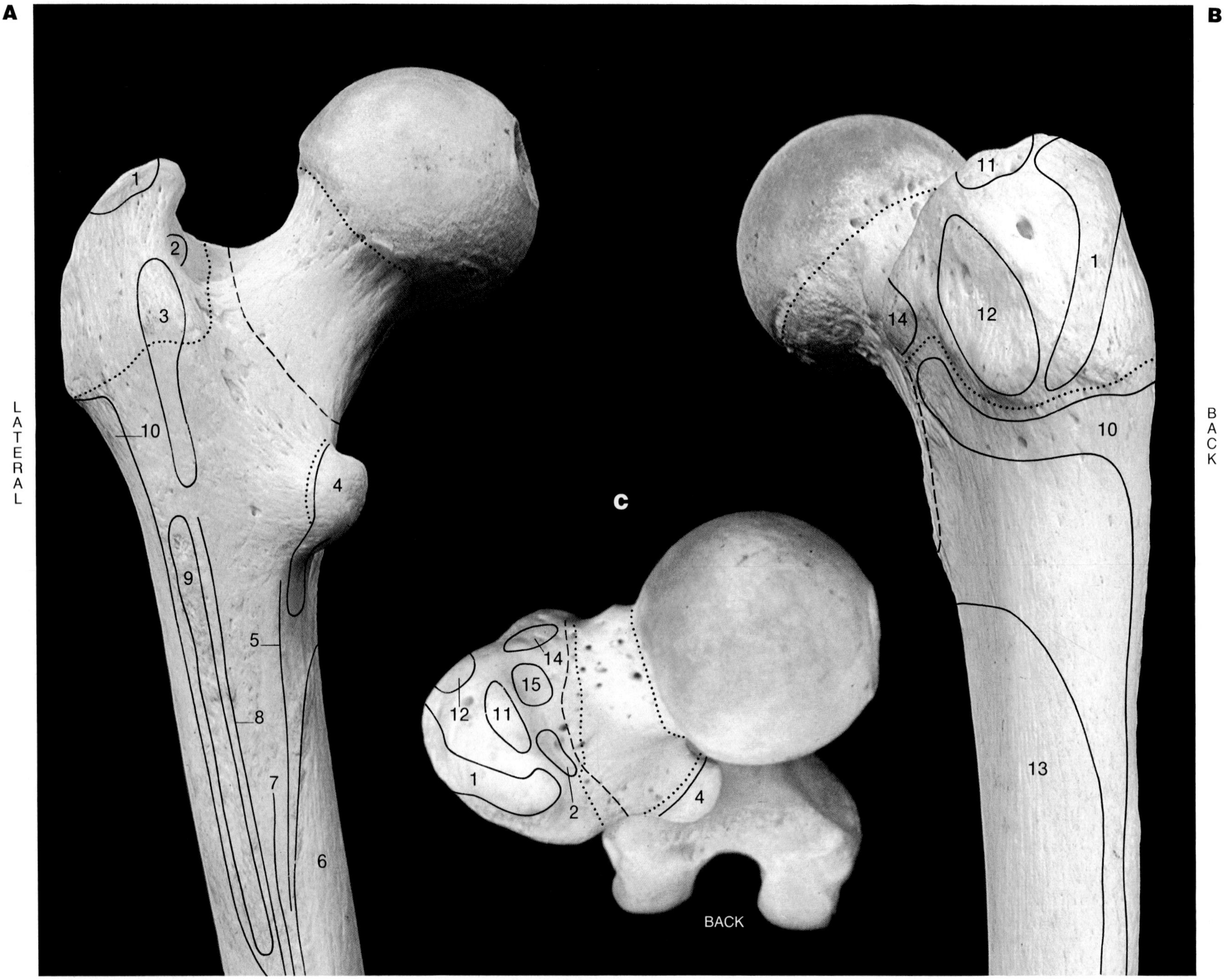

A

B

C

Left femur, upper end, A from behind, B from the lateral side, C from above.
Attachments

Dotted lines = epiphysial lines; interrupted line = capsule attachment of hip joint

● On the front of the femur (page 273) the capsule of the hip joint is attached to the intertrochanteric line, but at the back the capsule is attached to the neck of the femur and does not extend as far laterally as the intertrochanteric crest (page 272, A9).

1	Gluteus medius
2	Obturator externus
3	Quadratus femoris
4	Psoas major and iliacus
5	Pectineus
6	Vastus medialis
7	Adductor brevis
8	Adductor magnus
9	Gluteus maximus
10	Vastus lateralis
11	Piriformis
12	Gluteus minimus
13	Vastus intermedius
14	Iliofemoral ligament
15	Obturator internus

A

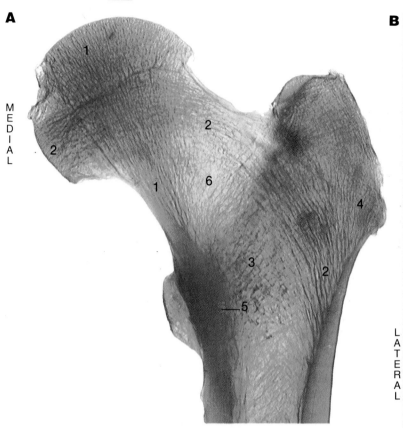

A Left femur, upper end, from the front

This is the posterior half of a cleared and bisected specimen, to show the major groups of bone trabeculae

1	From medial	⎫
2	From lateral	⎬ surface of shaft to head
3	From medial	⎫
4	From lateral	⎬ surface of shaft to greater trochanter
5	Calcar femorale	
6	Triangular area of few trabeculae	

● The calcar femorale (5) is a dense concentration of trabeculae passing from the region of the lesser trochanter to the under-surface of the neck.

B Left femur, shaft from behind

1	Gluteal tuberosity		4	Linea aspera
2	Lesser trochanter		5	Medial supracondylar line
3	Pectineal line		6	Lateral supracondylar line

● The rough linea aspera (4) often shows distinct medial and lateral lips; the lateral lip continues upwards as the gluteal tuberosity (1).

C Left femur, shaft, from behind. Attachments

1	Vastus lateralis		7	Adductor brevis
2	Quadratus femoris		8	Vastus medialis
3	Gluteus maximus		9	Adductor longus
4	Adductor magnus		10	Short head of biceps
5	Psoas and iliacus		11	Vastus intermedius
6	Pectineus			

● For diagrammatic clarity the muscle attachments to the linea aspera have been slightly separated.

B

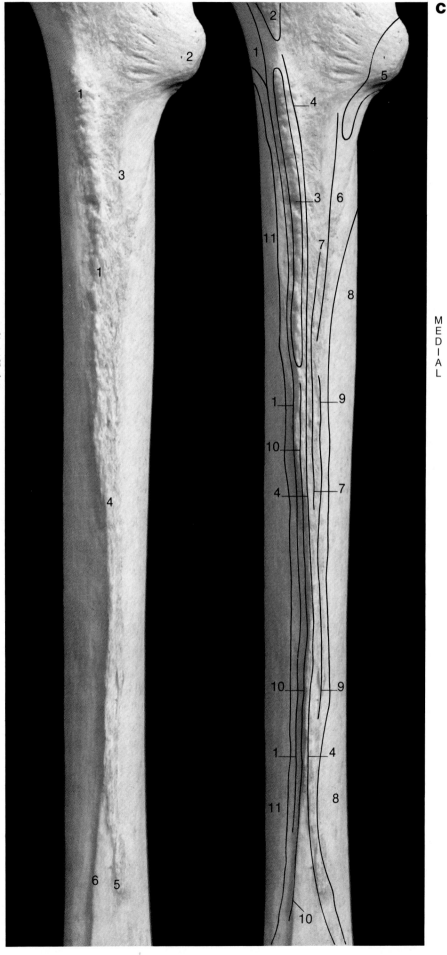

C

275

A

B

M E D I A L

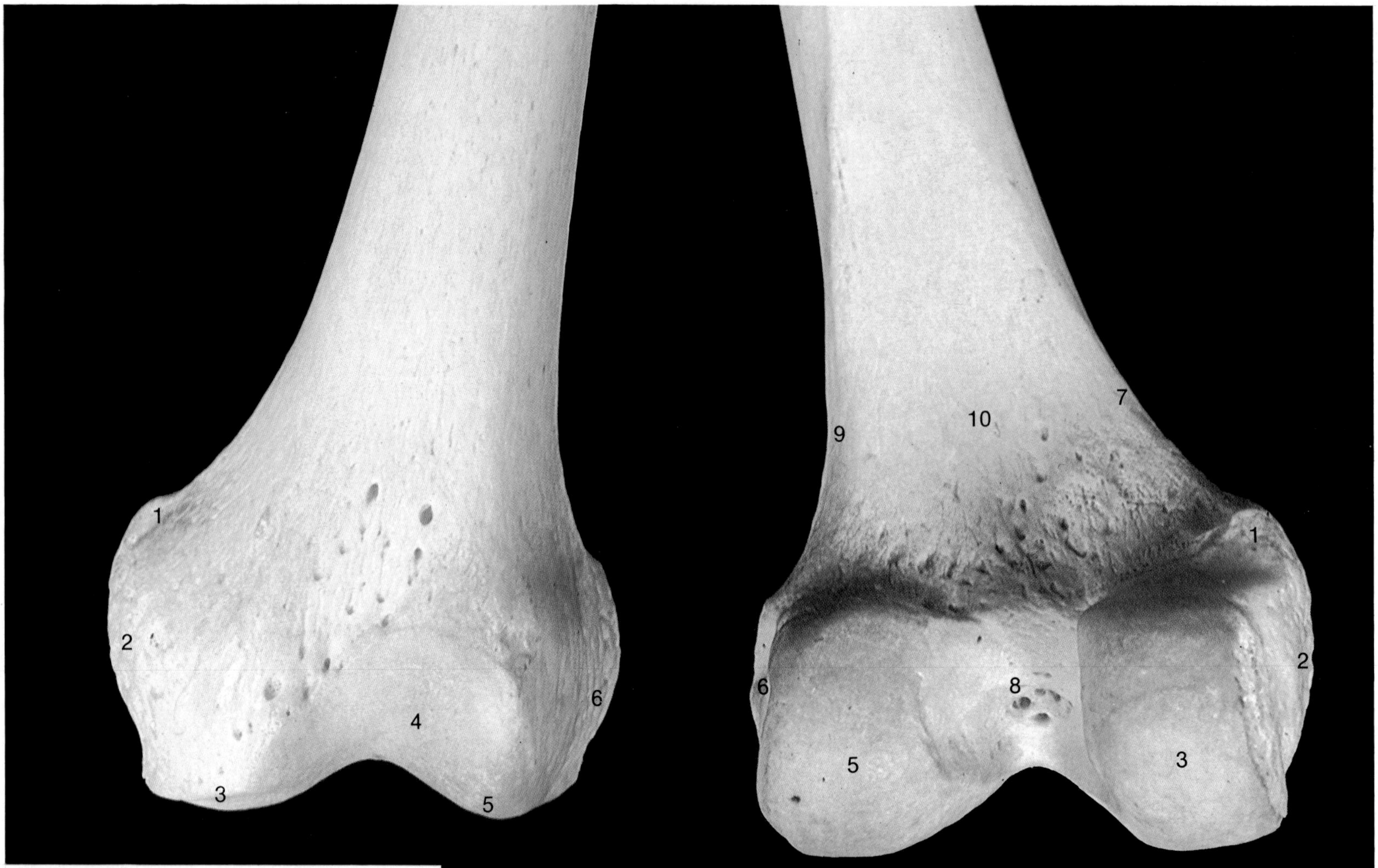

M E D I A L

Left femur, lower end, **A** from the front, **B** from behind, **C** from the medial side, **D** from the lateral side

1	Adductor tubercle
2	Medial epicondyle
3	Medial condyle
4	Patellar surface
5	Lateral condyle
6	Lateral epicondyle
7	Medial supracondylar line
8	Intercondylar fossa
9	Lateral supracondylar line
10	Popliteal surface
11	Impression for lateral head of gastrocnemius
12	Groove for popliteus tendon

● The condyles (3 and 5) bear the articular surfaces for the tibia, and project backwards (B3 and 5); the epicondyles (2 and 6) are the most prominent points on the (non-articular) sides of the condyles.

● The lower ends of the condyles (A3 and 5) lie in the same horizontal plane in order to rest squarely on the condyles of the tibia at the knee joint. The shaft therefore passes obliquely outwards and upwards from the the knee towards the hip.

B A C K

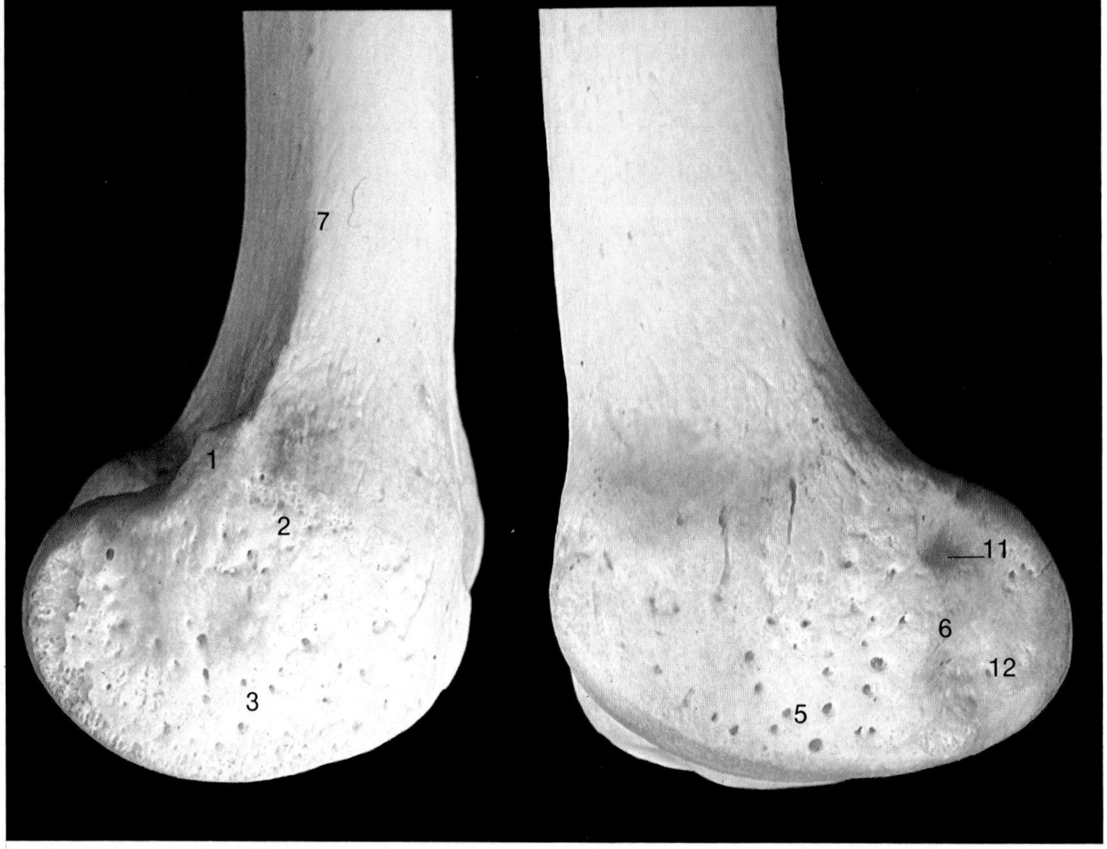

B A C K

C

D

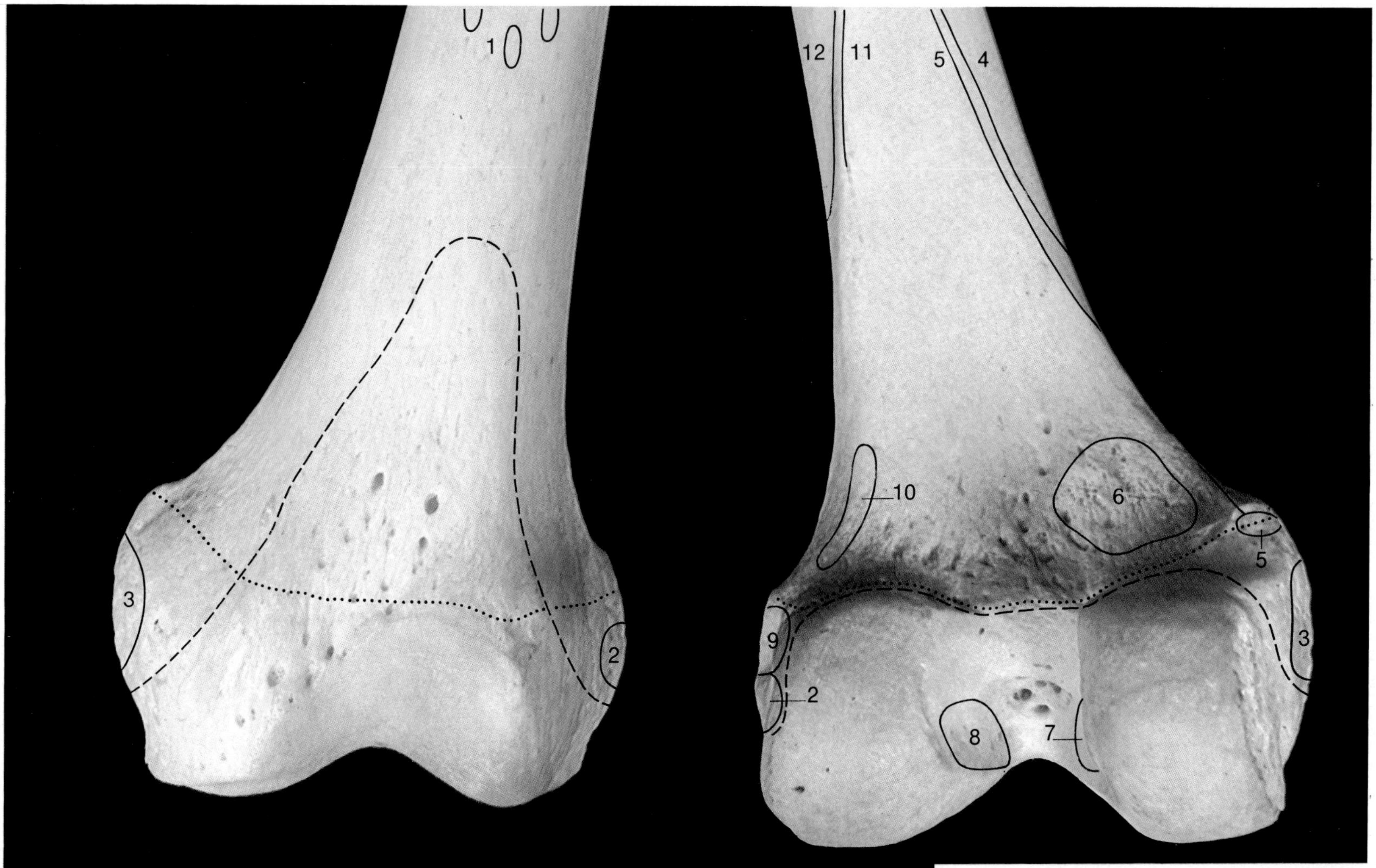

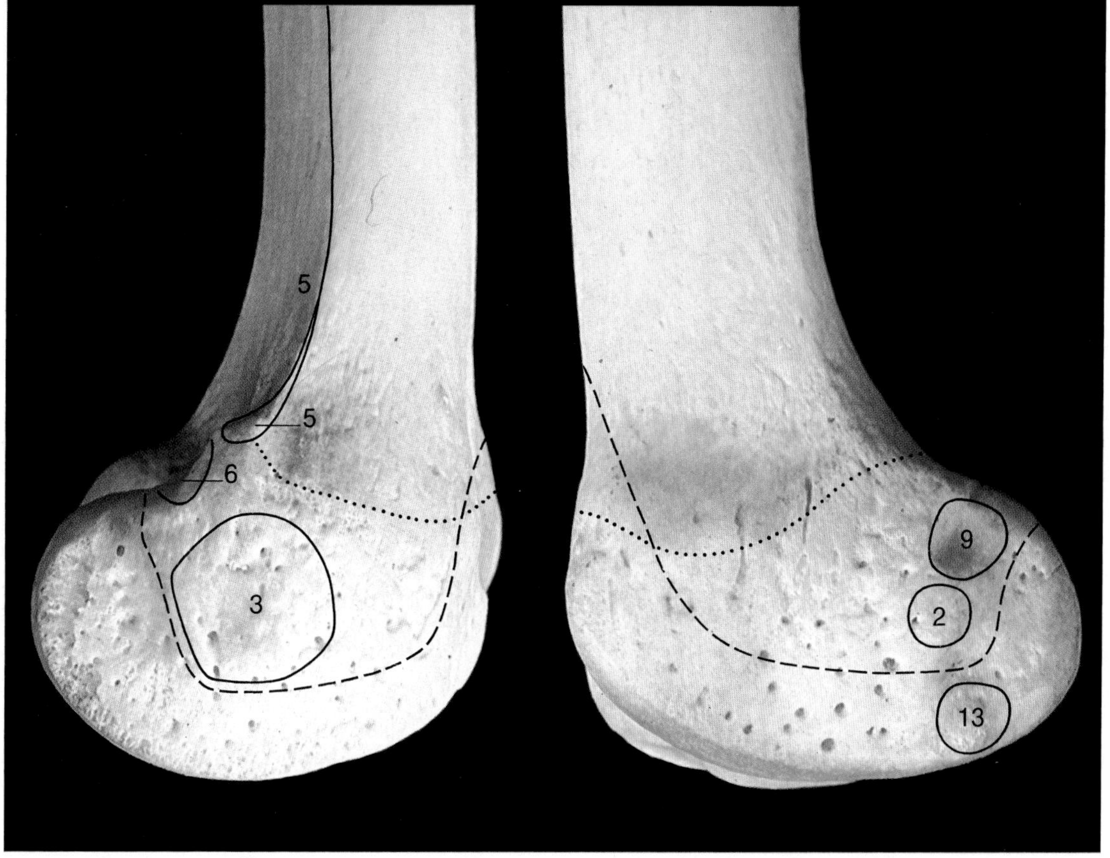

A

B

MEDIAL

MEDIAL

BACK

BACK

C

D

Left femur, lower end, A from the front, B from behind, C from the medial side, D from the lateral side. Attachments

Dotted lines = epiphysial lines; interrupted line = capsule attachment of knee joint

1	Articularis genu
2	Fibular collateral ligament
3	Tibial collateral ligament
4	Vastus medialis
5	Adductor magnus
6	Medial head of gastrocnemius
7	Posterior cruciate ligament
8	Anterior cruciate ligament
9	Lateral head of gastrocnemius
10	Plantaris
11	Short head of biceps
12	Vastus intermedius
13	Popliteus

● The medial head of gastrocnemius (B6) arises from the popliteal surface of the femur above the medial condyle and from the adjacent part of the capsule; the lateral head (D9) arises from an impression on the lateral surface of the lateral condyle above the lateral epicondyle (not from the popliteal surface of the femur) and from the adjacent part of the capsule.

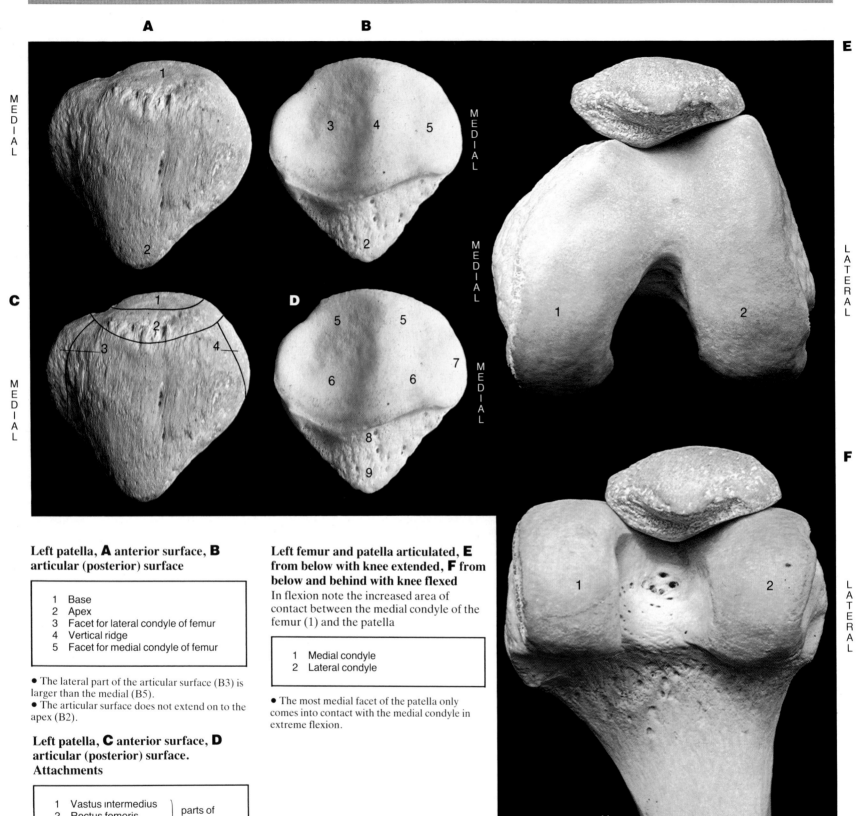

A **B** **E**

C **D** **F**

Left patella, A anterior surface, B articular (posterior) surface

1	Base
2	Apex
3	Facet for lateral condyle of femur
4	Vertical ridge
5	Facet for medial condyle of femur

● The lateral part of the articular surface (B3) is larger than the medial (B5).
● The articular surface does not extend on to the apex (B2).

Left patella, C anterior surface, D articular (posterior) surface. Attachments

1	Vastus intermedius	parts of quadriceps tendon
2	Rectus femoris	
3	Vastus medialis	
4	Vastus lateralis	
5	Facets for femur in flexion	
6	Facets for femur in extension	
7	Area for medial condyle in extreme flexion	
8	Area for infrapatellar fat pad	
9	Patellar ligament	

Left femur and patella articulated, E from below with knee extended, F from below and behind with knee flexed

In flexion note the increased area of contact between the medial condyle of the femur (1) and the patella

1	Medial condyle
2	Lateral condyle

● The most medial facet of the patella only comes into contact with the medial condyle in extreme flexion.

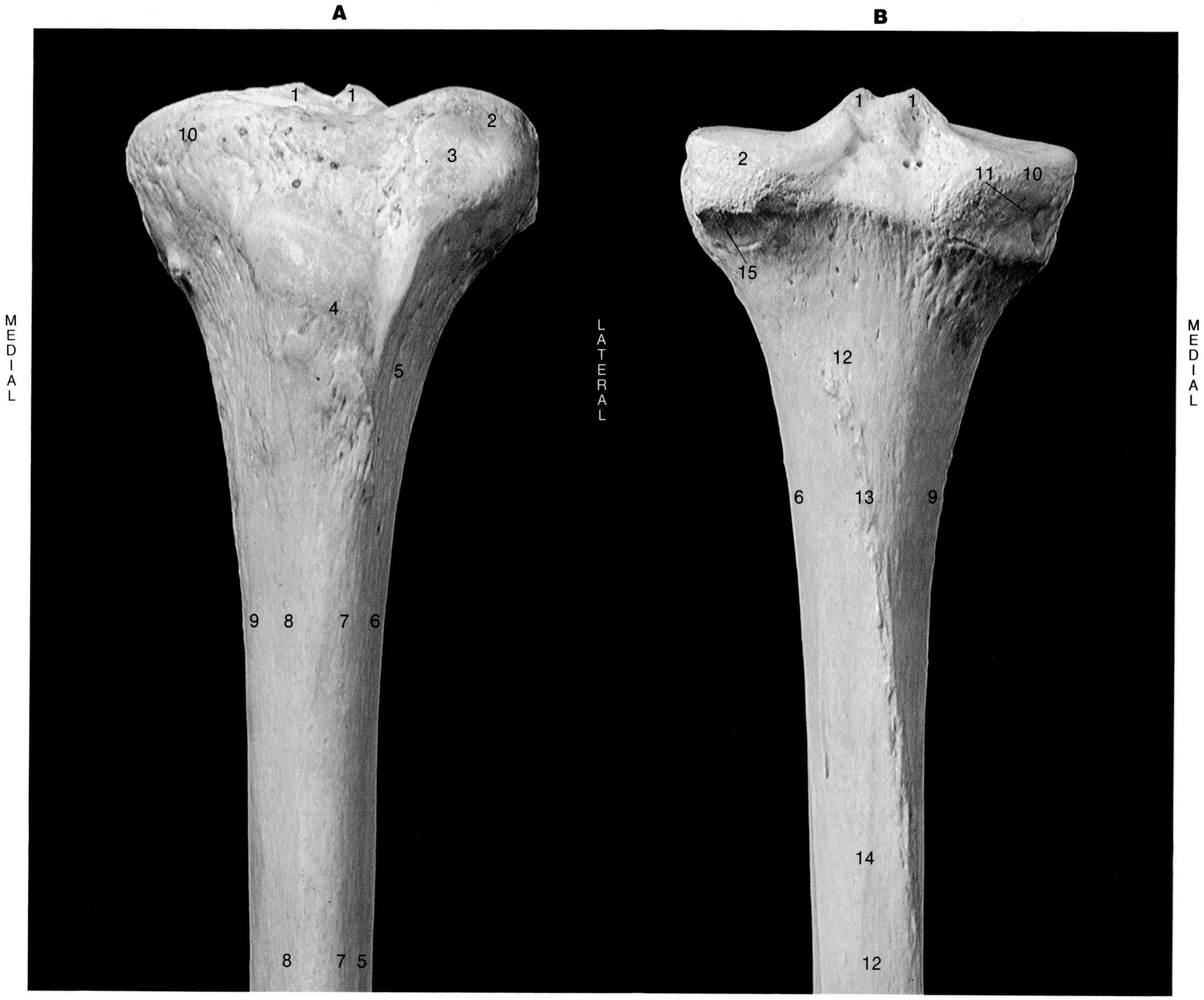

A

B

MEDIAL

LATERAL

MEDIAL

Left tibia, upper end, A from the front, B from behind

1	Tubercles of intercondylar eminence
2	Lateral condyle
3	Impression for iliotibial tract
4	Tuberosity
5	Lateral surface
6	Interosseous border
7	Anterior border
8	Medial surface
9	Medial border
10	Medial condyle
11	Groove for semimembranosus
12	Posterior surface
13	Soleal line
14	Vertical line
15	Articular facet for fibula

● The shaft of the tibia has three borders—anterior (7), medial (9) and interosseous (6)—and three surfaces—medial (8), lateral (5) and posterior (12).
● Much of the anterior border (7) forms a slightly curved crest commonly known as the shin. Most of the smooth medial surface (8) is subcutaneous. The posterior surface contains the soleal and vertical lines (13 and 14).
● The tuberosity (4) is at the upper end of the anterior border.

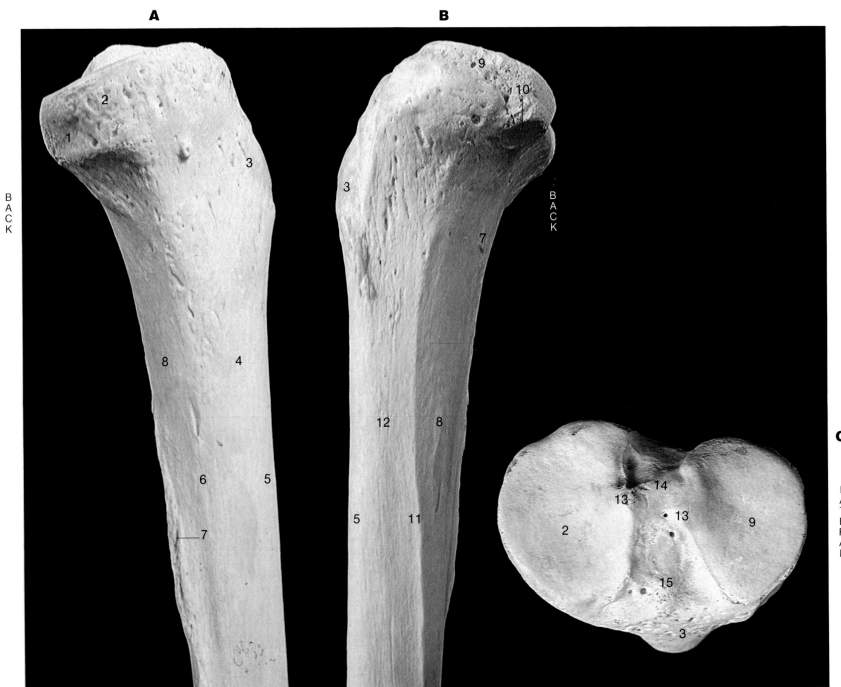

A   **B**

BACK   BACK   **C**

LATERAL

FRONT

Left tibia, upper end, A from the medial side, B from the lateral side, C from above

- The medial condyle (C2) is larger than the lateral condyle (C9).
- The articular facet for the fibula is on the postero-inferior aspect of the lateral condyle (B10).

1	Groove for semimembranosus
2	Medial condyle
3	Tuberosity
4	Medial surface
5	Anterior border
6	Medial border
7	Soleal line
8	Posterior surface
9	Lateral condyle
10	Articular facet for fibula
11	Interosseus border
12	Lateral surface
13	Tubercles of intercondylar eminence
14	Posterior intercondylar area
15	Anterior intercondylar area

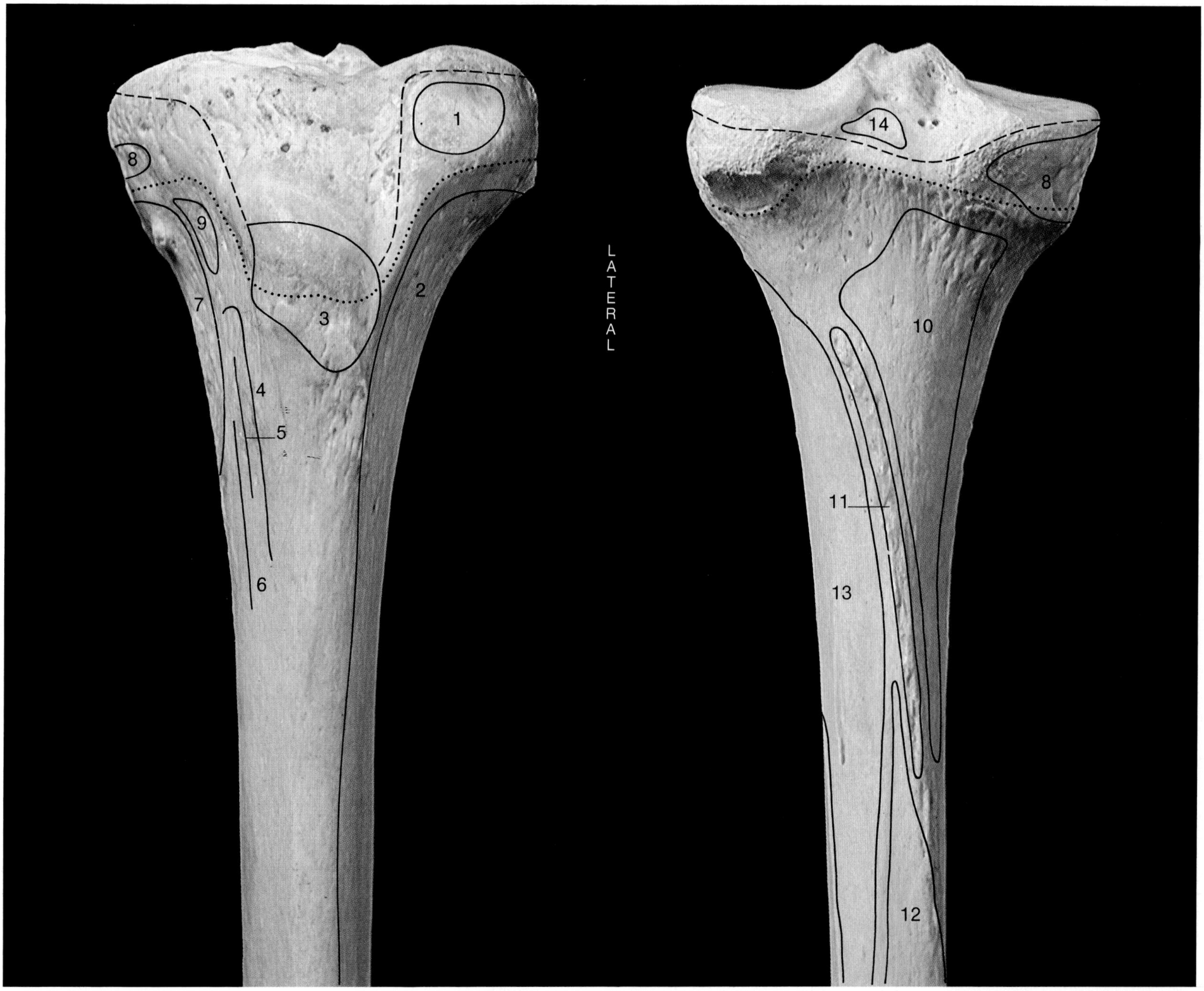

A

B

MEDIAL

LATERAL

MEDIAL

Left tibia, upper end, A from the front, B from behind. Attachments

Dotted lines = epiphysial lines; interrupted line = capsule attachment of knee joint

1	Iliotibial tract
2	Tibialis anterior
3	Patellar ligament
4	Sartorius
5	Gracilis
6	Semitendinosus
7	Tibial collateral ligament
8	Semimembranosus
9	Vastus medialis
10	Popliteus
11	Soleus
12	Flexor digitorum longus
13	Tibialis posterior
14	Posterior cruciate ligament

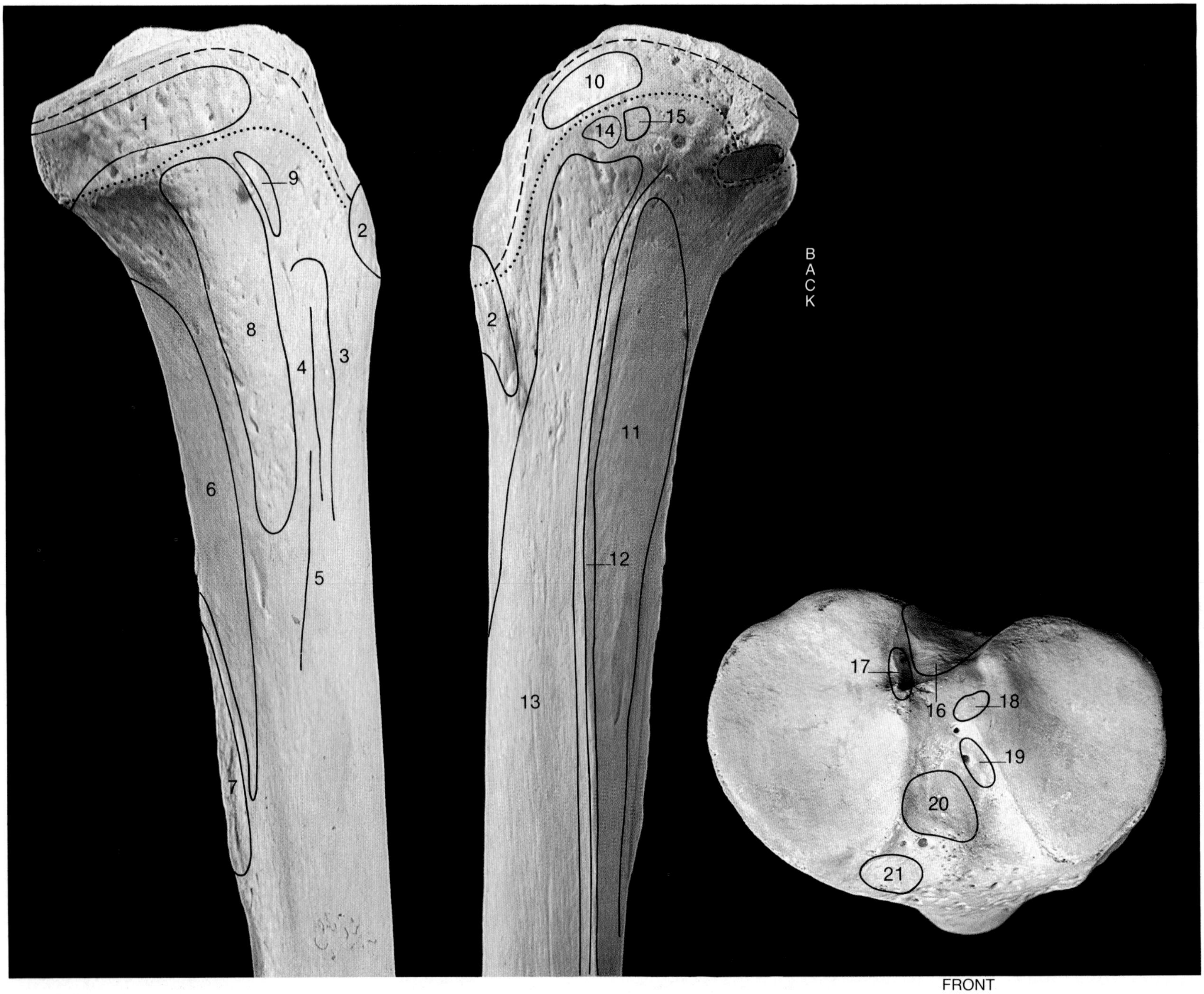

A

B

C

BACK

BACK

LATERAL

FRONT

Left tibia, upper end, A from the medial side, B from the lateral side, C from above. Attachments

Dotted lines = epiphysial lines; interrupted lines = capsule attachments of knee joint and superior tibiofibular joint

1	Semimembranosus	12	Interosseous membrane
2	Patellar ligament	13	Tibialis anterior
3	Sartorius	14	Extensor digitorum longus
4	Gracilis	15	Peroneus longus
5	Semitendinosus	16	Posterior cruciate ligament
6	Popliteus	17	Posterior horn of medial meniscus
7	Soleus	18	Posterior horn of lateral meniscus
8	Tibial collateral ligament	19	Anterior horn of lateral meniscus
9	Vastus medialis	20	Anterior cruciate ligament
10	Iliotibial tract	21	Anterior horn of medial meniscus
11	Tibialis posterior		

● Although arising mainly from the fibula (see page 285), extensor digitorum longus (B14) and peroneus longus (B15) have a small attachment to the tibia above tibialis anterior (B13).
● The horns of the lateral meniscus (C18 and 19) are attached close to one another on either side of the intercondylar eminence, but the horns of the medial meniscus (C17 and 21) are widely separated (see page 309).
● The tibial attachment of the anterior cruciate ligament (C20) is to the top of the intercondylar area, but the attachment of the posterior cruciate ligament (C16) extends 'over the top' on to the posterior surface.

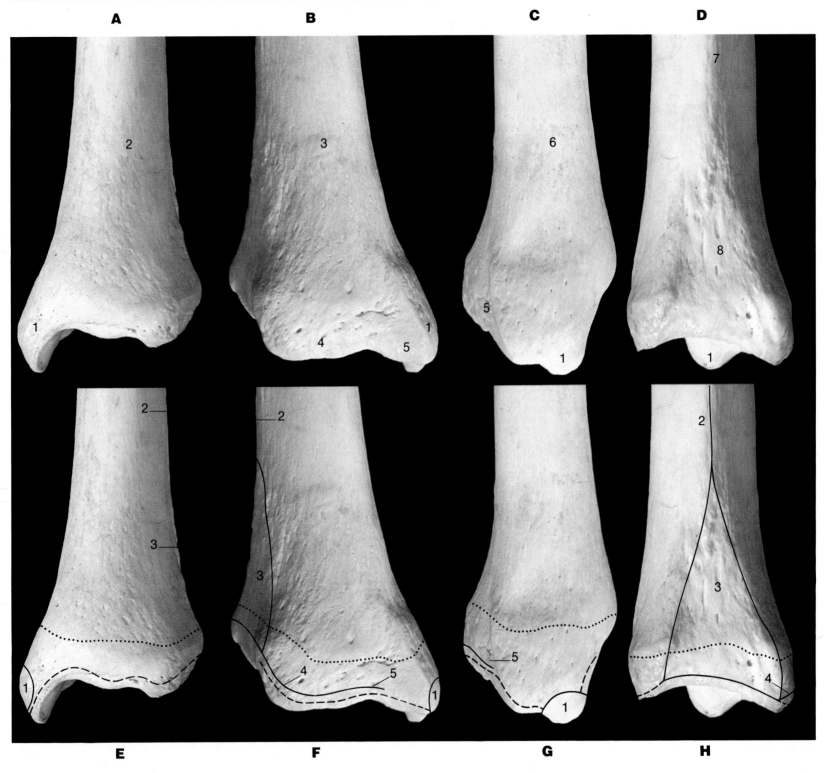

A B C D

E F G H

Left tibia, lower end, A from the front, B from behind, C from the medial side, D from the lateral side

1	Medial malleolus
2	Anterior surface
3	Posterior surface
4	Groove for flexor hallucis longus
5	Groove for tibialis posterior
6	Medial surface
7	Interosseous border
8	Fibular notch

● The lower end of the tibia has five surfaces—anterior, posterior, medial, lateral and inferior (for the inferior surface see page 286).
● The medial surface (C6) is continuous below with the medial surface of the medial malleolus (C1) (the lateral malleolus is the lower end of the fibula, see page 284).
● The fibular notch (D8) is triangular and constitutes the lateral surface of the lower end.

Left tibia, lower end, E from the front, F from behind, G from the medial side, H from the lateral side. Attachments

Dotted line = epiphysial line; interrupted line = capsule attachment of ankle joint

1	Medial collateral ligament
2	Interosseous membrane
3	Interosseous ligament
4	Posterior tibiofibular ligament
5	Inferior transverse ligament

● The medial collateral ligament (G1) is commonly known as the deltoid ligament.
● The lowest fibres of the posterior tibiofibular ligament (attached most medially to the tibia) are known as the inferior transverse ligament (F4 and 5).

283

A B C D

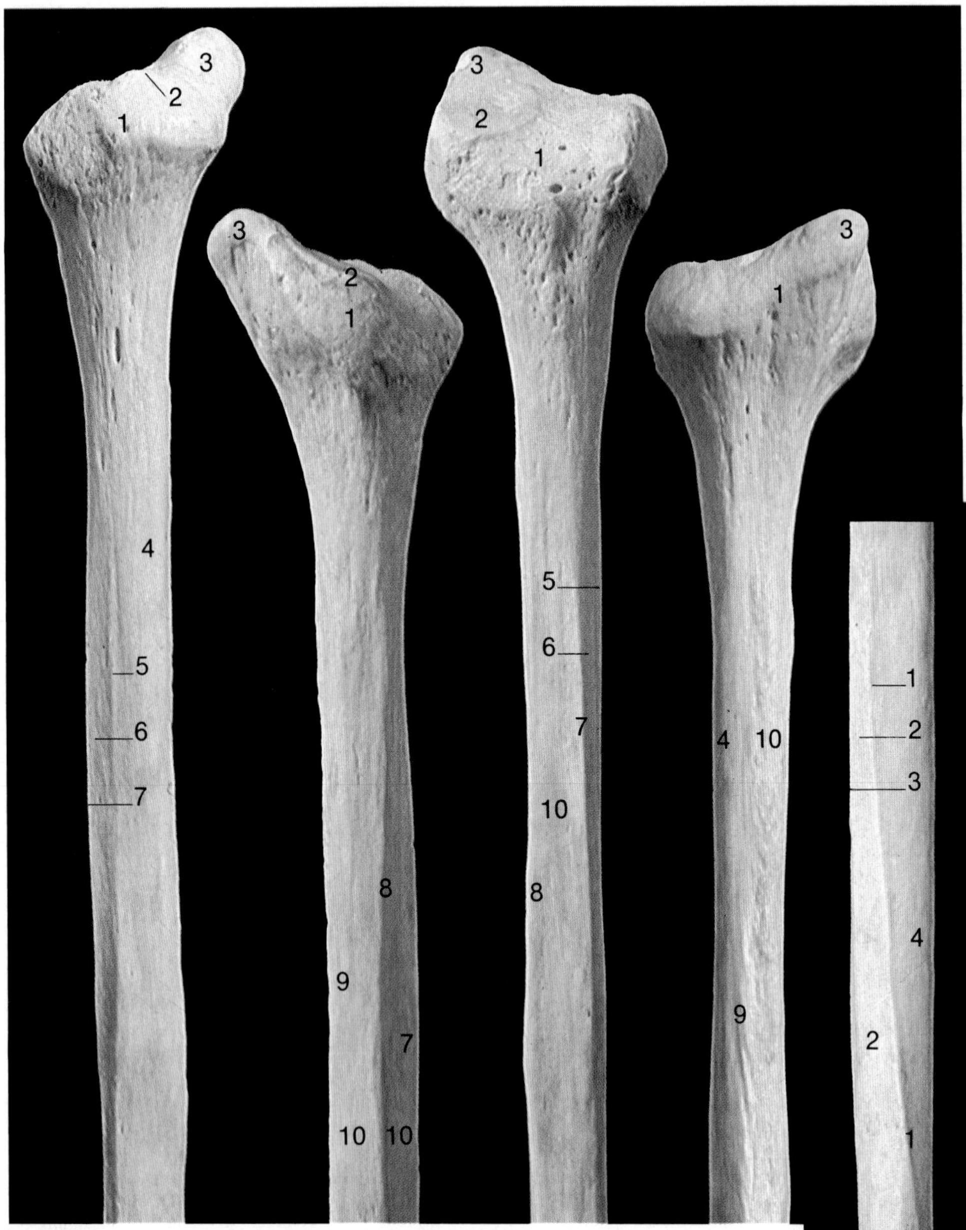

Left fibula, upper end, A from the front, B from behind, C from the medial side, D from the lateral side

1 Head
2 Articular facet on upper surface
3 Apex (styloid process)
4 Lateral surface
5 Anterior border
6 Medial surface
7 Interosseous border
8 Medial crest
9 Posterior border
10 Posterior surface

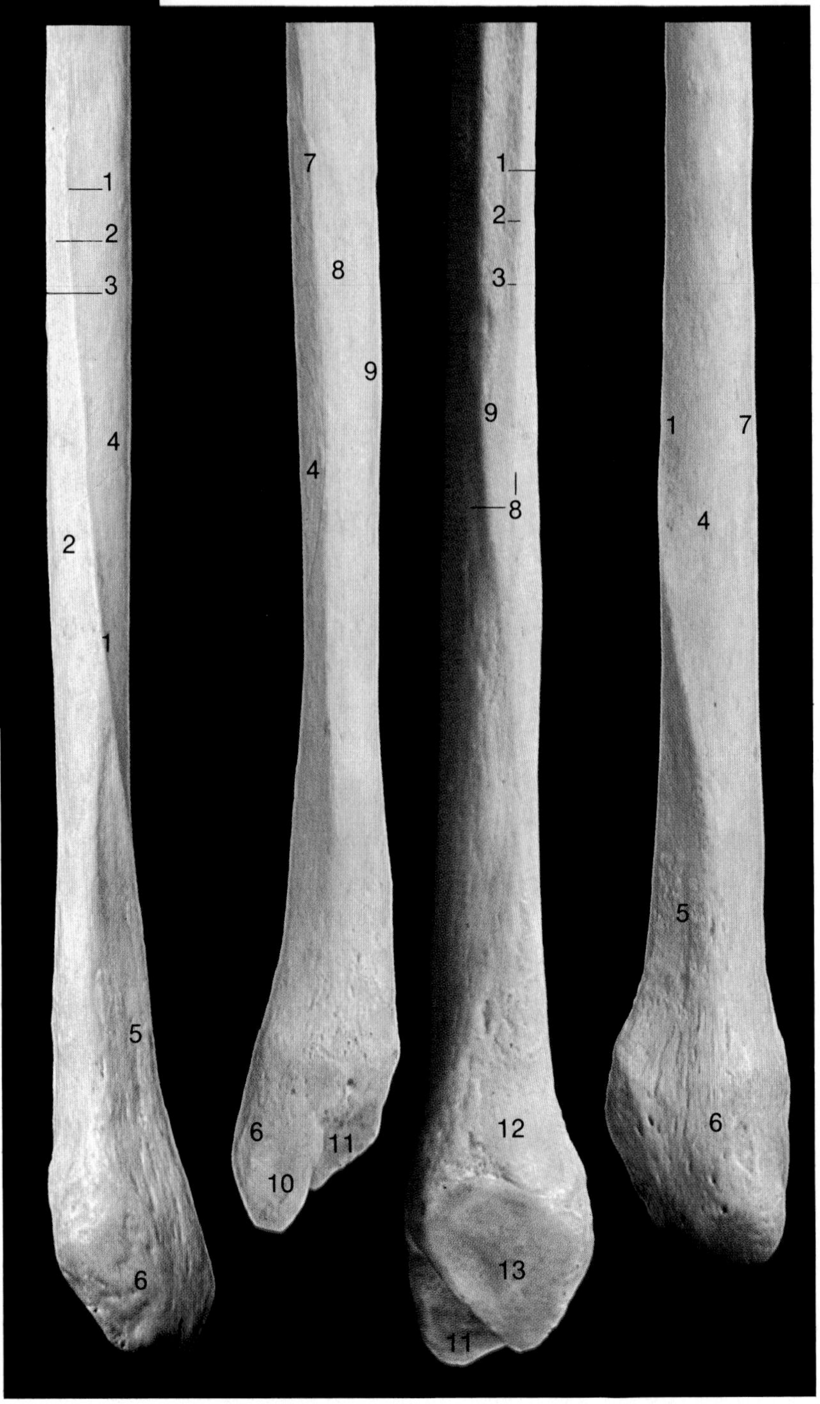

Left fibula, lower end, E from the front, F from behind, G from the medial side, H from the lateral side

1 Anterior border	8	Posterior surface
2 Medial surface	9	Medial crest
3 Interosseous border	10	Groove for peroneus brevis
4 Lateral surface	11	Malleolar fossa
5 Triangular subcutaneous area	12	Surface for interosseous ligament
6 Lateral malleolus	13	Articular surface of lateral
7 Posterior border		malleolus

● The fibula has three borders—anterior (A5), interosseous (A7) and posterior (B9)—and three surfaces—medial (A6), lateral (A4) and posterior (B10).
● At first sight much of the shaft appears to have four borders and four surfaces, but this is because the posterior surface (B10) is divided into two parts (medial and lateral) by the medial crest (B8).
● At the lower end the lateral surface (H4) comes to face posteriorly, so leaving the triangular subcutaneous area (H5) above the lateral malleolus (H6).
● The anterior border (E1) is easily identified by following it upwards from the apex of the triangular subcutaneous area (E5); the interosseous border (E3) is usually two or three millimetres behind the anterior border (although in the upper part of the shaft these two borders may fuse into one).
● The malleolar fossa (G11) is posterior to the articular surface (G13).

E F G H

284

A   **B**   **C**   **D**

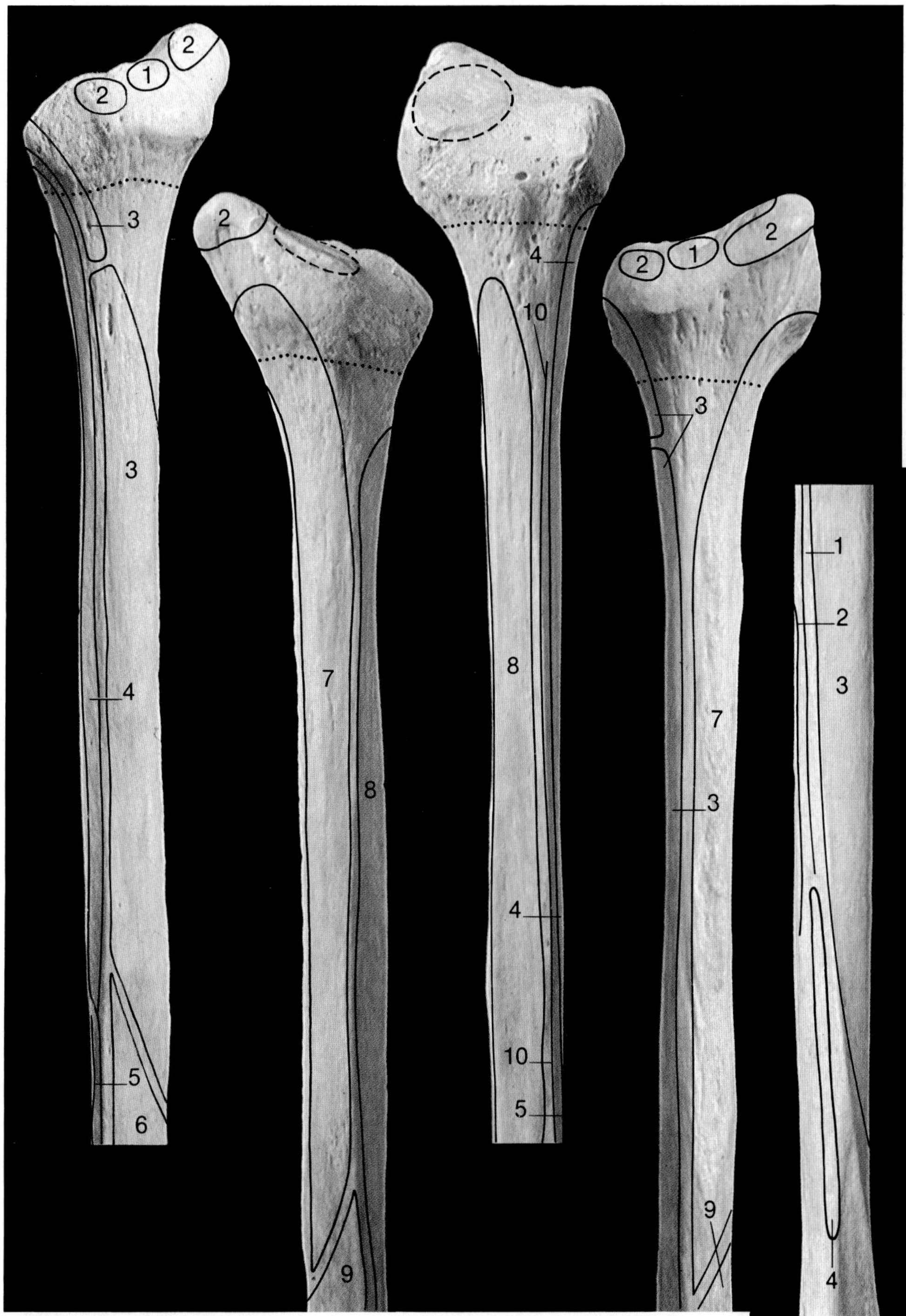

Left fibula, upper end, A from the front, B from behind, C from the medial side, D from the lateral side. Attachments

Dotted line = epiphysial line; interrupted line = capsule attachment of superior tibiofibular joint

1	Fibular collateral ligament	5	Extensor hallucis longus
2	Biceps	6	Peroneus brevis
3	Peroneus longus	7	Soleus
4	Extensor digitorum longus	8	Tibialis posterior
		9	Flexor hallucis longus
		10	Interosseous membrane

● The posterior surface (between the interosseous and posterior borders) gives origin to flexor muscles—soleus (B7) and flexor hallucis longus (B9) lateral to the medial crest, and tibialis posterior (B8) medial to the medial crest.

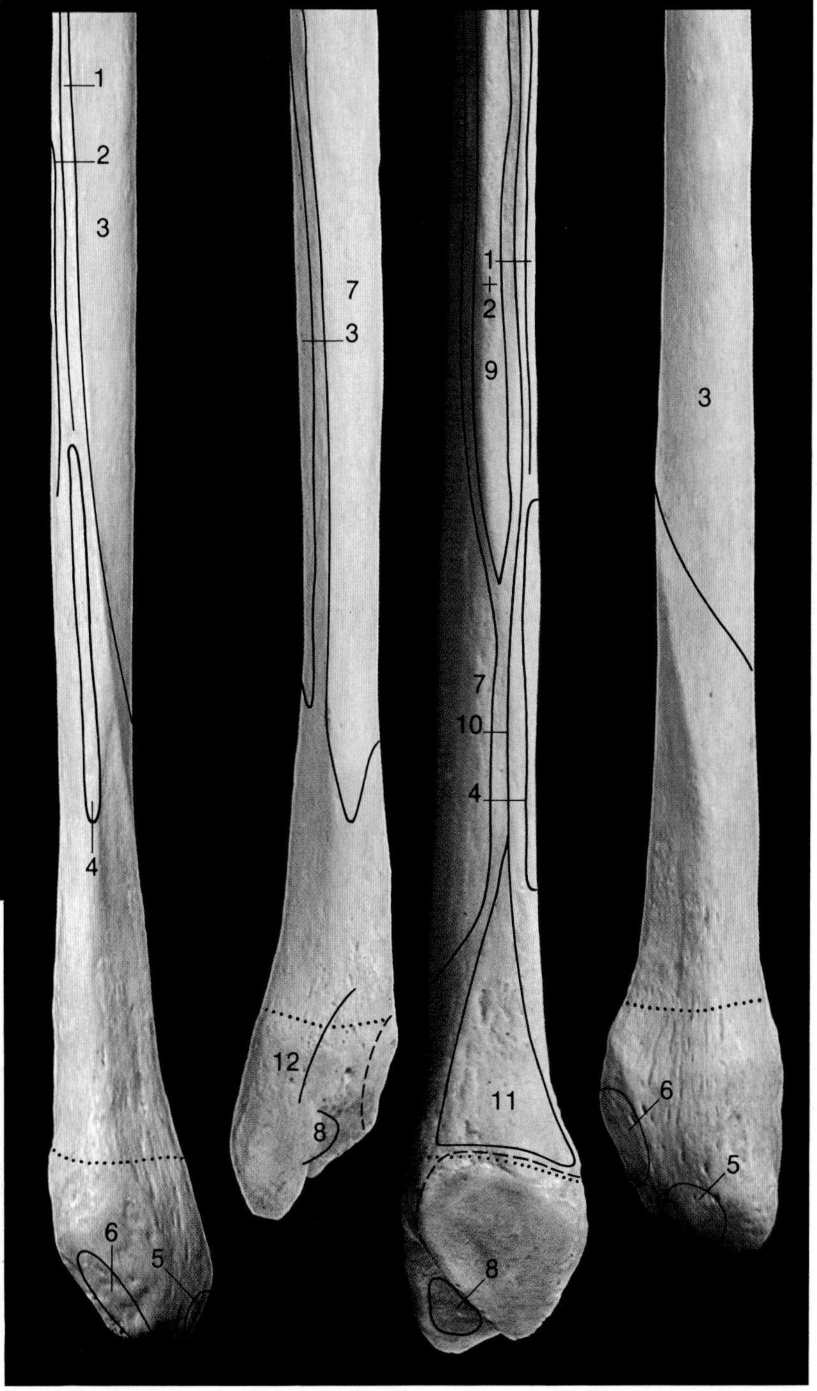

Left fibula, lower end, E from the front, F from behind, G from the medial side, H from the lateral side. Attachments

Dotted line = epiphysial line; interrupted line = capsule attachment of ankle joint

1	Extensor digitorum longus	7	Flexor hallucis longus
2	Extensor hallucis longus	8	Posterior talofibular ligament
3	Peroneus brevis	9	Tibialis posterior
4	Peroneus tertius	10	Interosseous membrane
5	Calcaneofibular ligament	11	Interosseous ligament
6	Anterior talofibular ligament	12	Posterior tibiofibular ligament

● The medial surface (between the anterior and interosseous borders) gives origin to extensor muscles—extensor digitorum longus (A4), extensor hallucis longus (A5) and peroneus tertius (E4).
● The lateral surface (between the anterior and posterior borders) gives origin to peroneus longus (A3) and peroneus brevis (A6).

E   **F**   **G**   **H**

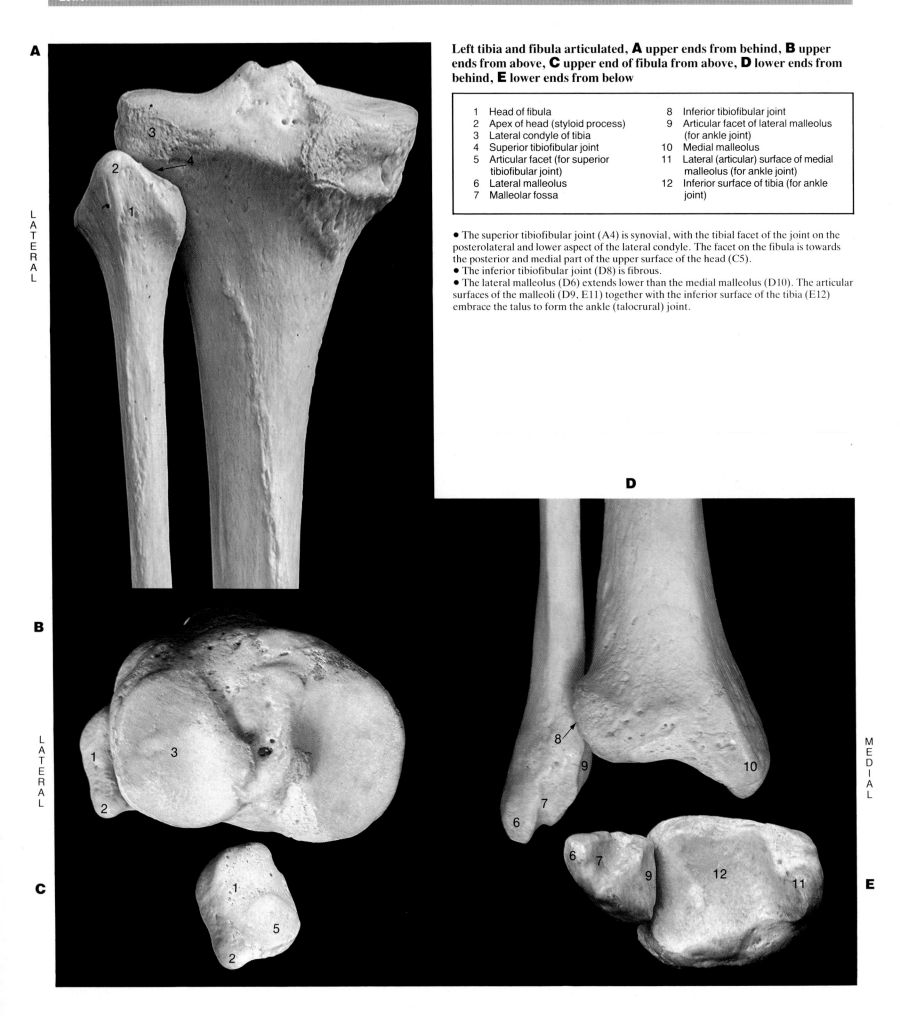

A

LATERAL

Left tibia and fibula articulated, A upper ends from behind, B upper ends from above, C upper end of fibula from above, D lower ends from behind, E lower ends from below

1	Head of fibula	8	Inferior tibiofibular joint
2	Apex of head (styloid process)	9	Articular facet of lateral malleolus
3	Lateral condyle of tibia		(for ankle joint)
4	Superior tibiofibular joint	10	Medial malleolus
5	Articular facet (for superior	11	Lateral (articular) surface of medial
	tibiofibular joint)		malleolus (for ankle joint)
6	Lateral malleolus	12	Inferior surface of tibia (for ankle
7	Malleolar fossa		joint)

● The superior tibiofibular joint (A4) is synovial, with the tibial facet of the joint on the posterolateral and lower aspect of the lateral condyle. The facet on the fibula is towards the posterior and medial part of the upper surface of the head (C5).
● The inferior tibiofibular joint (D8) is fibrous.
● The lateral malleolus (D6) extends lower than the medial malleolus (D10). The articular surfaces of the malleoli (D9, E11) together with the inferior surface of the tibia (E12) embrace the talus to form the ankle (talocrural) joint.

D

B

LATERAL

MEDIAL

C

E

A

B

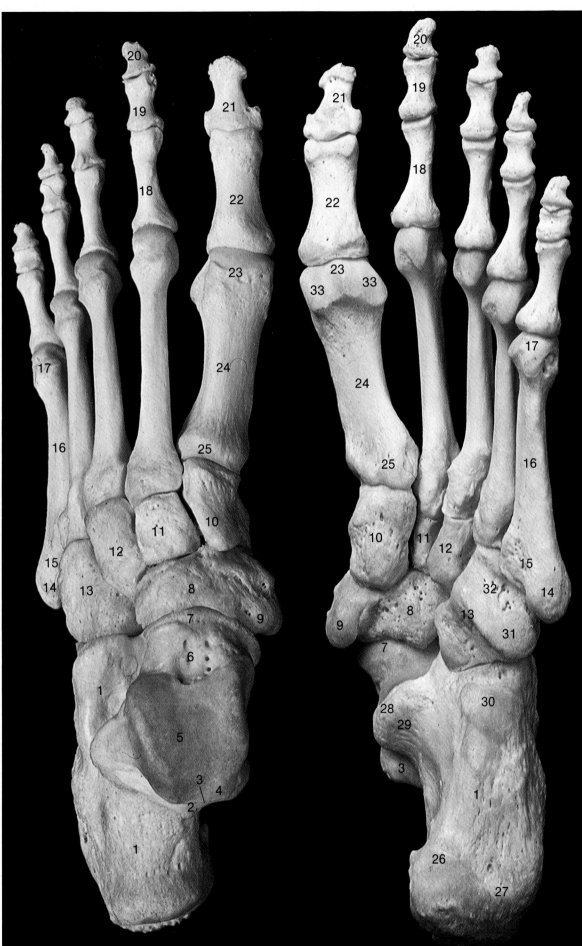

Bones of the left foot, A from above (dorsum), B from below (plantar surface)

1	Calcaneus
2	Lateral tubercle of talus
3	Groove on talus for flexor hallucis longus
4	Medial tubercle of talus
5	Trochlear surface of body of talus
6	Neck of talus
7	Head of talus
8	Navicular
9	Tuberosity of navicular
10	Medial cuneiform
11	Intermediate cuneiform
12	Lateral cuneiform
13	Cuboid
14	Tuberosity of base of fifth metatarsal
15	Base of fifth metatarsal
16	Shaft of fifth metatarsal
17	Head of fifth metatarsal
18	Proximal phalanx of second toe
19	Middle phalanx of second toe
20	Distal phalanx of second toe
21	Distal phalanx of great toe
22	Proximal phalanx of great toe
23	Head of first metatarsal
24	Shaft of first metatarsal
25	Base of first metatarsal
26	Medial process of calcaneus
27	Lateral process of calcaneus
28	Sustentaculum tali of calcaneus
29	Groove on calcaneus for flexor hallucis longus
30	Anterior tubercle of calcaneus
31	Tuberosity of cuboid
32	Groove on cuboid for peroneus longus
33	Grooves for sesamoid bones in flexor hallucis brevis tendons

Bones of the left foot, **A** from the medial side, **B** from the lateral side, **C** calcaneus from above, **D** talus from below, **E** calcaneus from behind

1	Medial process	
2	Medial surface	
3	Sustentaculum tali	
4	Anterior tubercle	
5	Lateral process	
6	Peroneal trochlea	
7	Posterior	talal
8	Middle	articular
9	Anterior	surface
10	Sulcus	
11	Posterior surface	
12	Groove for flexor hallucis longus	
13	Lateral tubercle	
14	Groove for flexor hallucis longus	
15	Medial tubercle	
16	Medial malleolar surface	
17	Neck	
18	Head	
19	Lateral malleolar surface	of talus
20	Posterior	calcanean
21	Middle	articular
22	Anterior	surface
23	Surface for plantar calcaneonavicular ligament	
24	Sulcus	
25	Tarsal sinus	
26	Navicular	
27	Tuberosity of navicular	
28	Medial	
29	Intermediate	cuneiform
30	Lateral	
31	First metatarsal	
32	Tuberosity of base of fifth metatarsal	
33	Cuboid	

Items 7, 8, 9, 10, 11, 12 — of calcaneus

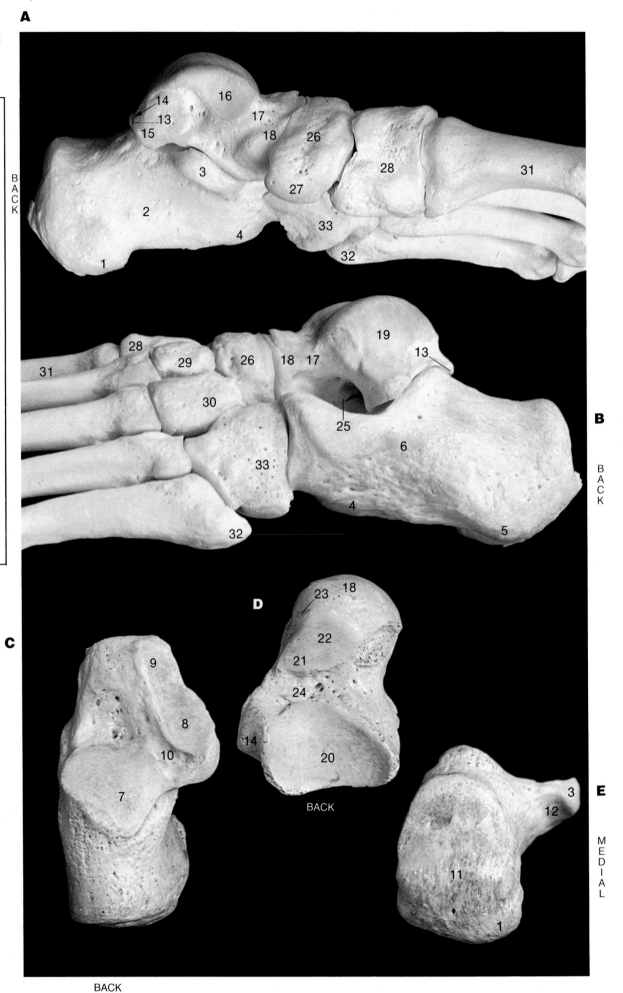

A   **B**

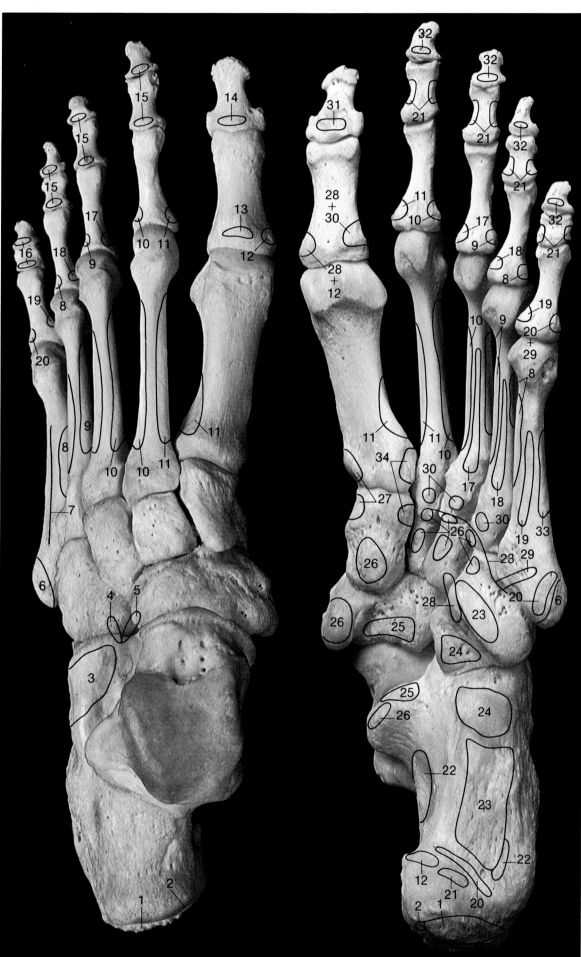

Bones of the left foot, A from above, B from below. Attachments

Joint capsules and minor ligaments have been omitted

1	Tendo calcaneus (Achilles' tendon)
2	Plantaris
3	Extensor digitorum brevis
4	Calcaneocuboid part of bifurcate ligament
5	Calcaneonavicular part of bifurcate ligament
6	Peroneus brevis
7	Peroneus tertius
8	Fourth ⎫
9	Third ⎬ dorsal interosseous
10	Second ⎪
11	First ⎭
12	Abductor hallucis
13	Extensor hallucis brevis
14	Extensor hallucis longus
15	Extensor digitorum longus and brevis
16	Extensor digitorum longus
17	First ⎫
18	Second ⎬ plantar interosseous
19	Third ⎭
20	Abductor digiti minimi
21	Flexor digitorum brevis
22	Flexor accessorius
23	Long plantar ligament
24	Plantar calcaneocuboid ligament
25	Plantar calcaneonavicular ligament
26	Tibialis posterior
27	Tibialis anterior
28	Flexor hallucis brevis
29	Flexor digiti minimi brevis
30	Adductor hallucis
31	Flexor hallucis longus
32	Flexor digitorum longus
33	Opponens digiti minimi (part of 29)
34	Peroneus longus

Left calcaneus, **A** from above, **C** from behind. **B** Left talus, from below

Curved lines indicate corresponding articular surfaces; capsules of talocalcanean and talocalcaneonavicular joints are shown by interrupted lines

1	Calcaneofibular ligament
2	Lateral ⎫
3	Medial ⎬ talocalcanean ligament
4	Tibiocalcanean part of deltoid ligament
5	Interosseous talocalcanean ligament
6	Inferior extensor retinaculum
7	Cervical ligament
8	Extensor digitorum brevis
9	Calcaneocuboid ⎫
10	Calcaneonavicular ⎬ parts of bifurcate ligament
11	Area for bursa
12	Tendo calcaneus (Achilles' tendon)
13	Plantaris
14	Area for fibrofatty tissue

● The interosseous talocalcanean ligament (5) is formed by thickening of the adjacent capsules of the talocalcanean and talocalcaneonavicular joints.

Secondary centres of ossification of left lower limb bones
D Hip bone, lower lateral part
E and **F** Femur, upper and lower ends
G and **H** Tibia, upper and lower ends
J and **K** Fibula, upper and lower ends
L Calcaneus
M Metatarsal and phalanges of second toe
N Metatarsal and phalanges of great toe

Figures in years, commencement of ossification → fusion.
P = puberty, B = ninth intra-uterine month. See introduction on page 106

● In the hip bone (D) one or more secondary centres appear in the Y-shaped cartilage between ilium, ischium and pubis. Other centres (not illustrated) are usually present for the iliac crest, anterior inferior iliac spine, and (possibly) the pubic tubercle and pubic crest (all P → 25).
● The patella (not illustrated) begins to ossify from one or more centres between the third and sixth year.
● All the phalanges, and the first metatarsal, have a secondary centre at their proximal ends; the other metatarsals have one at their distal ends.
● Of the tarsal bones, the largest, the calcaneus, begins to ossify in the third intra-uterine month and the talus about three months later. The cuboid may begin to ossify either just before or just after birth, with the lateral cuneiform in the first year, medial cuneiform at two years and the intermediate cuneiform and navicular at three years.
● The calcaneus (L) is the only tarsal bone to have a secondary centre.

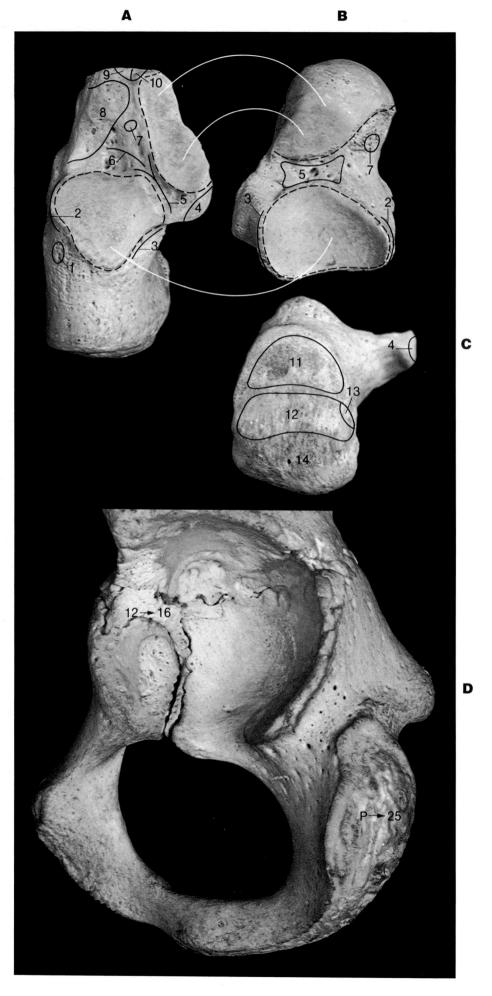

E

G

J

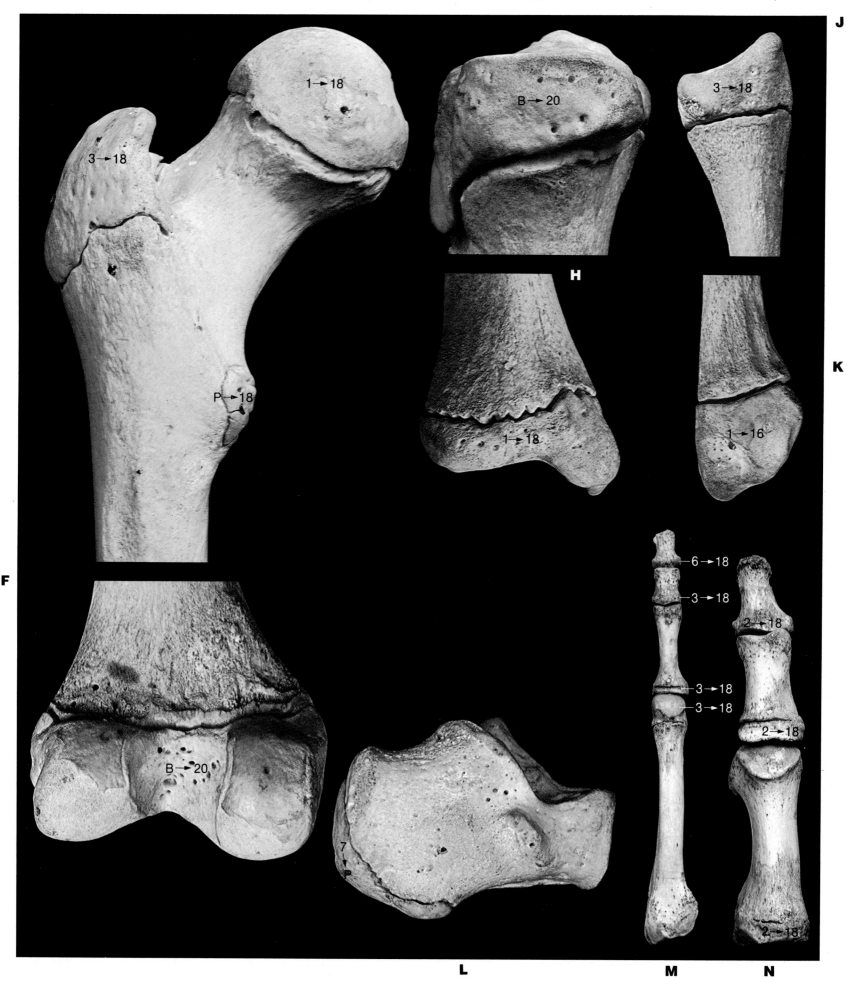

1→18

3→18

B→20

3→18

P→18

H

1→18

F

B→20

7↓
P

L

6→18

3→18

2→18

3→18

3→18

2→18

1→16

K

M

N

2→18

A Right gluteal region. Superficial nerves

Skin and subcutaneous tissue have been removed, preserving cutaneous branches from the first three lumbar (3) and first three sacral (13) nerves, the cutaneous branches of the posterior femoral cutaneous nerve (6) and the perforating cutaneous nerve (12). The curved line near the bottom of the picture indicates the position of the gluteal fold (fold of the buttock). The muscle fibres of gluteus maximus (5) run downwards and laterally, and its lower border does not correspond to the gluteal fold

1	Posterior layer of lumbar fascia overlying erector spinae
2	Iliac crest
3	Cutaneous branches of dorsal rami of first three lumbar nerves
4	Gluteal fascia overlying gluteus medius
5	Gluteus maximus
6	Gluteal branches of posterior femoral cutaneous nerve
7	Semitendinosus
8	Adductor magnus
9	Gracilis
10	Ischiorectal fossa and levator ani
11	Coccyx
12	Perforating cutaneous nerve
13	Gluteal branches of dorsal rami of first three sacral nerves

● The first three lumbar nerves and the first three sacral nerves supply skin over the gluteal region (by the lateral branches of their dorsal rami, 3 and 13) but the intervening fourth and fifth lumbar nerves do not have a cutaneous distribution in this region.

● The gluteal region or buttock is sometimes used as a site for intramuscular injections. The correct site is in the upper outer quadrant of the buttock, and for delimiting this quadrant it is essential to remember that the upper boundary of the buttock is the uppermost part of the iliac crest. The lower boundary is the fold of the buttock. Dividing the area between these two boundaries by a vertical line midway between the midline and the lateral side of the body indicates that the upper outer quadrant is well above and to the right of the label 5, and this is the safe site for injection—well above and to the right of the sciatic nerve which is displayed in the dissections opposite.

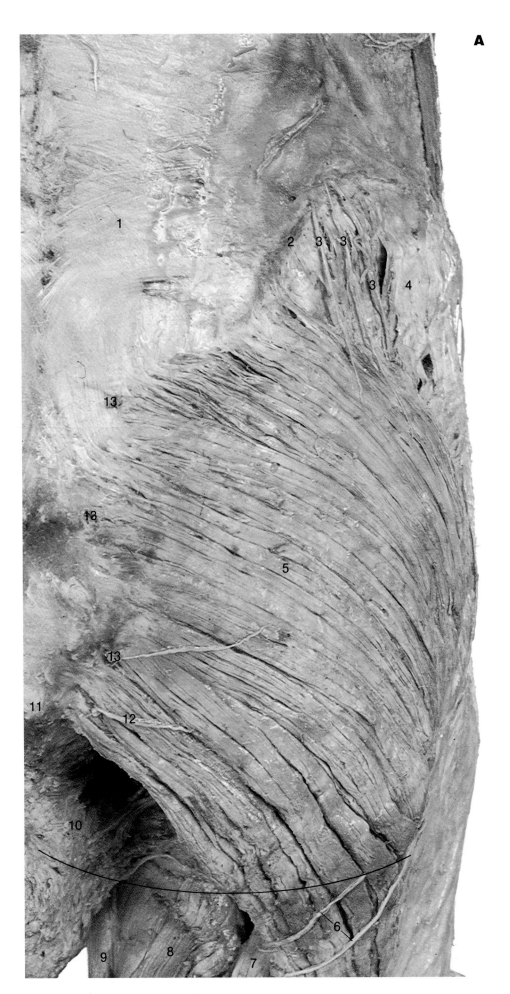

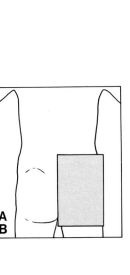

B

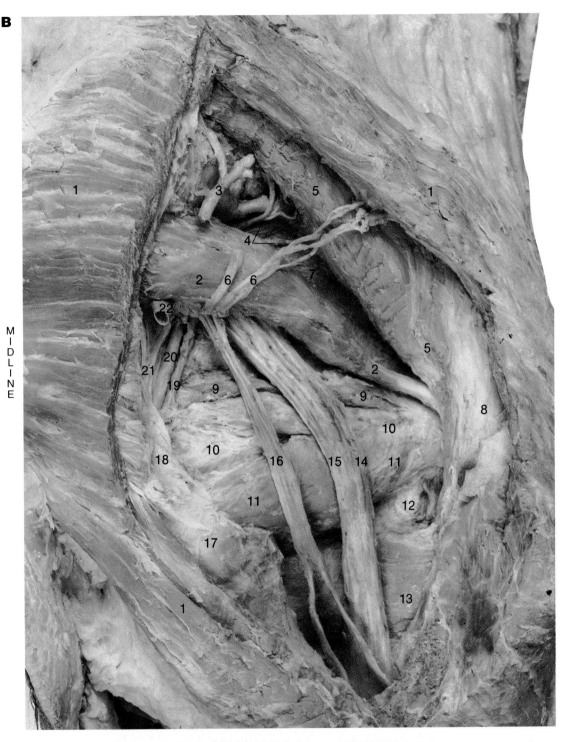

MIDLINE

C

Right gluteal region, **B** with most of gluteus maximus removed, **C** with the sciatic nerve displaced

The removal of the central part of gluteus maximus (1) displays piriformis (2) which is the guide to the surrounding structures. The superior gluteal artery (3) and nerve (4) are above it, running between gluteus medius (5) and minimus (7). The inferior gluteal nerve (6) and vessels (22) are below piriformis (2), and part of the nerve is seen entering gluteus maximus (1), the rest having been removed with the muscle. Also emerging below piriformis are the sciatic nerve (14 and 15) with the nerve to quadratus femoris (C23) under cover of it, the posterior femoral cutaneous nerve (16), and more medially the nerve to obturator internus (19), the internal pudendal artery (20) and the pudendal nerve (21). Obturator internus (10) with a gemellus on either side (9 and 11) and quadratus femoris (13) lie in that order below piriformis. In C the sciatic nerve has been displaced slightly laterally to show the underlying nerve to quadratus femoris (23, in front of the upper white marker; the lower marker is behind the nerve to obturator internus, 19)

1	Gluteus maximus
2	Piriformis
3	Superior gluteal artery
4	Superior gluteal nerve
5	Gluteus medius
6	Inferior gluteal nerve
7	Gluteus minimus
8	Greater trochanter of femur
9	Superior gemellus
10	Obturator internus
11	Inferior gemellus
12	Obturator externus
13	Quadratus femoris
14	Common peroneal } part of sciatic nerve
15	Tibial
16	Posterior femoral cutaneous nerve
17	Ischial tuberosity
18	Sacrotuberous ligament
19	Nerve to obturator internus
20	Internal pudendal artery
21	Pudendal nerve
22	Inferior gluteal artery
23	Nerve to quadratus femoris

● Emerging from the pelvis into the gluteal region above piriformis (2) are the superior gluteal nerve and vessels (4 and 3).

● Emerging from the pelvis into the gluteal region below piriformis are the inferior gluteal nerve and vessels (6 and 22), the sciatic nerve (14 and 15), the posterior femoral cutaneous nerve (16) and the nerve to quadratus femoris (23).

● Emerging from the pelvis below piriformis to enter the perineum are the pudendal nerve (21), the internal pudendal vessels (20) and the nerve to obturator internus (19), in that order from medial to lateral.

● The two parts of the sciatic nerve (common peroneal and tibial, 14 and 15) usually divide from one another at the top of the popliteal fossa (page 306) but are sometimes separate as they emerge beneath piriformis, and the common peroneal may even perforate piriformis.

● After curving laterally beneath piriformis the sciatic nerve lies midway between the ischial tuberosity (17) and the greater trochanter of the femur (8); these two bony points are surface markings for the upper part of the nerve as it passes centrally down the back of the thigh.

293

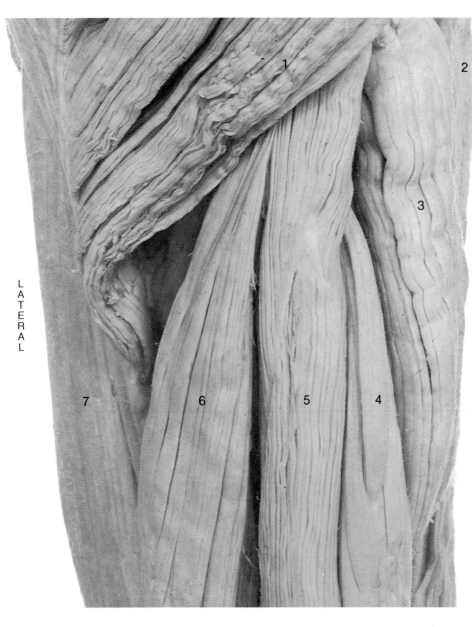

A

LATERAL

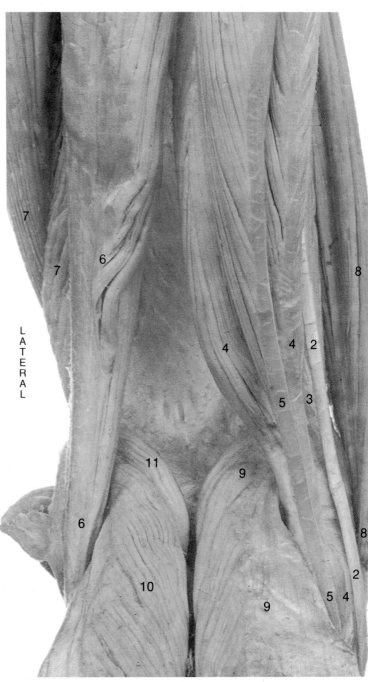

B

LATERAL

Back of the left thigh. Muscles, **A** in the upper part, **B** in the lower part bordering the popliteal fossa

All fascia, vessels and nerves have been removed. Biceps (6) passes downwards and laterally, forming in B the upper lateral boundary of the popliteal fossa. Semimembranosus (4) and semitendinosus (5) pass down on the medial side, forming in B the upper medial boundary of the popliteal fossa, where the tendon of semitendinosus (B5) overlies semimembranosus (B4)

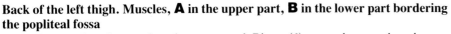

1	Gluteus maximus
2	Gracilis
3	Adductor magnus
4	Semimembranosus
5	Semitendinosus
6	Biceps
7	Vastus lateralis
8	Sartorius
9	Medial ⎱ head of
10	Lateral ⎰ gastrocnemius
11	Plantaris

● The long head of biceps (the part seen in A, 6), semimembranosus (4) and semitendinosus (5) are commonly called the hamstrings. The short head of biceps, which is under cover of the long head and arises from the back of the shaft of the femur and not from the ischial tuberosity (as the other muscles do), is not classified as a hamstring. The true hamstrings span both the hip and knee joint; they extend the hip and flex the knee.

● The origins of the hamstrings from the ischial tuberosity are under cover of the lower border of gluteus maximus (1), but are seen in C opposite, where gluteus maximus has been partly removed.

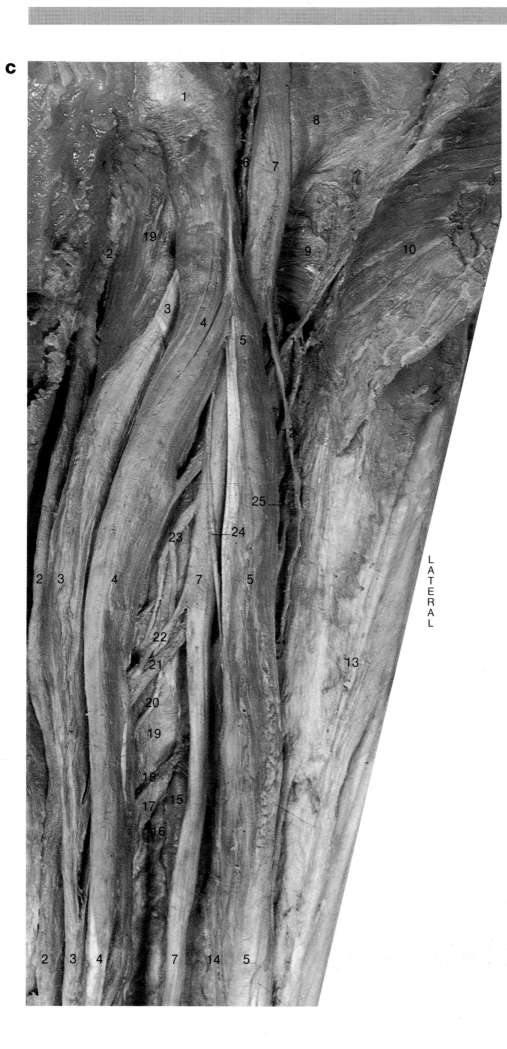

LATERAL

C Back of the right upper thigh

Gluteus maximus (10) has been reflected laterally and the gap between semitendinosus (4) and biceps (5) has been opened up to show the sciatic nerve (7) and its muscular branches

1	Ischial tuberosity
2	Gracilis
3	Semimembranosus
4	Semitendinosus
5	Long head of biceps
6	Anastomotic branch of inferior gluteal artery
7	Sciatic nerve
8	Quadratus femoris
9	Upper part of adductor magnus ('adductor minimus')
10	Gluteus maximus
11	First perforating artery
12	Nerve to short head of biceps
13	Iliotibial tract overlying vastus lateralis
14	Short head of biceps
15	Popliteal vein
16	Popliteal artery
17	Opening in adductor magnus
18	Fourth perforating artery
19	Adductor magnus
20	Nerve to semimembranosus
21	Third perforating artery
22	Nerve to semitendinosus
23	Nerve to semimembranosus and adductor magnus
24	Nerve to long head of biceps
25	Second perforating artery

● The only muscular branch to arise from the lateral side of the sciatic nerve (i.e. from the common peroneal part of the nerve—7, uppermost label near the top of the picture) is the nerve to the short head of biceps (12). All the other muscular branches—to the long head of biceps (24), semimembranosus (20), semimembranosus and adductor magnus (23) and semitendinosus (22)—arise from the medial side of the sciatic nerve (7, near the centre of the picture) (i.e. from the tibial part of the nerve).

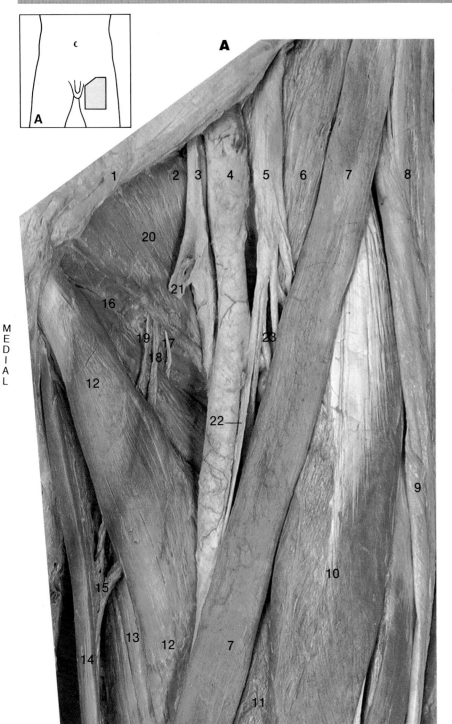

Left femoral region, **A** femoral vessels and nerve, **B** profunda femoris artery

The superficial vessels and nerves and the fascia lata have been removed to display in A the femoral vein (3), artery (4) and nerve (5) and the surrounding muscles. In B the femoral artery (4) has been displaced laterally to show the profunda femoris branch (24)

1	Inguinal ligament
2	Position of femoral canal
3	Femoral vein
4	Femoral artery
5	Femoral nerve
6	Iliacus
7	Sartorius
8	Fascia lata overlying tensor fasciae latae
9	Iliotibial tract overlying vastus lateralis
10	Rectus femoris
11	Vastus medialis
12	Adductor longus
13	Adductor magnus
14	Gracilis
15	Nerve and vessels to gracilis
16	Adductor brevis
17	Nerve to adductor brevis ⎫ from anterior
18	Nerve to adductor longus ⎬ branch of
19	Nerve to gracilis ⎭ obturator nerve
20	Pectineus
21	Great saphenous vein
22	Saphenous nerve
23	Muscular branches of femoral nerve overlying lateral circumflex femoral vessels
24	Profunda femoris artery
25	Medial circumflex femoral artery

• The boundaries of the femoral triangle are the inguinal ligament (1), the *medial* border of sartorius (7) and the *medial* border of adductor longus (12).
• The adjacent borders of pectineus (20) and adductor longus (12) are usually in contact with one another, but if they are not (as in this specimen) the anterior branch of the obturator nerve and its muscular branches (17 to 19) are visible in the floor of the triangle lying in front of adductor brevis (16).
• The femoral canal (2) is the medial compartment of the femoral sheath (removed) which contains in its middle compartment the femoral vein (3), and in the lateral compartment the femoral artery (4). The femoral nerve (5) is *lateral* to the sheath, not within it.
• The profunda femoris artery (24) arises from the posterolateral surface of the femoral artery (4) and so is under cover of it in A, but is shown in B when the parent vessel is displaced laterally.
• In the lower part of the femoral triangle the femoral vein (3) lies behind the artery (4) and both pass in front of adductor longus (12).
• The profunda femoris artery (24) passes behind adductor longus (as shown on page 298).

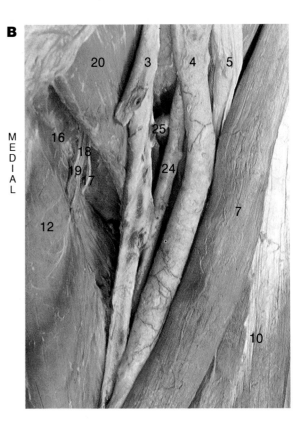

C Left obturator nerve

In this left femoral region, pectineus (6), adductor longus (1, lower label) and adductor brevis (7) have been detached from their origins and reflected laterally to display obturator externus (12) and the anterior (3) and posterior (11) branches of the obturator nerve

● The obturator nerve divides into its anterior and posterior branches when in the obturator foramen. The anterior branch emerges anterior to obturator externus, while the posterior branch pierces the muscle.

● The anterior branch of the obturator nerve (C3, A17 to 19) supplies adductor longus (A12 and 18), adductor brevis (A16 and 17) and gracilis (A14, 15 and 19).

● The posterior branch of the obturator nerve (C11) supplies obturator externus (C12) and part of adductor magnus (C10). (The rest of adductor magnus is supplied by the sciatic nerve—page 295, 23.)

1	Adductor longus
2	Superior ramus of pubis
3	Anterior branch of obturator nerve
4	Femoral vein
5	Femoral artery
6	Pectineus
7	Adductor brevis
8	Nerve and vessels to gracilis
9	Gracilis
10	Adductor magnus
11	Posterior branch of obturator nerve
12	Obturator externus

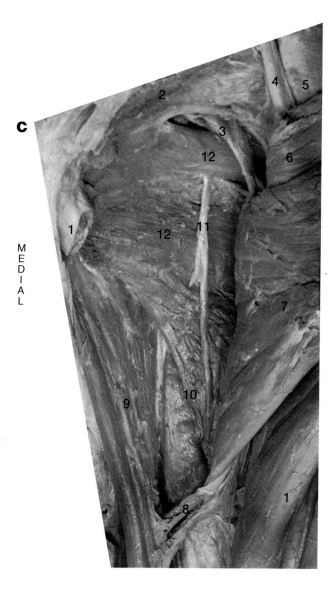

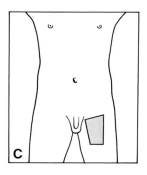

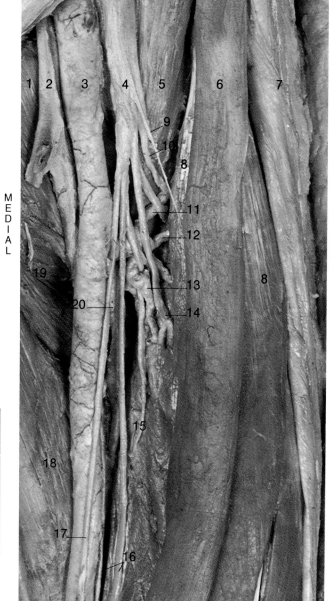

D Left femoral nerve

This is the same specimen as in A, but here sartorius (6) and rectus femoris (8) have been displaced laterally to open up the upper part of the adductor canal and show the lateral circumflex femoral vessels (11 to 13) and branches of the femoral nerve (4)

1	Pectineus	11	Ascending	⎫ branch of lateral
2	Femoral vein	12	Transverse	⎬ circumflex femoral
3	Femoral artery	13	Descending	⎭ artery
4	Femoral nerve	14	Nerve to vastus lateralis	
5	Iliacus	15	Vastus intermedius and nerve	
6	Sartorius	16	Vastus medialis and nerves	
7	Tensor fasciae latae	17	Saphenous nerve	
8	Rectus femoris	18	Adductor longus	
9	Nerve to sartorius	19	Adductor brevis and nerve	
10	Nerve to rectus femoris	20	Profunda femoris artery	

● The adductor canal extends from the apex of the femoral triangle to the opening in adductor magnus through which the femoral vessels pass (page 298).

● The canal, which is triangular in section, is bounded laterally by vastus medialis (D16), behind by adductor longus (D18) (and lower down by adductor magnus), and in front by sartorius (D6) which forms the roof of the canal.

● The contents of the canal are the femoral artery and vein (D3 and 2, with the vein lying deep to the artery), the saphenous nerve (D17) and the nerve to vastus medialis (D16, double in this specimen).

297

A Right femoral artery

In the upper part of the right thigh, all veins have been removed except for the uppermost part of the femoral vein (10), which is on the medial side of the femoral artery (9). The femoral nerve (8), whose femoral cutaneous branches have been removed, is lateral to the artery. Part of sartorius (3) has been resected to show the lateral circumflex femoral artery (11, here arising from the femoral artery) and the uppermost part of the adductor canal, which is the gutter behind the lower part of sartorius with vastus medialis (20) on the lateral side and adductor longus (18) medially. The profunda femoris artery (24) arises from the posterolateral side of the femoral artery (9) about 3 cm below the inguinal ligament. In the upper part of the adductor canal the saphenous nerve (25) lies in front of the nerve to vastus medialis (23)

1	Tensor fasciae latae
2	Lateral femoral cutaneous nerve
3	Sartorius
4	Iliacus
5	Superficial circumflex iliac artery (double)
6	Inguinal ligament
7	Superficial epigastric artery
8	Femoral nerve
9	Femoral artery
10	Femoral vein
11	Lateral circumflex femoral artery
12	Medial circumflex femoral artery
13	Pectineus
14	Superficial external pudendal artery (low origin)
15	Anterior branch of obturator nerve
16	Spermatic cord
17	Adductor brevis
18	Adductor longus
19	Gracilis
20	Vastus medialis
21	Vastus intermedius
22	Rectus femoris
23	Nerve to vastus medialis
24	Profunda femoris artery
25	Saphenous nerve
26	Nerve to rectus femoris
27	Descending ⎫ branch of
28	Transverse ⎬ lateral circumflex
29	Ascending ⎭ femoral artery

• The lateral circumflex femoral artery (11) is usually a branch of the profunda femoris (24), but frequently, as in this specimen, it arises directly from the femoral artery (9). It divides into ascending, transverse and descending branches (29, 28 and 27).
• The medial circumflex femoral artery (12) leaves the femoral triangle by passing backwards between pectineus (13) and the tendon of psoas (hidden behind the femoral artery, 9). It emerges in the gluteal region between the lower border of quadratus femoris and the upper border of adductor magnus (page 293).
• The femoral artery (9) with the femoral vein behind it (here removed) passes down the thigh *in front of* adductor longus (18).
• The profunda femoris artery (24) with the profunda femoris vein in front of it (here removed) passes down the thigh *behind* adductor longus (18) Above adductor longus the two veins lie between the two arteries. The upper border of adductor longus is seen separating the two arteries about 2 cm above the lower cut end of sartorius (3).

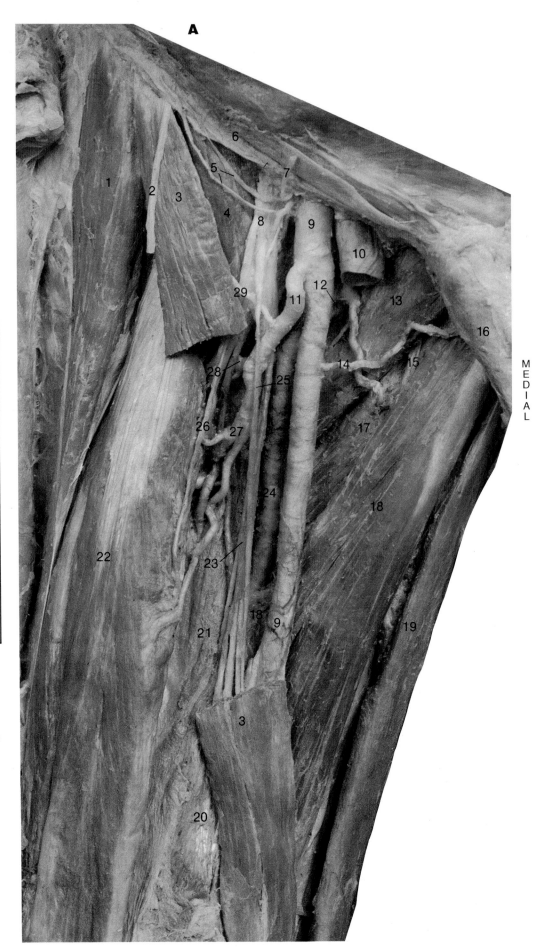

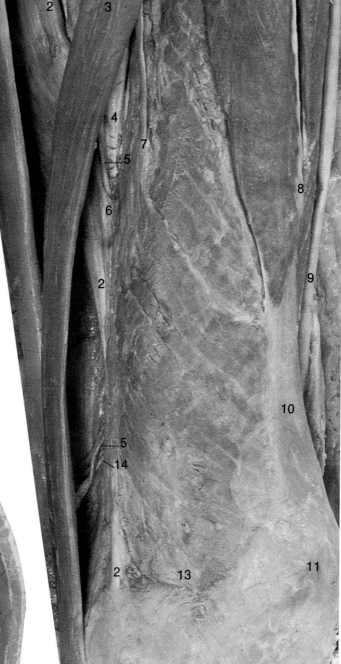

B

B Left lower thigh, from the front and medial side

The lower part of sartorius (3) has been displayed medially to open up the lower part of the adductor canal and expose the femoral artery (4) passing through the opening in adductor magnus (6) to enter the popliteal fossa behind the knee and become the popliteal artery (page 306)

1	Gracilis	9	Iliotibial tract
2	Adductor magnus	10	Quadriceps tendon
3	Sartorius	11	Patella
4	Femoral artery	12	Medial patellar retinaculum
5	Saphenous nerve	13	Lowest (horizontal) fibres of vastus medialis
6	Opening in adductor magnus	14	Saphenous branch of descending genicular artery
7	Vastus medialis and nerve		
8	Rectus femoris		

C Cross section of the left lower thigh

The section, viewed as when looking upwards from knee to hip, is at the level of the opening in adductor magnus (13) through which the femoral vessels (20) will pass to become the popliteal vessels. The vasti (1, 3 and 5) envelop the femur (2) at the sides and front, and rectus femoris (4) at this level has become narrow and tendinous. The femoral vessels (20) are between vastus medialis (1) and adductor magnus (12) and the profunda vessels (11) close to the back of the femur (2). The sciatic nerve (10) is deeply placed between biceps laterally (8 and 9) and semimembranosus medially (14)

1	Vastus medialis	11	Profunda femoris vessels
2	Femur	12	Adductor magnus
3	Vastus intermedius	13	Opening in adductor magnus
4	Rectus femoris	14	Semimembranosus
5	Vastus lateralis	15	Semitendinosus
6	Iliotibial tract of fascia lata	16	Gracilis
7	Lateral intermuscular septum	17	Sartorius
8	Short head of biceps	18	Great saphenous vein
9	Long head of biceps	19	Saphenous nerve
10	Sciatic nerve	20	Femoral vessels

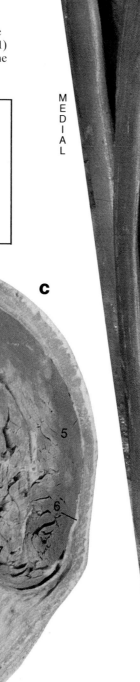

FRONT

C

MEDIAL

Right hip joint, **A** from the front, **B** from behind

All muscles except obturator externus (6) have been
removed to display the iliofemoral (8), pubofemoral (7) and
ischiofemoral (12) ligaments which reinforce the outside of
the capsule of the joint

1	Anterior inferior iliac spine
2	Inguinal ligament
3	Superficial inguinal ring and spermatic cord
4	Iliopubic eminence
5	Obturator canal
6	Obturator externus
7	Pubofemoral ligament
8	Iliofemoral ligament
9	Lesser trochanter
10	Intertrochanteric line and capsule attachment
11	Greater trochanter
12	Ischiofemoral ligament
13	Zona orbicularis
14	Intertrochanteric crest
15	Extracapsular part of neck of femur
16	Ischial tuberosity
17	Lesser sciatic notch and surface for obturator internus
18	Ischial spine

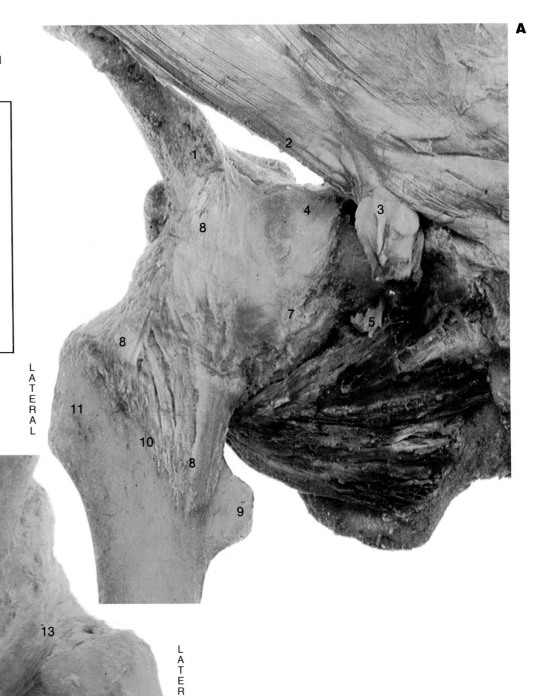

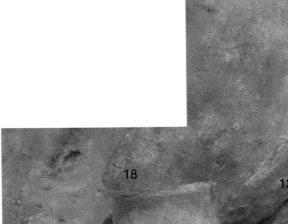

• The iliofemoral ligament (8) has the shape of an inverted Y. It and
the interosseous sacro-iliac ligament are the two strongest ligaments
in the body.

• Some of the fibres of the ischiofemoral ligament (12) help to form
the zona orbicularis—circular fibres of the capsule that form a collar
round the neck of the femur.

• Posteriorly the capsule is attached to the neck of the femur, not to
the intertrochanteric crest. (Anteriorly it is attached to the
intertrochanteric line.) See pages 273 and 274.

• Muscles producing movements at the hip joint:

Flexion: psoas and iliacus, with rectus femoris, sartorius, tensor
fasciae latae, pectineus and adductor longus and brevis.
Extension: gluteus maximus, semimembranosus, semitendinosus,
long head of biceps and the ischial part of adductor magnus.
Abduction: gluteus medius and minimus, with tensor fasciae latae and
piriformis.
Adduction: adductor longus, brevis and magnus, pectineus, gracilis
and quadratus femoris.
Medial rotation: anterior fibres of gluteus medius and minimus, and
psoas and iliacus.
Lateral rotation: obturator externus and internus and gemelli,
piriformis, quadratus femoris, gluteus maximus and sartorius.

C

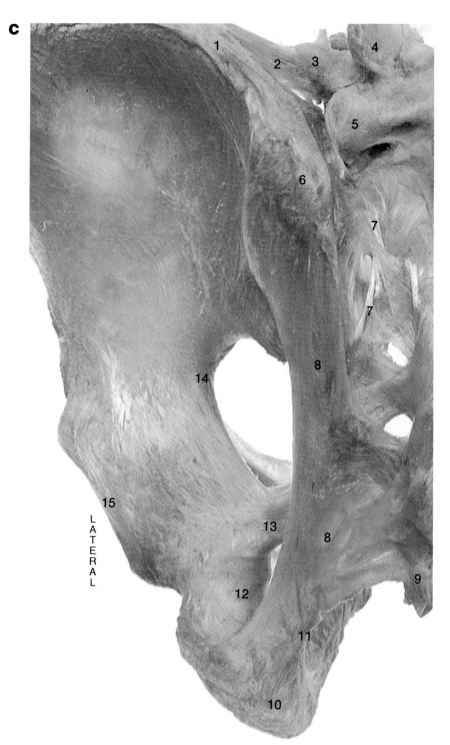

L A T E R A L

C **Left vertebropelvic and sacro-iliac ligaments, from behind**

All tissues except ligaments have been removed to show how the sacrotuberous and sacrospinous ligaments (8 and 13) bridge the greater and lesser sciatic notches (14 and 12), so converting them into foramina

1	Iliac crest
2	Iliolumbar ligament
3	Transverse process
4	Superior articular process } of fifth lumbar vertebra
5	Inferior articular process
6	Posterior superior iliac spine
7	Dorsal sacro-iliac ligaments
8	Sacrotuberous ligament
9	Coccyx
10	Ischial tuberosity
11	Falciform process of sacrotuberous ligament
12	Lesser sciatic notch
13	Sacrospinous ligament and ischial spine
14	Greater sciatic notch
15	Acetabular labrum

● The vertebropelvic ligaments are the iliolumbar (2), sacrotuberous (8) and sacrospinous (13) ligaments.
● The dorsal sacro-iliac ligaments (7) cover the interosseous sacro-iliac ligament.

● The acetabular labrum (6) is attached to the margin of the acetabulum and is composed of fibrocartilage.
● The transverse ligament (7) fills in the acetabular notch and the gap between the two ends of the labrum (6), and is composed of fibrous tissue, not fibrocartilage.
● The ligament of the head of the femur (8) extends from the transverse ligament (7) and the margins of the acetabular notch to the facet or pit on the medial side of the head of the femur. Like the transverse ligament it is composed of fibrous tissue.

D **Right hip joint with femur removed, from the right**

The femur has been disarticulated from the acetabulum and removed, leaving the acetabular labrum (6), transverse ligament (7) and the ligament of the head of the femur (8)

1	Reflected } head of rectus femoris
2	Straight
3	Pectineus
4	Adductor longus
5	Obturator externus
6	Acetabular labrum
7	Transverse ligament
8	Ligament of head of femur
9	Articular surface
10	Acetabular fossa (non-articular)

D

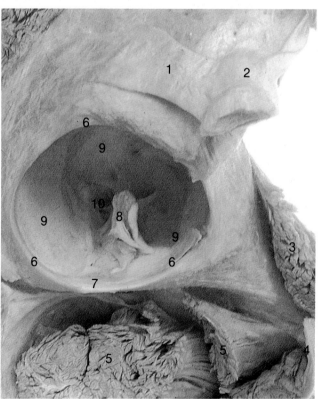

M E D I A L

A

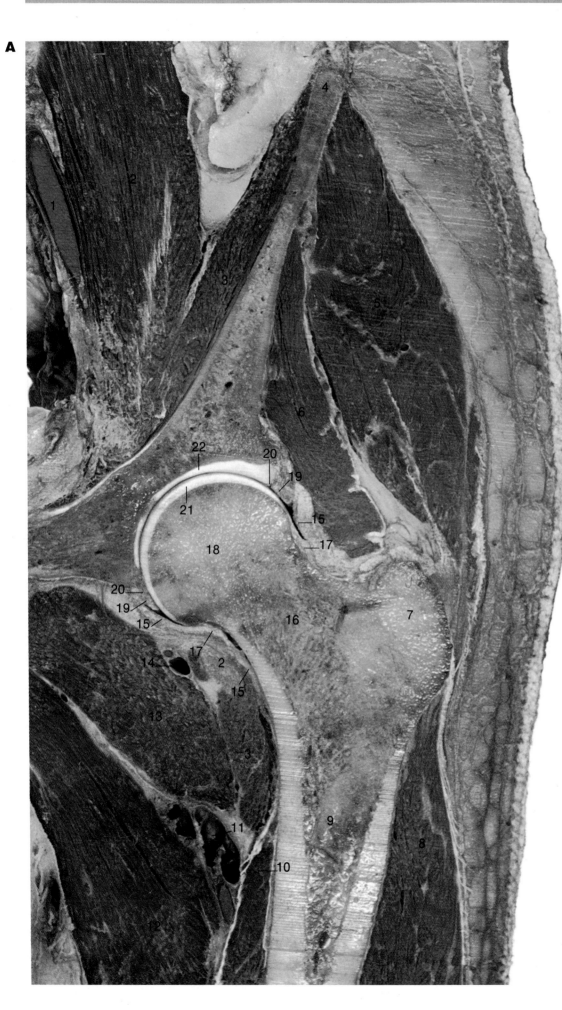

A Left hip joint, coronal section, from the front

The section has passed through almost at the centre of the head (18) of the femur and the centre of the greater trochanter (7). Above the neck of the femur (16), gluteus minimus (6) with gluteus medius (5) above it run down to their attachments to the greater trochanter (7), while below the neck the tendon of psoas (2) and muscle fibres of iliacus (3) pass backwards towards the lesser trochanter. The circular fibres of the zona orbicularis (17) constrict the capsule (15) round the intracapsular part of the neck of the femur

1	External iliac artery
2	Psoas major
3	Iliacus
4	Iliac crest
5	Gluteus medius
6	Gluteus minimus
7	Greater trochanter
8	Vastus lateralis
9	Shaft of femur
10	Vastus medialis
11	Profunda femoris vessels
12	Adductor longus
13	Pectineus
14	Medial circumflex femoral vessels
15	Capsule of hip joint
16	Neck of femur
17	Zona orbicularis of capsule
18	Head of femur
19	Acetabular labrum
20	Rim of acetabulum
21	Hyaline cartilage of head
22	Hyaline cartilage of acetabulum

● The convergence of gluteus medius and minimus (5 and 6) on to the greater trochanter is well displayed in this section. These muscles are classified as abductors of the femur at the hip joint, but their more important action is in walking, where they act to prevent adduction—preventing the pelvis from tilting to the opposite side when the opposite limb is off the ground.

B Radiograph of the left hip and sacro-iliac joints

In this standard anteroposterior view of the hip joint (4 and 5), much of the joint line of the sacro-iliac joint can also be seen (2)

1	Transverse process of fifth lumbar vertebra	
2	Sacro-iliac joint	
3	Anterior superior iliac spine	
4	Rim of acetabulum	
5	Head	
6	Neck	of femur
7	Greater trochanter	
8	Lesser trochanter	
9	Ischial tuberosity	
10	Superior pubic ramus	
11	Pectineal line	
12	Pubic tubercle	
13	Pubic symphysis	
14	First coccygeal vertebra	
15	Phleboliths in pelvic veins	
16	Ischial spine	
17	Sacrum	

● Phleboliths (15) are calcified plaques commonly seen in the walls of pelvic veins.

B

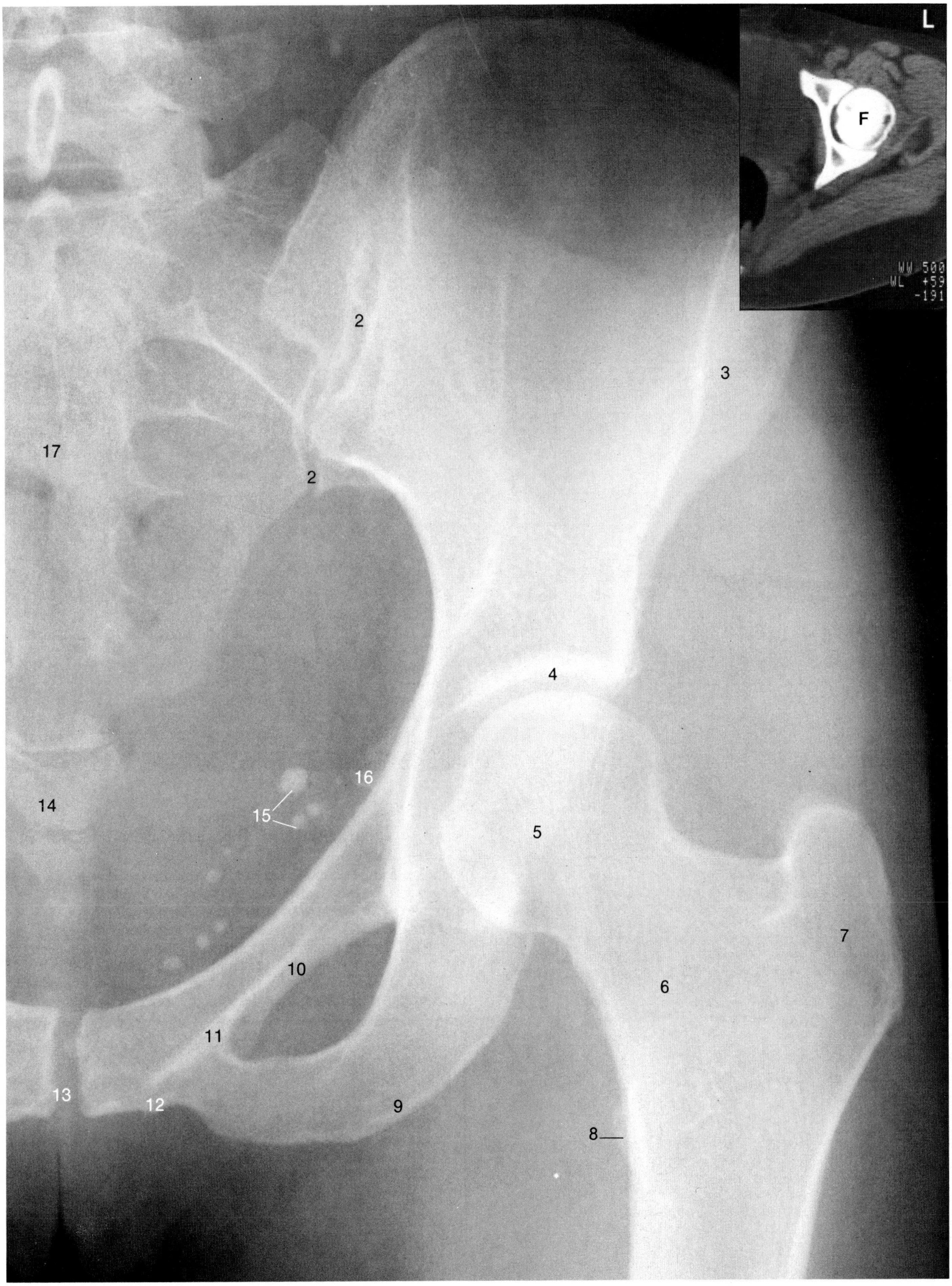

C

C CT scan of the left hip joint
In this scan of the left half of the pelvis the head of the femur (F) is shown in the acetabulum of the hip bone

303

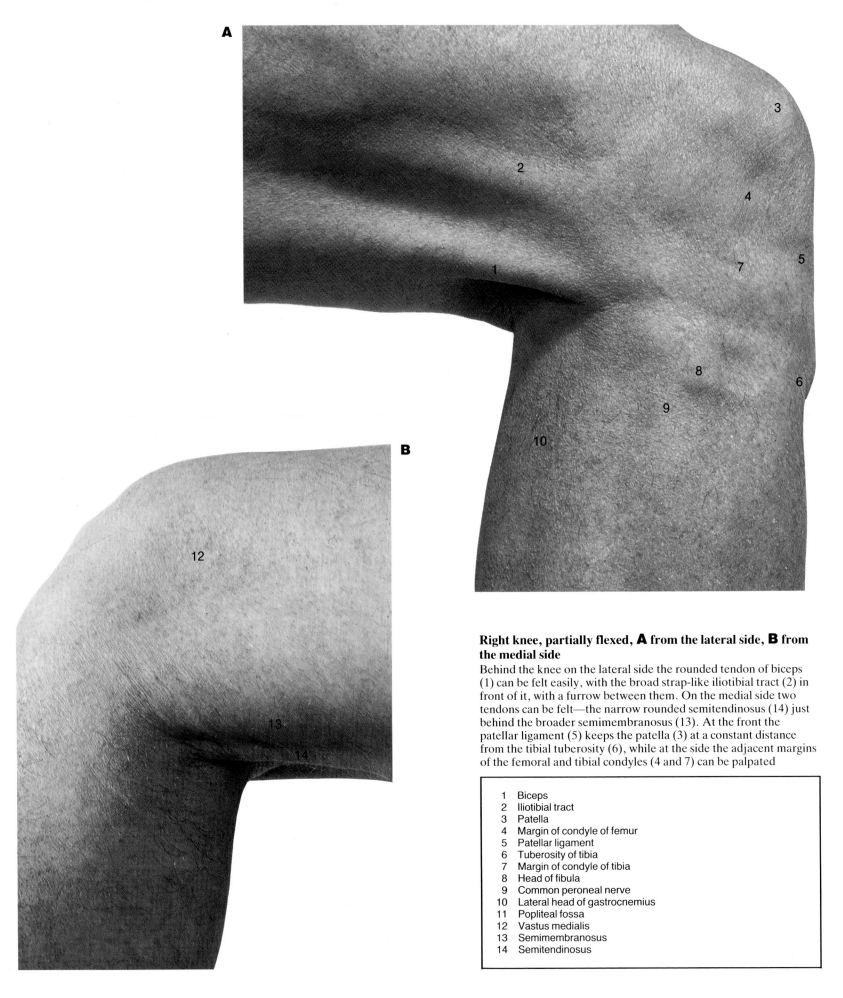

Right knee, partially flexed, A from the lateral side, B from the medial side

Behind the knee on the lateral side the rounded tendon of biceps (1) can be felt easily, with the broad strap-like iliotibial tract (2) in front of it, with a furrow between them. On the medial side two tendons can be felt—the narrow rounded semitendinosus (14) just behind the broader semimembranosus (13). At the front the patellar ligament (5) keeps the patella (3) at a constant distance from the tibial tuberosity (6), while at the side the adjacent margins of the femoral and tibial condyles (4 and 7) can be palpated

1	Biceps
2	Iliotibial tract
3	Patella
4	Margin of condyle of femur
5	Patellar ligament
6	Tuberosity of tibia
7	Margin of condyle of tibia
8	Head of fibula
9	Common peroneal nerve
10	Lateral head of gastrocnemius
11	Popliteal fossa
12	Vastus medialis
13	Semimembranosus
14	Semitendinosus

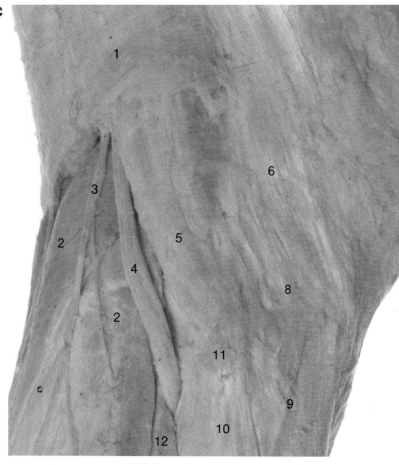

C Right knee, superficial dissection, from the lateral side

The fascia behind biceps (5) has been removed to show the common peroneal nerve (4) passing downwards immediately behind the tendon, and then running between the adjacent borders of soleus (12) and peroneus longus (10), under cover of which it lies against the neck of the fibula. Minor superficial vessels and nerves have been removed

1	Fascia lata
2	Lateral head of gastrocnemius
3	Lateral cutaneous nerve of calf
4	Common peroneal nerve
5	Biceps
6	Iliotibial tract
7	Patella
8	Attachment of iliotibial tract to tibia
9	Deep fascia overlying extensor muscles
10	Deep fascia overlying peroneus longus
11	Head of fibula
12	Soleus

● The iliotibial tract (6) is the thickened lateral part of the fascia lata (1). At its upper part the tensor fasciae latae and most of gluteus maximus are inserted into it; its lower end is attached to the lateral condyle of the tibia (8).

● Its subcutaneous position and contact with the neck of the fibula make the common peroneal nerve (4) the most commonly injured nerve in the lower limb.

D Right knee, superficial dissection, from the medial side

The great saphenous vein (5) runs upwards about a hand's breadth behind the medial border of the patella (1). The saphenous nerve (6) becomes superficial between the tendons of sartorius (4) and gracilis (7), and its infrapatellar branch (10) curls forwards a little below the upper margin of the tibial condyle

1	Patella
2	Vastus medialis
3	Branches of medial femoral cutaneous nerve
4	Sartorius
5	Great saphenous vein
6	Saphenous nerve
7	Gracilis
8	Semitendinosus
9	Medial head of gastrocnemius
10	Infrapatellar branch of saphenous nerve
11	Level of margin of medial condyle of tibia

● At the level of the knee joint the great saphenous vein (5) lies about a hand's breadth behind the medial border of the patella (1); this is the guide for the surface marking of the vessel.

● The saphenous nerve (6) becomes superficial by piercing the deep fascia between the lower ends of sartorius (4) and gracilis (7).

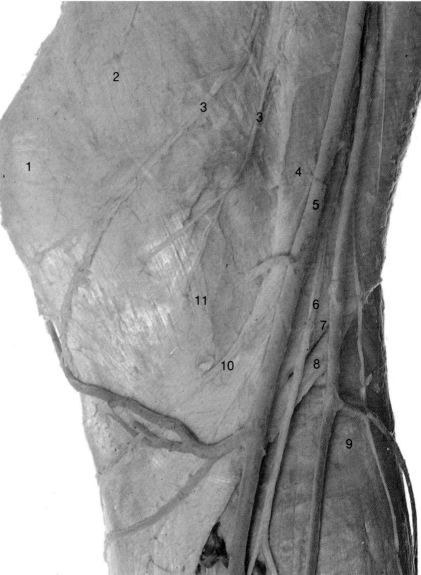

D

A

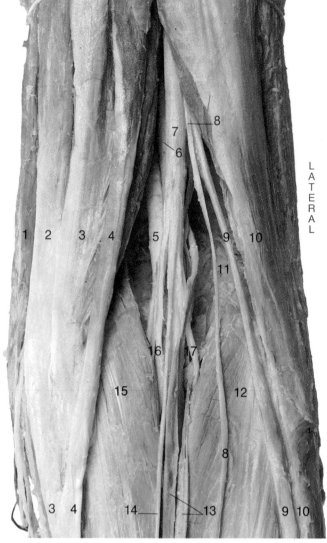

B

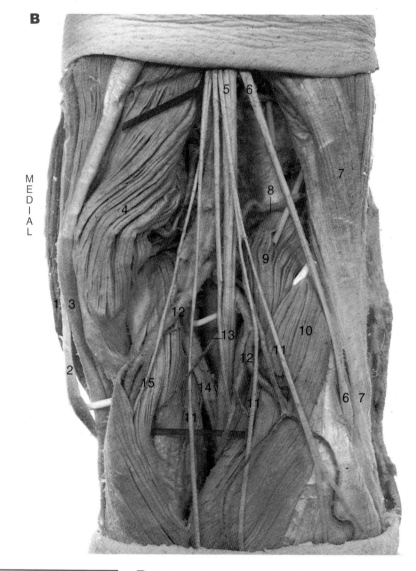

A Right popliteal fossa

The fascia that forms the roof of the diamond-shaped fossa and the fat within it have been removed but the small saphenous vein which pierces the fascia is preserved (13, double in this specimen). The main structures in the fossa are the tibial nerve (7), popliteal vein (6) and popliteal artery (5), which lie in that order from superficial to deep. The common peroneal nerve (9) passes laterally behind the posterior border of biceps. Semimembranosus (3) and semitendinosus (4) are on the medial side of the fossa, with the two heads of gastrocnemius (12 and 15) forming the lower boundaries

1	Sartorius
2	Gracilis
3	Semimembranosus
4	Semitendinosus
5	Popliteal artery
6	Popliteal vein
7	Tibial nerve
8	Lateral cutaneous nerve of calf
9	Common peroneal nerve
10	Biceps
11	Plantaris
12	Lateral head of gastrocnemius
13	Small saphenous vein (double)
14	Sural nerve
15	Medial head of gastrocnemius
16	Nerve to medial head ⎫
17	Nerve to lateral head ⎬ of gastrocnemius

B Right popliteal fossa. Vessels and nerves

Here the margins of the fossa have been displaced and markers hold various structures apart. The upper red marker passes between the tibial nerve (5) and the underlying popliteal vein (seen lower down, 14). The uppermost blue marker is behind an unlabelled muscular branch of the popliteal artery (seen lower down, 13). The middle blue marker is behind the superior lateral genicular artery (8), and the upper white marker between plantaris (9) and the lateral head of gastrocnemius (10). The lowest blue marker displaces the popliteal vein (14) medially to show the underlying popliteal artery (13). The lower red marker holds the two heads of gastrocnemius apart (10 and 15). The lower white marker (outside the fossa) is between the tendons of gracilis (2) and semitendinosus (3)

• The sural nerve (B11) has divided at an unusually high level into several branches. The peroneal communicating branch of the common peroneal nerve is not present.
• The principal structures in the middle of the fossa—the tibial nerve (B5), popliteal vein (B14) and popliteal artery (B13)—lie in that order from superficial to deep. The deep position of the artery makes palpation of its pulsation difficult.
• The most lateral branch of the sural nerve (B11) may here take the place of the lateral cutaneous nerve of the calf which normally arises from the common peroneal nerve.

1	Sartorius	9	Plantaris
2	Gracilis	10	Lateral head of gastrocnemius
3	Semitendinosus		
4	Semi-membranosus	11	Branches of sural nerve
5	Tibial nerve	12	Sural arteries
6	Common peroneal nerve	13	Popliteal artery
		14	Popliteal vein
7	Biceps	15	Medial head of gastrocnemius and nerve
8	Superior lateral genicular artery		

C

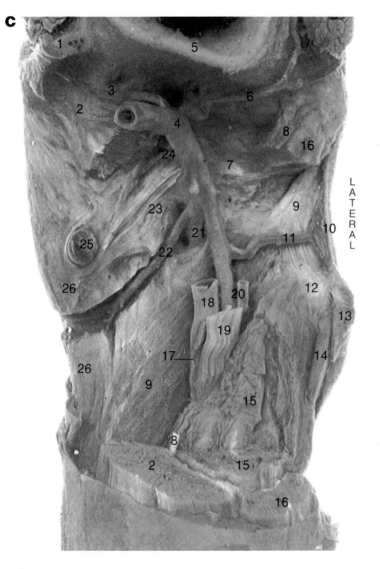

LATERAL

D

MEDIAL

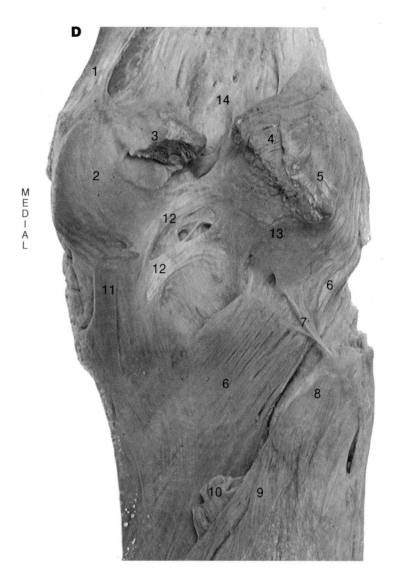

C Right popliteal fossa. Deep dissection of vessels

Most of the superficial muscles have been removed to show the branches of the popliteal artery (4). The knee is flexed so that the artery and the cut end of the femur (5) are seen 'end on'. The artery divides into anterior tibial (21) and posterior tibial (20) branches; usually the anterior tibial passes superficial to popliteus (9) but here the popliteal artery has divided at a high level and the anterior tibial has passed deep to the muscle. The upper pair of superior genicular arteries (3 and 6) run above the heads of gastrocnemius (2 and 16); the inferior pair (22 and 11) pass deep to the tibial and fibular collateral ligaments (26 and 10)

1	Adductor magnus
2	Medial head of gastrocnemius
3	Superior medial genicular artery
4	Popliteal artery
5	Popliteal surface of femur in section
6	Superior lateral genicular artery
7	Capsule of knee joint
8	Plantaris
9	Popliteus
10	Fibular collateral ligament
11	Inferior lateral genicular artery
12	Head of fibula
13	Biceps
14	Common peroneal nerve
15	Soleus
16	Lateral head of gastrocnemius
17	Nerve to popliteus
18	Popliteal vein
19	Tibial nerve
20	Posterior tibial artery and vein
21	Anterior tibial artery
22	Inferior medial genicular artery
23	Oblique popliteal ligament.
24	Middle genicular artery
25	Semimembranosus
26	Tibial collateral ligament

D Right popliteal fossa. Joint capsule and popliteal ligaments

The back of the capsule of the knee joint is shown (13 and 2), reinforced centrally by the oblique popliteal ligament (12) and forming the lower part of the floor of the fossa, with the popliteal surface of the femur (14) in the upper part of the floor

1	Adductor magnus
2	Capsule overlying medial condyle of femur
3	Medial head of gastrocnemius
4	Plantaris
5	Lateral head of gastrocnemius
6	Popliteus
7	Arcuate popliteal ligament
8	Head of fibula
9	Soleus
10	Popliteal vessels and tibial nerve
11	Semimembranosus
12	Oblique popliteal ligament
13	Capsule of knee joint
14	Popliteal surface of femur

● The oblique popliteal ligament (12) is derived from the semimembranosus tendon (11) and reinforces the central posterior part of the joint capsule (13); it is pierced by the middle genicular artery which passes through the capsule to supply the cruciate ligaments.
● The arcuate popliteal ligament (7) arches over popliteus (6) as it emerges from the capsule.

307

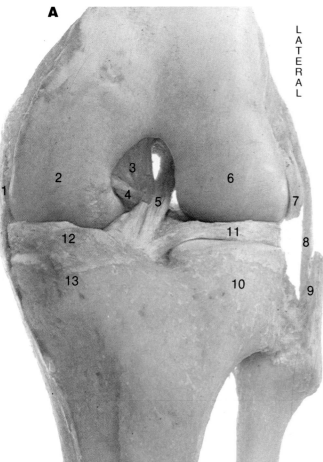

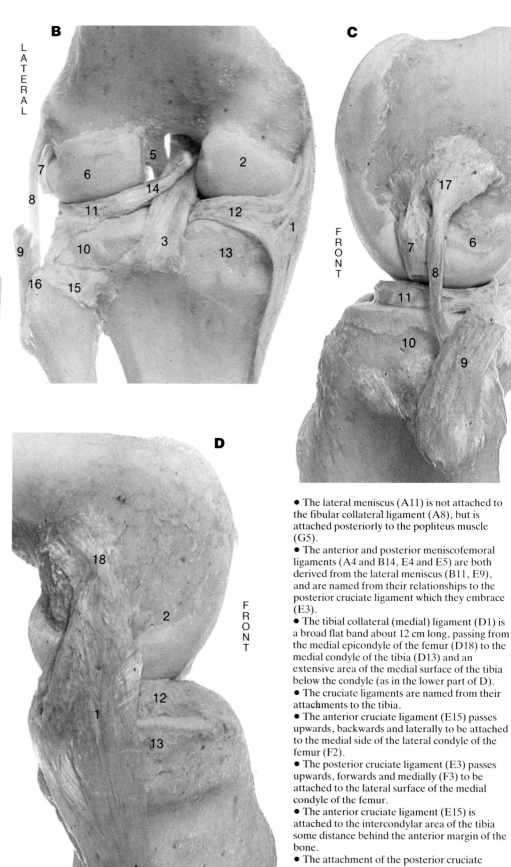

Left knee joint. Ligaments, A from the front, B from behind, C from the lateral side, D from the medial side

The capsule of the knee joint and all surrounding tissues have been removed, leaving only the ligaments of the joint, which is partially flexed

1	Tibial collateral ligament
2	Medial condyle of femur
3	Posterior cruciate ligament
4	Anterior meniscofemoral ligament
5	Anterior cruciate ligament
6	Lateral condyle of femur
7	Popliteus
8	Fibular collateral ligament
9	Biceps tendon
10	Lateral condyle of tibia
11	Lateral meniscus
12	Medial meniscus
13	Medial condyle of tibia
14	Posterior meniscofemoral ligament
15	Capsule of superior tibiofibular joint
16	Apex of head of fibula
17	Lateral ⎫ epicondyle of femur
18	Medial ⎭

● The fibular collateral (lateral) ligament (8) is a rounded cord about 5 cm long, passing from the lateral epicondyle of the femur (C17) to the head of the fibula just in front of its apex (B16), largely under cover of the tendon of biceps (C9).
● The medial meniscus (B12) is attached to the deep part of the tibial collateral ligament (B1). This helps to anchor the meniscus but makes it liable to become trapped and torn by rotatory movements between the tibia and femur.

● The lateral meniscus (A11) is not attached to the fibular collateral ligament (A8), but is attached posteriorly to the popliteus muscle (G5).
● The anterior and posterior meniscofemoral ligaments (A4 and B14, E4 and E5) are both derived from the lateral meniscus (B11, E9), and are named from their relationships to the posterior cruciate ligament which they embrace (E3).
● The tibial collateral (medial) ligament (D1) is a broad flat band about 12 cm long, passing from the medial epicondyle of the femur (D18) to the medial condyle of the tibia (D13) and an extensive area of the medial surface of the tibia below the condyle (as in the lower part of D).
● The cruciate ligaments are named from their attachments to the tibia.
● The anterior cruciate ligament (E15) passes upwards, backwards and laterally to be attached to the medial side of the lateral condyle of the femur (F2).
● The posterior cruciate ligament (E3) passes upwards, forwards and medially (F3) to be attached to the lateral surface of the medial condyle of the femur.
● The anterior cruciate ligament (E15) is attached to the intercondylar area of the tibia some distance behind the anterior margin of the bone.
● The attachment of the posterior cruciate ligament (E3) overlaps the posterior margin of the bone to extend on to the posterior surface (G7).
● The transverse ligament (small in E14; absent in A) connects the medial and lateral menisci anteriorly.

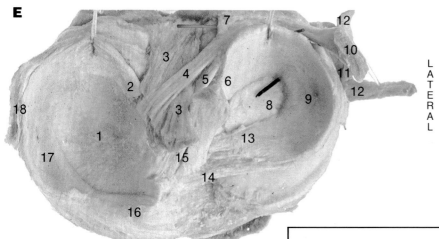

E

FRONT

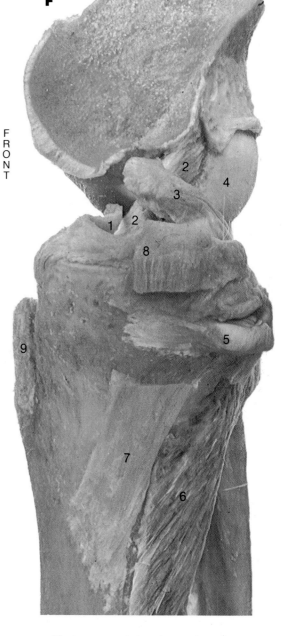

F

E **Left knee joint, from above with the femur removed**

This is the view looking down on the upper surface of the tibia after removing the femur by cutting through the capsule, the collateral ligaments (18 and 11), and the cruciate ligaments (15 and 3). The medial and lateral menisci (17 and 9) remain at the periphery of the articular surfaces of the tibial condyles (1 and 8). The horns of the menisci (2 and 16, 6 and 13) and the cruciate ligaments (15 and 3) are attached to the (non-articular) intercondylar area of the tibia. Compare with C on page 282

1	Medial condyle of tibia
2	Posterior horn of medial meniscus
3	Posterior cruciate ligament
4	Posterior ⎱ meniscofemoral
5	Anterior ⎰ ligament
6	Posterior horn of lateral meniscus
7	Attachment of lateral meniscus to popliteus (with underlying marker)
8	Lateral condyle of tibia
9	Lateral meniscus
10	Tendon of popliteus
11	Fibular collateral ligament
12	Tendon of biceps
13	Anterior horn of lateral meniscus
14	Transverse ligament
15	Anterior cruciate ligament
16	Anterior horn of medial meniscus
17	Medial meniscus
18	Tibial collateral ligament attached to medial meniscus

G

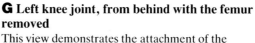

G **Left knee joint, from behind with the femur removed**

This view demonstrates the attachment of the lateral meniscus (5) to popliteus (4). There are markers underneath the attachment and behind the popliteus tendon

1	Head of fibula
2	Biceps
3	Fibular collateral ligament
4	Popliteus tendon
5	Attachment of lateral meniscus to popliteus
6	Anterior cruciate ligament
7	Posterior cruciate ligament
8	Posterior meniscofemoral ligament
9	Medial meniscus attached to tibial collateral ligament
10	Semimembranosus
11	Popliteus
12	Soleus
13	Interosseous membrane

F **Right knee joint, from the medial side with the medial femoral condyle removed**

Removal of the medial half of the lower end of the femur enables the X-shaped crossover of the cruciate ligaments to be seen: the anterior cruciate (2) is passing backwards and laterally, while the posterior cruciate (3) passes forwards and medially

1	Transverse ligament (displaced backwards)
2	Anterior cruciate ligament
3	Posterior cruciate ligament
4	Lateral condyle of femur
5	Semimembranosus
6	Popliteus
7	Tibial collateral ligament
8	Medial meniscus and attachment of tibial collateral ligament
9	Patellar ligament

A

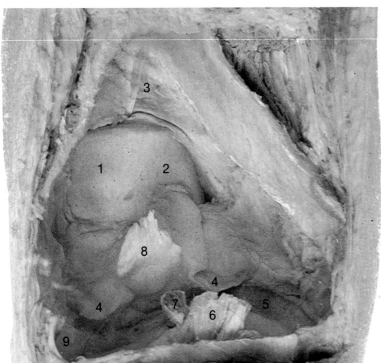

A Left knee joint, opened from behind with the femur removed

By looking into the joint from behind after removal of the femur, the articular surfaces of the patella (1 and 2) are seen, while below them are the alar and infrapatellar folds (4 and 8)

1	Lateral ⎫ articular surface of patella
2	Medial ⎭
3	Suprapatellar bursa (supported by glass rod)
4	Alar fold
5	Medial meniscus
6	Posterior ⎫ cruciate ligament
7	Anterior ⎭
8	Infrapatellar fold (ligamentum mucosum)
9	Lateral meniscus

● Below the patella (1 and 2) the synovial membrane is projected backwards by the infrapatellar fat pad, so forming the two alar folds (4) which have posterior free borders and a central infrapatellar fold (8). The latter is attached to the front of the intercondylar area of the femur. The folds with their contained fat occupy what would otherwise be the 'dead space' below the curved front parts of the femoral condyles.

B Left knee joint, from the medial side, with synovial and bursal cavities injected

The resin injection has distended the synovial cavity of the joint (6) and extended into the suprapatellar bursa (2), the bursa round the popliteus tendon (11) and the semimembranosus bursa (10)

B

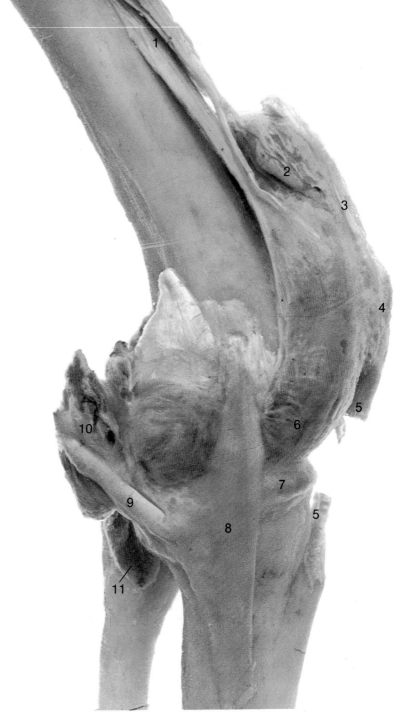

MEDIAL

FRONT

1	Articularis genu
2	Suprapatellar bursa
3	Quadriceps tendon
4	Patella
5	Patellar ligament
6	Capsule
7	Medial meniscus
8	Tibial collateral ligament
9	Semimembranosus
10	Semimembranosus bursa
11	Bursa of popliteus tendon

● The normal knee joint (the largest of all synovial joints) contains less than 1 ml of synovial fluid; the joint illustrated contains about 80 ml of injected resin which has distended the synovial cavity.

● The suprapatellar bursa (2) always communicates with the joint cavity. The bursa around the popliteus tendon (11) usually does so. The semimembranosus bursa (10) may do so.

● Muscles producing movements at the knee joint:

Flexion: semimembranosus, semitendinosus, biceps, gracilis, sartorius, gastrocnemius and popliteus.
Extension: vastus medialis, intermedius and lateralis, rectus femoris, and tensor fasciae latae and gluteus maximus acting via the iliotibial tract.
Medial rotation of leg: popliteus (when the leg is extended), semimembranosus, semitendinosus, gracilis and sartorius (when the leg is flexed).
Lateral rotation of leg: biceps (when flexed).

A

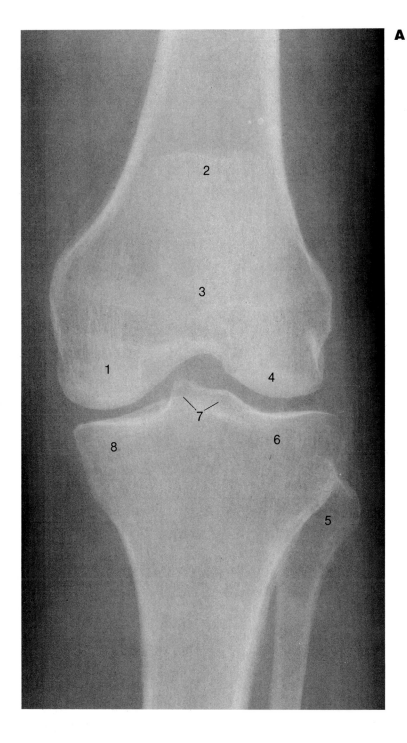

B

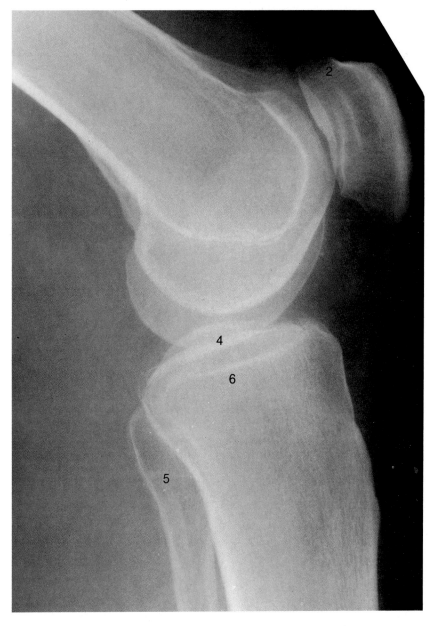

Radiographs of the left knee, A from the front, B from the lateral side in partial flexion

In A the shadow of the patella (2 and 3) is superimposed on that of the femur. The regular space between the condyles of the femur and tibia (1 and 8, 4 and 6) is due to the thickness of the hyaline cartilage on the articulating surfaces. In the side view the condyles (4 and 6) slightly overlap one another

1	Medial condyle of femur
2	Base ⎫ of patella
3	Apex ⎭
4	Lateral condyle of femur
5	Head of fibula
6	Lateral condyle of tibia
7	Tubercles of intercondylar eminence
8	Medial condyle of tibia

A

B

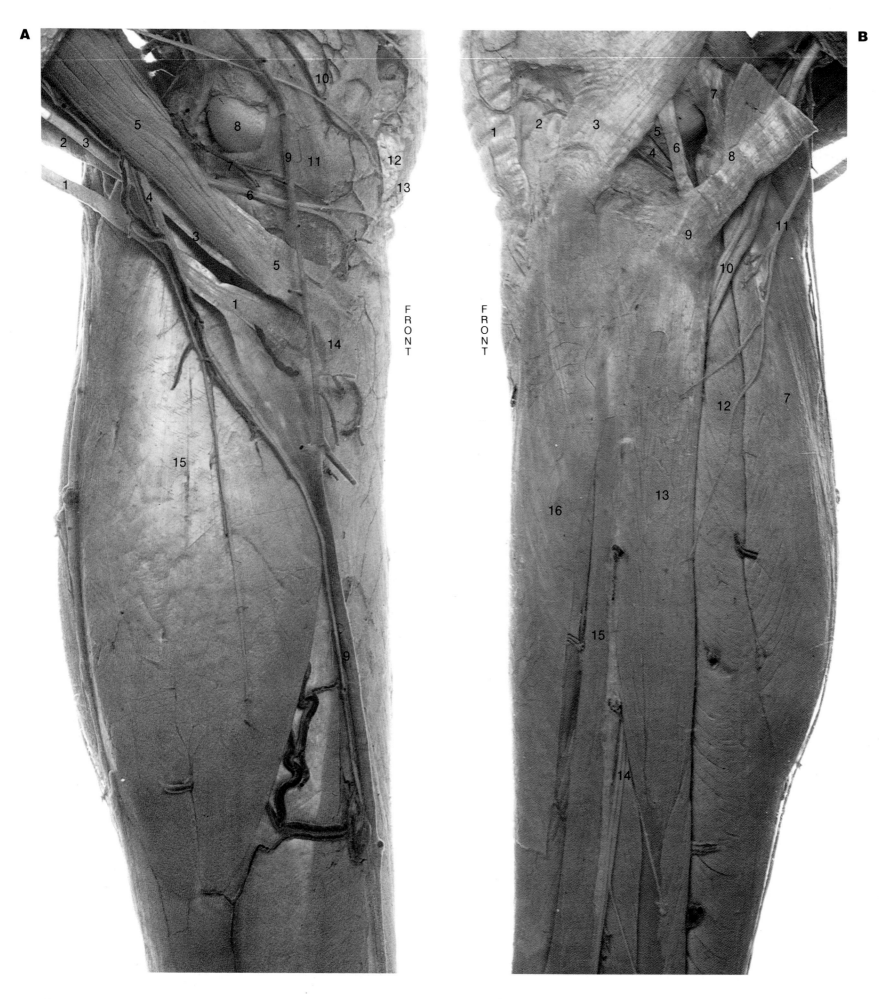

FRONT

FRONT

A Left knee and leg, from the medial side and behind

A small window has been cut in the capsule of the knee joint to show part of the medial condyle of the femur (8) and the medial meniscus (7). The tendons of sartorius (5), gracilis (3) and semitendinosus (1) gain attachment to the medial surface of the tibia (14). The saphenous nerve (4) becomes superficial between sartorius (5) and gracilis (3) and its infrapatellar branch (6) has pierced sartorius to run forwards immediately below the knee joint and the medial meniscus (7). The great saphenous vein (9) in the region of the knee is unusually small

1	Semitendinosus
2	Semimembranosus
3	Gracilis
4	Saphenous nerve and artery
5	Sartorius
6	Infrapatellar branch of saphenous nerve
7	Branch of saphenous artery overlying medial meniscus
8	Medial condyle of femur (part of capsule removed)
9	Great saphenous vein
10	Branches of superior medial genicular artery
11	Tibial collateral ligament
12	Infrapatellar fat pad
13	Patellar ligament
14	Medial surface of tibia
15	Medial head of gastrocnemius

B Left knee and leg, from the lateral side

A small window has been cut in the capsule of the knee joint to show the tendon of popliteus (5) passing deep to the fibular collateral ligament (6). The common peroneal nerve (10) runs down behind biceps (8) to pass through the gap between peroneus longus (13) and soleus (12). The superficial peroneal nerve becomes superficial between peroneus longus (13) and extensor digitorum longus (15)

1	Patellar ligament
2	Infrapatellar fat pad
3	Iliotibial tract
4	Lateral meniscus
5	Popliteus
6	Fibular collateral ligament
7	Lateral head of gastrocnemius
8	Biceps
9	Head of fibula
10	Common peroneal nerve
11	Lateral cutaneous nerve of calf
12	Soleus
13	Peroneus longus
14	Superficial peroneal nerve
15	Extensor digitorum longus
16	Fascia overlying tibialis anterior

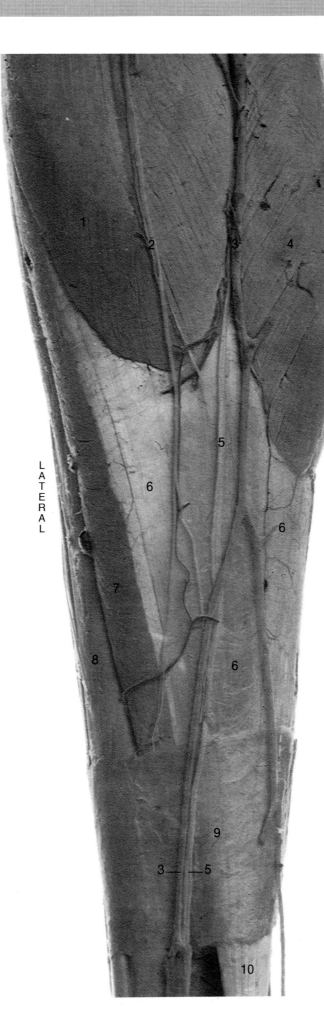

C Left calf, superficial dissection

Most of the deep fascia has been removed, but a small part has been preserved (9) to indicate that the superficial veins and nerves such as the small saphenous vein (3) and sural nerve (5) lie superficial to it

1	Lateral head of gastrocnemius
2	Lateral cutaneous nerve of calf
3	Small saphenous vein
4	Medial head of gastrocnemius
5	Sural nerve
6	Aponeurosis of gastrocnemius
7	Soleus
8	Peroneus longus
9	Deep fascia
10	Tendo calcaneus (Achilles' tendon)

● The medial head of gastrocnemius (C4) extends to a lower level than the lateral head (C1).

● Below knee level the great saphenous vein (A9) is accompanied by the saphenous nerve (A4).

● In the calf the small saphenous vein (C3) is accompanied by the sural nerve (C5).

● On the medial side of the upper leg, sartorius (A5), gracilis (A3) and semitendinosus (A1) all converge on to the medial surface of the tibia.

● On the lateral side of the upper leg, biceps (B8) converges on to the head of the fibula (B9), with the common peroneal nerve (B10) behind them. The nerve divides under cover of peroneus longus (B13) and in contact with the neck of the fibula into superficial and deep branches (page 314, A7 and 9).

● The two heads of gastrocnemius join a broad aponeurosis (C6) which lower down unites with the tendon of soleus (C7) to form the tendo calcaneus (Achilles' tendon, C10).

A

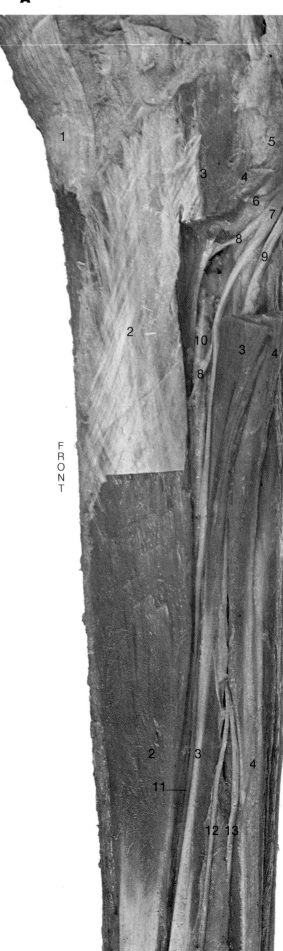

F
R
O
N
T

A Left leg, from the front and lateral side

Most of the deep fascia has been removed, and segments of extensor digitorum longus (3) and peroneus longus (4) have been cut out to display the deep (7) and superficial (9) branches of the common peroneal nerve just below the head of the fibula (5). The gap between tibialis anterior (2) and extensor digitorum longus (3) has been opened up to show the anterior tibial artery (10)

1	Tuberosity of tibia and patellar ligament
2	Tibialis anterior and overlying fascia
3	Extensor digitorum longus
4	Peroneus longus
5	Head of fibula
6	Recurrent branch of common peroneal nerve
7	Deep peroneal nerve
8	Branch to tibialis anterior
9	Superficial peroneal nerve
10	Anterior tibial artery overlying interosseous membrane
11	Extensor hallucis longus
12	Medial ⎫ branch of superficial peroneal nerve
13	Lateral ⎭

- The common peroneal nerve (page 312, B10) divides into its superficial and deep branches (A9 and A7) below the lateral side of the head of the fibula (A5), where it lies in contact with the neck of the bone under cover of peroneus longus (A4). Just before dividing into its two main branches it gives off a small recurrent branch (A6) (to the knee and superior tibiofibular joints).
- The deep peroneal nerve (A7) supplies the muscles of the anterior compartment of the leg—tibialis anterior (A2 and B2, to which two branches are shown here, A8), extensor digitorum longus (A3 and B6), extensor hallucis longus (A11 and B3) and peroneus tertius (page 321, C7).
- The superficial peroneal nerve (A9) supplies the muscles of the lateral compartment—peroneus longus (A4) and peroneus brevis (under cover of peroneus longus in A, but its lower end is seen at D7). After supplying the peroneal muscles, the nerve pierces the deep fascia between extensor digitorum longus and peroneus longus (A3 and 4), and divides into medial and lateral (cutaneous) branches (A12 and 13).

B Left lower leg and ankle, from the front and lateral side

The deep fascia has been removed to show the order of the structures in front of the ankle: from medial to lateral, tibialis anterior (2), extensor hallucis longus (3), anterior tibial vessels (4), deep peroneal nerve (5) and extensor digitorum longus (6)

1	Medial malleolus
2	Tibialis anterior
3	Extensor hallucis longus
4	Anterior tibial vessels
5	Deep peroneal nerve
6	Extensor digitorum longus
7	Medial branch of superficial peroneal nerve
8	Lateral malleolus

- On the front of the ankle the *extensor hallucis* longus tendon (B3) is immediately adjacent to the *tibialis anterior* tendon (B2). Behind the medial malleolus it is the *flexor digitorum* longus tendon (D1) that lies immediately adjacent to the *tibialis posterior* tendon (D12).

B

M
E
D
I
A
L

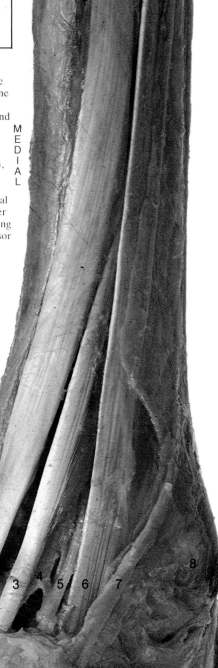

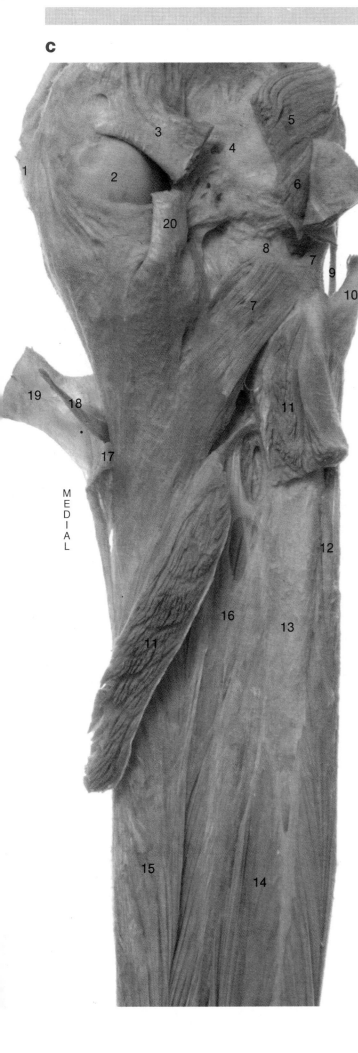

C

MEDIAL

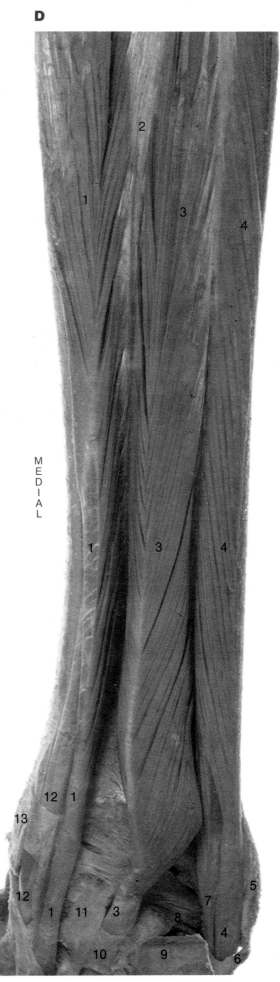

D

MEDIAL

C Right popliteal fossa and upper calf

All vessels and nerves and most parts of the superficial muscles have been removed to show popliteus (7) and the deep muscles of the calf—tibialis posterior (16), flexor digitorum longus (15) and flexor hallucis longus (14)

1	Tibial collateral ligament
2	Medial condyle of femur
3	Medial head of gastrocnemius
4	Capsule of knee joint
5	Plantaris
6	Lateral head of gastrocnemius
7	Popliteus
8	Attachment of popliteus to lateral meniscus
9	Fibular collateral ligament
10	Biceps
11	Soleus
12	Peroneus longus
13	Posterior surface of fibula (soleus removed)
14	Flexor hallucis longus
15	Flexor digitorum longus
16	Tibialis posterior
17	Semitendinosus
18	Gracilis
19	Sartorius
20	Semimembranosus

D Right lower calf and ankle

All vessels and nerves have been removed to show the order of the structures behind the ankle: from medial to lateral behind the medial malleolus (13), tibialis posterior (12), flexor digitorum longus (1), posterior tibial vessels and tibial nerve (11) and flexor hallucis longus (3). Behind the lateral malleolus (5), peroneus brevis (7) lies against the bone with peroneus longus (4) behind it

1	Flexor digitorum longus
2	Fascia overlying tibialis posterior
3	Flexor hallucis longus
4	Peroneus longus
5	Lateral malleolus
6	Superior peroneal retinaculum
7	Peroneus brevis
8	Posterior talofibular ligament
9	Tendo calcaneus (Achilles' tendon)
10	Part of flexor retinaculum
11	Position of posterior tibial vessels and tibial nerve
12	Tibialis posterior
13	Medial malleolus

• Tibialis posterior (C16, D12) is the deepest muscle of the calf.
• Flexor hallucis longus (C14, D3), although passing to the great toe on the *medial* side of the foot, arises from the fibula (C13) on the *lateral* side of the leg.

A

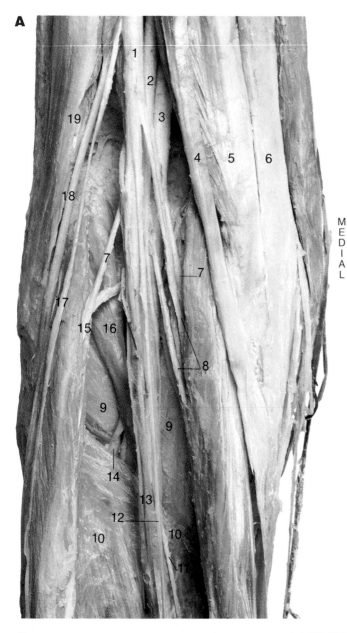

B

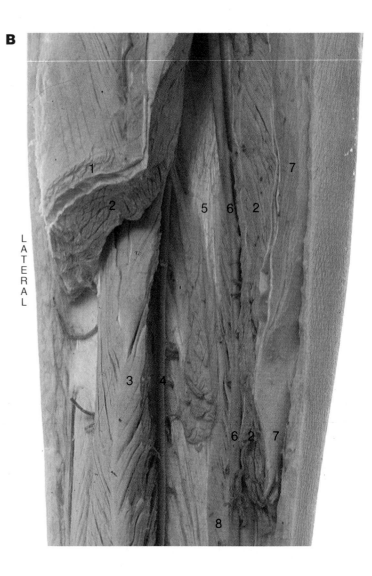

A Left popliteal fossa and upper calf

Gastrocnemius has been incised longitudinally and
the two heads (8 and 15) split apart to reveal
plantaris (16) and its thin tendon (11), popliteus
(9) and the upper part of soleus (10). The sural
nerve (12) and small saphenous vein (13) remain
in the midline and obscure the lower part of the
tibial nerve (1)

1	Tibial nerve
2	Popliteal vein
3	Popliteal artery
4	Semitendinosus
5	Semimembranosus
6	Gracilis
7	Sural artery
8	Medial head of gastrocnemius and nerves
9	Popliteus
10	Soleus
11	Plantaris tendon
12	Sural nerve
13	Small saphenous vein (double)
14	Nerve to soleus
15	Lateral head of gastrocnemius and nerve
16	Plantaris
17	Lateral cutaneous nerve of calf
18	Common peroneal nerve
19	Biceps

B Left calf. Deep dissection of muscles and arteries

In the middle of the calf most of gastrocnemius (1
and 7) and soleus (2) have been removed with
nerves and veins. The peroneal artery (4) runs
down the medial crest of the fibula between flexor
hallucis longus (3) and tibialis posterior (5). The
posterior tibial artery (6) runs down behind the
tibia on tibialis posterior (5) and flexor digitorum
longus (8) and under cover of soleus (2). Compare
with the cross section in D

1	Lateral head of gastrocnemius
2	Soleus
3	Flexor hallucis longus
4	Peroneal artery
5	Tibialis posterior
6	Posterior tibial artery
7	Medial head of gastrocnemius
8	Flexor digitorum longus

● Flexor hallucis longus, going to the great toe on the
medial side of the foot, arises from the fibula on the
lateral side of the leg; the tendon crosses to the medial
side in the sole (page 320, B).

316

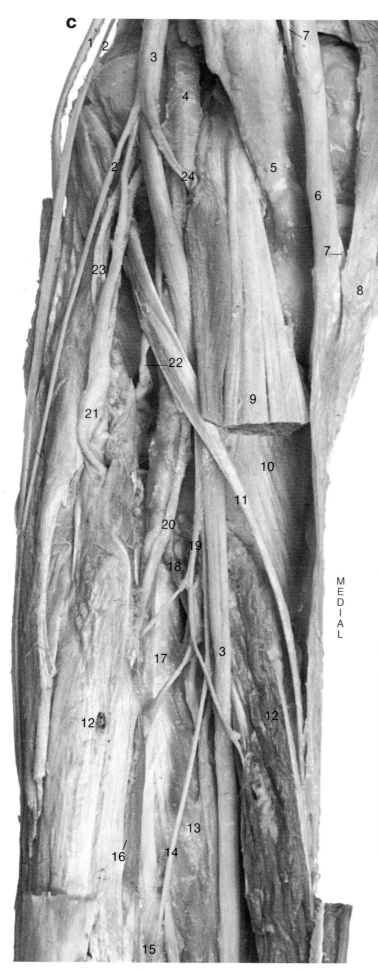

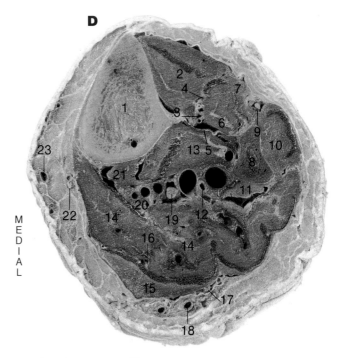

C Left popliteal fossa and calf. Deep dissection

Soleus (12) has been bisected in the midline and displaced to each side to show the branches of the tibial nerve (3). (The knee joint was injected with orange resin and the capsule removed.)

1	Common peroneal nerve
2	Sural nerve (double origin)
3	Tibial nerve
4	Popliteal artery
5	Semimembranosus
6	Semitendinosus
7	Gracilis (displaced laterally at upper end)
8	Sartorius
9	Medial head of gastrocnemius
10	Popliteus
11	Plantaris
12	Soleus
13	Flexor digitorum longus
14	Nerve to flexor hallucis longus
15	Flexor hallucis longus
16	Peroneal artery
17	Fascia over tibialis posterior
18	Posterior tibial artery
19	Nerve to deep surface of soleus
20	Nerve to tibialis posterior
21	Nerve to superficial surface of soleus
22	Nerve to popliteus
23	Nerve to lateral head of gastrocnemius
24	Nerve to medial head of gastrocnemius

D Cross section of the left leg, from below

The section is viewed looking from the ankle to the knee. Behind the interosseous membrane (5), tibialis posterior (13) is the deepest of the calf muscles, with the tibial nerve (19) behind it and the posterior tibial vessels (20) more medially, between flexor digitorum longus (21) and soleus (14). The peroneal artery (12) is adjacent to flexor hallucis longus (11) behind the fibula (8). Note the (unlabelled) large veins within and deep to soleus (14; see note). In the anterior compartment, the anterior tibial vessels (3) and deep peroneal nerve (4) are between tibialis anterior (2) and extensor hallucis longus (6)

1	Tibia
2	Tibialis anterior
3	Anterior tibial vessels
4	Deep peroneal nerve
5	Interosseous membrane
6	Extensor hallucis longus
7	Extensor digitorum longus
8	Fibula
9	Superficial peroneal nerve
10	Peroneus longus and brevis
11	Flexor hallucis longus
12	Peroneal artery
13	Tibialis posterior
14	Soleus
15	Gastrocnemius
16	Plantaris tendon
17	Sural nerve
18	Small saphenous vein
19	Tibial nerve
20	Posterior tibial vessels
21	Flexor digitorum longus
22	Saphenous nerve
23	Great saphenous vein

● The deep veins of the calf, deep to and within soleus, are a site for potentially dangerous venous thrombosis.

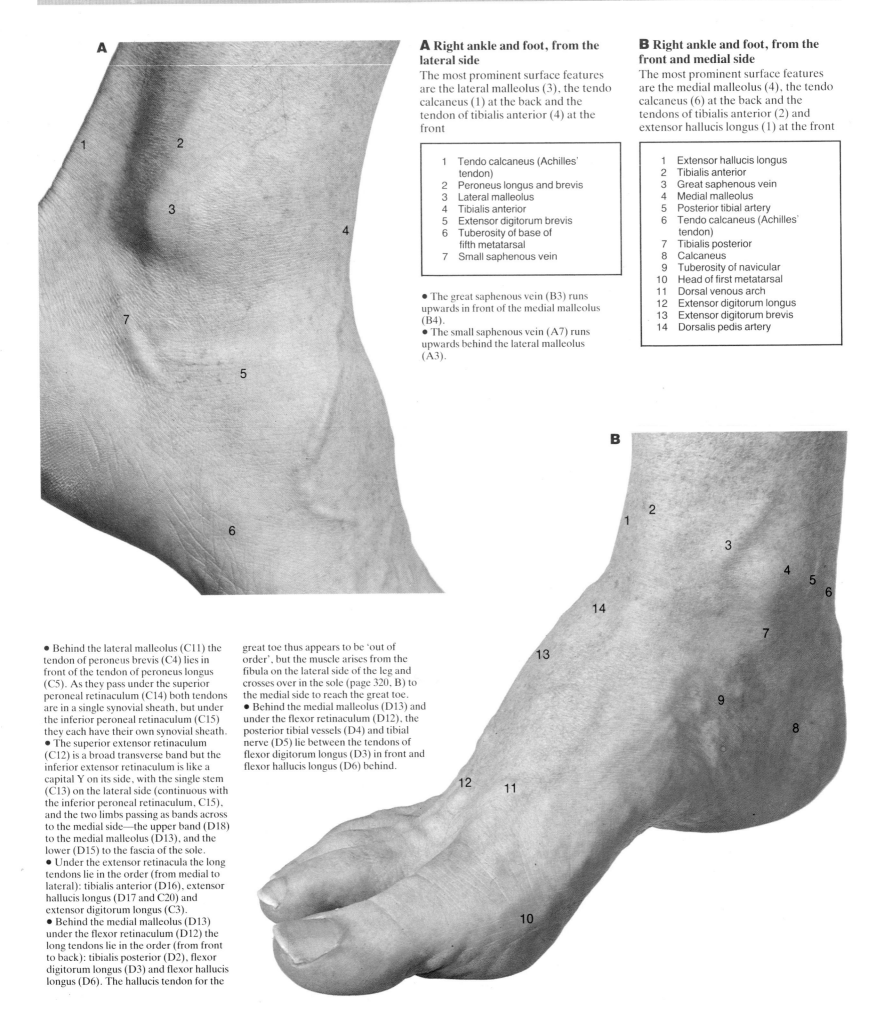

A Right ankle and foot, from the lateral side

The most prominent surface features are the lateral malleolus (3), the tendo calcaneus (1) at the back and the tendon of tibialis anterior (4) at the front

1	Tendo calcaneus (Achilles' tendon)
2	Peroneus longus and brevis
3	Lateral malleolus
4	Tibialis anterior
5	Extensor digitorum brevis
6	Tuberosity of base of fifth metatarsal
7	Small saphenous vein

● The great saphenous vein (B3) runs upwards in front of the medial malleolus (B4).
● The small saphenous vein (A7) runs upwards behind the lateral malleolus (A3).

B Right ankle and foot, from the front and medial side

The most prominent surface features are the medial malleolus (4), the tendo calcaneus (6) at the back and the tendons of tibialis anterior (2) and extensor hallucis longus (1) at the front

1	Extensor hallucis longus
2	Tibialis anterior
3	Great saphenous vein
4	Medial malleolus
5	Posterior tibial artery
6	Tendo calcaneus (Achilles' tendon)
7	Tibialis posterior
8	Calcaneus
9	Tuberosity of navicular
10	Head of first metatarsal
11	Dorsal venous arch
12	Extensor digitorum longus
13	Extensor digitorum brevis
14	Dorsalis pedis artery

● Behind the lateral malleolus (C11) the tendon of peroneus brevis (C4) lies in front of the tendon of peroneus longus (C5). As they pass under the superior peroneal retinaculum (C14) both tendons are in a single synovial sheath, but under the inferior peroneal retinaculum (C15) they each have their own synovial sheath.
● The superior extensor retinaculum (C12) is a broad transverse band but the inferior extensor retinaculum is like a capital Y on its side, with the single stem (C13) on the lateral side (continuous with the inferior peroneal retinaculum, C15), and the two limbs passing as bands across to the medial side—the upper band (D18) to the medial malleolus (D13), and the lower (D15) to the fascia of the sole.
● Under the extensor retinacula the long tendons lie in the order (from medial to lateral): tibialis anterior (D16), extensor hallucis longus (D17 and C20) and extensor digitorum longus (C3).
● Behind the medial malleolus (D13) under the flexor retinaculum (D12) the long tendons lie in the order (from front to back): tibialis posterior (D2), flexor digitorum longus (D3) and flexor hallucis longus (D6). The hallucis tendon for the great toe thus appears to be 'out of order', but the muscle arises from the fibula on the lateral side of the leg and crosses over in the sole (page 320, B) to the medial side to reach the great toe.
● Behind the medial malleolus (D13) and under the flexor retinaculum (D12), the posterior tibial vessels (D4) and tibial nerve (D5) lie between the tendons of flexor digitorum longus (D3) in front and flexor hallucis longus (D6) behind.

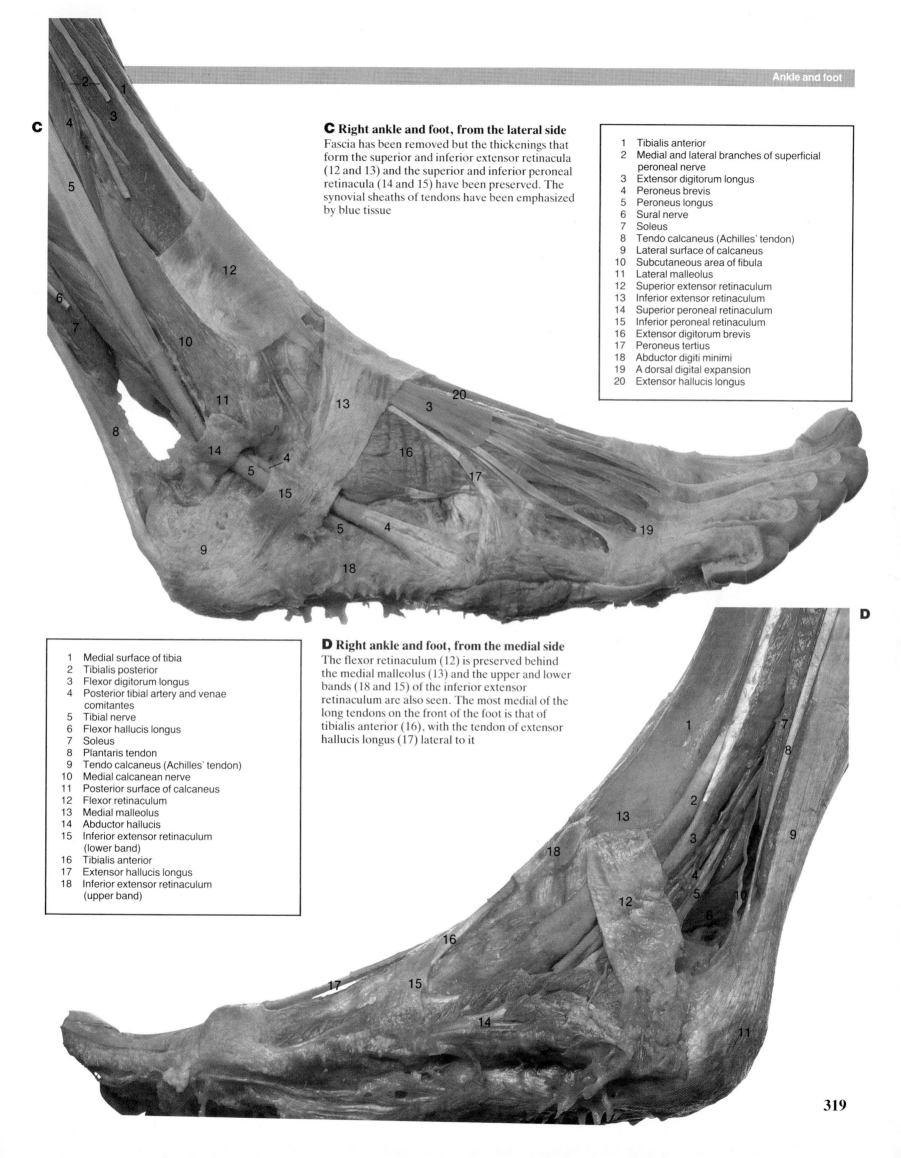

C Right ankle and foot, from the lateral side
Fascia has been removed but the thickenings that form the superior and inferior extensor retinacula (12 and 13) and the superior and inferior peroneal retinacula (14 and 15) have been preserved. The synovial sheaths of tendons have been emphasized by blue tissue

1 Tibialis anterior
2 Medial and lateral branches of superficial peroneal nerve
3 Extensor digitorum longus
4 Peroneus brevis
5 Peroneus longus
6 Sural nerve
7 Soleus
8 Tendo calcaneus (Achilles' tendon)
9 Lateral surface of calcaneus
10 Subcutaneous area of fibula
11 Lateral malleolus
12 Superior extensor retinaculum
13 Inferior extensor retinaculum
14 Superior peroneal retinaculum
15 Inferior peroneal retinaculum
16 Extensor digitorum brevis
17 Peroneus tertius
18 Abductor digiti minimi
19 A dorsal digital expansion
20 Extensor hallucis longus

D Right ankle and foot, from the medial side
The flexor retinaculum (12) is preserved behind the medial malleolus (13) and the upper and lower bands (18 and 15) of the inferior extensor retinaculum are also seen. The most medial of the long tendons on the front of the foot is that of tibialis anterior (16), with the tendon of extensor hallucis longus (17) lateral to it

1 Medial surface of tibia
2 Tibialis posterior
3 Flexor digitorum longus
4 Posterior tibial artery and venae comitantes
5 Tibial nerve
6 Flexor hallucis longus
7 Soleus
8 Plantaris tendon
9 Tendo calcaneus (Achilles' tendon)
10 Medial calcanean nerve
11 Posterior surface of calcaneus
12 Flexor retinaculum
13 Medial malleolus
14 Abductor hallucis
15 Inferior extensor retinaculum (lower band)
16 Tibialis anterior
17 Extensor hallucis longus
18 Inferior extensor retinaculum (upper band)

319

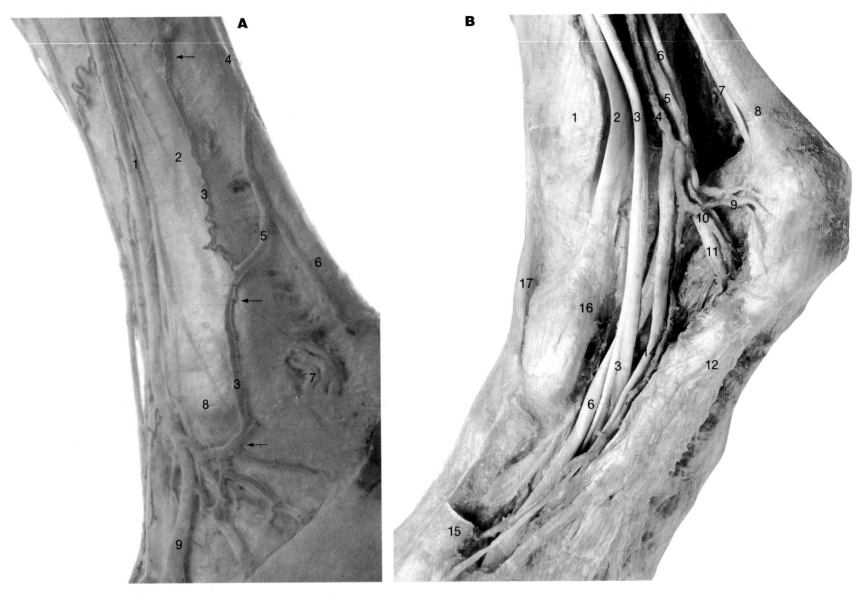

A Right lower leg and ankle, from the medial side and behind

The deep fascia remains intact apart from a small window cut to show the position of the posterior tibial vessels and tibial nerve (7). The great saphenous vein (1) runs upwards in front of the medial malleolus (8) with the posterior arch vein (3) behind it. The arrows indicate common levels for perforating veins

1	Great saphenous vein and saphenous nerve
2	Tibialis posterior and flexor digitorum longus underlying deep fascia
3	Posterior arch vein
4	Small saphenous vein
5	Communication with small saphenous vein
6	Tendo calcaneus (Achilles' tendon)
7	Posterior tibial vessels and tibial nerve
8	Medial malleolus
9	Dorsal venous arch

B Right ankle and sole, from the medial side and below

The foot is in plantar flexion, and the flexor retinaculum and most of abductor hallucis (15) have been removed to show how the tendon of flexor hallucis longus (6) passes deep to flexor digitorum longus (3) in the sole to run towards the great toe

1	Medial malleolus
2	Tibialis posterior
3	Flexor digitorum longus
4	Posterior tibial artery
5	Tibial nerve
6	Flexor hallucis longus
7	Plantaris tendon
8	Tendo calcaneus (Achilles' tendon)
9	Calcanean nerves and vessels
10	Lateral plantar artery
11	Lateral plantar nerve
12	Plantar aponeurosis overlying flexor digitorum brevis
13	Medial plantar artery
14	Medial plantar nerve
15	Abductor hallucis
16	Tuberosity of navicular
17	Tibialis anterior

● The perforating veins are communications between the superficial veins (above the deep fascia) and the deep veins (below the fascia). The commonest sites for them are just behind the tibia (where indicated by the arrows in A), behind the fibula and in the adductor canal. These communicating vessels possess valves which direct the blood flow from superficial to deep; venous return from the limb is then brought about by the pumping action of the deep muscles (which are all below the deep fascia). If the valves become incompetent or the deep veins blocked, pressure in the superficial veins increases and they become varicose (enlarged and tortuous).
● The posterior arch vein (A3) unites some of the perforating veins and usually drains into the great saphenous.

C

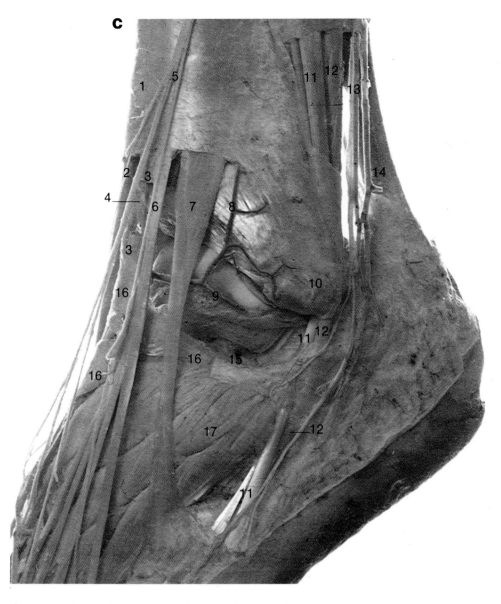

D

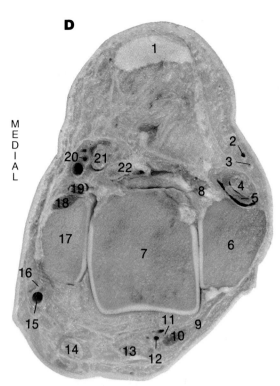

C Left ankle and foot, from the front and lateral side

The foot is plantar flexed and part of the capsule of the ankle joint has been removed to show the talus (9). The tendons of peroneus tertius (7) and extensor digitorum longus (6) lie superficial to extensor digitorum brevis (17). The sural nerve and small saphenous vein (13) pass behind the lateral malleolus (10)

● Muscles producing movements at the ankle joint:
Dorsiflexion: tibialis anterior, extensor digitorum longus, extensor hallucis longus and peroneus tertius.
Plantar flexion: gastrocnemius, soleus, plantaris, tibialis posterior, flexor digitorum longus, flexor hallucis longus, peroneus longus and peroneus brevis.

1	Deep fascia forming superior extensor retinaculum
2	Tibialis anterior
3	Extensor hallucis longus
4	Anterior tibial vessels and deep peroneal nerve
5	Superficial peroneal nerve
6	Extensor digitorum longus
7	Peroneus tertius
8	Perforating branch of peroneal artery
9	Anterior lateral malleolar artery overlying talus (ankle joint capsule removed)
10	Lateral malleolus
11	Peroneus brevis
12	Peroneus longus
13	Small saphenous vein and sural nerve
14	Tendo calcaneus (Achilles' tendon)
15	Tarsal sinus
16	Inferior extensor retinaculum (partly removed)
17	Extensor digitorum brevis

D Cross section of the left ankle

This section, looking down from above, emphasizes the positions of tendons, vessels and nerves in the ankle region. The talus (7) is in the centre, with the medial malleolus (17) on the left of the picture and the lateral malleolus (6) on the right. The great saphenous vein (15) and saphenous nerve (16) are in front of the medial malleolus, with the tendon of tibialis posterior (18) immediately behind it. The small saphenous vein (2) and the sural nerve (3) are behind the lateral malleolus, with the tendons of peroneus longus (4) and peroneus brevis (5) intervening. At the front of the ankle the dorsalis pedis vessels (12) and deep peroneal nerve (11) are between the tendons of extensor hallucis longus (13) and extensor digitorum longus (10). Behind the medial malleolus (17) and tibialis posterior (18), the posterior tibial vessels (20) and tibial nerve (21) are between the tendons of flexor digitorum longus (19) and flexor hallucis longus (22)

1	Tendo calcaneus (Achilles' tendon)
2	Small saphenous vein
3	Sural nerve
4	Peroneus longus
5	Peroneus brevis
6	Lateral malleolus of fibula
7	Talus
8	Posterior talofibular ligament
9	Peroneus tertius
10	Extensor digitorum longus
11	Deep peroneal nerve
12	Dorsalis pedis artery and venae comitantes
13	Extensor hallucis longus
14	Tibialis anterior
15	Great saphenous vein
16	Saphenous nerve
17	Medial malleolus of tibia
18	Tibialis posterior
19	Flexor digitorum longus
20	Posterior tibial artery and venae comitantes
21	Tibial nerve
22	Flexor hallucis longus

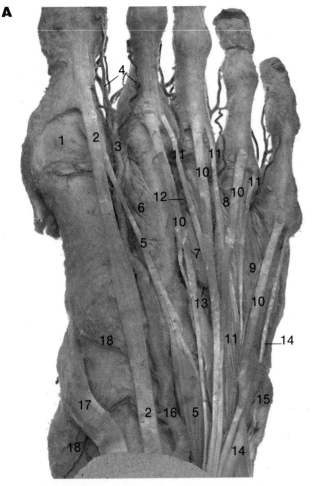

A

A Dorsum of the right foot

Fascia and superficial nerves have been removed to show tendons and arteries

1	First metatarsophalangeal joint	11	Extensor digitorum brevis
2	Extensor hallucis longus	12	Second dorsal metatarsal artery
3	First dorsal metatarsal artery	13	Arcuate artery
4	Digital arteries	14	Peroneus tertius
5	Extensor hallucis brevis	15	Tuberosity of base of fifth metatarsal and
6	First ⎫		peroneus brevis
7	Second ⎬ dorsal interosseous	16	Dorsalis pedis artery
8	Third ⎪	17	Tibialis anterior
9	Fourth ⎭	18	Tarsal arteries
10	Extensor digitorum longus		

● Extensor digitorum longus (10) sends its tendons to the four lateral toes, while extensor digitorum brevis (11) sends its tendons to the four medial toes; the part of extensor digitorum brevis that goes to the great toe is often known as extensor hallucis brevis (5).

B Right talocalcanean and talocalcaneonavicular joints

The talus has been removed to show the articular surfaces of the calcaneus (23, 24 and 25), talus (27) and plantar calcaneonavicular ligament (26)

1	Dorsal venous arch	15	Sural nerve
2	Tibialis anterior	16	Tendo calcaneus (Achilles' tendon)
3	Extensor hallucis longus	17	Abductor hallucis
4	Dorsalis pedis artery and vena comitans	18	Flexor hallucis longus
5	Deep peroneal nerve	19	Posterior tibial vessels and medial and
6	Extensor digitorum longus		lateral plantar nerves
7	Extensor digitorum brevis	20	Flexor digitorum longus
8	Calcaneonavicular part of bifurcate	21	Tibialis posterior
	ligament	22	Deltoid ligament
9	Cervical ligament	23	Posterior ⎫ articular surface
10	Interosseous talocalcanean ligament	24	Middle ⎬ on calcaneus
11	Inferior extensor retinaculum	25	Anterior ⎭ for talus
12	Peroneus brevis	26	Plantar calcaneonavicular ligament
13	Peroneus longus	27	Articular surface on navicular for talus
14	Small saphenous vein		

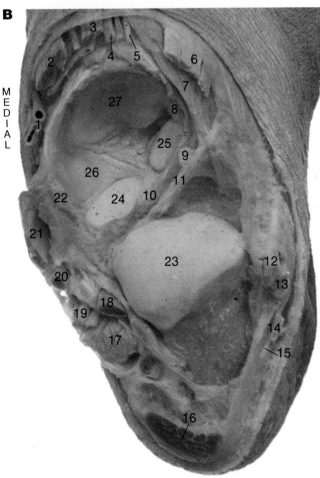

B

MEDIAL

BACK

● There are two joints beneath the talus (page 290, A and B). The more posterior is the talocalcanean joint, between the posterior articular surfaces of the calcaneus and talus; this joint is sometimes known anatomically as the subtalar joint.
● The more anterior joint, the talocalcaneonavicular, is between (a) the middle and anterior articular surfaces of the talus and calcaneus and the upper surface of the plantar calcaneonavicular ligament, all of which constitute the talocalcanean part of the joint, and (b) the head of the talus and the posterior articular surface of the navicular, which constitute the talonavicular part of the joint. The two parts of the joint share one synovial cavity.
● Do not confuse the talocalcanean joint with the talocalcanean part of the talocalcaneonavicular joint.

● Clinicians sometimes use the term subtalar joint as a combined name for both the talocalcanean and talocalcaneonavicular joints, because it is at both these joints beneath the talus at which most of the movements of inversion and eversion of the foot occur.
● Muscles producing inversion of the foot: tibialis anterior and tibialis posterior.
● Muscles producing eversion of the foot: peroneus longus and peroneus brevis.
● The deltoid ligament (C3) is the medial ligament of the ankle joint. On the lateral side of the joint there are three separate ligaments—anterior and posterior talofibular (D12 and E23) and calcaneofibular (D14).

F Sagittal section of the left foot, from the right

The section is through the medial side of the foot, passing through the great toe and first metatarsal (17), medial cuneiform (15), navicular (13), talus (3) and calcaneus (6)

1	Tibia	13	Navicular
2	Tibiotalal part of ankle joint	14	Cuneonavicular joint
3	Talus	15	Medial cuneiform
4	Talocalcanean (subtalar) joint	16	First tarsometatarsal (cuneometatarsal)
5	Interosseous talocalcanean ligament		joint
6	Calcaneus	17	First metatarsal
7	Tendo calcaneus (Achilles' tendon)	18	Sesamoid bone
8	Flexor accessorius	19	Metatarsophalangeal joint of
9	Flexor digitorum brevis		great toe
10	Plantar aponeurosis	20	Proximal phalanx
11	Plantar calcaneonavicular ligament	21	Interphalangeal joint
12	Talonavicular part of	22	Distal phalanx
	talocalcaneonavicular joint		

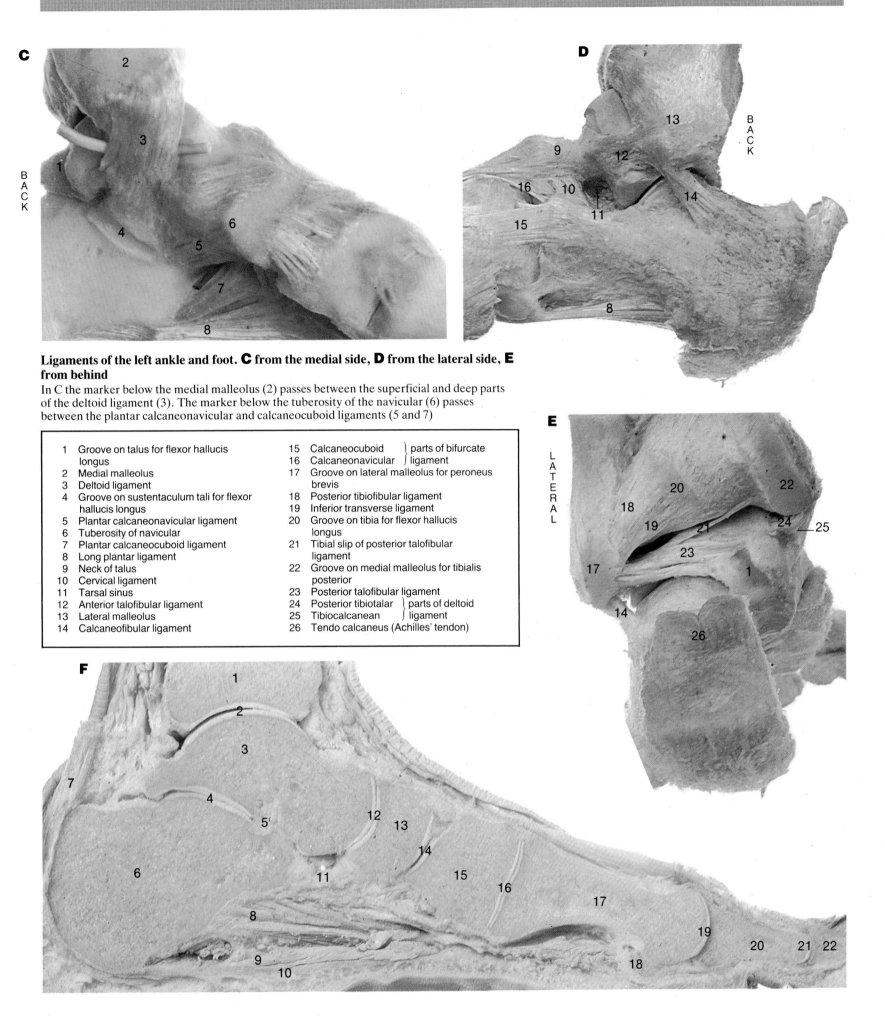

Ligaments of the left ankle and foot. C from the medial side, D from the lateral side, E from behind

In C the marker below the medial malleolus (2) passes between the superficial and deep parts of the deltoid ligament (3). The marker below the tuberosity of the navicular (6) passes between the plantar calcaneonavicular and calcaneocuboid ligaments (5 and 7)

1	Groove on talus for flexor hallucis longus	15	Calcaneocuboid ⎫ parts of bifurcate
2	Medial malleolus	16	Calcaneonavicular ⎭ ligament
3	Deltoid ligament	17	Groove on lateral malleolus for peroneus brevis
4	Groove on sustentaculum tali for flexor hallucis longus	18	Posterior tibiofibular ligament
5	Plantar calcaneonavicular ligament	19	Inferior transverse ligament
6	Tuberosity of navicular	20	Groove on tibia for flexor hallucis longus
7	Plantar calcaneocuboid ligament	21	Tibial slip of posterior talofibular ligament
8	Long plantar ligament	22	Groove on medial malleolus for tibialis posterior
9	Neck of talus	23	Posterior talofibular ligament
10	Cervical ligament	24	Posterior tibiotalar ⎫ parts of deltoid
11	Tarsal sinus	25	Tibiocalcanean ⎭ ligament
12	Anterior talofibular ligament	26	Tendo calcaneus (Achilles' tendon)
13	Lateral malleolus		
14	Calcaneofibular ligament		

323

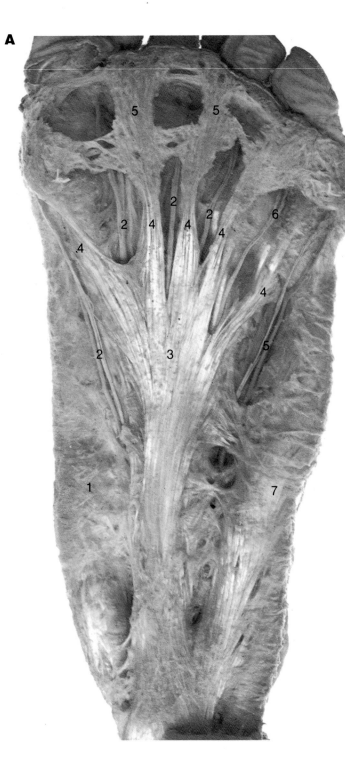

A Sole of the left foot. Plantar aponeurosis

Skin and connective tissue of the sole have been removed to show the tough central part of the plantar aponeurosis (3) which divides into slips (4) for each toe, and thinner medial and lateral parts overlying abductor hallucis (1) and abductor digiti minimi (7) respectively

1	Medial part of aponeurosis overlying abductor hallucis
2	Digital branches of medial plantar nerve and artery
3	Central part of aponeurosis overlying flexor digitorum brevis
4	Digital slip of central part of aponeurosis
5	Superficial stratum of digital slip of aponeurosis
6	Digital branches of lateral plantar nerve and artery
7	Lateral part of aponeurosis overlying abductor digiti minimi

B Sole of the left foot, with the plantar aponeurosis removed

The central muscle is flexor digitorum brevis (19), and passing forwards from beneath its borders are various digital vessels and nerves (such as 24 and 11) which arise from the medial and lateral plantar vessels and nerves still largely under cover of the muscle

1	Plantar digital nerve of great toe	12	Fourth dorsal interosseous
2	Plantar digital nerves of first cleft	13	Third plantar interosseous
3	Superficial transverse metatarsal ligament	14	Plantar digital nerve of fifth toe
4	Fibrous flexor sheath	15	Flexor digiti minimi brevis
5	First lumbrical	16	Abductor digiti minimi
6	Second lumbrical	17	Deep branch of lateral plantar nerve
7	Third lumbrical	18	Lateral plantar artery
8	Fourth lumbrical	19	Flexor digitorum brevis
9	Third plantar metatarsal artery	20	Plantar aponeurosis
10	A superficial digital branch of medial plantar artery	21	Abductor hallucis
		22	Flexor hallucis brevis
11	Fourth common plantar digital nerve	23	Flexor hallucis longus
		24	First common plantar digital nerve

C Sole of the left foot, with flexor digitorum brevis removed

Flexor accessorius (11) joins the lateral side of flexor digitorum longus whose tendon to the little toe (1) is the most clearly seen. One of the cut tendons of flexor digitorum brevis is labelled at 4. The medial and lateral plantar nerves (10 and 12) are now displayed; their accompanying arteries have been removed. The deep branch of the lateral plantar nerve (15) reaches the deeper part of the sole by curling round the lateral border of flexor accessorius (11)

1	Fourth tendon of flexor digitorum longus (fourth lumbrical absent)	9	Abductor hallucis
		10	Medial plantar nerve
2	Common plantar digital branch of lateral plantar nerve	11	Flexor accessorius
		12	Lateral plantar nerve
3	Transverse head of adductor hallucis	13	Long plantar ligament
4	Third tendon of flexor digitorum brevis (cut)	14	Abductor digiti minimi
		15	Deep branch of lateral plantar nerve
5	Second lumbrical and common plantar digital branch of medial plantar nerve	16	Second plantar interosseous
		17	Fourth dorsal interosseous
6	Oblique head of adductor hallucis	18	Third plantar interosseous
7	Flexor hallucis brevis	19	Flexor digiti minimi brevis
8	Flexor hallucis longus		

B

C

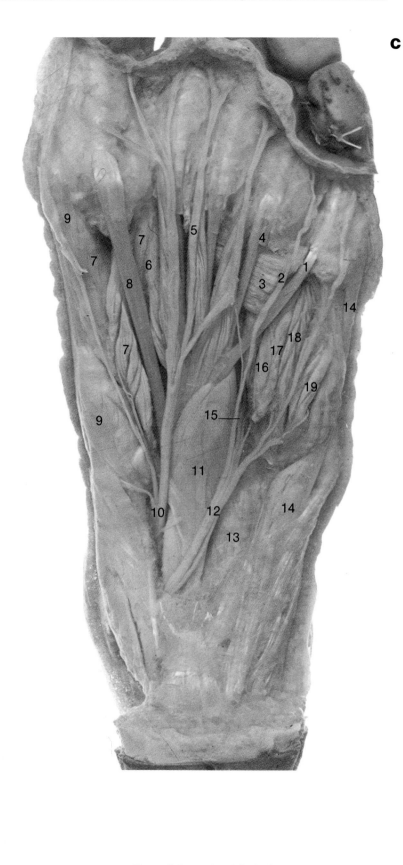

• Flexor digitorum brevis in the foot corresponds to flexor digitorum superficialis in the upper limb: their tendons split to allow the tendons of flexor digitorum longus to pass through, and the phalangeal attachments of the tendons are similar in hand and foot.
• The medial plantar nerve (C10) normally supplies abductor hallucis (C9), flexor digitorum brevis (B19), flexor hallucis brevis (C7) and the first lumbrical (B5; in C, unlabelled adjacent to 6). All the other muscles of the sole are supplied by the lateral plantar nerve (C12).

325

A

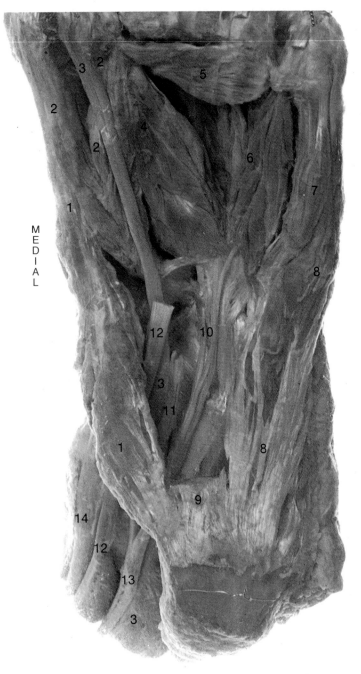

B

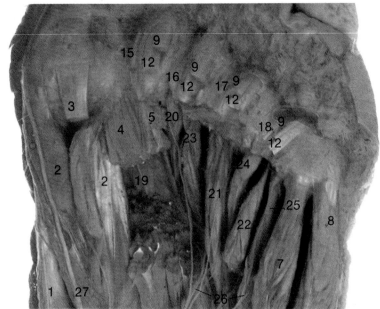

C

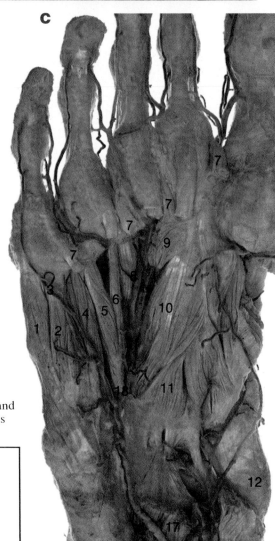

Sole of the left foot. Deep muscles, **A** adductor hallucis, **B** interossei

Most of the flexor muscles and tendons have been removed to show in A the two heads of adductor hallucis (4 and 5), and in B (which corresponds to the front part of A) the dorsal interossei (19 to 22) and plantar interossei (23 to 25), with the ends of the lumbricals (15 to 18). Many of the muscular filaments from the deep branch of the lateral plantar nerve (26) are preserved

1	Abductor hallucis	15	First	
2	Flexor hallucis brevis	16	Second	lumbrical
3	Flexor hallucis longus	17	Third	
4	Oblique	18	Fourth	
5	Transverse } head of adductor hallucis	19	First	
6	Interossei	20	Second	dorsal interosseous
7	Flexor digiti minimi brevis	21	Third	
8	Abductor digiti minimi	22	Fourth	
9	Flexor digitorum brevis	23	First	
10	Deep branch of lateral plantar nerve	24	Second } plantar interosseous	
11	Medial plantar nerve	25	Third	
12	Flexor digitorum longus	26	Branches of deep branch of lateral plantar nerve	
13	Tibial nerve	27	Plantar digital nerve of great toe	
14	Tibialis posterior			

D

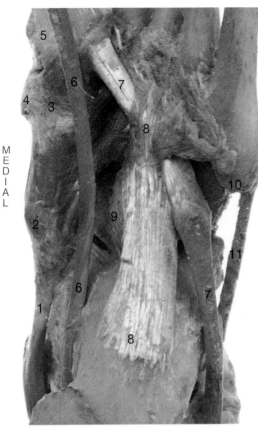

MEDIAL

D Sole of the left foot. Ligaments and tendons

The anterior end of the long plantar ligament (8) forms with the groove of the cuboid (E7) a tunnel for the peroneus longus tendon (7) which runs to the medial cuneiform (3) and the base of the first metatarsal (5). Peroneus brevis passes to the tuberosity of the base of the fifth metatarsal (10). The main attachment of tibialis posterior (1) is to the tuberosity of the navicular (2), while tibialis anterior is attached to the medial cuneiform (3) and the base of the first metatarsal (5)

1	Tibialis posterior
2	Tuberosity of navicular
3	Medial cuneiform
4	Tibialis anterior
5	Base of first metatarsal
6	Flexor hallucis longus
7	Peroneus longus
8	Long plantar ligament
9	Plantar calcaneocuboid ligament
10	Tuberosity of base of fifth metatarsal
11	Peroneus brevis

● Tibialis anterior (D4) is attached to the medial sides of the medial cuneiform and base of the first metatarsal (D3 and 5); peroneus longus (D7) is attached to the lateral sides of the same bones.
● The plantar calcaneonavicular ligament (E11), commonly called the spring ligament, is one of the most important in the foot. It stretches between the sustentaculum tali (E9) and the tuberosity of the navicular (E13), blending on its medial side with the deltoid ligament of the ankle joint and supporting on its upper surface (page 322, B26) part of the head of the talus.
● The plantar calcaneocuboid ligament (D9), commonly called the short plantar ligament, is largely covered by the long plantar ligament (D8).

C Sole of the right foot. Plantar arch

Most of the flexor muscles and tendons have been removed to show the lateral plantar artery (15) crossing flexor accessorius (17) to become the plantar arch (18) which would lie deep to the flexor tendons

1	Abductor digiti minimi
2	Flexor digiti minimi brevis
3	Plantar digital artery
4	Third plantar interosseous
5	Fourth dorsal interosseous
6	Second plantar interosseous
7	Lumbrical
8	Plantar metatarsal artery
9	Transverse } head of adductor hallucis
10	Oblique } head of adductor hallucis
11	Flexor hallucis brevis
12	Tuberosity of navicular
13	Abductor hallucis
14	Medial plantar artery and nerve
15	Lateral plantar artery
16	Flexor digitorum brevis
17	Flexor accessorius
18	Plantar arch

● Unlike the palm of the hand which has superficial and deep arterial arches (pages 133 and 136), the sole of the foot has one plantar arch (C18), formed by the lateral plantar artery anastomosing with the dorsalis pedis artery which enters the sole by passing between the two heads of the first dorsal interosseous muscle. The arch gives off plantar metatarsal arteries (as at C8), and these divide to form the plantar digital vessels.

E

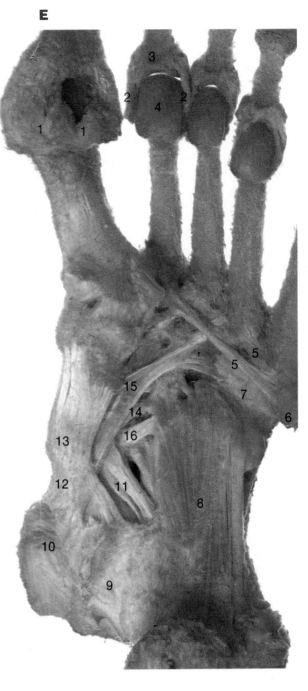

E Sole of the left foot. Ligaments

The anterior end of the long plantar ligament (8) has been removed to show the groove for peroneus longus on the cuboid (7). The tibialis posterior tendon (12) is attached to the tuberosity of the navicular (13). The deltoid ligament of the ankle joint is labelled (10) where it passes from the lower margin of the medial malleolus to the sustentaculum tali (9) of the calcaneus

1	Sesamoid bone
2	Collateral ligament of metatarsophalangeal joint
3	Base of proximal phalanx
4	Head of second metatarsal
5	Plantar metatarsal ligament
6	Tuberosity of base of fifth metatarsal
7	Groove on cuboid for peroneus longus
8	Deep fibres of long plantar ligament
9	Groove on sustentaculum tali for flexor hallucis longus
10	Deltoid ligament
11	Plantar calcaneonavicular ligament
12	Tibialis posterior
13	Tuberosity of navicular
14	Plantar cuneonavicular ligament
15	Fibrous slip from tibialis posterior
16	Plantar cuboideonavicular ligament

A

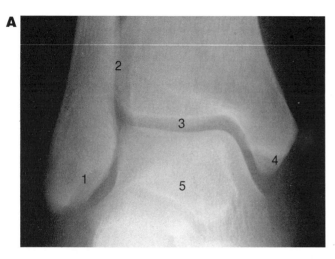

Radiographs of the ankle and foot, A from the front, B from the side, C from above

The side view in B shows a small calcanean spur (about 2 cm below the label 7)

- The talus (A5) is embraced on either side by the two malleoli; the lateral malleolus of the fibula (1) extends about 1 cm lower than the medial malleolus of the tibia (4).
- The calcaneocuboid joint (B9, C9) and the talonavicular part of the talocalcaneonavicular joint (B13, C13) together form the midtarsal joint.
- For notes on the joints beneath the talus see page 322.

C

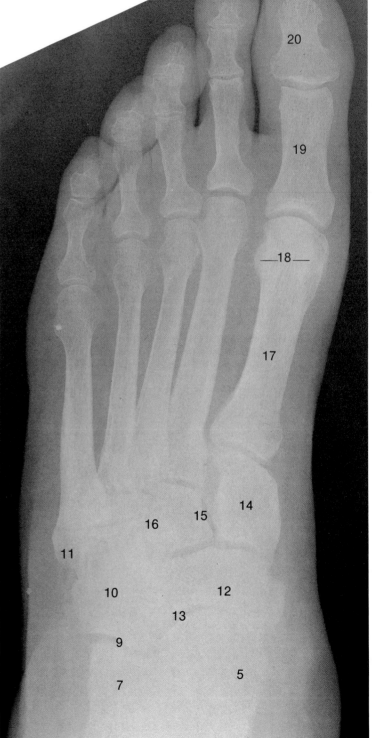

1	Lateral malleolus	12	Navicular
2	Inferior tibiofibular syndesmosis	13	Talonavicular part of
3	Ankle joint		talocalcaneonavicular joint
4	Medial malleolus	14	Medial
5	Talus	15	Intermediate } cuneiform
6	Talocalcanean (subtalar) joint	16	Lateral
7	Calcaneus	17	First metatarsal
8	Tarsal sinus	18	Sesamoid bones in flexor hallucis brevis
9	Calcaneocuboid joint	19	Proximal } phalanx of great toe
10	Cuboid	20	Distal
11	Tuberosity of base of fifth metatarsal		

B

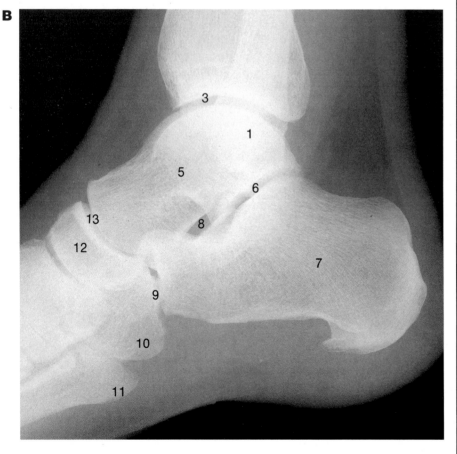

Appendix

Skeleton

The left forearm is in the position of supination, the right in pronation

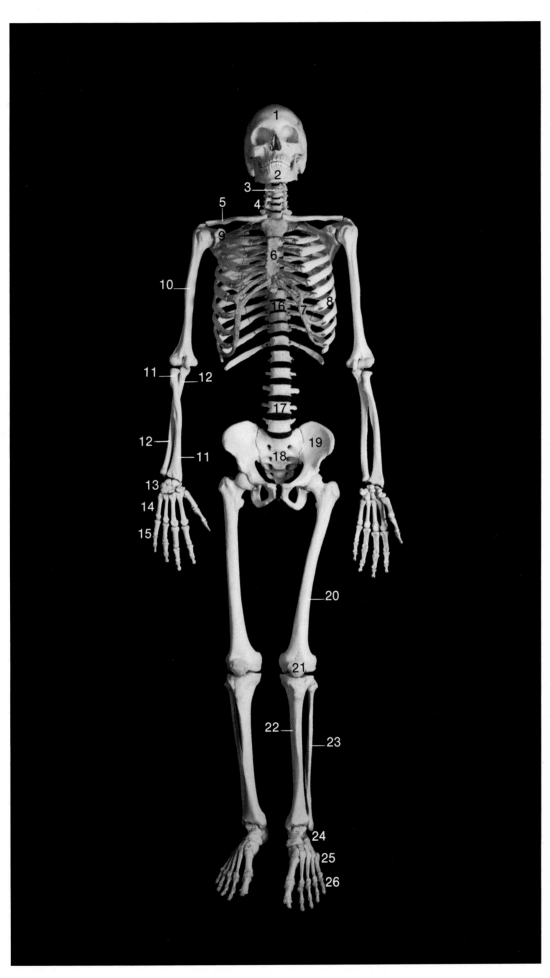

1	Skull
2	Mandible
3	Hyoid bone
4	Cervical vertebrae
5	Clavicle
6	Sternum
7	Costal cartilages
8	Ribs
9	Scapula
10	Humerus
11	Radius
12	Ulna
13	Carpal bones
14	Metacarpal bones
15	Phalanges of thumb and fingers
16	Thoracic vertebrae
17	Lumbar vertebrae
18	Sacrum
19	Hip bone
20	Femur
21	Patella
22	Tibia
23	Fibula
24	Tarsal bones
25	Metatarsal bones
26	Phalanges of toes

Arteries

Some major arteries, from the front

1	Superficial temporal a.
2	Facial a.
3	Internal carotid a.
4	External carotid a.
5	Common carotid a.
6	Brachiocephalic trunk
7	Internal thoracic a.
8	Vertebral a.
9	Subclavian a.
10	Axillary a.
11	Brachial a.
12	Radial a.
13	Ulnar a.
14	Deep palmar arch
15	Superficial palmar arch
16	Heart
17	Coronary a.
18	Aorta
19	Pulmonary trunk
20	Pulmonary a.
21	Coeliac trunk
22	Left gastric a.
23	Splenic a.
24	Common hepatic a.
25	Superior mesenteric a.
26	Renal a.
27	Inferior mesenteric a.
28	Common iliac a.
29	Internal iliac a.
30	External iliac a.
31	Femoral a.
32	Profunda femoris a.
33	Popliteal a.
34	Anterior tibial a.
35	Posterior tibial a.
36	Dorsalis pedis a.
37	Plantar arch

Veins

Some major veins, from the front

(The pulmonary veins enter the left atrium at the back of the heart and are not shown)

1	Internal jugular v.
2	External jugular v.
3	Subclavian v.
4	Axillary v.
5	Brachial v.
6	Basilic v.
7	Cephalic v.
8	Median forearm v.
9	Brachiocephalic v.
10	Superior vena cava
11	Azygos v.
12	Liver
13	Hepatic v.
14	Portal v.
15	Splenic v.
16	Inferior mesenteric v.
17	Superior mesenteric v.
18	Renal v.
19	Inferior vena cava
20	Common iliac v.
21	Internal iliac v.
22	External iliac v.
23	Femoral v.
24	Profunda femoris v.
25	Great saphenous v.
26	Popliteal v.
27	Small saphenous v.

Arteries

Veins

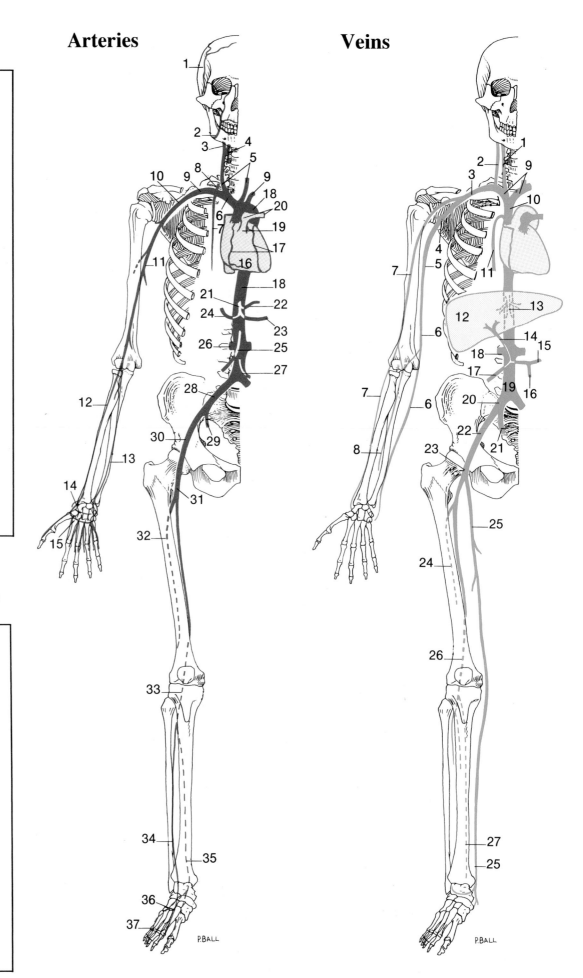

P.BALL

P.BALL

Nerves

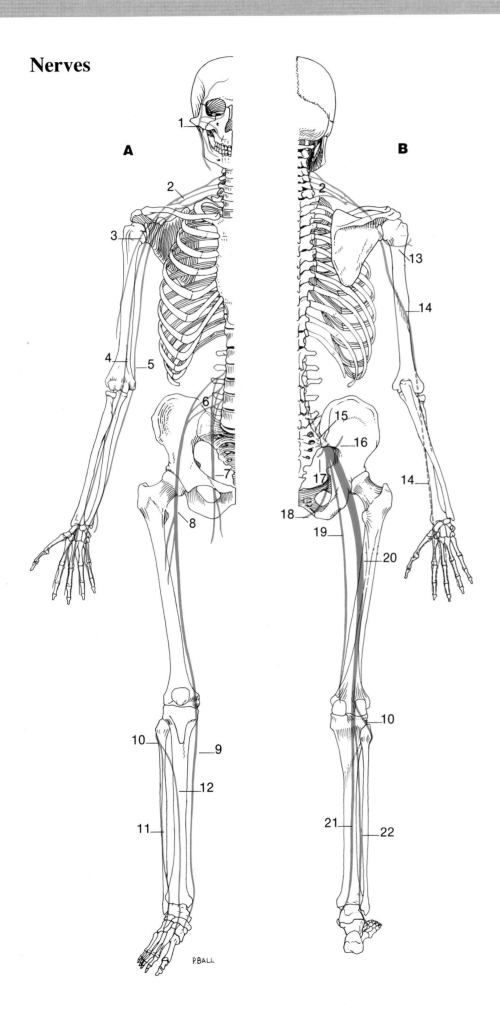

A

B

P.BALL

Nerves

The facial nerve and some major branches of the brachial, lumbar and sacral plexuses, **A** from the front, **B** from the back

1	Facial n.
2	Brachial plexus
3	Musculocutaneous n.
4	Median n.
5	Ulnar n.
6	Lumbar plexus
7	Obturator n.
8	Femoral n.
9	Saphenous n.
10	Common peroneal n.
11	Superficial peroneal n.
12	Deep peroneal n.
13	Axillary n.
14	Radial n.
15	Sacral plexus
16	Superior gluteal n.
17	Inferior gluteal n.
18	Pudendal n.
19	Posterior femoral cutaneous n.
20	Sciatic n.
21	Tibial n.
22	Sural n.

331

The reference lists of vessels and nerves have been arranged for quick identification of parent trunks and branches. Thus, the left common carotid artery is one of the three branches of the arch of the aorta, while the right common carotid is one of the branches of the brachiocephalic trunk.

The arrows indicate a continuity (instead of branching) with a change of name.

The generally accepted standard pattern has been given. For common variations, which are particularly frequent among veins, reference should be made to standard texts. (The articular and vascular branches of nerves have been omitted.)

The inclusion of items in these lists does not necessarily imply that they are illustrated in the atlas; many of the smaller and less important items are not shown but have been included in the lists for reference purposes.

For skull foramina, two lists are given: one for the principal foramina and their contents, which most students would be expected to know, and another giving more specialized details for those who require them.

Arteries

AORTA AND BRANCHES

Ascending aorta → arch of aorta → thoracic aorta → abdominal aorta

Ascending aorta

Right coronary
  Conus
  Sinuatrial nodal (55%)
  Atrial
  Right marginal
  Posterior interventricular
    Septal
  Atrioventricular nodal (90%)
Left coronary
  Anterior interventricular
    Conus
    Diagonal
    Septal
  Circumflex
    Sinuatrial nodal (45%)
    Atrioventricular nodal (10%)
    Atrial
    Left marginal

Arch of aorta

Brachiocephalic trunk
  Right common carotid
    Right internal carotid
    Right external carotid
  Right subclavian → axillary → brachial
  Thyroidea ima (occasional)
Left common carotid
  Left internal carotid
  Left external carotid
Left subclavian → axillary → brachial

Thoracic aorta

Pericardial
Right bronchial
Oesophageal
Mediastinal
Phrenic
Posterior intercostal (3 to 11)
  Left bronchial (from third)
Subcostal

Abdominal aorta

Coeliac trunk
Superior mesenteric
Inferior mesenteric
Middle suprarenal
Renal
  Inferior suprarenal
Testicular (ovarian)
Inferior phrenic
  Superior suprarenal
Lumbar
Median sacral
Common iliac
  Internal iliac
  External iliac → femoral

CAROTID ARTERIES AND BRANCHES

Internal carotid

Caroticotympanic
Pterygoid
Cavernous
Hypophysial
Meningeal
Ophthalmic
  Central of retina
  Lacrimal
    Lateral palpebral
    Zygomatic
    Recurrent meningeal
  Muscular
    Anterior ciliary
  Long posterior ciliary
  Short posterior ciliary
  Supra-orbital
  Posterior ethmoidal
  Anterior ethmoidal
  Anterior meningeal
  Medial palpebral
  Supratrochlear
  Dorsal nasal
Anterior cerebral
  Striate (and others)
Middle cerebral
  Striate (and others)
Posterior communicating
Anterior choroidal

External carotid

Ascending pharyngeal
Superior thyroid
  Infrahyoid
  Sternocleidomastoid
  Superior laryngeal
  Cricothyroid
Lingual
Facial
  Ascending palatine
  Tonsillar
  Glandular
  Submental
  Inferior labial
  Superior labial
    Septal
  Lateral nasal
Occipital
Posterior auricular
Superficial temporal
  Transverse facial
Maxillary → sphenopalatine
  Deep auricular
  Anterior tympanic
  Middle meningeal
  Accessory meningeal
  Inferior alveolar
    Dental
    Mylohyoid
    Mental
  Deep temporal
  Pterygoid
  Masseteric
  Buccal
  Infra-orbital
    Anterior superior alveolar
    Dental
  Posterior superior alveolar
    Dental
  Greater palatine
    Lesser palatine
  Pharyngeal
  Artery of pterygoid canal

SUBCLAVIAN ARTERY AND BRANCHES

Subclavian → axillary → brachial

Vertebral
  Spinal
  Meningeal
  Anterior spinal
  Posterior spinal
  Posterior inferior cerebellar
Internal thoracic
  Pericardiacophrenic
  Mediastinal
  Thymic
  Sternal
  Perforating
    Mammary
  Anterior intercostal
  Musculophrenic
  Superior epigastric
Thyrocervical trunk
  Inferior thyroid
    Ascending cervical
    Inferior laryngeal
    Glandular
    Pharyngeal
    Oesophageal
    Tracheal
  Suprascapular
  Superficial cervical
Costocervical trunk
  Superior intercostal
  Deep cervical
Dorsal scapular

Basilar (union of vertebrals)

Pontine
Labyrinthine
Anterior inferior cerebellar
Superior cerebellar
Posterior cerebral

AXILLARY ARTERY AND BRANCHES

Axillary → brachial

Superior thoracic
Thoraco-acromial
  Acromial
  Clavicular
  Deltoid
  Pectoral
Lateral thoracic
  Lateral mammary
Subscapular
  Circumflex scapular
  Thoracodorsal
Anterior circumflex humeral
Posterior circumflex humeral

Brachial

Profunda brachii
  Posterior descending
  Radial collateral
Nutrient
Superior ulnar collateral
Inferior ulnar collateral
Radial
  Radial recurrent
  Palmar carpal
  Superficial palmar
  Dorsal carpal
  Dorsal metacarpal
    Dorsal digital
  First dorsal metacarpal
  Princeps pollicis
  Radialis indicis
  Deep palmar arch
    Palmar metacarpal
    Perforating
Ulnar
  Anterior ulnar recurrent
  Posterior ulnar recurrent
  Common interosseous
    Anterior interosseous
      Median
    Posterior interosseous
      Interosseous recurrent
  Palmar carpal
  Dorsal carpal
  Deep carpal
  Superficial palmar arch
    Common palmar digital
      Palmar digital

SOME BRANCHES OF THE ABDOMINAL AORTA

Coeliac trunk

Left gastric
  Oesophageal
Common hepatic
  Hepatic
    Cystic
  Gastroduodenal
    Right gastro-epiploic
    Superior pancreaticoduodenal
    Supraduodenal
  Right gastric
Splenic
  Pancreatic
  Short gastric
  Left gastro-epiploic

Superior mesenteric

Inferior pancreaticoduodenal
Jejunal and ileal
Ileocolic
  Ascending
  Anterior caecal
  Posterior caecal
  Appendicular
  Ileal
Right colic
Middle colic

Inferior mesenteric

Left colic
Sigmoid
Superior rectal

Internal iliac

Anterior trunk
  Superior vesical
  Inferior vesical
  Middle rectal
  Uterine
  Vaginal
  Obturator
  Internal pudendal
    Inferior rectal
    Perineal
    Artery of the bulb
    Urethral
    Deep artery of the penis (clitoris)
    Dorsal artery of the penis (clitoris)
  Inferior gluteal
Posterior trunk
  Iliolumbar
  Lateral sacral
  Superior gluteal

External iliac → femoral

Inferior epigastric
  Cremasteric
  Pubic (accessory obturator)
Deep circumflex iliac

333

FEMORAL ARTERY AND BRANCHES

Femoral → popliteal

Superficial epigastric
Superficial circumflex iliac
Superficial external pudendal
Deep external pudendal
Profunda femoris
  Lateral circumflex femoral
  Medial circumflex femoral
  Perforating
Descending genicular

Popliteal

Sural
Superior genicular
Middle genicular
Inferior genicular
Anterior tibial → dorsalis pedis
  Posterior tibial recurrent
  Anterior tibial recurrent
  Anterior medial malleolar
  Anterior lateral malleolar
  Dorsalis pedis → plantar arch
    Tarsal
    First dorsal metatarsal
      Dorsal digital
    Arcuate
      Dorsal metatarsal (2–4)
        Dorsal digital
Posterior tibial
  Circumflex fibular
  Peroneal
    Nutrient
    Perforating
    Communicating
    Lateral malleolar
    Calcanean
  Nutrient
  Communicating
  Medial malleolar
  Calcanean
  Medial plantar
    Superficial digital
  Lateral plantar → plantar arch
    Superficial digital
    Plantar metatarsal
      Common plantar digital
        Plantar digital
      Perforating

Veins

TRIBUTARIES OF MAJOR VEINS

SUPERIOR VENA CAVA

Superior vena cava

Left brachiocephalic
  Left internal jugular
  Left subclavian
  Left vertebral
  Left supreme (first posterior) intercostal
  Left superior intercostal (2–4)
  Inferior thyroid
  Thymic
  Pericardial
Right brachiocephalic
  Right internal jugular
  Right subclavian
  Right vertebral
  Right supreme (first posterior) intercostal
Azygos
  Right superior intercostal (2–4)
  Right posterior intercostal (5–11)
  Right subcostal
  Right ascending lumbar and/or lumbar azygos
  Right bronchial
  Oesophageal
  Pericardial
  Mediastinal
  Vertebral venous plexuses
  Hemi-azygos
    Left ascending lumbar and/or lumbar azygos
    Left subcostal
    Left posterior intercostal (9–11)
    Oesophageal
    Pericardial
    Mediastinal
    Vertebral venous plexuses
  Accessory hemi-azygos
    Left posterior intercostal (5–8)
    Left bronchial
    Oesophageal
    Pericardial
    Mediastinal
    Vertebral venous plexuses

INFERIOR VENA CAVA

Inferior vena cava

Common iliac (right and left)
Fourth lumbar (right and left)
Third lumbar (right and left)
Testicular (ovarian) (right)
Renal (right and left)
Suprarenal (right)
Inferior phrenic (right and left)
Hepatic (right, middle and left)
(Upper lumbar veins join ascending lumbar.
  Left testicular or ovarian and suprarenal veins
  join left renal)

INTERNAL JUGULAR VEIN

Internal jugular

Inferior petrosal sinus
Pharyngeal
Lingual
Facial
Superior thyroid
Middle thyroid

EXTERNAL JUGULAR VEIN

External jugular

Posterior auricular
Posterior branch of retromandibular
Occipital
Posterior external jugular
Suprascapular
Superficial cervical
Anterior jugular

RETROMANDIBULAR VEIN

Retromandibular

Superficial temporal
Maxillary
Transverse facial
Pterygoid plexus
  Middle meningeal
  Greater palatine
  Sphenopalatine
  Buccal
  Dental
  Deep facial
  Inferior ophthalmic
Anterior branch to join facial
Posterior branch to external jugular

FACIAL VEIN

Facial

Supratrochlear
Supra-orbital
Superior ophthalmic
Palpebral
External nasal
Labial
Deep facial
Submental
Submandibular
Tonsillar
External palatine (paratonsillar)

GREAT SAPHENOUS VEIN

Great saphenous

Dorsal venous arch
Perforating
Accessory saphenous
Anterior femoral cutaneous
Superficial epigastric
Superficial circumflex iliac
Superficial external pudendal
Deep external pudendal
(Small saphenous vein communicates with great
  saphenous but usually drains to popliteal
  vein)

CARDIAC VEINS

Coronary sinus

Great cardiac
Middle cardiac
Small cardiac
Posterior of left ventricle
Oblique of left atrium

Anterior cardiac

Venae cordis minimae

DURAL VENOUS SINUSES

Posterosuperior group

Superior sagittal
Inferior sagittal
Straight
Transverse
Sigmoid
Petrosquamous
Occipital

Antero-inferior group

Cavernous
Intercavernous
Inferior petrosal
Superior petrosal
Sphenoparietal
Basilar
Middle meningeal veins

HEPATIC PORTAL SYSTEM

Portal vein

Superior mesenteric
  Jejunal and ileal
  Right gastro-epiploic
  Pancreatic
  Pancreaticoduodenal
  Ileocolic
    Caecal
      Appendicular
  Right colic
  Middle colic
Splenic
  Pancreatic
  Short gastric
  Left gastro-epiploic
  Inferior mesenteric
    Left colic
    Sigmoid
    Superior rectal
Left gastric
Right gastric
  Prepyloric
Paraumbilical (to left branch)
Cystic (to right branch)

PORTAL-SYSTEMIC ANASTOMOSES

Oesophageal branches of the left gastric vein with the hemi-azygos vein
Superior rectal branch of the inferior mesenteric vein with the middle and inferior rectal veins (internal iliac)
Paraumbilical veins of the falciform ligament with anterior abdominal wall veins
Retroperitoneal colonic veins with posterior abdominal wall veins
Bare area of the liver with diaphragmatic veins

Lymphatic system

THORACIC DUCT AND CISTERNA CHYLI TRIBUTARIES

Thoracic duct

Left jugular trunk
Left subclavian trunk
Left bronchomediastinal trunk

Right lymphatic duct

Right jugular trunk
Right subclavian trunk
Right bronchomediastinal trunk

Cisterna chyli

Left lumbar trunk
Right lumbar trunk
Intestinal trunks

LYMPH NODES OF THE HEAD AND NECK

Deep cervical

Superior (including jugulodigastric)
Inferior (including jugulo-omohyoid)

Draining superficial tissues in the head

Occipital
Retro-auricular (mastoid)
Parotid
Buccal (facial)

Draining superficial tissues in the neck

Submandibular
Submental
Anterior cervical
Superficial cervical

Draining deep tissues in the neck

Retropharyngeal
Paratracheal
Lingual
Infrahyoid
Prelaryngeal
Pretracheal

LYMPH NODES OF THE UPPER LIMB AND MAMMARY GLAND

Draining the upper limb

Axillary
  Apical
  Central
  Lateral
  Pectoral (anterior)
  Subscapular (posterior)
Infraclavicular
Supratrochlear
Cubital

Draining the mammary gland

Pectoral
Subscapular
Apical
Parasternal
Intercostal

LYMPH NODES OF THE THORAX

Draining thoracic walls

Superficial
  Pectoral
  Subscapular
  Parasternal
  Inferior deep cervical
Deep
  Parasternal
  Intercostal
  Phrenic
  Diaphragmatic

Draining thoracic contents

Brachiocephalic
Posterior mediastinal
Tracheobronchial
  Paratracheal
  Superior tracheobronchial
  Inferior tracheobronchial
  Bronchopulmonary
  Pulmonary

LYMPH NODES OF THE ABDOMEN AND PELVIS

Lumbar

Pre-aortic
  Coeliac
    Gastric
      Left gastric
      Right gastro-epiploic
      Pyloric
    Hepatic
    Pancreaticosplenic
  Superior mesenteric
  Inferior mesenteric
Lateral aortic
  Common iliac
  External iliac
  Internal iliac
  Inferior epigastric
  Circumflex iliac
  Sacral
Retro-aortic

LYMPH NODES OF THE LOWER LIMB

Superficial inguinal
  Upper
  Lower
Deep inguinal
Popliteal

335

Nerves

CRANIAL NERVES AND BRANCHES

I Olfactory (from olfactory mucous membrane)

II Optic (from retina)

III Oculomotor

Superior ramus (to superior rectus and levator palpebrae superioris)

Inferior ramus (to medial rectus, inferior rectus, inferior oblique and ciliary ganglion)

IV Trochlear (to superior oblique)

V Trigeminal

Ophthalmic
  Lacrimal
  Frontal
    Supratrochlear
    Supra-orbital
  Nasociliary → anterior ethmoidal → external nasal
    Internal nasal (from anterior ethmoidal)
    Ciliary ganglion
    Long ciliary
    Infratrochlear
    Posterior ethmoidal
Maxillary → infra-orbital
  Meningeal
  Pterygopalatine
    Orbital
    Palatine
    Nasal
    Pharyngeal
  Zygomatic
  Posterior superior alveolar
  Middle superior alveolar
  Anterior superior alveolar
  Palpebral ⎫
  Nasal ⎬ (from infra-orbital)
  Superior labial ⎭
Mandibular
  Meningeal
  Nerve to medial pterygoid (and tensor veli palatini and tensor tympani)
  Anterior trunk
    Buccal
    Masseteric
    Deep temporal
    Nerve to lateral pterygoid
  Posterior trunk
    Auriculotemporal
    Lingual
    Inferior alveolar
      Mental

VI Abducent (to lateral rectus)

VII Facial

Greater petrosal
Nerve to stapedius
Chorda tympani
Posterior auricular (to occipitalis and auricular muscles)
Nerve to posterior belly of digastric
Nerve to stylohyoid
Temporal ⎫
Zygomatic ⎪ to frontalis and
Buccal ⎬ muscles of facial
Marginal mandibular ⎪ expression
Cervical ⎭

VIII Vestibulocochlear

Cochlear (from coils of cochlea)
Vestibular (from utricle, saccule and ampullae of semicircular ducts)

IX Glossopharyngeal

Tympanic
  Lesser petrosal
Carotid
Pharyngeal
Muscular (to stylopharyngeus)
Tonsillar
Lingual

X Vagus

Meningeal
Auricular
Pharyngeal (to muscles of pharynx and soft palate except stylopharyngeus and tensor veli palatini)
Carotid body
Superior laryngeal
  Internal laryngeal
  External laryngeal (to cricothyroid)
Right recurrent laryngeal (to muscles of larynx except cricothyroid)
Cardiac (cervical)
Cardiac (thoracic)
Left recurrent laryngeal (to muscles of larynx except cricothyroid)
Pulmonary
Oesophageal
Anterior trunk
  Gastric
  Hepatic
Posterior trunk
  Coeliac
  Gastric

XI Accessory

Cranial root (to muscles of palate and possibly larynx via vagus)
Spinal root (to sternocleidomastoid and trapezius)

XII Hypoglossal

Meningeal
Descending (upper root of ansa cervicalis, from first cervical nerve joining lower root from second and third cervical nerves, to form ansa and supply sternohyoid, sternothyroid and superior and inferior bellies of omohyoid)
Nerve to thyrohyoid (from first cervical nerve)
Muscular (to geniohyoid and muscles of tongue except palatoglossus)

SOME HEAD AND NECK NERVE SUPPLIES

All the muscles of	Supplied by	Except	Supplied by
Pharynx	Pharyngeal plexus	Stylo-pharyngeus	Glosso-pharyngeal nerve
Palate	Pharyngeal plexus	Tensor veli palatini	Nerve to medial pterygoid
Larynx	Recurrent laryngeal nerve	Crico-thyroid	External laryngeal nerve
Tongue	Hypoglossal nerve	Palato-glossus	Pharyngeal plexus
Facial expression (including buccinator)	Facial nerve		
Mastication	Mandibular nerve		

CERVICAL PLEXUS AND BRANCHES

Lesser occipital C2
Great auricular C2, 3
Transverse cervical C2, 3
Supraclavicular C3, 4
Phrenic (to diaphragm) C3, 4, 5
Communicating (with vagus and hypoglossal nerves and superior cervical sympathetic ganglion)
Muscular (to rectus capitis lateralis, rectus capitis anterior, longus capitis and longus colli, and by lower root of ansa cervicalis (descending cervical) to sternohyoid, sternothyroid and inferior belly of omohyoid) C1, 2, 3

TYPICAL THORACIC NERVE BRANCHES

Thoracic spinal nerve

Dorsal ramus
  Medial
  Lateral
Ventral ramus → anterior cutaneous
  Recurrent
  Collateral
  Lateral cutaneous
    Posterior
    Anterior

BRACHIAL PLEXUS AND BRANCHES

Supraclavicular branches
From the roots
  To scalenes and longus colli C5, 6, 7, 8
  To join phrenic nerve C5
  Dorsal scapular (to rhomboids) C5
  Long thoracic (to serratus anterior) C5, 6, 7

From the upper trunk
  Nerve to subclavus C5, 6
  Suprascapular (to supraspinatus and
    infraspinatus) C5, 6

Infraclavicular branches
From the lateral cord
  Lateral pectoral (to pectoralis major and
    minor) C5, 6, 7
  Musculocutaneous C5, 6, 7
  Lateral root of the median C(5), 6, 7

From the medial cord
  Medial pectoral (to pectoralis major and
    minor) C8, T1
  Medial root of the median C8, T1
  Medial cutaneous of arm C8, T1
  Medial cutaneous of forearm C8, T1
  Ulnar C(7), 8, T1

From the posterior cord
  Upper subscapular (to subscapularis) C5, 6
  Thoracodorsal (to latissimus dorsi) C6, 7, 8
  Lower subscapular (to subscapularis and teres
    major) C5, 6
  Axillary C5, 6
  Radial C5, 6, 7, 8, T1

Musculocutaneous C5, 6, 7
Muscular (to coracobrachialis, biceps and
  brachialis)
Lateral cutaneous of forearm

Median C(5), 6, 7, 8, T1
In the arm
  To pronator teres (occasional)
In the forearm
  Muscular (to pronator teres, flexor carpi
    radialis, palmaris longus and flexor
    digitorum superficialis)
  Anterior interosseous (to flexor pollicis
    longus, flexor digitorum profundus and
    pronator quadratus)
  Palmar cutaneous
  Communicating (with ulnar nerve)
In the hand
  Muscular (to abductor pollicis brevis, flexor
    pollicis brevis, opponens pollicis and the
    two lateral lumbricals)
  Common palmar digital
    Palmar digital

Ulnar C(7), 8, T1
Muscular (to flexor carpi ulnaris and flexor
  digitorum profundus)
Palmar cutaneous
Dorsal
  Dorsal digital
Superficial terminal
  Nerve to palmaris brevis
  Common palmar digital
    Palmar digital
Deep terminal (to abductor digiti minimi,
  opponens digiti minimi, flexor digiti
  minimi brevis, adductor pollicis, all the
  interossei and the two medial lumbricals)

Axillary C5, 6
Muscular (to deltoid and teres minor)
Upper lateral cutaneous of arm

Radial C5, 6, 7, 8, T1
Muscular (to triceps, anconeus,
  brachioradialis, extensor carpi radialis longus
  and brachialis)
Posterior cutaneous of arm
Lower lateral cutaneous of arm
Posterior cutaneous of forearm
Superficial terminal
  Dorsal digital
Deep terminal (posterior interosseous)(to
  extensor carpi radialis brevis, supinator,
  extensor digitorum, extensor digiti minimi,
  extensor carpi ulnaris, extensor pollicis
  longus, extensor indicis, abductor pollicis
  longus and extensor pollicis brevis)

LUMBAR PLEXUS AND BRANCHES

Muscular (to psoas major and minor, quadratus
  lumborum and iliacus) T12, L1, 2, 3, 4
Iliohypogastric (to part of internal oblique and
  transversus abdominis) L1
Ilio-inguinal (to part of internal oblique and
  transversus abdominis) L1
Genitofemoral L1, 2
  Genital branch (to cremaster)
  Femoral branch
Lateral cutaneous of thigh L2, 3
Femoral L2, 3, 4
  Nerve to pectineus
  Anterior division
    Intermediate femoral cutaneous
    Medial femoral cutaneous
    Nerve to sartorius
  Posterior division
    Saphenous
    Nerves to quadriceps femoris
Obturator L2, 3, 4
  Anterior branch
    Muscular (to adductor longus, adductor
     brevis and gracilis)
  Posterior branch
    Muscular (to obturator externus and
     adductor magnus)
Accessory obturator (occasional)(to pectineus)
  L3, 4

SACRAL PLEXUS AND BRANCHES

Nerve to quadratus femoris and inferior gemellus
  L4, 5, S1
Nerve to obturator internus and superior gemellus
  L5, S1, 2
Nerve to piriformis S(1), 2
Superior gluteal (to gluteus medius and minimus
  and tensor fasciae latae) L4, 5, S1
Inferior gluteal (to gluteus maximus) L5, S1, 2
Posterior femoral cutaneous S2, 3
Sciatic L4, 5, S1, 2, 3
  Muscular (to biceps, semitendinosus,
    semimembranosus and adductor magnus)
  Tibial L4, 5, S1, 2, 3
    Muscular (to gastrocnemius, plantaris,
     soleus, popliteus, tibialis posterior, flexor
     digitorum longus and flexor hallucis
     longus)
    Sural
    Medial calcanean
    Medial plantar
     Common plantar digital
      Plantar digital
     Muscular (to abductor hallucis, flexor
      digitorum brevis, flexor hallucis brevis
      and first lumbrical)
    Lateral plantar
     Muscular (to flexor accessorius and
      abductor digiti minimi)
     Superficial
      Muscular (to flexor digiti minimi brevis,
       and fourth dorsal and third plantar
       interossei)
      Common plantar digital
       Plantar digital
     Deep (to adductor hallucis, first to third
      dorsal and first and second plantar
      interossei, and second to fourth
      lumbricals)
  Common peroneal L4, 5, S1, 2
    Recurrent
    Lateral cutaneous of calf
    Peroneal communicating
    Superficial peroneal
     Muscular (to peroneus longus and
      peroneus brevis)
     Medial dorsal cutaneous
     Intermediate dorsal cutaneous
      Dorsal digital
    Deep peroneal
     Muscular (to tibialis anterior, extensor
      hallucis longus, extensor digitorum
      longus, peroneus tertius and extensor
      digitorum brevis)
     Dorsal digital
Perforating cutaneous S2, 3
Pudendal S2, 3, 4
  Inferior rectal (to external anal sphincter)
  Perineal
    Posterior scrotal (labial)
    Muscular (to perineal muscles and levator
     ani)
  Dorsal nerve of penis (clitoris)
Nerves to levator ani and coccygeus S3 and 4
Pelvic splanchnics (nervi erigentes) S2, 3, (4)

Muscles

MUSCLES OF THE HEAD

Muscles of the scalp
Epicranius
  Occipitofrontalis
  Temporoparietalis

Muscles of the nose
Procerus
Nasalis (compressor and dilator naris)
Depressor septi

Muscles of the eyelids
Orbicularis oculi
Corrugator supercilii
Levator palpebrae superioris (see Muscles of the Orbit)

Muscles of mastication
Masseter
Temporalis
Lateral pterygoid
Medial pterygoid

Muscles of the mouth
Levator labii superioris alaeque nasi
Levator labii superioris
Zygomaticus minor
Zygomaticus major
Levator anguli oris
Mentalis
Depressor labii inferioris
Depressor anguli oris
Buccinator
Orbicularis oris
Risorius

MUSCLES OF THE NECK

Superficial and lateral muscles
Platysma
Sternocleidomastoid
Trapezius (see upper limb)

Anterior vertebral muscles
Longus colli
Longus capitis
Rectus capitis anterior
Rectus capitis lateralis

Lateral vertebral muscles
Scalenus anterior
Scalenus medius
Scalenus posterior

Suprahyoid muscles
Digastric
Stylohyoid
Mylohyoid
Geniohyoid

Infrahyoid muscles
Sternohyoid
Sternothyroid
Thyrohyoid
Omohyoid

MUSCLE GROUPS IN HEAD AND NECK

Muscles of the pharynx
Superior constrictor
Middle constrictor
Inferior constrictor
Stylopharyngeus
Palatopharyngeus
Salpingopharyngeus

Muscles of the palate
Palatoglossus
Palatopharyngeus
Tensor veli palatini
Levator veli palatini
Musculus uvulae

Muscles of the larynx
Cricothyroid
Posterior crico-arytenoid
Lateral crico-arytenoid
Transverse arytenoid
Oblique arytenoid
Aryepiglottic
Thyro-arytenoid and vocalis
Thyro-epiglottic

Muscles of the tongue
Extrinsic
  Genioglossus
  Hyoglossus and chondroglossus
  Styloglossus
  Palatoglossus
Intrinsic
  Superior longitudinal
  Inferior longitudinal
  Transverse
  Vertical

Muscles of the orbit
Levator palpebrae superioris
Orbitalis
Muscles of the eyeball
  Superior rectus
  Inferior rectus
  Medial rectus
  Lateral rectus
  Superior oblique
  Inferior oblique

MUSCLES OF THE TRUNK

Suboccipital muscles
Rectus capitis posterior major
Rectus capitis posterior minor
Obliquus capitis inferior
Obliquus capitis superior

Deep muscles of the back
Splenius capitis
Splenius cervicis
Erector spinae
  Iliocostalis
  Longissimus
  Spinalis
Transversospinalis
  Semispinalis
  Multifidus
  Rotator
Interspinal
Intertransverse

Muscles of the thorax
External intercostal
Internal intercostal
Innermost intercostal
Subcostal
Transversus thoracis
Levatores costarum
Serratus posterior superior
Serratus posterior inferior
Diaphragm

Muscles of the abdomen
Anterolateral muscles
  External oblique
  Internal oblique
  Cremaster
  Transversus abdominis
  Rectus abdominis
  Pyramidalis
Posterior muscles
  Psoas major
  Psoas minor
  Iliacus
  Quadratus lumborum

Muscles of the pelvis
Piriformis
Obturator internus
Levator ani
Coccygeus

Muscles of the perineum
Anal muscle
  External anal sphincter
Urogenital muscles
  Superficial transverse perinei
  Bulbospongiosus
  Ischiocavernosus
  Deep transverse perinei
  Sphincter urethrae

MUSCLES OF THE UPPER LIMB

Connecting limb and vertebral column
Trapezius
Latissimus dorsi
Levator scapulae
Rhomboid major
Rhomboid minor

Connecting limb and thoracic wall
Pectoralis major
Pectoralis minor
Subclavius
Serratus anterior

Scapular muscles
Deltoid
Subscapularis
Supraspinatus
Infraspinatus
Teres minor
Teres major

Muscles of the upper arm
Biceps brachii
Coracobrachialis
Brachialis
Triceps

Muscles of the forearm
Anterior forearm muscles
Superficial flexor group
Pronator teres
Flexor carpi radialis
Palmaris longus
Flexor carpi ulnaris
Flexor digitorum superficialis
Deep flexor group
Flexor digitorum profundus
Flexor pollicis longus
Pronator quadratus
Posterior forearm muscles
Superficial extensor group
Brachioradialis
Extensor carpi radialis longus
Extensor carpi radialis brevis
Extensor digitorum
Extensor digiti minimi
Extensor carpi ulnaris
Anconeus
Deep extensor group
Supinator
Abductor pollicis longus
Extensor pollicis brevis
Extensor pollicis longus
Extensor indicis

Muscles of the hand
Thenar group
Abductor pollicis brevis
Flexor pollicis brevis
Opponens pollicis
Adductor pollicis
Lumbricals (four)
Dorsal interossei (four)
Palmar interossei (four)
Hypothenar group
Palmaris brevis
Abductor digiti minimi
Flexor digiti minimi brevis
Opponens digiti minimi

MUSCLES OF THE LOWER LIMB

Muscles of the iliac region
Psoas major
Psoas minor
Iliacus

Muscles of the gluteal region
Gluteus maximus
Gluteus medius
Gluteus minimus
Piriformis
Obturator internus
Superior gemellus
Inferior gemellus
Quadratus femoris
Obturator externus

Muscles of the thigh
Anterior femoral group
Tensor fasciae latae
Sartorius
Quadriceps femoris
Rectus femoris
Vastus lateralis
Vastus medialis
Vastus intermedius
Articularis genu
Medial femoral group
Gracilis
Pectineus
Adductor longus
Adductor brevis
Adductor magnus
Posterior femoral group
Biceps femoris
Semitendinosus
Semimembranosus

Muscles of the leg
Anterior muscles
Tibialis anterior
Extensor hallucis longus
Extensor digitorum longus
Peroneus tertius
Lateral muscles
Peroneus longus
Peroneus brevis
Posterior muscles
Superficial group
Gastrocnemius
Soleus
Plantaris
Deep group
Popliteus
Flexor hallucis longus
Flexor digitorum longus
Tibialis posterior

Muscles of the foot
Dorsal muscle—extensor digitorum brevis
Plantar muscles
First layer
Abductor hallucis
Flexor digitorum brevis
Abductor digiti minimi
Second layer
Flexor accessorius
Lumbricals (four)
Third layer
Flexor hallucis brevis
Adductor hallucis
Flexor digiti minimi brevis
Fourth layer
Dorsal interossei (four)
Plantar interossei (three)

Skull foramina

PRINCIPAL FORAMINA AND CONTENTS
(For a more detailed list, see pages 340 to 341)

Supra-orbital foramen
Supra-orbital nerve and vessels

Infra-orbital foramen
Infra-orbital nerve and vessels

Mental foramen
Mental nerve and vessels

Mandibular foramen
Inferior alveolar nerve and vessels

Optic canal
Optic nerve
Ophthalmic artery

Superior orbital fissure
Ophthalmic nerve and veins
Oculomotor, trochlear and abducent nerves

Inferior orbital fissure
Maxillary nerve

Sphenopalatine foramen
Sphenopalatine artery
Nasal branches of pterygopalatine ganglion

Foramen rotundum
Maxillary nerve

Foramen ovale
Mandibular and lesser petrosal nerves

Foramen spinosum
Middle meningeal vessels

Foramen lacerum
Internal carotid artery (entering from behind and emerging above)
Greater petrosal nerve (entering from behind and leaving anteriorly as the nerve of the pterygoid canal)

Carotid canal
Internal carotid artery and nerve

Jugular foramen
Inferior petrosal sinus
Glossopharyngeal, vagus and accessory nerves
Internal jugular vein (emerging below)

Internal acoustic meatus
Facial and vestibulocochlear nerves
Labyrinthine artery

Hypoglossal canal
Hypoglossal nerve

Stylomastoid foramen
Facial nerve

Foramen magnum
Medulla oblongata and meninges
Vertebral and anterior and posterior spinal arteries
Accessory nerves (spinal parts)

339

Skull foramina (detailed list)

INSIDE THE SKULL

MIDDLE CRANIAL FOSSA

Optic canal: in the sphenoid between the body and the two roots of the lesser wing
Optic nerve
Ophthalmic artery

Superior orbital fissure: in the sphenoid between the body and the greater and lesser wings, with a fragment of the frontal bone at the lateral extremity
Oculomotor, trochlear and abducent nerves
Lacrimal, frontal and nasociliary nerves
Filaments from the internal carotid (sympathetic) plexus
Orbital branch of the middle meningeal artery
Recurrent branch of the lacrimal artery
Superior ophthalmic vein

Foramen rotundum: in the greater wing of the sphenoid
Maxillary nerve

Foramen ovale: in the greater wing of the sphenoid
Mandibular nerve
Lesser petrosal nerve (usually)
Accessory meningeal artery
Emissary veins (from cavernous sinus to pterygoid plexus)

Foramen spinosum: in the greater wing of the sphenoid
Middle meningeal vessels
Meningeal branch of the mandibular nerve

Venous (emissary sphenoidal) foramen: in 40% of skulls, in the greater wing of the sphenoid medial to the foramen ovale
Emissary vein (from the cavernous sinus to the pterygoid plexus)

Petrosal (innominate) foramen: occasional, in the greater wing of the sphenoid, medial to the foramen spinosum
Lesser petrosal nerve (if not through foramen ovale)

Foramen lacerum: between the sphenoid, apex of the petrous temporal and the basilar part of the occipital
Internal carotid artery (entering from behind and emerging above)
Greater petrosal nerve (entering from above and behind, and leaving anteriorly as nerve of pterygoid canal)
Nerve of pterygoid canal (leaving through anterior wall)
A meningeal branch of the ascending pharyngeal artery
Emissary veins (from the cavernous sinus to the pterygoid plexus)

Hiatus for the greater petrosal nerve: in the tegmen tympani of the petrous temporal, in front of the arcuate eminence
Greater petrosal nerve
Petrosal branch of the middle meningeal artery

Hiatus for the lesser petrosal nerve: in the tegmen tympani of the petrous temporal, about 3 mm in front of the hiatus for the greater petrosal nerve
Lesser petrosal nerve

ANTERIOR CRANIAL FOSSA

Foramina in the cribriform plate of the ethmoid
Olfactory nerve filaments
Anterior ethmoidal nerve and vessels

Foramen caecum: between the frontal crest of the frontal bone and the ethmoid in front of the crista galli
Emissary vein (between nose and superior sagittal sinus)

POSTERIOR CRANIAL FOSSA

Internal acoustic meatus: in the posterior surface of the petrous temporal
Facial nerve
Vestibulocochlear nerve
Labyrinthine artery

Aqueduct of the vestibule: in the petrous temporal about 1 cm behind the internal acoustic meatus
Endolymphatic duct and sac
A branch from the meningeal branch of the occipital artery
A vein (from the labyrinth and vestibule to the sigmoid sinus)

Jugular foramen: between the jugular fossa of the petrous temporal and the occipital bone
Glossopharyngeal, vagus and accessory nerves
Meningeal branches of the vagus nerve
Inferior petrosal sinus
Internal jugular vein
A meningeal branch of the occipital artery

Hypoglossal canal: in the occipital bone above the anterior part of the condyle
Hypoglossal nerve and its (recurrent) meningeal branch
A meningeal branch of the ascending pharyngeal artery
Emissary vein (from the basilar plexus to the internal jugular vein)

Condylar canal: occasional, from the lower part of the sigmoid groove in the lateral part of the occipital bone to the condylar fossa on the external surface of the occipital bone behind the condyle
Emissary vein (from the sigmoid sinus to occipital veins)
A meningeal branch of the occipital artery

Mastoid foramen: in the petrous temporal near the posterior margin of the lower part of the sigmoid groove, passing backwards to open behind the mastoid process
Emissary vein (from the sigmoid sinus to occipital veins)
A meningeal branch of the occipital artery

Foramen magnum: in the occipital bone
Apical ligament of the dens of the axis
Tectorial membrane
Medulla oblongata and meninges (including first digitations of denticulate ligaments)
Spinal parts of the accessory nerves
Meningeal branches of the upper cervical nerves
Vertebral arteries
Anterior spinal artery
Posterior spinal arteries

IN THE BASE OF THE SKULL EXTERNALLY

Foramen lacerum
Foramen ovale
Foramen spinosum
Jugular foramen } see INSIDE THE SKULL
Hypoglossal canal
Condylar canal
Mastoid foramen
Foramen magnum

Inferior orbital fissure—see IN THE ORBIT

Lateral incisive foramen: opens into the incisive fossa, in the midline at the front of the hard palate
Nasopalatine nerve
Greater palatine vessels

Greater palatine foramen: between the maxilla and the palatine bone at the lateral border of the hard palate behind the palatomaxillary fissure
Greater palatine nerve and vessels

Lesser palatine foramina: two or three, in the inferior and medial aspects of the pyramidal process of the palatine bone
Lesser palatine nerves and vessels

Palatovaginal canal: between lower surface of the vaginal process of the root of the medial pterygoid plate and the upper surface of the sphenoidal process of the palatine bone
Pharyngeal branch of the pterygopalatine ganglion
Pharyngeal branch of the maxillary artery

Vomerovaginal canal: occasional, medial to the palatovaginal canal, between the upper surface of the vaginal process of the root of the medial pterygoid plate and the lower surface of the ala of the vomer
Pharyngeal branch of the sphenopalatine artery

Petrosquamous fissure: between the squamous temporal and the tegmen tympani
Petrosquamous vein

Petrotympanic fissure: between the tympanic part of the temporal bone and the tegmen tympani
Chorda tympani
Anterior ligament of the malleus
Anterior tympanic branch of the maxillary artery

Cochlear canaliculus: in the petrous temporal, at the apex of a notch in front of the medial part of the jugular fossa
Perilymphatic duct
Emissary vein (from the cochlea to the internal jugular vein or inferior petrosal sinus)

Carotid canal: in the inferior surface of the petrous temporal
Internal carotid artery
Internal carotid (sympathetic) plexus
Internal carotid venous plexus (from the cavernous sinus to the internal jugular vein)

Tympanic canaliculus: in the inferior surface of the petrous temporal, on the ridge of bone between the carotid canal and the jugular fossa
Tympanic branch of the glossopharyngeal nerve
Inferior tympanic branch of the ascending pharyngeal artery

Mastoid canaliculus: in the inferior surface of the petrous temporal, on the lateral wall of the jugular fossa
Auricular branch of the vagus nerve

Stylomastoid foramen: between the styloid and mastoid processes of the temporal bone
Facial nerve
Stylomastoid branch of the posterior auricular artery

IN THE ORBIT

Superior orbital fissure }
Optic canal } see INSIDE THE SKULL

Frontal notch or foramen: in the supra-orbital margin of the frontal bone one finger's breadth from the midline
Supratrochlear nerve and vessels

Supra-orbital notch or foramen: in the supra-orbital margin of the frontal bone two finger's breadths from the midline
Supra-orbital nerve and vessels

Anterior ethmoidal foramen: in the medial wall of the orbit between the orbital part of the frontal bone and the ethmoid labyrinth
Anterior ethmoidal nerve and vessels

Posterior ethmoidal foramen: occasional, 1 to 2 cm behind the anterior ethmoidal foramen
Posterior ethmoidal nerve and vessels

Zygomatico-orbital foramen: in the orbital surface of the zygomatic bone
Zygomatic branch of the maxillary nerve

Nasolacrimal canal: at the front, lower, medial corner of the orbit formed by the lacrimal bone and maxilla
Nasolacrimal duct

Inferior orbital fissure: towards the back of the orbit, between the maxilla and the greater wing of the sphenoid
Maxillary nerve
Zygomatic nerve
Orbital branches of the pterygopalatine ganglion
Infra-orbital vessels
Inferior ophthalmic veins

Infra-orbital canal: in the orbital surface of the maxilla
Infra-orbital nerve and vessels

MISCELLANEOUS

Infra-orbital foramen: the anterior opening of the infra-orbital canal, in the maxilla below the infra-orbital margin
Infra-orbital nerve and vessels

Mental foramen: on the outer surface of the body of the mandible below the second premolar tooth or slightly more anteriorly
Mental nerve and vessels

Mandibular foramen: on the inner surface of the ramus of the mandible, overlapped anteriorly and medially by the lingula
Inferior alveolar nerve and vessels

Foramina in the infratemporal (posterior) surface of the maxilla
Posterior superior alveolar nerves and vessels

Pterygomaxillary fissure: between the lateral pterygoid plate and the infratemporal (posterior) surface of the maxilla, and continuous above with the posterior end of the inferior orbital fissure
Maxillary artery (entering pterygopalatine fossa)
Maxillary nerve (entering inferior orbital fissure)
Sphenopalatine veins

Sphenopalatine foramen: at the upper end of the perpendicular plate of the palatine between its orbital and sphenoidal processes and (above) the body of the sphenoid; in the medial wall of the pterygopalatine fossa (viewed laterally through the pterygomaxillary fissure) and lateral wall of the nasal cavity (viewed medially)
Nasopalatine and posterior superior nasal nerves
Sphenopalatine vessels

Foramina in the perpendicular plate of the palatine
Posterior inferior nasal nerves

Pterygoid canal: at the root of the pterygoid process of the sphenoid in line with the medial pterygoid plate, leading from the anterior wall of the foramen lacerum to the posterior wall of the pterygopalatine fossa (and only clearly seen in a disarticulated sphenoid)
Nerve of the pterygoid canal
Artery of the pterygoid canal

Musculotubular canal: at the lateral side of the apex of the petrous temporal, at the junction of the petrous and squamous parts, and divided by a bony septum into upper and lower semicanals
Tensor tympani (upper semicanal)
Auditory tube (lower semicanal)

Parietal foramen: in the parietal bone near the posterosuperior (occipital) angle
Emissary vein (from the superior sagittal sinus to the scalp)

341

Index

Page numbers refer to items in notes as well as those illustrated

A

357

Window on the World

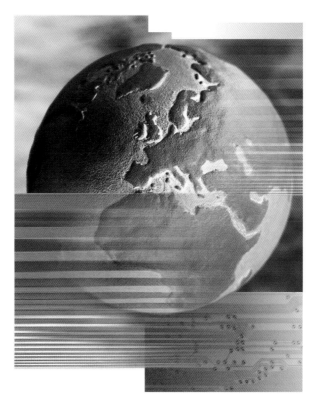

When we pray
God works

Daphne Spraggett with
Jill Johnstone

paternoster
Lifestyle

Contents

Introduction

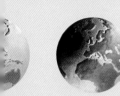

Muskaan and I slipped off our shoes outside a simple village church in India. We joined the sari-clad ladies sitting together on the floor on one side of the church and chatted with them until the service began.

The pastor began by thanking God for his great love and for sending his Son Jesus to die on the cross so that we might be forgiven our sins and have our hearts made clean. He thanked God that Jesus is our special friend who is always ready to help everyone who trusts in him. I was excited because wherever we go in the world we meet people who love Jesus and belong to his great family.

The pastor then prayed for the people in the village and the millions of others in India who know nothing about God's love. And I was reminded that although there are more than 2,015,743,000 Christians in the world, there are many more people who have never heard about God's love or that he sent Jesus to be their Savior. How will they hear about him? I don't know, but I do know that God wants us – you and me – to pray for them.

About this book

There are about 230 countries in our world, and the people who live in them belong to thousands of smaller groups that speak different languages and have different customs. These are all called people groups. In India alone there are at least 4,635 people groups and 1,652 different languages.

In this book you will read about some of these countries and people groups. There are chapters, too, about special groups like missionaries' children, street children and refugees. Each chapter has stories, information and pictures to help you learn a little about them. When you have read a chapter, find out more about the country or people group by reading books and magazines, watching news and educational programs on TV, looking on the Internet and asking questions. The more you know and understand, the better you can pray!

God has answered lots of prayers since the first edition of this book was written, so I have included some things to thank God for. As you pray, keep your eyes and ears open for the answers. Your prayers are helping to change countries, people groups, situations and individuals. That's exciting! And remember to thank God for answering your prayers.

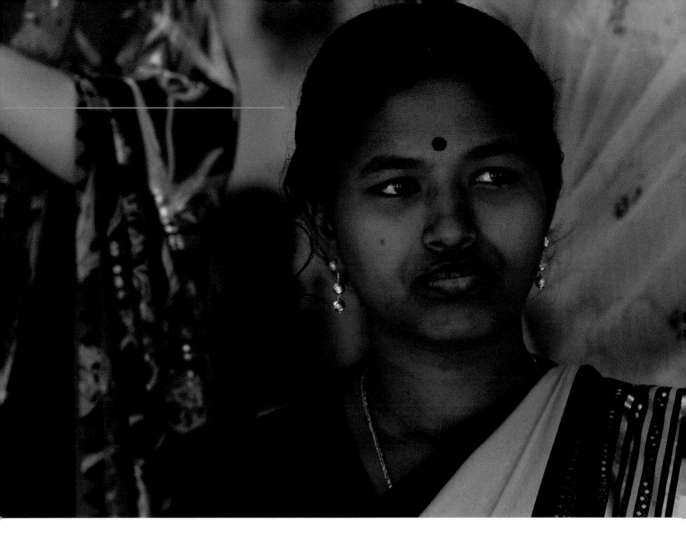

Why should we pray?

People often say that God could work without our prayers because he is the King of kings and Lord of lords. So why should we pray? In Luke 10:2 Jesus told his disciples, "Ask the Lord of the harvest to send out workers into his harvest field." God wants us to pray because he wants us to share in his work in the world.

Some of the countries in this book have been changed, or are being changed, because people prayed and went on praying – sometimes for years and years. Albania, China, Mongolia and Russia are just a few of them.

To help you pray

Prayer is simply talking with God. We can pray anywhere, at any time and about anything. We don't have to use special words, close our eyes or put our hands together. I often pray when I'm walking or working or when I wake up in the middle of the night.

Remember, the more we pray and learn to listen to God, the more we get to know and love him. He wants us to pray because, when we do, we are working with him to change the world.

There are times when we pray but God doesn't seem to answer our prayers. Sometimes it's because we've done things that haven't pleased him. If we've said or done things to hurt others or been selfish or forgotten to help others, we have to make these things right and ask God to forgive us. Then he hears and answers our prayers (Psalm 66:18).

We have to remember, too, that Satan wants people and countries to belong to him and not to God. He even tempted Jesus to do things his way, not God's way (Matthew 4:1–11). So don't give up, but keep praying!

When nothing seems to happen, remember that prayer is like planting a seed in the ground. For weeks and months you may see nothing, but a lot is happening underground. Keep on trusting God, because one day you will see the answer to your prayers (Matthew 21:22) just as one day you'll see the plant begin to grow.

So … let's pray and work with God to change the world!

To Help You

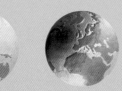

■ On pages 198 to 209 there are short chapters telling you a little about animism, Buddhism, Christianity, Hinduism, Islam and Judaism.

■ You will find the meanings of difficult words in this book in the Word List on pages 214 to 217.

■ There is a map of the world on pages 112 and 113.

■ On page 210 you will find some ideas to help you, your family and Sunday school get involved in missionary work now.

■ If you want to learn more about the countries and people groups you are praying for, turn to pages 212 and 213 where there is a list of Christian agencies who might be able to help you. This is what to do:

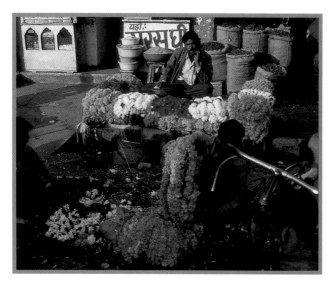

● If you want to ask about a people group, find out first what country or countries they're in. Then look at the list on page 212 to see which agencies may be able to help you.

● If it is listed, look on their web site.

● If you write a letter, don't ask about more than one or two people groups or countries at a time. Say what you want to know, and why. Ask what materials they have and tell them how you will use it (for example, at home, Sunday school or club).

● Make sure that you write at least a month before you need materials or information. (This is important because they could have lots of requests at the same time, or they might need to send your letter to someone else to answer.) Remember that it costs money to help you, so be ready to pay for what they send you.

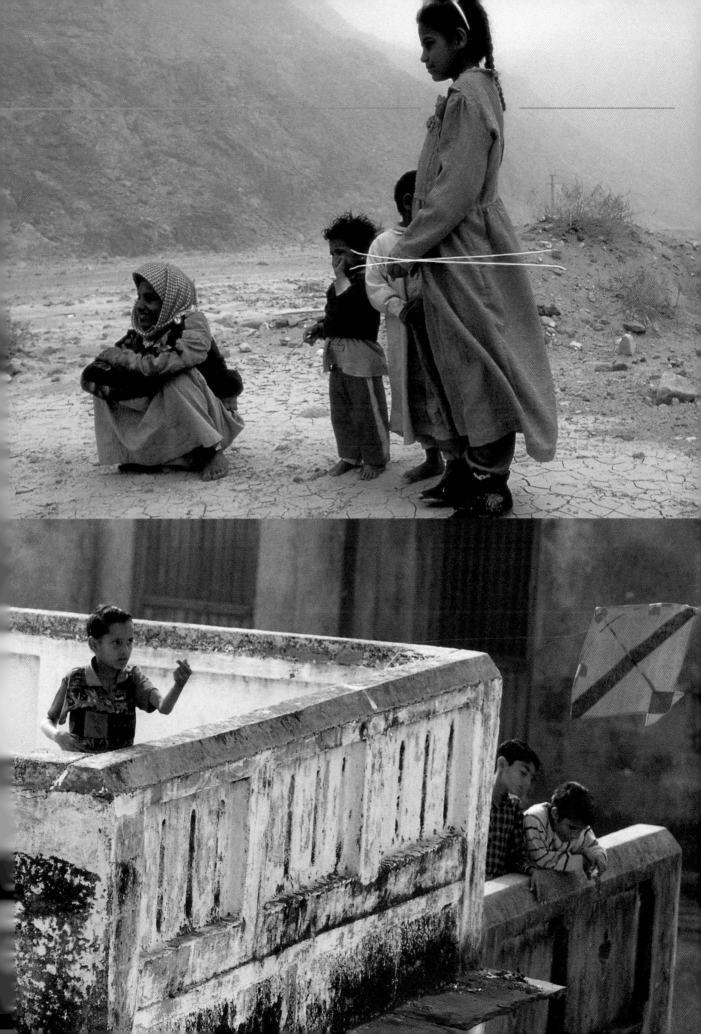

Afghanistan

A Country at War with Itself

Mountains and deserts
Afghanistan, a land of great mountains and scorching desert, is in the heart of Central Asia. The climate is harsh with hot, dry summers and bitterly cold winters.

Invasions and war
Fierce battles have been fought in Afghanistan for hundreds of years. The Persians, ancient Greeks, Mongols, Turks and, much later, the British and the Soviets, have all invaded Afghanistan. To make matters worse, there has always been fighting between the many different tribes in the country.

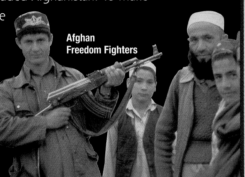

Afghan Freedom Fighters

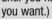

Fact file

Area: 251,825 sq. mi. (a little more than twice the size of the British Isles)

Population: 22,720,416

Capital: Kabul

Religion: Islam

Languages: Pushto; Dari

Chief exports: Carpets; fruit; cotton; gemstones; opium

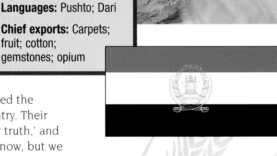

In 1978, the Soviet Union invaded Afghanistan and millions of Afghans fled to Iran and Pakistan. In 1988, the Soviets withdrew their forces.

No peace
"Why don't we have peace? What's it like to live without fighting?" Saud asked his father.

"Unfortunately, I don't know what that's like either," his father replied. "The most recent fighting started when the Communists came. We fought a *jihad* against them."

"What's a *jihad*?" asked Saud.

"It's a holy war that we as Muslims fight to defend our country against people who don't worship Allah. Many of us became *mujahidin* guerrillas to get rid of the Communists. A guerrilla fights for a special cause against the government, and a *mujahidin* guerrilla fights for the cause of Islam," his father told him. "Our *jihad* was successful, and the Communists left in 1989. But each group of

mujahidin wanted to have all the power. So the fighting went on.

Then, in 1996, a group called the Taliban took over the country. Their name means 'seekers after truth,' and there's much less fighting now, but we have to follow lots of very strict Islamic rules."

"That's why girls aren't allowed to go to school, isn't it?" Saud asked. "Someone said that in the boys' school we have to spend a lot more time studying the Koran than they used to. I can't go up to the next class unless I pass my Islamic exams."

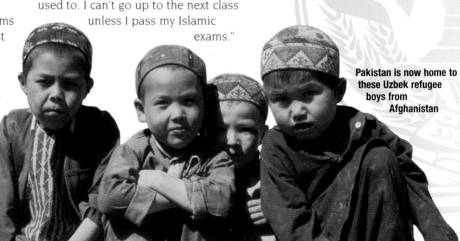

Pakistan is now home to these Uzbek refugee boys from Afghanistan

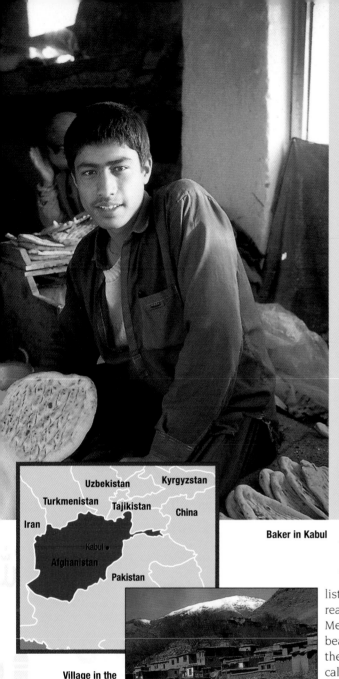

You can read more about the Hazara and Uzbek people on pages 76 and 174

To help you pray for Afghanistan

You can thank God for:

- the secret believers in Afghanistan.
- the New Testaments translated into Pushto and Dari.
- the aid workers caring for those who are injured, blind, poor, sick and needy.

You can ask God:

- to bring peace to this war-torn land.
- to help and protect those who are translating the Scriptures into other languages spoken in Afghanistan.
- to give understanding to people who listen to Christian radio broadcasts, often in secret, so that they can know Jesus and the peace he brings.
- that the different groups who are fighting for power will realize that they are destroying both their country and their people.

Baker in Kabul

Village in the mountains

"Yes, the Taliban have changed what you have to study and they closed all the girls' schools in Kabul. And it's because of the Taliban that your mother can't work or go out without covering herself with a *chaderi*. She also has to have one of the men from our family with her wherever she goes. Women whose husbands and sons have died in the fighting often don't have enough money to buy food for their children," Saud's father explained. "If we kept strictly to all the rules we wouldn't watch television, listen to music or read foreign books. Men have to grow beards and wear these long shirts, called *shalwar kamiz*, over baggy trousers. Your little sister isn't even supposed to play with dolls or teddies because they look like living beings."

Help for victims of war

Six-year-old Ramazan saw a truck loaded with sacks of wheat coming down the street. He ran to gather a few grains that had trickled out from a hole in one of the sacks. He was all alone. His parents and brother had been killed when a mortar shell destroyed their house.

There are many children like Ramazan. Aid workers from around the world are working in Afghanistan to help the poor, orphans and sick and hungry children, as well as those who have been blinded or badly injured during the 20 years of war.

God answers prayer

Ten days after being burnt in an accident, Hyerloh's feet were blistered and infected, and they felt like they were still on fire. An aid worker stopped when she heard him cry out from his father's shop, "Please help me!" She didn't have any medicine, but she prayed that God would heal his feet.

Three weeks later, she saw Hyerloh again. "Look! look!" he exclaimed. "My feet are all better!" There was no sign that they had been so badly burned.

"That's wonderful! Let's thank God for answering our prayers and healing you," the lady said to Hyerloh. She told him about Jesus, God's son, who loved him and had healed many people while he lived on earth.

Albania

God Answers Prayer

One of Europe's poorest countries

The Albanians call their country Shqiperi, "the land of the eagle," and they have a double-headed eagle on their flag. That's not surprising, because if you climbed the rugged mountains in Albania you would see many eagles circling overhead.

Albania has many natural resources, including chrome, oil, natural gas, copper and iron – so it could be a rich country. But it's actually one of Europe's poorest countries. How could this be?

Selling peppers in the market

Italy

Yugoslavia

Macedonia

• Tirane

Albania

Greece

Dark days

In 1944 Albania became a Communist country. For the next 41 years a man called Enver Hoxha ruled Albania. He didn't allow Albanians to travel abroad or have things like cars and fridges. He forced them to live with very little food and few supplies. People couldn't worship in mosques or churches, say prayers or own Muslim or Christian books. Parents were even forbidden to give their children Muslim or Christian names.

God's people all around the world heard about the sad situation there, but they weren't allowed to go to Albania, so they prayed. And, after many years of praying, in 1991 the Communist government was forced to resign. Immediately people from other countries were ready to take supplies into Albania. Christians were ready, too, to share Jesus' love with the

people of Albania.

They were shocked to discover the terrible conditions in which many Albanians were living. Hospitals were poorly equipped and had no medicines. The people often didn't have enough money to buy food for their families. Sad, starving children filled orphanages and children's homes, with very few people to care for them.

Sometimes aid workers felt like they were stepping back in time. Out in the countryside villages had no electricity or running water. In Tirana, the capital, there were more donkey carts and bicycles than cars.

God's light

The new government allowed Christians and Muslims to worship and speak about their beliefs. Before the Communists came to power, Albania

Fact file

Area: 11,100 sq. mi.

Population: 3,113,434

Capital: Tirana

Language: Modern Albanian

Religion: Islam

Chief exports: Iron ore; petroleum; fruit; vegetables

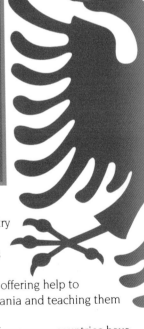

was the only Muslim country in Europe. Now Muslims from other countries are offering help to people in Albania and teaching them about Islam.

Christians from many countries have helped care for children in orphanages and shared the good news and hope of Jesus with many Albanians. Now there are several thousand Albanians, mainly young people, who follow Jesus.

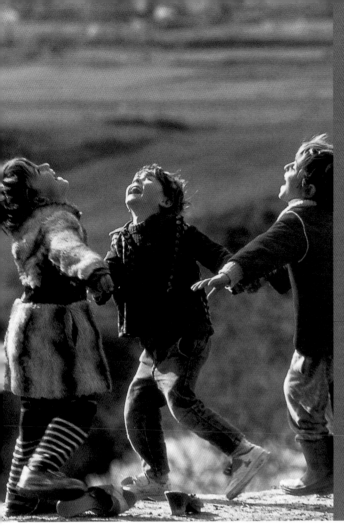

To help you pray for Albania

You can thank God for:

- each Albanian boy, girl and grownup who follows Jesus.
- the way that Albanian Christians, even though they are poor themselves, showed his kindness and love to the refugees from Kosovo by helping and caring for them.

You can ask God:

- to encourage all Christians to learn more about him and to share his love with everyone.
- to teach Christians that even though many of them are poor, he blesses all those who give to others.
- to help Christian workers get jobs for the refugees so that they will have enough money to care for their families.
- to give his strength to leaders in the churches as they teach people from the Bible and encourage them to follow Jesus.
- to bring peace and hope to the people of Albania and give them leaders who will rule the country wisely and fairly.

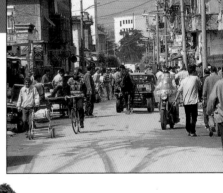

Street in Tirana, the capital of Albania

You can speak Albanian

Hello is "Tungjatjeta" (toon-jat-yeta)

How are you? is "Se jeni?" (see-yenee)

Where are you going? is "Ku po shkoni?" (koo-paw-shkawnee)

Goodbye is "Mirupafshim" (meer-oo-pafsheem)

Showing God's love

Although they were very poor themselves, the Albanian Christians wanted to help these refugees. In Tirana, the churches gave them food, water, clothing and love. Other Christians provided homes for mothers with young babies.

Niki and his family were refugees. Niki had been born with a hole in his heart and the journey from Kosovo had made him very weak. He had to be carried everywhere. Christians caring for Niki and his family prayed that God would work a miracle and send help for him. One day, there was a fax from the International Red Cross. "Bring Niki to Tirana tomorrow," it said. "We've found a group who will pay for his medical treatment." Two days later Niki had a successful operation in Paris. God answered prayers for Niki's physical heart to be healed. With Jesus in their hearts, Niki and his family will live forever.

More dark days

In 1997, thousands of Albanians lost all their money and blamed the government. People lost their homes and belongings. There was so much crime that thousands of people fled the country. Many Christian workers also had to leave Albania for a while.

A year later war broke out in Kosovo, a province of nearby Yugoslavia. Although the Serbs claimed Kosovo for themselves, most of the people living there are Albanians. The Serbs killed hundreds of Kosovar Albanians and destroyed their homes. Thousands of them fled into Albania to escape.

Collecting water with a donkey

Azeri

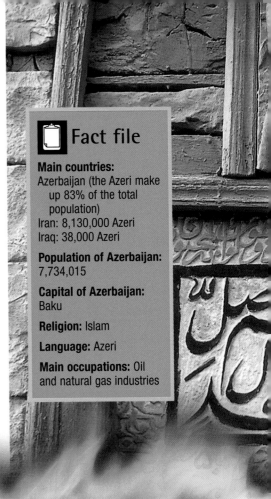

The Fire Guardians

Farzali lives in the city of Baku, the capital of a country on the Caspian Sea called Azerbaijan. His people, the Azeri, are Muslims. A people called the Armenians, who have a Christian background, also live in Azerbaijan. During the 1990s there was fighting between the Azeri and the Armenians, and many Armenians left the country.

Are we Muslims?
Farzali was excited when his friend Babeli invited him to come to his house after school. "I'll ask my mother, but I'm sure I can come," he said. "I'm so glad there isn't any more fighting with the Armenians. I used to get so scared, and my mother never let me go anywhere without my big brother!"

📋 Fact file

Main countries:
Azerbaijan (the Azeri make up 83% of the total population)
Iran: 8,130,000 Azeri
Iraq: 38,000 Azeri

Population of Azerbaijan: 7,734,015

Capital of Azerbaijan: Baku

Religion: Islam

Language: Azeri

Main occupations: Oil and natural gas industries

Do you know?

- Before oil was discovered in the Gulf States, more than half the world's oil supplies came from oil fields near Baku.

- The people of Azerbaijan built the first oil tanker in the world and the first oil pipeline (which was made of wood).

- Natural gas leaks from the earth in Azerbaijan, causing fires that burn spontaneously.

- Azerbaijan was once a republic of the old Soviet Union and is now a member of the Commonwealth of Independent States.

Babeli nodded. "My mother was the same. I loved going to Samweli's house to play, but she never wanted me to go because his family was Armenian. She said they would try to make me a Christian. Samweli and his family had to go to live in Armenia when the fighting got really bad. I miss him. Do you think it's so bad to be a Christian?"

Farzali frowned. "I think it would be terrible. My great-grandfather says it's unforgivable for an Azeri to become a Christian."

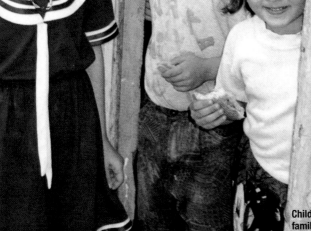

Children from a Christian family

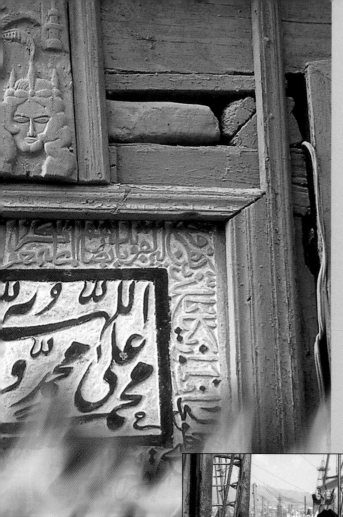

![hand icon]

To help you pray for the Azeri

You can thank God for:

- the fact that the fighting has stopped between the Azeri and the Armenians.
- the few Azeri Christians.
- the New Testament and children's Bible in their language.

You can ask God:

- to send Christians to Azerbaijan to teach what the Bible says.
- to show the Azeri people that only Jesus can give them the holiness and purity they want so much.
- to help the Christians planning Azeri radio broadcasts to answer the questions Azeri people have about Jesus.
- to bring Azeri to believe in Jesus.

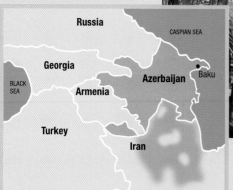

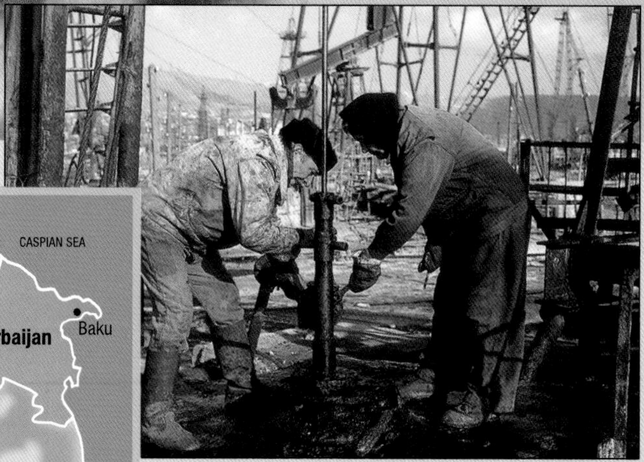

Map showing Russia, Georgia, Armenia, Azerbaijan, Baku, Turkey, Iran, Black Sea, Caspian Sea

Workers on an oil field in Azerbaijan

Fire guardians

The ancient Greeks called the Azeri "fire guardians" because they worshipped fire. Farzali's cousin even wore a fire-red dress on her wedding day. Farzali was confused and wondered which was true – the old Azeri religion, Islam or the Christian religion? He knew they couldn't all be true.

Clean and pure

Azeri want to be made clean and pure, but only Jesus can do that for them. Few Azeri people have heard about Jesus, but now the New Testament and a children's Bible have been printed in their language, and they can listen to Christian radio. Now is the time to pray that Jesus will take away Farzali's confusion.

"Why do they make such a big fuss?" Babeli asked. "My family all say we're Muslims, but we never go to the mosque."

Farzali wasn't sure if his family were Muslims or not. His great-grandfather certainly was, and he read the Koran every evening. But his father never read it. He was more concerned about politics and money. He said that the government was rich because of all the oil, but most of the people were still poor.

The next day, Farzali went with his father and great-grandfather to visit his uncle's farm. Farzali loved his great-grandfather. He was over 100 years old, but he was still very strong.

Farzali's uncle told them, "Today is a special day when we speak with our ancestors and bathe in the river that flows from the mountains. Before the Azeri became Muslims we worshipped fire and our ancestors. A few of us still keep some of these ancient ceremonies."

Farzali bathed in the river. Even great-grandfather lowered himself into the cold water. Farzali wondered if he really was in touch with his ancestors.

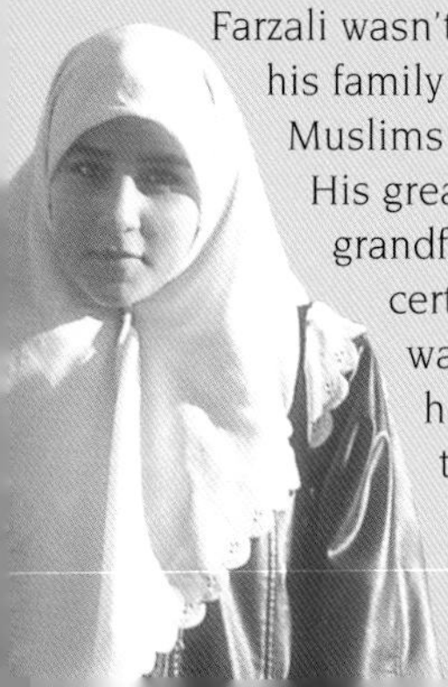

Muslim schoolgirls in Azerbaijan

Balinese

From the Island of the Gods

A beautiful island

Anne thought Bali was the most beautiful place she'd ever seen. It had sandy beaches, brightly colored flowers, rice fields of green and gold and thousands of temples. She could see the mountains in the distance – some of them were volcanoes. She had even seen a performance of the graceful legong dances, which tell the stories of gods and demons, witches and kidnapped princesses. The dancers had worn dresses of gold, scarlet and green, with headdresses glittering with gold and bright, tropical flowers on their shiny black hair. And all the Balinese people she'd met had such gentle, smiling faces.

It's no wonder that more than 1,500,000 tourists visit Bali, a small island in the long necklace of Indonesian islands, each year. Visitors often call it "the island of the gods" or "the last paradise."

Invitation to the gods

There are thousands of temples on Bali, because the Balinese are Hindus and worship many gods. The Balinese had many gods long before they became Hindus, and they still worship these gods, too. Every day they give small offerings to the spirits of their ancestors who have died. They believe it's very important to be on their good side.

At the beginning of every year (the year in Bali is only 210 days long), the Balinese hold a special feast for the gods. At this feast they bring their gods out from their shrines and invite them to live in objects made of wood, stone and coins for a while. The people ask the gods to join them in feasting and dancing for ten days. At the end of that time, the gods are put back in their shrines until the next ceremony.

Spirits of the ancestors

The Balinese believe that the spirits of their gods and ancestors live in the mountains. When they build their houses, they make sure that the room with the altar for the spirits faces the mountains.

The Balinese are very concerned about what happens to them when they die. Sometimes a family will save money for several years so they can build an elaborate funeral tower and hold a cremation ceremony.

They believe that the soul of the dead person can't take its place with the spirits of all the other ancestors in the mountains until after such a ceremony.

Jesus' power

There aren't many Balinese Christians yet. Sometimes their Hindu neighbors treat Christians badly because they're afraid that their gods will be angry if people follow Jesus.

Eight-year-old Nyoman was afraid. Some people in the village had done mean things to his family because

Traditional dancers

Bali ● Bedugul
BALINESE
INDIAN OCEAN   Nusa Peneda
Nusa Dua

PACIFIC OCEAN

Philippines

Malaysia

Indonesia

Java

Do you know?

The Balinese have a legend that says that their beautiful island was once flat and nothing would grow there. When the island of Java became Muslim, the Hindu gods moved the short distance to Bali. They needed mountains where they could live, so they created some. Then water from these mountains made the island fertile.

they're Christians. "Why won't they let us have water for our fields? They don't want to have anything to do with us. What did we do wrong?" he asked his parents. "The other kids make fun of me and won't play with me. They even said that some night, when I'm asleep, the gods will come and punish me because I don't follow them."

"Don't be afraid, Nyoman," his father replied. "Jesus has promised that he'll always be with us. He's more powerful than anything or anyone who wants to harm us. People in the village think the gods are angry because we've become Christians. They want us to turn back to our old gods. But we know that with Jesus we don't have to fear their gods. Jesus will look after us even when we're asleep. Let's pray, Nyoman, and ask him to take away your fears."

Christians often try to show Jesus' love to their Hindu neighbors by helping them in practical ways. They want them to know that Christianity isn't a boring religion that belongs to white people, so Christians are beginning to tell Bible stories the Balinese way, through dance and mime.

One by one, Balinese are coming to know Jesus as the friend who is always with them. And those who follow Jesus are praying that many more Balinese will realize Jesus is far greater and more powerful than all the thousands of gods they keep in their shrines and bring out on special occasions.

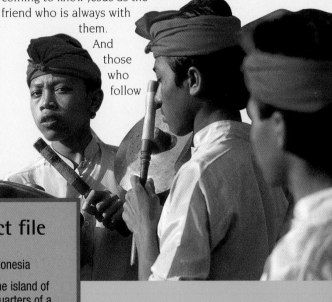

 Fact file

Country: Indonesia

Location: The island of Bali (three-quarters of a mile east of Java)

Numbers: About 2,000,000

Languages: Balinese; Indonesian

Religions: Hinduism; animism

Occupations: Mainly farmers growing rice, maize and coffee; weaving and wood carving

 To help you pray for the Balinese

You can thank God for:

- the Balinese who are coming to know Jesus as their friend.
- the Bible translation in Balinese.
- the groups that are using Balinese-style dance and mime to tell the Christian story.

You can ask God:

- to help Christians show Jesus' love to their Hindu friends and neighbors.
- to show the Balinese that he is so much more powerful than all the gods they worship.
- to help Christians like Nyoman know that evil spirits can't harm them when they trust in Jesus.
- for whole families to come to know Jesus so that children can learn about Jesus when they're young.

Lake temple

Baloch

Carpet Weavers of Pakistan

Fact file

There are about 5 million Baloch.

Three million of them live in Pakistan, with about 1.5 million in Karachi. Others live in Iran, Oman and other Gulf States.

Hard work

Abdullah tossed the freshly cut wheat onto the bullock cart. "Not a bad harvest this year," he thought. He looked over at his grandfather, with his wrinkled face and white beard, wearing his turban and long homespun shirt over baggy trousers. Abdullah knew his grandfather was glad he was there to help, because he couldn't manage the small farm on his own anymore.

Abdullah's father and his brother Ghaus had gone to the city of Karachi to find work. Even though Abdullah was only 12 years old, they left him in charge of doing most of the farm work. It was especially difficult because of the fierce heat in the summer and the bitter cold in the winter.

Warm quilts for sale in the bazaar

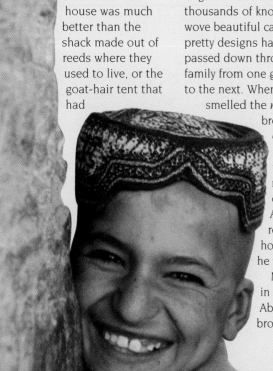

The old bullock plodded into the high-walled courtyard leading to the house Abdullah's father had built. The house was much better than the shack made out of reeds where they used to live, or the goat-hair tent that had been his grandfather's home.

Abdullah's sisters were sitting at the carpet looms, where they worked most of the day. Their nimble fingers had to tie thousands of knots as they wove beautiful carpets. The pretty designs had been passed down through the family from one generation to the next. When he smelled the *nan* (wheat bread) and curry his mother was making for dinner, Abdullah realized how hungry he was.

Meanwhile, in Karachi, Abdullah's brother Ghaus lay half-conscious in the gutter. His father hadn't seen him for months, but he didn't want the rest of the family to know. Every day, as soon as he finished work at his kebab stall on a busy street, he went looking for his son. Like thousands of other young people, Ghaus was taking drugs. His father was afraid that by the time he found him it might be too late to help him.

A rich province … but a needy people

Abdullah's farm is in Balochistan, one of the four provinces in Pakistan. Balochistan has natural gas, copper, iron ore and coal, and there are lots of fish in the sea. But the Baloch people feel that the Pakistan government neglects them. They complain that Pakistan's other provinces use most of Balochistan's natural gas. They desperately need better roads and railways, clean water supplies and good health care and schools. Some Baloch people would like Balochistan to become an independent country.

Because they're poor and feel neglected, lots of Baloch have left the country areas to find work in Karachi or overseas. Since

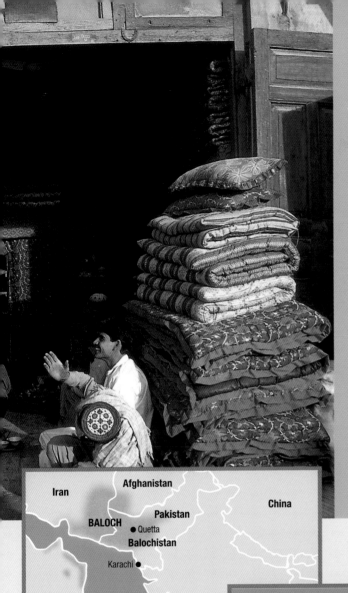

To help you pray for the Baloch

You can thank God for:

● the New Testament in Balochi.

You can ask God:

● for whole Baloch families – women and girls as well as men and boys – to follow Jesus.

● for Christians from other countries to teach reading and provide the Baloch with health care.

● to send caring Christians to reach out to the drug addicts in Karachi and show them that Jesus can help them.

● that the few Baloch Christians will tell others what Jesus has done for them.

● to help the team preparing radio broadcasts.

● that many Baloch will listen to the Christian radio broadcasts.

Iran
Afghanistan
Pakistan
China
BALOCH
● Quetta
Balochistan
Karachi ●
India

Do you know?

A Baloch proverb

"Strong water can flow uphill." (The powerful can do anything.)

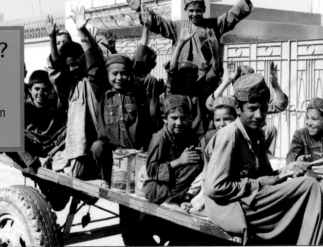

Friendly Baloch boys

there aren't many schools in the mountainous countryside, very few Baloch learn to read.

The Baloch like to listen to programs in their own Baloch language from Radio Quetta (the capital of Balochistan). Some have started to tune in to Christian programs in Baloch and have written to the radio station to find out more about Jesus and what he taught.

The country of Pakistan is strongly Muslim. It's difficult for Christians to get into Balochistan to talk about Jesus, but about 15 young Baloch men have decided to follow Jesus. Christians find that their Baloch friends listen carefully when they explain the Bible to them. And the Baloch now have the New Testament in their own language.

How can Christians help the Baloch? They need jobs, health care and reading lessons. Christians can show Jesus' love by trying to meet some of these needs. God recently healed some sick Baloch when Christians prayed for them. This miracle showed them that Jesus is all-powerful, and they decided to follow him.

21

Bangladesh

One of the Poorest Countries on Earth

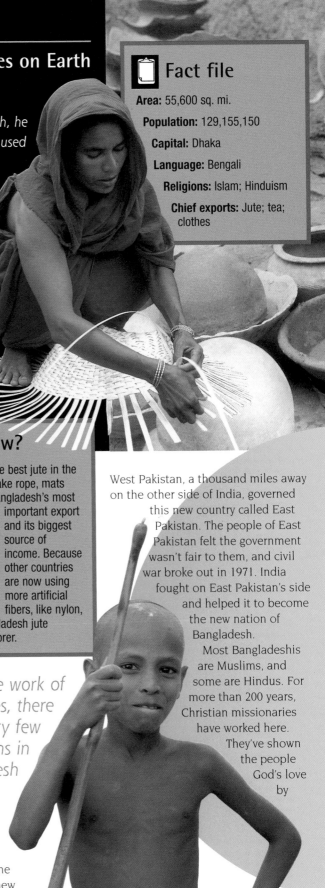

Fact file

Area: 55,600 sq. mi.

Population: 129,155,150

Capital: Dhaka

Language: Bengali

Religions: Islam; Hinduism

Chief exports: Jute; tea; clothes

Homeless

"What are going to do now?" Chandra cried. Scared to death, he sat close to his father on the pile of mud where their house used to be. He held a squawking chicken that was struggling to escape. Aziz, his father, gripped a small basket of rice. That was all they had managed to save when floodwaters from the huge Brahmaputra River, along with pounding rain and strong winds, had destroyed their home.

"We'll start again, somehow," Aziz sighed. "The floods bring fresh soil so we can grow good crops, but the winds and heavy rains destroy everything. They kill people and take our homes and our cattle. Oh, if only I knew what's happened to your mother and little sister. We can only hope they're safe somewhere." Aziz tried to reassure Chandra, fighting back his own tears.

Floods and cyclones

Almost half of Bangladesh is made up of low-lying islands, most of them less than nine feet above sea level. It rains in Bangladesh for about six months every year – from May to October. Every year when the snows on the Himalayan Mountains melt, the water comes rushing down the mighty Ganges, Brahmaputra and Meghna rivers to the ocean. Every year the rivers burst their banks and flood the countryside, bringing fresh soil to the land. Every year homes and fields are washed away, and animals and people die. When a cyclone hits the country, the chaos and destruction are terrible.

It's no wonder that Bangladesh is one of the poorest countries in the world. There are so many rivers, so little land and so many people that it's also one of the most crowded countries on earth. Everyone, from the smallest child to the oldest grandfather, has to work hard just to live.

Do you know?

Bangladesh grows the best jute in the world. It's used to make rope, mats and sacks. Jute is Bangladesh's most important export and its biggest source of income. Because other countries are now using more artificial fibers, like nylon, instead of jute, Bangladesh jute farmers are even poorer.

Despite the work of missionaries, there are still very few Christians in Bangladesh

A new nation

The country we call Bangladesh was once a part of India. In 1947, it became the eastern part of the new Muslim nation of Pakistan.

West Pakistan, a thousand miles away on the other side of India, governed this new country called East Pakistan. The people of East Pakistan felt the government wasn't fair to them, and civil war broke out in 1971. India fought on East Pakistan's side and helped it to become the new nation of Bangladesh.

Most Bangladeshis are Muslims, and some are Hindus. For more than 200 years, Christian missionaries have worked here. They've shown the people God's love by

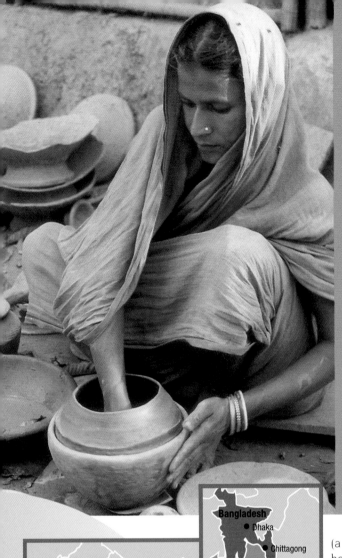

To help you pray for Bangladesh

You can thank God for:

● the work of groups like Tearfund and Tearcraft.

● every Christian who is showing God's love to the people of Bangladesh.

You can ask God:

● to help the leaders of Bangladesh to be honest, wise and fair to both rich and poor people.

● to help Christians show God's love to the people of Bangladesh.

● that every young man and woman studying in Bible school will learn how to teach others about Jesus.

● to bring Christians to care for the many homeless children in Bangladesh.

● that men would have respect for women and stop violence against them.

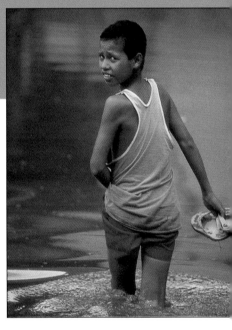

Walking through flood water

Bangladesh
● Dhaka
● Chittagong
BAY OF BENGAL

India
Bangladesh

BAY OF BENGAL

(a part of Tearfund) helps many people there to earn a living. Maybe you've seen some of the beautiful jewelry or carvings from Third World countries like Bangladesh. You may even have bought a jute *sika* or a handmade card for your mother.

In Bangladeshi homes, *sikas* are used like shelves. It's quite easy to make a *sika*, but growing the jute and getting it ready for use is very hard work.

Shaheen and his family grow jute in one of their fields. "It grows in water, like rice," he explains, "but it's much taller than rice. A good crop will grow between nine and 12 feet high. The jute fibers are found inside each stalk.

"When it's time for harvest, the men and boys cut down the heavy stalks and bring them home by boat or ox-cart. The women arrange them in big, round stacks to dry. It smells terrible! When the jute is dry, everyone in the family has to help beat the stalks, until all the fibers come loose. Finally, it has to be spun.

teaching their children, caring for sick people and setting up hospitals and schools. They've done everything possible to help those suffering as a result of the many natural disasters, but there are still very few Bangladeshi Christians.

God uses many ways to help his people

About 25 years ago, a Christian visiting Bangladesh wanted to do something to help the poor people there. He realized that the Bangladeshis could use local materials to make items to sell in other countries. Now Tearcraft

"Christian groups often buy the jute and sell it to village women and girls who make *sikas*, bags and mats. My wife and daughters like making these things, and they're paid for everything they produce. Life has been so much easier since these groups started to help us. Sometimes, when they come to buy the things my family has made, they tell us about God's love and that he sent his Son Jesus to die on a cross for us and be our Savior. It's a wonderful story, and we'd like to know more about Jesus."

Beja

Frightened by the Evil Eye

What about the future?

Amna watched her grandmother carefully. Amna hoped she would be as wise as her grandmother someday. As they sat together on the palm matting outside their wooden house, her grandmother dropped five cowrie shells. She looked closely at the shape they made on the ground. Then she shook her head and scooped them up again.

"What's the matter?" Amna asked anxiously. "What do the shells say?" She knew that her family needed some good luck right now because her older sister, Khadija, was going to be married after the Idd (a Muslim festival). Khadija was worried. She was only 12 years old, and their parents had arranged her marriage to her cousin Ahmed.

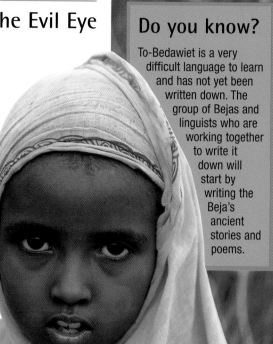

"What's Ahmed like?" Amna asked Khadija, who was sitting behind her on the mat, patiently braiding Amna's frizzy hair. "Have you ever met him?"

"He's been here to talk about our marriage and drink *jabana* (Beja coffee) with our brothers, but I've never met him," Khadija replied. "He must be really old because he's been working for our uncle in Khartoum for a long time. It'll be so strange to go to live with his mother and sisters on the other side of town. I'll be very lonely without you, Amna." After the wedding Khadija had to stay with Ahmed's family, but because of their marriage customs she still wouldn't meet Ahmed face to face for another year.

Sometimes Khadija and Amna sit and listen to the conversation between their brothers. "I don't like it when they talk about the war between the north and south of the country," Amna said. "And I wish our eldest brother didn't have to go away to Eritrea just so he wouldn't get called into the army." Her brothers used a lot of Arabic words, and Amna wished they would just talk in their own language, To-Bedawiet, so she could understand what they were talking about.

Bound by fear

The Beja (*bay-juh*) are a group of tribes living in the eastern part of Africa that borders the Red Sea coast and stretches from southern Egypt through northern Sudan to

Map labels:
Egypt
Saudi Arabia
BEJA
RED SEA
Sudan
AFRICA
Eritrea
Ethiopia

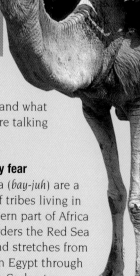

Beja nomad under a *howdah*

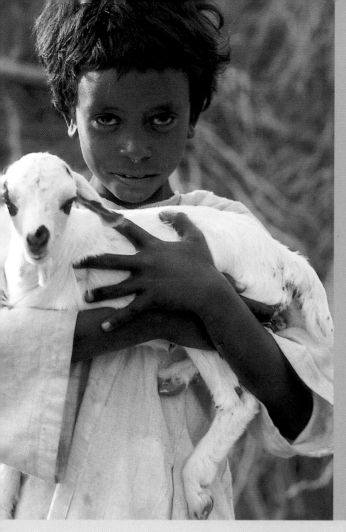

Fact file

Countries: Northern Sudan; southern Egypt; Eritrea

Numbers: About 2,000,000

Occupations: Most are nomadic herdsmen, but many are settling in towns and villages.

Eritrea. There are about two million Beja. They have lived as nomads in this hot, dry, desert land and the windy Red Sea Hills for more than 4,000 years, looking for pasture for their herds of camels, cattle, sheep and goats. But it's a harsh place to live, and now some Beja are settling in the towns and villages. They keep to themselves and don't easily make friends with strangers.

The Beja are Muslims, but few of them really understand the Muslim faith or pray and fast according to the Muslim law. They're afraid of the evil eye and *jinns* (evil spirits) which, they believe, want to harm them. Life is very hard for the Beja because of their fear and superstition, as well as drought, famine and war.

Only a few Beja people have ever become Christians. In 1978, some Christian missionaries were given permission to bring medical care to the Beja. The Beja didn't want the missionaries to be there, and the local Beja leaders forced them to leave. The missionary team started to work in another area, but they were forced to leave again.

Grinding *dura* (sorghum)

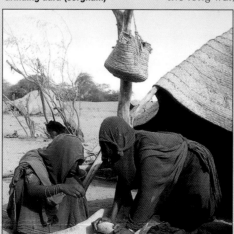

A new friend

One day, as she was buying milk from the donkey man, Amna made a new friend. Nora came from a place hundreds of miles away, in the south of Sudan. Her father had been killed in the long war, and now she helped her mother selling tea by the roadside. They needed to earn money to buy food for the family and pay for her brothers to go to school.

Amna missed her sister so much that she was especially glad to have a new friend. "Nora," she asked, "what do the shells say about your future? Will you have to get married soon? Will our brothers be safe?"

Nora squeezed her hand. "Amna, please don't worry. God loves us all, and we can trust him to take care of us. We don't have to be worried and scared of the spirits all of the time. You're my friend, and I want you to know Jesus, who's my best friend."

Jesus died for the Beja as well as for you and me. Will the Beja listen to the message God wants them to hear? Will they ever know Jesus as their friend? Your prayers can help make this happen!

25

Bhutan

Land of the Thunder Dragon

The thunder dragon

Sangay had been looking forward to going to his first Buddhist festival, but now that he was finally there he was scared. Monks were dancing around wearing big ugly masks with bulging eyes and sharp teeth, and he didn't want them to get too close.

"Why is there a picture of a fire-breathing dragon on the flag and on the temple walls?" he asked.
Sangay's mother told him the story of the thunder dragon. "Have you heard the dragon roar when there's a storm?" she asked. "A very long time ago, there was a monk who wanted to build a monastery. When he found a good place to build this monastery, he heard thunder. He thought the thunder was a dragon roaring, so he named his monastery Druk, which means 'Thunder Dragon.' So our country is called Druk Yul, 'the Land of the Thunder Dragon,' and we are called Drukpas, 'the dragon people.'"

Sangay's parents are farmers. Because the land is covered with mountains and hills, they grow their rice and wheat in special terraced fields, which are flat areas built into the sides of the hills. Sangay helps his parents in the fields and with their goats. Sangay's big brother lives away from home in a town where he goes to school. Sangay would like to go to school with his brother, but it would cost too much money for them both to go. So Sangay stays home to help on the farm and is learning to read and write at a small school in the local monastery.

Snow leopards and festivals

Bhutan, the land of the Thunder Dragon, is a small country between China and India in the Himalaya mountains. The southern part of Bhutan is warm and humid, while in the northern part it's very cold. The Himalayas are the

highest mountains in the world, and snow and ice always cover them. In the valleys between the mountains there are forests and mighty rivers. Black bears, tigers, red pandas and snow leopards are just a few of the rare animals found in Bhutan.

Fact file

Area: 18,200 sq. mi.

Population: 2,123,970

Capital: Thimphu

Language: Dzongkha

Religion: Buddhism

Chief export: Timber

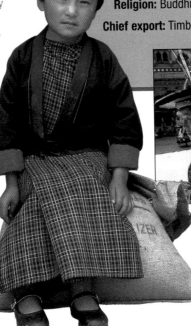

Dancers at a festival

Bhutan is a Buddhist kingdom, and the colorful temple festivals are important occasions

26

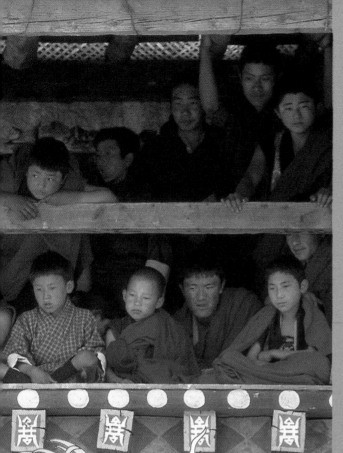

 To help you pray for Bhutan

You can thank God for:

- Christians from other countries who work in Bhutan.
- Christian parents and teachers who tell children about God's love and teach them how to be like Jesus.
- the people who are translating the New Testament into Dzongkha and other languages spoken in Bhutan.

You can ask God:

- to lead children who are sent to study in Christian schools in India to know Jesus.
- to bring Bhutanese students studying in other countries to meet Christians who will share the good news about Jesus with them.
- to give Christians in Bhutan the courage to share God's love with others.
- to help the people and leaders to be able to adjust to new ways.

Young Buddhist monks watching a festival performance

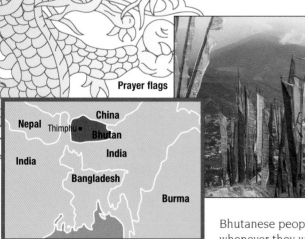

Prayer flags

Nepal
China
Thimphu
Bhutan
India
India
Bangladesh
Burma

Since Bhutan is a Buddhist kingdom, religion, culture and traditions play a big part in the peoples' lives. Buddhist religious ceremonies are held for every occasion.

Although it seems very strange to us, some men in Bhutan have several wives and some women have several husbands. The king of Bhutan, Jigme Singya Wangchuck, married four sisters on the same day. The Bhutanese people can visit the king whenever they want to, to ask him a question or talk with him. About 30 people go to see him each day. The king wears a knee-length tunic called the *kho*. All Bhutanese men must also wear the *kho* whenever they leave the house. The women wear the *kira*, a dress made from one piece of cloth with a wide belt and fastened at the shoulders.

Talking about Jesus

When the king saw the crime and other bad things happening around the world, he decided to try to protect his people from these things. So he let the people in Bhutan watch videos and listen to the radio, but no one was allowed to watch television until 1999. The king realized that what we watch and listen to affects the things we do, the way we treat other people and the way we think.

It's very expensive to travel in Bhutan, and only a few people are allowed to visit the country each year. Experts from other countries help Bhutan with medical care, farming and engineering. Some of these people that come to help are Christians, but they aren't allowed to talk to others about their faith in Jesus. No one knows how many Christians there are in Bhutan, but many people pray for Bhutan and we can see how God is answering those prayers. In the southern part of the country there are small groups of Christians. In Thimphu, the capital, there are house churches where people meet together secretly.

Bijago

Who Believe in a Great Spirit who Punishes Them

Temples and idols

The Bijagos Islands belong to Guinea-Bissau, a small West African country. The islands, with their white, sandy beaches, palm trees and brightly colored birds, are very beautiful. But the Bijago people are very poor. Many live in round houses made of mud with thatched roofs that are very dark inside. Since they can't grow good crops, they don't get enough to eat and they're sick most of the time, and their cattle are very weak.

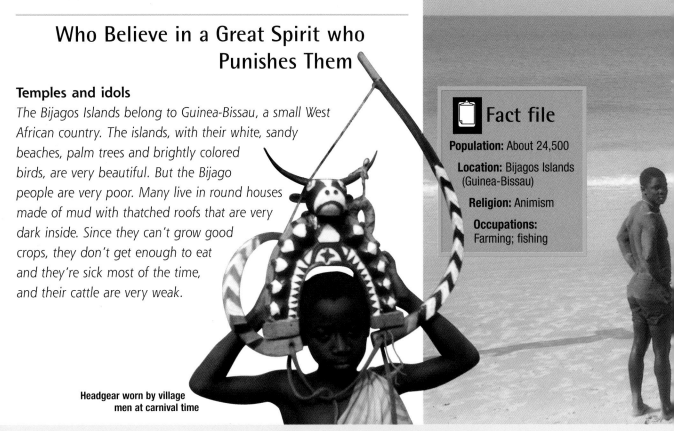

Headgear worn by village men at carnival time

The Bijago are animists. They believe in a Great Spirit who made them but who won't help them and sends punishment and disaster instead. They build temples of mud and thatch with altars in the middle surrounded by the fetishes and carved idols that the people worship. The Bijago are afraid of the *iran* (evil spirits) and hope that if they sacrifice animals and perform special ceremonies, these spirits won't harm them.

Moving house … again!

"Why do we have to move to the island of Rubane every single rainy season?" Carlos complained. "Why can't we live here all the time? Why do we have to sacrifice an animal before we cut down the forest to make our fields? And why do we have

to go there to plant our rice anyway?"

Carlos stood beside his father, asking question after question. His father had sharpened his *machete*, a big broad knife, and now he was catching the chickens and putting them into a woven palm-branch basket. Carlos glanced across at his mother. She was collecting all the pots and pans, the kerosene lamp, her grass skirts and everything else the family would need for the next six months. Everyone in the village was busy packing their belongings and gathering everything from their babies to their pigs and chickens.

"It's our custom, Carlos," his father said. "Rubane is a sacred place belonging to our village. The *iran* won't let us build our homes there, and they'll send

Do you know?

A Bijago woman chooses the man she wants to be her husband and proposes to him by giving him food. She builds a house and then invites him to live with her there.

You can speak Bijago

Hello (a greeting that means "You have got up!") is "Mensuxuque" (men-soots-ook-e)

Hello (the reply, which means "Yes, I have got up!") is "Ee nhensuxuque" (ee nee-en-soots-ook-e)

Goodbye is "Tosoxa" (toe-soets-a)

trouble and sickness to our village if anyone dies there. That's why the witch doctor sacrifices an animal even before we start to cut down the forest. Don't you

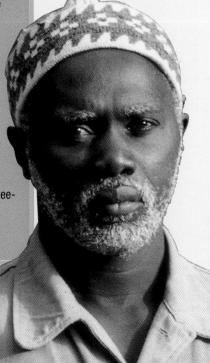

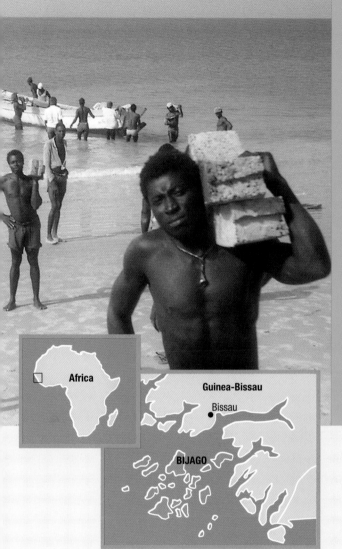

Africa

Guinea-Bissau

Bissau

BIJAGO

To help you pray for the Bijago

You can thank God for:

- the Bijago Christians.
- the Bible translated into Bijago.
- the practical help that organizations like Tearfund have given to the Bijago.

You can ask God:

- to help the Bijago pastors and evangelists as they teach their people that he is far greater and stronger than the *iran*.
- to bring more pastors and evangelists to travel from island to island, teaching the people about Jesus.
- for Sunday school teachers to help children to know and follow Jesus.
- to help Bijago students at Bible school.

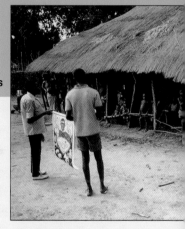

Telling people about Jesus

remember that he gave us a piece of the meat to cook in the part of the forest where we made our fields last year? We call that 'paying the ground.' The *iran* will definitely harm us if we don't do that."

The port was a very noisy place that day. People scrambled to find places for themselves and their belongings in the small dugout canoes that they would paddle across to Rubane Island. Before long, the village was deserted.

They wouldn't be back for another six months.

Jesus helps a whole village!

Forty years ago, the village of Ancarave, on the island of Uno, was just like any other Bijago village. People and animals were sick. They got their water for drinking, cooking and washing from a dirty, slimy pool.

The witch doctors made offerings to the *iran*, but nothing improved. One day some Christian visitors came to the island. "You don't have to be afraid of the *iran*," they told the people. "The priests and witch doctors make sacrifices, but you still get sick and don't have enough

to eat. Your children and animals still die. God is far more powerful than any of the *iran*. He loves you so much that he sent his only Son, Jesus, as a sacrifice for you – so that you never have to make sacrifices again. If you trust in Jesus, he'll help you." Some of the people began to follow Jesus, but the village chief was afraid, so he went on following the *iran*.

These Christians translated the Bible into the Bijago language and, in 1973, Tearfund helped them dig a well. The people could hardly believe what a difference having clean, fresh water made. The village chief began to understand that Christians dug the well, but it was really God who had helped them. He became a Christian and burned all his

idols. The Bijago Christians danced and sang for joy. Other villages saw what Jesus had done for the people of Ancarave and wanted to follow him, too. Now there are Christians on other islands as well.

When civil war broke out in Guinea-Bissau in 1998, many Bijago who lived on the mainland returned to the islands. Some were strong Christians who helped lead the churches, but the Bijago still need more evangelists and pastors who will live among them and teach them about God's love.

Bulgaria

Dreams, Miracles and Life-giving Water

Fact file

Area: 42,800 sq. mi.

Population: 8,225,045

Capital: Sofia

Official language: Bulgarian

Religions: Eastern Orthodox Christianity; Islam

Chief exports: Machinery; food; wine; shoes; iron; steel; textiles

Christians

If you looked at a map, you would find Bulgaria in the southeast corner of Europe – beside the Black Sea. If you looked in a history book, you would read that Bulgaria was a Communist country from 1944 until 1989. If you asked a pastor in Bulgaria, he would tell you what it was like during those years when the government tried to stop people from going to church. He might even tell you that he was put in prison.

"Then what happened?" you ask.

"Well," the pastor says, "when the Communists stopped controlling the government, we hoped we'd be free to worship God. But this didn't last long.

"Most Bulgarians belong to the Eastern Orthodox Church, and the new socialist government decided that this was the religion of Bulgaria. They said that all other Christian churches were sects.

"We've tried to help the poor and care for orphans and the sick and elderly. We run camps for children and give food to the hungry. But people have accused some of our workers of wrongdoing and vandalized our churches. We have to remind ourselves that we're doing this to show Jesus' love and not get discouraged."

Muslims

If you asked one of the million and a quarter Muslims living in Bulgaria about his country, he would tell about their suffering, too. "The Communist government closed most of our mosques. We weren't allowed to wear our traditional clothes or use Muslim names – which we'd been doing for a long time before the Communists ever arrived!

"Many Bulgarian Turks and Gypsies are also Muslims. They are often very poor and live in crowded slums. It's hard for them to find work. Many of the schools are closed now, but even before that lots of Muslim children had stopped going to school because their parents couldn't buy them clothes or books. They said it wasn't worth going because there wouldn't be jobs for them when they'd finished. It's sad to see children with no hope for the future."

God has used dreams and miracles to teach the people about Jesus

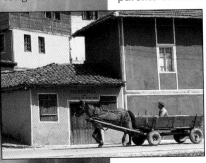

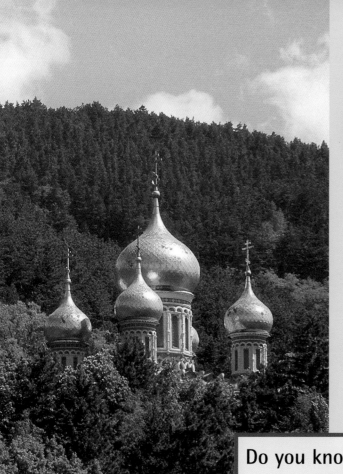

To help you pray for Bulgaria

You can thank God for:

- each person in Bulgaria who follows Jesus.
- the dreams and miracles that help people understand who he is.
- Scripture Union, Child Evangelism Fellowship and other groups working with children.

You can ask God:

- to show Muslim Turks that they can follow Jesus and still be Turkish.
- to help the different people groups love, understand and respect each other.
- to show churches and Christian groups how to work together.
- for church leaders and pastors to have good Bible training.

Children in national costume

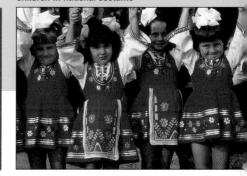

Do you know?

Bulgarian Turks now have a Turkish New Testament written in the Cyrillic (Russian-style) alphabet. For example, the Turkish word for child, which is "çocuk" (*chaw-juk*) in our alphabet, would be "уодужк" in Cyrillic. And the word for girl is "kiz" (*kerz*), or "къз."

Dreams

Ahmed is a Bulgarian Turk who was taught that it was important to serve Allah. So he learned to read Arabic and studied the Koran, where he read about Jesus. When he was about 11 years old, Ahmed had a dream about Jesus.

"God and Jesus came to my house," he remembers. "Jesus offered me a jar of water, but I wouldn't take it until he promised he would never leave me."

Then, when Ahmed was about 20, a man gave him an old Turkish Bible. Ahmed read it, but he didn't really understand it. So he wrote to the man who had given him the Bible. The man came to see Ahmed, but he wasn't a Christian so he couldn't explain what the Bible meant.

"I wanted to know about Jesus, but no one could help me," Ahmed said. "Then I prayed and opened my Bible. I read the story in John 4 about the Samaritan woman who met Jesus at the well. He offered her life-giving water. I finally understood my dream from all those years ago. From then on, I knew what it was like not to be thirsty inside, and I followed Jesus."

Asking for water: A miracle!

Güngüler (*gyoon-gyoo-lezh*) is a Gypsy girl who lives with her family in a city slum in Bulgaria. Every day she has to clean and cook and look after her little brother and sister while her mother goes out to work. Güngüler was born dumb and couldn't speak a word for the first nine years of her life. Her Muslim family often prayed to Allah and took her to Muslim teachers to heal her, but Güngüler still couldn't talk.

When some Christians visited the slum where Güngüler lived, she squeezed into the crowded room and listened to their stories about Jesus healing the blind, the deaf and the dumb. She wondered if Jesus could heal even her. The Christians prayed for Güngüler, and God worked a miracle. For the first time in her life, Güngüler spoke. "May I please have a drink of water?" she asked.

Her mother couldn't believe her ears when Güngüler ran up to her, calling, "I can talk! Jesus healed me!" Her whole family were amazed and filled with joy. They wanted to learn all about this God who had healed Güngüler, and they decided to follow Jesus as well.

Although God doesn't always perform miracles when we pray, miracles do show people who don't know God how powerful and loving he is. All around the country, Bulgarians, Turks and Gypsies are coming to know Jesus as their friend. But they don't always understand the Bible well enough to put what it says into practice in their lives.

Buryat

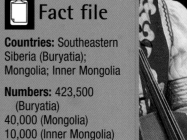

Buddhists in Siberia

Punishment for sin

"What a great film!" Bator exclaimed. "I've never seen anything like it. Do you think it's true that God loves everyone so much that he sent his only Son to earth? Imagine sending him as a baby!"

"I couldn't believe how good Jesus was. I wish I could be like that, never doing anything wrong," said Temudjin. "And he was so smart, too. I was really sad when they put him on that cross. What if he really did die to take the punishment for our sins so that we can be clean before God?"

Bator and Temudjin sat on a bench outside a Buddhist temple. Brightly-colored prayer flags fluttered over the monastery, and the boys could hear the sound of gongs and the monks chanting inside the temple.

Prayer flags

Temudjin let his prayer beads slip, one by one, through his fingers. Earlier that morning he and his uncle had gone to the temple and set the prayer wheels spinning. "It's so different from Buddhism," Temudjin said. "My uncle says if we do bad things we have to be punished for our own sins. And we have to go on suffering for them each time we're reborn."

"Well, I'm going to read the book about Jesus that the teacher gave me," said Bator. "I want to know more about him. Come on – I'll race you home!"

A page from history

Bator and Temudjin are Buryats (*boor-yahts'*). They live in Buryatia (*boor-yaht'-ee-yah*), in southeastern Siberia. For hundreds of years the Buryats were nomads, breeding horses and cattle in the wide valleys between the forest-covered mountains. Several centuries ago Buryats, particularly those living to the east of Lake Baikal, became Buddhists. But they kept many of their old animistic beliefs as well. Buryat boys went to school at the Buddhist monasteries, and many of them became monks.

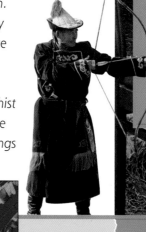

All this changed after the Russian Revolution. By the end of the 1930s, the Communists had forced the Buryats to settle in villages and had set up government-run schools for the children. They closed the monasteries and the people were no longer allowed to be Buddhists. They even destroyed a lot of their shrines and religious books.

There were more changes in 1989, when the Communists lost power.

Buddhist monastery

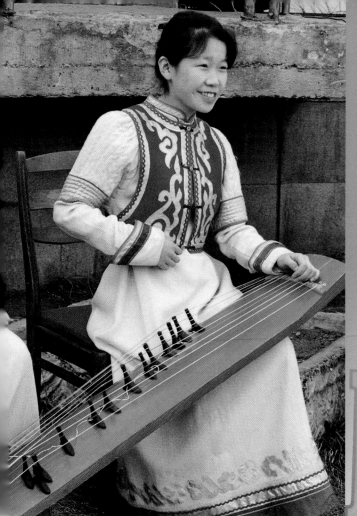

 To help you pray for the Buryat

You can thank God for:

● Buryats in Buryatia and Mongolia who follow Jesus.

● the translation of the New Testament into Buryat.

You can ask God:

● to show Buryats that only Jesus can take away sin and give them eternal life.

● for Christians helping in schools, farming and health care to show the Buryats how much God loves them.

● to show the Buryats that the Dalai Lama is not God, but only a man.

● that many Buryats will choose to follow Jesus.

● that Christians will pray for the Buryats to know Jesus.

Poster for *Jesus* film in Ulan Ude

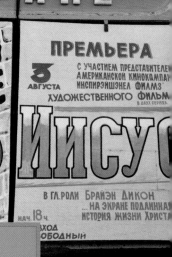

Then, in 1991, the Dalai Lama, the Buddhists' spiritual leader, was allowed to visit Ulan Ude, the capital of Buryatia. He told the people to put all the years of atheistic Communism behind them and return to their Buddhist beliefs. Many Buryats have done just that, and now a lot of Buddhist monks are trained there to take the message of Buddhism around the world.

Another page from history

In 1817, the tsar (king) of Russia gave three English missionaries permission to travel to Siberia. He even gave them land and money to help them in their work among the Buryats. "Why do you want to help the Buryats? We certainly don't think much of them!" said

the Russians living in the region. The Buryats also wondered why the missionaries had come, and only 20 of them ever became Christians. Those missionaries translated the whole Bible into the Buryat language. Since then the Buryat script has been changed several times, and now no one can read their translation.

Then, in 1841, the tsar said that the missionaries had to leave. The Russian Orthodox Church set up its own mission to the Buryats and built churches, but there were still very few Buryat Christians.

A presentation to guests

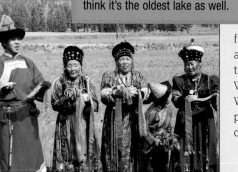

Today

Today a few more Buryats, in all the countries where they live, are following Jesus, who died to take away their sins. The *Jesus* film has been shown in a lot of places and some people have started work on a new translation of the Bible.

Do you know?

Lake Baikal contains as much water as all the Great Lakes of North America put together, which makes it the biggest freshwater lake in the world. It's also the deepest lake in the world, and experts think it's the oldest lake as well.

What's the future like for young Buryats like Bator and Temudjin? People from different cults, sects and other religions are all trying to get their attention. What will they choose? Who will they follow? Your prayers can help them to decide.

33

Chad

Where the Lake is Drying Up

Too little rain

It hardly ever rains in Chad, so when it does rain little children take off their clothes and run into the streets, laughing and splashing in the puddles. The frogs come out to catch termites and people catch the termites, too – fried termites make a delicious snack!

Lake Chad, in the southwest of the country, used to be much bigger and full of fish. Today, the lake is drying up because so many people and cattle are using the water and there isn't enough rain each year to fill it again.

Fact file

Area: 495,750 sq. mi.

Population: 7,650,980

Capital: N'Djamena

Languages: French (spoken by the educated); Chad Arabic (60%); and 124 other languages

Main religions: Islam; Christianity

Chad is in the middle of north Africa, hundreds of miles from the sea. There are so few roads and so much desert, that it's very hard to get things like food and clothes and farming supplies from other countries. Because of this, as well as civil wars, infertile soil and lack of rain, Chad is one of the poorest countries in the world.

Many tribes and languages

Jill, a missionary in Chad, tells us what it's like to live there. "I learned two different languages when I came here: French and Chad Arabic, which most people know.

But different tribes speak over 100 different languages. So I also learned one of these tribal languages so I could talk to even more people.

"Chad is divided into three parts, just like its flag. In the north there are the cold, windy Tibesti Mountains and the Sahara Desert. In the central part there's dry grassland, which provides food for the camels, goats and sheep of the nomads. The south gets more rain, and cotton and dates grow well there.

"The people in each area are different, too. In the south there are quite a lot of Christians, but in the north and central parts of Chad most people are Muslims or follow their own traditional religions. Many of them wear charms, or little bags with bits of bark, hair or other 'magic' things inside, to protect them from sickness and other troubles. Muslims also wear charms with verses from the Koran inside. When people become Christians, they burn their charms because Jesus is stronger than any other power and they don't need to be afraid any more."

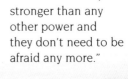

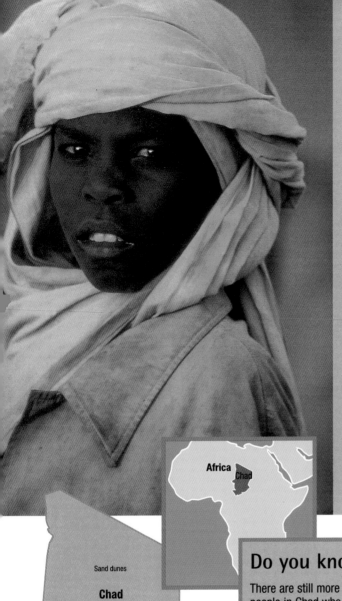

To help you pray for Chad

You can thank God for:

● every missionary who has gone to Chad to tell the people about Jesus' love.

● each Chadian who has decided to follow Jesus.

You can ask God:

● for more missionary doctors, nurses, teachers, Bible translators and farming specialists to go Chad to show people God's love.

● to help the missionaries' children in Chad who sometimes find it hard to live there.

● to remind people to read the Christian booklets and listen to the cassettes they are given and to help them understand who Jesus is.

● to show people in Chad that trusting in their charms will never really help them, but that Jesus promises to help everyone who trusts in him.

● to send enough rain each year so that crops will grow well and the people and their animals will have enough food to eat.

Africa Chad

Sand dunes

Chad

Dry grassland

Thick bush

Chad is divided into three different parts, just like its flag

Mission to Chad

Naomi and her sisters are Dutch and live in N'Djamena, the capital of Chad, with their missionary parents. "We do have a few Chadian friends,"

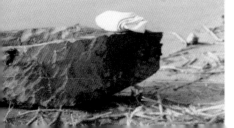

Do you know?

There are still more than 70 groups of people in Chad who don't have any part of the Bible in their own language and who don't have a Christian or missionary living among them. How would you have learned about Jesus if there were no Christians who spoke your language?

Naomi said, "but sometimes other children make fun of us. And we don't like mosquitoes, sandstorms or being sick. But it is fun living in such a different place. None of our Dutch friends can see camels, donkeys and men wearing turbans pass by their houses!

"Some of the missionaries here take care of children in orphanages or sick people. Others are translating the Bible into some of the different languages. There's a special school in N'Djamena where Chadians can learn English, and our parents teach some of them how to make sandals they can sell in the market. We have lots of visitors, and our parents always tell them about God's love and give them Christian tapes and books.

"Brahim, who's about 12, comes to our house a lot. He'd like to go to school, but he has to work selling donuts so that he and his grandmother can buy food. He brings donuts to our house, and we always give him something to eat and talk to him about Jesus. One day he asked us to read him a story, so we told him the story of Jesus blessing the little children. He loved the story, but when we told him it was from the Bible he was really scared. His friends had told him that he'd get into trouble with the Muslim teachers if they found out he went into a Christian's house. He ran to the sink and washed his hands and ears because he'd touched a Bible and listened to the story. Then he left without even waiting to be paid for the donuts! We're all praying that someday Brahim will forget his fear and love and follow Jesus."

Children of the Streets

Homeless, Unwanted Children all around the World

Russia

"Get out!" Anton's mother screamed. "And don't come back until you have some money!" Anton ran out of the house, scared that his mother would beat him. He was hungry, cold and sick. His parents couldn't find jobs, and they spent what little money they had on alcohol. Anton is only nine years old. He's tired of trying to get food by begging and stealing. He'll probably get caught some day, and he's afraid. There are thousands of other children like Anton, living on the streets of St. Petersburg, Russia.

Street children in Delhi, India live in these pipes

Aid worker on the streets in South America

Project Hope is a Christian organization reaching out to street children in St. Petersburg. Every day, workers invite children on the streets to their shelter. They give them food, showers and clothing. If they're sick, they can see a doctor. They can learn skills like carpentry and how to repair shoes and use computers. More than that, Project Hope teaches these children about God's love for them.

India

"Rupee! Rupee! Give me!" Little Ram stuck out a dirty, empty hand. His big brown eyes pleaded for just one of the hundreds of passengers to give him a coin so he could buy a *chapatti* to eat. He hadn't eaten all day, and he was so hungry. Ram's parents are both dead, and he has no one to take care of him. At night he huddles with other homeless boys on the street. Ram is just one of the two million children living on the streets in India.

Colombia

Señor Jaramillo, a rich businessman in Bogota, Colombia, saw a little homeless girl killed when she was running to pick up an empty box. It changed his life. He was shocked to find out that many homeless children live in the city sewers. Now he puts on scuba-diving gear and goes down into the sewers every night, searching for these children. He gives food, clothes, education and jobs to as many of them as he can.

South American street children

South Africa

There was a time when Johannes couldn't remember anything except being miserable. His

What else can you do?

Find out if there is an organization in your area that helps the homeless. There are probably homeless people and families in the city nearest to where you live. How could you show the love of Jesus in a practical way to these people? Perhaps you could collect food, clothing, books or toys through your church or school to help those who do not have as much as you do. Or you could help to raise money to send to organizations helping street children in other parts of the world.

parents were always fighting and drinking. There was never enough food, and they beat him. He was sure they didn't want him, so he left home to live on the streets of Johannesburg. He started taking drugs, trying to escape from the pain of life. He stole or begged for food and drugs.

A few years later, he was invited to the Emmanuel shelter for street children.

"I never knew there were such kind people who wanted to help children like me," Johannes said with a smile. "I'm going to school and I've decided to follow Jesus, who loves all children. I thank God for protecting me and helping me."

Helping the homeless

In almost every country and major city in the world, millions of children are living on the streets. There may be as many as 200 million street children in the world today. That's almost as many as all the people living in the United States! Every one of these children feels lonely and unloved.

Some of these children are orphans, others live on the streets because they're afraid of drunken parents, abuse and hunger. Many of them sleep in cardboard boxes in railway stations and doorways, under bridges and even in sewers. It's often difficult to help them because they quickly learn to steal, fight, use drugs and even kill to survive. In some countries the police beat them and even shoot them.

These children need places of safety where people will take care of them and love them. Please pray that these hurt and lonely children will get help and feel Jesus' love. Many of these children are your age and even younger. As you pray for them, remember to thank God for your own home and family.

Young people at the Emmanuel shelter, South Africa. Johannes holds the coke bottle.

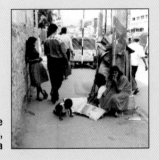

Home on the street, Colombo, Sri Lanka

To help you pray for homeless children

You can thank God for:

- the street children who have been shown love and kindness and who have begun to learn that they really do matter.

- the people who work with street children.

- Christians who give money to organizations to provide food and shelter for street children.

You can ask God:

- to bring these unwanted and unloved children to know Jesus as their friend who is always with them.

- to use each shelter, training project and camp to help street children learn that there can be more to life than living on the streets.

- to make governments realize that it's important to do all they can to protect children from the difficult – and often terrible – things so many of them have to face.

- to show boys and girls who have loving families, homes and toys, and who can go to school, how they can help children who have none of these good things.

China

God is at Work

So many people!

China is the third largest country in the world, after Russia and Canada, and it's almost the same size as Europe. About one-fifth of the world's people live in China, which means that more people live there than in any other country. There are at least 56 different people groups living in China. You can read more about some of these groups in this book – including the Hui, Dai Lu, and Tibetans.

About two-thirds of the people in China work as farmers. Rice is the most important crop, but they also grow fruit, vegetables, tea and cotton. China's towns and cities are big and bustling, and Shanghai is one of the biggest cities in the world.

A fortune cookie

Fact file

Area: 3,696,100 sq. mi.

Population: 1,262,556,787

Capital: Beijing

Main language: Mandarin Chinese

Religions: Buddhism; folk religions; Islam

Economy: China grows more rice and rears more pigs than any other country in the world. Industries include iron and steel manufacture, machinery, vehicles, ships, clothes and toys.

The door is slammed shut

In 1949, the Communist Party took control of China. They wanted to make China a country where everyone was equal, where nobody was either rich or poor. The Communists took land from wealthy landowners and set up big collective farms for the peasants to work on. They built big factories to produce iron, steel and heavy machinery and formed a huge army, but many people were still poor.

The Communists also wanted to get rid of all religions in China. Christian missionaries were forced to leave China in 1950. For 140 years, missionaries had shared the good news of Jesus with the people in China. Had all those years of work been for nothing? What would happen to the Christians they left behind? Would they remember all they had been taught and remain faithful? Would the pastors be allowed to teach and preach about Jesus?

The door into China slammed shut. For the next 30 years it was almost impossible for Christians outside to get news of their friends in China. All around the world Christians prayed for China. And God answered their prayers in an amazing way.

God opens the door

As they faced persecution, many of the Chinese Christians stood firm for Jesus. Their churches were closed down, and during the Cultural Revolution (1966–90) some of their leaders were killed. Others were put in prison or sent far away to work in prison camps. Life would have been much easier and safer for these Christians and their families if they had just said that they didn't believe in Jesus anymore. But they never turned their backs on Jesus.

The Chinese eat their food with chopsticks.

中华人民共和国万岁   世界人民大团

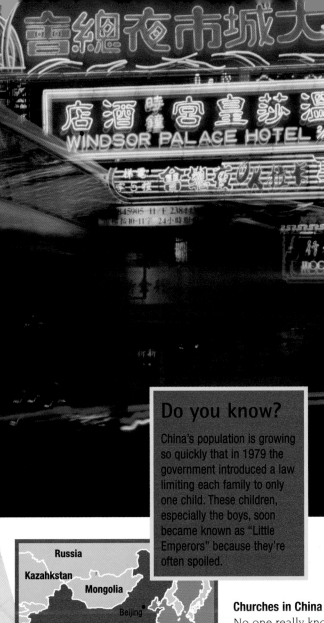

To help you pray for China

You can thank God for:

- the millions of Chinese people who know Jesus as their friend, and all the Christians who shared God's love with others even when they were suffering themselves.

- Christians around the world who never gave up praying for the Chinese people.

You can ask God:

- that many children will hear about Jesus from their friends and families and that soon it will be possible for every church to have a Sunday school.

- to help Christians show Jesus' love by always being ready to give whatever they can to those who are in need.

- that soon there will be enough good seminaries, Bible schools and training courses where church pastors and leaders can study the Bible and learn how to teach and care for the people in their churches.

- that many young people and students at universities will come to know him.

- for leaders in China who will rule this huge country wisely and fairly.

Do you know?

China's population is growing so quickly that in 1979 the government introduced a law limiting each family to only one child. These children, especially the boys, soon became known as "Little Emperors" because they're often spoiled.

When the government tried to get rid of religion in China, the church grew instead

Churches in China

No one really knows how many Christians there are in China today, but there are millions more than there were when the missionaries left.

There are all sorts of church groups in China. Some of the churches in the towns and cities have huge congregations, but in the countryside many churches meet in homes. Although the churches have a lot more freedom, there are still restrictions. Bibles are now being printed in China, but there are still not enough for everyone who wants one.

There are other restrictions, too. Yang is nine years old. His parents are Christians, and he likes to listen as they read the Bible and pray. Yang usually begs his father to read him another story from the Bible. "Can I have some of my friends over to hear the stories, too?" he pleads.

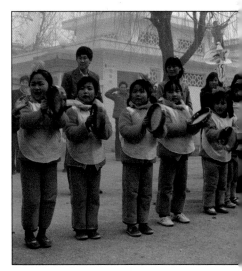

Quietly, in their homes, they talked about Jesus and the help and strength he gave them. They also shared his love with other people, especially those who were poor or sick. Instead of disappearing, as the Communists planned, the church in China grew.

When the door into China began to open at last, Chinese people from other parts of the world visited their families there. Some were Christians who secretly carried Bibles with them. They brought back the great news that the church was growing.

"You know we're not supposed to teach the Bible to young people," his father says with a smile. "But if one or two of your friends came sometimes, I could tell them Bible stories too. Go and get one of them now, but be quiet about it!"

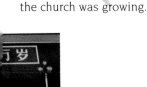

Colombia

Light shines in the darkness

Hope for the poor …

Maria held her little brother's hand and dragged him through the crowd of children waiting for a sandwich and a cup of hot chocolate. Maria and Carlos hadn't eaten anything since the day before. That sandwich tasted so good, and the hot chocolate really warmed them up.

Maria and Carlos live with their mother in a small, dark room in a slum area of Bogotá, the capital of Colombia. Their mother is addicted to drugs and their father is in prison. Sometimes Maria earns a little money by washing cars or sorting through trash for bottles and papers that she can sell. Sometimes she steals food so that she and Carlos can eat.

Figure from San Augustin Archeological Park

There are lots of children like Maria and Carlos in Colombia's cities. Some have come from the countryside with their families, trying to escape from the violence of guerrilla activities and drug cartels. They usually don't have any money and can't find work, so they get poorer and poorer. It's easy to turn to crime when you're starving and have nothing.

A few Christian organizations run centers to help these people. They invite children to their centers, where

Family living in a slum, Bogotá

Fact file

Area: 439,735 sq. mi.

Population: 42,321,361

Capital: Bogotá

Language: Spanish. The Amerindian peoples also speak 65 different languages.

Coffee

Religion: Christianity (Roman Catholic, but with a growing evangelical church)

Chief exports: Oil; coal; emeralds; coffee; bananas

Colombians are learning that Jesus gives hope to the poor, the rich, and the prisoners

they can have a bath, clean clothes and food. Children can also play games and even learn to read there. But, best of all, children like Maria and Carlos are learning that God loves them.

Colombia is the fourth largest country in South America, and 100 years ago it was one of the poorest. A lot of people are still very poor, but others have made a lot of money from coffee, oil production and trade with other countries. Colombia is rich in gold, platinum and emeralds. There's a huge illegal trade in drugs as well, which is often the cause of terrible violence. "So many people think of Colombia as a place of begging, stealing, smuggling, killing, dying and drugs," a friend in Colombia said. "Although violence is unfortunately a part of life in Colombia, it's also a beautiful land. And most Colombians

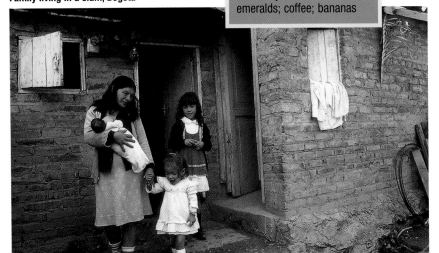

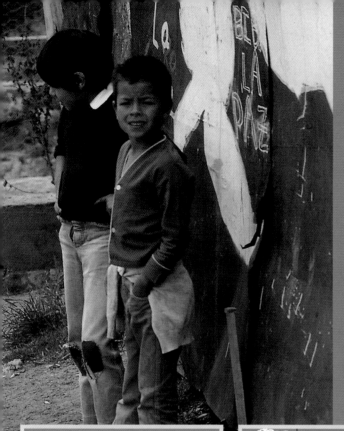

![hand icon] To help you pray for Colombia

You can thank God for:

- the people showing God's love and care to children in city slums.
- all of the prisoners who have asked Jesus to forgive them for the bad things they've done.

You can ask God:

- that people in Colombia who are hurt, afraid, poor, lonely and angry will discover Jesus' love, help and comfort.
- to stop the violence and drug trade in Colombia.
- to give Christian government leaders the wisdom and courage to speak out for what's right.
- to protect pastors as they talk about Jesus' love in areas where there's a lot of violence.
- that all Colombian Christians will work together to share Jesus' love with others.

Do you know?

Colombia is the largest producer of coal in South America. It also produces half the world's emeralds and is the world's second largest producer of coffee. It has 1,721 species of birds – the highest recorded number in any country in the world.

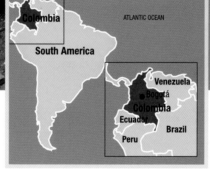

are warm and loving people. Evangelical Christians used to be persecuted for their faith, but now more people than ever are following Jesus."

... and hope for the rich

Juliana has everything she wants. She goes to a private school and plans to go to university. She spends most weekends with her grandparents in the country and every summer she visits her cousins in the United States. Her father is a wealthy lawyer. When her parents got divorced, Juliana was so sad … but she didn't know who to talk to.

One of Juliana's friends at school saw how upset she was and invited her to go to church with her. "Whenever I'm sad," she told Juliana, "I talk to Jesus and he listens and answers my prayers." Juliana's parents

are Catholics but, like many Colombians, they hardly ever go to church. Juliana went to church with her friend and found out that it was true that Jesus would always help her. She's praying that her parents will know Jesus someday, too.

... and hope for those in prison

Until recently, Medellin was one of the most violent cities in Colombia. It has a maximum security prison called Bellavista, or "Beautiful View," which is full of thieves, murderers and drug pushers. But something amazing is happening in the prison.

Several years ago, a man who had been a prisoner came to know Jesus. His life was changed so completely that he went back to tell the prisoners about Jesus. A lot of them have asked God to forgive their sins and to make them new people. Now they're

studying in their own Bible school in prison, and every day they meet to sing and talk about what God has done for them. These services are broadcast on a radio program called "A Cry of Hope." People outside the prison listen to the programs and are coming to know Jesus, too. Once a month, the children of prisoners are allowed to visit their fathers. The prisoners who have come to know Jesus want their children to know about him, too. The children were very excited one visiting day when they were all given a book called "The Gospel for Kids."

Men and women, boys and girls – whether they are poor or rich – are discovering that God loves them. They're praying that, as God changes lives, their country will become a peaceful place where people can live without fear.

Cuba

The Church is Growing

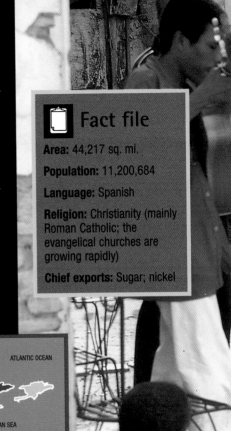

Sugar and slaves

In 1492, Christopher Columbus discovered the beautiful Caribbean island of Cuba and claimed it for Spain. Spaniards settled there and established sugar plantations. They shipped thousands of West Africans across the Atlantic Ocean to work as slaves on these plantations. Today, many Cubans are descendants of those slaves.

Sugar made a lot of people very wealthy, and by 1959 Cuba was one of the richest countries in Latin America. The beautiful beaches and the luxury of cities like Havana attracted many tourists from North America.

But not everyone was rich. Thousands of very poor people needed better homes and enough food and clothing for their families. They couldn't even afford to send their children to school.

USA

ATLANTIC OCEAN

GULF OF MEXICO

Mexico

Cuba

CARIBBEAN SEA

PACIFIC OCEAN

Havana

Cuba

Preparing the famous Havana cigars

There are still not enough Bibles in Cuba for all those who want one

Revolution and education

On 1 January 1959, Fidel Castro and his guerrillas overthrew the government. They wanted to make Cuba a better country. They made sure that every child went to school and adults were taught to read, too.

Roberto was eight years old when the revolution took place. "We went to school in a small hut," he said. "My family was very poor. We didn't have shoes, our clothes were ragged and old, and I was very hungry most of the time. I was excited because they told me if I learned to read I'd get a good job. Then I could have more to eat and better clothes to wear."

He smiled sadly. "Everyone goes to school now, and there are more doctors and a lot of us have better houses than we used to have, but the revolution didn't really help us very much. The United States stopped trading with us because we were Communists. The Russians did help us, but they're not helping us any more. I'm still very poor. Medicine is

Fidel Castro (center) with Cuban church leaders

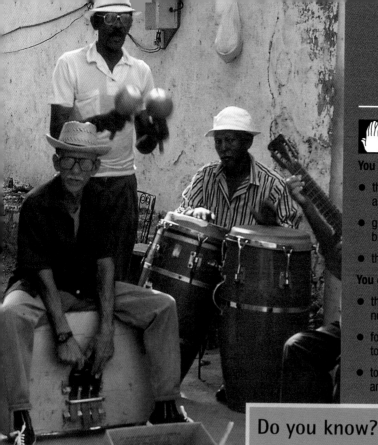

 To help you pray for Cuba

You can thank God for:

- the public meetings that Christians were allowed to hold in 1998 and 1999.
- greater freedom for Bibles to be printed in Cuba and to be brought in from other countries.
- the many Cubans who are coming to know Jesus.

You can ask God:

- that people who have suffered because they follow Jesus will not be angry but will forgive those who hurt them.
- for more Bibles, books and teachers to train leaders and pastors to help all the new churches.
- to help the many people in Cuba who don't have enough food and other things we take for granted.
- that when Cuba is no longer a Communist country, the new government will lead the country wisely.

Young woman and child who have received the Scriptures

Do you know?

As in other Communist states, the Cuban government tried to get rid of Christianity but couldn't. Christians have been persecuted, arrested, imprisoned or forced to leave the country. Despite this, many Christians have stood firm for Jesus. Although persecution is still taking place, thousands of people, especially young people, are coming to know Jesus.

scarce, food is rationed and my children often go hungry and don't have good clothes.

"Right after the revolution, a lot of wealthy people left Cuba and went to live in the United States. Since then, thousands have tried to escape in small boats. Cuba is my home and it's very beautiful, but there are so many problems here it's hard to know where to start."

Cuba for Christ!

Although Cuba is now a secular country, almost half the people are Roman Catholics. After the revolution in 1959, police informers seemed to be everywhere. Because they wouldn't stop following Jesus, Christians were often persecuted and put in prison, where they were treated very badly.

Maria, a young Cuban woman, describes what it's like to be a Christian there. "In the 1980s, the evangelical churches started to grow – and they're still growing. A lot of Cubans, especially young people and children, have discovered the joy of

knowing Jesus as their friend. Christians all over Cuba meet together in churches and homes. They're so excited to share the good news about Jesus. Everyone wants a Bible, but there aren't enough to go around. We're so grateful to people who bring them into the country and for organizations that send them. The government's allowing us to print some Bibles here now, but there still aren't enough! Christians have a little more freedom to meet together now. But there are still restrictions, and our pastors and leaders are still threatened and churches are closed down.

"In 1998, the Pope visited Cuba. Thousands of people joined him to worship God in an open-air service in Havana. A year later, the evangelical churches were allowed to hold 19

huge open-air meetings in cities all across Cuba. It was so exciting to hear thousands of people shouting, 'Cuba for Christ!' There were 100,000 people at the rally in Havana, and President Fidel Castro and several members of the government sat in the front row.

"We thank God for the Christians around the world who are praying for Cuba. Please keep praying that the people of Cuba will know and love Jesus."

Dai Lu

From the Land of Twelve Thousand Rice Fields

Xishuangbanna

In the Yunnan Province of southwest China, near the borders with Myanmar and Laos, there's a region called Xishuangbanna (Shish-wang-banna). This is the home of the Dai Lu people. Fifty years ago, monkeys, elephants, tigers, bears, deer and even peacocks lived in the thick green forests that covered the high mountains. Since then, they've cut down almost half the forest to make room for more people – especially for the Han Chinese, who have come to live in the area. Cutting down the forest has affected the climate. This means the rainfall has decreased and rivers have been drying up.

The Dai Lu people build their houses on stilts out of wood, bamboo and thatch. Pigs and hens make themselves at home under the houses.

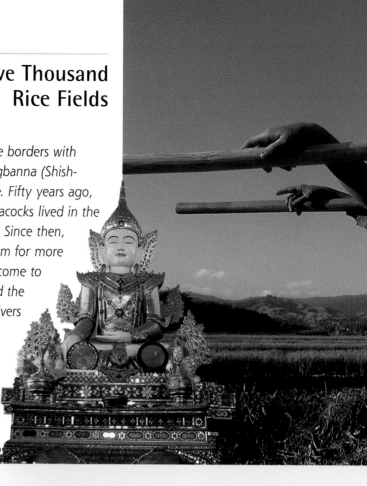

Shrine at a Dai Buddhist temple

The Dai Lu grow coconut palms, banana, papaya and mango trees, pineapples and peppers all around their houses. And there are more paddy fields (fields where rice is grown) than you can count, because Xishuangbanna means "the land of twelve thousand rice fields."

Help for another life?

The Dai Lu people are Buddhists, and there's a temple in every village. Most children go to schools run by the government now, but seven-year-old Artuk's parents decided to send him to the temple for his schooling. Artuk tried to be brave as he waved goodbye to his parents and left with his big brother, who was taking him to the temple. He wondered what it would be like to live

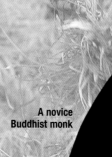

A novice Buddhist monk

there for three whole years.

Forty other little boys were already there. "It's your turn to have your head shaved," a monk told Artuk. "And here's the robe you'll wear every day," he said, handing Artuk an orange robe.

"Will you teach us how to read?" Artuk asked. "Yes, we'll start tomorrow," replied the monk. "You'll learn to read the sacred Buddhist scriptures so you can earn merit for yourself and for your whole family. This will help you in your next life."

Artuk knew Buddhists believe that when they die they're reborn as another person or animal. This is called reincarnation. Artuk also knew that all the good things he did would help him in his next life. But he was frightened

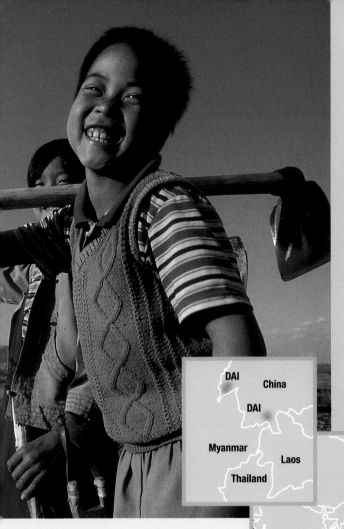

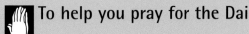

✋ To help you pray for the Dai

You can thank God for:

- the few Dai Lu Christians.

- each person working on translating the Bible.

You can ask God:

- to help the Dai Lu understand that doing good things will never get them to heaven.

- to show them that the only way to stop worrying about sin and evil spirits is to follow Jesus.

- to show the Dai Lu that following Jesus will make them even happier than remembering their old stories.

- that Han Chinese Christians in Yunnan will show the Dai Lu how much God loves them.

- that some day there will be churches in every town where the Dai Lu live.

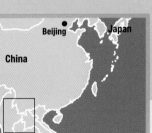

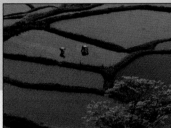

Paddy fields

sometimes – what if he ever did something wrong? What would happen to him in the next life?

The good guy wins again

"Tell us the story of the Water Throwing Festival! Please!" the children all begged their father after dinner one night. The Dai Lu people love to tell stories and, like many of their stories, this one is about how the good guy wins and the bad guy loses.

"All right," their father said. "Once upon a time, a powerful demon-king ruled our people. He made life very hard for them. He had seven wives, but the youngest one, Yu Xiang (*yoo shang*), was a kind and gentle person. She didn't like to see anyone suffer. 'I wish the demon-king would die,' she thought, 'so the Dai Lu people can be free from his evil power.'

"The demon-king loved Yu Xiang very much, and one day he told her his biggest secret. 'My power is in the single white hair on my head,' he said, 'I can only be defeated if it is pulled out

and tied around my neck.' That night, when he was fast asleep, Yu Xiang pulled out that white hair, tied it tightly around his neck, and cut off his head.

"Everyone was so happy that the demon-king was dead! But as soon as his head touched the ground, it burst into flames and burned up everything it touched. At last, brave Yu Xiang was able to pick up the head. When she did, the fire stopped. But when she put it down, the fire started again. 'Quick, quick!' the people shouted as they threw water over Yu Xiang to put out the fire and wash away the blood. Now, when we celebrate the Water Throwing Festival and have fun throwing water at each other, we remember this

story. The water we throw makes us pure and clean and keeps us from harm."

There are only a few Dai Lu Christians. Most of the Dai Lu people don't know that doing good things or throwing water can never make their hearts clean or help them go to heaven. Who will tell them the best story of all, that God sent his only Son, Jesus, to defeat all of the evil powers? How will the Dai Lu know that the only way to have a pure, clean heart is to follow Jesus? Who will tell Artuk that he doesn't have to worry about the bad things he does if he tells Jesus he's sorry? How will he know that there's no other life after he dies, unless he knows Jesus and goes to heaven?

📋 Fact file

Numbers: About 614,300 in China

Locations: Yunnan Province of China; others in Myanmar, Thailand and Laos

Language: Dai

Religions: Buddhism; animism

Occupations: Farmers; traders

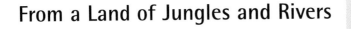

Dayak

From a Land of Jungles and Rivers

The omen bird

The villagers following Idjam along the jungle trail stopped when their leader cried out. "I can hear the omen bird. Look, there it is!" Idjam said. "It's warning us about something – let's go home. This must not be a good day to plant the rice fields. We'll come back tomorrow."

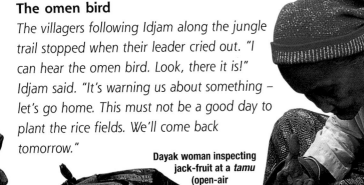

Dayak woman inspecting jack-fruit at a *tamu* (open-air market)

Do you know?

Dayak fathers train their young sons to hunt animals in the jungle. The father buys live chickens for his family to eat and shows his son how to kill them so that he won't be afraid to kill an animal.

A white man comes

Hanji is the teacher in a village school. He remembers how frightened he was when the first missionary came to his village. "I was just a little boy," he smiles, "and I'd never seen a white person before."

Idjam wondered what was wrong as he hurried back to the village. They had offered a sacrifice to the spirits before cutting down the jungle for fields. They left some trees on the hilltop for visiting spirits to rest on. The ash left from burning the trees and undergrowth should guarantee a good harvest. But the appearance of the omen bird meant the spirits were angry.

Idjam and the villagers set out for their fields again the next day. They didn't hear the omen bird and were soon at work. Using sharp-pointed sticks, the men and boys made holes in the ground between the burnt-out tree stumps. The women and girls followed, dropping a few rice seeds into each hole. At harvest time the men cut down the

rice with a knife, a few stalks at a time. The women gather the rice, put it in a square basket and then pound it to remove the husk.

Most Dayak live along the riverbanks and in the jungle areas of Kalimantan in central Borneo. While there are some Christians among them, most are still animists. They live in constant fear of evil spirits hiding in rocks, trees, rivers, caves and on the mountains, waiting to hurt them.

Dayak hunter with blowpipe

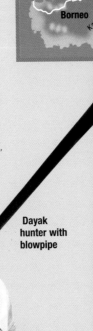

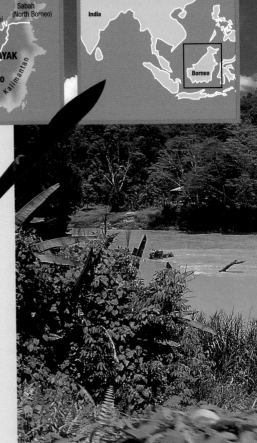

Map labels: JAVA SEA, Brunei, Sabah (North Borneo), Sarawak, DAYAK, Borneo, Kalimantan, China, India, Borneo

"Night after night he told us about Jesus, God's Son. He told us that Jesus had power over all the evil spirits. I was afraid of those spirits, so I decided to follow Jesus. Some of my friends did, too. At first the older men were afraid the spirits would be angry because we burned all our charms, but when nothing bad happened to us some of them became Christians too.

"The missionaries taught us to read, and it was great to be able to read stories about Jesus. Some of us went to Bible school and became evangelists to our own people. I opened the school here in this village."

Empty schools and churches

Hanji shook his head as he looked over at a group of boys playing in the river. "They should all be in school," he said, "but no one makes them go. Parents want their children to stay at home and help feed the chickens and pigs, look for food, or take care of their little brothers and sisters. Sometimes the children themselves decide they just don't want to come to school. That's too bad, because the Dayak way of life is changing and it's important to know how to read and write. Some children do come every day because they want to go to high school and even university.

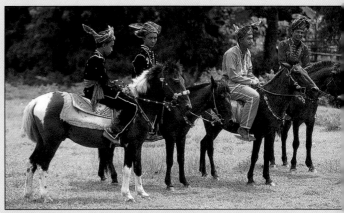
Bajau Dayak horsemen at the weekly *tamu* (open-air market) in Sabah

"It's hard to help people understand that going to church is important, too – even though almost half the people in this village say they're Christians, some of them think they don't need to go to church. The girls like to come to Sunday school and sing and learn Bible stories, but usually the boys would rather play or go fishing. I keep praying that these children and their parents will want to learn more about Jesus and what it's really like to follow him."

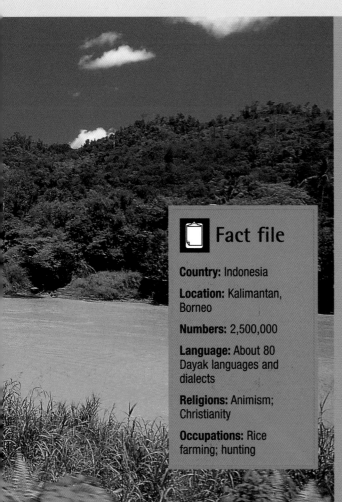

 To help you pray for the Dayak

You can thank God for:

● Dayaks who are no longer afraid of the spirits because they trust Jesus.

● Dayaks who have studied at Bible school.

You can ask God:

● that church leaders will help others to know and follow Jesus.

● for more Christians to teach the Dayaks to read and write.

● for the Dayaks to want to read the Bible and learn more about God.

● to help young Dayak Christians who leave their villages to find good churches and Christian friends.

● to help Christians understand that it's important to go to church and Sunday school.

Fact file

Country: Indonesia

Location: Kalimantan, Borneo

Numbers: 2,500,000

Language: About 80 Dayak languages and dialects

Religions: Animism; Christianity

Occupations: Rice farming; hunting

A river in the jungle at the northern tip of Borneo. Many of Borneo's rivers are now muddy due to logging erosion.

Djibouti

One of the Hottest Places on Earth

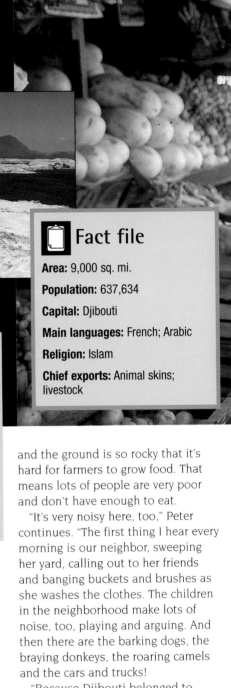

Leaves or people?

"I'm not taking off," announced the pilot. *"The plane's overloaded and we'll never get over the mountain."* The passengers on board the flight to Djibouti were angry.

"How can we be overloaded?" someone asked a flight attendant. *"DC9s hold 72 passengers, and there are only 40 of us."*

"We're overloaded with eight and a half tons of khat, *but if we refuse to take it ..."* The flight attendant drew her finger across her throat. Khat *is a leaf that people use as a drug. People that chew it feel dreamy and don't want to eat. Khat is big business in Djibouti, and the airline makes a lot more money carrying* khat *than people.*

At last the plane took off, leaving behind two Somali ladies and a big pile of luggage. Even so, the plane just barely cleared the mountains near the end of the runway.

Lake Assal

Fact file

Area: 9,000 sq. mi.

Population: 637,634

Capital: Djibouti

Main languages: French; Arabic

Religion: Islam

Chief exports: Animal skins; livestock

Do you know?

Lake Assal, in the center of Djibouti, is 509 feet below sea level and is the lowest place in Africa. The water in the lake is even saltier than the Dead Sea in Israel and 10 times saltier than the water in the ocean. When the water dries up in the hot sun, islands of salt are formed which float on top of the water.

When the plane landed at Djibouti's main airport, crowds of drug dealers pushed, pulled and yelled for their *khat*. As soon as they had it, they rushed into the city to their waiting customers. Soon there were thousands of people throughout the city with their cheeks bulging with *khat* leaves. Many of them sat chewing peacefully, forgetting how poor they were, or how hungry.

A really hot place

Peter lives in the city of Djibouti, the capital, with his missionary parents. "It's one of the hottest places on earth," he says. "It's usually much too hot to sleep at night, especially since we have to sleep under mosquito nets. There's almost never any rain,

Almost all Djiboutians are Muslims, but a few have decided to follow Jesus

Cooking pancakes

and the ground is so rocky that it's hard for farmers to grow food. That means lots of people are very poor and don't have enough to eat.

"It's very noisy here, too," Peter continues. "The first thing I hear every morning is our neighbor, sweeping her yard, calling out to her friends and banging buckets and brushes as she washes the clothes. The children in the neighborhood make lots of noise, too, playing and arguing. And then there are the barking dogs, the braying donkeys, the roaring camels and the cars and trucks!

"Because Djibouti belonged to France for almost 100 years before it

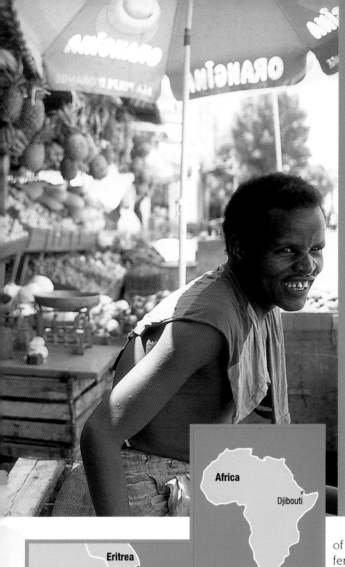

To help you pray for Djibouti

You can thank God for:

● every missionary working in Djibouti.

● every Christian in Djibouti.

You can ask God:

● that missionaries teaching English will be able to tell their students about Jesus.

● that through their teaching, Bible translation, medical work, agriculture and youth work, missionaries can talk to those who want to know more about Jesus.

● to provide food for all the poor people in Djibouti.

● that Djiboutians will understand the message of the Bible.

● for missionaries' children to tell their Djiboutian school friends about Jesus.

Africa

Djibouti

Marketplace in the evening

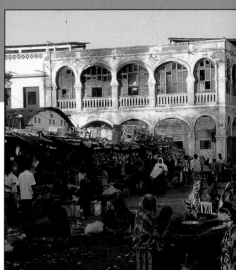

Eritrea

Ethiopia

Gulf of Tadjoura

Djibouti

Djibouti town

Somalia

became an independent country in 1977, French is one of the main languages. Before we came to live in Djibouti, my parents had to learn French. I go to a French school and have lots of Djiboutian friends. Most of my friends want to learn English as well, and some of them study in the English language school where my father's a teacher. One of my favorite things to do is play soccer with my friends. They're all Muslims, but sometimes they ask me questions about who Jesus is."

Peter always loves going with his father to visit their Afar friends in Tadjoura. "We have to cross the Gulf

of Tadjoura on the ferry to get there. It's lots of fun. There's only room for 12 cars, but most people are foot passengers. You wouldn't believe some of the things they take with them. There are always big boxes of groceries, crates of soft drinks, furniture and even huge bags of clothes to sell in the markets. The passengers usually include some sheep and goats, too. Everyone always seems to enjoy the trip."

Nomads and refugees

Djibouti is a small African country on the Gulf of Aden. On the map it looks a bit like a boomerang. It has a long coastline and borders with Eritrea, Ethiopia and Somalia. The two main groups of people living in Djibouti used to be enemies – the Afars in the north and the Issas in the south. Almost all the people were nomads, moving around the harsh desert and mountains with their herds of sheep, goats, cattle and camels. It's a hard

way of life. Although many people still live as nomads, a lot of them have moved into the capital, which is a major seaport, hoping to find work. Refugees from civil wars in Ethiopia and Somalia have settled there, too, but a lot of people are poor and have no work.

Almost all Djiboutians are Muslims, but a few have heard about Jesus and decided to follow him. Some of the refugees from Ethiopia are also Christians. They pray (sometimes all night long!) for their own people and for the people of Djibouti. They ask God that these people will follow Jesus.

Dogon

Sharing the Good News

Cliff caves

If you gaze straight up the cliff face, you will see a tiny moving figure. That's Oumar, swinging dangerously on a rope. He doesn't dare look down! He climbs hundreds of feet to reach caves hollowed out of the cliff. He is collecting pigeon dung to sell as fertilizer at the market. Oumar's people are called the Dogon. They live in a part of Mali, western Africa that is very rocky. The fertilizer helps them to grow as much food as they can on the few fields they have. If you look directly behind you, you can see the Sahara Desert, where nothing grows. So every bit of soil is precious to the Dogon. The Dogon even bury their dead in caves high up in these cliffs.

The Dogon wear masks decorated with cowrie shells

When Oumar is safely down again, he'll tell you how he loves all of the ceremonies that are part of Dogon life. He can't wait until he is older to learn to dance on colorful stilts wearing a mask of cowrie shells and hibiscus.

Dogon dancers on stilts

How would you tell Oumar about Jesus?

Oumar has been learning about Dogon tribal beliefs since he can remember. He probably wouldn't understand at first if you told him about Jesus. But there are some truths in the Bible that would help Oumar understand.

If a Dogon person does something wrong, the elders (the leaders) may make that person leave the village. This is a terrible punishment, because it means they have to start

life again all by themselves. But if they admit that they were wrong and want to be forgiven, they have to bring a goat or sheep to the edge of the village. The elders kill or sacrifice the animal and make a trail of blood to the door of this person's home. Then the people of the village accept the person who did wrong.

So you could tell Oumar about how God teaches us in the Bible that sin makes us unfit to go to heaven, just as his people believe sin makes a person unfit to live in the village. But killing a goat or sheep

won't get us into heaven. God's own Son Jesus, who the Bible calls "the Lamb of God," sacrificed himself for us. Jesus died on the cross so that we can be forgiven for all the bad things we've done and be acceptable to God. All we need to do is believe in him and be truly sorry. Then God will accept us into heaven to live with him always.

Praying for rain

The land where the Dogon live is very dry, but they need rain for the crops. One year, despite all the sacrifices the spirit worshippers made and the chanting of Muslims, rain

Cliff village

MEDITERRANEAN SEA

Sahara Desert

Mali

Africa

Bamako • **DOGON**

ATLANTIC OCEAN

Do you know?

The region of the Bandiagara cliffs in Mali where the Dogon live is a world heritage site. These cliffs protect many ancient archeological structures (houses, altars and *toguna*, or meeting places). People have lived in these cliffs for at least 1,000 years.

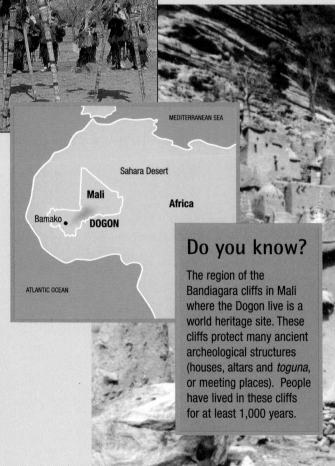

didn't come. A visitor told the elders in one village, "When Christians pray, their God answers their prayers. Why don't you ask them to pray for you? I'm sure their God will send rain." The elders weren't too sure, but they talked with some Christians.

"Yes, we'll pray," the Christians told them, "but only if you stop all your sacrifices. Then when the rain comes everybody will know that our God sent it." The leaders agreed, the Christians prayed and the rain came.

The spirit worshippers immediately ran out to make sacrifices. The rain stopped. The elders realized they had broken their promise. "We're sorry," they said. "Please pray again. Our crops are dying, and we will be hungry." God sent plenty of rain so that Oumar and his people would know that God hears and answers our prayers.

It's hard to forgive others as God forgave us

There are about half a million Dogon, and more than 15,000 of them have come to know Jesus. The nomadic Fulani people live in the same part of Mali with the Dogon. The Dogon Christians don't always tell the Fulani about Jesus, though, because their cattle ruin the Dogon crops.

The Dogon know that God forgave them – and some have forgiven the Fulani. There is even a church among the Fulani now. Missionaries and Dogon pastors even hold a Bible school for Fulani Christians.

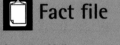

Fact file

Country: Mali

Numbers: About 500,000

Religions: Animism; Islam; Christianity

To help you pray for the Dogon

You can thank God for:

- the New Testament that has been translated into Dogon.

- the Dogon Christians who are sharing the good news about Jesus with the nomadic Fulani people.

You can ask God:

- to send enough rain for the crops to grow well so that the Dogon will have enough food for their families and some to sell in the market as well.

- to help the teams of Dogon Christians who are being trained to take the good news of Jesus' love to other Dogon people.

- to provide the resources for Dogon women to be trained, too, so that they can teach the Bible to other Dogon women and children.

- to help the team translating the Old Testament finish a translation that everyone will be able to understand easily.

- to provide plenty of books and teaching materials in Dogon for the new Doundou Ebon-Ezer Bible School.

51

Druzes

Followers of a Secret Religion

The big secret

Do you find it hard to keep secrets? The Druzes have an important secret they've kept for almost a thousand years!

The Druzes live in the mountains of Lebanon, Syria, Israel and Jordan. Most of them are farmers who have olive groves and cherry and apple orchards on the hillsides and grow vegetables in their carefully tended gardens. Everyone has lots of work to do, but they still have plenty of time to visit with friends and family. Some Druzes live in the towns now as well. Wherever they are and whatever they do, the Druzes are known as hardworking people who can be trusted.

Their big secret is their religion. They keep what they believe to themselves and never share it with outsiders. Many people have tried to find out what they believe, but the Druzes often mislead them. Their religion has to be kept a secret.

Druze shrine where St Luke's tomb is claimed to be

No one can ever become a Druze – you must be born one. They believe that when they die, their souls immediately enter newborn Druze babies. That's the only way a person can become a Druze. A Druze should only marry another Druze, but if they marry someone of another faith their children will not be Druzes.

There are only a few people who know all the secrets about their religion. They are the 'Uqqal, the "Informed" or "Knowledgeable Ones." Both men and women can become 'Uqqal, but they must be at least 40 years old and have spent long periods of time studying the secrets of their religion. They are the only ones who are allowed to study the "Book of Wisdom," the Druze scriptures.

Knowledgeable Ones

On Thursday evenings, everyone in a Druze village meets in the *khilwa*, or meeting place. Let's talk to Samir and Salim as their parents join the other villagers. The women are all wearing long dresses, either dark blue or black, and white veils.

"Like most Druzes, our parents are 'Ignorant Ones', or *Juhhal*," Salim said quietly. "In the meeting room the women sit in one part of the room and the men sit in another."

"There's our uncle. He's an 'Uqqal," Samir whispered as a tall man walked by. "His white turban is a symbol of purity. He has to live by much stricter rules than our parents. He can't drink wine or smoke tobacco. He sometimes eats with us, but he always checks that we've bought everything or grown it ourselves. He wouldn't eat it if he thought the food had been stolen. They discuss all the village matters at the meeting,

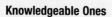

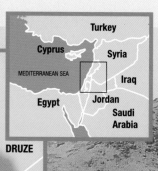

Fact file

Estimated numbers: 300,000 – 450,000

Countries: Most live in Syria and Lebanon. There are smaller groups in Israel and Jordan.

then the *Juhhal*, including our parents, have to leave. But our uncle will stay with the *'Uqqal* for secret meditation and to learn more about Druze beliefs."

Lessons to learn

"All the children in the village have to go to the meeting hall, too," added Samir. "We're taught many things, especially how we should live and how important it is to be honest and truthful, particularly to other Druzes. We must never tell anyone else about our Druze beliefs, or believe in anything else like Islam or Christianity. That's hard for

some of us, especially when we go to a Christian school."

The children are taught to always be ready to help each other and look after strangers, like Ali, who come to their village for help.

Bandits in Syria were hunting Ali, but he knew that he would find shelter in the chief's home in a Druze village. When the armed bandits came looking for Ali, the village chief walked out to greet them.

"Where's Ali? Give him up to us right now!" the bandits demanded. "We know

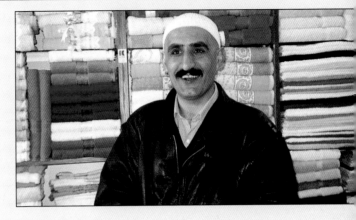

he's here. If he gives us money, he can live!"

"I am a Druze," the chief replied calmly. "This man has come to my home for shelter, and we will fight to the death to protect him!"

As the bandits raised their rifles, the Druze villagers fired shots at

them. The bandits ran away. The chief smiled. He had protected Ali.

The Druzes are waiting for Al-Hakim, the founder of their religion, to return to earth as their savior. But God wants the Druzes to trust in Jesus, the true Savior he has sent.

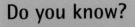

Do you know?

The Druze "Book of Wisdom" is written by hand and every copy is guarded carefully in a secret place. Only "Knowledgeable Ones" are allowed to study the "Book of Wisdom."

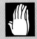 ## To help you pray for the Druzes

You can thank God for:

- Christian schools and orphanages where Druze children are shown his love and can learn about Jesus.

- the many good things, such as being honest and truthful and caring for others, that Druze children learn.

You can ask God:

- to show children like Samir and Salim that studying the secret beliefs of the Druzes will never bring them eternal life.

- that Christians will make friends with Druze people and help them to understand that God wants the Druzes to be his friends, too.

- that many Druzes will be willing to read the Bible, and discover the truth about Jesus and his love.

- to send Christians to tell the Druzes that Jesus is the true Savior sent from God.

- to help the few Druze Christians to never doubt their faith in Jesus; to help them as their lives completely change – from keeping their religion a secret to sharing with everyone the great news about all that Jesus did when he died and rose again.

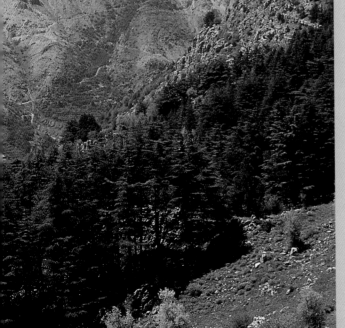

Mountains in Lebanon

Egypt

Light Shines in the Darkness

"I wonder what we'll find today?" Dirty and ragged, Faud and Ramzi sit on top of the big pile of trash in their father's donkey-cart. As the tired old donkey plods along the busy Cairo street, cars, trucks and buses honk their horns as they pass. Every morning, Faud and Ramzi go with their father to collect trash from the city streets, offices and apartment blocks.

Faud and Ramzi's family lives in a crowded slum called "Garbage City" on the outskirts of Cairo, the capital of Egypt. When they get home, Faud and Ramzi carefully sort through the trash. They make piles of paper and cardboard, plastic and glass – they can make a little money selling these to factories for recycling. They leave the rest to the pigs, dogs and cats to paw through for food. Faud and Ramzi are used to the dirt and smell. After all, they've lived there all their lives.

Fact file

Area: 385,227 sq. mi. (96% of the country is desert)

Population: 68,469,695

Capital: Cairo (It is the largest city in the Middle East and Africa)

Language: Arabic

Religions: Islam (87.57%); Christianity (11.93%)

Chief export: Oil

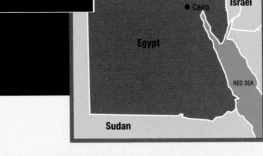

MEDITERRANEAN SEA

Israel

● Cairo

Egypt

RED SEA

Sudan

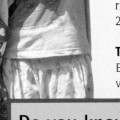

A church in a cave near Cairo can seat 20,000 people

There are more than a million people in Cairo like Faud, Ramzi and their parents who scratch a living from the trash of the 15 million other people who live there. About half the people in Cairo are very poor, but there are also a lot of rich people, including at least 200,000 millionaires.

Teaching the poor

But some of the people in slum villages are finding hope through learning about Jesus. Farouk and Ali, two Coptic Christians (Coptic is an ancient name for Egyptian), go almost every day to the village where Faud and Ramzi live. "Why do you go there?" a friend asked them. "Aren't you afraid you'll get sick from all the trash?"

"The Bible says that God cares for the poor and needy," Farouk said, "and God wants us to care for them, too. That's why we go to the slums. The people there need all the help we can give them. Our church helps these people when they're sick, and we've set up a school where the children can learn to read. Come with us and meet some of the children."

Faud and Ramzi and the other children rushed over to Farouk and his friends as soon as they arrived. "It's time for our reading lesson," Farouk told them. "Go and get your books." Faud and Ramzi and some of the other children ran to their little

Do you know?

The Egyptians built the pyramids more than 4,000 years ago as tombs for the pharaohs. They are the only one of the seven wonders of the ancient world that still survives.

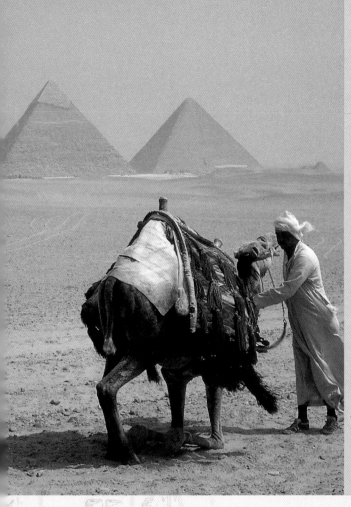

To help you pray for Egypt

You can thank God for:

- Christians who go into the slums to help the poor.
- the *Jesus* film and Christian radio and television programs in Arabic.
- Christian bookshops and the work of the Bible Society.

You can ask God:

- that young people who learn about Jesus in Sunday schools, youth clubs and summer camps will decide to follow him.
- that as Christians study the Bible, their love for Jesus will grow.
- that Christians will always follow Jesus, even when they're persecuted.
- for those who don't know Jesus to see his love, joy and peace shine through Christians.

The pyramids, tombs built by ancient Egyptians

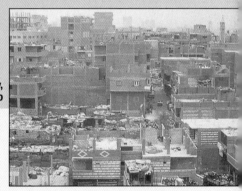

Garbage City, Cairo

huts and came back with their books. They were so excited to be learning to read. "Sometimes we bring Bible story books or tapes for them to listen to as well," Farouk told his friend.

There's a church in a cave on the mountainside beyond Garbage City. It can seat 20,000 people. "Many people from the slums are coming to know Jesus there," Farouk said. "They're discovering that even though they're so poor, they're important to God. In Psalm 113:7 it says that God 'raises the poor from the dust and lifts the needy from the ash heap,' and that's happening here."

An ancient church

A lot of stories in the Bible take place in Egypt. In Acts 2, in the New Testament, it says that there were Egyptians in the huge crowd in Jerusalem on the day of Pentecost. They heard Peter talk about God's love in sending Jesus, who would forgive their sins. Those Egyptians took the Christian faith back to their own country. The

Coptic church grew. It wasn't long before almost all Egyptians were Christians, and they were sending out missionaries to North Africa and Europe.

In AD 642, Arab Muslims invaded Egypt. Christians were forced to become Muslims, and thousands were persecuted and martyred. Egypt became a Muslim country. But the Coptic church never completely disappeared.

Today there are about nine million Coptic Christians living in Egypt. They have to have permission from the president himself to repair their churches or build new ones. They're often persecuted for their faith, but they're still finding ways to help people and share God's love.

The Sphinx

Ethiopia

Land of Refugees and Singing Christians

Ato is excited!

Seven-year-old Ato clapped his hands and jumped for joy. He had never been to school and he couldn't believe that some Christians had offered him a chance to go to the school they had started in his village. Ato's family used to be farmers in the highlands of Ethiopia, but they had moved to a slum in Addis Ababa, the capital city. Ato's mother had told him stories about life on the farm and about how hard it was to grow enough food for the family – especially when there were terrible droughts. His two sisters had become sick and died on the farm because there wasn't enough healthy food for them to eat. Ato also knew about the civil war that had been fought in his country and about how people from all over the world had sent food to help them. Life had been very difficult for his family on the farm, but life in the city was not much better and they were still very poor. For Ato, to go to school was a great opportunity for a better life.

Fact file

Area: 427,000 sq. mi.

Population: 62,564,875

Capital: Addis Ababa

Main language: Amharic, but 123 other languages are spoken

Main religions: Christianity; Islam

Chief exports: Coffee; animal skins; oil-seed

The story so far

The first Christians came to Ethiopia about AD 300 and Orthodox Christianity became the state religion for the next 1,700 years. During the nineteenth and twentieth centuries, many Protestant missionaries worked in Ethiopia. They told people about Jesus, taught them to read and write and cared for the sick. But there are still people in some parts of Ethiopia who have never heard about Jesus.

A Communist government took over the country of Ethiopia in 1974. During the civil war that followed, many

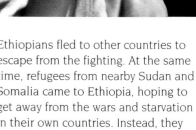

Do you know?

Ethiopia may hold the key to a great mystery! The ark of the covenant was the most holy object belonging to the ancient Israelites. The ark was a small box with a gold lid. Inside it were the stone tablets with the Ten Commandments that God gave to Moses on Mt. Sinai (you can read more about how the Israelites made the ark in Exodus 25). The ark was in the temple in Jerusalem until it disappeared in 587 BC when the Babylonians captured Jerusalem. Many Ethiopians believe that the ark of the covenant was smuggled out of the confusion and taken to Axum in Ethiopia. They claim that the ark is still there, in a small, closely guarded chapel.

Ethiopians fled to other countries to escape from the fighting. At the same time, refugees from nearby Sudan and Somalia came to Ethiopia, hoping to get away from the wars and starvation in their own countries. Instead, they only found more fighting and famine in Ethiopia. Aid agencies worked in the refugee camps to help the homeless, starving and dying people.

There have been Christians in Ethiopia for nearly 2,000 years

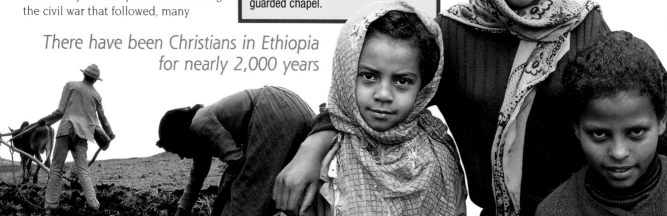

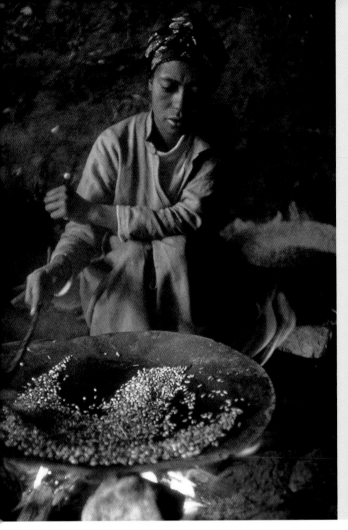

To help you pray for Ethiopia

You can thank God for:

● the thousands of Ethiopians who are Christians.

● the Christians who are helping to show God's love as they bring food, medical care, education, clean water and new ways of farming to people in need.

● each small Bible school.

You can ask God:

● to protect Ethiopian Christians who are helping to translate the Bible into their own language, and to help them to write clearly and accurately.

● to help every pastor and evangelist to be faithful in the way they live as well as in the words they speak.

● to help Ethiopian Christians work together and show those who belong to different people groups that Jesus loves them all.

● to bring peace to Ethiopia and nearby countries so that refugees can return to their own homes.

Ethiopia has many needs and is one of the world's poorest countries

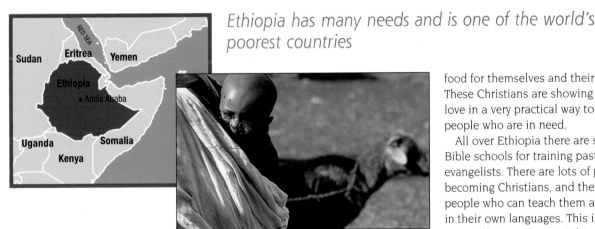

The Communist government imprisoned Christian leaders and closed churches, and many missionaries had to leave the country. In spite of this, the church grew larger and larger. When the Communist government was overthrown in 1991, it was discovered that thousands of Ethiopians had come to know Jesus as their friend. The Christians in Ethiopia love to sing. They often sing going along the road to market or washing their clothes by the river, and everywhere they go they tell others how Jesus died to give them eternal life.

Some Ethiopian Christians are working among people groups in their country who have never heard of the God who loves them. Some are helping missionaries with Bible translation and others are teaching children or working in health care projects. Some are trying to bring clean water to all the villages, and still others are starting agricultural projects to help people grow enough food for themselves and their families. These Christians are showing God's love in a very practical way to many people who are in need.

All over Ethiopia there are small Bible schools for training pastors and evangelists. There are lots of people becoming Christians, and they need people who can teach them about God in their own languages. This is especially important in Ethiopia, where 123 different languages are spoken!

Ethiopia continues to have many needs. There are still refugees who cannot go back to their own countries. The people still suffer from war and drought, and Ethiopia is one of the poorest countries in the world. Although some people are well educated and have good jobs and nice homes, many children never go to school and their families, like Ato's family, are very poor.

Falashas

Black Jews from Ethiopia

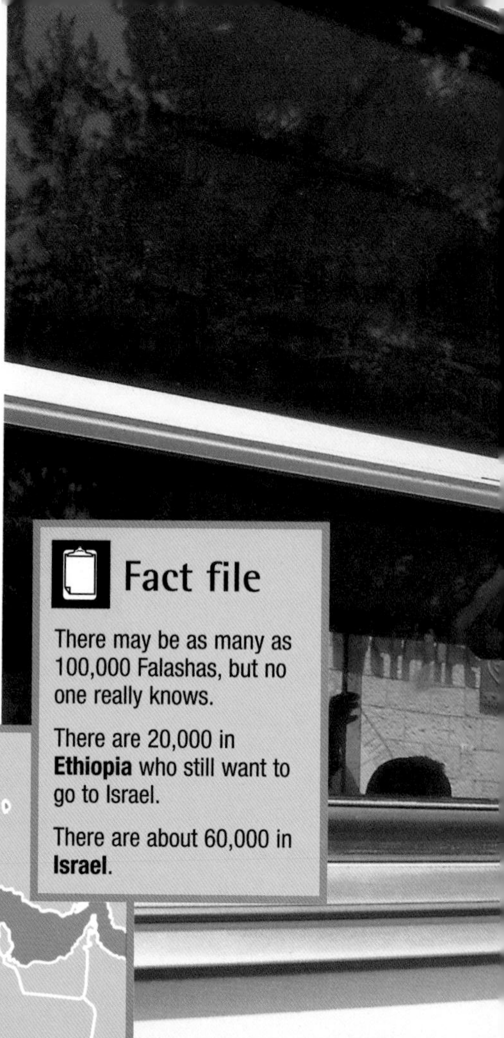

"The House of Israel"

The Falashas (fah-lah-shuhz) are black Jews who have lived in Ethiopia for a very long time. The word falasha means "stranger" in the Amharic language of Ethiopia, but they call themselves Beta Israel, or "the House of Israel."

Some people think the Falashas may be descendants of Jews who returned to Ethiopia with Menelik, the legendary son of King Solomon and the Queen of Sheba – but no one really knows. The Falashas follow the Jewish faith, keep the Sabbath and obey the laws from the first five books of the Bible.

📋 Fact file

There may be as many as 100,000 Falashas, but no one really knows.

There are 20,000 in **Ethiopia** who still want to go to Israel.

There are about 60,000 in **Israel**.

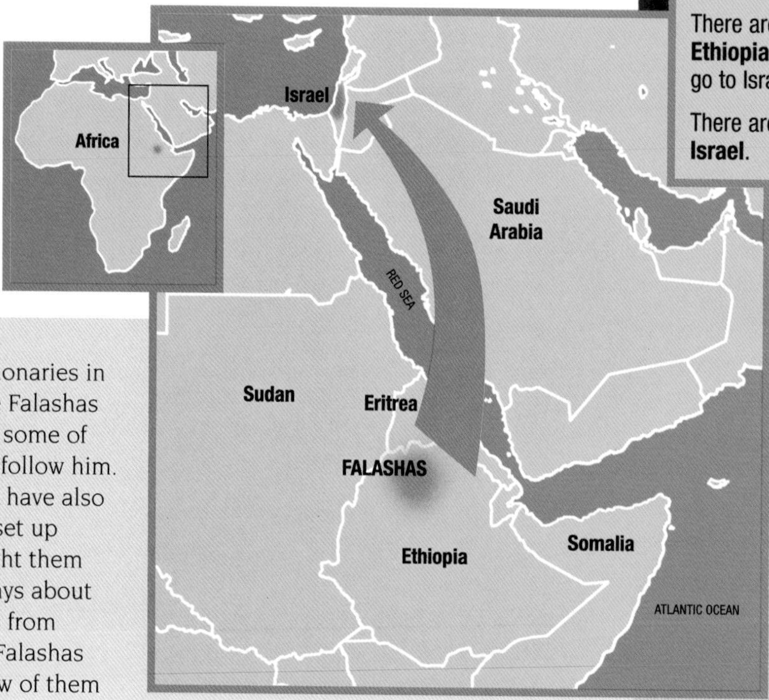

Christian missionaries in Ethiopia told the Falashas about Jesus, and some of them decided to follow him. The missionaries have also helped the sick, set up schools and taught them what the Bible says about Jesus. When Jews from Europe told the Falashas about Israel, a few of them decided to go there.

Map labels: Africa, Israel, Saudi Arabia, RED SEA, Sudan, Eritrea, FALASHAS, Somalia, Ethiopia, ATLANTIC OCEAN

Operation Moses

During the Communist revolution in Ethiopia in the 1970s and 1980s, the Falashas suffered a lot because they believed in God.

"It was terrible," Abraham remembers. "I was only a little boy. There was civil war in Ethiopia and, to make matters worse, we were starving because there was no rain to make our crops grow. Our animals died, too. My family joined thousands of others in the long walk to a refugee camp in Sudan. It took us ten days, and a lot of children and old people died on the way. We hoped that, once we reached the camps, we'd be able to go to Israel. The Bible says that the Jewish people will to return to Israel someday, and we thought maybe that day had come.

Falasha boys outside a school in Jerusalem

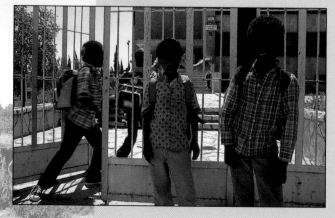

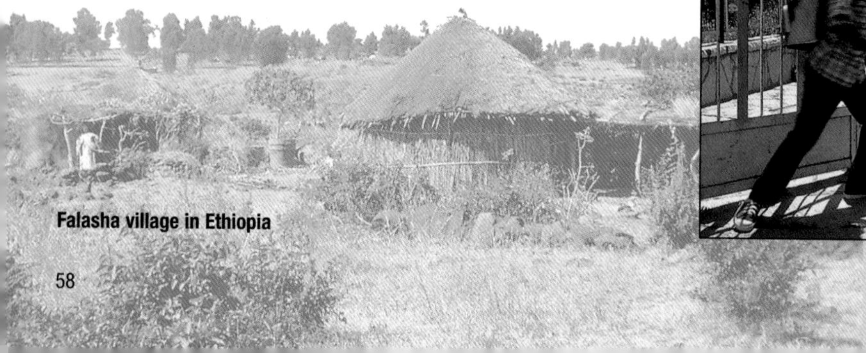

Falasha village in Ethiopia

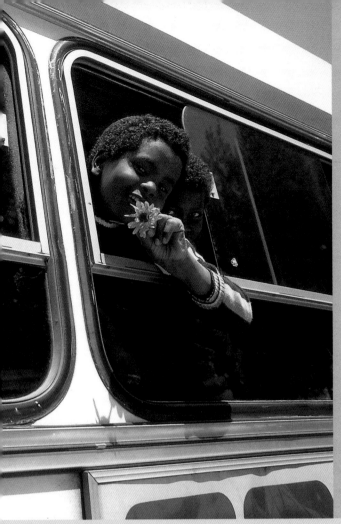

 ## To help you pray for the Falashas

You can thank God for:

- every Ethiopian Jew who has come to know Jesus.

- the Israeli government, who rescued so many Ethiopian Jews and gave them a fresh start in Israel.

You can ask God:

- to show the Falashas that their journey to God does not end in Israel, but that he has a home in heaven for all who believe in Jesus.

- to help the Ethiopian Jews as they adjust to life in Israel.

- for the children to do well at school and for the older people to adjust to their new life.

- to give the Falashas good friends in Israel.

- for the Falashas to hear that Jesus loves them and wants them to follow him.

Falasha children on a school bus in Jerusalem, Israel

"We were very excited when we heard that the Israelis had arranged a secret rescue plan called 'Operation Moses.' They crammed us all onto planes, which was scary since most of us had never been on a plane before."

That was in 1984. About 13,000 Ethiopian Jews were flown to Israel, but the flights were stopped when the story leaked out.

Operation Solomon

For those left behind in Ethiopia, life became even more difficult. The civil war was even worse, and there was famine in the country again. Jews, along with everyone else, had to obey new laws. "These laws were hard for us," Hailu said, "especially since markets could only be held on Saturdays, the Jewish

Sabbath. Like thousands of other Jews, my family moved from the countryside to Addis Ababa, the capital city. We registered with the Israeli Embassy there, hoping we could go to Israel. We had to wait a long time and sold everything we owned so that we could buy food. We were so glad that the Israelis and some Christians helped us.

"By 1991, the Communist government only controlled Addis Ababa and the area around the city. The rebel armies were getting closer to the city, and the Israelis were afraid that there would be a lot of killing and looting and the Ethiopian Jews would be blamed for it.

"The Israelis had secret talks with the Ethiopian government and the rebels. The government finally agreed to let Israeli planes

fly in to get us, and the rebels promised not to attack the city for a few days.

"All the seats had been taken out of the planes," Hailu remembers, "and we weren't allowed to take any luggage so they could carry more people. In just 30 hours, 14,400 Ethiopian Jews were flown to Israel – and several babies were born on the way! 'Operation Solomon' was kept secret until we all landed in Israel."

"In Ethiopia," Hailu continued, "we lived in small villages and worked as farmers, potters, iron workers or weavers. Everything was so different in Israel. My family lived in a big apartment building with electricity, running water, flush toilets, elevators and new kinds of food. But we soon felt at

home, especially once we learned to speak Hebrew."

Some of the Ethiopian Jews in Israel have been Christians for several generations, and a few others have come to know Jesus more recently. Please pray that many more Ethiopian Jews in Israel will meet Messianic Jews (followers of Jesus) who will tell them about Jesus.

Do you know?

The New Testament talks a lot about the Jews. They're the descendants of the Israelites of the Old Testament. Although the Jews in Jesus' day rejected him, God wants us to take the gospel to the Jews so that they can follow Jesus and live forever.

Fiji

A Nation of Islands

The beautiful islands of Fiji, with their warm sunny beaches, are located in the South Pacific Ocean to the east of Australia. Although there are more than 300 islands, only 112 of them are inhabited. Vitu Levu and Vanua Levu, the two main islands, were formed from volcanoes and their steep mountain slopes are covered with forests. Suva, the capital of Fiji, is the biggest city in the whole of the South Pacific region.

Fiji is a fertile country. If you look carefully at the coat of arms on Fiji's flag you will see sugar cane, a coconut palm, a cocoa pod and bananas. Two of the country's main exports are sugar and copra (dried coconut). Coconut oil is extracted from the copra and used to make many different things – including soap, shampoo and margarine.

Fact file

Area: 7,050 sq. mi.

Population: 816,905

Capital: Suva

Main religions: Christianity; Hinduism; Islam

Official language: English

Chief exports: Sugar; copra; gold; fish

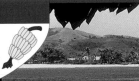

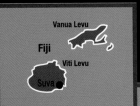

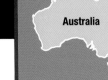

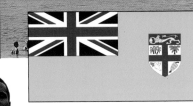

Sharing the good news

You will also see a dove of peace, a Christian symbol, on the coat of arms on Fiji's flag. Christians came to Fiji over 150 years ago to tell the people there about Jesus. Fijian Christians believed the good news of Jesus was too wonderful to keep to themselves, and many of them set out on dangerous journeys in deep-sea canoes to tell people on other Pacific islands about God's love. And so another symbol of Christianity in Fiji is a deep-sea canoe.

Many years ago, there was a missionary called Dr. Brown who wanted evangelists from Fiji to go with him to Papua New Guinea to tell people there about Jesus. Dr. Brown asked for volunteers at the pastors' training college, but he thought no one would be willing

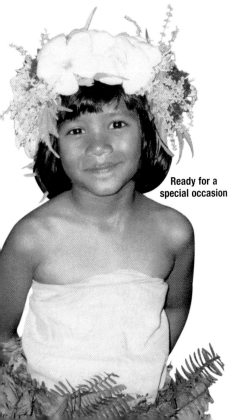

Ready for a special occasion

Presidential guard

to go because thousands of people in Fiji had just died from measles. He was very surprised when every one of the 84 students said they would go with him! One of their leaders stood up and said, "Our minds are made up. We have given ourselves to God's work. If we live, we live. If we die, we die." They were willing to risk everything to tell others that Jesus died on the cross so that we can be forgiven for the bad things we've done and have eternal life.

Indians of Fiji

About 100 years ago, people from India were brought to Fiji to work on the sugar plantations. Now there are almost as many Indians as Fijians in

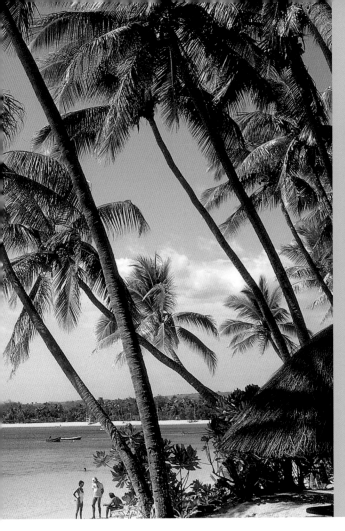

 ## To help you pray for Fiji

You can thank God for:

- all the Christians in Fiji.
- the Indians who know Jesus.
- the friendships between Fijian Christians and Indians.
- the many Chinese people who come to work in Fiji for a few years and the young people from other islands who study there.

You can ask God:

- to resolve the political situation peacefully, restore democracy to the island and help the government leaders to always be fair.
- to help Fijians and Indians learn to live at peace with one another and to forgive each other.
- to bring many Indian boys and girls to know and love Jesus at Sunday school.

Do you know?

The International Date Line passes between the islands of Fiji. This means that Fiji is one of the first countries in the world to welcome each new day.

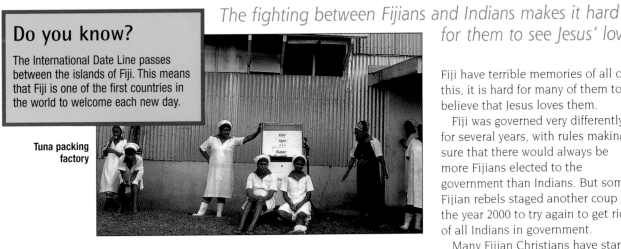

Tuna packing factory

The fighting between Fijians and Indians makes it hard for them to see Jesus' love

the country. Most of these Indians are Hindus, Muslims or Sikhs.

Fiji was a British colony for almost 100 years. After Fiji became a country with its own government in 1970, many ethnic Fijians were afraid that the Indians would take over their country. They were upset when the Fiji Labour Party, which tried to bring Indians and Fijians together, won the national elections in 1987. There were more Indians than Fijians in the

newly elected government, so the army tried to get rid of this government.

Some Fijians were angry with the Indians and did things that were very wrong. Some of them set fire to mosques and temples belonging to the Indians. But Christian leaders spoke out against these terrible actions. The Indian people felt angry and afraid, and many of them left Fiji. Because the Indians who still live in

Fiji have terrible memories of all of this, it is hard for many of them to believe that Jesus loves them.

Fiji was governed very differently for several years, with rules making sure that there would always be more Fijians elected to the government than Indians. But some Fijian rebels staged another coup in the year 2000 to try again to get rid of all Indians in government.

Many Fijian Christians have started to pray for people all over the world who haven't heard about Jesus, and some have become missionaries in other countries. Although they want to share the love of Jesus with those in their own country too, the uncertain political situation will probably make it even harder for Indians to accept Jesus. And it will also be harder for those Indians who have accepted Jesus already to live as Christians in Fiji.

Garifuna

Descendants of Slaves and Carib Indians

"Look what I've got!"

The man checking security at a small Caribbean airport rummaged through Roger's suitcase. He pulled out a book. "What's this? What language is it?" he demanded in Spanish. "It's not Spanish."

"It's a Garifuna (gah-ree-foo-na) New Testament," Roger replied. "Garifuna? That's my language!" the man exclaimed. "I've seen a Spanish Bible, but I've never seen a book in Garifuna. I'd love to learn how to read it. Where can I get a copy of this?"

"I'm afraid they're all sold out," Roger explained. "This is my only copy." "Please let me have it," the man pleaded. He was so excited when Roger gave it to him. He clutched the New Testament and showed it to everyone, shouting, "Look what I've got!"

Do you know?

Although most of them speak Spanish and some can read it, Garifuna is the "language that speaks to their hearts." One Garifuna minister was so delighted with his New Testament that he said, "May we chew God's word, swallow it and let it enter into our veins!"

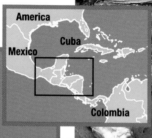

The Garifuna New Testament has been reprinted since Roger gave his last copy to this man several years ago. Nearly all of the Garifuna speak Spanish, the language of the countries in which they live. But they speak their own language among themselves. Now they're learning to read in their own language and, as they read the New Testament and their teachers explain it to them, a lot of them are deciding to follow Jesus.

The Old Testament has now been translated into Garifuna as well.

Shipwrecked slaves

The Garifuna, or Black Caribs, are descendants of slaves that British and Spanish boats brought from Africa in the seventeenth century. Sometimes these boats were shipwrecked and the slaves escaped. Their masters set other slaves free. Many of them settled on St. Vincent in the Windward Islands, where they married Carib Indians.

Because they caused some trouble, the British shipped them all off to the island of Roatan, far away across the Caribbean Sea, in 1797. Eventually they made their way to South America, where they settled in villages along the coasts of Belize, Honduras and Guatemala. A lot of them still make their living by fishing and farming.

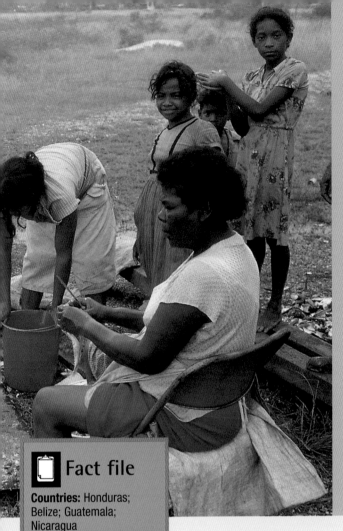

To help you pray for the Garifuna

You can thank God for:

- the Garifuna Bible, both Old and New Testaments.
- each Garifuna who has come to know Jesus.

You can ask God:

- that the Garifuna will read and understand the whole Bible.
- to give patience to those teaching people to read the long and complicated words in Garifuna.
- to use the *Jesus* film to bring more Garifuna people to know him.
- to take away their fear of evil spirits as the Garifuna turn to Jesus.
- to send people to train Garifuna Christians to become pastors, leaders and evangelists.

Fact file

Countries: Honduras; Belize; Guatemala; Nicaragua

Numbers: About 100,000

Languages: Spanish; Garifuna

Religion: Animism

Occupations: Farming; fishing

They took their own African and Carib beliefs with them, and soon added Catholicism to the mixture. Nearly all Garifuna children are baptized into the Roman Catholic Church, but they also wear a ribbon tied around their wrist to protect them from evil spirits. They believe there are spirits living all around them and put a cross over the doorway of their houses to protect the family from harm. They believe dreams, crying chickens and howling dogs are all omens that foretell the future.

Jesus is alive!

Although many Garifuna knew a few stories about Jesus, very few of them understood who he really is and why God sent him to earth. There was great excitement when missionaries showed the *Jesus* film in Garifuna in a field outside one village. Two hundred people came to watch.

In the film, Jesus speaks to a small child in Garifuna, "Hello. What are you doing?" "Nothing," the child replies.

"He knows our greeting," the people cried in delight, clapping their hands. "He speaks Garifuna!" They watched the film with great excitement, talking with one another about what they saw and heard.

"Who wouldn't believe in Jesus?" one lady said to her friend. "Did you see how he healed the blind man?"

"Look!" some men exclaimed. "They fish like we do. We know what it's like to fish all night and catch nothing. When Jesus told them to put their nets back in the sea, they had a great catch! Amazing! And Jesus calmed that storm, too. Lots of people we know have died in storms like that. He must be more powerful than all the spirits of the sea if he can do that! He must be worth following."

As they watched Jesus dying on the cross, many of the people wept. At the end of the film, 35 people said they wanted to follow Jesus. More people came to watch the film the next night, and even more decided to follow him.

Many of the Garifuna want to hear God's word and learn how to follow him. The churches are growing. A missionary working with the Garifuna said, "It's great to know so many children are praying for the Garifuna." God is answering our prayers so let's keep praying that many more Garifuna will come to know Jesus.

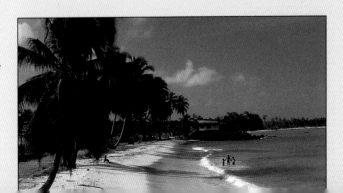

Gonds

Forest-dwellers of Central India

"Who can help us?"

"What else can we do?" The people in Lion village were very worried. Lots of people were sick, and several had died. "What about the medicine man?" someone asked. "We've been to him," someone else said. "He prayed to the spirits and made sacrifices and offerings to them, but it only made things worse." "I don't know why the spirits are treating us like this," another person said sadly.

"Let's go talk to the Christians and their teacher," someone suggested. "They say their God is more powerful than all our spirits. Maybe he can stop this sickness."

Right: Dressed for a Gond wedding

Pakistan
• Delhi
India
GOND
• Nagpur
ARABIAN SEA
BAY OF BENGAL

So they went to the missionary. "Can you help us?" they asked.

"I'll pray for you, and so will all the Christians in the village," said the Indian missionary. "Our God is greater than any other god or spirit. He promises that he will hear and answer our prayers. He can heal this sickness."

As the missionary and the Christians prayed together, God healed ten people in Lion village! "It's true that the God of the Christians is greater than the spirits," the people said. "We want to follow him."

A forest village

Lion village is deep in the forests of central India, and the villagers belong to the Gond tribe. There are many different tribes in India, but the Gonds are one of the largest. Although the Indian government classifies them as Hindus, most of them are animists. They believe that evil spirits wait in the fields and forests, looking for ways to harm them. The Gonds make sacrifices to these spirits, hoping they will leave them alone.

Many of the Gonds work as farmers. They keep some cattle and grow millet, maize, wheat and beans. They make their simple homes from bamboo and timber with roofs of leaves. The houses have only one or two rooms. In one room there will be a few wooden stools and a hammock or two, and some cooking pots in the kitchen.

Many older Gonds can't read or write, and so other people often cheat them when they sell things in the towns. The Indian government wants to help them, and in some places it has set up schools where Gond children can study.

> ### Do you know?
> The Gonds have two important gods. They believe one was born six months before the world was created, and the other six months after. They have other gods as well, and each family has its own god.

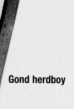

Gond herdboy

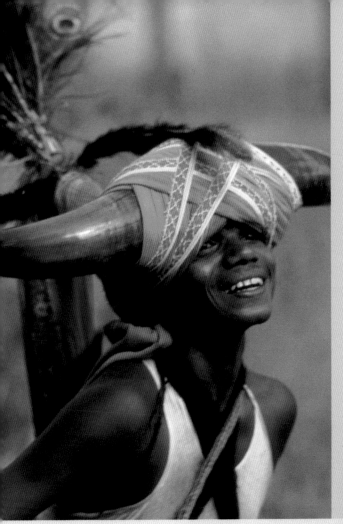

To help you pray for the Gonds

You can thank God for:

- every Gond who is following Jesus.

- Gond Christians who are studying the Bible and learning how to tell others about Jesus.

You can ask God:

- that lots of Gond boys and girls will decide to follow Jesus, who is always with them and helps them when they're afraid.

- to show the Gonds that he is far more powerful than all the gods and spirits they fear and worship.

- to keep the Indian missionaries safe as they travel to Gond villages.

- to help those who are translating the Bible into Gondi, which is a difficult language, so that everyone can understand it.

- that there will be a church in every Gond village.

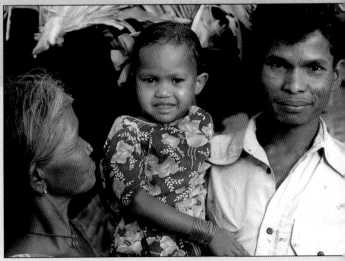

Lion village

Because of the amazing miracle of healing, many of the people who live in Lion village are Christians. Let's go with an Indian missionary to visit them. Since there aren't any roads for cars or buses, we'll travel in a bullock cart. "It will take us all day to get there," the missionary warns us. "And the cart doesn't have springs or comfortable seats, so you'll probably feel a bit sore as we bump along the rough trails. It's a long way, but you might prefer to walk! Since we'll have to travel very slowly through the forest, you'll have plenty of time to see all the birds, and maybe even a bear or a tiger!"

Everyone in Lion village is excited to see us, and

Fact file

Country: Central India

Numbers: About 12,700,000 (they're the biggest tribal group in Central India)

Language: Gondi, but they often speak the language of other peoples who live in the same areas.

Religions: Animism; Hinduism

Occupations: Farmers; laborers; businessmen

they make us feel at home. "Since we started to follow Jesus," someone tells us, "he's changed our lives and made us into new people." "Yes," someone else says, "we used to be afraid of the spirits all the time, but now we know they don't have

any power over us. Jesus gives us joy and peace." Someone else is eager to tell us about the miracle. "We know Jesus cares for us," he said, "because when everyone in the village was sick, only Jesus had the power to make us well. Now we want to learn as much as we can about him. And we want others to know Jesus, too."

New life for the Gonds

Some of the Gond Christians are going to special training centers to learn what the Bible says and how to share the good news about Jesus with their own people. They're reaching out to more villages, but there are still a lot of villages where the people have never heard of Jesus. Please help change the world for the Gonds by praying for them.

Greece

Home of the First Olympic Games

A visit to church

Like a lot of Greek boys, nine-year-old Dimitris had only been to church a few times. Every time he went with his grandmother, she bought him a candle, lit it and told him to bow down in front of a picture of a saint. These pictures, called icons, were everywhere in the church. Dimitris made the sign of the cross, kissed the picture and left the candle beside it. As they stood listening to the church service, Dimitris saw the joy on his grandmother's face.

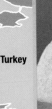
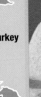

Greek Orthodox priests

Another way of worship

Dimitris and his grandmother saw a group of young people singing and handing out booklets on the street one day. Dimitris wanted to listen, but suddenly a man started to shout at the group and some of the people who had taken the booklets dropped them.

"What's happening? Why is the man so angry?" Dimitris asked his grandmother. "The music was really good – and they were singing about Jesus. What's wrong with that?"

"They're evangelicals," she told him. "Almost all Greeks belong to the Greek Orthodox Church – even though most of them don't go to church very often. A lot of Greeks, like that man shouting, think the evangelicals are heretics because they don't belong to the Orthodox Church or follow our traditional way of worshipping God. Your uncle goes to an evangelical church. He says it's a very simple place with no icons, statues or candles to help them worship God. The people who go there talk about Jesus as their friend who is with them always. I just wish we could all get along as we worship the same God in different ways."

Sharing the good news

The evangelical church in Greece is small and not very popular. Some evangelicals have even been put in prison for talking about Jesus. As well as holding meetings in their churches, they preach on the streets, sing, put on plays, give out booklets and help those in need. Some groups publish and sell Christian books, and now there are two Bible schools.

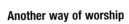

Spinning yarn

c. 1400 BC Earliest record of Greek mythology	c. 776 BC Race in Olympia	c. 450 BC "Golden Age" of Greek ar	c. 400–300 BC Aristotle/Plato/ Socrates

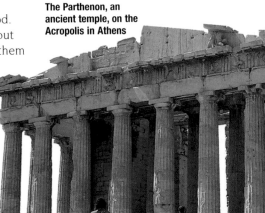

The Parthenon, an ancient temple, on the Acropolis in Athens

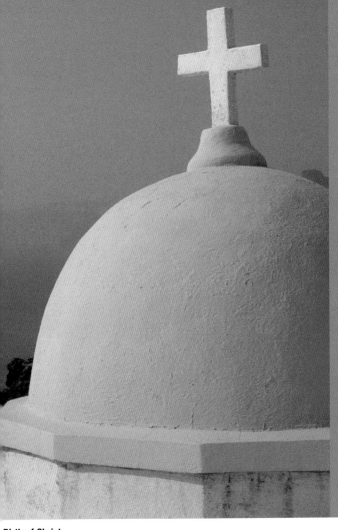

To help you pray for Greece

You can thank God for:

- every Greek who knows and follows Jesus.

- Christian books, cassettes, papers and radio broadcasts that explain who Jesus is and what he has done to save us.

You can ask God:

- to help all who call themselves Christians to work together and be an example of Jesus' love.

- to encourage young people to be brave and not afraid as they talk to people on the streets about Jesus.

- that young people going to university will meet Christians who are filled with joy because they follow Jesus.

- to keep the "Morning Star" safe as it sails from island to island and to give the crew courage as they share the good news about Jesus.

- that Christian tourists visiting Greece will have opportunities to share Jesus' love with the people they meet.

Olympic gold medal

Birth of Christ

C. AD 50 Paul preaches to the Greeks	**1054** The beginning of the Eastern Orthodox Church	**1829** Greece became independant
C. AD 60 New Testament written in Greek		**1896** First modern Olympic Games

2004 Olympic Games return to Greece

There are hundreds of islands in the beautiful blue waters of the Ionian and Aegean Seas surrounding Greece. The boat "Morning Star" visits these islands with teams of

Do you know ?

Greece was the first country in Europe to hear the gospel, which was preached to them by the apostle Paul himself (about AD 50). The people are proud that the original New Testament was written in the Greek language. In Acts 16, 17 and 18 we read how God called Paul to take the good news about Jesus to Greece.

evangelists. Angry protesters have tried to stop them from preaching on some of the islands, and sometimes the evangelists have been arrested. But people on other islands welcome the "Morning Star," and some have decided to follow Jesus because the evangelists have explained the truth of the Bible to them. Some of these people had always gone to church but never heard that Jesus is our friend and savior who is with us all the time.

Living history

Our world would be a very different place without the art, literature, theater, science and philosophy that came from Greece. A lot of ideas that people have today are based on what the great Greek philosophers said thousands of years ago. You may also

know some of the myths about the Greek gods Zeus, Apollo, Athena and others.

Sports have always been important to the Greeks, too. The first Olympic game, a running race, was held in the Greek town of Olympia in the eighth century BC as part of a religious festival. The first modern Olympic Games were held in Athens in 1896, and again in 2004. They take place in a different country every four years.

Greece has beautiful beaches, ancient ruins, islands and mountain villages that haven't changed for centuries. More than nine million tourists visit Greece every year. But Greece still needs missionaries who will talk to people like Dimitris and his family about Jesus.

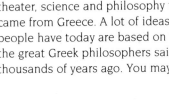

Greenland

The Largest Island in the World

An Eskimo boy

Eight-year-old Sigssuk snuggled into bed. He was tired, but much too excited to sleep. His father had taken him on his first ever seal-hunt today, and they'd caught two seals. He dreamed of becoming a great hunter someday!

Sigssuk is an Eskimo, or Inuit, and lives with his family on the northwest coast of Greenland. Hunting is a very important part of their lives. Almost as soon as he'd learned to walk, Sigssuk's father had given him a puppy and a toy whip so he could learn to train his own dog. His father also built him a special kayak (canoe), which he hung from a beam in the house so that it was just a few inches from the ground. Sigssuk had great fun sitting in it and learning how to control it with a small paddle.

Every summer, when it's daylight all the time, Sigssuk goes with his family on camping trips. He catches little auks (seabirds) in a net. They cook and eat some of the birds, but they put the rest in a special sealskin sack to save for food in the winter.

Fact file

Area: 840,020 sq. mi.; 85% of the land is a glacial ice cap

Population: 56,156

Capital: Nuuk

Languages: Greenlandic; Danish

Religion: Christianity

Chief exports: Fish and fish products

The sun never rises during the long, dark winter months in Greenland. During the winter Sigssuk goes to the village school, where he learns to read and write. School is much more exciting when some of the men teach them about hunting and show them how to build their own kayaks and sledges. It's usually too cold for Sigssuk and his friends to play outside in the winter. So they stay inside and play games, watch television and videos and listen to the grown-ups tell stories about hunting expeditions.

Greenland is the largest island in the world. It belongs to Denmark, but Greenland has governed itself since 1979. Most of the country lies inside the Arctic Circle, and an enormous ice sheet covers a lot of it. Some, like Sigssuk and his family, are Eskimos. But most Greenlanders are descendants of Eskimos who have married European settlers. Nearly all of them live in small towns on the south and west coasts, where they make a living from fishing and hunting.

Greenland may be a cold, dark place – but Jesus brings warmth and light

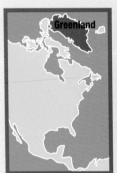
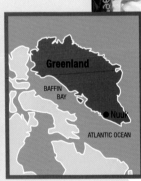

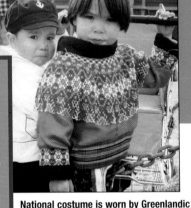
National costume is worn by Greenlandic children on special occasions

The first Christians

Erik the Red, a Norseman from Iceland, first discovered Greenland about 1,000 years ago. He called the country Greenland – even though it's covered in ice – to persuade his family and friends to join him there. A group of brave men, women and children set sail across the stormy seas. They took their horses, cows and sheep with them. Erik's son, Leif the Lucky, became a Christian on a visit to Norway. When he returned to Greenland he told everyone about Jesus and a lot of people became Christians.

A missionary from Denmark went to Greenland in 1721, hoping to find that the descendants of those first settlers were Christians. But no one in Greenland followed Jesus anymore. Other settlers came from Denmark

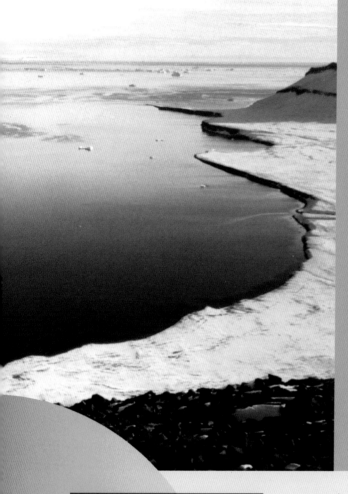

To help you pray for Greenland

You can thank God for:

- the *Jesus* film in Greenlandic.
- camps where children can learn about Jesus.
- the new translation of the Bible in Greenlandic.

You can ask God:

- to show the people that being a Christian means far more than going to church once a year.
- to help Christians encourage one another to always follow Jesus.
- for Christians to go to the Discipleship Training School to study the Bible and learn to tell others about Jesus.
- that many in Greenland who are sad and lonely will discover that Jesus really is alive and ready to help them when life is difficult.

Boys enjoying themselves at the Christian camp run by the Ebenezer church in Nuuk

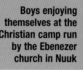

Do you know?

The ice sheet covering Greenland averages nearly 5,000 feet in depth. If the ice ever melted, all the oceans of the world would rise about 20 feet!

ancestors to help him.

One day, Olaf heard that the first movie in Greenlandic, a film about Jesus, was going to be shown in Nuuk. Olaf and his family couldn't wait to see it. As Olaf watched the *Jesus* film, he realized that Jesus died on the cross to take away all the bad things he had done. He wanted Jesus to give him a clean new life.

Now Olaf and

his family really are following Jesus.

Several evangelical organizations in Greenland hold special meetings and camps for both children and adults. When Niels became a Christian at one of these camps he knew it would be very hard to be a real Christian at home because all his friends drank alcohol and took drugs. It's never easy to be different from everyone else! Even some of those who go to Bible schools and special training courses to learn about Jesus find it hard to keep following Jesus once they return to their homes.

and Norway, and the Greenlanders started to follow Jesus again and were baptized. They built churches in almost every little town and village, and the Bible was translated into the Greenlandic language.

The *Jesus* film

Olaf and his family live in Nuuk, the capital of Greenland. Like many Greenlanders, they call themselves Christians and always go to church at Christmas time. But when Olaf fell and broke his arm, his mother stitched a charm inside his coat to keep him safe and asked the spirits of her

Cutting up a whale

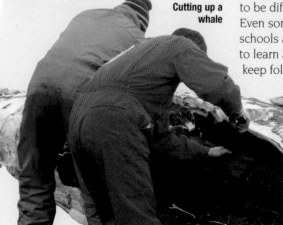

Guinea-Bissau

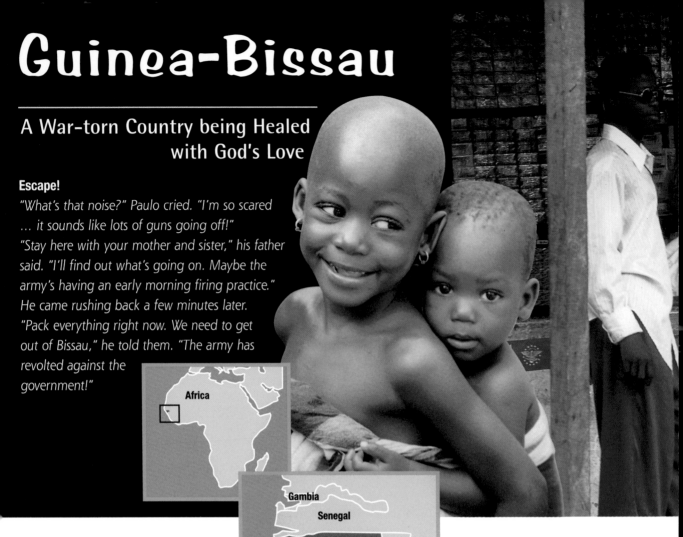

A War-torn Country being Healed with God's Love

Escape!

"What's that noise?" Paulo cried. *"I'm so scared ... it sounds like lots of guns going off!"*

"Stay here with your mother and sister," his father said. *"I'll find out what's going on. Maybe the army's having an early morning firing practice."* He came rushing back a few minutes later. *"Pack everything right now. We need to get out of Bissau,"* he told them. *"The army has revolted against the government!"*

They grabbed what belongings they could and joined thousands of people trying to escape from the fighting in the city. Paulo's mother carried his little sister and Paulo ran beside his father, afraid that he might get lost on the way. Every taxi and truck that passed them was already filled with people, so they walked and walked until they reached safety.

Sharing God's love

"I'm tired and hungry," Paulo complained when they finally sat down to rest under a mango tree. "Where are we going to stay?" As they were sitting there wondering what to do, a man came by. "Come to my house," he said. "You can stay with me." The man was a Christian, and his house was already packed with other refugees. "You can stay here as long as there's enough rice in my house," he said.

When food supplies began to arrive in Bissau from other countries, pastors, Bible school students and other Christians helped give it out. As they gave food to the people, they told them about the love of Jesus. Pastors talked about God's love and care over the radio. They also helped with peace talks between the two sides in the fighting.

This revolt on Sunday, June 7th, 1998 came as a surprise to Paulo and his family and most people in Bissau. The airport was closed down, along with the post office, schools and most of the stores. The civil war lasted for 11 months.

Paulo's family returned to Bissau

Many people learned about Jesus' love during the war when Christians helped those who were suffering

Do you know?

Many people in Guinea-Bissau are afraid of evil spirits. When twins are born, they're sometimes left outside to die because the witch doctor tells the parents that one of the babies is a spirit baby. That's changing now because Christians are explaining to parents that both twins are special and precious to God.

after the war. They, along with many others, found that their house had been destroyed and their belongings stolen. But they couldn't afford to fix or replace anything since they had scarcely enough money to buy food! Through the Christian love of the man

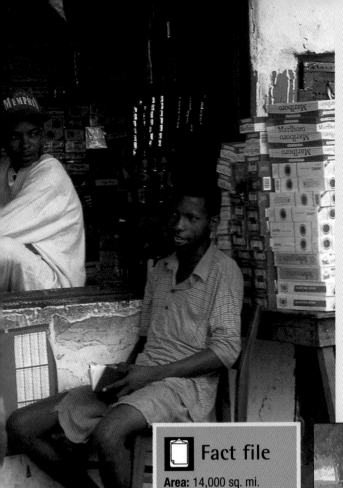

To help you pray for Guinea-Bissau

You can thank God for:

- the Christians who opened their homes to people fleeing from the fighting.
- Christian radio broadcasts and the *Jesus* film.

You can ask God:

- to help each new Christian to want to know Jesus more and more.
- to give patience to those helping adults learn to read.
- to provide enough money for those who want to go to Bible school to learn to teach others about God.
- that the tribes in Guinea-Bissau, who live in fear of evil spirits, will realize that Jesus is more powerful.
- that the leaders will rule the country fairly and wisely.

Fact file

Area: 14,000 sq. mi.

Population: 1,179,000

Capital: Bissau

Main languages: Portuguese; Creole

Main religions: Animism; Islam; Christianity

Main products: Peanuts; cashew nuts; cotton

Crushing cashew fruit. The juice is used to make a drink.

You can speak Creole

Good morning is "Bon dia" (bon dee-a)

How are you? is "Kuma di kurpu?" (Koo-ma dee koor-poo)

See you later is "Te logu" (Te log-oo)

who took them in when they were refugees, Paulo and his family learned that Jesus is their friend and helps them when life is really hard. Many other men and women, boys and girls also came to know Jesus. So now there are new groups of Christians in places where there were no Christians before the war. They have seen God's love at work. His love has filled their hearts, and they want to share that love with others.

A poor country

Guinea-Bissau is a small country in West Africa, between Senegal in the north and Guinea in the south. It's one of the poorest countries in the world. Portugal ruled Guinea-Bissau for many years, but in 1974, after a long war, the country became independent.

Most of the country is on the African mainland. Mangrove swamps and marshes cover the land along the coast, where rice grows. Further inland are rain forests and *savanna* where people grow peanuts, mangoes, beans and cotton. Offshore, out in the Atlantic Ocean, are the forest-covered Bijagos Islands.

Many languages

Although it's a small country, more than 25 people groups live in Guinea-Bissau. Each group has its own language, but most people speak Creole – a mixture of Portuguese and local African languages. The New Testament has been translated into the Balanta, Bijago, Mandingo and Papel languages, and the whole Bible has now been translated into Creole.

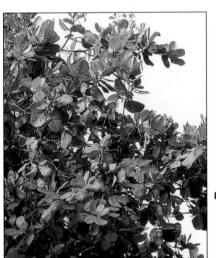

Cashew tree

Gypsies

Nomads of the World

Who are the Gypsies and where do they come from? About 1,200 years ago, large groups of people began moving out of the region that we call the Punjab in northwest India and northeast Pakistan. As they went, they earned their living as musicians and entertainers, horse traders, blacksmiths and craftsmen.

Today, there may be as many as 40 million Gypsies living all over the world – in more than 40 countries and on every continent. Many of them are still nomads, moving from place to place, often following their traditional work. Although most Gypsies speak the language of the people among whom they live, most of them also speak one of the 20 or more Romany dialects. There are many different groups of Gypsies, each with a slightly different dialect and lifestyle.

for the Gypsy people. But God has been answering prayers, and since 1950 thousands of Gypsies in many parts of the world have become Christians.

Inside a Gypsy caravan in the UK

Because Gypsies have kept their own way of life and have never become a part of the countries where they live, they are often despised, disliked and neglected. As they tend to move from one place to another, few of their children go to school long enough to learn to read or write.

Gypsy children are well loved. If your parents were Gypsies you would be sure to know to be respectful to older people and not to talk to strangers. You would also learn the many Gypsy rules about cleanliness. You would live in a caravan and help to keep it spotless. You would only be allowed to eat certain kinds of food. For example, Muslim Rom Gypsies eat chicken, but not pork. But Kaale Rom Gypsies from Finland think chickens are dirty. Some

Gypsies eat hedgehogs, while others think they're unclean. If you were a Gypsy you would learn many traditional dances and songs. If you were invited to a wedding, you might be there feasting and dancing for three whole days!

Are you a "Gorgio"? That is what Gypsies call those who aren't Gypsies. In 1901 there was a Gypsy called Rodney Smith who preached about Jesus to "Gorgios" in Britain and South Africa. Thousands of them became Christians. When people asked Rodney Smith why he wasn't preaching to his own people, he told them that the time had not yet come

Do you know?

In the parable of the great banquet (Luke 14:15–24), a man prepared a party for all his guests. But when those he had invited refused to come, the master told his servant to "Go out to the roads and country lanes and make them come in, so that my house will be full." Many leaders of the Gypsy Christians believe that they are these last guests, coming to Jesus now.

Gypsy site in London, UK

Clara's discovery

Clara was twenty years old. She lived with her parents in their Gypsy caravan. Sometimes as a child she had gone to school, but she had never learned to read. One night she was very upset after an argument with her parents.

Although she had heard about God's love for her, she didn't know very much about him. That night she asked God to help her read the Bible so that she would know the right way to live. She was very disappointed because nothing seemed to happen.

The next morning, when she was helping her mother clean the caravan, she found an old Bible. She opened it and was amazed to discover that she could read it! Excitedly she told her mother, who couldn't believe it until Clara read to her.

A few weeks later Clara began to understand what Jesus had done for her, and she put her trust in him. Ever since then, she has been telling people about God's special gift to her and, more importantly, about his gift of forgiveness and her new life in Jesus.

Gypsies worldwide

Life is often very difficult for Gypsies, but God's Holy Spirit is bringing many of them hope and peace. European Gypsies are sending money to help Gypsies in India and Madagascar, and going as missionaries to Gypsies in Argentina and Russia. Gypsy Christians from France have gone to many different countries to tell other Gypsies about God's love. Gypsy evangelist Tom Wilson has said, "We Gypsies are a nation of evangelists; we can't help gossiping the gospel."

Romanian Gypsies

Gypsy children baptized at the Great Dorset Steam Fair in the UK

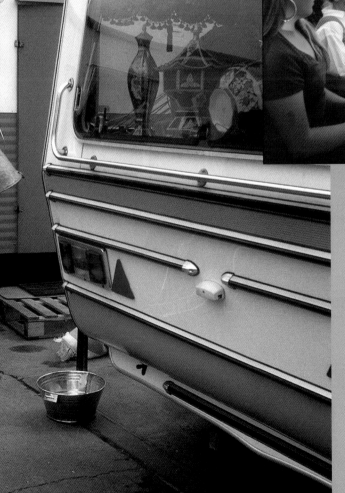

To help you pray for Gypsies

You can thank God for:

- European Gypsies who are telling other Gypsies throughout the world about God's love and salvation.

- Gypsy Bible schools where Gypsies can learn more about Jesus and how to read the Bible.

- the Christian radio broadcasts that are made especially for Gypsies.

- the Gypsies who have started their own churches where they feel at home and can worship him in their own way.

You can ask God:

- to help Christians who are translating the Bible into the Romany languages to use the right words so that Gypsies will be able to understand God's word.

- to lead "Gorgio" Christians to be willing to help Gypsies when they are despised, to make friends with them and to help their children learn to read.

- to fill Gypsy Christians with love and joy and the readiness to always "gossip the gospel."

Haiti

The Land Freed by Slaves

The country of Haiti occupies the western third of a beautiful island in the Caribbean Sea called Hispaniola. The other two thirds of the island form the Dominican Republic. More than 200 years ago, Haiti's French rulers brought people from West Africa and made them work as slaves in Haiti. These slaves rebelled against the French rulers and fought for their freedom for 13 years. On January 1st 1804, the whole country was declared independent. It was the first Black republic in the world.

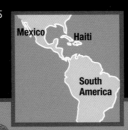

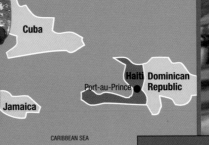

Mexico · Haiti · South America · Cuba · Jamaica · Haiti Port-au-Prince · Dominican Republic · CARIBBEAN SEA

Fact file

Area: 10,580 sq. mi.

Population: 8,222,025

Capital: Port-au-Prince

Main languages: French (official); Haitian Creole

Main religions: Christianity; spiritism; voodoo

Chief exports: Coffee; sugar

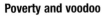

Poverty and voodoo

Sadly, Haiti has not really been a free country since 1804. One dictator after another has ruled Haiti. One was known as "Baby Doc" Duvalier. It is thought that while he was in power he stole millions of dollars from his poverty-stricken country.

Haiti is the poorest country in the western world. Although there are some very rich Haitians, the majority are poor farmers, descendants of those black slaves from Africa. Because they long for a better life with freedom from riots, fear and poverty, many have tried to make the dangerous journey to the United States in small boats.

Although most Haitians would say that they are Christians, not very many of them really know Jesus. Many Haitians practice voodoo, which involves worshipping spirits. This disobeys God's first commandment not to worship any other gods (Exodus 20:3). Because evil spirits can

People in Haiti have never really known peace or prosperity

take control of people who worship them and make them do strange and frightening things, these people are full of fear and sadness.

The witch doctor's son

Gerard, the son of a wealthy witch doctor, liked to listen to Christian radio broadcasts at boarding school. Some of Gerard's friends were surprised when they found him listening to a Christian radio station.

"Aren't you going to be a witch doctor some day?" they asked.

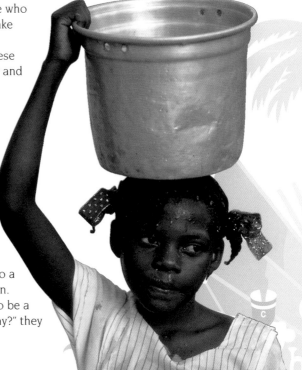

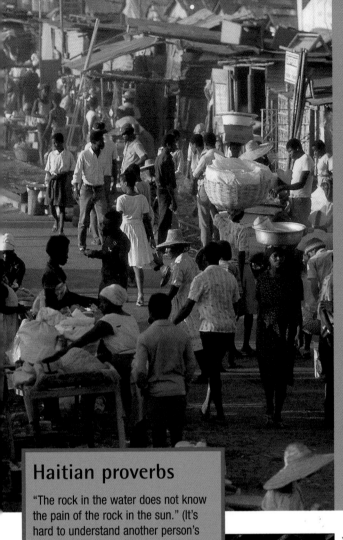

 To help you pray for Haiti

To help you pray for Haiti

You can thank God for:

- the Christians in Haiti who are filled with joy and who share Jesus' love with others.

- the missionaries in Haiti who are teaching young people about Jesus.

You can ask God:

- to give people the strength to stop practicing voodoo.

- to send people to help the adults and children in Haiti who are poor, sick, hurt, afraid and hungry.

- to help everyone who hears about Jesus on the Christian radio stations to understand what is said.

- to help the missionaries know how to explain God's love clearly to people in Haiti.

- to send leaders who will rule the country wisely and with justice and kindness.

Haitian proverbs

"The rock in the water does not know the pain of the rock in the sun." (It's hard to understand another person's problems.)

"However bad today has been, tomorrow could be better."

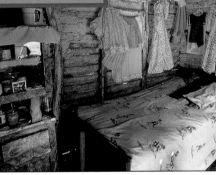

Interior of a Haitian home

"Yes, just like my father," he answered, "but the music they play is really good and the Bible studies are so interesting. I've never heard anything like it before!"

His father was furious when he discovered Gerard and his sister listening to a Christian radio station at home. "Don't you ever listen to that station again!" he shouted. "If you become a Christian, I'll drive you out of the house with a whip!"

Not long after this, Gerard became

very sick. His father tried to cure him with traditional medicine, chanting and drum-beating. But none of it did any good. Gerard's sister, listening to Christian radio when her father wasn't around, heard the story about Elijah. "Men who worshipped other gods shouted and danced around all day trying to get their gods to answer them. But nothing happened. Then God answered Elijah's prayer by sending fire down on his sacrifice, even though it was soaked with water!" she told Gerard. "Why don't you pray to the Christians' God and ask him to make you better?"

"I don't know how to pray to their God. I don't even know how to become a Christian," Gerard said sadly.

"Write to the missionaries and ask them," his sister insisted. "I'll get you some paper and a pen."

Gerard didn't quite understand the reply he received from the missionaries. He was still very sick, but he decided to go to the radio station. He had to walk part of the way and he had to sit down a lot to rest by the side of the road. When he arrived, they gave Gerard medicine and explained how to become a Christian. Gerard wanted to know Jesus so much that he wasn't afraid of his father anymore. He asked Jesus to forgive his sins and be his friend.

You can read more about Elijah in your Bible, in 1 Kings 18.

Although fighting and poverty are part of everyday life in Haiti, Haitian ministers, missionaries and radio stations are telling people about the love of Jesus. And some people, like Gerard, are finding that Jesus can forgive them for the bad things they've done and help them through their problems.

Hazara

Descendants of Genghis Khan's Army

A story from history

Almost 800 years ago Genghis Khan, the powerful leader of the Mongols, sent some of his men into Central Asia. But the people really didn't want them there! So, the story says, the ruler seized them, burned their beards and sent them back to Genghis Khan. Genghis Khan was very angry that this ruler dared to insult his men, so he and his mighty Mongol army invaded Central Asia to punish him. The Hazara claim that they're descendants of that great Mongol army. With their slanted eyes and round, flat faces, they do look like Mongolians. Even their language, which is a Persian dialect, has many Mongol words.

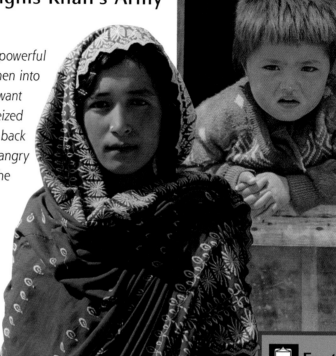

Life in Hazarajat

In Afghanistan, the Hazara live in a region called Hazarajat. For most of the year they live in small village houses built of mud bricks. The houses have flat roofs, which are ideal for drying mulberries, grapes and peaches in the hot summer months. The Hazara then store the dried fruit for eating during the long, cold winters. Wealthier people live in large houses that look like walled fortresses. All the animals belonging to the family –

dogs, donkeys, goats, sheep, hens, and even the cow – live in the courtyards of these big houses.

Abdul is a Hazara refugee living in Quetta, in Pakistan. Abdul smiles sadly when he remembers his country. "During the summer months we took our sheep and goats up to the high valleys in the mountains where there's plenty of grass for them to eat. The boys and young men had to watch the animals very carefully. I remember driving away many wolves and eagles who tried to snatch the smaller animals! While we were in the mountains we lived in *yurts* (tents) made from reed mats. The women and girls milked the animals. They churned some of the milk and used it to make balls of *crut* (hard cheese) for the winter.

Do you know?

As Shi'ite Muslims, the Hazara are very religious and follow very strict rules. They will eat a meal with Christians or Jews because they're people with a Holy Book. They don't like eating with Buddhists or Communists because they don't have such a book.

Fact file

Countries: Afghanistan; Pakistan; Iran

Numbers: 2,324,000 live in Afghanistan

Others live as refugees in Pakistan and northern Iran.

"It's very cold in the winter time, and we always hope for lots of snow because it's our only source of water. We call it 'Afghan gold,' because without snow our rivers dry up, our crops die and we starve."

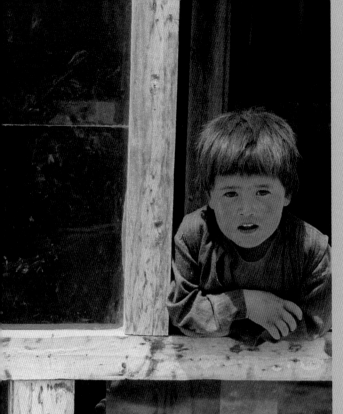

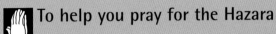
To help you pray for the Hazara

You can thank God for:

● each Hazara Christian.

● Christian radio programs in Dari, a language that most Hazara people know.

You can ask God:

● to show the Hazaras that they are important to him.

● to help those who have been crippled, blinded, orphaned or who have lost everything.

● to send Christians to share Jesus' love with Hazara refugees living in Pakistan.

● that Hazara people will read the New Testament in Dari and decide to follow Jesus.

● to help Hazara Christians, wherever they are, to tell others about Jesus.

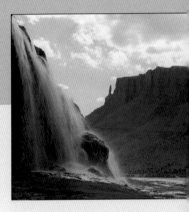

A refugee

Once I asked Abdul why he left Afghanistan.

"The more powerful Pushtuns and Tajiks look down on us," Abdul said. "Some Hazaras have gone to live in the cities. It seems natural enough that they would want a better way of life for themselves and their children. Instead, the Hazaras in the cities found they had to work very hard for very little money. Then, in 1979, thousands of Hazaras demonstrated against the government and a lot of them were taken as prisoners. It is as if they disappeared from the face of the earth – they've never been heard from since.

"A year later, the Soviet army arrived. They burned our houses and fields. Muslim soldiers, the *mujahidin*, were also fighting for power. There wasn't much left for us to live for. My father sent me across the mountains here to Quetta where many other Hazaras live. He wanted me to keep on studying."

Abdul looked around him, frightened, and then came closer. "I studied English," he said, "because I knew that would help me get a good job. It did, and I started to work in a hospital. Some people I worked with invited me to join an English club, where I learned about Jesus, the Son of God. Sometimes it just amazes me that he loves even the homeless and the poor. And that means Jesus loves the Hazara." Abdul whispered, "I'm a follower of Jesus. If the *mujahidin* knew that, they would kill me. Please pray for me."

A few months later, Abdul was forced to return to Hazarajat. The *mujahidin* were hunting for him and several other new Christians.

In 1996, a Muslim group called the Taliban took over the country, defeating some of the *mujahidin* groups. At first people thought they would bring peace, but thousands of Hazaras have suffered under their rule. One reason is that the Hazara are Shi'ite Muslims and not Sunni Muslims, like most other people in Afghanistan.

Please pray that God will help Abdul and the other Hazara Christians be faithful to Jesus – no matter what.

Herero

Children of the Omumborumbonga Tree

Questioning the tree

The Herero people, who live in Namibia, South West Africa, have a legend that, at the beginning of time, a man and woman came out of the Omumborumbonga tree. This is a large, twisted, ancient-looking tree that grows in the dry bush country where the Herero graze their cattle.

The man was called Mukuru, the first ancestor, and his wife was Kamungarunga. Even today, when some Herero pass the Omumborumbonga tree, they will bow, put a bunch of grass into the branches and ask it questions.

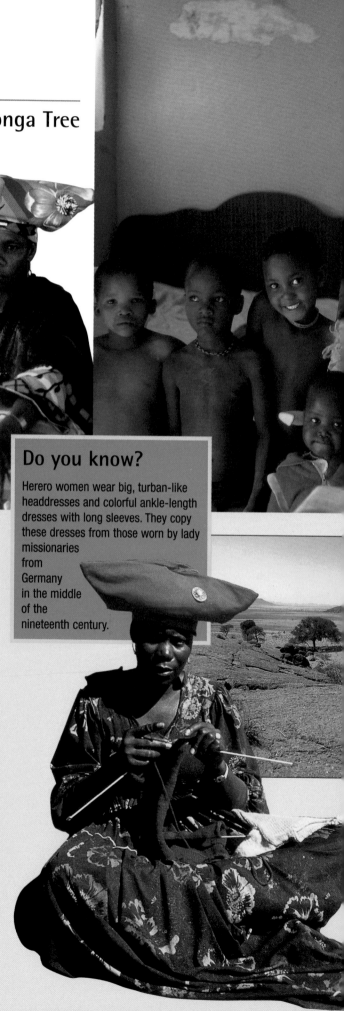

Africa

Angola

HERERO

Botswana
● Windhoek

Namibia

South Africa

Do you know?

Herero women wear big, turban-like headdresses and colorful ankle-length dresses with long sleeves. They copy these dresses from those worn by lady missionaries from Germany in the middle of the nineteenth century.

The Herero believed that a god named Karunga was present everywhere and that people had souls that went to heaven after death. They wanted to say and do only good things so they could go to Karunga as clean and fresh as the rain. Karunga, they believed, sent a flood to punish people for quarreling. Do these ideas sound familiar? It isn't surprising that the Herero people quickly understood when missionaries told them about God the creator who is everywhere, and about heaven, Adam and Eve and the great flood of Noah. But they were amazed to learn that we don't have to be clean and pure before we can talk to Jesus. They could hardly believe that if we do or think or say something wrong, we can ask him to forgive us. He's the only one who can make us clean.

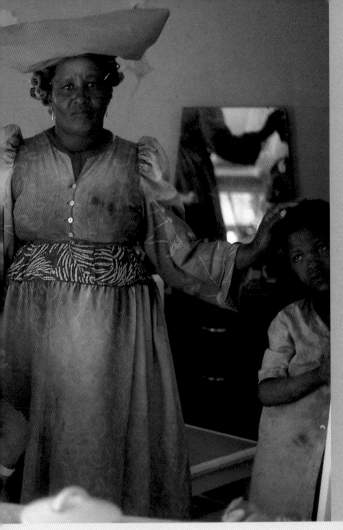

 To help you pray for the Herero

You can thank God for:

- each Herero Christian.
- the Herero Bible.

You can ask God:

- to help evangelists explain to children who are poor, unhappy or afraid that God loves them.
- to send teachers to help people know Jesus and follow only him.
- to help each Herero Christian who is studying at Bible school.
- that Herero Christians will forgive those who have hurt them, particularly during the war for independence from South Africa, just as Jesus forgave them.
- to help Herero Christians care for refugees and those who have no work.

 Fact file

Main country: Namibia, with a smaller group in Botswana

Numbers: About 181,000 (Namibia); 18,000 (Botswana)

Main religions: Christianity; traditional African religion

Traditional occupation: Cattle breeding

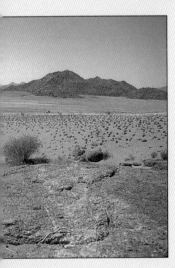

Holy fire

Some of the Herero people still follow their old beliefs. They have many taboos that sometimes make people afraid – for example, they aren't supposed to look at twins or at their chief in case something really bad happens to them. They worship their dead relatives at a sacred fire and believe that if that fire ever went out, the tribe would die out, too.

Alphonso and Poppi, a young Herero couple, had come to know Jesus as their savior and friend. On their wedding day, they refused to worship at the sacred fire. The village elders were very angry with them because they were afraid that some terrible disaster would come to the village. "We can't worship at the fire," Alphonso and Poppi said, "because we belong to Jesus. The Bible tells us that as Christians we must worship God and follow only him."

Maybe they'll be brave and tell lots more people about Jesus like Ananias did. Ananias was a poor Herero shepherd who went to South Africa in 1945 to preach about Jesus. Full of joy and love for Jesus, he was the first Herero missionary.

War and peace

Between 1904 and 1907 there was a terrible war in Namibia as the people fought for independence from Germany. More than 70,000 of the Herero people were killed or died in the desert and only 20,000 were left alive. It has taken them many years to recover from that war, but now there are as many Herero as there were then. Most live in Hereroland, East Namibia, while some live near the capital, Windhoek. South Africa governed Namibia from 1920 until 1990, but Namibia fought for freedom from the apartheid laws (that kept black and white people apart). In 1990, Namibia became an independent country.

The first missionaries translated the New Testament into the Herero language, and the whole Bible was completed in 1988. Please pray that as Herero men, women, boys and girls read the Herero Bible, they will come to know that they really are sons and daughters of the living God.

Hui

Chinese Descendants of Warriors and Merchants from Arabia

Dumplings and noodles

"Come and eat momo (dumplings) with us," my friends invited me, "or you could have lamien (noodles). We're going to a Hui (whey) restaurant. The food's great, but whatever you do don't ask for pork, because they're Muslims."

As we walked along the busy street in a city in north central China I saw people who looked Chinese and who dressed like most of the other people I'd seen here. But the men had white caps on their heads, and the women were wearing short veils of fine black or dark green cloth.

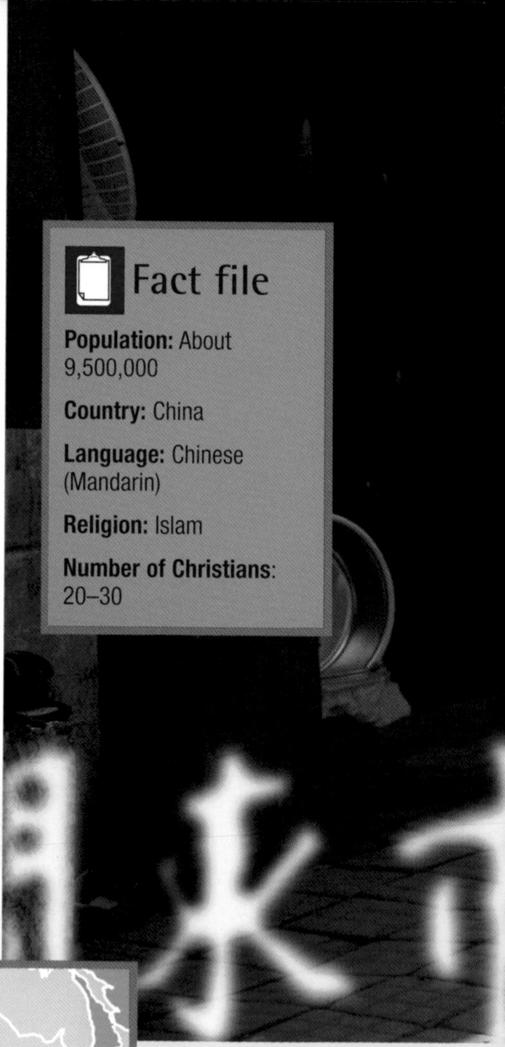

Fact file

Population: About 9,500,000

Country: China

Language: Chinese (Mandarin)

Religion: Islam

Number of Christians: 20–30

"These are Hui people," my friends told me. "They live in this part of the city near the main mosque. We'll bring you back here on Friday so you can see the hundreds of men come to the mosque to pray and listen to the sermon."

Merchants and warriors

Who are the Hui? Where did they come from and why are they Muslims?

More than a thousand years ago, hundreds of Arab and Persian merchants made the long journey along the Silk Road, right across Asia to China. Arab warriors also came to China to help Chinese emperors fight against their enemies. Still more Arabs traveled to China by sea. Many of them never returned to their homelands.

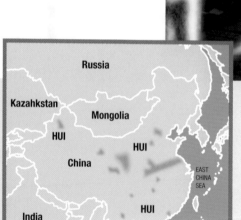

These men were Muslims, and they were proud of their Arab background. Wherever they settled in China they built mosques, married local Chinese women and brought their children up as Muslims. They became known as the Hui.

Hui Muslims live in different places all across China. In the country they often work as farmers. In towns and cities they

Friday prayers

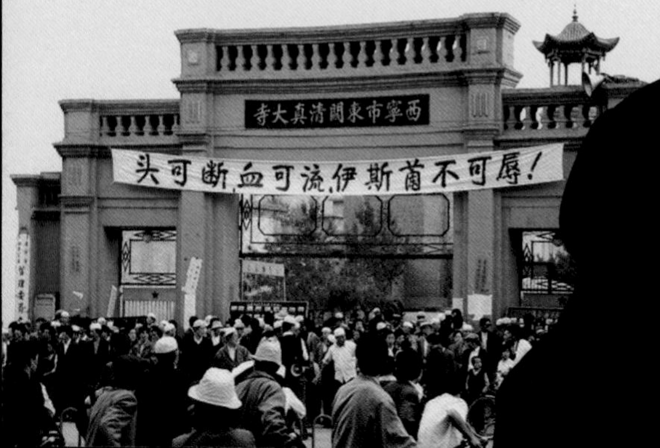

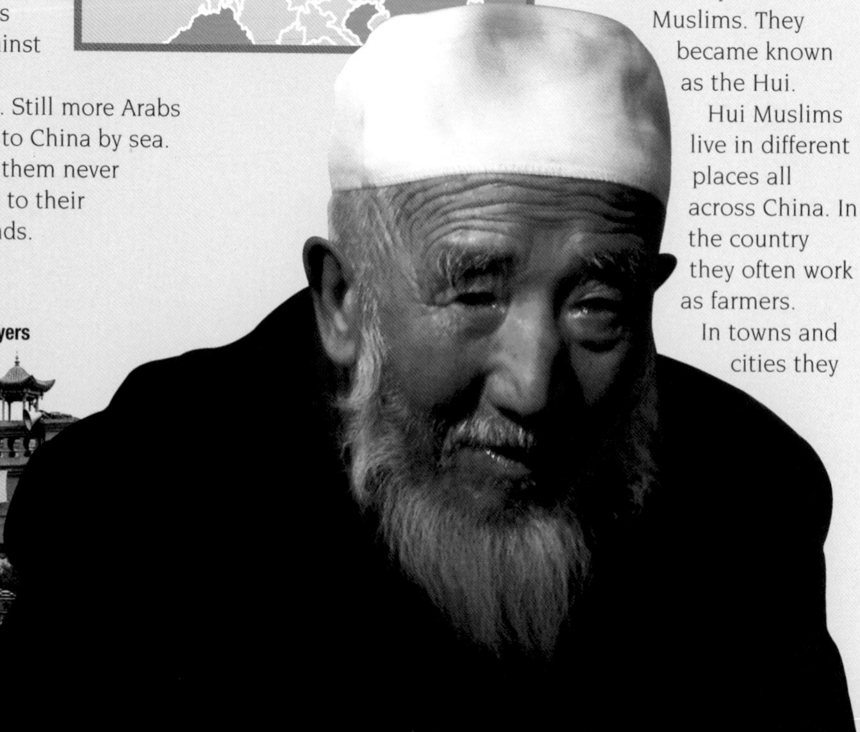

寺大清閣東市等西

头可断血可流伊斯菌不可辱!

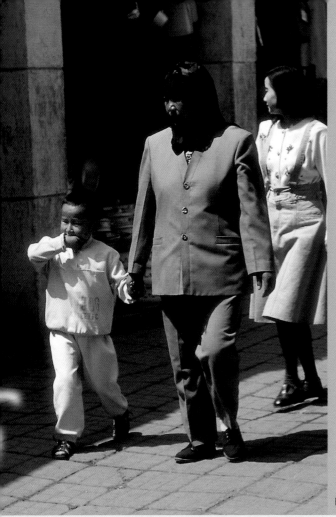

To help you pray for the Hui

You can thank God for:

- the Hui Christians.
- those who prepare Christian radio broadcasts.

You can ask God:

- to help Hui children and young people to understand that they will never know his love simply through keeping their traditions, customs and laws.
- that many Hui people will tune in to Christian radio stations and discover for themselves that they can only have hope and eternal life by trusting in Jesus.
- that when the Hui receive Christian leaflets or booklets, they will read them and learn about Jesus' love for them.
- that Han Chinese Christians will make friends with Hui people and share God's love and care with them.
- that many people around the world will pray that Hui people will come to know him as their savior and friend.

Hui women wear short black or green veils

---

live around their mosques. A lot of them work in their own Hui shops and restaurants, but most of them have jobs like anyone else.

In many parts of China the Hui seem no different from the Han, the people we usually think of as being Chinese. These Hui speak Mandarin, have Chinese names and look and dress like them. But they are different. They are Muslims.

There are more than nine and a half million Hui in China. Many of them live in north central China, where the Chinese government has set up a special region for them called the Ningxia (*ning-shia*) Hui Autonomous Region. About a third of the people who live in this region are Hui. There they can follow their own religion and culture.

Learning Arabic
Liang is a young Hui boy. His father goes to the mosque every Friday and has even been on pilgrimage (H*ajj*) to Mecca. "Sometimes I go to watch the men pray," Liang said, "but I don't think I want to go to the mosque with them yet, because there aren't many other boys and young men who go. I'm quite happy to follow our other Islamic customs, though.

"My father wants me to learn to read Arabic so I can read the Koran. We speak Mandarin Chinese at home, but we use a few Arabic words as well. I've

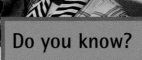

seen Arabic words written on the walls of the mosque. The writing looks beautiful, but I think it's going to be hard to learn. I'm still learning to write Chinese ... that's hard enough!"

There are very few Hui Christians – perhaps no more than 20. The Hui's traditions are very important to them, and probably only a quarter of them have ever heard about Jesus. How will they hear about the Savior who loves them and wants them to follow him? Who will tell them?

Restaurant worker

Do you know?
The Hui are the largest of the ten Muslim people groups in China. About three-quarters of them have never even heard about Jesus.

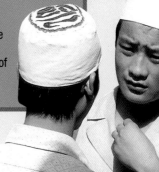

Iceland

On the Edge of the Arctic Circle

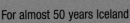

Land of fire and ice

Iceland is a large island, about 500 miles north of Scotland. It's called the land of fire and ice because it has a lot of active volcanoes as well as huge glaciers and ice fields that cover large areas. Much of the ground is black with volcanic ash and rocks. Iceland also has the largest lava bed on earth. In 1963, some fishermen out in their boats were amazed when the sea seemed to be boiling. A few weeks later, a volcano under the sea erupted, shooting steam, fire and ash high into the air. In a very short time, the volcano became the new island of Surtsey.

Workers in a fish processing factory

Icelandic girl in traditional costume

Do you know?

For almost 50 years Iceland has welcomed refugees from countries like Hungary, Vietnam and the Balkans. Because it's such a small country, it can only invite a few. Some who come had never heard of Iceland before, but when they arrive they receive a very warm welcome and plenty of help. When they've lived there for five years, they can apply for Icelandic citizenship.

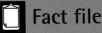

Fact file

Area: 39,768 sq. mi.

Population: 280,969

Capital: Reykjavik

Religion: Christianity (Lutheran)

Chief exports: Fish and fish products; aluminum

Because Iceland is nearly as far north as the Arctic Circle, it's almost never dark during the summer. But it's dark almost all the time in the winter, when people stay inside their snug, warm houses to read, tell stories and play games like chess. Most of the houses in Reykjavik (*raik-ya-vik*), the capital of Iceland, get their heat from hundreds of hot springs that occur there naturally.

1,000 years of Christianity

"Please tell me a story," Erik asked as he sat down beside his father. "Tell me how Iceland became a Christian country." His father smiled. He loved to tell this story.

"We've been a Christian country now for a thousand years," Erik's father began. "It all started a long time ago when the first settlers came to Iceland. They were great adventurers and made long and dangerous journeys across the sea. Some came

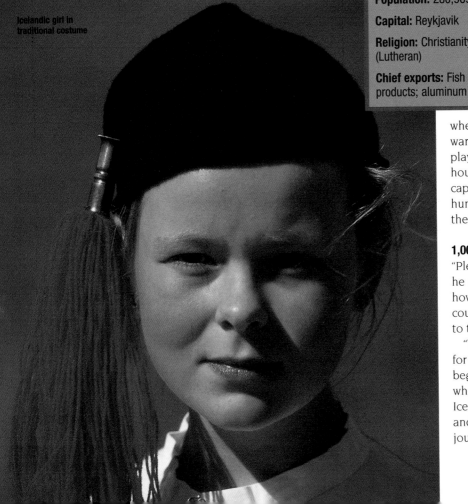

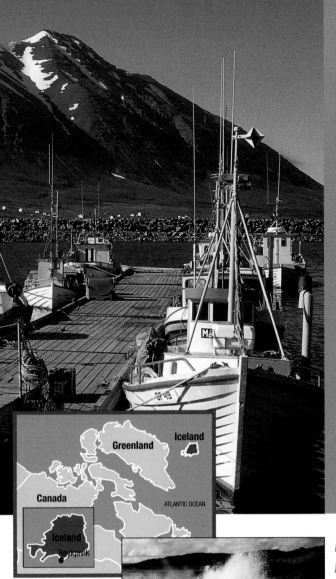

To help you pray for Iceland

You can thank God for:

- each Icelander who is discovering that Christianity is far more than just a part of their tradition.

- the new translation of the Bible.

- university students who are deciding to follow Jesus.

You can ask God:

- that a lot of children will choose to follow Jesus at Christian camps.

- that those who study in the Bible school will share the good news about Jesus wherever they go.

- that there will be more pastors and evangelists who will teach the Bible clearly.

- to help those who follow Jesus to tell others about him.

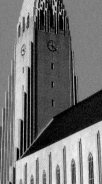

Geysers (right), and sulphurous gases escaping from the ground (below) are evidence of Iceland's volcanic activity

Iceland chose to be a Christian country more than a thousand years ago

Christian country or go on following the old gods. So they called a special meeting in the year AD 1000. They elected a man everyone respected very much and gave him the huge responsibility of choosing for them. He chose to follow Jesus and, for the past thousand years, Iceland has been a Christian country. In nearly every home, families have always met together every night to pray and read the Bible … just like we do."

"Hardly any of my friends at school go to church except when there's a wedding, a baptism or a funeral," Erik said, "but a lot of them still say the Lord's Prayer at home every day."

"That's right," his father replied. "Nearly everyone in Iceland would call themselves Christians because it is part of our culture and tradition."

"That's why my friends think the Christian camp I go to in the summer sounds fun, but they don't want to go. They never want to come to church with me when I invite them, either. They don't understand when I tell them that Jesus is my friend, who promises to be with me all the time," Erik said. "Are we still a Christian country, then?"

"Well," said his father, "some of us are praying that God will make the whole country excited about following Jesus. We've seen God beginning to answer those prayers. We have a new edition of the Bible that everyone can understand, some of the churches have been running a three-month Bible school, and Christians are telling others the good news about Jesus. Some people from here have even gone to tell people in other countries about Jesus."

from Norway, while others were Norsemen who had married Christian women. They brought the good news of Jesus with them, and soon almost half the people in Iceland had decided to follow Jesus. There were still a lot of people who followed the old Norse gods like Thor and Odin.

"Our ancestors knew they had to choose whether we should become a

India

Land of a Million Gods

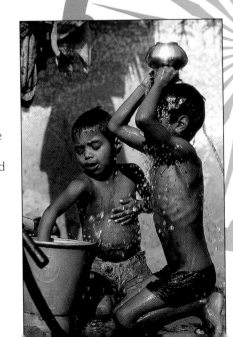

A festival

"Come on, wake up!" Sanjay said, shaking his brother. "It's almost dawn. The sadhus are already on their way down to the river. It's time for us to go!" Sanjay and his brother had spent the last two nights huddled together beside a small dung fire waiting for this very moment. All around them were the tents of millions of people who had also come for the Maha Kumbh Mela.

Hindu artist holding her image of a god

Colored dyes for sale at a bazaar

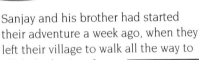

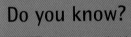

Fact file

Area: 1,237,060 sq. mi. (about a third the size of the United States)

Population: 1,013,661,777 (almost four times the number of people living in the United States)

Capital: New Delhi

Languages: Hindi; English and 16 other official languages including Urdu, Tamil and Telegu. Altogether, there are 1,652 languages!

Religions: Hinduism (about 78%); Islam (about 12%); Christianity (about 3%); Sikhism (1.92%)

Chief exports: Gems; jewelry; cotton; textiles; clothes; tea

Sanjay and his brother had started their adventure a week ago, when they left their village to walk all the way to Allahabad, "city of God." They were going to the great *mela*, or festival, at the holy place where the Ganges and Yamuna Rivers meet.

Sometimes a farmer had given the two boys a ride on his bullock cart. And once or twice they'd traveled a few miles on crowded buses. But mostly they had walked – along the hot and dusty paths and roads.

As they finally neared the river, Sanjay and his brother were caught up in the huge crowd of pilgrims. Everyone was pushing, slipping and sliding, dodging sacred cows and wandering goats, on their way down to the river. At last they reached the mighty river and stepped into the water. Sanjay faced the rising sun and poured water over himself, hoping that the water's flow would wash his sins away.

Do you know?

Experts say that by the year 2020 there will be more people living in India than in any other country in the world.

The Maha Kumbh Mela is one of India's great religious festivals. Although it is held every four years, it only comes to this sacred place every twelfth year. Hindus, whether high or low caste, rich or poor, come from all over India, hoping to wash away their sins in the Ganges. Most of them have never heard that Jesus is the only one who can truly wash their sins away and make their hearts clean.

A million gods

Indians are very religious. Most are Hindus, but others are Muslims, Christians, Sikhs, Buddhists, Jains or animists. Wherever you go in India,

Most missionaries in India today are Indians, telling their own people about Jesus

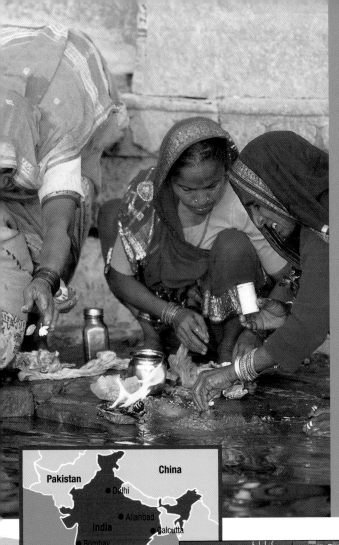

To help you pray for India

You can thank God for:

- every Indian Christian.

- the thousands of missionaries and preachers, from other countries as well as from India, who have told people there about Jesus.

- Indian missionaries.

- the Christians working among the millions of people who are poor and homeless, blind and sick, drug addicts and lepers.

You can ask God:

- that both adults and children would read and understand the millions of Scripture portions, New Testaments and booklets that are given out each year.

- that many Indians will listen to the Christian radio programs beamed into India and follow Jesus.

- that one day Jesus will truly be king, the one and only God, over all India.

Women preparing offerings

Map showing: China, Pakistan, Delhi, Allahbad, India, Calcutta, Bombay, Sri Lanka

The cow is a sacred animal in the Hindu religion and is often seen in the streets

you will find temples and shrines. There are more than a million Hindu gods. Some of these gods are very important and are worshipped all over India. Every day the Hindu priest has to wake up the gods in his temple, bathe them with milk and honey, dress them, offer them food and pray to them.

When people worship at a temple they bring offerings of food or flowers for the brightly painted gods. They ring the temple bell to make sure the god or goddess is awake. Even after they have made their offerings and prayed, they're still never sure the god will be kind to them.

Sharing the good news

Christian missionaries have worked in India for hundreds of years. One of the best known is William Carey, who went to India more than 200 years ago. He lived there for almost 40 years, translating the Bible into several Indian languages and teaching many people to follow Jesus.

There aren't many missionaries from other countries who can get visas to work in India now, but that doesn't mean that there aren't missionaries there. Although militant Hindus have threatened and attacked some of them, thousands of Indian missionaries and Christians are bravely talking to people about Jesus. They work in towns and cities, in hospitals, schools and churches. Some are helping the millions of people who have no homes and live on the streets. Others go into the thousands of villages. They give out Christian books, show films about Jesus and teach children to read.

But there are still millions of people in India who have never heard about Jesus. India is a country with a million gods and a billion people. But there is only one God ... who loves every single one of those billion people.

An Island Nation

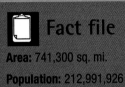

📋 Fact file

Area: 741,300 sq. mi.

Population: 212,991,926

Capital: Jakarta

Language: Indonesian

Religions: Islam (87%); Christianity (9.6%); Hinduism (1.9%)

Chief exports: Oil; gas; timber; rubber; textiles

700 languages!

The country of Indonesia has at least 13,500 islands. That means that if you tried to visit a different one every day, it would take you 37 years to visit them all! The islands are spread out over an area of the Indian and Pacific Oceans as large as the United States. Java, where 60% of Indonesians live, Sumatra and Sulawesi are three of the biggest islands. There are about 213 million people living in Indonesia. They belong to so many different people groups that about 700 different languages are spoken. (You can read about the Balinese, Dayak, Minangkabau and Sundanese in this book.) At school everyone has to learn Indonesian, the national language.

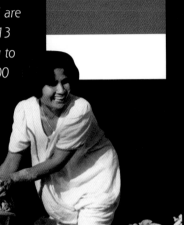

For almost 350 years, the Dutch ruled most of Indonesia. But the country declared its independence in 1945. War broke out in 1965, when Communists tried to take over the country.

Choosing a religion

Petrus, who was eight years old then, still remembers how frightened he was. "There were the Communists fighting on one side," he said, "and Muslims on the other. The Muslims didn't want the Communists to take control, so they killed anyone they thought might be a Communist. We just wanted peace. Then everything changed when the government defeated the Communists. They brought back an old law that said everyone had to choose a religion.

A lot of people were animists, who had no real religion. Some chose to become Muslims, Hindus or Buddhists. My father had seen how kind and forgiving Christians were to others during the war, so he decided we should become Christians. About two million people chose Christianity as their religion, but a lot of us didn't really understand what being a Christian meant. We were glad that missionaries and evangelists taught us how to follow Jesus."

There has been terrible fighting in Indonesia, but Christians there are reaching out with God's love

Do you know?

Indonesia has the fourth largest number of people of any country in the world — after China, India and the United States.

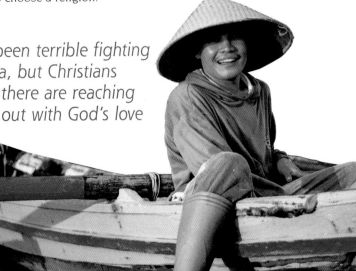

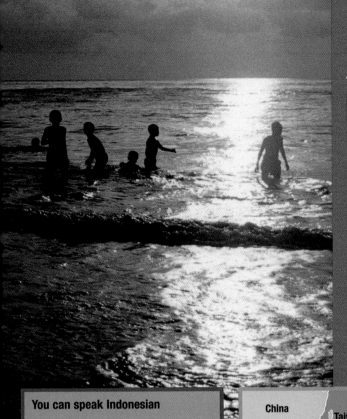

To help you pray for Indonesia

You can thank God for:

● all the Indonesians who know and love Jesus.

● Bible colleges where Indonesians can study to become evangelists, pastors and missionaries.

You can ask God:

● to send evangelists and missionaries to every inhabited island in Indonesia to tell people about Jesus.

● for pastors and church leaders to teach the truth of the Bible.

● that all Christians will want to learn more about Jesus and how they can follow him.

● that he will help Christians forgive those who hurt them, instead of trying to hurt them back.

● that the government will lead the many different peoples wisely and fairly.

You can speak Indonesian

Good morning is "Selamat pagi"
  (si-**lah**-mat **pah**-ghee)
Goodbye is "Selamat tinggal"
  (si-**lah**-mat **tin**-gahl)
Please is "Tolong" (**toh**-long)
Thank you is "Terima kasih"
  (**te**-ree-mah **kah**-see)
Yes is "Ya" (yah)
No is "Tidak" (tee-**dak**)

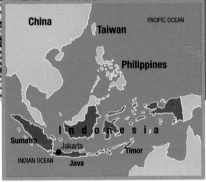

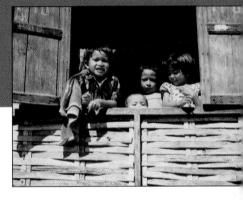

Trouble in the islands

"What happened then?" we ask him. "Is there peace now?"

"Indonesia isn't a peaceful nation," Petrus tells us, "and we have lots of problems. A man named Suharto was president for 32 years, but people were tired of him being so unfair. He resigned in 1998. We could be a rich country, but some people are wealthy while millions of others don't have enough food to eat.

"The government would like us to think of ourselves as one people instead of many people groups. They want us to be one nation, with one language and with a belief in God. But some parts of the country, like Aceh in Sumatra and Ambon in Maluku, want independence. There has been terrible fighting in these places and in East Timor, which voted to become independent, and a lot of people have been killed. Some Muslims want Indonesia to become a Muslim nation with Muslim laws. They're afraid that a lot more people will become Christians, so they've burned down churches and stoned and killed Christians. It's sad that, in some places, Christians have done the same things to Muslims."

The good news

"Are churches still telling people the good news about Jesus?" we ask. "With so much persecution, maybe people won't even want to hear about him."

"Let me tell you a story," Petrus says. "A boy called Enjang was six years old when he started to study the Koran. He got really scared when he read about hell. His uncle showed him where he could read about Isa, Mary's son. Enjang loved reading about Isa and realized that Isa is the Muslim name for Jesus. Little by little, Enjang began to love Jesus. He started to tell other Muslim children about him, but that made their parents very angry. Enjang's own brother was so angry that he made him leave his home. But Enjang knew that Jesus loved him so much that he told people about Jesus wherever he went.

"Because of people like Enjang, the church in Indonesia is growing. We're praying that soon every part of our country will hear about God's love. Christians are sharing the good news about Jesus in lots of different ways. They're helping people who have been hurt in the violence or who have lost their homes and jobs. They're praying that people will forgive each other for all the bad things that have been done and that our country will live in peace. Please pray for us, too."

Iraq

Between the Tigris and Euphrates Rivers

A Bible land

Did you ever wonder where in the world the Bible begins? Genesis 2 talks about a place called Mesopotamia, between the Tigris and Euphrates rivers. Hundreds of years later, the Jewish people were taken into exile in Babylon (you can read about this in 2 Kings). Both Mesopotamia and Babylon were part of the country that is now called Iraq. It was in Babylon that Daniel served Nebuchadnezzar and Balshazzar and went into the lions' den. And, hundreds of years after that, people from Mesopotamia were in Jerusalem on the day of Pentecost and heard the disciples speak about Jesus in their own language (in Acts 2, in the New Testament).

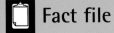

📋 Fact file

Area: 169,238 sq. mi.

Capital: Baghdad

Population: 23,114,884

Official languages: Arabic; Kurdish in the Kurdish region

Religion: Islam

Chief export: Oil

Woman selling produce at a market in Baghdad

These people took the good news about Jesus back to their own country. Although Iraq is now a Muslim country, there are people there who know and love Jesus.

Iraq is a large, oil-rich Arab republic in the Middle East. Almost three-quarters of the people living there today are Arabs. Kurds live in the northern mountain region, and a people known as the Marsh Arabs live in the south.

A troubled land

"I just can't believe this," Paul said as he showed his father a magazine. "The United Nations says that between five and six thousand children are dying every month in Iraq. How can this be happening?"

"It's a sad story,"

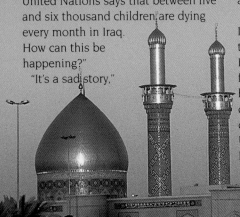

Paul's father said. "Iraq has had problems for a long time. In July 1958, the king and prime minister were killed during a violent revolution. After several coups, a man called Saddam Hussein came to power in July 1979.

"In 1980, Iraq invaded Iran. They had been fighting over control of a waterway to the Persian Gulf for a long time. Millions of Iraqi and Iranian people were killed. The war lasted for eight years, but no one really won."

"But if that war ended in 1988, why are so many children still dying?" Paul asked.

"Well," his father continued, "in 1990, Iraq invaded Kuwait. Among other things, Iraq accused Kuwait of stealing oil from oil fields along the border between the two countries. Many countries, including the United States and Britain, took part in the short but terrible Gulf

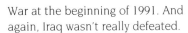

War at the beginning of 1991. And again, Iraq wasn't really defeated.

"Not long after that, the Kurds in the north of Iraq, who want a country of their own, revolted again. Many Kurds were killed and their homes destroyed. It was awful to watch long lines of Kurdish refugees on television as they trudged hopelessly across snow-covered mountains, away from the ruins of their villages. And far away in the south of the country, where the Tigris and Euphrates rivers meet, the Marsh Arabs were being driven out of the swamps which had been their home for hundreds of years. A lot of them died, and

Do you know?

Mesopotamia, "the land between the rivers," was the birthplace of civilization. Agriculture, animal farming and writing were all first developed here.

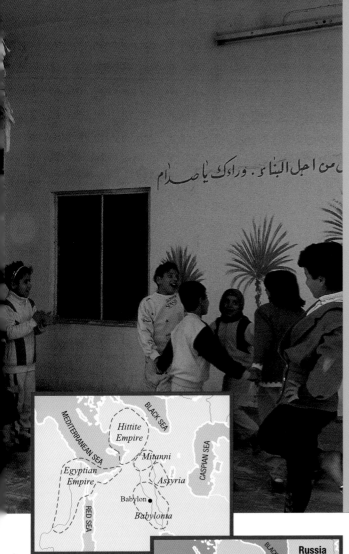

اِنّنا من اجل البناء . ورائك يا صدام

To help you pray for Iraq

You can thank God for:

- every person who has discovered that, no matter what happens, Jesus loves them and helps them.

- the thousands of Bibles and New Testaments that have been sent into Iraq.

- Christian radio broadcasts in Arabic and Kurdish, and the *Jesus* film.

You can ask God:

- that enough food and medicine will reach the people who need it.

- to send people to take care of all the children who are hungry, sick or dying.

- that Iraqi Christians training to become church leaders will return to help the churches in Iraq.

- for a government that will lead Iraq towards peace and rebuild the country.

Children sing praises to Saddam Hussein at an orphanage

Ancient world in 1350 BC

Iraqi soldier during the Gulf War

The good news of Jesus

Paul sat quietly for a few minutes. "Are there any Christians in Iraq?" he asked.

"Yes, some have gone to other countries as refugees," his father said. "When the Gulf War started, the evangelical church in Baghdad decided to meet every day to pray and read the Bible together. Muslims joined them sometimes, and some of them became Christians. Surprisingly, the *Jesus* film has been shown several times on national television. Christians used to be persecuted in Iraq. But now, perhaps because they've suffered so much, people want to hear about Jesus and his love."

"Can they buy Bibles there?" Paul asked.

"Thousands of Bibles and New Testaments have been brought in from

only a few have been able to continue their way of life."

"That's terrible," Paul said. "Is anything being done?"

"Other nations didn't want Saddam Hussein and the Iraqi government to ever be able to form such a strong army again. So they stopped trading with Iraq. Iraq is allowed to sell a certain amount of oil in exchange for food, but most people are very poor. There isn't enough food or medicine. That's why so many children are dying. A lot of people think we should start trading with Iraq again because it's ordinary people, especially children, who are suffering most. I read that some Iraqis have become very rich, and that Saddam Hussein has at least 50 palaces. It seems so unfair."

Jordan," his father told him. "The government has also given permission for Arabic Bibles and Christian children's books to be published in Baghdad and for thousands of New Testaments to be given to Christian children in state schools. The churches need trained pastors and leaders, but training is expensive."

"Isn't there anything we can do?" Paul asked.

"The Bible tells us that God loves the poor, the homeless and the downtrodden. The situation is too big for us, but not for God. We can pray that, in the midst of their suffering, people in Iraq will experience Jesus' love and care."

Israel

The Holy Land of Jews, Christians and Muslims

The Promised Land

"Why do people say that Israel is the homeland of the Jewish people?" Tanya asked her father. *Tanya's family are Messianic (Christian) Jews who emigrated to Israel from Russia.*

"It's a long story that started thousands of years ago," her father replied. *"This is the 'Promised Land' God gave to his people, the Hebrews, and it was here that famous kings like Saul, David and Solomon lived. Jesus was born and lived and died here, so it's special to Christians. And Muslims believe that Mohammed traveled from Jerusalem to heaven on his winged horse to speak with God. So Jews, Christians and Muslims all call it the Holy Land."*

The Dome of the Rock, Jerusalem

Conquered

"A long time ago, this land was called Palestine. Every time another country invaded Palestine, Jews left the country – sometimes just a few, but often quite a lot left at a time. They settled in almost every country on earth but, wherever they went, they were usually persecuted. And they longed and prayed for the day when they could return to their own land – but not many ever returned.

"After the Arabs conquered Palestine in AD 641, Arab Muslims settled here. Twelve centuries passed by.

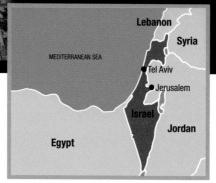

Lebanon
Syria
MEDITERRANEAN SEA
Tel Aviv
Jerusalem
Israel
Jordan
Egypt

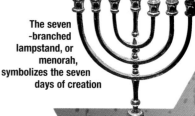

The seven -branched lampstand, or menorah, symbolizes the seven days of creation

Arab and Jewish Christians are setting an example of how to live together as part of God's family

Orthodox Jews praying at the Western Wall in Jerusalem

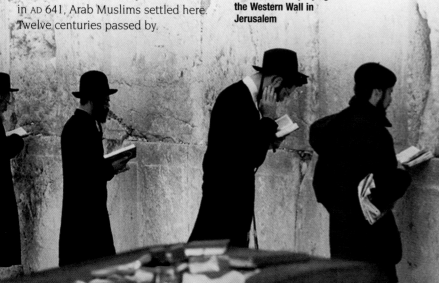

Then, at the end of the nineteenth century, some Jews arrived from Europe and started farming. More and more Jews returned to Palestine, but it wasn't really their own country. In 1922, Britain was asked to govern the country. It split the country in two. The eastern part was put under Arab rule, and Jews were allowed to settle in the west."

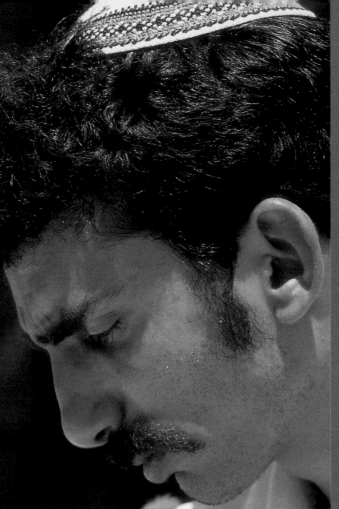

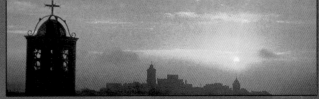

To help you pray for Israel

You can thank God for:

- the *Jesus* video in both Hebrew and Arabic that explains how Jesus really is the promised Messiah.
- Christian books, magazines and Sabbath (Sunday) school materials.

You can ask God:

- for many in Israel, both Arabs and Jews, to come to know Jesus as the true Messiah, the Son of God.
- to help Messianic (Christian) Jews and Arab Christians learn to trust each other.
- that Israeli and Arab Christian parents will teach their children to love Jesus.
- that tourists in Israel will not only visit historic places but will also pray for the country.
- for peace and understanding between Arabs and Jews in Israel.

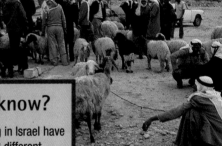

Palestinians at a sheep market in Beersheba

A new State

"Was that the beginning of the State of Israel?" Tanya asked.

"Not exactly," her father said. "It wasn't until 1948 that the United Nations voted to divide the western part of the country into a Jewish State and an Arab State. And on May 14th, 1948, the new Jewish State of Israel was formed. Ever since, thousands of Jews have come to Israel from countries all around the world."

"I have friends at school from Europe, America, Asia and Africa. If we didn't all have to learn Hebrew, we'd never understand each other!" Tanya said.

"Yes, it's wonderful to see Jews from all these different places returning to Israel," her father said. "But because so many people are coming to live here, there isn't enough work for everyone."

"Is that why you work in a laboratory now, even though you were a doctor in Russia?" Tanya asked.

"That's right," her father said, "And I'm grateful to have a job."

"What about the Arabs?" asked Tanya.

"During the more than 50 years since the Jews were given their own country there have been wars and a lot of fighting between Jews and Arabs," her father said sadly. "Thousands of Arabs have had to leave their homes. They're still looking for a country of their own. It's sad that we can't all learn to live together, but some of our leaders are trying to work towards peace."

Christians

"Some of the kids at school say I can't be a Jew because I'm a Christian," Tanya said. "Why do they say that?"

"The Old Testament tells us about God's promise of a Savior," her father said. "A lot of Jewish people are longing for this Savior, or Messiah, to come and bring peace to his people. But they don't understand that *Yeshua* (Jesus) is the Messiah that God promised. That's why some of them

Do you know?

The Jews living in Israel have come from 102 different countries. One person in every six has come from Russia, so stores often have signs in Hebrew, English, Arabic and Russian.

feel we can't be Jews if we follow *Yeshua*."

"Aren't there some Arabs living in Israel who are Christians, too?" Tanya asked. "There are only Jewish Christians in our church."

"There are whole villages of Arab Christians, but we don't often meet them," her father replied. "A friend of mine recently went with some other members of his church to visit an Arab church. It was a big step, because usually there isn't much friendship between Jews and Arabs. He said they were kind, and made them feel at home. As he told me about their visit, I thought about what the Bible says in Galatians 3:28: 'we are all one in Christ Jesus.' If we follow Jesus, we're all members of one family – God's family."

Japan

Land of the Rising Sun

Japan is a chain of four main islands and about 4,000 smaller islands in the North Pacific Ocean. Mountains and hills cover many of the islands, and most of Japan's nearly 130 million people live crowded on the narrow plains along the coasts.

The rising sun on Japan's flag symbolizes the sun goddess. The Japanese call their country "Nippon," which means "the land of the sun." The Japanese tradition is that their emperor descended from the sun goddess and was himself a god. He was made emperor in a special ceremony as part of a secret meeting with the sun goddess. Emperors used to be very powerful, but the emperor today has little power and his role is mainly ceremonial.

The cherry blossom has special significance in Japan

Fact file

Area: 145,870 sq. mi.

Population: 126,714,220

Capital: Tokyo

Language: Japanese

Religions: Shinto; Buddhism (but freedom of religion is guaranteed)

Chief exports: Machinery; vehicles; ships; electronic equipment; textiles

Do you know?

The islands of Japan are really the tops of a huge range of mountains under the Pacific Ocean. Some of them are volcanoes! Every year, about 1,500 earthquakes are recorded in Japan. Most of them are minor, but once in a while a very strong one causes a lot of damage.

Shinto

The main religion of Japan is called Shinto, "the way of the gods." Its followers worship the emperor, the sun, Mount Fuji, the fox god, the snake god, spirits of water and fire and many other things. Children visit Shinto shrines to learn more about their culture and beliefs.

If the influence of Shinto becomes really strong, people could be stopped from preaching about Jesus. This has happened before. Shintoists can't understand why Christians refuse to worship at Shinto shrines, since they don't see a problem with worshipping more than one god. Many Japanese people feel that if they became Christians and worshipped only Jesus, they would be turning against their family and culture.

There are even more Japanese Buddhists than Shintoists. Although many people don't really believe in Buddhism, they're afraid to give it up.

The flag of Japan shows the rising sun, symbol of the sun goddess

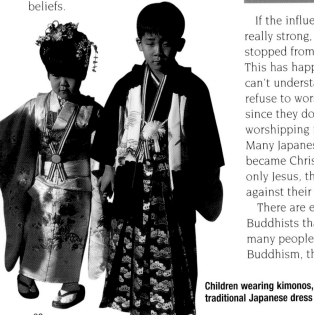

Children wearing kimonos, traditional Japanese dress

Lighting a candle at a shrine

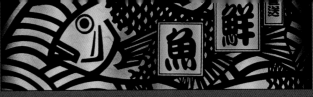

To help you pray for Japan

You can thank God for:

- the freedom of religion the Japanese have, and that some have chosen to follow Jesus.
- every Christian who has shared God's love with the people of Japan.

You can ask God:

- to show Japanese pastors and evangelists and missionaries from other countries the best ways to help the people of Japan understand that God loves them and wants them to follow him.
- to help each Christian be brave enough to worship only Jesus and never bow down to idols.
- that many people will learn that he is the one and only Creator-God who loves them and sent Jesus to save them.
- for Christians to have such joyful hearts that wherever they are – at home, or school or work – others will want to discover that joy for themselves.
- that many people will go into Christian bookstores to buy Bibles and books to help them learn how to follow him.

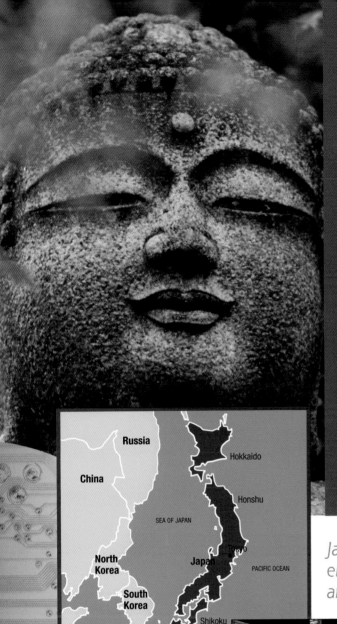

Japan makes more cars and electronic toys and products than any other country

Too many lessons!

In the Japanese culture it's very important to be successful, and children have to work hard in school if they want to do well.

Toshio was angry. "I don't want to take classes after school," he complained. "I want time to ride my bike or just play computer games! Why do I have to work all night?"

"Shhh, Toshio! Your father will hear you. Only studying will get you into college and a good job."

"I don't care, and I don't see why he does either – a good job hasn't made him happy. He's always at work. I want to have fun with my friends."

"If you don't pass all your exams, what will our neighbors think of us?" Toshio's mother sighed. Toshio ran out of the house. He felt like crying. His mother was always worrying about what other people might think.

Not all Japanese think like Toshio. Although they have a long day at school, and compulsory school clubs afterwards, many still take extra classes at night to make sure they pass their exams! Some sleep very few hours.

Japan makes more cars and electronic appliances than any other country in the world. The Japanese use thousands of robots to do the work in their factories, clean sewers, wash windows and pick oranges.

The family shrine

Japanese people often live to be very old. Toshio's mother takes care of his great-grandmother, who is very religious. She worships at the family shrine every day, and she scolds Toshio's mother for not doing so.

Jolas

Who Pray to the Spirits in Poems

Praying to the spirits

Ampa's week-old baby brother squirmed as a Jola elder shaved his head. The old man was chewing betel nut and spat some of his red saliva on the baby's head. "This will protect the baby's heart," he said. Then the old man blew and prayed into the baby's tiny ears. They also sacrificed a chicken to please the spirits so that they would look after the baby.

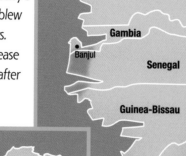

Set free from evil spirits

"Tell me again about how happy you were when I was born!" Five-year-old Samuel smiled at his mother, who was cuddling his baby sister.

His mother Mariama smiled back at him. "It is a story with a happy ending," she said. "When your big sister was born, I was overjoyed.

Ampa stood and watched this ceremony for his little brother and remembered when he was 10 years old and very sick. His father had asked the priest to pray to the spirits for him. The priest prayed a poem he made up. He told the spirit that Ampa was sick and that his father had brought palm wine and a chicken as a gift. In his poem he asked one spirit to tell another spirit, and so on, until eventually a spirit told the creator god. Ampa didn't really understand how all of this talking to the spirits worked. He had heard about some missionaries who said they could talk directly to the true Creator God. Ampa thought that would be amazing … if it was really true.

The Jolas

Most Jolas are farmers who grow rice, vegetables and groundnuts (peanuts). They live in the West African countries of Senegal, Gambia and Guinea-Bissau. Ampa's family lives in Gambia, which is one of the smallest countries in Africa. Gambia is a narrow strip of land (rarely more than 30 miles wide) that runs along either side of the Gambia River for about 300 miles. Apart from its Atlantic coast, Gambia is completely surrounded by Senegal.

You can speak Jola

Hello is "saafi" (sah-fee)

Peace is "kasuumaay", which you use to ask how someone is, or tell them you are okay (kah-soo-my)

Goodbye is "ukatoolaal" (oo-kah-tolal)

Do you know?

Jola kings always wear long red gowns and tall red felt hats to worship their gods. No one else who worships the Jola gods is allowed to wear red or to sit on a stool after a king has sat on it. So, wherever he goes, a Jola king carries a small stool with him. He also carries a brush made of palm leaves, which is the symbol of his authority. Whatever he touches with it belongs to him.

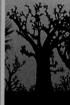

She was so beautiful, and I knew that when she was old enough she would help me look after the house. Then I had another baby, a little boy. I was very happy because I knew your father and his family would be pleased. But the baby died, and everyone was very sad.

"Soon I was expecting another baby. Your father's family took me to the *marabout*, the local holy man, who told them I'd been cursed by evil spirits.

He said I had to change my name and keep out of the spirits' way. When the baby was born, the *marabout* tied charms around his hands, waist and neck to protect him from the evil spirits. But he died, too."

Mariama's family had sent her away from her home in Senegal because they believed she had been cursed. "In Sibanor," she said, "a small village in Gambia, I met a Jola Christian who invited me to church. There I heard about Jesus, who loves and cares for everyone who follows him, and who is much more powerful than any evil spirit.

"I came back to Senegal, and before long there was another baby on the way.

My family took me to the *marabout* again, who gave me a special charm so the baby wouldn't die. I went back to Sibanor because I knew the nurses at the Christian hospital there would look after me and my baby. You were that precious baby, Samuel. One day I took you to the church and the elders prayed for you and gave you the name Samuel. I took off all the charms you were wearing, and from then on I trusted Jesus to look after you."

"What happened then?" Samuel asked.

"I asked Jesus to be my friend," his mother said. "My family was very angry and afraid, but God helped me to follow him. Now he has

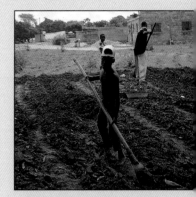
Preparing the ground for planting

given me another beautiful baby daughter. I'm glad that I can serve God in the church as a deaconess. There are only a few Jolas who are Christians, Samuel, and I pray that our people and the rest of our family will come to know Jesus, too."

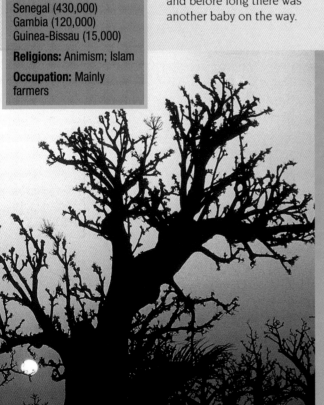
Sunset in the "bush"

To help you pray for the Jolas

You can thank God for:

● the Jolas who are following Jesus.

● the beautiful songs and poems Jola Christians make up to worship him.

● the Sunday schools and youth clubs where children learn about Jesus.

You can ask God:

● for Christians to be faithful to Jesus even when others get angry because they're following him.

● to help the Jola Christians share his love and power with others.

● to bring many more Jolas to trust in Jesus and be free from the power of evil spirits.

● that Jola Christians would become evangelists, pastors and leaders in their churches.

Kal-Tamashaq

Blue-veiled Guardians of the Sahara

Famine of no hope

The Kal-Tamashaq, or "the people of Tamashaq", live in the Sahara Desert. Let's talk to Amud, who's hoeing between the millet plants over there in the hot sun. "Our lives are very different now," Amud told us. He pulled his long blue veil across his mouth as he spoke. "Slaves used to work in our gardens while we traveled across the desert with our camels, herds and families. Then came the worst famine we'd ever seen. There wasn't any rain for six years, and lots of people and animals starved to death. We called it 'the famine of no hope.' Now we're poor and we don't have slaves to grow our millet and vegetables. At least I still have my own tent."

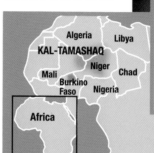

KAL-TAMASHAQ

Algeria · Libya
Mali · Niger · Chad
Burkino Faso · Nigeria

Africa

A nomad's tent

We look over at Amud's ragged, oval tent made of leather. "That tent has been my home for a long time. When I was young, we used to carry our tents and belongings from place to place on the backs of our camels. We were so proud that we were called 'the Lords of the desert.' In our own language we call ourselves *Imashagan*, which means 'noble and free.' But now, sometimes, we feel like God has abandoned us."

Fact file

The Kal-Tamashaq are often called Tuaregs, which is the French name for them.

Countries where they live:
Niger (1,094,000)
Mali (683,000)
Burkina Faso (85,500)

There are others living in Algeria, Libya, Mauritania and Tunisia.

Religion: Islam

Language: Tamashaq

Proud nomads

The Kal-Tamashaq are descendants of the Berbers of North Africa. Hundreds of years ago, the Arabs drove them out of their homeland and south into the Sahara Desert and the Sahel. Even though they were treated this way, the Tamashaq were strong and powerful. They weren't afraid of anyone. It wasn't long before they forced the black Africans, who lived in the lands where they settled, to become their slaves.

The Kal-Tamashaq became very rich. They spent their days raiding, trading and herding. They moved through the desert with their herds of camels, cattle, sheep and goats. Traders gave the Kal-Tamashaq money or other valuables to guide and

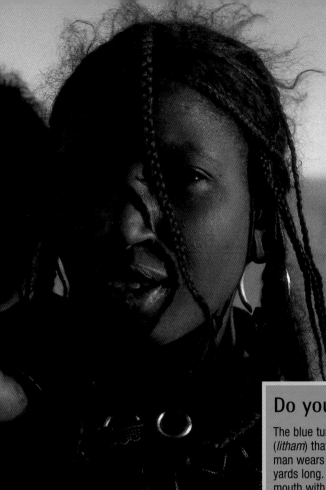

 ## To help you pray for the Kal–Tamashaq

You can thank God for:

- the few Tamashaq who follow Jesus.
- the parts of the Bible that have been translated into Tamashaq.

You can ask God:

- to help the many Tamashaq people who are very poor.
- that Christian workers would show his love and care to the Tamashaq.
- for more evangelists, pastors and missionaries who can show the Tamashaq that they're important to him and who can teach Christians how to follow Jesus.
- to give Tamashaq Christians the courage to tell others about how he has helped them.
- to send enough rain each year so they'll have enough food for themselves and their animals.

Do you know?

The blue turban and veil (*litham*) that the Tamashaq man wears is about six yards long. He covers his mouth with his veil when he meets anyone he respects, and when he eats he uses his left hand to lift the veil from his mouth.

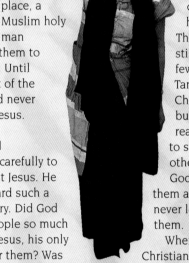

protect them as they traveled across the Sahara between west and north Africa. Everyone was afraid of these blue-veiled guardians of the desert, but they weren't afraid of anyone.

When France took control of large areas of West Africa in the nineteenth century, they banned raiding, which had always been a part of the Tamashaq way of life. They also enforced the boundaries between countries, so the Tamashaq couldn't move freely from place to place. The proud Tamashaq weren't so powerful anymore.

No longer powerful

The last 50 years have been very hard for the Kal-Tamashaq. When Mali became independent from France in 1960, the black Africans in the south of the country took over. The Tamashaq fought the government in a civil war. They were defeated, and many of them were killed. The harsh climate defeated them, too. There's never much rain in the Sahel, but since "the famine of no hope" (which lasted from 1968–74), there have been lots of droughts and famine, and thousands of people have died. Many Tamashaq had to abandon their nomadic life and go to refugee camps, where they sometimes felt they were treated unfairly.

The Tamashaq are Muslims, but because they moved around so much they didn't build many mosques, and most of them don't keep Ramadan. But when they moved to a new place, a Muslim holy man traveled with them to pray for them. Until recently, most of the Tamashaq had never heard about Jesus.

Not abandoned

Biga listened carefully to the tape about Jesus. He had never heard such a wonderful story. Did God really love people so much that he sent Jesus, his only Son, to die for them? Was he powerful enough to actually change people's lives? Would he really help them every day? When Biga decided to follow Jesus, some people laughed at him for following the white man's religion. But it didn't take them long to realize that Biga was a different person because God had changed him.

There are still only a few Tamashaq Christians, but they really want to show others that God loves them and will never leave them.

When Christian organizations started to send food and aid to the Tamashaq, the Christians made sure that the neediest people got their share. "How can we follow Jesus, too?" some of them wanted to know. "Life is very hard, but now we know that God hasn't abandoned us!"

Kazakhstan

Nomads, Space and Jesus

Kazakhstan is a large Central Asian country stretching from the Caspian Sea in the west to China in the east. High grassy plains called steppes roll across the northern part of the country, but there are dry, sandy deserts in the south. In the east, towards Kazakhstan's border with China, are the soaring Altai and Tien Shan Mountains.

For many centuries, the Kazakh people were nomads. They never lived in one place for very long but traveled across the steppes with their herds of cattle, sheep, horses and camels looking for pasture. About a hundred years ago, Russia conquered Kazakhstan. Thousands of Russians then came to live in Kazakhstan, forcing the Kazakh nomads off their land. Many nomads were made to live in villages and towns, but others fled to China with their animals.

Do you know?

Astana, the name of the new capital of Kazakhstan, simply means "capital." At one time this city was called Akmola, meaning "tomb."

Kazakh proverbs
"Those who seek find; those who ask receive." (That's almost the same as the words of Jesus in Matthew 7:7–8!) "The five fingers aren't all the same." (Everybody is different.)

Fact file

Area: 1,049,150 sq. mi.

Population: 18,588,000

Capital: Astana (until 1995, Almaty was the capital)

Language: Kazakh is the official language, but people speak Russian whenever they are doing business.

Religions: Islam; Russian Orthodox

Chief exports: Oil; wheat; wool

Kazakh nomads

Some Kazakhs are hearing about Jesus on their radios

The Russian settlers planted wheat on the land that had been used for grazing animals, and they started to mine iron and lead. In 1957 *Sputnik* I, the world's first space rocket, was launched from Baykonur in Kazakhstan.

Kazakhstan is once again independent from Russia. It could be a wealthy country because there is so much oil, coal and gold, and it has the world's largest chrome mine, but many Kazakhs are very poor. A few people have all the money, and there are lots of people who can't find jobs. Many children don't bother going to school, and there is more and more crime.

The Kazakhs are Muslims, but many of them are afraid of evil spirits. Christians are telling Kazakhs about God's love and about how they don't have to be afraid if they ask Jesus to protect them. Christian radio broadcasts and the *Jesus* film are also sharing the truth about Jesus with Kazakhs.

A Bactrian camel

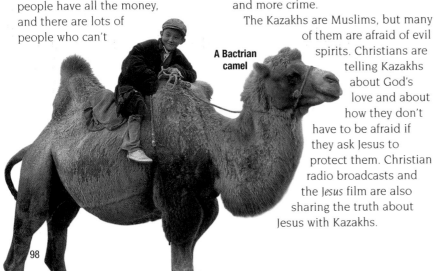

"No one cares about me!"

Aibek shivered. He wanted to cry. No one in the bazaar was interested in a little boy begging for food. He should have been at school but he was much too hungry, cold and miserable. At home there was never enough food for him and his five brothers and sisters. His

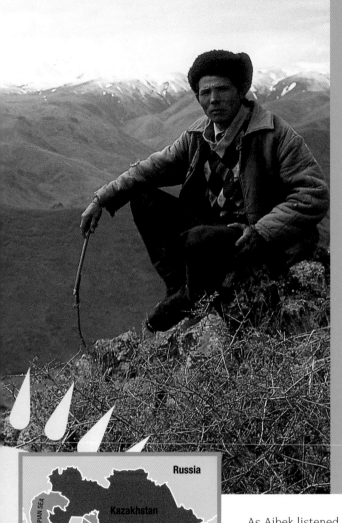

To help you pray for Kazakhstan

You can thank God for:

● Kazakhs who are becoming Christians and who want to share Jesus' love with their friends and families.

● Christians who have gone to Kazakhstan to tell the people about Jesus.

● the New Testament and some other parts of the Bible that have been translated into Kazakh.

You can ask God:

● to build Christian churches and fellowships throughout Kazakhstan where people can worship God and learn more about being Jesus' followers.

● to help Kazakh Christians to be brave and tell their friends, families and co-workers about Jesus.

● to send more Christian workers to Kazakhstan so that as many Kazakhs as possible will hear about God's love for them.

● to use the Christian radio broadcasts and the *Jesus* film to tell more people about Jesus.

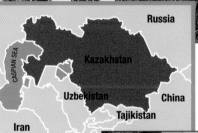

Russia
Kazakhstan
CASPIAN SEA
Uzbekistan
China
Tajikistan
Iran

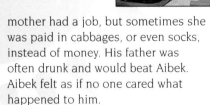

Muslim prayers

As Aibek listened, he realized that someone *did* care about him. God loved him so much that he sent his Son Jesus to die on the cross so that Aibek could be forgiven for all the bad things he had done and go to be with God in heaven one day. In heaven there would be no hunger, cold or beatings. Aibek learned that Jesus would always be with him and be ready to hear his prayers. Aibek decided that following Jesus should be the most important thing in his life.

One very cold day, when there was no electricity, he told his mother and brothers and sisters that he was going to pray. As he said "Amen," the electricity came on again. Aibek is excited because he knows Jesus loves him and he wants his family and friends to know Jesus, too.

mother had a job, but sometimes she was paid in cabbages, or even socks, instead of money. His father was often drunk and would beat Aibek. Aibek felt as if no one cared what happened to him.

One day Aibek's big sister came home and said, "I've decided to become a Christian. Come along to the meetings with me to hear about Jesus." Aibek didn't know what a Christian was, but he went with her and had fun singing. It was warm in the meeting room, so he stayed to listen to the Bible stories.

God heals a little girl

Nurgal went up to her big sister Akmaral and whispered in her ear. A little later, Akmaral stood up in the meeting and said, "Nurgul would like us to ask Jesus to make the painful sores on her hands and feet go away."

Every day for two weeks Akmaral prayed for her. At first Akmaral was not sure that God would heal Nurgul but, as she prayed, her faith grew.

One day Nurgul told her, "It doesn't hurt any more! The sores are gone!"

Kurds

Sharing the Good News

Persecuted and ill-treated

There are probably about 30 million Kurds. They have their own culture, traditions and languages. But they don't have a country of their own. Most of them live in the rugged, mountainous area in the heart of the Middle East. Although this region is often called Kurdistan, "the land of the Kurds," it doesn't belong to them but to the countries of Turkey, Iran, Iraq and Syria.

The governments of these countries have often treated the Kurds cruelly and persecuted them. They want them to forget they are Kurds and to think of themselves as ordinary citizens of the countries where they live. Because of this, the Kurds have often been involved in long and violent struggles. In Iraq they have been bombed and attacked with poison gas.

Kurdish guard

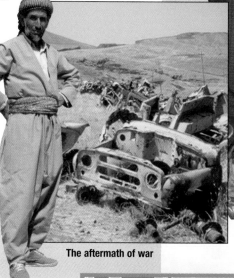

The aftermath of war

A refugee in northern Iraq
Khaled clapped his hands and jumped for joy. He had finally passed his English exam so he could move up to the next class.

When Khaled was younger, a bomb hit his home in Kirkuk. He

Kurdish trader

In 1991, thousands of Kurdish refugees died while fleeing from Iraq to Turkey and Iran. There are about 15 million Kurds living in Turkey. Nearly all of them live in the eastern area of the country that is part of Kurdistan. Some are refugees from Iraq, but for most of them this is their homeland. They have often been ill treated. Until 1991, the Turkish government wouldn't even allow them to have books in their own language.

Hearing the good news

The Kurds are Muslims. For a long time Christians have wanted to take the message of Jesus' love to them, but it's been difficult to visit the areas where they live. In the past few years, Christians have been allowed to give food, medicine and other

aid to the Kurds in northern Iraq. The Kurds there often want to hear stories about Jesus.

Thousands of Kurds have left their homelands and settled in other countries. Although they often work for very low pay in these other places, they feel life is safer for them and better for their families. Some Kurds in Turkey have become Christians while studying the Bible, and others elsewhere are hearing the good news about Jesus and following him.

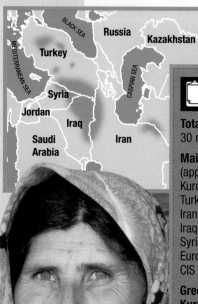

Fact file

Total worldwide: About 30 million

Main countries
(approximate numbers of Kurds):
Turkey (15 million)
Iran (7 million)
Iraq (4 million)
Syria (1.5 million)
Europe (850,000)
CIS (400,000)

Greet your friends in Kurdish: Good day is "Roj bas" (rawzh baash) (roj = day; bas = good)

has terrible scars on his face where he was burned. His parents fled to Kurdish Iraq with Khaled and his ten brothers and sisters. Thanks to the help of some aid workers, Khaled was able to start school. His father is too ill to work, so every day after school Khaled and his brothers have to work selling cigarettes, candy or sunflower seeds.

Because he was so tired from working and had so little time to study, it wasn't surprising that he failed his English exam. But he really wanted to pass it. A Christian family invited him to come to their home to study English. Every day for two weeks Khaled walked nearly five miles, in the summer heat, to their house. It was worth it, because he passed his exam. Now he and two of his brothers have English lessons with this family every week. These Christians pray that Khaled and his family will come to know Jesus.

A refugee in Europe

One day some soldiers came to the Kurdish village in Turkey where Serhat lived. They destroyed all the houses in the village, including theirs.

Serhat's father decided they should go to Germany. They traveled by bus, then by boat, and finally on foot. They were so glad to finally cross the border into Germany. The Germans took them to a refugee camp where they had to wait for permission to stay in Germany.

Serhat was always delighted when visitors came to the camp to play with the children, especially those who spoke Turkish, which he understood. They

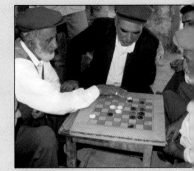

told stories about Jesus, who loves children and wants to be their friend. Serhat had never heard about Jesus before. His new friends gave him a cassette of Christian songs written for children. He listened to these songs again and again and watched the *Jesus* video. Is it really true, he wondered, that Jesus offers a new life to all who trust in him?

Do you know?

It is thought that the Kurds are descendants of the Medes, who are mentioned in the Bible (for example in Daniel, chapters 5 and 6).

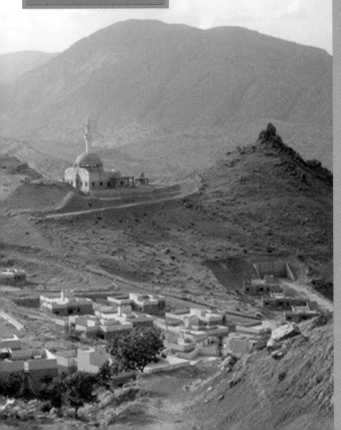

To help you pray for the Kurds

You can thank God for:

- the translation of the New Testament into Sorani Kurdish, and for the translations into each of the main Kurdish dialects that will be completed soon.

- the *Jesus* video, radio broadcasts and Christian song and message cassettes.

You can ask God:

- that wherever Kurdish refugees are living, Christians will help them, and that through their help many Kurds will come to know Jesus as their friend.

- that many Kurds will hear the good news that Jesus offers new life to all who trust in him.

- that governments of all the countries where Kurds are living, and particularly those in the Middle East, will treat them fairly.

- to help children who are hurt and confused by the way in which they and their families have been treated.

- to show Christian workers the best ways to show Jesus' love and care to the Kurds.

A Kurdish village in Iraq

Kyrgyz

Who Live in a Land of Snow-capped Mountains

A Kyrgyz hero

Aigul thought about last night's thanksgiving feast for her uncle. She had especially loved the exciting stories the storyteller had told about Manas, the ancient Kyrgyz hero.

Had Manas really lived, Aigul wondered? Had he really learned to ride a horse as soon as he could walk? And become a mighty warrior by the time he was nine years old and rescued his father from the enemies who had captured him? Was he really the leader of all the nomadic tribes in Central Asia? Whether the stories were true or not, Aigul knew that all the Kyrgyz took great pride in their great warrior-hero.

Aigul wasn't too pleased when her father killed a sheep for the feast. He explained that they had to shed blood to show how grateful they were that her uncle, who had been seriously ill, was well again.

A Kyrgyz shepherd

The Good Shepherd

Aigul remembered another amazing story she had heard the week before. Teachers from another country had visited their school and told them that God had sent his only Son, Jesus, into the world to be born as a baby. "When he grew up," the visitors said, "he told the people that he was the Good Shepherd. He wanted them to follow him so he could look after them. He even said he would give his life for the people who followed him. And he did. Cruel men hated him so much that they killed him. But, because he was the Son of God, he rose from the dead to live forever. He's still the Good Shepherd and

Her uncle carved up the sheep's head and gave different parts to the guests. "Eat this eye, so your sight will improve!" he said as he gave an eye to an old man. He gave the youngest guest an ear, saying, "This is to remind you to listen to your elders!"

Shepherds and sheep

Manas performed his amazing deeds long ago, when the Kyrgyz were nomads. They used to ride on horseback in the valleys of the snow-clad Tien Shan (or "Heavenly") Mountains with their herds of sheep, goats, yaks and camels. They lived in *yurts*, round tents made from thick, heavy felt. The Kyrgyz haven't been nomads for a hundred years, but the symbol of the top of a

yurt in the middle of the Kyrgyz flag reminds the people of their history.

Animals are still important to Aigul's people. As long as a family owns a cow and a few sheep and goats, no one thinks of them as poor. Several families join together to employ a shepherd to look after their animals. The shepherd leads the animals from pasture to pasture, and the sheep actually know the shepherd's voice and follow him.

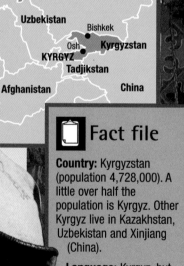

Fact file

Country: Kyrgyzstan (population 4,728,000). A little over half the population is Kyrgyz. Other Kyrgyz live in Kazakhstan, Uzbekistan and Xinjiang (China).

Language: Kyrgyz, but many speak Russian as well.

Religion: Islam

Occupations: About 80% of Kyrgyz work in some sort of farming.

wants us to follow him, too."

"Manas died a long time ago," Aigul thought, "but even though Jesus died, the teachers say he rose from the dead and is still alive today! I wonder if I could follow him?"

Changes

Bishkek, where Aigul lives, is the capital of Kyrgyzstan (*Ker-ger-stan*), a small Muslim republic in Central Asia. It's a modern city with broad, tree-lined streets and colorful parks. During most of the twentieth century, Kyrgyzstan was under Russian or Soviet rule.

Russian settlers took over a lot of the best land and forced many of the nomadic Kyrgyz to settle on big collective farms. Although the Russians made it possible for everyone to go to school for free, they changed the way the Kyrgyz language was written from Arabic letters to the Cyrillic script used in Russia. The Communist rulers also banned the teaching of religion and closed mosques and churches. Kyrgyz Muslims and Russian Christians sometimes met in secret, but often children grew up knowing only what their grandparents taught them about Allah or Jesus. Very few Kyrgyz had ever even heard of Jesus.

In 1991, Krygyzstan once more became on independent country. Christians from other countries arrived to offer their help and

Traditional headdress

Do you know?

At a feast there's always plenty to eat. The Kyrgyz national dish, called *besh-barmak*, is made from mutton mixed with noodles. Its name means "five fingers," because the Kyrgyz used to eat it with their hands!

to tell the Kyrgyz about God's love for them. Some have started to follow Jesus, the Good Shepherd, who takes care of them.

Hunting with a hawk

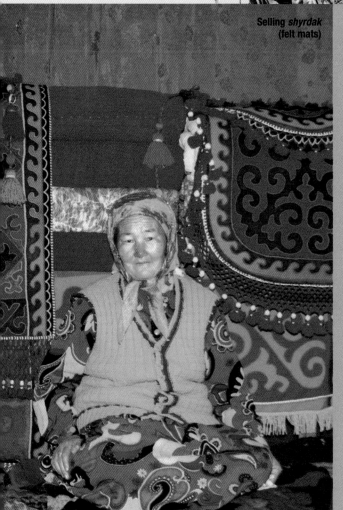

Selling *shyrdak* (felt mats)

To help you pray for the Kyrgyz

You can thank God for:

- every Kyrgyz man, woman, boy and girl who has started to follow Jesus.

- the New Testament and children's Bible in the Kyrgyz language.

- the Christian bookstore in Bishkek.

You can ask God:

- to help all the local Christians, whether they are Kyrgyz, Russian, German or from some other country, to work together and love one another.

- for Christians to tell Kyrgyz boys and girls about Jesus through songs and stories.

- that as the Kyrgyz church grows, pastors and church workers will teach Christians how to obey God and how to tell others about Jesus.

- to give the leaders of Kyrgyzstan wisdom as they govern this country which has few natural resources and where many people are poor and don't have jobs.

Lesotho

The Switzerland of Africa

Lesotho is a small country completely surrounded by the Republic of South Africa. If you visited Lesotho you would see lots of mountains, fast-flowing streams and rushing rivers. Although it's thousands of miles away, Lesotho reminds some people so much of Switzerland that they call it "the Switzerland of Africa." Because it's usually cool and damp in Lesotho, the people wrap up in warm, colorful blankets. They wear cone-shaped hats made of woven grass on their heads.

Most of the two million people living in Lesotho are Basotho, and they speak a language called Sesotho. Because there aren't enough jobs in Lesotho, many men go to South Africa to work in the gold mines.

Children walking to school

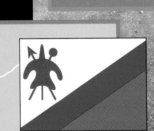

Lesotho · Maseru

South Africa

Shepherd boys

In many countries boys go to school while the girls stay at home to help their families, but not in Lesotho. A lot of Basotho boys, especially those from poor families in the country, begin to look after flocks of sheep and goats and herds of cattle when they're only seven years old. Wool from the sheep and mohair, which is made from goats' hair, are two of Lesotho's main exports. That means that the animals are very valuable.

Imagine what it would be like to be a shepherd boy in Lesotho. You would spend many weeks away from home, all by yourself, looking after the sheep and goats in the mountains. In the summer it rains, and in the winter it's very cold. The frost and snow might feel even colder because you wouldn't have a warm house or fire or even dry clothes to wear. What would you think about during the long, dark nights? What would you do if thieves or wild animals came to steal or kill your animals? You would be in big trouble if you weren't able to keep all the animals safe. If something happened to one of your sheep, your family might not have enough food to eat. You can read in the Bible about the adventures of another shepherd boy – the story of David and Goliath is in the Old Testament, in 1 Samuel 17. David knew that God would keep him safe in every situation.

Some of the shepherd boys who know how to read and write are learning how to teach their friends who are also

Would you walk many miles to learn about the Bible? Lots of Lesotho church leaders do!

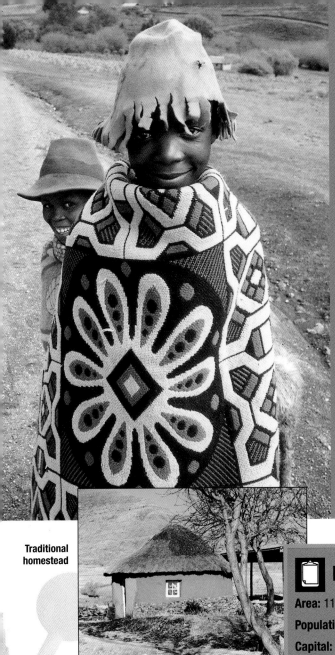

Traditional homestead

To help you pray for Lesotho

You can thank God for:

- the many people in the capital city, Maseru, who are coming to know Jesus as their friend.
- all the boys and girls who are learning about Jesus through Scripture Union.
- new Christians who go into mountain villages to share the good news of Jesus' love with others.

You can ask God:

- to protect MAF pilots as they fly into remote villages with supplies and medical care and share Jesus' love with people there.
- to keep the shepherd boys safe and bring many of them to know Jesus, a friend who is with them all the time.
- to help the Christian leaders with their Bible lessons so that they will know how to teach others about Jesus.
- to look after the men who have to go to South Africa to work in the mines to earn money for their families, and to keep their families at home safe.

MAF airplane

Fact file

Area: 11,740 sq. mi.

Population: 2,152,553

Capital: Maseru

Main languages: Sesotho; English

Religion: Christianity (mainly Roman Catholic)

Chief exports: Wool; mohair; diamonds; livestock

shepherds. The boys who know how to read will be able to get better jobs in Lesotho when they grow up.

In the towns, most of the boys and girls go to school. An organization called Scripture Union is teaching many of the children about Jesus.

Teachers who ride on horseback

Most Basothos belong to the Roman Catholic or the Lesotho Evangelical Church, but many of them don't really understand that Jesus died to forgive their sins. Missionaries are training church leaders to explain to the people what the Bible says. The missionaries send these leaders homework to do, and once a month they travel many miles (on horseback, by bus or on foot!) to attend a special class.

There are lots of villages scattered throughout the mountains. Christian workers, often riding on horseback, visit these villages to tell the people about Jesus. They have also shown the *Jesus* film to thousands of people in Lesotho. Many people watch this film about Jesus' life and teaching, the miracles he did and his death on the cross, and they ask Jesus to be their friend.

A flying ambulance

The Missionary Aviation Fellowship (MAF) has built 40 runways throughout Lesotho. Their planes carry supplies to areas that are difficult to get to, and sometimes they fly patients to the hospital. "It was lots of fun but kind of scary flying in the plane," recalls Mokeane, a little Basotho boy. "I broke my arm and an MAF pilot flew me to the hospital in Maseru. I loved looking out of the plane to see all the little rivers and trees! It only took us 25 minutes to get there. If we had gone on horseback and bus, it would have taken nine or ten hours!"

Lobi

Who File their Teeth to Points

Children who vanish

Sie watched the long line of people hurrying down the road. There were children, some not much bigger than himself; women carrying cooking pots and sacks of food on their heads; men cracking whips so that everyone moved quickly. He shivered as he heard the cries of the children. These cries are heard only once every seven years, at the time of the joro. Sie was afraid. He was too young this time, but he knew his turn was coming.

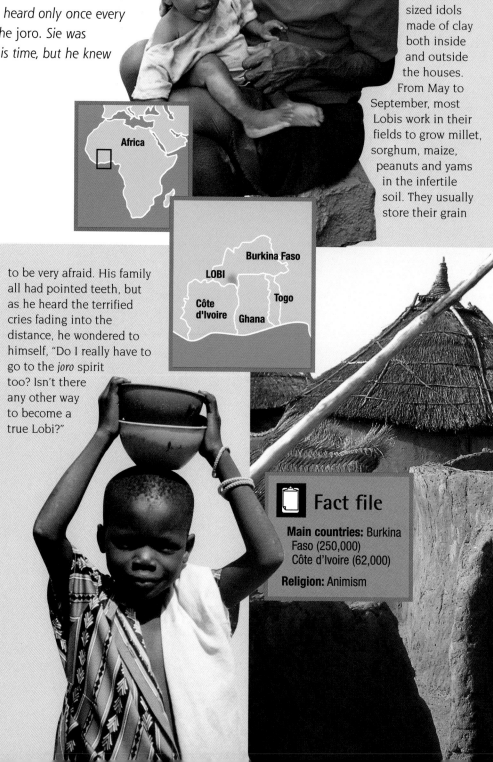

Africa

Slaves no more
The homes of the Lobis are big and built of mud, and the inner rooms are very dark because there are no windows. There are life-sized idols made of clay both inside and outside the houses. From May to September, most Lobis work in their fields to grow millet, sorghum, maize, peanuts and yams in the infertile soil. They usually store their grain

Burkina Faso

LOBI

Côte d'Ivoire

Togo

Ghana

The *joro* is the initiation ceremony of the Lobi people who live in Burkina Faso in West Africa. Tribal leaders take children who are seven years old and older from their parents and go into the bush for two or three months. After many frightening tests of bravery, each child is brought before a large idol of the *joro*, the evil spirit who controls the initiation. The children's teeth are then filed to points as a sign that they are true Lobis. Some children never return, and their families aren't allowed to ask what happened to them. It is enough to know that the *joro* spirit took them.

Although anyone who has been through the *joro* is forbidden to talk about it to those who haven't been initiated, Sie knew enough

to be very afraid. His family all had pointed teeth, but as he heard the terrified cries fading into the distance, he wondered to himself, "Do I really have to go to the *joro* spirit too? Isn't there any other way to become a true Lobi?"

📋 Fact file

Main countries: Burkina Faso (250,000) Côte d'Ivoire (62,000)

Religion: Animism

on the flat roofs of their houses in round bins which have cone-shaped covers made of thatch.

There are very few Lobis who are Christians, but more and more are coming to know Jesus. There are 80 churches and meeting places in Burkina Faso where Christians worship on Sundays. One of these churches is in Nako, near the main center where the initiation ceremonies take place. About 100 Christian Lobi men and women have been trained to share the good news about Jesus with their people and teach them to follow him. They're also telling other animistic and Muslim peoples in Burkina Faso about Jesus.

The New Testament was translated into Lobi and published in 1985. Although most children and young people are learning to read, only one Lobi adult out of every 10 can read.

Perhaps Sie will not have to go to the *joro* to become a true Lobi. Each time the initiation ceremonies are

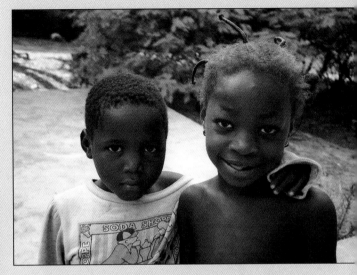

Do you know?

Many years ago, Lobi women had their faces scarred to make them look so ugly that slave traders wouldn't want them. They pierced holes in both lips and inserted round pieces of wood into them. A few women still wear lip rings.

held, Christians pray that the spirits will lose their power over the people. There are signs that God is answering these prayers. Please join them in praying that the slaves of the *joro*, who takes life, will become the children of God, who gives life!

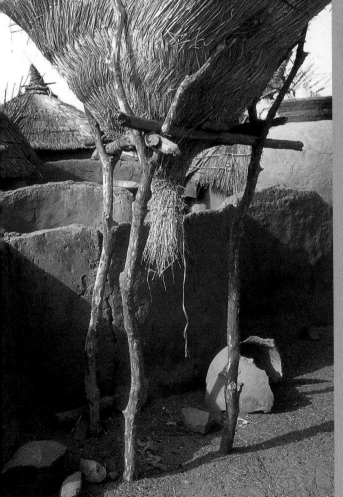

 ## To help you pray for the Lobi

You can thank God for:

- the Lobi New Testament.
- Christian Lobis studying at Bible school.
- Christians leading camps and programs for young people.

You can ask God:

- that Lobis learning to read will read the New Testament for themselves.
- to help those translating the Old Testament into Lobi to find the right words so the meaning is clear.
- that young people will understand that they don't have to be afraid of the *joro* if they trust in Jesus.
- that the church in Nako will become so strong that the initiation ceremonies will come to an end.

Where Christians Gave up their Lives for Jesus

A bird's-eye view

If you look at a map of Africa, you'll see a long, narrow island in the Indian Ocean about 250 miles off the coast of southeast Africa. This is Madagascar. It's the fourth largest island in the world, more than twice the size of the state of Colorado.

Peter is on an airplane about to take off from Mahajanga, on the west coast. Let's fly over the island with him to see what it's like. "There are fields of rice and sweet potatoes, and quite a few cattle, on this part of the island," he tells us. Soon we're flying over the large central plateau where most of the people live.

Manambold Gorge

Fact file

Area: 226,650 sq. mi.

Population: 15,941,727

Capital: Antananarivo

Official languages: Malagasy; French

Religions: Christianity; traditional religions

Chief exports: Coffee; cloves; vanilla; sugar

Christians in Madagascar are teaching people about Jesus in hospitals, prisons and schools

"The hills and steep valleys of the plateau used to be covered in forests," Peter says, "but the people have cut down a lot of the trees for firewood and clear a new patch of land every year to grow their crops. Since these forests have been cut down, the heavy rains wash away a lot of the red soil each year. This is called erosion, and it makes it more difficult to grow crops in the soil." Now we see a big city on a mountain. "Look," Peter says, "there's Antananarivo, the capital city. Look for the old churches and palaces."

Suddenly, it looks like the land is disappearing from under us as we leave the central plateau and fly across the forests of the eastern plain to the coast. A lot of the forest has been cleared for farming here, too. "Most of the people in Madagascar are very poor," Peter says. "There isn't

much rain in some places in the west, so the crops don't grow well. Cyclones pass through Madagascar nearly every year, destroying the forest and crops and causing flooding. There aren't many good roads, so it's difficult to get help to the people who need it most."

Risking their lives for Jesus

Almost 200 years ago, two brave Welshmen took the good news about Jesus to Madagascar. They brought their wives and babies with them, but

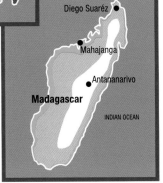

Africa

Diego Suaréz

Mahajanga

Antananarivo

Madagascar

INDIAN OCEAN

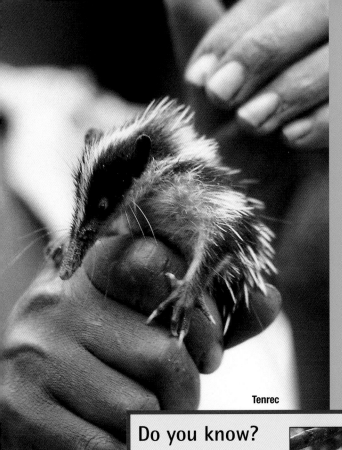

Tenrec

To help you pray for Madagascar

You can thank God for:

- every missionary and church leader.
- the groups that teach young people about Jesus.
- the Malagasy Bible Society.

You can ask God:

- to help Christians today to be faithful to Jesus.
- for many young people to know Jesus and to tell others about him, too.
- for Christians to go to places where the people have never heard about Jesus.
- that Christian radio programs will reach many people with the good news about Jesus.

Do you know?

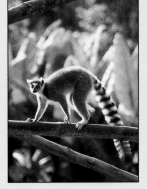

There are many different plants and animals found only in Madagascar. These include lemurs (relatives of monkeys), tenrecs and the Malagasy mongoose. Some of them are in danger of dying out because they live in the forests that are being destroyed.

Lemur

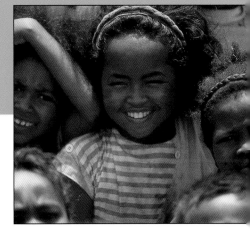

a few months later only one, David Jones, was still alive. It would have been very easy for him to go back to Wales and forget all about the people of Madagascar! But he knew God wanted them to hear about Jesus, so he stayed. He set up a little school, and the king's son was one of his first students. There were no books because their language, Malagasy, had never been written down. When other missionaries joined David Jones, they put the language into writing and taught the children and their parents to read and write. They taught them about Jesus, too, and translated the Bible into Malagasy. A lot of people asked Jesus to be their savior and friend.

Then a new ruler, Queen Ranavalona, decided that the people of Madagascar should worship their dead kings and queens. She said that anyone who worshipped or prayed to

Jesus would be put to death.

Many of the Christians met secretly – in houses, caves or on mountaintops – to pray and read the Bible. The queen had thousands of them tortured and killed because they wouldn't stop following Jesus. She reigned for 33 years, but when she died there were far more Christians than when her cruel reign began. God is so much more powerful than any human ruler.

Remembering God's help

Although more than half the people in Madagascar are Christians, many of them want to worship other gods as well as being Christians – but it doesn't work.

Some of the Christians do love and follow Jesus, just as the Malagasy

martyrs did long ago. Lots of young people, too, are learning about Jesus and following him. Some of them work with the Malagasy Bible Society, which trains them to tell others about Jesus. They bring the Bible to people in hospitals, prisons and schools. They know it's important for people to have the Bible and read and understand what it says. Some of these volunteers teach reading with special Bibles for people just learning to read.

But there are still people groups in Madagascar who have never heard of Jesus because their villages are so remote and there aren't any roads into the mountain areas where they live. Please pray that someday they, too, will hear about him and put their trust in him.

Maldives

Beautiful Islands in the South Indian Ocean

Holiday paradise

Peter's father pulled a world atlas down from the bookshelf and opened it to show him the map of India. "Look, Peter," he said, pointing to a chain of tiny islands in the Indian Ocean. "These are the Maldives. I thought we could go there this summer. We'll have to fly to India and then about 300 miles southwest to get there." He traced the chain of islands with his finger. "We won't be able to see all the islands, though – see how they stretch right down here to the equator? That's about 500 miles." He handed Peter a travel magazine. "See for yourself how beautiful they are."

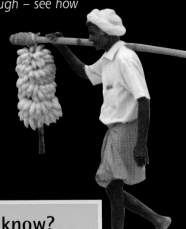

Fact file

Land area: 115 sq. mi.

Population: 286,223

Capital: Malé

Language: Divehi

Religion: Islam

Economy:
Fishing; tourism

"Wow!" exclaimed Peter. "Coral islands! Coconut trees! And sandy beaches! The islands look like they're floating in the sea." Peter started to read the magazine. "I can hardly wait to go! We'll have to bring our snorkels, and we'll do lots of swimming … oh, and wind surfing! And scuba diving!"

Every year, thousands of people visit the Maldives to bask in the sun and swim in the clear blue sea. They stay in hotels built for tourists, but often the only Maldivians they meet are those who work in the hotels.

Over 1,000 islands

"Hey Dad," Peter said a few nights later, "I've been reading more about the Maldives. Did you know that there are at least 1,200 little islands, but only 202 of them are inhabited? Most of the islands are so flat that if the sea level rose only a little, they would be flooded. That's why their government is really concerned about global warming.

Do you know?

Although the Maldives are very beautiful, some Maldivians believe that Allah, the Muslim god, sent all the *jinns* of the world to live in their islands.

Decorated ceramic

"Malé, the capital island, is less than a square mile in area. It must be very crowded with 60,000 people living there! The international airport is on the nearby island of Hulule."

"Very good," his father replied, "I've found out a few things too. The people call themselves Div*e*hi, which means 'islanders.' Their language is called Div*e*hi, too … and they write from right to left! Most children go to school, and in Malé there are schools where the children study in English. If they want to go to college or university they have to go to another country.

"Boat building is an important business, and more than a third of the people are fishermen. Some people say the Maldives is among the 20 poorest countries in the world. They must be very glad to have the money they earn from tourists."

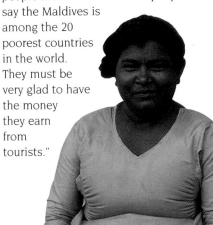

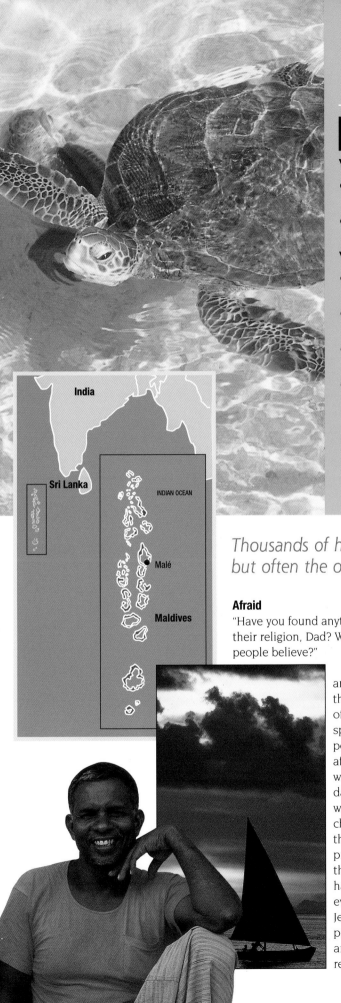

To help you pray for the Maldives

You can thank God for:

- the parts of the Bible that have already been translated into *Divehi*.

- the Christian radio broadcasts that are being beamed into the islands.

You can ask God:

- to take away any fear that Christians working there may have and to give them joy as they share his love by caring for others.

- for Maldivians to discover that through trusting in Jesus they can be set free from fear and the power of evil spirits.

- to lead Maldivians studying in other countries to meet Christians who will share God's love with them.

- that the leaders of the country will allow each person to worship in the way he or she chooses.

India

Sri Lanka

INDIAN OCEAN

Malé

Maldives

Thousands of holiday-makers visit the Maldives every year but often the only Maldivians they meet are hotel workers

Afraid

"Have you found anything out about their religion, Dad? What do the people believe?"

"The Maldivians are Muslims, but they're also afraid of *jinns*, or evil spirits. Many people are so afraid that they won't go out after dark. They often wear blue glass charms around their necks to protect them from the *jinns*. We don't have to be afraid of evil spirits because Jesus is more powerful than they are. Do you remember what we read in church on Sunday about Jesus casting out demons in Luke 4:31–36? Jesus will always protect us."

Peter shivered. "I know, but all this talk about evil spirits is scary. Aren't there any Christians there?"

His father shook his head. "Only a few," he said. "The government doesn't allow missionaries, but Christians from other countries do go there to work. They can read the Bible and pray in private, but they can't speak about Jesus to Maldivian people. Some foreign Christians have been expelled from the country and some Maldivian Christians put in prison. It's not easy to be a Christian when that happens!"

"But Jesus can change the world, can't he?" asked Peter. "Let's start praying that the people of the Maldives will hear the good news that Jesus saves them and protects them from evil spirits."

World Map

Countries which are featured in this book are shown in red.
People groups are shown in orange.

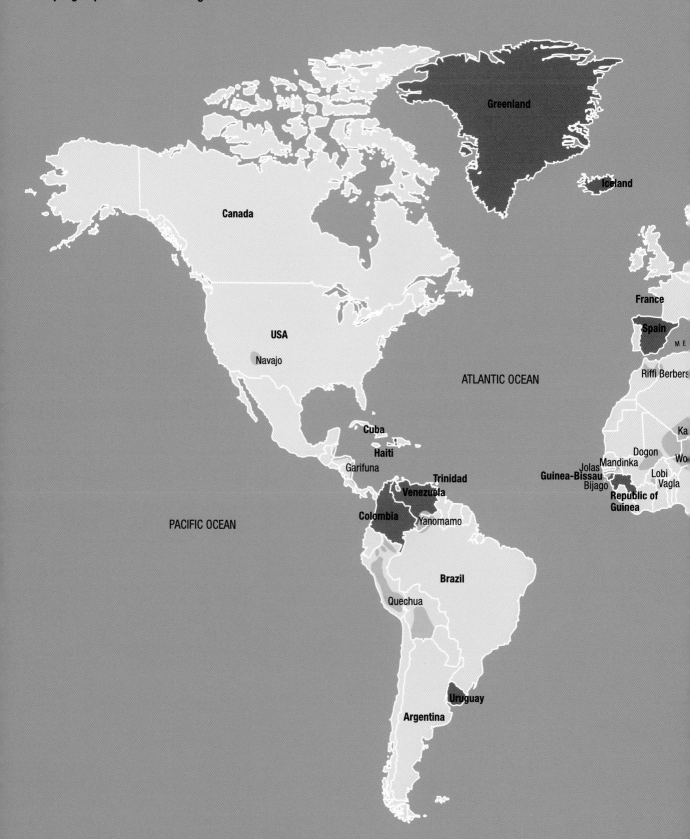

Greenland

Iceland

Canada

USA

Navajo

ATLANTIC OCEAN

France

Spain

M E

Riffi Berbers

Ka

Cuba

Haiti

Garifuna

Dogon

Wo

Mandinka

Jolas

Lobi

Trinidad

Guinea-Bissau

Vagla

Venezuela

Bijago

Republic of
Guinea

Colombia

Yanomamo

PACIFIC OCEAN

Brazil

Quechua

Uruguay

Argentina

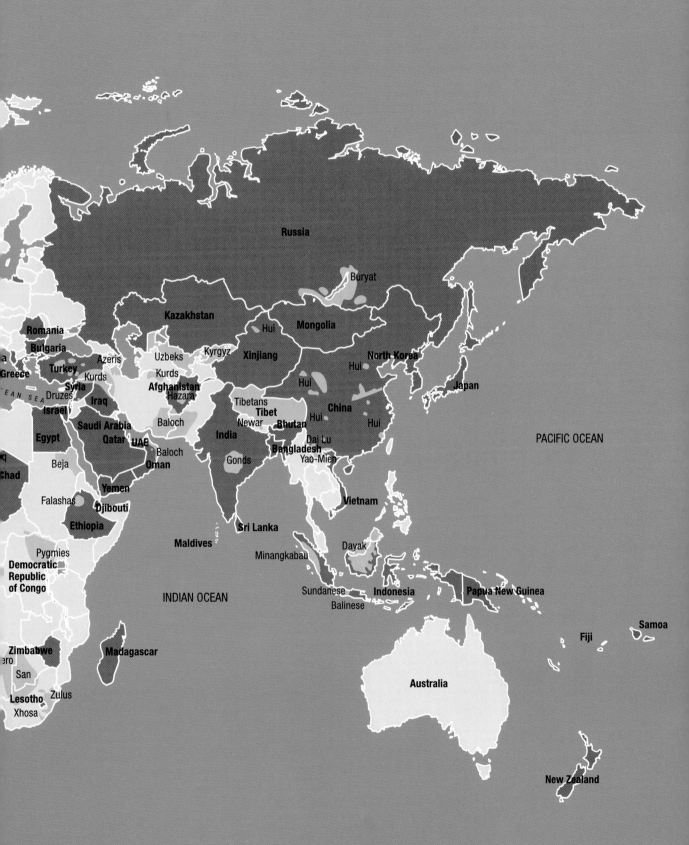

Russia

Buryat

Kazakhstan

Hui   Mongolia

Romania   Kyrgyz
Bulgaria   Uzbeks   Xinjiang   North Korea
                Azeris   Hui
Greece   Turkey   Kurds   Hui   Japan
        Syria   Kurds   China
EAN SEA Druzes   Afghanistan   Hui
Israel   Iraq   Hazara   Tibetans   PACIFIC OCEAN
                                          Tibet   Hui
        Saudi Arabia   Baloch   Newar Bhutan   Hui
Egypt   Qatar   UAE   India   Dai Lu
        Oman   Baloch   Bangladesh Yao-Mien
Beja   Gonds
q
Chad
        Yemen   Vietnam
Falashas   Djibouti
        Ethiopia   Sri Lanka
                        Maldives   Dayak
Pygmies   Minangkabau
Democratic   INDIAN OCEAN
Republic   Sundanese   Indonesia   Papua New Guinea
of Congo   Balinese

                                                                    Samoa
                                                            Fiji
Zimbabwe   Madagascar
ero
San   Australia
Lesotho   Zulus
Xhosa

                                                    New Zealand

Mandinka

Who Hope Charms Will Keep Them Safe

Charms for a baby

Nene cuddled her baby son. Outside her mud and thatch house, the village people were singing and dancing. The marabout (Muslim teacher) had come, and Nene had paid him to tie ten jujus (charms) around her baby's arms, neck and waist. She hoped these would keep him safe from sickness and evil spirits. Nene was very worried. The charms hadn't worked for her other three babies, who had all died. Nene had wanted to take the children to the Christian nurse at the nearby clinic, but her husband wouldn't let her. "If you do," he told her, "they'll make you take off the jujus and burn them. That's against our Mandinka ways, and the children wouldn't be protected from the evil spirits.

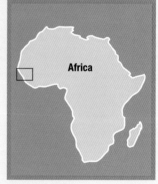

Fact file

Location: Gambia and Senegal

Numbers: 513,200 (Gambia) 310,000 (Senegal)

Religion: Islam

Language: Mandinka

Occupations: Farming; trading

Senegal

Gambia

Banjul

MANDINKA

Senegal

MANDINKA

Africa

The *marabout* makes *jujus* by writing verses from the Koran on bits of paper. Then he sews them into little leather pouches and hangs them on a string. The Mandinka believe that the power of these *jujus* comes from Allah, the Muslim God.

Followers of Islam

Almost half the people living in the small West African country of Gambia are Mandinkas. Many centuries ago, they left their homeland in Mali and traveled west in search of better farmland. Eventually they settled in Gambia and the surrounding countries.

The Mandinkas were animists. Traders passing through the region converted some of them to Islam, but a lot of the Mandinkas continued to follow their traditional religion. Now most Mandinkas say they are Muslims, like nearly all the other people in Gambia. But many of them are still afraid of the spirits.

"I'm so afraid!"

Oumar sat near the fire and listened to the grown-ups tell scary stories about beautiful women who were really witches and sold children for meat. He had lots of strange dreams and was scared to go anywhere in the dark.

"I'm always afraid," he told his mother one day. "I can't even sleep. I wish there was a god who was more powerful than the bad

114

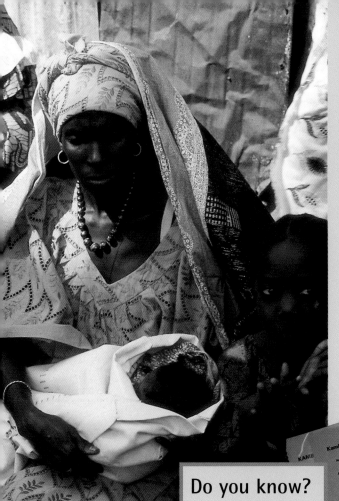

To help you pray for the Mandinka

You can thank God for:

- the Mandinka New Testament.

- the clinics, youth centers and other places where people can feel God's love and learn about him.

- the Mandinkas who are helping to translate the Old Testament.

You can ask God:

- that Mandinkas who are learning to read will understand what the Bible says.

- to help Mandinka Christians to always follow Jesus, help others and tell them about God's love and care.

- to show the Mandinkas that he is far greater and more powerful than all the gods and spirits that they fear.

- to send more missionaries to Gambia to help the Mandinkas and to tell them about Jesus.

Mandinka Scriptures

Do you know?

Only two out of every ten Mandinka people can read. So programs teaching them to read are very important.

witches and spirits and who would take care of me."

"We're Muslims, Oumar," she said. "We believe in the great God Allah. He'll help you." So Oumar learned as much as he could from the Muslim teachers. He prayed five times every day and fasted during the month of Ramadan, but he was still afraid.

Oumar wanted to do well in school so he could get a good job and help his mother. At the Catholic high school he learned about the Lord Jesus Christ, the Son of God. Oumar was confused. "I wonder which is true?" he asked himself. "Islam or Christianity?"

Oumar started to study the Bible through a correspondence course. He wanted to prove that Jesus was not really the Son of God so he could know that

Islam was true. But he was surprised to learn that Jesus really was the one who could take away his fears. Oumar wanted to follow this God more than anything else, but he was afraid his mother would be very angry. Oumar knew that he had finally found the truth. He had to make a choice to follow Jesus or be afraid forever.

Oumar told his teacher that he wanted to follow Jesus. Now he knows that Jesus is always with him and helps him when he's afraid. His mother was angry with him at first, but when she saw the change in Oumar's life, and that he wasn't afraid anymore, she wanted to follow Jesus too.

Showing God's love

There aren't many Mandinka Christians yet, but missionaries are showing them God's love and helping them in a lot of different ways. They provide medical care, reading classes (there are even special classes in prisons), and youth centers where young people can learn new skills.

There's a Mandinka New Testament, and a team translating the Old Testament. The missionaries pray that a lot more Mandinkas will put their trust in Jesus, who will take away their fears.

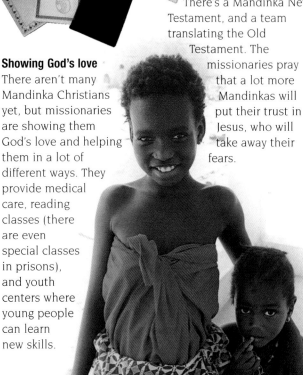

Minangkabau

The People of the Water Buffalo

The weak triumphs over the strong

The Minangkabau (mee-nahng-kah-bow) people, who live in West Sumatra in Indonesia, enjoy telling a legend about the water buffalo. (Minang means "winning," and kabau means "water buffalo.") About 600 years ago, the king of the nearby island of Java tried to conquer West Sumatra. The people of West Sumatra knew they weren't strong enough to win a war, but they had another idea.

Pick your best water buffalo to fight our best buffalo," they told the king. "If your buffalo wins, we'll serve you; but if ours wins, you must never attack us again." The Javanese king agreed and found the biggest, fiercest water buffalo in Java. He was sure they would win!

Do you know?

All Minangkabau children learn two languages. They speak Minangkabau at home, but at school they speak Indonesian, the national language.

China

Malaysia

MINANGKABAU

Sumatra

I n d o n e s i a

INDIAN OCEAN

On the day of the contest, this enormous buffalo stomped out onto the field. The Javanese army laughed and laughed when they saw the buffalo the people of West Sumatra sent out onto the field. It was just a tiny calf. How ridiculous to think such a little creature could beat their giant!

What the Javanese didn't know was that their enemy had a sneaky plan. For three days, the West Sumatrans had kept the baby buffalo away from its mother and her milk. As you can imagine, he was very hungry indeed. They had also tied sharp knives to his head. When the calf saw the big water buffalo, he thought it was his mother and rushed towards it. He pushed his head under the Javanese buffalo's belly, searching for milk. As he did so, the knives on his head cut into the big animal again and again. Bellowing with pain, the big buffalo ran away and finally fell down dead!

"Minang kabau!" the West Sumatrans shouted. "Our buffalo is the winner!" Since then, the people of West Sumatra have called themselves the Minangkabau because they're proud that they were so smart. They even make points shaped like the horns of a water buffalo on the roofs of their houses.

The Bible is full of true stories like this, where the weak triumphs over the strong. One of the best known is the story of David and Goliath (you can read about this in I Samuel 17 in the Old Testament).

The family name

The surnames of most people in the world come from their father's

Planting rice in a paddy field

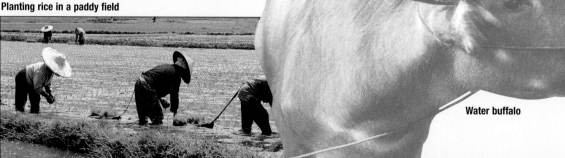

Water buffalo

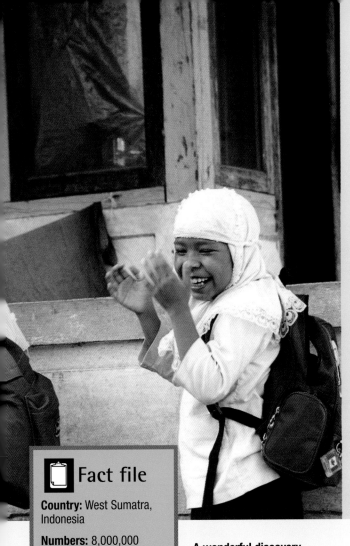

To help you pray for the Minangkabau

You can thank God for:

- the Minangkabau who know Jesus.
- Christian radio programs.
- the New Testament in Minangkabau.

You can ask God:

- for more Christians to share the good news about Jesus with the Minangkabau.
- to show these people that they can be Christians and still be Minangkabau.
- that Minangkabau all over the world will meet Christians and hear about Jesus.
- that the government and local people will be fair to the Minangkabau Christians and not hurt them.

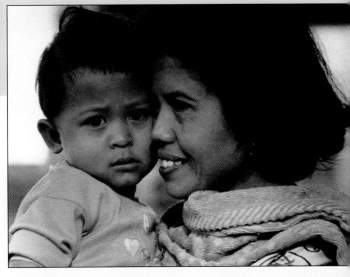

Fact file

Country: West Sumatra, Indonesia

Numbers: 8,000,000

Occupations: Rice farming; business; restaurant owners

family – yours is probably the same. But the Minangkabau use the mother's name. They're unusual in other ways, too. The men are leaders within the bigger family (called a clan) and in the village, but it's the women who own the rice fields and houses. Because they don't own land, the men often leave their villages to find work in the towns, only returning to help at harvest time. Some of them never go back, which is why there are Minangkabau in every part of Indonesia. A lot of them open restaurants, where they serve their very hot spicy food called Nasi Padang.

A wonderful discovery

There are about eight million Minangkabau. About four million of them live in the mountain region of West Sumatra, and the rest are scattered throughout Indonesia. Almost all of them are Muslims, but many of them still also believe that spirits living in the forests and mountains cause sickness and trouble. Those who become Christians know that they'll probably lose their jobs, their families will disown them, and they may even be thrown into prison. The government even closed down a hospital, that was helping a lot of people, just because it was run by Christians. And nearly all the copies of the New Testament in Minangkabau were taken and burned soon after they were printed.

There are only about 200 Minangkabau Christians. How will the rest of the Minangkabau hear the good news about Jesus? God will answer your prayers to make that happen. Some hear about Jesus as they listen to radio broadcasts. Some, like Pak Iman, hear about him when they work in other parts of Indonesia or the world.

On a business trip in America, Pak Iman found a Bible in his hotel room. He had never seen one, but he started to read it and then took it home with him. For six years, Pak Iman read the Bible and watched the Christians where he worked. He finally decided to follow Jesus, but he was afraid to tell his wife and children. He was surprised and happy to discover that his wife had been reading the Bible, too, and that she and their children all wanted to become Christians. God is answering prayers for the Minangkabau.

117

Missionary Kids

Belonging to Two Worlds

Two countries

"What's America like?" Paul asked his friend David. "I was only four the last time we were there. Were you scared to go there?"

David remembered how confused he felt when they arrived at JFK Airport in New York. Everything was so big, exciting and a bit frightening. Riding on the moving sidewalks and going up and down escalators had been fun, but there were so many people rushing around that he made sure he kept close to his father.

"Yes, I was a bit scared," David admitted, "even though I knew I'd be seeing my grandparents and all the rest of our family. I wondered how I'd get along with them, but they made me feel right at home. We had lots of treats, like hamburgers at MacDonald's and going to Disney World … that was awesome!"

Two schools

"What about school?" Paul asked. "Our school here is so small, and all the teachers are our friends. We're just like a big family and we do everything together. Maybe I won't find any friends in America."

"I know how you feel," David said. "At first my new school seemed too big.

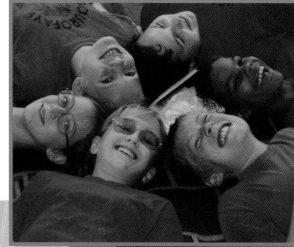

Paul and David are both nine years old, and they go to a small, international boarding school for MKs (missionaries' kids) in West Africa. David and his family recently returned from a year of "home leave" in America, and Paul and his family are about to go home.

Paul grinned. "I can't wait for things like that, and television. There'll be lots of big stores and things to buy, but I probably won't know what to choose! What's the food like? Is it very different?"

David laughed. "Well, I missed peanut stew!" he said. "But there were lots of other good things to eat. We hardly ever have ice cream here, but we could have it every day in America if we wanted! In hundreds of different flavors! I didn't like shopping in the big malls at first. They were too big and there were so many things to choose from that I couldn't decide what I wanted. But it was great being able to buy the newest computer games and bring them back here – especially now that we have electricity all the time."

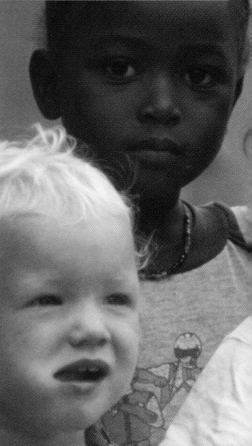

There were almost as many kids in my class as we have in the whole school here. I wondered whether I'd make friends, and if the other kids would think I was weird because I didn't know much about life in America. I wondered whether I would know as much as the kids in my class did. But I didn't need to worry, because sometimes I even got the best grades in my class. And it was great having enough kids for a soccer team!

"My class really liked hearing about Africa – the different animals, village life and my African friends. They liked hearing about our school here, too. I told them about the fun we have, and about our games and sports and some of the tricks we play on each other. They wanted to hear about our visits to the cotton fields and markets. I told them about some of the difficult things as well, like the heat and insects, how much I miss my parents at the beginning of each term, and how sick I felt when I had malaria. I told them how lonely I am sometimes when I go home to the village during school holidays because even though I still play with my African friends, it's not the same since I've gone away to school. My life is so different from theirs because they never leave the village except to go to their fields or to the market.

"They couldn't believe that we studied the Bible every day and had our own church service on Sundays – and that we actually enjoyed it! Most kids I met didn't even go to Sunday school."

Two cultures

MKs have lots of unusual experiences. Their parents often teach them at home until they're old enough to go away to school. Sometimes they travel a lot and live in fascinating places. They meet all sorts of people and have friends from all around the world. But they can also feel very lonely. "It's really hard to say goodbye to friends who go on home leave or move to other places," said an MK called Mary, "but we stay in touch through letters and e-mail. MKs understand each other, because none of us really belong to the country where we grow up. And we don't always feel at home in the country our parents call 'home.' Sometimes we feel like we don't really belong anywhere, although we seem to belong everywhere. But we can understand other people, no matter where they come from."

If you know a missionary family, you could be a friend to the children. You could write to them about the things you do so that when they come home everything won't seem quite so strange. They'll write to you, too, and tell you about their school and the things they do.

To help you pray for missionary kids

You can thank God for:

● the friends MKs have from different countries.

● their missionary parents, who show Jesus' love and care to others.

● schools where MKs can study and learn the same things as children in their home countries.

You can ask God:

● to help MKs find friends and not to feel lonely.

● to keep them safe and well.

● to help them adjust when they return to their home countries.

● that they can use their experiences to understand and help others.

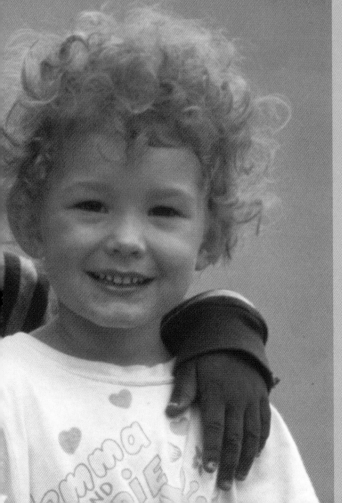

Mongolia

Very Hot or Very Cold

From mountains to desert

The country of Mongolia is sandwiched between Russia and China. In the north you will find windswept mountains, plains, forests and lakes, but the Gobi Desert in the south is a vast wilderness of sand and gravel. The winters are long and cold, but the summers are very hot. There are only a few towns in Mongolia. More people are moving into these towns, but most people still live in the country. Those who still follow the traditional way of life move to the pastures in the mountains during the summer with their flocks of sheep, goats, camels, yaks and horses. In the cold winter months they move down to the grassy plains. Their homes are felt-covered gers, or tents, which they take with them. The gers protect them from both heat and cold.

Do you know?

Most Mongolians learn to ride a horse almost as soon as they learn to walk. Each year at the Nadam Festival, on July 11, they can show off their horse-riding skills in long races across the steppes. These young jockeys retire by the time they're 12 years old.

Fact file

Area: 604,250 sq. mi.

Population: 2,662,020

Capital: Ulaanbaatar

Language: Khalkh Mongolian

Religion: Buddhism

Chief exports: Minerals; meat; wool

Buddhism and Communism

For many centuries Mongolia was a Buddhist country and most families sent their eldest sons to be Buddhist monks. Few people were ever allowed to preach about Jesus there, and those who did rarely met anyone who wanted to learn anything about him.

In 1924 Mongolia became a Communist republic and, for the next 65 years, Mongolia was closed to the outside world. The Communist government destroyed many of the Buddhist monasteries and banned religion. In 1990 a miracle happened: the Communist government lost power and the people were given the freedom to choose which religion they would follow. Some returned to Buddhism, but others became Christians.

Growing up in Mongolia

Jill was excited to meet a Mongolian student and had lots of questions about this mysterious country. Udbal grew up in Ulaanbaatar, Mongolia's capital. "It's the only large city in the country," she told Jill. "Some people live in apartments, but many still prefer to live in *gers*. In the city, you'll often see tall buildings and *gers* next to one another. The city *gers* have electricity, but they don't have running water. My parents both worked, so my brothers, sisters and I helped carry water, chop wood, shop, cook and clean."

Jill wanted to know if it was true that they drank fermented horses' milk. Udbal laughed. "Mares' milk, yes. It becomes fizzy after a few days and is very refreshing. We make cheese from the milk of sheep and

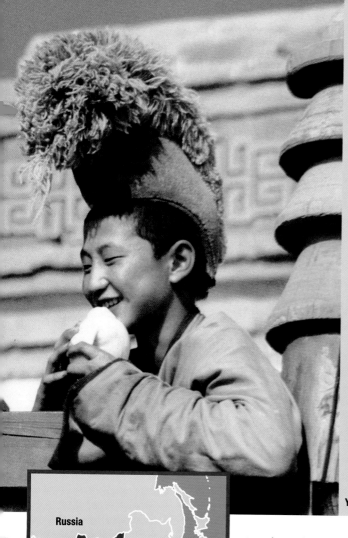

✋ ## To help you pray for Mongolia

You can thank God for:

- those Mongolians who have come to know Jesus.
- the New Testament in Mongolian.

You can ask God:

- for Mongolian Christians to share God's love.
- to help students in Bible school.
- that Mongolians will read and understand the New Testament.
- to help those translating the Old Testament.
- to bring help for the poor and the sick, especially the street children.

Nomad woman

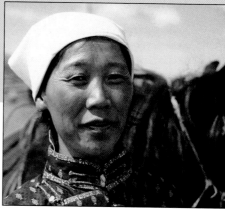

Young monks

In the city, you'll often see tall buildings and gers next to one another

Russia

Mongolia • Ulaanbaatar

Japan

China

A group of tent-like homes called *gers*

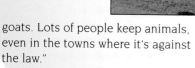

goats. Lots of people keep animals, even in the towns where it's against the law."

"Did you learn about Buddhism as a child?" Jill asked her.

"It was never mentioned at school, and the Communists only allowed one Buddhist monastery to stay open. My father is an atheist and doesn't believe in God. When I was little I wondered about the world: Who made

it? Where do people come from? How can there be no God, as the Communists say? Most children wonder about these things, but when we asked questions, we were told to be quiet."

Jill wanted to know how Udbal became a Christian. "When I was at school," she answered, "a man from overseas asked me to help translate the New Testament. I thought it was a children's book because of the exciting stories. Gradually I realized it was a special book about God and his son Jesus. I believed what the Bible said, and I began to trust in Jesus."

New Christians

The church in Mongolia has grown in the years since 1990. By 1999, there were more than 30 churches. Most of them are in Ulaanbaatar, but there are churches in the other towns as well. Lots of young people have become interested in Christianity through seeing the *Jesus* film, and many have decided to follow him. Now there is a Bible school, where young Christians can study and train to be leaders in the churches.

The New Testament has been translated into Mongolian and printed in the Russian alphabet. It's also being printed in the Mongolian alphabet. Some of the Old Testament has already been translated and the whole Bible should be published soon.

Navajo

Craftsmen of the American West

Skilled workmen

The Navajo (nah-vuh-hoh) are the largest group of American Indians in the United States. They live in the western states of Arizona, New Mexico and Utah. Although most of them now live in modern houses, almost every family still has at least one "hogan." The hogan is a traditional one-room home made of wood and mud or stone. A Navajo storyteller explains the hogan like this: "Long, long ago, our Holy People told us that the door of the hogan must always face east towards the rising sun. Inside, there's a special place for everyone and everything. The area for the mother and her little children is on the north side, the father and older boys use the south side for their things and any special guests are honored with a place on the west. We hang our belongings from nails in the walls or tuck them into crevices in the walls or up in the domed ceiling."

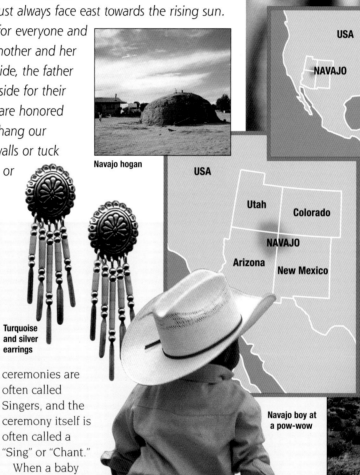

USA

NAVAJO

Navajo hogan

USA

Utah

Colorado

NAVAJO

Arizona

New Mexico

Turquoise and silver earrings

Navajo boy at a pow-wow

The Navajo are very artistic. They color wool with dyes made from desert plants and then use it to weave beautiful rugs on handmade looms. They also make beautiful silver and turquoise jewelry. The Navajo medicine men use an amazing mixture of pollen, corn meal, crushed flowers, charcoal and ground minerals to make sand paintings for their ceremonies. Today, the Navajo make framed sand paintings to sell to art collectors and tourists.

Ceremonies, songs and celebrations

As part of their religion, Navajo memorize and recite songs and chants. Some ceremonies last for nine days, and they can't make any mistakes. The Navajo who perform these ceremonies are often called Singers, and the ceremony itself is often called a "Sing" or "Chant."

When a baby laughs out loud for the first time there's a special celebration for the whole family, and the person who made the child laugh pays for the party! It's no wonder visitors are careful to ask if the babies have laughed out loud yet before playing with them, because grandparents, uncles, aunts and cousins are all included in the celebration. During the party, the guests all walk past the mother and baby, and the baby gives each one a piece of rock salt. Salt was always a prized item for the Navajo, and by giving it

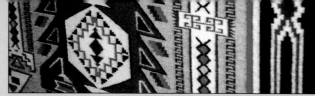

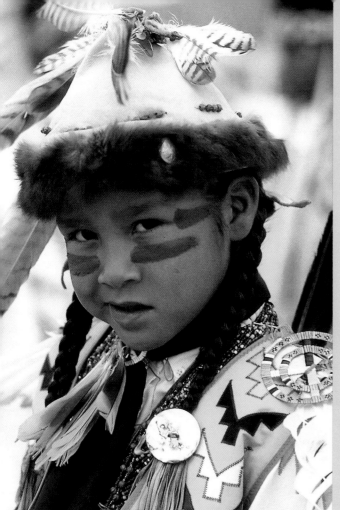

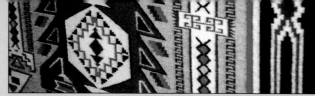

To help you pray for the Navajo

You can thank God for:

- the Navajo Bible.
- every Navajo pastor and church leader.

You can ask God:

- to help older people as they learn to read, and to give their teachers patience.
- that the Navajo who can't read will listen to the Bible on tape.
- that Navajo Christians will share Jesus' love with their families and friends.
- to help them spread the message about Jesus in America and other countries.
- that all Christian leaders in the Navajo Nation will be wise and faithful.

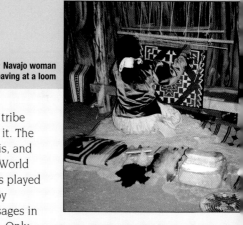

Navajo woman weaving at a loom

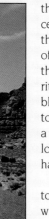

Monument Valley

away the mother is teaching her child to be generous and share with others. This is important to the Navajo, because to be stingy is to be a bad Navajo.

The Navajo are afraid of evil spirits and witches, and they're always trying to be careful not to make the spirits angry by doing wrong things. They have special ceremonies to heal themselves from the power of evil, "Sings" to protect them from harm, and other rituals to ask the spirits to bless them. When Christians told the Navajo that there is a God who is good and loves them, they found it hard to understand.

Today, Navajo are coming to know Jesus as their friend who sets them free from the fear of evil spirits. Pastors and teachers are helping them to understand God's love. They're also learning to sing the praises of the one true God, who doesn't mind if they make mistakes when singing.

The Bible in Navajo

Because the Navajo language is one of the most difficult languages in the world to learn, very few people outside the tribe know how to speak it. The Americans knew this, and during the Second World War Navajo soldiers played an important role by sending radio messages in their own language. Only those who were meant to receive them could understand them.

Although it's a very difficult language, the Navajo are the only North American tribe with the whole Bible in their own language. It took 40 years to translate and was published in 1986. One of the translators was a blind Navajo man, Geronimo Martin. He knew English and had learned to read Braille. As he read an English Braille Bible with his fingers, he translated it aloud into Navajo, and other people recorded his words. It's amazing to think that a blind man was able to help his own people see the truth of Jesus by giving them the Bible.

Many older Navajo speak only their own language and have never been to school. Some are now being taught to read, but learning to read when you are older is very difficult. The Navajo like to listen to stories, so Geronimo's wife and some other Navajo Christians are reading the Navajo Bible aloud and making cassettes for them.

New Zealand

Aotearoa: Land of the Long White Cloud

Kiwis

New Zealand has two main islands that are simply called the North Island and the South Island. It's a beautiful country with long, sandy beaches, rolling hills, steep mountains, volcanoes, giant trees and hot, bubbling pools and springs. Some plants, animals and birds that live in New Zealand aren't found anywhere else in the world. One of them is the kiwi, a large bird that isn't able to fly but looks like a hen. "Kiwi" is also a nickname for New Zealanders. The people love sports and are known all over the world for their skill in rugby, cricket and water sports.

Maori wood carving

Fact file

Area: 103,500 sq. mi.

Population: 3,861,905

Capital: Wellington

Language: English

Religion: Freedom of religion, but mainly Christian

Chief exports: Meat; dairy products; wool; fruit

Do you know?

In the North Island there are four active volcanoes and it's a common sight to see geysers and clouds of steam rising from hot bubbling springs that well up from volcanic rocks in the area.

You can greet one another in Maori
Hello is "Tena koe" (**Ten**-a kway)
Goodbye is "Haere ra"
  (hy-**air**-ay rah)

Maoris

The Maori name for New Zealand is Aotearoa, which means the "land of the long white cloud." It's usually not too hot or too cold in New Zealand, and there's plenty of rain, so it's an ideal place for sheep farming. There are three and a half million people living there, along with more than 45 million sheep: that's over twelve sheep to every person!

Most of the people living in New Zealand are descendants of British and European settlers, but about 10% are Maoris. Twelve or more centuries ago, the Maoris traveled vast distances from the Pacific islands of Polynesia. They came in 60-foot-long canoes, each carved from a single log. They built beautiful meeting places in New Zealand, where the tribes still meet. On special occasions they cook food in leaves buried in the ground between hot stones. Sweet potatoes, cabbage, beef, lamb and pork taste delicious cooked this way.

When the settlers arrived from Britain and Europe in the

There are more than twelve sheep for every person living in New Zealand!

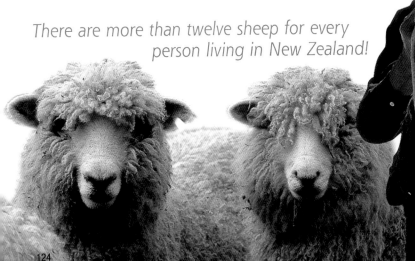

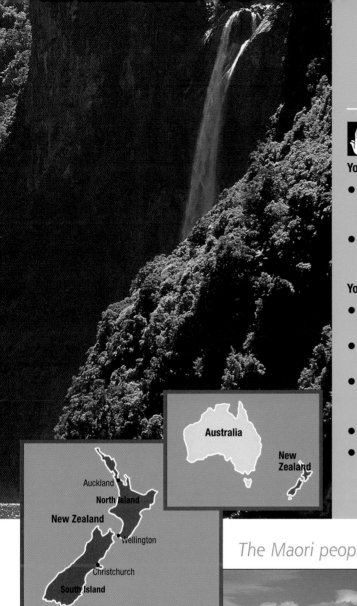

To help you pray for New Zealand

You can thank God for:

- the many Christians in New Zealand who know Jesus and want to tell others that Jesus loves them and died on the cross to take away their sins.

- each Christian who volunteers to teach Bible-in-school classes and to run camps, after-school clubs and other activities so that children will learn to follow Jesus.

You can ask God:

- to help Christians talk about Jesus in a loving, caring way to people of other faiths.

- that as Maoris bring back some of their old customs and traditions, Maori Christians will be faithful in following Jesus.

- for Christians to give money to Bible schools so that Maori and Kiwi evangelists, pastors and missionaries can be trained to teach about Jesus.

- to bring many people in New Zealand to follow Jesus.

- for all Christians in New Zealand to love and care for each other, because they all belong to God's family.

Australia

New Zealand

Auckland
North Island
New Zealand
Wellington
Christchurch
South Island

City skyline, Auckland

Long boat, Matauri Bay

The Maori people came to live in New Zealand more than 1,000 years ago

Many countries, many faiths

Although many people in New Zealand say they are Christians, only one person out of nine reads the Bible regularly. Few of them believe that Jesus is the only way to God. People of different faiths have come to live in New Zealand from many other countries. Some are refugees; others have come seeking work. Among them are Buddhists and Muslims from South East Asia, Hindus from Fiji and Confucians from Hong Kong. They have brought their own religions with them and have set up their own places of worship.

Maori cooking pits

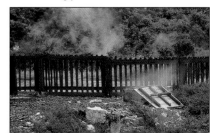

nineteenth century, they fought fiercely with the Maori people over land. A lot of Maori people lost the land where their people had lived for hundreds of years. In school, Maori children were often punished for speaking their own language instead of English, until their leaders demanded their rights. "We've been here more than 1,000 years, so why shouldn't we speak our own language?" they asked. Now Maori artists, painters, craftsmen and film producers are reviving old customs and traditions, and children often learn their history in action songs. Some Maoris have become strong Christians, and some are studying in Bible schools.

Newars

Who Have a Living Goddess

Fact file

Country: Nepal

Location: Kathmandu Valley, but there are also Newars scattered throughout Nepal.

Numbers: About 400,000

Language: Newari

Religions: Buddhism; Hinduism

Occupations: Businessmen; tradesmen; craftsmen; farmers

The Kathmandu Valley

"Look! The Himalayas! They're even higher than I thought they'd be. Do you think we'll see Mount Everest?" We gazed out of the plane's window at the distant snow-covered mountains that straddle the northern border of Nepal. We had already flown over the Terai, the flat, fertile plain along Nepal's southern border with India. Below us now, encircled by mountains, we could see the towns and villages, rivers, green fields and temples of the Kathmandu Valley. In a few minutes we would be landing at Kathmandu, Nepal's capital city.

The people in the fertile Kathmandu Valley grow rice, corn, wheat and many different fruits and vegetables. The cities of Kathmandu, Patan, Bhaktapur and Kirtipur are full of ancient Hindu temples and huge Buddhist stupas (shrines). There are also lots of houses and palaces with beautifully carved wooden doors and shutters.

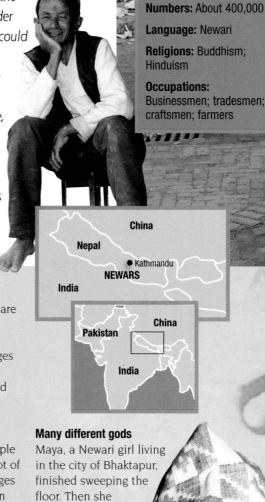

The door shuts … and opens again

Nepal is proud of being the only Hindu kingdom in the world. But the people have actually mixed their Hindu beliefs with Buddhism and animism. In 1816, after a war with the British over the borders of the Terai, Nepal shut itself off from the rest of the world. For many years, Christians on India's border with Nepal told the Nepalis they met about Jesus. And they prayed for the day when they could go into Nepal.

At last, after a short revolution in 1951, Christians were among the first to go in to help the new king and his country. At first, Nepalis who became Christians were often put in prison. But democracy was introduced in 1991, and since then Christians have had greater freedom to worship God. Now there are more than 250,000 Christians in Nepal! But there are still many villages all over Nepal where the people have not yet heard about God's love.

Many different peoples

Almost 100 different people groups live in Nepal. A lot of them live in remote villages in deep river valleys or on the sides of mountains. There are very few roads in these areas – only rough, narrow trails. If these people need food, medicine or anything else, men or donkeys have to carry it in to them.

The Newars are one of Nepal's people groups. About half of them live in the Kathmandu Valley, and the rest live throughout the country.

Many different gods

Maya, a Newari girl living in the city of Bhaktapur, finished sweeping the floor. Then she picked up the empty brass water pot and joined some other girls going to the water tank. Talking and laughing, they passed temples where people were worshipping and making offerings to the gods. In the city square,

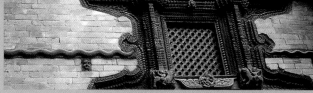

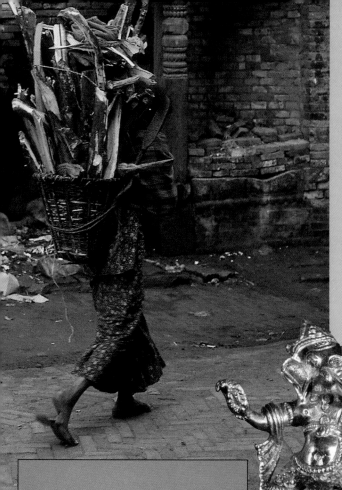

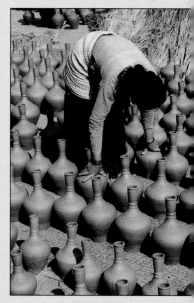

To help you pray for the Newars

You can thank God for:

- every person in Nepal who loves and follows Jesus.
- the Christian books available in several of the languages spoken in Nepal.

You can ask God:

- that many Newari children will hear about Jesus and understand that he is the only God.
- that Newars will discover that Jesus is far more powerful than all the gods they worship.
- that Christians visiting the Kathmandu Valley will talk to Newari people about Jesus.
- that many young Newars, especially those who will lead their country someday, will come to know and follow Jesus.
- that many more Christians will go to Nepal to tell the Newars and the other people groups about Jesus.

Ganesh, the Hindu elephant god

The Himalayas

Do you know?

The Newars worship hundreds of gods, and they set aside over 150 special days each year to worship them.

potters were forming new pots on their wheels. At the water tank, Maya washed herself and then filled the pot.

As she went back into her house, Maya looked up at the figure of Ganesh, the Hindu elephant god. The Newars believe that Ganesh brings wealth and wisdom to their homes. Maya knew that Newars were supposed to be Buddhists and worship Buddha. But they worshipped other gods too, so she wasn't sure if they were Hindus as well.

"Why do we have so many gods everywhere?" Maya asked her mother. They were mixing red vermilion powder, rice and flower petals to make offerings for the Buddha and the other gods in their house and at the temple. "We have gods for every part of our lives," her mother told her. "There's a god for everything you need."

The Living Goddess

As she helped her mother, Maya asked her to tell the story of the Living Goddess.

"The Newari girl who is chosen to be Kumari, the Living Goddess, always comes from a family belonging to the gold and silver-smith's caste," Maya's mother told her. "She's only five years old when she's chosen, and she has to be perfect in every way. She has to pass lots of difficult and frightening tests to show that she really is the Living Goddess. Once she has been chosen, she always wears beautiful clothes and jewels and lives in Kathmandu, in Kumari Bahal, the House of the Living Goddess. People worship her, and even the king comes to her for advice. She doesn't stay a goddess forever, though. When she reaches her teens she becomes an ordinary person again. That must be quite hard for her. Be glad you're an ordinary Newari girl, Maya!"

Clay pots drying at Bhaktapur

Kumari is only a goddess for a few years. But Jesus has always been God, and always will be God. And he promises that he'll always be with those who follow him.

North Korea

Following a God-king

 Fact file

Area: 46,540 sq. mi. (slightly smaller than England)

Population: 24,039,193

Capital: Pyongyang

Language: Korean

Religions: Buddhism; Confucianism (but it is a Communist state)

Chief exports: Coal; iron; copper; oil; grain

A first god-king

Once upon a time, says a Korean legend, Hwanung, the son of the Great Creator, decided to come down from heaven and become king of everything he could see. As he looked around at the beautiful country he heard a bear praying. "Make me into a human being," it said. "I'm tired of being a bear."

Hwanung felt sorry for the bear and told it to eat 20 pieces of garlic and some mugwort (a plant with a bitter taste) and stay in a cave for 100 days. The bear obeyed, and turned into a woman!

The woman longed for a son and gave birth to Tangun. According to the legend, Tangun was the first king of Korea, thousands of years ago. He reigned for more than 1,000 years and his people worshipped him.

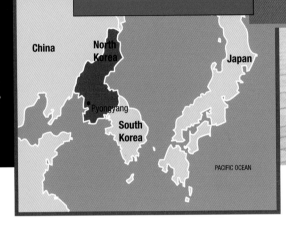

A second god-king

Not long ago, there was another man who thought he was a god-king. In 1945, when Korea was divided into two separate countries – North Korea and South Korea – at the end of World War II, Kim Il Sung, the "Great Leader," came to power in North Korea.

At that time there were so many Christians in North Korea that Pyongyang, the capital city, was sometimes called the "Jerusalem of Korea."

But Kim Il Sung expected everyone to worship him. He made everyone wear a badge with his picture. Every building in Pyongyang had his picture above the doorway. All over the city, there were posters of Kim Il Sung. And high on a hill outside the city, he built a 330-foot-tall statue of himself with his arms outstretched, smiling down on the city.

No other god

The "Great Leader" was a Communist and wanted to get rid of every trace of religion in North Korea. He had all the church buildings destroyed, and nearly three million Koreans were killed, including thousands of Christians.

At school, the teachers showed the children a little black book and asked,

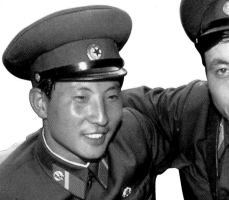
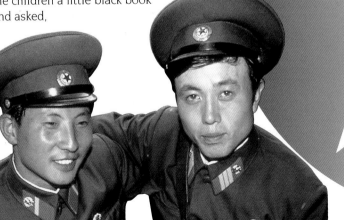

North Korean soldiers

128

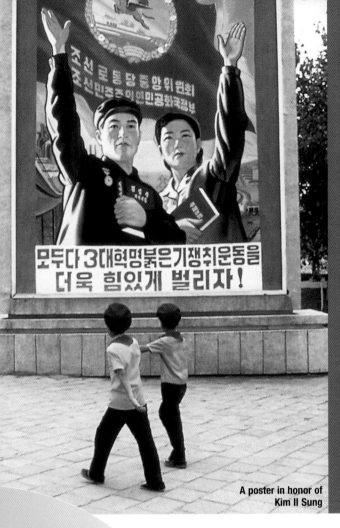

A poster in honor of
Kim Il Sung

To help you pray for North Korea

Remember that many people there have never heard of Jesus because the country has been closed to the outside world for more than 50 years.

You can thank God for:

● the many secret believers in North Korea.

You can ask God:

● that the Christians will know he is near them despite the threat of punishment or even death if they are betrayed.

● that Christian businessmen who visit North Korea, and those who take food into the country, will speak of Jesus' love.

● that Christians will help the children abandoned on the streets.

● to prepare the hearts of North Koreans for the day when the good news about Jesus can once more be shared openly.

● to work a miracle in the hearts of Kim Il Yong and his government so that they will know that he alone is God.

● for Christians around the world to pray faithfully until people can once more share the gospel in North Korea.

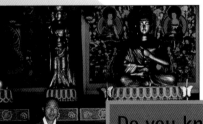

Buddhist monastery

Do you know?

Just north of the demilitarized zone which separates North and South Korea is a beautiful mountain region which can be visited by boat. Christians often go on the journey to pray for North Korea.

"Are there any books like this hidden in your house? Search for them, even in your parents' bedroom, then tell us." Some children did find that book and told their teachers. They never saw their parents again. The little black book was the Korean Bible.

Some brave people continued to follow Jesus and met in secret to worship him. They knew they couldn't worship another god. Two million people fled to South Korea, but Kim Il Sung attacked the South, too. Everyone was afraid. Korea was no longer like its name "Chosun," the "Land of Morning Calm."

The children were taught to worship Kim Il Sung. They sang, "He is our Great Leader and we keep his image in our hearts." You can read in the Bible (in Daniel chapter 3) about some other people who were expected to worship an image. They refused, and God protected them.

Death of the god-king

In 1994 Kim Il Sung died. The people wept because the one who had made himself their god was dead. His son, Kim Jong Il, the "Dear Leader," took his place.

But floods, hail and drought destroyed the crops. People starved. Aid agencies were allowed to bring food into the country, but the government arranged how it was distributed. It is thought that at least two million people died from starvation during the next five years or risked their lives escaping into China.

The one true God

Christians have tried all sorts of ways to tell the people of North Korea about God's love. They've beamed in radio broadcasts, although most radios in North Korea can receive only government broadcasts. They've even sent Christian literature to North Korea by balloon, and in plastic envelopes that they've thrown into the ocean.

In South Korea, many Christians are praying that the North Koreans will see that they've been worshipping a false god. God is answering their prayers. There are now three official churches and more than 500 registered "church-service houses" where people can meet for prayer, as well as many more underground churches.

129

Oman

Where Oil has Replaced Frankincense

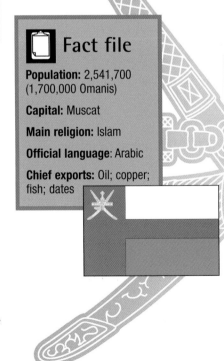

Frankincense tree in the desert

Guardian of the Straits

David had so many questions he wanted to ask Uncle Jack. His favorite uncle had worked in so many interesting places, and for the last year he'd been working in Oman. "Where's Oman? And what's it like living there?" he asked. "Let's have a look," Uncle Jack said as he pulled a map from his briefcase. "See, it's here on the eastern side of the Arabian Peninsula. Its coastline stretches along the Arabian Sea and the Gulf of Oman and it has land borders with Saudi Arabia, Yemen and the United Arab Emirates.

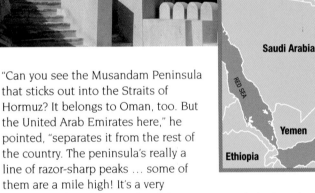

"Can you see the Musandam Peninsula that sticks out into the Straits of Hormuz? It belongs to Oman, too. But the United Arab Emirates here," he pointed, "separates it from the rest of the country. The peninsula's really a line of razor-sharp peaks … some of them are a mile high! It's a very important place, because from there Oman protects the 20,000 ships, many of them oil tankers, which pass through the Straits of Hormuz each year from the Persian Gulf."

Past and present

"What's the rest of Oman like?" David asked. "And what about the people who live there?"

"It's almost twice as big as the state of New York, but only about two and a quarter million people live in Oman – compared with almost 20 million in New York. The one and a half million local Omani people are all Arabic-speaking Muslims. But about a third of the people living in Oman are guest workers from other countries. A lot of them are from India, Pakistan or Bangladesh and work in low-paid jobs. Others, like myself, are experts in our professions who go there to train Omanis. I work with people in the oil industry.

"When I flew over Oman," Uncle Jack continued, "all I could see were bare, rocky mountains, oil wells in the sandy desert, and a few green oases. As we came in to land at Muscat I could see gardens and fields all along the coast, where most of the people live. I even caught a glimpse of the twin forts built into cliffs on either side of the bay. There are actually over 1,000 forts in the country.

"Oman is a rich country now because of oil, but a long time ago it was frankincense that made people in Oman wealthy."

Fact file

Population: 2,541,700 (1,700,000 Omanis)

Capital: Muscat

Main religion: Islam

Official language: Arabic

Chief exports: Oil; copper; fish; dates

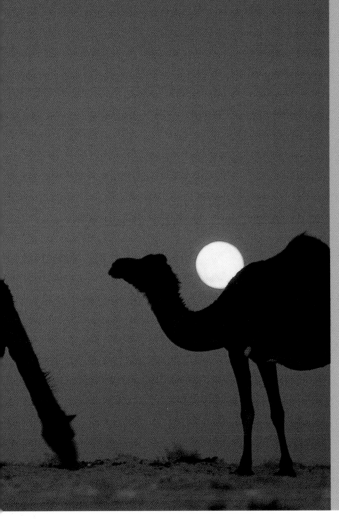

To help you pray for Oman

You can thank God for:

- the few Omani Christians.
- the Bibles in Arabic that have been given to some Omanis.

You can ask God:

- for Christians working in Oman to have opportunities to talk with their Omani friends about Jesus.
- to send Arab Christians to Oman who can clearly explain the good news about Jesus to the Omani people.
- that many Omanis will listen to Christian radio and television shows.
- to encourage Arab Christians to write books that will help children understand who Jesus is.
- for Christians in the west to show God's love and care to Omani students studying in their countries.

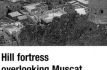

Hill fortress overlooking Muscat

Life is much more comfortable for Omanis now, but they still don't know the peace and love of Jesus

A new day

"If oil has made Oman rich," said David, "what was it like before?"

"By the 1950s, Oman had become the poorest country in Arabia," Uncle Jack said. "Even when oil was discovered in the 1960s the ruler, Sultan Sa'id, didn't use the money to modernize his country right away. He even told people they weren't allowed to ride bicycles or wear sunglasses. So many Omanis went to other countries to find work, and those left behind weren't very happy. In 1970, Sultan Qaboos took control from his father. He told the people: 'Oman in the past was in darkness ... but a new day will rise.'"

"What does that mean?" asked David.

"Well," said Uncle Jack, "there were only three schools in Oman in 1970,

and one hospital. Today, there are many modern hospitals, hundreds of schools and a university. The government has built good roads, new harbors and airports. There are new industries and many people now own expensive cars, mobile phones and televisions. The government wants Omanis to be trained so that they will become the experts in the industries in their own country. I suppose the new day means that Omanis have a better life and hope for the future."

Christian guest workers

"If Omanis are Muslims, does that mean there aren't any Christians there?" David asked.

Do you know?

There's an amazing network of underground and surface irrigation canals in Oman. They're called *falaj*, and some are over nine miles long and nearly 400 feet deep. They were built over 1,000 years ago! Some have been restored and are in use today.

"There are a few," Uncle Jack replied. "Missionaries built the first hospital, clinics and schools in Oman, and so the people really respect them. Most Christians in Oman are guest workers who want to tell Omanis about Jesus. They can meet together to worship God. But only about 40 Omanis have ever become Christians, and those who do follow Jesus know that their families, friends and the authorities will be angry and try to stop them. You can pray that an even greater 'new day' will come for the people of Oman, when they'll see the light of Jesus' love, forgiveness and new life."

"Tok Pisin"

Papua New Guinea (PNG for short) occupies half of the world's second largest island (there's a country called Irian Jaya on the other half). If you wanted to visit someone in another part of PNG, you would have to climb steep mountains, cross fast-flowing rivers and trek through tropical jungle! You wouldn't need a car, since there aren't many roads outside the towns. There are lots of small airstrips around the country, but even if you did have a plane it would still be hard to travel because many of the airstrips need to be repaired.

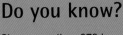

Do you know?

Since more than 870 languages are spoken in PNG, each language is spoken, on average, by about 6,000 people. That would be a bit like each town having its own language!

Speak "Tok Pisin"
(If you say the words out loud, you will see how much they sound like English.)
Good morning is "Moninnau" (**moh-nin-nau**)
Goodbye is "Lukim-yu" (**look-im-yoo**)
Please is "Plis" (pliss)
Thank you is "Tenku" (**tank**-yoo)

There are over 800 different groups of people in PNG – and each group speaks its own language! Even people living in valleys quite close to one another often don't speak the same language. It's a good thing everyone also speaks "Tok Pisin," a kind of pidgin, or simplified, English. Everyone can also read the Bible which has been translated into "Tok Pisin."

Sometimes in PNG everyone in a village becomes a Christian all at once! Although this seems wonderful, very often people don't really try to change to be more like Jesus. Instead, they carry on with their traditional witchcraft and fighting. But many who are truly following Jesus are working together to teach people what God says, so they will learn to live at peace with one another.

Fear of spirits

One day John, a missionary in PNG, had a haircut and some of his hair fell on the ground. "Don't leave your hair there," his friend Aiyako warned him. "A witch doctor could use it to put a curse on you."

Another day Aiyako and John were eating with people from a different tribe. "Don't leave any food on your plate," whispered Aiyako. "Someone might use it to attack us through the spirits."

A church in Papua New Guinea

📋 Fact file

Area: 178,703 sq. mi.

Population: 4,806,640

Capital: Port Moresby

Official languages: English; Tok Pisin

Main religions: Christianity; animism

Chief exports: Gold; coffee; timber; copper

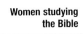

Women studying the Bible

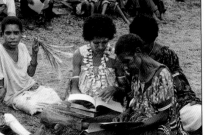

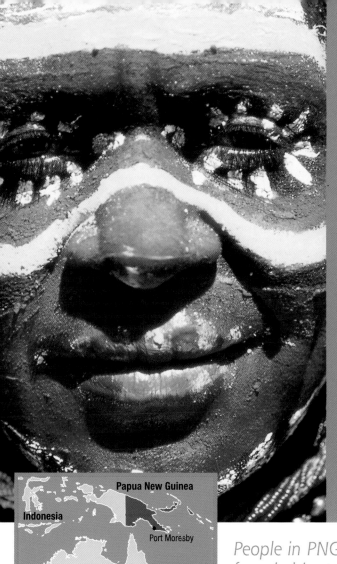

To help you pray for PNG

You can thank God for:

- the New Testament that has now been translated into "Tok Pisin" as well as into several other languages spoken in PNG.

- teachers who are helping people learn to read in their own languages so that they can read the New Testament.

- Christians from PNG who have gone to other countries to share God's love with other men and women, boys and girls.

You can ask God:

- to help Christian leaders in churches and in the government be a good example to those they serve.

- to help pastors to faithfully teach the Bible to their people so that they will learn to follow and obey Jesus and not be afraid of spirits.

- to give people understanding when they watch the *Jesus* film in their own language so they will know that the Bible is not a fairy tale but is about real people and God's son, Jesus.

- to encourage people to keep the airstrips in good repair so that books and other goods can arrive safely in the remote parts of the country.

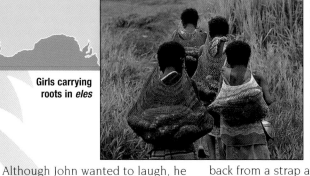

Girls carrying roots in *eles*

People in PNG carry everything in bags – from babies to Bibles!

Although John wanted to laugh, he knew Aiyako was really scared and he felt sorry for him. John explained that the Bible tells us that when we trust in God we don't need to be afraid of anything. God is bigger and stronger than anything that could hurt us. Thousands of people in PNG are full of the same sorts of fears.

Carrying babies in bags

Most people in PNG carry their belongings in net bags. One of the people groups, the Nabak, call this bag an *ele*. They hang these bags from the walls and use them as drawers or shelves. A Nabak boy carries everything in an *ele* slung over his shoulder, and his sister's *ele* hangs down her back from a strap around her head. Mothers even carry their babies in *eles* on their backs.

Nabak women sometimes make the bags from tree bark, but often they use strands from the yucca plant. First they pull the yucca plant through a slit in a big piece of bamboo to scrape off the outside part, which is green. Then they spread the strands that are left out in the sun to dry. When the strands are dry enough, the women make them into a coarse thread. They rub cold ashes from the fire on their thighs and roll the strands back and forth across their thighs until they form a thread. It takes a long time to make thread this way, so it's not surprising that it takes several weeks to make just one bag. When they have enough thread, the women start "crocheting" the bag with needles made from the bones of the wings of bats and flying foxes.

God's *ele*

People all around the world have prayed for PNG, and God has been changing the country. Pastors are teaching the people what God says in the Bible so they can learn to love and serve God in everything they do. Hundreds of Nabak people now have a special *ele* for carrying their Nabak New Testament. Christians from PNG are going all over the world to tell others about Jesus. God is using these people as his *ele* to carry the good news of Jesus around the world.

133

Pygmies

Children of the Forests of Central Africa

Hunting in the forest

"You'll be ready to come hunting with us soon," Mateke's father told him. Mateke tried to hide his excitement. He couldn't wait to go hunting with the men rather than taking care of his little brother and gathering fruit, nuts, leaves and grubs. He was so proud that every arrow he'd shot at the tree stump that morning had hit the target. He and his friend Matedu spent a lot of time shooting at big spiders, rats and frogs, and it had paid off.

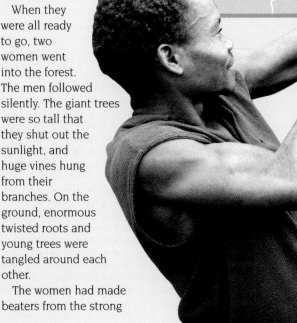

Mateke watched as the men got ready to go hunting. They dipped their sharpened arrows into poison from the bark of the *anga* tree. Then they dried the arrows over the fire.

When they were all ready to go, two women went into the forest. The men followed silently. The giant trees were so tall that they shut out the sunlight, and huge vines hung from their branches. On the ground, enormous twisted roots and young trees were tangled around each other.

The women had made beaters from the strong stems and leaves of the *mangunga* plant. They beat the ground, calling out to frighten the animals and make them run towards the hunters. What would the men catch today? Monkeys? Birds? Or maybe a deer? Mateke's mouth watered as he thought of the delicious stew his mother would make.

A decorated bow

New huts

Mateke looked around at his village. There were nine small huts. He had heard the men say that they would have to move again soon, because there weren't many animals left in that part of the forest.

Every time they move, the Pygmies collect their few belongings – their bows and arrows, knives and cooking pots – and travel into the forest. When they find a good place, the men clear the trees and the women build new huts by bending long, thin tree branches to make a small dome. Then they cover the dome with large *mangunga* leaves, leaving a small opening for a door. They don't need any furniture –just a mattress made of *mangunga* leaves.

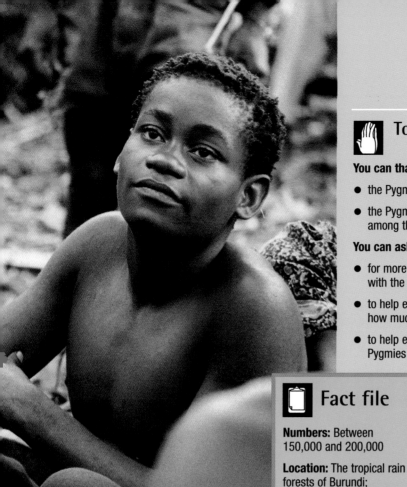

Fact file

Numbers: Between 150,000 and 200,000

Location: The tropical rain forests of Burundi; Cameroon; Central African Republic; Democratic Republic of Congo; Gabon; Peoples' Republic of Congo and Rwanda.

Occupation: Semi-nomadic hunter-gathers

Languages: Bantu or Sudanic dialects; the languages of the people they mix with.

God's book

"Do you think the preacher will find us again when we move?" Mateke asked Matedu. "I hope so," Matedu said. "I love listening to his stories about the God who made us. Do you remember how we all hid in the forest the first time he came? I can't believe we were afraid of him!"

"I remember that," Matedu said, "and he knew that we needed salt, so he

A Pygmy house

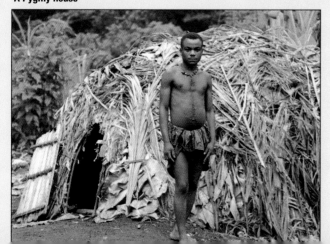

brought us some. He asked my father if he ever prayed to God."

"Yes," Mateke remembered. "And your father said that he did. He told the preacher that the forest is our God and our father and mother. It gives us all we need – houses, food and clothing – and when a big storm comes, it protects us."

"And then the preacher showed my father 'God's book' that says there's only one God," Mateke said. "I still remember how amazed I was when the preacher told us that God made our forest, the trees, the animals, and even us. He told us about how we've all broken God's laws. But God wants us to follow him, so he sent his Son called Jesus. I'm so glad that Jesus died for all of us, and that he forgives us if we ask him to. My father says his heart tells him it's true."

Mateke and Matedu are Pygmies. There are about ten different Pygmy groups living in the forests of central Africa. They're nomadic hunters and gather food from the forest. They also trade meat and honey with neighboring peoples for things they need like salt, clothing, tools and vegetables. Mateke's tribe lives in the great Ituri forest of northeast Congo. Although Pygmies live in the forests far away from anyone else, they're hearing the good news about Jesus and learning to follow him. Some Pygmies are going to school now, and a few are studying in Bible schools to become pastors and evangelists. It's not easy for them to leave their homes to go to school and live in buildings when they've lived in the forests all their lives. But they want to learn how to tell their people about God's love.

Qatar

The Thumb of the Arabian Gulf

Serving guests

Six-year-old Ahmed felt important. He was old enough now to help his father entertain his guests in the majlis, a room set apart for male visitors. Dressed in his thaub (ankle-length shirt) and embroidered cap, he carefully served coffee to his father's guests, speaking only when spoken to.

Ahmed was very interested in their conversation. His father had a special guest today – a foreigner from America who had just started working in his father's company.

Do you know?

Qatar has the third largest natural gas reserve in the world. Only Russia and Iran have bigger reserves.

"Thank you very much," said Jim, the man from America, when Ahmed handed him his coffee. Jim asked Ahmed how old he was and what he liked to do. Ahmed liked Jim. Because he was only a child, none of the other men ever spoke to him.

A wealthy country

Ahmed's country, Qatar, sticks out like a thumb into the Arabian Gulf. It's a small desert country, with a population of about 600,000. Ahmed was used to seeing foreigners, since only a quarter of the people living in his country are true Qataris – the rest are guest workers from other countries. But he had never talked to one before.

"Yes, we feel at home here. It's nice to have our own newspaper, radio and TV channel," Jim was saying. Ahmed knew that his father sometimes thought these foreigners felt too much at home in Qatar, especially when they wore jeans, tee shirts and shorts in public.

Soon the men were talking about oil again. "Did you know that most of the

people living in Doha, the capital, moved here after 1940, when oil was discovered?" his father asked Jim.

"Yes," added one of the other men, "life's very different here since they found all those reserves of natural gas offshore. Our country is so wealthy now that it provides free schooling and medical care, and even free housing for the poor."

"What did people do for work before oil was discovered?" Jim asked.

"Most Qataris tried to make a living from fishing, camel herding and pearl diving. Our main trade items used to be pearls and guano, a kind of manure

The few Qatari Christians all live outside Qatar

📋 Fact file

Area: 4,247 sq. mi.

Population: 599,065

Capital: Doha

Language: Arabic

Religion: Islam

Chief exports: Oil; gas; fertilizers

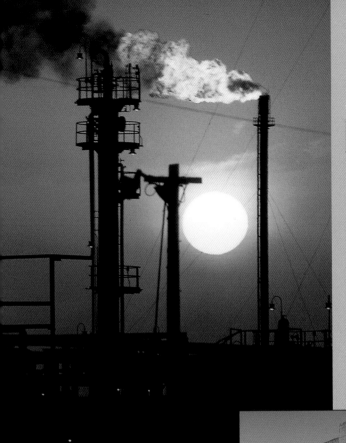

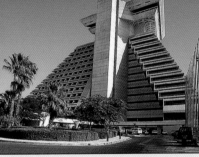

Modern buildings reveal Qatar's wealth

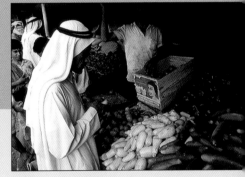

At the *souk* (market)

produced by sea birds that makes very good fertilizer," one of the men explained.

"Is there any farming in Qatar?" Jim wanted to know.

"Yes, but it's difficult," Ahmed's father told him. "There isn't much land, it's too hot and water is scarce. But now that sea water is being distilled to remove the salt, the farmers have more water. The government provides the farmers with free seeds and fertilizers to help them grow more and better crops. There are even some experimental farms that use greenhouses to keep plants cool, not warm!"

"How does the government work?" asked Jim.

"Well," said one of the men, "the ruling Sheikh chooses most of the leaders from his own family. He doesn't have to explain his actions to anyone, but he does have to keep Islamic law and listen to the Muslim religious leaders."

"Has life changed a lot for young people since the country became rich?"

Jim asked. There was a long silence. Ahmed's older brothers wanted their freedom and liked speeding around the desert in their cars and drinking illegally. His father had even beaten one of his brothers because he hadn't said the Muslim prayers. But Ahmed also knew his brothers were afraid of the future, of not passing their exams, and of punishment by Allah or their parents because of bad habits and not keeping Islamic laws. How could his father tell a stranger all this?

As a Christian, Jim really wanted to tell his host that riches don't bring peace, happiness or hope for the future. He remembered the story of the first known Qatari believer.

One day in 1985, some young evangelists in England met a man from Qatar and talked to him about Jesus. Afterwards, since they didn't know anything about Qatar, they looked it up

in the book *Operation World*. "Wow!" one of them said. "It says there are no known Qatari believers! Let's pray for that man – he could be the first."

He was, but the evangelists didn't realize how much suffering their new friend would go through when he gave up Islam and decided to follow Jesus. His wife divorced him, his children were taken away and he wasn't allowed to return to Qatar. Since then, a few other Qataris living outside the country have come to know Jesus. They've suffered for their faith, but they all agree it's worth sacrificing everything for the hope and freedom they have in Jesus.

Jim prayed that one day he would know his host well enough to tell him that only through trusting in Jesus would he know real freedom, peace and hope.

Quechua

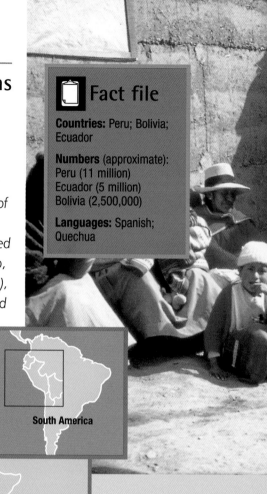

Children of the Incas

Fact file

Countries: Peru; Bolivia; Ecuador

Numbers (approximate):
Peru (11 million)
Ecuador (5 million)
Bolivia (2,500,000)

Languages: Spanish; Quechua

Living on a mountain

"Hey, Pedro, how much further do we have to climb to get to your house?" John panted. *"I'm out of breath!"*

"Not much further," Pedro grinned. *"Only about an hour!"* Pedro is a Quechua boy whose family lives in a village in the Andes Mountains of Peru. Wrapped in warm ponchos, the two boys continued climbing along the steep path. As they walked, Pedro pointed out small terraced fields of maize, wheat and potatoes as well as sheep, alpacas (which are bred for their fine soft fleece), llamas and a condor. *"You might be surprised when you see my house,"* Pedro told his new friend. *"It only has one room, with a dirt floor. We don't have electricity or running water, either. But you'll be very welcome, and my mother's a great cook!"*

South America

Ecuador

Peru

QUECHUA

Bolivia

SOUTH PACIFIC OCEAN

Chile

At last they reached Pedro's village. "Here it is," Pedro said, as he stopped at a small thatched hut built of stone. "Come on in." Soon they were eating maize and potatoes that Pedro's mother had cooked over a fire in the corner of the hut. "A lot of Quechua are poor," Pedro said, "but we have some sheep, a few llamas and a little land.

Because a lot of our people don't have any land, they go down to the cities. Even if they do find jobs, they don't earn much and usually have to live in the slums."

The Incas

There are about ten million Quechua people in Peru. They are descended from the Incas, who built huge terraces, great palaces and temples and an amazing network of roads and cities. The Incas were also famous for their beautiful gold jewelry and pottery. They believed that their king, or Inca, was the sun and that they themselves were the children of the sun and the moon. By the sixteenth century, the Inca Empire spread from Ecuador to Chile – over 2,000 miles. In 1532, when the Spaniards reached Peru looking for new lands and gold, they found two Inca leaders and their followers quarrelling over who should be the next king. Because the Incas were fighting among themselves, a small group of Spanish soldiers was able to defeat them quickly and take everything from them – their country and

"We have the Bible in our own language"

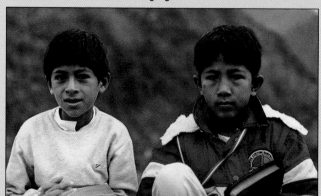

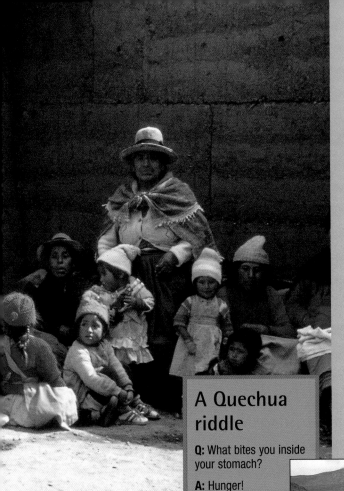

![hand icon] ## To help you pray for the Quechua

You can thank God for:

- Quechua men, women and children who are learning to know Jesus, the Good Shepherd.

- answering prayers to break the power of the Shining Path. Pray that they will never again be able to hurt people.

- Quechua Christians who, when they were wrongly accused and put in prison, shared Jesus' love with other prisoners.

- Romulo Saune's widow and her work sharing Jesus' love with the women she teaches.

You can ask God:

- that each Quechua Christian will always follow Jesus, no matter what happens.

- to provide training programs to show Quechua Christians how to teach young people about Jesus.

- that every person in the Quechua villages turning to Jesus will read the Bible and follow him faithfully.

A Quechua riddle

Q: What bites you inside your stomach?

A: Hunger!

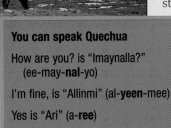

Llama, kept as a pack animal and for its wool

You can speak Quechua

How are you? is "Imaynalla?" (ee-may-**nal**-yo)

I'm fine, is "Allinmi" (al-**yeen**-mee)

Yes is "Ari" (a-**ree**)

No is "Mana" (**ma**-na)

their rich gold and silver mines. The Spanish brought their Catholic faith to Peru. Today, nearly 500 years later, most of the Quechua people belong to the Roman Catholic Church. But when they need help, they usually turn to priests who still follow their old Inca religion.

Prayer for a troubled country

There have been a lot of problems in Peru since it became independent in 1821. In the 1980s and early 1990s, a Communist guerrilla group called the Shining Path terrorized and killed more than 20,000 people in the mountains. Christians started a movement in 1989 to pray for peace in Peru, and God has been answering the prayers of people around the world.

A good shepherd

When he was a little boy, Romulo Saune looked after his family's sheep. When he came to know and follow Jesus, his favorite verses in the Bible were about Jesus, the Good Shepherd, who gave his life for his sheep (us). (You can read this story in your Bible in the Gospel of John, chapter 10.) Romulo became a well-known Christian leader and spent his life helping his Quechua people. He loved to tell them about Jesus, the Good Shepherd. He knew how important it was for his people to have the Bible in their own language, and so he translated it into one of the Quechua dialects.

The Shining Path guerrillas hated Romulo. Even though he knew it was

dangerous, Romulo often visited Christians in remote mountain villages because he loved them and wanted them to learn more about Jesus. One day in September 1992, as he was returning home, Shining Path guerrillas killed Romulo and four others who were with him. He was another good shepherd who had given his life for his sheep, the Quechua.

Is that the end of the story? No, because God has been answering the prayers of Christians in Peru and around the world. Romulo Saune's widow teaches women so they can read the Bible for themselves. And high up in the Andes Mountains, whole Quechua villages like Pedro's are coming to know Jesus, their Good Shepherd, and are learning to follow him.

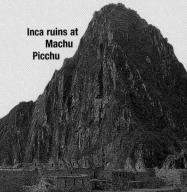

Inca ruins at Machu Picchu

Refugees

Looking for Help and Safety

Homeless ... Sierra Leone

"Run, run as fast as you can!" screamed 12-year-old Finda. "We have to get away from here!" She ran with her baby brother in her arms as her frightened little brothers and sister ran after her. They came home from playing to find that Sierra Leonean rebels had murdered their mother, and their father had disappeared. For seven days Finda led the little ones through the forest to a refugee camp in the neighboring country of Guinea.

But Guinea is a poor country and can't really help refugees like Finda. There's no water in the camp, so Finda has to walk three miles to get water three times every day. She also has to look for firewood in the forest. Sometimes she's able to earn a little money to buy food for the family. Her brothers and sister go to school in the camp, but she's too busy looking after them to go herself.

Refugees from Sierra Leone at a camp in Guinea

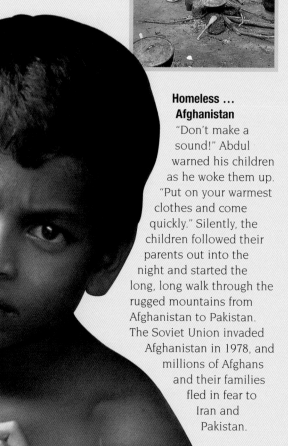

Refugee child in Sri Lanka

Homeless ... Afghanistan

"Don't make a sound!" Abdul warned his children as he woke them up. "Put on your warmest clothes and come quickly." Silently, the children followed their parents out into the night and started the long, long walk through the rugged mountains from Afghanistan to Pakistan. The Soviet Union invaded Afghanistan in 1978, and millions of Afghans and their families fled in fear to Iran and Pakistan.

Abdul and his family and many others made their homes in tents in refugee camps. Even though that war is over, a lot of refugees are afraid to go home because there's still fighting in Afghanistan.

Homeless ... Sri Lanka

Sri Lanka is a beautiful place. But a terrible civil war is being waged there. "I was only five years old when the Tamil Tiger guerrillas demanded a separate state for Tamils in the north of Sri Lanka," Mohan said sadly. "That happened in 1986. We lived in Jaffna, and there was a lot of fighting there. My family fled by boat to India, but we decided to return home as soon as it seemed more peaceful. When we arrived back, the fighting was worse than ever. We fled again, away

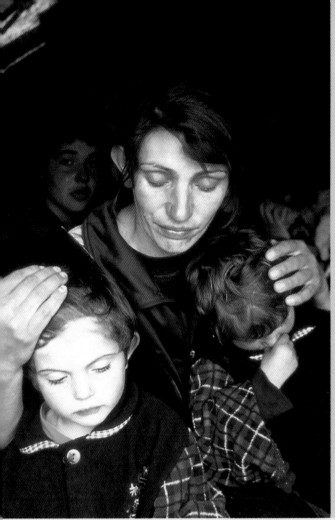

To help you pray for refugees

You can thank God for:

- organizations like the United Nations High Commission for Refugees (UNHCR) who do so much to help refugees.
- churches helping refugees to settle in new countries where things seem strange at first.

You can ask God:

- that many Christians will show God's love to the millions of sad and hurting refugees.
- for caring people to look after refugee babies and children.
- for people to comfort refugee children who feel lonely and frightened because they are lost or their parents have died.
- that governments will help make refugees feel welcome.
- to bring peace to troubled countries so that many refugees can return to their own homes.

Refugees from Kosovo in Albania

from the fighting. I lost my parents and I've wandered around the country ever since, trying to keep out of the way of the fighting. More than anything, I just want my family and to feel safe."

40 million refugees
As you sit in your own comfortable home, can you imagine what it would be like to be a refugee, having to flee from your home and country, hoping to find a place where you could feel safe?

There are about 40 million refugees in the world, and at least half of them are children. That's a big number – more than twice the population of Australia! Refugees are frightened to stay in their own country because of racial hatred, religious

persecution or war. They leave everything behind and try to find a new life somewhere else.

Some have had to leave their homes and villages and find a place to live in another part of their own country. People all over the world have lost their homes because of floods in Bangladesh, volcanoes in Turkey, drought in the Sahel of Africa and hatred and violence in Colombia. These refugees look for another place where they will be safe and have food, care and hope for the future.

Jesus, a refugee
There have always been refugees. History is full of them. In the book of Exodus in the Bible we can read the story of the Israelites' escape from slavery in Egypt. Joseph and Mary,

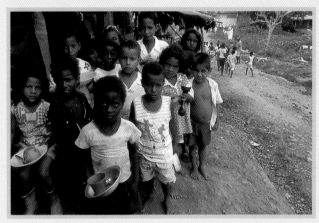

Feeding program in Colombia

with baby Jesus, were refugees when they fled to Egypt from cruel King Herod.

The Bible says that we should care for the poor, the suffering and the refugees. In Matthew 25:34–40, Jesus tells us that those who feed the hungry, give water to the thirsty, provide clothes for those who have none,

look after the sick and visit those in prison do all these things for him. You can pray for refugees all around the world. You might also think of some practical ways to follow Jesus' command to help refugees.

Republic of Guinea

Where Missionaries were Banned

Rich, but poor

Guinea, in West Africa, is one of the poorest countries in the world. Crops like rice, coffee, bananas and oranges grow easily there. Iron, gold and diamonds are found there. Guinea is also the world's second largest producer of a mineral called bauxite, which is used in making aluminum. Guinea used to be one of France's richest colonies. But when it became independent in 1958, the president wanted Guinea to become a Communist country. Guinea is still trying to recover from the consequences of Communism and the president's harsh and foolish decisions.

Fact file

Area: 95,000 sq. mi. (a little smaller than the state of Nevada)

Population: 7,430,346

Capital: Conakry

Official language: French, but there are 8 national languages and another 20 spoken in the country.

Religions: Islam; animism

Chief exports: Bauxite; fruit; coffee; diamonds

More than three-quarters of the people living in Guinea are Muslims. Although missionaries worked there when it was a French colony, very few people became Christians. In 1967, the president forced almost all the missionaries to leave. The missionaries prayed for the millions of people in Guinea who had never heard about the God who loves them. God answered their prayers. In 1984, when the president died, missionaries were allowed to return to Guinea. Even before that, though, God was at work. The people had become so poor that a lot of them went to work in other African countries so they could buy food and clothes for their families. Sometimes these people heard about Jesus.

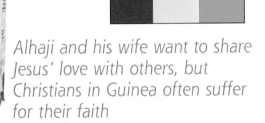

Alhaji and his wife want to share Jesus' love with others, but Christians in Guinea often suffer for their faith

Looking for God

Alhaji was a Muslim. He wanted to know more about God, so he prayed, fasted and studied the Koran. He was a tailor, and when he went to live in Gambia he quickly found work sewing

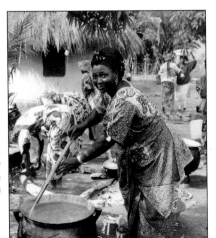

Preparing the celebration feast for the opening of the church

for some missionaries. They gave him a book to read, but he couldn't understand it because it was in English (Guinea is French-speaking, Gambia is English-speaking).

Alhaji learned to read English just so he could know what the book said! The book told him about Jesus, the Son of God. The missionaries also gave him a Bible, which he started to read as well as the Koran. He prayed that God would show him the right way. One day he read John 3:16: "God loved the world so much that he gave his only Son, so that whoever believes in him will have everlasting life." When he read that, he realized that the Bible is the true word of God, and he decided to follow Jesus.

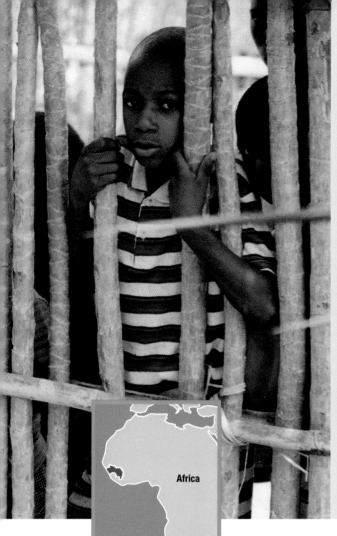

 To help you pray for Guinea

You can thank God for:

- Christians like Alhaji.
- Christian youth centers and training projects.

You can ask God:

- that Christians in Guinea will always show others how Jesus loves and cares for them.
- for more missionaries to share the good news about Jesus.
- that lots of children will follow Jesus, even when others make fun of them.
- that many forest people will realize that worshipping spirits and the devil brings fear, but following Jesus brings peace and joy.
- to show Muslims that Jesus is God.

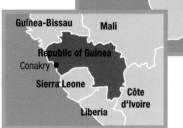

Africa

Guinea-Bissau Mali

Republic of Guinea
Conakry •

Sierra Leone
                        Côte
                        d'Ivoire
        Liberia

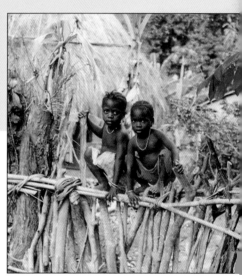

God works miracles

When Alhaji told his wife, she was angry. She left him and went back to Guinea. He was very sad, but he didn't stop studying the Bible or following Jesus or praying for his wife. Then God worked a miracle. Alhaji's wife decided to follow Jesus, too, and went back to live with him. They decided to return to Guinea to tell their people about the God of the Bible who loves them all.

When they reached their village, Alhaji told them about God's love and everyone welcomed them at first. They built a house, set up a little tailor's shop, and Alhaji started to teach six young men to make clothes. They studied the Bible with him and

wanted to trust in Jesus, but they all turned back to Islam. Alhaji didn't give up. He knew that God would help him explain the truth about Jesus.

After a while, 15 people had decided to follow Jesus. But each one of them had to leave his own home because of that decision. Alhaji looked after all of them and taught them how to make a living as tailors. He also taught them all about the Bible. Some of the people in the village were very angry, especially when the Christians decided to build a church. They persecuted them and tried to stop them, but God is in control of everything and, in March 2000, the church opened.

The Sacred Forest

The people of the forest region of Guinea are animists. Some belong to the Sacred Forest cult and say they have been "born again" through the devil's mouth. When the leader of the cult comes into the village, everyone is supposed to hide indoors. When the son of one village chief became a

Christian, he refused to hide. This made his father, who was afraid of what would happen, very angry. "I belong to Jesus," the son said, "And he has set me free from the devil's power. He'll keep me safe." The chief was amazed when nothing happened to his son. "It must be true that this Jesus really is more powerful than all the spirits we fear!" he exclaimed.

New life in Jesus

Like Alhaji and the son of the village chief, others in Guinea have decided to follow Jesus. They want everyone to know the good news that Jesus is the Son of God who loves them and sets them free from fear.

Riffi Berbers

Berbers of the Rif Mountain Range

A sacrifice and a feast

Jamina, a ten-year-old Riffi (Reef-ee) Berber girl from north Morocco, was busy helping her mother prepare for the feast of Eid el-Kabir. This is a special day when Muslims sacrifice a sheep and then eat it to celebrate Abraham's willingness to sacrifice his son Ishmael, and God's provision of a sheep to sacrifice instead. Are you thinking that the son was Isaac, not Ishmael? You're right! (You can read the Bible story in Genesis 22.) Muslims believe that it was Ishmael, from whom all Arab people are descended, that Abraham took to Mount Moriah.

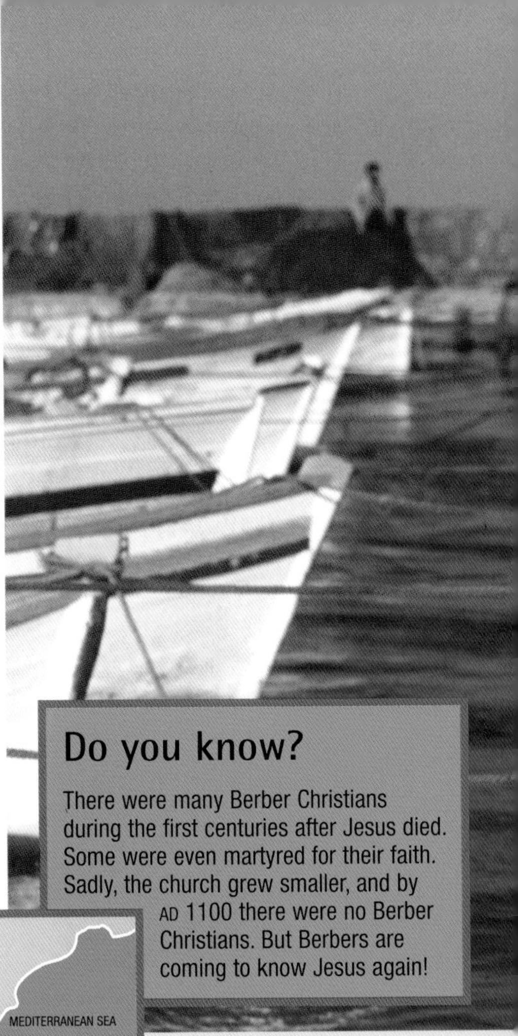

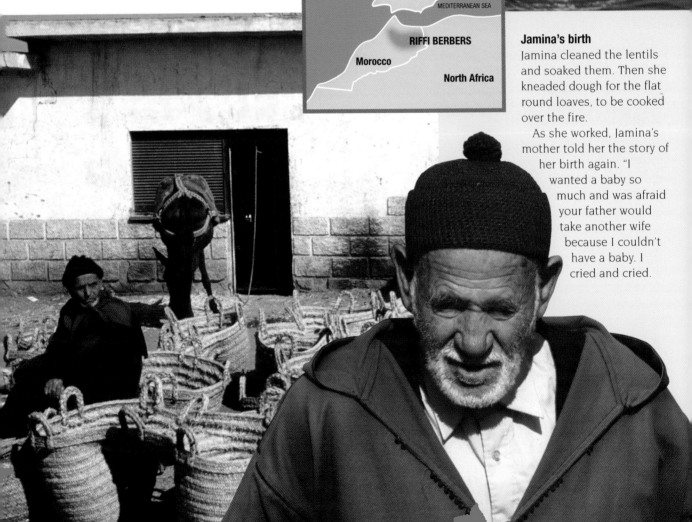

Do you know?

There were many Berber Christians during the first centuries after Jesus died. Some were even martyred for their faith. Sadly, the church grew smaller, and by AD 1100 there were no Berber Christians. But Berbers are coming to know Jesus again!

Map labels: ATLANTIC OCEAN · Spain · MEDITERRANEAN SEA · RIFFI BERBERS · Morocco · North Africa

Jamina's birth

Jamina cleaned the lentils and soaked them. Then she kneaded dough for the flat round loaves, to be cooked over the fire.

As she worked, Jamina's mother told her the story of her birth again. "I wanted a baby so much and was afraid your father would take another wife because I couldn't have a baby. I cried and cried.

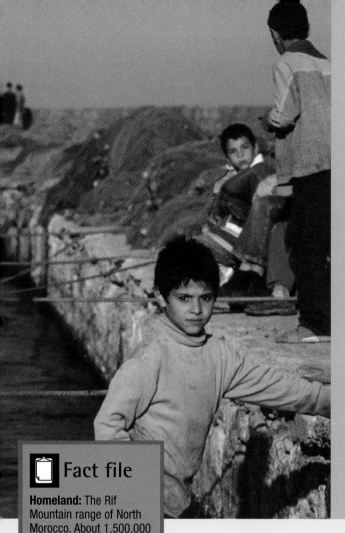

To help you pray for the Riffi

You can thank God for:

- Christian radio broadcasts in Arabic and Riffi and the Bible correspondence courses.

- Christian films that have been dubbed in Riffi, and for cassettes in Riffi of stories from the Old Testament.

You can ask God:

- to help the people producing the Christian radio broadcasts and dramatized stories to make them really interesting.

- that those who listen to the broadcasts will find them easy to understand.

- that the teachers for the Bible correspondence courses will know how to answer the questions the students ask about Jesus.

- to help Christian parents encourage their children to learn Bible passages just as Muslim children learn passages from the Koran.

- to fill each Riffi Christian with such love and joy that their friends will want to know Jesus as well.

Fact file

Homeland: The Rif Mountain range of North Morocco. About 1,500,000 Riffi live there.

Occupation: Mainly farming

Other countries where they live: France, Netherlands, Belgium, Spain, Germany and England, where they have gone to look for work.

Then my mother took me to a saint's tomb where I was told to jump three times through the window. Not long after that, I had a beautiful baby!" Jamina's mother is very superstitious, like a lot of Riffi Muslims. Few of them have heard that God promises to help us. You can read about how God does this in the story of Hannah in the Old Testament, in 1 Samuel 1.

No school today!
Mohammed, Jamina's little brother, was glad it was Eid el-Kabir so he didn't have to go to school and study Arabic. Some boys made fun of him for making mistakes when reciting from the Koran. Like most Riffi girls, Jamina had only been to school for three years. Her mother needed her at home to fetch water and wood, look after her baby sister (whom she carried on her back), clean and work in the fields.

Jamina's father had prepared the sheep for the sacrifice. Her brother and sister blew up the sheep's lungs like a balloon and were laughing and shouting. Jamina was looking forward to eating meat. Usually they ate just bread and olive oil, and sometimes lentils or sardines.

Jamina's father worked in Spain, but he had come home for the feast. He loved his family and always made sure they had enough money. He had lots of interesting stories to tell. This time he had seen a film about Jesus. "Muslims believe Jesus was a prophet," he said, "but the film showed us how good he was and it said he was the Son of God. But I'm not sure why he died. I'd like to know more about him."

Arab rulers
The original people in North Africa were called Berbers. There are three main groups of Berber people in Morocco, including the Riffi Berbers, whose home is in the Rif Mountain range.

Almost all Berbers are Muslims. There are more than two million Riffi Berbers, but only about 40 are Christians.

Moroccan market

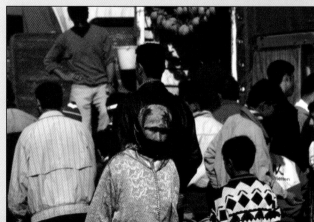

Romania

Free at Last

A ride on the train

Imagine you're taking a train ride through Romania. You see flat land and farms, thick forest, high mountains (with wolves and bears!), deep gorges and the River Danube, the longest and most important river in Romania. You could wear a tee shirt in the summer, but you'd want lots of warm clothes in the winter.

A Romanian grandfather sits next to you on the train, telling stories about how this beautiful country used to be a wonderful place to live. Romania used to be famous for its fine flour and wines.

Romanian Orthodox church

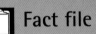

Fact file

Area: 91,700 sq. mi.

Population: 22,326,500

Capital: Bucharest

Language: Romanian

Religion: Orthodox Christian

Chief exports: Petroleum products; heavy machinery

"But it's not like that anymore," he says, "not since Ceausescu."

"Who's Ceausescu?" you ask. And he tells you a sad story …

"For 24 years," he begins, "a Communist dictator called Nicolae Ceausescu ruled Romania. He and his family lived in luxury, but the rest of us were often hungry, cold and very afraid. People in villages were forced to leave their homes, and their land was made into big farms owned by the government. Unwanted children, orphans and the sick and elderly were neglected. Ceausescu sold the fuel and food we needed desperately to other countries to pay his debts.

"But God was still with us," the man continues. "A brave Christian pastor called Laszlo Tokes spoke out when villages were destroyed and Christians were persecuted. He and his wife were arrested and beaten by the secret police, and the windows of their church and home were smashed. Thousands of church members and their friends gathered to protest. The protest quickly spread and turned into a revolution.

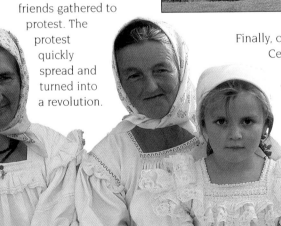

Finally, on Christmas night, 1989, Ceausescu was overthrown."

"Did life get better for everyone then?" you ask hopefully.

"I'm afraid not," the old man says sadly. "Even today, many people are still very poor, without proper food or shelter. Thousands of children your age still live on the streets. But God is helping

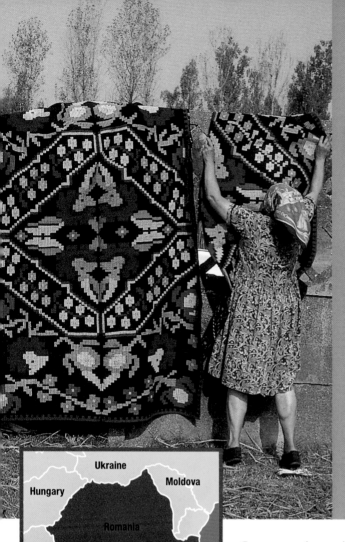

To help you pray for Romania

You can thank God for:

- the Christians from Romania and other countries who are showing Jesus' love and care to the thousands of destitute orphans and street children and to the homeless, sick and elderly.

- all of the Romanians who are learning to follow Jesus.

You can ask God:

- to give the government leaders wisdom as they rule the country, so that everyone in need will receive help.

- to help Christians in Romania learn to forgive, love and trust one another after the many years of persecution.

- to show people from other countries working with churches in Romania the best ways to help them grow and glorify God.

- to give wisdom to church leaders in Romania as they teach the Bible and reach out to those who have no hope.

- to provide for each Romanian who is studying at Bible school to become a pastor.

Can you imagine not having a Bible – and giving up your most prized possessions to get one?

You can speak Romanian

Hello is "Salut" (sah-**loot**)

Goodbye is "La revedere" (lah reh-veh-**dair**-ay)

Please is "Va rog" (vah-**rog**)

Thank you is "Multumesc" (mool-tsoo-**mesk**)

us to rebuild our lives. After Ceausescu was gone, people all around the world found out about the conditions here during those 24 years. Many churches and other groups brought in truckloads of food, clothes and other supplies. Nurses and care workers came to love and look after the many children in the orphanages.

"I will tell you one more story," he says, "to help you remember that even when everything seems very dark, God brings light to people."

"Ceausescu didn't like Christians. He picked on them, put them in prison and even killed them for believing in God. But the church still grew because people found strength through trusting in God. One day, an

American Christian visiting Romania was sitting in his car waiting for a friend. A woman holding a brown paper bag asked him for something and showed him the bag, but he didn't understand. Finally, his Romanian friend arrived. 'She's asking for a Bible,' he said, with tears in his eyes. 'In the bag are her best clothes. She wants to exchange them for a Bible. That's all she has to give.'"

Construction in Bucharest

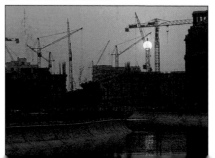

The Romanian grandfather turns to you. "How many Bibles do you have in your house?" he asks.

You can't remember and look away, ashamed at what you take for granted.

"Ah," he smiles, "Then you probably can't even imagine this woman's joy when she received that Bible. And, of course, she was able to keep her best clothes too.

"Just after the revolution, there was a cartoon version of the Bible shown on TV called 'Superbook.' A million people in Romania saw this and wrote asking for books and Bibles. Since the revolution, at least a thousand churches have been started. Christian schools, colleges, Bible schools, bookstores and radio stations have also been set up. More and more Romanians are coming to know Jesus every day."

"What can I do to help?" you ask.

"Please pray for us," he said.

147

Russia

A Thousand Years of Christianity

Christ is risen!

"Christ is risen!" The priest called out in the crowded church. "He is risen indeed!" the people replied. Olga was glad to be in church with her grandmother on Easter Sunday. She couldn't help smiling when she saw the joy on her grandmother's wrinkled face. Olga admired her grandmother's strong faith in Jesus, even when life was difficult and she had so little money for food and rent.

As they left the church, with its golden, onion-shaped domes, Olga said, "I can't imagine what it must have been like when churches were closed. Was it really against the law for children to learn Bible stories?"

They sat together on a park bench, and Olga's grandmother told her the story.

Do you know?

Russia is the largest country in the world. It takes seven days to travel by the Trans-Siberian Railway from Vladivostok in the east to Moscow in the west. It's a distance of 5,600 miles, which makes it the longest train journey in the world.

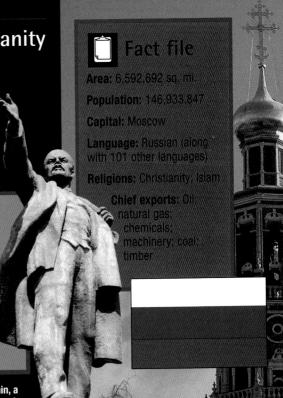

Statue of Lenin, a
Communist leader of
Russia

Choosing a religion

"Yes, it's hard to believe now, isn't it?" Olga's grandmother said. "I suppose it all started more than a thousand years ago, when a prince called Vladimir lived in this country. He wanted our country to follow a great religion and decided to find out all he could about Judaism, Islam and Christianity. There's a legend that says that, in AD 988, Prince Vladimir saw a light shining over the city of Kiev. He thought this bright light came from Jesus Christ, and he decided to follow him. So Russia became a Christian country. Poor peasants, rich nobles, and even the tsar (king) himself, worshipped God in the same way. The way we worship God in the Orthodox Church has never changed.

"Although some Russians were rich, most were very poor. At the beginning of the twentieth century, workers felt they weren't being treated fairly. Finally, in a revolution in 1917, a group called the Bolsheviks drove the ruler, Tsar Nicholas II, and his family from power. They took control of the government and all the farms and factories. They turned Russia into a Communist country. Life became harder than ever before."

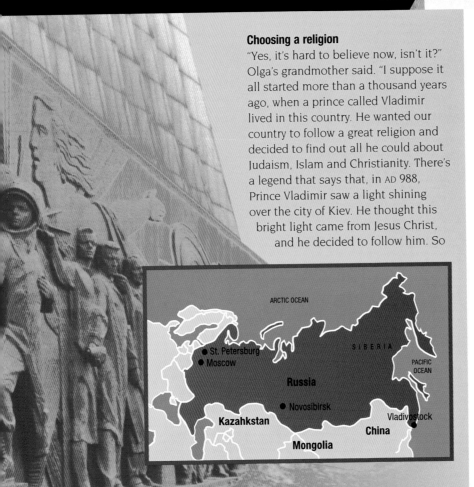

For 70 years Russians were taught atheism, but now people are hearing about Jesus

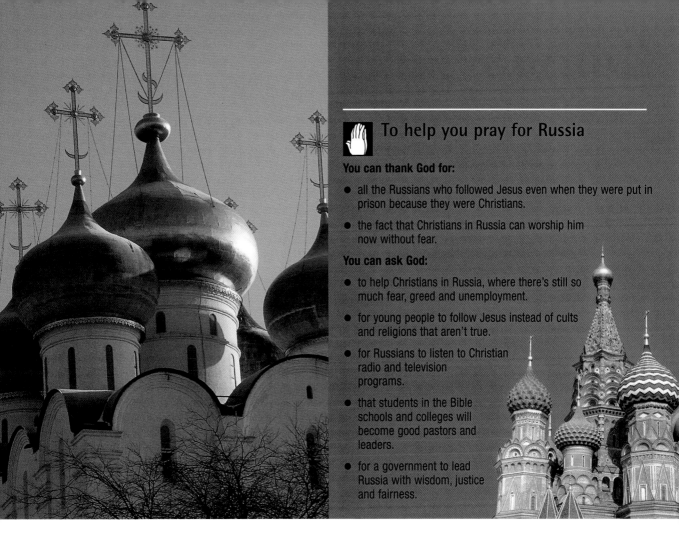

To help you pray for Russia

You can thank God for:

- all the Russians who followed Jesus even when they were put in prison because they were Christians.

- the fact that Christians in Russia can worship him now without fear.

You can ask God:

- to help Christians in Russia, where there's still so much fear, greed and unemployment.

- for young people to follow Jesus instead of cults and religions that aren't true.

- for Russians to listen to Christian radio and television programs.

- that students in the Bible schools and colleges will become good pastors and leaders.

- for a government to lead Russia with wisdom, justice and fairness.

Religion banned

"What happened to the churches?" asked Olga.

"Religion was banned," her grandmother replied. "Very few people had Bibles and most churches were closed down. Our beautiful church was turned into a cowshed. I was very sad – until I remembered that Jesus was born in a stable.

"There were a lot of us who didn't want to stop worshipping God. But the secret police closely watched the few churches that the government allowed to stay open. Many Baptists and other groups formed 'underground' churches that met in secret, often outdoors. The secret police often found them and took away their pastors. Some of them were tortured, put in prison or sent far away to Siberia, in the east of Russia. Although the Communists made life very hard for Christians and punished many of them, they just couldn't get rid of Christianity."

"I'm glad it's different now," Olga said as she looked up at her grandmother and smiled. "We can go to church and have our own Bibles, and I learn about Jesus at school and at Sunday school. What happened to make it all change?"

New freedom

"In 1985, Mikhail Gorbachev was elected as General Secretary of the Communist Party. He knew many things were wrong in our country and started to make changes," Olga's grandmother answered. "He lifted the ban on religion and started to give us back some of the church buildings.

"In 1988, Christian leaders from around the world came to Russia to celebrate a thousand years of Christianity here! Since then, we've been free to worship God again."

"Some of my friends go to Baptist churches," Olga told her grandmother. "They said that sometimes Christians from other countries visited their churches when the government tried to get rid of religion in our country. They said that people all around the world were praying for us. God must have heard their prayers."

"That's right," her grandmother said. "Since 1991, a lot of Christians have come to help the churches. Even though we can buy Bibles now, a lot of people still don't know what it says. They were taught atheism for 70 years, and now followers of all sorts of cults and religions have come into our country and are trying to get people to follow them. We still need prayer, and we need people who can teach us to follow Jesus."

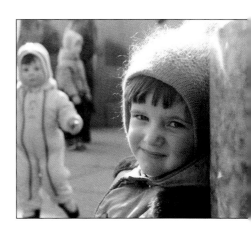

Samoa

A Land Founded on God

Daily prayers

At the end of Ben and Mary's first day on Samoa, they heard church bells ringing. It sounded like they were ringing all over the island. "We have to be very quiet now," their hostess Tili whispered. "It's the time for prayer. Every day, when the church bells ring at dusk, everyone in Samoa stops what they're doing to pray and read the Bible. Let's go back to my house – we can be quiet there." Samoan houses are called fales, and they're all open to the sea breezes. Samoans only lower the canvas sides of their houses in very bad weather.

Fact file

Area: 1,093 sq. mi. made up of the two large islands of Savai'i and Upolu and seven very small islands

Population: 180,070

Capital: Apia

Official Languages: Samoan; English

Major Religions: Christianity (Congregationalism, Roman Catholicism, Methodism)

Savai'i

Apia Upolu

Samoa

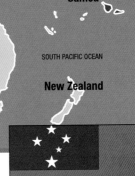

Australia

Samoa

SOUTH PACIFIC OCEAN

New Zealand

An island nation

Samoa, which was called Western Samoa until 1997, is one of the island nations in the South Pacific Ocean. Most Samoans live on the two main islands, Savai'i and Upolu. There are also seven much smaller islands. These mountainous islands were formed thousands of years ago when volcanoes in the South Pacific erupted. Mangoes, coconuts, pineapples and breadfruit (which grow on a tree but taste like potatoes) grow all over the fertile valleys. Coral reefs surround the islands, and there are lots of fish, shellfish and turtles.

A missionary king

"Are all the people in Samoa Christians?" Mary asked Tili later. "Is that why everyone has to stop to pray and read the Bible every day?"

"It's been almost 200 years since people in Samoa first heard about Jesus," she told them. "One of our chiefs became a Christian when he was visiting Tonga, another island nation in the South Pacific. When he came back to Samoa, he wanted everyone to know about Jesus. Lots of Samoans decided to follow Jesus. The King of Tonga even sent people to teach the people here how to follow Jesus. Missionaries came from other countries, too, and soon there were thousands of Christians all over the islands. And there were

Almost all Samoans go to church, but not all of them really understand how to follow Jesus

churches in every town and village. We wanted more and more people to know Jesus, so Samoan missionaries sailed to other Pacific islands to tell them about God's love."

"That's amazing! Are the Samoans still excited about following Jesus?" Ben asked.

"Most Samoans would say they're Christians," Tili replied, "but not all of

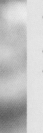

To help you pray for Samoa

You can thank God for:

- the Samoans who have told other people in the South Pacific about Jesus.
- the time Samoans have every day to pray and read the Bible.

You can ask God:

- to help the churches in Samoa teach families how they can all follow Jesus.
- that people will listen to the daily Christian radio broadcasts.
- that Samoans will realize that following Jesus is more important than going to church just because everyone else is going.
- to help young people find true happiness in knowing Jesus.
- to help Samoan Christians from the different churches work together.

Climbing a palm tree

them really follow Jesus. Some still want to practice old Samoan customs and ceremonies that honor evil spirits as well. And for some people, being a Christian is just part of our culture. Nearly everyone goes to church on Sundays and to two services during the week as well as to the early morning prayer meeting. We're still sending missionaries to other places, but here in Samoa Christians from all the different kinds of churches need to learn to work together."

Founded on God

"We heard that thousands of Christians from all the different churches in Samoa took part in a March for Jesus," Mary said.

"Yes," said Tili. "It was a very special event. Even members of the government marched. Their motto is, 'The whole government is founded on God.' But I wish all of our people were really 'founded on God.' We were very glad that people from all the different church groups took part in the march. That doesn't always happen."

"What about young people?" Ben asked. "I've heard that a lot of them leave Samoa. You must be sad to see them go."

"Most Samoans don't have a lot of money, but we're happy people and proud to be independent," Tili said. "But a lot of young people are leaving the country because they think they'll find a more exciting life and earn more money in countries like Australia and New Zealand. Some also go to American Samoa, which is just 60 miles to the

In a *fale*

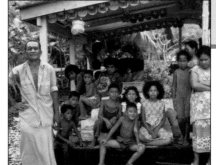

Do you know?

Samoans hold lots of feasts. They wrap the food in leaves and cook it among hot stones, then announce what each delicious dish is before they place it before the guests. Guests wear turtle shell combs, coral necklaces, coconut shell brooches and *lapa lapas*, skirts worn by both men and women. And, despite the heat, men wear shirts, ties and jackets in church but have bare feet and wear *lapa lapas* instead of trousers.

east. The people there are much richer than we are. But although they have their own government, they're not independent like we are because they're ruled by the United States.

"Sometimes," Tili continued, "there doesn't seem to be the love, joy and peace we might expect in a country where nearly everyone says they're a Christian."

151

San

Bushmen of the Kalahari Desert

Rescue in the desert

A hundred years ago, a missionary named Frederick Arnot was traveling through the Kalahari Desert in Botswana to reach the Zambezi River. He and his African helpers were almost fainting from thirst, but they struggled towards a water hole and knelt by its side. They could almost taste the water … but it was completely dry. They lost all hope and some of them collapsed, unconscious, on the sand. Without water they could not go on. They knew they might die.

A group of San Bushmen had seen them from a distance. They ran over and began to dig furiously, scooping up handfuls of sand. Their leader took several lengths of reed and slid them into the hole. Carefully he pushed the reeds, skillfully jointed together, into the ground. After sucking and blowing for some time, he smiled – water!

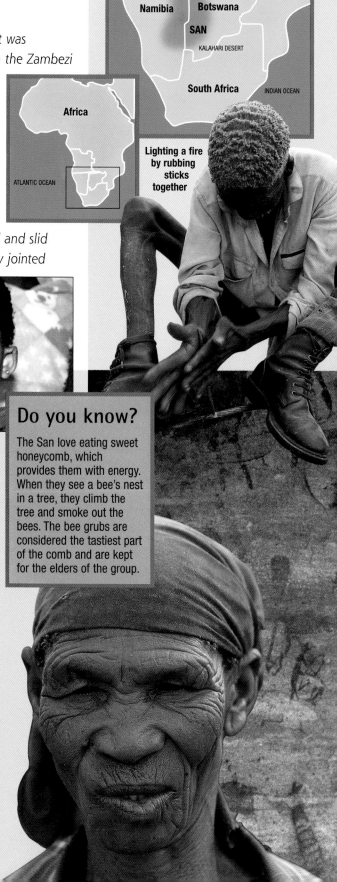

Lighting a fire by rubbing sticks together

He began to suck steadily on the reed, and as the water rose slowly up the stem he spat it into a tortoise shell. Ten minutes later the shell was full. He gently poured this precious water over Arnot's tongue and down his throat until Arnot was able to swallow. For six hours, the sweating Bushmen worked without stopping to get water for the whole group. Then, without waiting for thanks, the Bushmen left as silently as they had come.

In those days, the people who lived around them wanted the Bushmen's land for themselves and hunted them like wild animals. Having received nothing but cruelty from others, the Bushmen still saved the lives of strangers. As a result of their kindness, and because he saw how God had looked after them, Tinka, Arnot's chief guide, became a Christian. Most Bushmen live in fear of the spirit world. But their painful history and their kind ways would help them to understand the forgiveness and love of Jesus, who sacrificed himself to save others who didn't always treat him as they should.

Do you know?

The San love eating sweet honeycomb, which provides them with energy. When they see a bee's nest in a tree, they climb the tree and smoke out the bees. The bee grubs are considered the tastiest part of the comb and are kept for the elders of the group.

Poisoned arrows

It scarcely ever rains in the Kalahari Desert, and not much besides thorn bushes and coarse grass grows there. Wild animals such as giraffes, lions, impala and wildebeest roam the desert.

When the San moved around the desert hunting wild animals and gathering roots and berries, they built shelters of branches, twigs and grass and ate what they killed the same day. They could go without food or water for long periods, which was a great advantage as they often had to follow animals for long distances before killing them. The San hunted the animals with poisoned arrows.

The Bushmen used to roam freely over southern and eastern Africa. They left beautiful rock paintings, which tell us about their beliefs, the animals they hunted and their way of life. As they were able to find fewer and fewer places of safety from white men and other African tribes, most had to give up their nomadic lifestyle and change their ways to fit in with life on farms or in towns. The Botswana government is doing all it can to help them settle and give them land rights, water and education.

There are about 30 different San dialects. Many of their words contain click sounds, made with the tongue against the teeth or roof of the mouth. One click is like the sound we make to urge on a horse, another is like a "tut tut" of disapproval. An organization called Language Recordings has put Bible talks on tape in some Bushmen dialects,

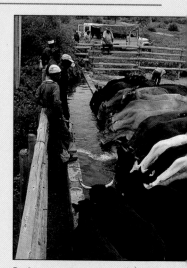
Bushmen cowboys on a cattle drive in Namibia

and missionaries are telling them the good news about Jesus. Not all San have heard about Jesus, but some have decided to follow him.

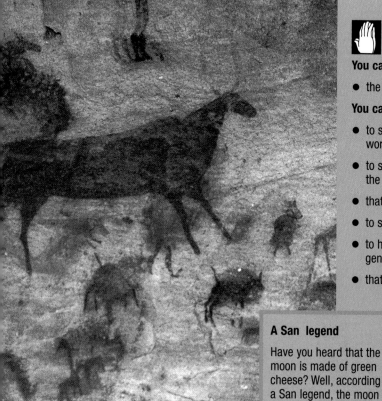

To help you pray for the San

You can thank God for:

- the work of Language Recordings.

You can ask God:

- to show the San that he can set them free from fear of the spirit world.

- to send missionaries who will understand, love and teach the San.

- that the leaders of the San will follow Jesus.

- to send people to learn the San dialects and translate the Bible.

- to help the San settle on farms and in towns without losing their gentle ways.

- that the San will always be ready to help others.

A San legend

Have you heard that the moon is made of green cheese? Well, according to a San legend, the moon is an ostrich feather, thrown up into the sky by a mantis (insect)!

Saudi Arabia

The Birthplace of Mohammed

Pilgrimage

"It's nearly time for the Hajj," Hassan told his son Abdul. *"You're 12 years old now, so this year you'll be coming with me on pilgrimage to Mecca."*

Abdul was excited about traveling hundreds of miles from Riyadh, where they lived, to Mecca. Riyadh may be the royal capital and the largest city in Saudi Arabia, but Mecca is the birthplace of Mohammed himself.

Abdul had been studying Islam for years, and he knew that the Hajj was one of the five pillars, or duties, of their religion. Every Muslim should make this pilgrimage at least once, if possible. Abdul's father had already been three times.

"I can hardly wait to go," Abdul told his father. *"Tell me what it's like."*

📋 Fact file

Area: 830,000 sq. mi.

Capital: Riyadh

Other major cities: Jeddah; Mecca; Medina

Population: 21,606,691

Official language: Arabic

Religion: Islam

Chief export: Oil (Saudi Arabia has the biggest oil deposits in the world.)

Do you know?

Although Saudi Arabia is a desert, if you fly over it you'll see green fields that look like enormous wheels. They're watered by huge sprinklers that rotate from the center of the field. Because of this system, farmers can grow wheat, barley, tomatoes and melons in the middle of the desert!

"More than two million Muslim pilgrims from all over the world travel to Mecca every year during the *Hajj*. Everyone wears the same white robe to show that we're all equal in the sight of Allah," Hassan explained. "After our ritual washing and prayer we go to the *Kaaba* and walk around it seven times, keeping it on our left. As we walk around it we have to touch and, if we can, kiss the black stone in the *Kaaba*."

"The *Kaaba's* very old, isn't it?" Abdul asked. "We read in the Koran that Abraham built it at the place where Allah provided water for Hagar and Ishmael in the desert." (You can read in the Bible, in Genesis 21, how God spoke to Hagar and provided water for her and Ishmael.)

"That's right," Hassan said, "and when Allah told Mohammed that all Muslims should turn towards Mecca when they worship him, Mohammed took all the idols out of the *Kaaba* and made it into a holy place. A new black silk cover is put over it every year.

"After we walk around the *Kaaba* seven times, we have to run between two sacred pillars seven times, praying as we go. And the next day we go to the Plain of Arafat, about 10 miles outside Mecca, to hear the special sermon. There are so many pilgrims, we probably won't be able to hear everything. So we'll take our radios so we can listen to the sermon as it's broadcast. Afterwards we'll collect small pebbles and throw them at three stone pillars to get rid of the evil that's inside us. Then, on our way home, we'll visit the Tomb of Mohammed in Medina."

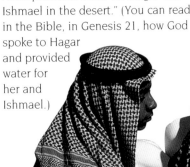

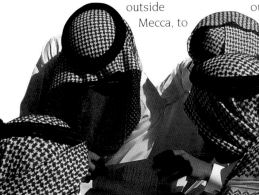

Students at the Petroleum University

154

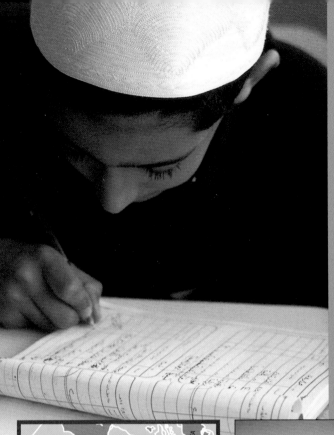

 To help you pray for Saudi Arabia

You can thank God for:

- Christian radio and television programs in Arabic that can be received in Saudi Arabia.
- the few Saudis who are following Jesus.
- Christian guest workers in Saudi Arabia.

You can ask God:

- that Saudi and other Arab Christians will help each other follow Jesus.
- that Saudis who go to other countries to work or study will meet Christians who will tell them about Jesus.
- to help guest workers share their faith with other guest workers.
- to use every Bible, Christian book or video taken into Saudi Arabia to bring someone to know Jesus.

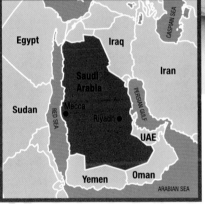

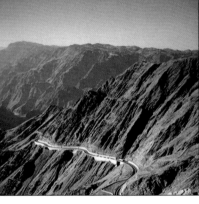

Asir Mountains

In Saudi Arabia Christians from other countries often have to meet in secret

Keeping Islam in and Jesus out

Mohammed wanted everyone in Arabia to follow Islam. Shortly after his death in AD 672, the authorities forced every Christian and every Jew to leave Arabia. Today, Islam is the only religion officially allowed inside Saudi Arabia because the government considers itself the keeper of Islam. The religious police make sure that everyone keeps the Islamic laws and that women dress in the right way. They also make sure that all the stores close when the call for prayer booms out five times each day from minarets all over the country.

Maybe someday Abdul will meet Christians who will explain to him that keeping strict laws and following certain customs can never take away our sins. Only Jesus can do that.

Wouldn't Abdul be amazed to learn that he could come to Jesus at any time and know that, wherever he is, God will hear and answer his prayers?

An oil-rich desert

The kingdom of Saudi Arabia is a hot, dry, desert country covering most of the Arabian Peninsula. A strong Arab leader, Ibn Saud, brought together all the nomadic tribes who lived there to create the new Islamic kingdom of Saudi Arabia in 1932. The king's word is law, and the large royal family controls everything.

When oil was discovered, Saudi Arabia became powerful and wealthy. Countries all around the world wanted to buy their oil. Some of the money from oil has been used to build better houses for the people, to set up

schools and universities, to make roads across the desert and to develop industries. The Saudi Arabian government sends huge sums of money to Muslim organizations in other countries to help them publish Muslim literature, train Muslim missionaries and build huge mosques.

Guest workers

Thousands of people from other countries come to Saudi Arabia as guest workers. Some work for the oil companies, and others work as laborers, housemaids and nurses. There are Christians among them, but they often have to meet in secret.

Spain

A Land of Contrasts

A big problem

"Come on, Carlos," José said impatiently as they made their way between the busy sidewalk cafés to the entrance of the subway station. They pushed to the front of the crowd listening to a group of young people playing guitars and singing. The boys didn't want to miss the story. "I hope it'll be about one of the people Jesus healed, just like he healed your brother Juan!" Carlos said excitedly.

José and Carlos live in Madrid, the capital of Spain. A lot of people are moving into the city because they're poor and tired of farming. They think it will be easy to get work in the city, but there aren't enough jobs. And, because they have so little money, they're forced to live in very small, crowded apartments.

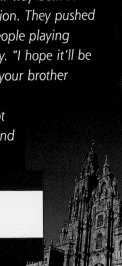

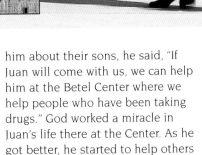

When José and his family came to live in Madrid they stopped going to church, because they said they didn't believe in God anymore. They had no work, no faith, and soon José's brothers were stealing and taking drugs. "There's nothing else to do," they complained. One of José's brothers died and another, Juan, became very sick. Their parents didn't know what to do. They felt so alone, and no one seemed to care what happened to them.

One night they stopped at a Christian meeting being held outdoors. A man saw their sad faces and asked if he could help them. When they told him about their sons, he said, "If Juan will come with us, we can help him at the Betel Center where we help people who have been taking drugs." God worked a miracle in Juan's life there at the Center. As he got better, he started to help others who came to the Center. He learned that Jesus is alive and has the power to heal. Jesus forgave him for all the bad things he had done and gave him the strength not to take drugs anymore. Juan had a new life following Jesus!

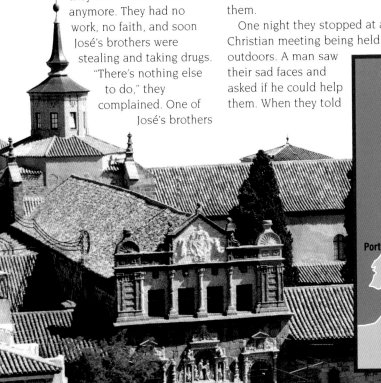

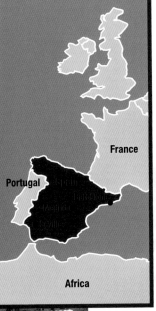

France

Portugal

Africa

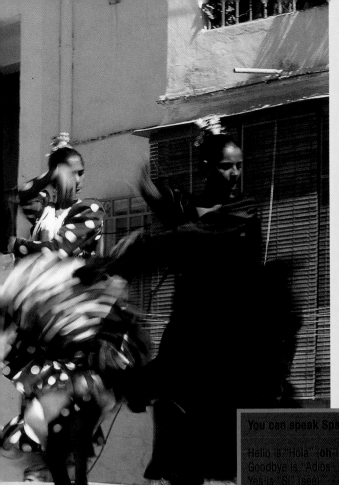

To help you pray for Spain

You can thank God for:

- the freedom to preach the good news about Jesus in Spain.

- centers like Betel, which care for drug addicts and share Jesus' love.

You can ask God:

- that people will realize that Jesus is alive and ready to help them.

- for more missionaries, pastors and evangelists to tell people about Jesus and help them to follow him.

- that lots of children will go to the children's clubs and learn about Jesus.

- to help children when others laugh at them or refuse to play with them because they follow Jesus.

- that a lot of people will listen to Christian radio and television programs.

You can speak Spanish

Hello is "Hola" (oh-lah)
Goodbye is "Adios" (ad-ee-os)
Yes is "Sí" (see)
No is "No" (no)
Please is "Por favor" (por fa-vor)
Thank-you is "Gracias" (gra-see-as)

Many people in Spain are coming to know Jesus as a friend who is with them always

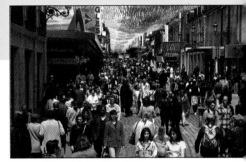

Crowded Madrid shopping street

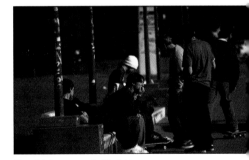

Spanish teenagers in Madrid

A feast day

But it's not only drug addicts who need to know about Jesus. Although many people in Spain are still Roman Catholic, there's no longer an official religion. A lot of people have stopped going to church or only go on special occasions, but they still love to celebrate "feast days" of the saints.

In Lidia's village, everyone worked hard cleaning the street and preparing for the feast day of their village saint. When the church bells rang, Lidia and her family went to the church for Mass. Lidia looked at the statue of Christ on the cross and remembered her cousin Marta telling her that she had come to know Jesus as her special friend through a *Club de Amigos* (Friends' Club). Marta had been so excited to tell her that Jesus is alive. Lidia thought that sounded

wonderful, too, and really wanted to know Jesus like her cousin did. "When I visit Marta," she thought, "maybe I can go to the club with her and find out how I can have him as my friend, too."

The church service was soon over. Outside the church, the band started to play. Young men carried gold-covered statues of their saint and Jesus. Everyone joined in the parade and Lidia forgot about her cousin for a while as she and her friends joined in the feasting and dancing.

People in need

The sunny country of Spain lies in the southwest corner of Europe. With its castles, church steeples, colorful fiestas, beautiful beaches and delicious food, it's no wonder many people think of holidays when they

think of Spain! There are people with great needs in Spain but in towns and villages across the country there are some who are discovering that when they ask Jesus to be their friend, he is with them always and helps them all the time.

Sri Lanka

Island of Beauty and Battle

Golden beaches

Sri Lanka, just south of India, is a beautiful sunny island with many golden beaches lined with palm trees. There are plenty of fish in the sea and all around the coast there are villages where fishermen live. It's a fertile country, too, and all sorts of things grow here – tea, rubber, rice, spices, coconuts and tropical fruits. It's no wonder that almost half the people are farmers. Others work in factories making clothes that are sold around the world. Colombo, the capital, is a busy city and the streets are often jammed with bicycles, small three-wheeled taxis, cars, buses and bullock carts. About 17 million people live in Sri Lanka. Twelve million of them are Sinhalese, who are mostly Buddhists. Another three million are Tamils, whose ancestors came from India. The Tamils are mainly Hindus. There are about a million Muslim Moors, and several other smaller groups of people with different backgrounds and beliefs.

Fact file

Area: 25,330 sq. mi.

Population: 18,827,054

Capital: Colombo

Main languages: Sinhala; Tamil

Major religions: Buddhism; Hinduism

Chief exports: Tea; rubber; textiles; gem stones

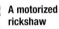

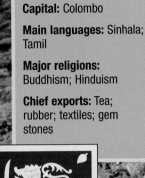

A motorized rickshaw

Violence

Since 1980, there has been lots of violence in Sri Lanka and thousands of people have been killed. Some Tamils believe that the government, made up mainly of Sinhalese, has treated them unfairly. In the north and east of the island, Tamil guerrillas are fighting government forces to make a separate country for themselves. Some have even planted bombs in the city of Colombo.

Many children in Sri Lanka have lost their parents in the fighting and live on the streets. Some are involved in the violence, others are abused or abandoned, and some have to work long hours in dangerous jobs to earn a little bit of money.

There is another battle going on, too. Some Buddhists are very angry when Christians tell others about

Do you know?

There is buried treasure in Sri Lanka! Sri Lanka has an important gem industry. Some of the gems are mined in the mountains, but some are mined in the paddy (rice) fields. A little shelter with a thatched roof in the middle of a field often covers a mineshaft. Deep in these mines, people find rubies, emeralds, agate, onyx and other stones. They're often polished, ready to be sold, in homes around the fields.

God's love. They have burned down homes and churches to make the Christians afraid so they'll stop sharing the good news about Jesus. But the Christians have stayed and others have started to follow Jesus.

Once Sri Lanka was called a pearl because of its shape, but today it reminds people of a tear. Only Jesus, through the power of the Holy Spirit, can bring peace to this island.

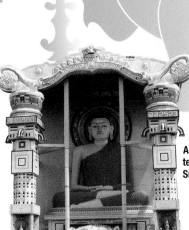

A Buddhist temple in Sri Lanka

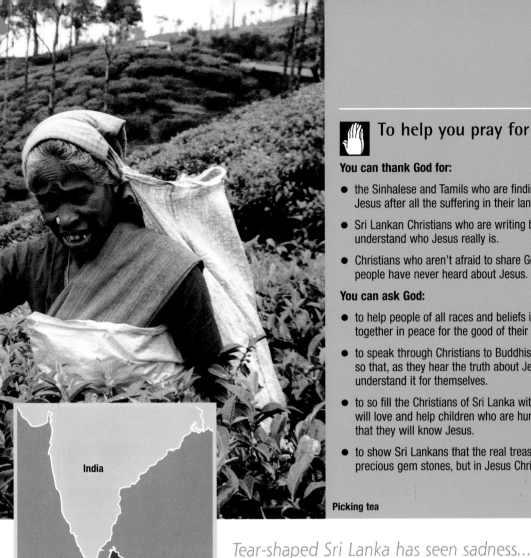

To help you pray for Sri Lanka

You can thank God for:

- the Sinhalese and Tamils who are finding a new way of life with Jesus after all the suffering in their land.
- Sri Lankan Christians who are writing books to help Buddhists understand who Jesus really is.
- Christians who aren't afraid to share God's love in villages where people have never heard about Jesus.

You can ask God:

- to help people of all races and beliefs in Sri Lanka learn to live together in peace for the good of their country.
- to speak through Christians to Buddhists, Hindus and Muslims so that, as they hear the truth about Jesus, they will believe and understand it for themselves.
- to so fill the Christians of Sri Lanka with Jesus' love that they will love and help children who are hurt or lonely or abused so that they will know Jesus.
- to show Sri Lankans that the real treasure is not in their precious gem stones, but in Jesus Christ.

Picking tea

India

Colombo
Sri Lanka

Tear-shaped Sri Lanka has seen sadness... but it's also pearl-shaped, a treasure to God

A church in the country

As we drove along the narrow dirt road, Pastor Mahess, who was with us in the van, told us his story. "When I first came to work here," he said, "the Buddhist monks told the people they weren't allowed to listen when I told them about God and his love for them. I tried to help the people, but they burned down my house. I kept telling the people that God wants to help them. One day, a man whose son was very sick came to see me. The doctor couldn't make him better. The monks at the temple couldn't help him either. I prayed for the boy and he got better. Soon the boy's whole family was following Jesus."

The van stopped beside a large, simple stone house. There was a crowd of men and women, boys and girls waiting outside. "This is the church," Mahess said, "and my home."

Everyone went into the church to worship God.

At the end of the service a little girl held my hand and gave me a shy smile. "Please pray for me," she said. "My name is Kumari. I'm nine years old and I live with my aunt because my mother and father have gone away to work. Sometimes I think they've forgotten me, but I'm glad I can come to church where everyone treats me as part of their family."

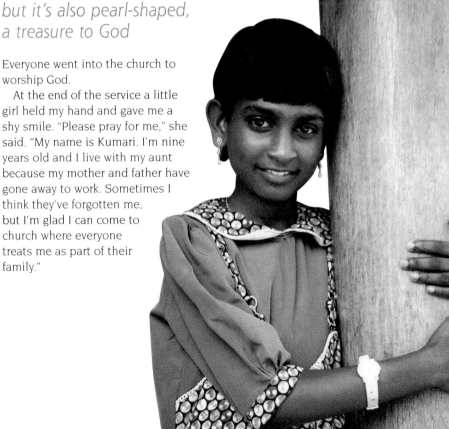

Sundanese

From Beautiful West Java

Can the gods help?

"Why do I always forget everything I've learned?" Paru wondered. "I can never remember the passages from the Koran I'm supposed to memorize. I feel so stupid. Even my little brother can learn them."

Paru was walking home, up the path between the steeply terraced rice fields. Every time he walked this path, he was amazed when he looked up at the high volcanic mountains that everyone called the "home of the gods." "The gods must have been happy with the offerings we made before we planted our fields this year, because the rice, corn, tea and hot peppers are all growing well," Paru thought. "I wish the gods would help me remember those verses from the Koran … but they never do."

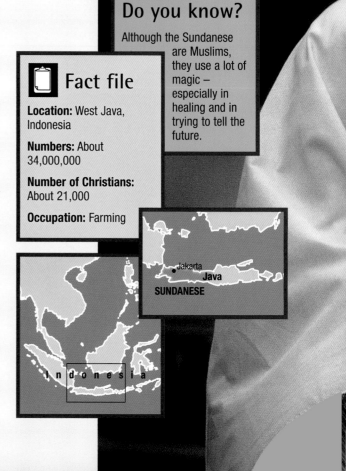

The early Dutch missionaries set up the Pasundan churches, and a lot of the 21,000 Sundanese Christians today belong to these churches. Many of them say they're Christians because their parents and grandparents were Christians. Not all of them really know what it means to have Jesus as their friend and savior, and so they're not really interested in telling their Muslim neighbors about Jesus.

Music and drama

Christians in other parts of Indonesia want to show the Sundanese that Christianity is not just a

Java, the home of the Sundanese, is the most important island of Indonesia. Jakarta, the capital of Indonesia, is on Java's northwestern coast. About 34 million Sundanese live in beautiful West Java, and millions of them, like Paru, have never heard about Jesus. Most Sundanese are Muslims, but long before they became Muslims they worshipped their own gods. When people from India brought Hinduism and Buddhism to Java in the fifth and sixth centuries AD, the Sundanese began to worship the gods of those religions as well. Even though they're Muslims now, many of them still worship the gods that they believe live in the mountains.

Christian villages

When the Dutch colonized Java in the nineteenth century, a few missionaries wanted to help the Sundanese. They set up clinics, schools and churches and tried to teach them about God's love, but the Dutch government didn't really want them there. The Sundanese didn't want them, either. And they certainly didn't want to hear about Christianity, because it was the religion of the Dutch, who had taken over their land and were telling them how they had to live.

In those days, Sundanese who did become Christians were often persecuted. So the missionaries built special villages for the new Christians. Some of these villages still exist, but they are no longer completely Christian.

Do you know?

Although the Sundanese are Muslims, they use a lot of magic – especially in healing and in trying to tell the future.

📋 Fact file

Location: West Java, Indonesia

Numbers: About 34,000,000

Number of Christians: About 21,000

Occupation: Farming

Jakarta
Java
SUNDANESE

Indonesia

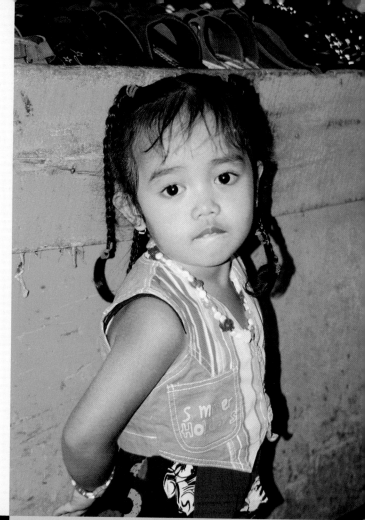

western religion. They use Sundanese drama and music to tell Bible stories so that the people will understand that God loves them, too.

One evening, two young people stopped Sita and her friends as they were walking along a busy street in Jakarta. "Come and watch this story," they invited them. "It's about why God in heaven sent his only Son to earth."

"What an amazing story," Sita told them afterwards, "and I think everyone could understand it because it was just like our Sundanese plays. The Christian's God must be really powerful to be able to bring his Son back to life again after he was killed. I'd like to know

more about their God."

A few months later, Sita decided to follow Jesus. But her family was very angry. "What do you mean, you've become a Christian?" shouted her brother. "You can't be a Christian! We're Sundanese, and that means we're Muslims." Sita was sad because her family was so angry, but she knew she had to follow Jesus, the one true God.

Please pray for the Sundanese. More and more of the people, like Sita, are becoming Christians. But there are so many Sundanese and lots of them, like Paru, have never heard the good news about Jesus.

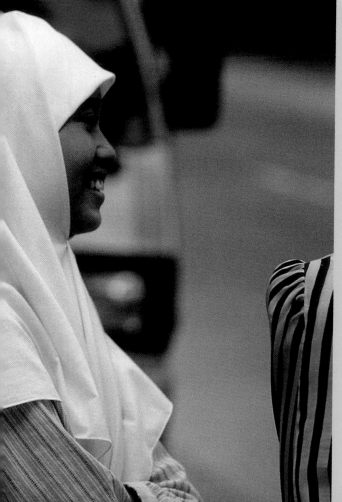

To help you pray for the Sundanese

You can thank God for:

- Indonesian Christians who are telling the Sundanese about Jesus.
- every Christian in the Pasundan churches.
- Sundanese Christians like Sita, who follow Jesus even when it's very difficult.

You can ask God:

- to send Christians to the villages to tell children like Paru that Jesus is more powerful than all the gods in the mountains, and that Jesus promises to help everyone who trusts in him.
- to use the Christian drama and music programs to show the Sundanese that they can be Christians.
- that many Sundanese people will listen to the Christian radio programs and understand what it means to be a Christian.
- for many more people around the world to pray for the Sundanese.

Syria

A Modern Country but an Ancient Land

What's a Christian?

"What do you mean you've become a Christian?" Maria asked her brother Ibrahim. "Of course you're a Christian. You've always been a Christian, just like the rest of our family. We belong to a church, don't we? There have been Christians here in Damascus since New Testament times."

"Yes, that's true," Ibrahim said. "It even says in Acts 9 that Saul (Paul) came here to Damascus to arrest the Christians because he didn't want the faith to spread to other places. He knew how easily that could happen because travelers and traders came here from far and wide and would take the good news about Jesus with them. It's a good thing God spoke to him before he ever reached Damascus. And after Saul became a Christian, he himself took the good news about Jesus to lots of other places.

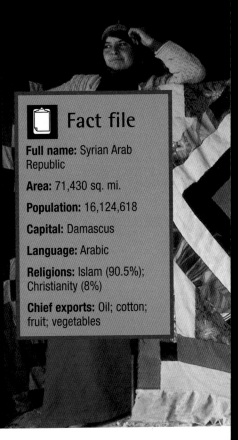

Fact file

Full name: Syrian Arab Republic

Area: 71,430 sq. mi.

Population: 16,124,618

Capital: Damascus

Language: Arabic

Religions: Islam (90.5%); Christianity (8%)

Chief exports: Oil; cotton; fruit; vegetables

"But Maria," Ibrahim continued, "when I went to study in Aleppo, I met Christians who were really excited about their faith. They told me that I could know Jesus as a special friend and they taught me to study the Bible for myself. It's an amazing book! Will you come to a Bible study group with me? My friends have a really good video, too, about the life of Jesus."

"I'll come," Maria said. "You're so excited about it … I wish I could know Jesus like you do."

An ancient land

Damascus, the capital of modern Syria, is an ancient city. It may even be the oldest city in the whole world! You can find Damascus in the very first book in the Bible, in Genesis chapters 14 and 15. You can also read there about the River Euphrates, which flows through Syria and has been dammed to provide hydroelectric power for the country.

Syria has been a secular country since

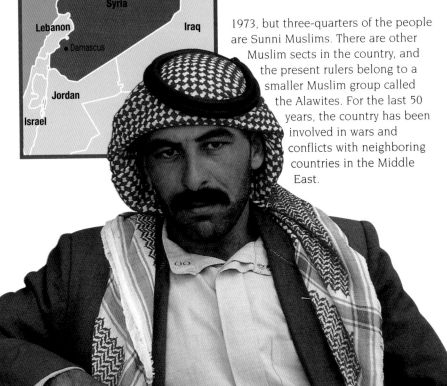

There have been Christians in Syria since New Testament times

1973, but three-quarters of the people are Sunni Muslims. There are other Muslim sects in the country, and the present rulers belong to a smaller Muslim group called the Alawites. For the last 50 years, the country has been involved in wars and conflicts with neighboring countries in the Middle East.

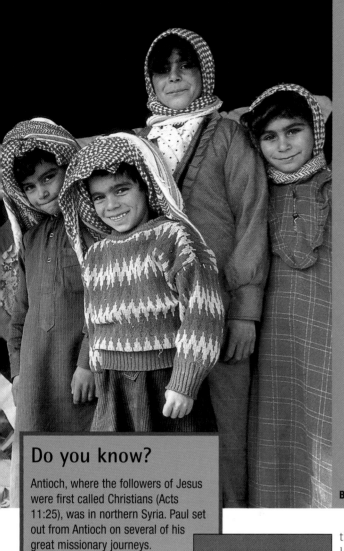

Bedouin family

To help you pray for Syria

You can thank God for:

- the freedom Syrian Christians have to meet together to worship.
- the work of the Bible Society in providing Bibles and Christian books.

You can ask God:

- that those who follow Jesus will help others who only say they're Christians to really know and follow him, too.
- that many people will watch the *Jesus* video and understand God's love.
- to help Christians live so that other people will see their joyful, caring lives and want to know Jesus, too.
- that Christians will share the good news about Jesus with their Muslim friends when they have opportunities to do so.
- for wise government and peace in Syria and neighboring countries, especially Israel and Lebanon.

Do you know?

Antioch, where the followers of Jesus were first called Christians (Acts 11:25), was in northern Syria. Paul set out from Antioch on several of his great missionary journeys.

Not just some old book

There are Orthodox and Armenian churches in almost every town in Syria. There are some Protestant churches too, but there aren't enough pastors and Christian workers to lead them. Although Christians make up only a small part of Syria's population, they have a lot of freedom. They can go to church whenever they want, and radio and television stations broadcast Christian programs at Christmas and Easter. They can buy Christian books and Bibles, and a lot of people watch the *Jesus* video in Arabic. Many Christians are highly respected in Syria and have good jobs as merchants, teachers, doctors and lawyers. Others work for the government and in the armed forces.

A lot of Christians in Syria are finding out that the Bible isn't just a big, old book of stories about things that happened a long time ago. As they read it, they realize that it's the word of the living God. The Bible has lots to say to people today. They're excited about it and many, like Ibrahim and Maria, are coming to really know Jesus for the first time.

Christians and Muslims

For 1,300 years, both Muslims and Christians have lived in Syria. "We live in the Christian part of Damascus, and that's where our friends are," Ibrahim explains. "We meet Muslims at work and at school, but we really don't understand each other, so it's very hard to talk about our faith.

"I have a few Muslim friends, and I try to show them who Jesus is by the way I live. I want them to see that Jesus has made my life pure and clean, and that he fills me with joy. Some of my Christian friends don't understand why I want my Muslim friends to know Jesus, and my Muslim friends are afraid they'll be persecuted if they become Christians. But I want all my family and friends to know Jesus, who makes our lives new when we trust in him."

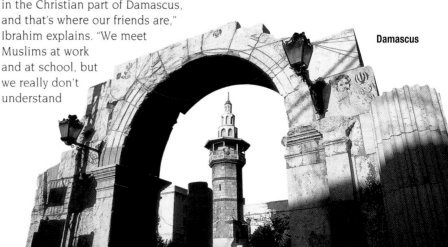

Damascus

Tibetans

Following their God-king

A mysterious world

The Himalayan and Kun Lun Mountains surround the Tibetan plateau like a gigantic wall, and for hundreds of years few people ever visited it. Tibet was like a mysterious world. Now visitors can fly into Lhasa, the capital city, or travel through the country on roads built by the Chinese.

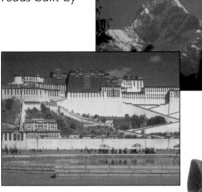

The Potala in Lhasa where the Dalai Lama lived and studied

Do you know?

Tsampa is the most important part of any Tibetan meal. Tibetans make *tsampa* by roasting barley, grinding it into flour, and then mixing it with salted tea and butter made from yak milk. All of the fat in yak milk helps the people stay healthy in the extremely cold climate in Tibet.

The Tibetan plateau, the highest and largest on earth, is often called "the roof of the world." It covers an area of 714,300 square miles and averages over 15,000 feet above sea level.

The Buddhist religious leaders used to also be the political leaders (this is called a theocracy). The officials and priests were looked upon as royalty, but most ordinary people were treated like slaves. They even had to stick out their tongues when they met important people to show they didn't have demons inside them! Some Tibetans still do this as a sign of respect.

The Dalai Lama

The Dalai Lama is the most important priest, or "lama," and the leader of the Tibetan people. Tibetans believe that the Dalai Lama is a god-king, and that when he dies his soul is "reborn" in a baby. So as soon as the Dalai Lama dies, the search begins for the next Dalai Lama – a

Fact file

Location: About 2,000,000 Tibetans live in central Tibet. Another 2,500,000 live in the western Chinese provinces of Qinghai, Sichuan and Gansu.
As many as 450,000 live in exile in India, Nepal, Bhutan and Sikkim, and some live in North America and Europe.

Religion: Tibetan Buddhism

Language: Tibetan, but most also speak the language of the country in which they live.

baby boy born within 18 months of his death.

Tenzin Gyatso (*Ten-zin Chi-at-zo*), the present Dalai Lama, was born in 1935 in a farmhouse hundreds of miles from Lhasa. Although he wasn't even two years old, he had to pass certain tests

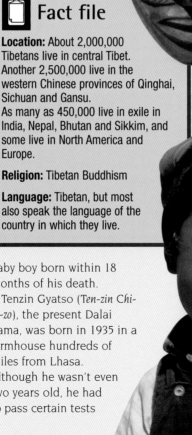

Tibetan mask

Tibetan nomad child

to see if he was the new Dalai Lama. In one test, a number of objects were put in front of him. Some of them had belonged to the previous Dalai Lama. Everyone watched anxiously while Tenzin Gyatso pointed out exactly what had belonged to him. The new Dalai Lama had been found!

Thousands of five-year-old Tibetan boys used to enter monasteries to become monks and learn the Buddhist scriptures. Tenzin Gyatso, too, was only five years old when he was taken to Lhasa to be

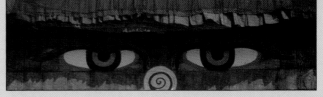

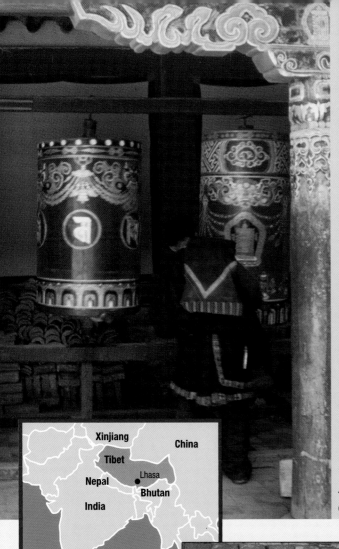

To help you pray for the Tibetans

You can thank God for:

- the Tibetans who follow Jesus instead of a human god-king.
- the modern translation of the New Testament in Tibetan.
- the Christians who have helped Tibetan nomads when floods and other disasters have killed their flocks of yaks, sheep and goats.

You can ask God:

- for Chinese Christians and others to be able to travel freely throughout Tibet to tell people about God's love and care.
- that many Tibetans will listen to Christian radio programs, understand what they hear and follow Jesus.
- to show Tibetans that although the Dalai Lama is their leader and a very good man, he is only a man and not a god.
- to help many Tibetans discover that Jesus is the true King of kings and God over all.

Tibetans spinning prayer wheels outside a temple

Spinning yarn with a traditional wheel

enthroned in the Potala, the most important monastery in Tibet, and to begin his studies. Buddhist monks taught him everything they could about Buddhism. He wasn't allowed to leave the Potala except to visit another monastery. He must have been lonely without his family or other children to play with. Someone gave him a pair of binoculars, and he loved watching people out on the streets. He could see pilgrims twirling prayer wheels on their way to the temples to make offerings, prayer flags fluttering on the roofs, and officials arriving at the Potala on horseback.

The end of peace

In 1950, the Chinese army invaded Tibet and set up a Communist government. Monasteries, as well as the ancient Buddhist scriptures, were destroyed. The Chinese killed thousands of Tibetans. Thousands more fled across the high mountain passes to India and Nepal. In 1959, the Dalai Lama was forced to flee to Dharamsala, in India, where he still lives. He has visited many countries around the world to ask for help to free Tibet from China's rule. He was awarded the Nobel Peace Prize in 1989 for his work promoting world peace.

The Tibetans are still devoted to their god-king, and want Tibet to be a free and independent country. Monks have led demonstrations against the government, but the Chinese have stopped them. Lots of changes have taken place in Tibet. Priests don't have the power they once had. There are more Chinese in Lhasa now than Tibetans. Chinese has taken the place of Tibetan as the official language. Although more children are able to go to school now, a lot of their lessons are in Chinese.

Following the King of kings

There are only a few Tibetan Christians. For over a hundred years, missionaries have been telling Tibetans living in countries on the border with Tibet about Jesus. Tibetans living around the world are hearing about Jesus, the King of kings and God above all other gods.

Trinidad

Carnival and Calypso

A carnival

It's Mardi Gras, or Shrove Tuesday, and time for the carnival in Port-of-Spain, the capital of Trinidad! Thousands of men, women, boys and girls crowd the streets, and people are dancing to the beat of the steel drums, wearing beautiful costumes that sparkle and glitter in the sun.

Everyone taking part in the carnival has spent weeks preparing to play mas, *or masquerade. They've made elaborate costumes, practiced music and written funny calypso songs. And it's all over at midnight, because tomorrow is Ash Wednesday, the start of the Christian season of Lent.*

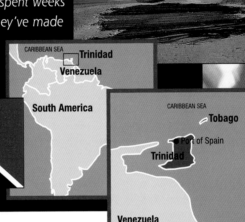

CARIBBEAN SEA — **Trinidad**

Venezuela

South America

CARIBBEAN SEA

Tobago

Port of Spain

Trinidad

Venezuela

Fact file

Area: 2,000 sq. mi.

Capital: Port of Spain

Population: 1,294,958

Languages: English; Hindi; French; Spanish

Religions: Christianity (Roman Catholic and Protestant); Hinduism; Islam

Chief exports: Oil; steel products; sugar cane; cocoa; coffee; fruit

Lots of festivals

People in Trinidad celebrate lots of festivals. In November they celebrate *Divali*, the Hindu festival of lights, when candles shine from hundreds of thousands of little clay pots while people spend the night feasting and dancing. Another Hindu festival, *Phagwa*, or New Year, takes place in March. During this festival, people celebrating on the streets throw red food dye at each other!

Muslims in Trinidad have festivals, too. On *Hosay* they remember the murder of two warrior brothers, Hosein and Hassan. They carry models of Hosein's tomb through the streets to the beat of drums and chanting, then they feast all evening and dance all night. The next day, they throw the "tombs" into the sea as a sign of burial.

Some of these traditions might seem a bit strange to us, but have you ever thought what someone from a faraway country might think if they saw you decorating a Christmas tree or blowing out candles on a birthday cake? Different cultures have special ways of having fun and celebrating what's important to them.

Trinidad and Tobago

Trinidad is one of two main islands making up the Republic of Trinidad and Tobago. Trinidad is the most southerly of all the Caribbean islands and is only about 4 miles from Venezuela. While some people are poor, the money from oil, natural gas, pitch and steel industries has given Trinidadians a higher standard of living than most people in countries near them.

People from all over the world

Although it was late at night, nine-year-old Earl was sitting outside his house with his father. He was too excited to sleep after the carnival. "I love festivals," he said. "Why do we have so many?"

"Because Trinidadians all come from different parts of the world," his father replied. "Most of us have our roots in Africa, India and Europe, but some come

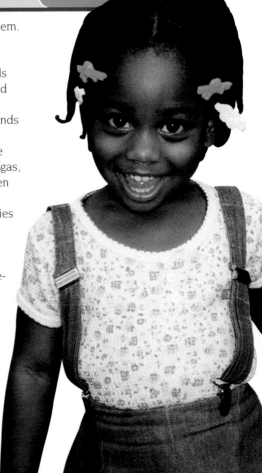

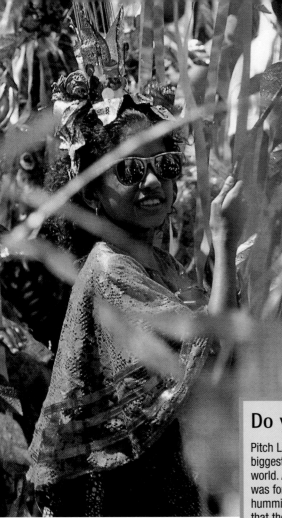

You can thank God for:

● Christian radio and TV programs.

● Christians who are teaching children about Jesus in schools and in churches.

● Christian bookstores.

You can ask God:

● to help the different peoples of Trinidad live together in peace.

● that the Prime Minister and government will be wise and fair to everyone.

● that Christians will tell others the good news about Jesus.

● that the churches will help a lot more Trinidadians come to know Jesus.

Do you know?

Pitch Lake, in the south of Trinidad, is the biggest natural source of asphalt in the world. A local legend says that the lake was formed when a chief killed a sacred hummingbird. This made the gods so angry that they drowned his whole village in pitch.

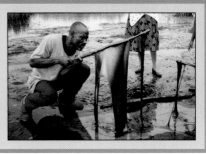

from the Middle East, China and even South America. When people came to Trinidad from all those different places, they brought their cultures and religions – and festivals – with them."

"Why did they all come to Trinidad?" Earl asked.

"Oh, it all started a long time ago," his father said. "Christopher Columbus discovered this island in 1498. I've heard some people say that when he sailed near the southeast coast he saw three mountain peaks that reminded him of the Holy Trinity, so he named the island Trinidad.

"The island belonged to Spain after that, but there weren't many people

Playing *mas*

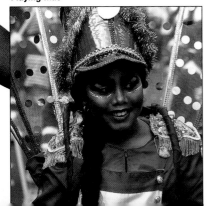

living here until the eighteenth century, when Catholic refugees from French colonies settled here. They planted sugar and cacao plantations and brought slaves from Africa to work for them. They tried to force the slaves to forget their African religions and become Catholics. In 1797, the British captured Trinidad and it became a British colony."

"What happened when the British came?" asked Earl.

"Well, the government finally did away with slavery in 1834, but the plantation owners still needed workers. This time they brought people from India, promising them that after they had worked on the plantations for five years they could have a free trip home. Many of these Indians decided to stay in Trinidad after five years, and they were given small plots of land for themselves. Some of them were Muslims, but most were Hindus. Both have kept their own religion and culture.

"Whether we came from Africa, India, Europe or somewhere else, we're all Trinidadians and we like to join in the different festivals. Do you remember singing those words in our national anthem, 'here every race and creed find an equal place'? That's a great thought, but unfortunately I don't think it's always true. Sometimes there are tensions between the people of different races."

As Earl listened to his father, he thought about the church he went to each Sunday with his family. He loved the singing and learning stories from the Bible. And he knew that the problems between people in Trinidad would make Jesus sad.

Even though more than half the people of Trinidad say they're Christians, most of them don't really follow Jesus. If Trinidadians of every race followed Jesus, the rejoicing in heaven would be better than any festival!

Turkey

One Country on Two Continents

Istanbul is the only city in the world on two different continents. The smaller, western part of the city is in Europe, but the rest is in Asia. An important channel of water called the Bosphorus, which links the Black Sea to the Mediterranean Sea, separates the two parts of the city. Every day, thousands of people cross this waterway on their way to and from work. Some cross on the bridges that rise high above the water while others ride across on the busy ferryboats.

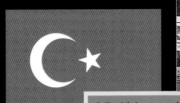

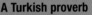

Map showing: BLACK SEA, Istanbul, BOSPHORUS, Russia, Ankara, Georgia, Turkey, MEDITERRANEAN SEA, Syria, Iraq

Bridge over the Bosphorus

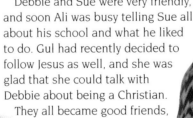

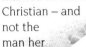

Fact file

Area: 300,948 sq. mi.

Population: 66,590,940

Capital: Ankara

Language: Turkish

Religion: Islam

Chief exports: Textiles; leather clothing; iron; steel; fruit

A Turkish proverb
It's impossible to have a rose without thorns. (Even the nicest things always have a catch.)

A Turkish drink to make
Put 2 tablespoons of plain (or Greek) yogurt in a glass of cold water. Add a little salt and mix well.
This drink, called Ayran (*eye-ran*), is very refreshing. Turkish children often buy it at MacDonald's to drink with a hamburger.

There are only a few Turkish Christians, but their numbers are growing year by year

New friends

Gul and her little brother Ali were very excited. They were going to meet Debbie and Sue, friends of their older sister, Aysha, who lived in America. Aysha had shocked the family three years ago by telling them that she had decided to follow Jesus. Although her parents were upset when Aysha stopped following Islam and became a Christian, they saw that her faith had given her a new love and respect for them. A little later she had married an American Christian – and not the man her parents had chosen for her to marry. Gul and Ali could hardly imagine what Aysha's friends would be like.

Debbie and Sue were very friendly, and soon Ali was busy telling Sue all about his school and what he liked to do. Gul had recently decided to follow Jesus as well, and she was glad that she could talk with Debbie about being a Christian.

They all became good friends, and Debbie and Sue visited them often. Before long, Gul and Ali's parents became interested in the message

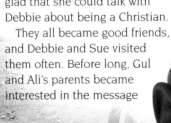

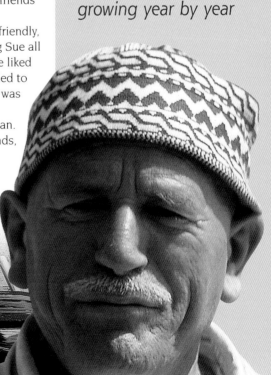

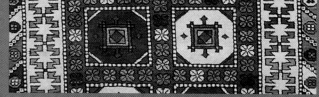

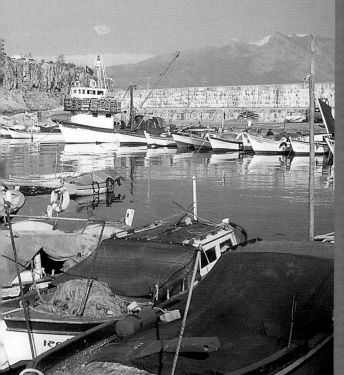

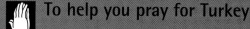

Devastation caused by the 1999 earthquake

You can speak Turkish

Hello is "Merhaba" (**mer**-hah-ba)
Goodbye is "Hoşçakal" (**hosh**-ja-kal)
Please is "Lütfen" (**lewt**-fen)
Thank you is "Teşekkür ederim"
    (tesh-e-**kewr** ed-e-rim)
Yes is "Evet" (eh-**vet**)
No is "Hayir" (hi-**yerh**)

of the Bible, too. They watched a video about the life of Jesus that really made them think about who Jesus was and why he came to die on the cross. Debbie and Sue gave them a New Testament. They read the Gospels, the stories of Jesus' life, and they began to understand more about God's love. Then they, too, decided to follow Jesus.

Earthquake!

In August 1999, a terrible earthquake destroyed many homes near Istanbul. Thousands of people died or were badly hurt, and everyone was very frightened. Christians from the small Protestant churches joined together to provide food and to help as many people as they could.

For several days, rescuers dug frantically in the rubble. At last they gave up hope of finding anyone else still alive. But as bulldozers started to clear the rubble, rescuers discovered Murat, a seven-year-old boy, trapped deep under a huge pile of bricks and concrete. He had been buried alive for nine days.

"It's a miracle," said the doctors who examined Murat. "It's so hot here in August, we don't know how anyone could live so long in this heat without water."

"But I did have water," Murat insisted. "Every evening, a nice man came to visit me and brought me bread and water." His family was puzzled. They had been sure Murat was dead and they knew no one could have visited him because he was buried so deep under the rubble.

Was this a miracle? Did an angel visit Murat? Does God have a special plan for Murat, who should have died but was wonderfully saved?

Telling others about Jesus

Because the 66 million Turks are almost all Muslims, it isn't easy for the few who follow Jesus to tell others about him. Although the law doesn't say that people can't become Christians, some Turkish Christians have been prevented from meeting together to worship God. Others have lost their jobs and some have even been put in prison because they believe in Jesus. Now many more families just like Gul's and Ali's are taking an interest in Christianity. Several thousand people are studying the Bible through correspondence courses, and Christians like Debbie and Sue are always ready to help those who want to learn more.

Christians have shown God's love to others as they helped those who were hungry, hurt and homeless as a result of the earthquake. Because of their kindness, more people are coming to know about Jesus' love for them.

United Arab Emirates

More Foreigners than Locals

Seven small states

At one time seven Arab sheikhs (chiefs) in the Arabian Gulf area each ruled their own independent states, which were called sheikhdoms or emirates. In 1971, the seven small sheikhdoms joined together to become the United Arab Emirates (or UAE for short). Each sheikh continues to have power in his own state, but they all meet together regularly to make decisions which affect the whole region. Abu Dhabi is the largest emirate and its capital city is also the capital of the UAE. Oil is found in five of the emirates, and the money from this has changed the country rapidly.

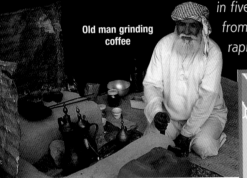

Old man grinding coffee

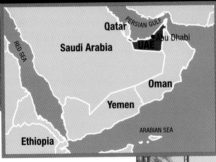

Qatar · PERSIAN GULF · Abu Dhabi · Saudi Arabia · UAE · RED SEA · Oman · Yemen · ARABIAN SEA · Ethiopia

Simple villages in the desert have become modern cities. Harbors, once the haunt of pirates, smugglers and Arab *dhows* (trading boats) are now ports for huge oil tankers, and the airports handle millions of passengers a year.

Oil and sand

A popular pastime in the UAE is watching camel races and bullfights (in which bulls wrestle with each other). One bull usually shows quite quickly that it's stronger, and the other turns and runs – with its owner hanging on to its tether! Some sheikhs also hunt with falcons in the desert.

Most of the UAE is hot, dry desert, but a little rain falls in the eastern mountains. Farmers can grow vegetables, dates and limes where the land is irrigated. The government has spent some of the money from selling oil on removing the salt from sea water so that it can be used to irrigate crops, keep cattle and provide beautiful fountains and green parks in the cities.

There are presently about four foreign workers to every local person, but that's expected to change. Most people in the UAE can now have a good education, so nationals are beginning to replace foreigners in skilled occupations.

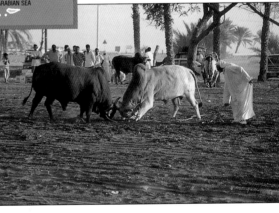

Bull fight – a typical Friday afternoon's entertainment

Christian hospitals

When the UAE was a poor country, Christian workers provided the only medical care available and saved many lives. Today modern hospitals and clinics are available to everyone, but the few remaining Christian medical centers are still popular because of the staff's love and care.

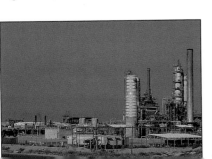

Oil refinery

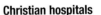

Oil has brought riches to the UAE, but not happiness or hope for the future

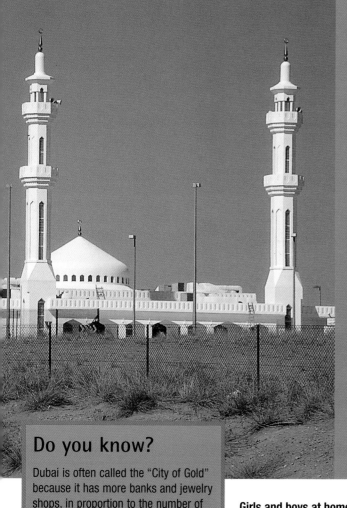

 To help you pray for the UAE

You can thank God for:

- the many guest workers who have come to know Jesus as their friend and savior while working in the UAE.

- the Christian hospitals and medical centers that continue to care for those who come to them.

- Christian radio and television broadcasts that can be received in the UAE.

You can ask God:

- to help Christian guest workers please him by the way they live.

- to show people in the UAE that wealth doesn't bring true happiness, but that Jesus offers forgiveness, joy and peace to all who trust in him.

- to help Christian doctors, nurses and midwives as they treat their patients and share his love.

- to bring children to know Jesus as their special friend.

Do you know?

Dubai is often called the "City of Gold" because it has more banks and jewelry shops, in proportion to the number of people who live there, than any other city in the world.

A proverb from UAE

"Too many captains sink the ship," which is just like our saying, "Too many cooks spoil the broth."

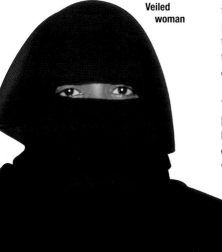

Veiled woman

Girls and boys at home

As in other Muslim countries, men can have more than one wife. So children in a family may have the same father but a different mother. When they grow up, many young men go to other countries to study, but only a few girls get that opportunity.

Sharifa adjusted her headscarf. She was now nine years old, and she had to wear it whenever she went out. "I'm not looking forward to having to wear the black cloak and veil when I'm thirteen," she confided to her friend one day.

"I'm not, either," her friend said. "Boys seem to have more fun. They can play soccer and go out with their friends. We don't get to do anything except play at home or go visiting with our mothers."

"At least we can go to school. I'd like to be a teacher some day like my sister," Sharifa said. "Did I tell you my father's arranging her marriage? She says she'd rather choose her own husband."

Christian guest workers

The discovery of oil has made the country rich, but that hasn't given the people happiness or hope for the future. Even the best Muslims can never be sure that God has forgiven their sins and accepted them.

Christians working in the UAE are allowed to meet and worship as long as they don't invite Muslims to their meetings. They could be sent back to their own countries or put in prison for talking about Jesus to a Muslim.

Birthday party at a Christian hospital

Uruguay

Where Christmas Day is Called "Family Day"

Taxicab evangelists

Ricardo slumped down on the back seat of the taxi. He had just been fired from his job, and he was miserable. He knew it was his own fault. But what could he do now? There weren't enough jobs for all the people looking for work. He never should have left his father's farm to work in the city.

The taxi driver switched on the radio. "Whatever problem you have right now," the voice on the radio was saying, "God is ready to help you. He loves you and sent Jesus to die on the cross for you and take away your sins. Trust in him, and you'll discover he's a friend who is with you all the time." Ricardo sat up to listen.

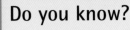

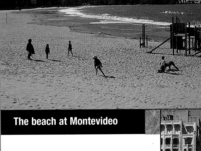

The beach at Montevideo

Fact file

Area: 68,000 sq. mi.

Population: 3,337,058 (almost half live in Montevideo)

Capital: Montevideo

Language: Spanish

Religions: Roman Catholic; secular

Chief exports: Meat; leather; wool; textiles

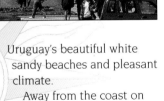

Montevideo

"It's true," the taxi driver said as he saw Ricardo's interest. "Since I came to know Jesus as my savior and friend, my life has changed completely." The driver explained to Ricardo how his life, his family and his attitudes to things had changed, how God had answered his prayers and how he felt hope and peace with Jesus in his life. Ricardo agreed to think about it and read the Bible the driver gave him. "Maybe," he thought, "losing my job isn't the end of the world. Maybe there's hope after all."

In Montevideo, Uruguay's capital, more than 60 taxi drivers have become Christians. They meet together to pray and read the Bible, and every day they share the good news of Jesus with their passengers.

Tourists and cowboys

Uruguay, the smallest country in South America, is sandwiched between Brazil and Argentina. Tourists from around the world come to enjoy

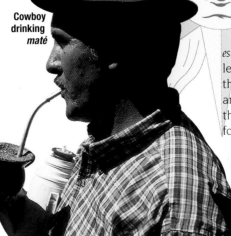

Cowboy drinking *maté*

Uruguay's beautiful white sandy beaches and pleasant climate.

Away from the coast on the rolling grassy plains and low hills, cowboys raise cattle and sheep on huge farms called *estancias*. A lot of people, like Ricardo, leave the countryside because they think they'll be able to get better jobs and earn more money in the cities. But there aren't enough jobs in the cities for everyone.

An empty place

Most Uruguayans are descendants of settlers from Spain and Italy. Early in the twentieth century, many of them turned their backs on Roman Catholicism. Even

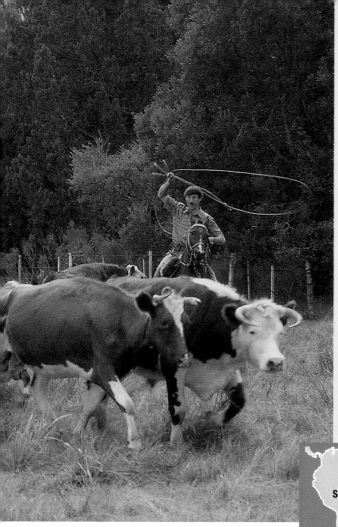

 To help you pray for Uruguay

You can thank God for:

- Uruguayans who are listening to the good news about Jesus.
- the groups sharing the gospel in many different places.
- evangelistic teams from Brazil and Argentina telling people in Uruguay about Jesus.

You can ask God:

- that Christians will share their faith with others.
- that Christians working with young people will show them how to follow Jesus.
- to show the people that practicing spiritism and witchcraft can never make them happy.
- to use Christian books and radio broadcasts to help people follow Jesus.

South America

ATLANTIC OCEAN

Paraguay

Brazil

Uruguay

Argentina

Montevideo

ATLANTIC OCEAN

Many Uruguayans are discovering that there's an empty place in their lives when they don't believe in God

Christmas Day lost its name and became "Family Day." A lot of people who thought God didn't matter became agnostics.

Everyone in Uruguay goes to school, and many people go on to study at universities. Most people thought that a good education, a good job and a good pension were far more important than God. They're surprised when they find out this isn't true. There isn't enough work for everyone to have a good job, and there is more crime and violence.

About half of all Uruguayans say they're Catholics, but many of them never go to church. Instead, they're listening to Mormons and Jehovah's Witnesses who go from door to door talking about their beliefs, which are not true to the Bible. Others are listening to spiritists (who contact spirits), and children often wear

charms, which they think will keep evil spirits from harming them. The people of Uruguay are discovering that there's an empty place in their lives when they don't believe in God.

God answers prayer

Twelve-year-old Gonzalo heard an evangelist speaking about Jesus and decided to follow him. He wanted to learn all he could about God, Jesus and the Bible, and for the next two years he went to a young people's club.

But Gonzalo's father belonged to a group that practiced a kind of witchcraft called Macumbas. One day he got angry with Gonzalo and told him he could never go to church again. Gonzalo decided he should obey his father, even though he didn't want to. The boys in the club prayed for Gonzalo. Three weeks later, his father

changed his mind. Gonzalo came back to the club, and the boys thanked God for answering their prayers so quickly.

Books and Bibles

Carlos and his friends got permission to set up a bookstall in the public square, the busiest spot in town. People stopped to look at the Christian books and Bibles and Carlos and his friends were busy selling books and explaining the gospel. They were so pleased to be able to share the truth about Jesus with so many people who wouldn't otherwise have heard about him. The Christian Literature Crusade also has a specially equipped van to take books all around the country.

In almost every town, Christian churches are growing as Christians share their faith and talk to their friends about Jesus.

Uzbeks

Is Jesus More than the Christians' Prophet?

Who is Jesus?

Akmal and Timur were bored. The two eight-year-old boys lay in the shade of a leafy mulberry tree on a summer afternoon. "It's too hot to play soccer with Zahid and the others in the school yard," grumbled Akmal. "It's too far to go to the river for a swim and I don't have any money for the pool. There's nothing to do."

"Let's go over to my uncle's house and watch a video," suggested Timur. "Maybe he has some new ones. He's got air-conditioning, so at least we can stay cool."

"OK," said Akmal, "anything's better than sitting here doing nothing."

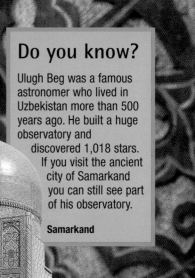

Do you know?
Ulugh Beg was a famous astronomer who lived in Uzbekistan more than 500 years ago. He built a huge observatory and discovered 1,018 stars. If you visit the ancient city of Samarkand you can still see part of his observatory.

Samarkand

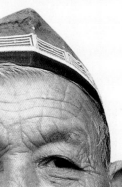

Uzbek family

The two boys wandered down the hot, dusty street until they reached Timur's uncle's house. Timur's aunt was busy making bread, but she gave the thirsty boys some cold tea to drink. "You can watch a video with your cousins while I finish baking," she said.

"Hey, here's a new one called 'Iso' (Jesus). I wonder what it's about?" Timur put it in the VCR. They watched the video in silence for a few minutes.

"I don't like movies without gangsters and gunfights or karate," Akmal said doubtfully.

"Hey, look, that guy who was paralyzed can walk now!" Timur said.

"Yeah, and now that girl who was dead is alive again! Wouldn't it be great to be able to do that? I wonder who this guy Jesus

is. Is he real? Does it say on the video case?" Akmal asked.

"No, not really ... oh, look! Why are they putting him on that cross? What did he do? Rewind it – I want to know why they're trying to kill him," Timur exclaimed.

"He just said he was king."

"What? Oh ... no! Why doesn't he do another miracle and just get down from there?" Akmal asked. "I can't believe they let him die in the movie. I thought he was a god or something who couldn't die. Wait ... there he is again! He didn't die! Oh, I knew he wouldn't!"

"But why did he die

first?" Timur asked. "He did really die, didn't he? Why didn't he just escape? I'm glad he's alive, anyway."

"They just said he had to die to be punished for all the things everyone ever did wrong. You don't think that includes us, do you?"

"It says so ..." said Timur thoughtfully. "Do you think it's a true story? I wish it was. I'd like to meet Jesus and find out how he did those things. He seems like he'd be nice to talk to."

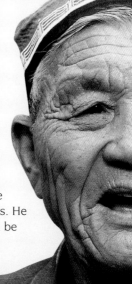

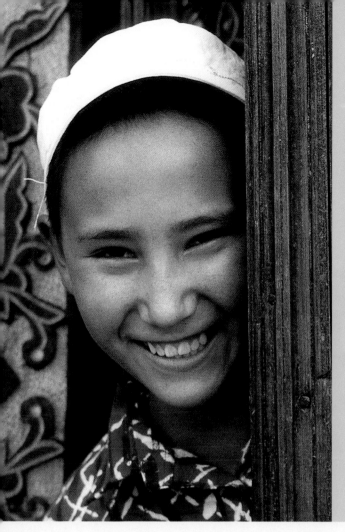

 ## To help you pray for the Uzbeks

You can thank God for:

- all Uzbek Christians.
- the *Jesus* video in Uzbek.

You can ask God:

- for Uzbeks, both atheists and Muslims, to search for the forgiveness and peace that only Jesus can give.
- to take away any fear the Christians feel as they share Jesus' love and concern with their friends and families.
- that as Uzbek Christians read the New Testament, they will come to know Jesus better.
- to help the people producing Christian radio broadcasts.
- that Christians from other countries will share the good news about Jesus with the people in Uzbekistan.

That night Timur told his father about the video and asked if he knew who Jesus was. "Oh, he's the Christians' prophet," he replied, "but I don't know any more about him than that. If you're so interested in religion, go and ask your grandfather to tell you about our prophet Mohammed. We Uzbeks are Muslims, not Christians."

Timur decided he would go back to his uncle's the next day and watch the video again. He wanted to know more about Jesus.

In the vegetable market in Tashkent

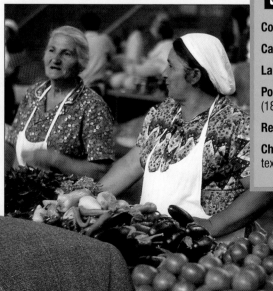

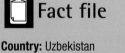 ## Fact file

Country: Uzbekistan

Capital: Tashkent

Language: Uzbek

Population: 24,317,851 (18,500,000 are Uzbeks)

Religions: Islam; atheism

Chief exports: Cotton; textiles; gold; natural gas

No religions!

For almost 70 years, Uzbekistan was part of the former Soviet Union. The Communist government made it very difficult for the Uzbek Muslims and Russian and German Christians who lived there to practice their religions. They weren't allowed to teach their beliefs in schools, mosques or churches, and very few people had copies of the Koran or the Bible. Most young Uzbeks, like Timur, only knew about Islam from the little they heard at weddings, birth ceremonies and funerals.

Freedom once more

When the Soviet Union broke up in 1991, Uzbekistan once again became an independent country. Many Uzbeks have returned to their Muslim faith. But there are still lots of problems in Uzbekistan. The people hoped their new freedom would mean that they would have a better life. Instead, more than a million people have no jobs and there are many cotton growers who work hard in the hot sun all day for very little money.

There are more than 23 million Uzbeks, but only about 500 believe in Jesus. Some Christians from other countries have gone there to work, but they often have to share the good news about Jesus quietly.

175

Vagla

People of the Talking Drums

The fable of the drum

Once upon a time there was a Vagla man who kept getting lost while he was out hunting, and his son had to spend a lot of time looking for him. One day, when out searching for his father, the son reached a river where he heard drumming and singing. He listened carefully, wondering if his father was nearby.

A crocodile lying on the bank offered to take him out into the river to see who was drumming. As he sat on the crocodile's back, the boy looked down into the water and saw people dancing to the drums. "Have you seen my father?" the boy asked them.

"No, he's not here," they replied, "but we'll help you. You can have our drums, and you can beat them whenever your father is lost in the forest. Then he'll be able to find his way back to the village."

Traditional dancer

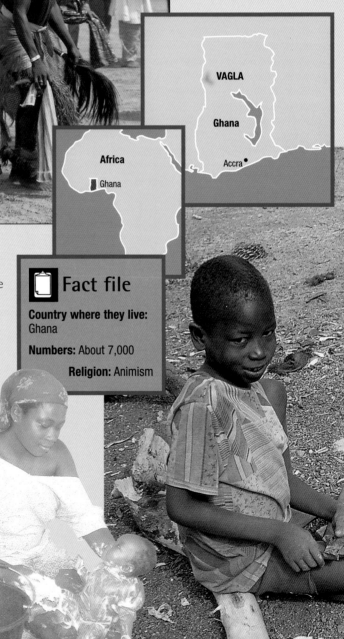

The boy never had to search for his father again. In fact, the drums sent such clear messages over long distances that the village elders began to use them for the whole village.

Communication

A Vagla chief told this fable to encourage young people in his tribe who were learning to read and write in their own language. He wanted them to understand that what they were doing would help the whole tribe – just as the talking drums do.

Vagla people can use drums to send messages because their language is musical. If someone says a word in a high-pitched tone, it means something different from saying it in a low-pitched one. This makes it possible to beat out messages in musical notes so that everyone can understand what is being "said" by the drums.

Wouldn't this be a great way to make God's message clear to the whole tribe!

The god Kiipo

The Vagla people live in northwest Ghana. There are only about 7,000 of them. They worship a god called Kiipo. The priest of Kiipo sacrifices sheep and cattle to this god at a special rock near the village of Sonyo. They hope that, because they do this, Kiipo will give them enough food and keep them safe from enemies and the evil spirits that they believe lurk in the bush. Every village has its own priest to make special sacrifices of chickens to these spirits to keep them from harming anyone.

Rooftop business

A Vagla village is made up of ten or more rectangular houses, each with a courtyard. The houses are

Africa

Ghana

VAGLA

Ghana

Accra

📋 Fact file

Country where they live: Ghana

Numbers: About 7,000

Religion: Animism

all joined together under one roof and this strong flat roof is used as a street. A lot of village life takes place up on the rooftop and Vagla men, wearing colorful cotton garments, meet there to talk business. They have to remember never to sit or stand still on the ladders leading up to the roof because they believe the spirits also climb up and down between the yard and the rooftop.

Vagla Christians

Nearly all Vagla Christians are young men who still work with their fathers on family farms. Since they don't earn any money, they can't give much to pay a pastor's wages. Because their houses are linked together, it's very obvious if someone wants to live or believe in a different way from everyone else. Relatives and village elders often try to force new Christians to take part in the ceremonies and sacrifices to Kiipo.

Translators have finished the Vagla New Testament and are working on the Old

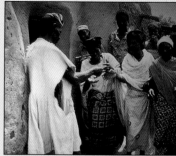

A group of Christians

Testament. Several Vagla Christians have already been to Bible school and have become pastors and evangelists among their own people. Please pray that they will learn how to use fables, proverbs and even the talking drums to make God's message clear to the whole tribe.

Do you know?

Christians are setting Bible songs to Vagla music. One person who works among the Vagla says that there's a song played on seven antelope horns that sounds like a traffic jam! Although their kind of music might sound like just a lot of noise to us, it's very special to the Vagla. And the Vagla might think the music you like to listen to sounds a bit strange, too!

Children on their way to Sunday school

 ## To help you pray for the Vagla

You can thank God for:

- the New Testament that has been translated into Vagla and the work that is well underway on the translation of the Old Testament.

You can ask God:

- to keep young Vagla Christians faithful to him even when their families try to force them to worship Kiipo.

- that as they learn to read the New Testament, Vagla Christians will discover more about his love, power and the way they should live.

- to help Vagla Christians write stories, fables, songs and books which will explain the Christian message to their people.

- to show Vagla Christians just how important it is to teach their children to know Jesus.

- to demonstrate his power to the village elders and priests of Kiipo, so that they will know that he is more powerful than their god or the evil spirits.

- to help Vagla Christians share the good news about Jesus with their friends.

- that Vagla Christians who are helping with the translation of the Old Testament will be enthusiastic and thorough in their work and that the translation will soon be completed.

Children making their own toys

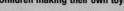

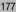

Venezuela

"Little Venice"

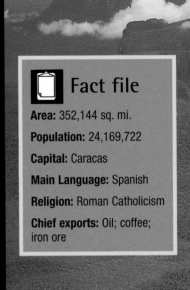

Oil and Indians

"My company's sending me to Venezuela for six months," Jim and Claire's father told them one evening. *"While I'm there, you can all come for a vacation!"* Jim and Claire were so excited, they tried to find out all they could about Venezuela.

Jim found an encyclopedia. *"It says here,"* he said, *"that Venezuela is the most northerly country in South America and has miles of sandy beaches. It also has mountains, plains, tropical jungles and more than 20 national parks."*

Bird of paradise flower

Fact file

Area: 352,144 sq. mi.

Population: 24,169,722

Capital: Caracas

Main Language: Spanish

Religion: Roman Catholicism

Chief exports: Oil; coffee; iron ore

Caracas · Trinidad · Venezuela · Guyana · Colombia · Brazil

Rain forest

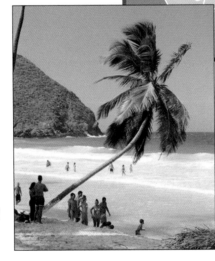

Claire was reading another book. "It also has some of the biggest oil fields in the world," she said. "They're at the north end of Lake Maracaibo. The Goaro Indians, who build their houses on stilts over the water, live nearby. When the first European explorers saw their villages they called the region Venezuela, 'little Venice,' because the Italian city of Venice is also built on water."

"That was a long time ago," Jim added. "It says here that most Venezuelans live in cities now. Some of them are very rich and live in huge houses with bars on the windows, alarm systems and guard dogs to protect them from thieves. But not everyone's rich. A lot of Venezuelans live in cramped houses made of metal, bits of wood and plastic. I wonder if all the children go to school, or just the ones from rich families?"

"This book says that schools are free," Claire said, "and that nearly all the children go to school. Some even start when they're only three years old. But a lot of children from poor families

drop out because their families think it's more important for them to earn a little money than to study."

Missionary to the Indians

Five months later, Jim and Claire were in Caracas, the capital city of Venezuela. One day Jacinto, a Venezuelan missionary, came to visit the family. Jim and Claire had lots of questions for Jacinto. "How did you

Some Venezuelans bargain with dead saints for jobs, health and money

become a missionary?" "Where are you working?" "What do you do?" they wanted to know.

Jacinto smiled. "I learned about Jesus and decided to follow him when I was in college. Then a friend took me to a camp where I met some missionaries working among Indians in this country. The government doesn't usually let missionaries from other countries live among them because they're afraid that they'll bring diseases and harm the Indians. But I could live with them, and I wanted to

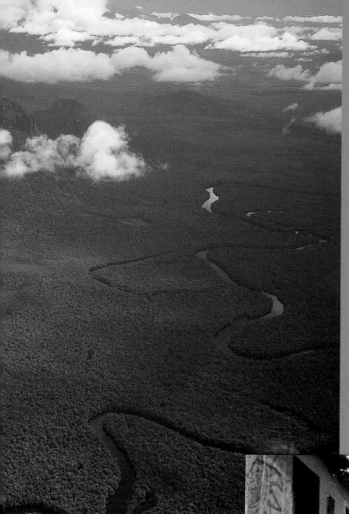

![hand icon] **To help you pray for Venezuela**

You can thank God for:

- the *Jesus* video and its powerful message.

- Christians who go to Indian villages to share the good news about Jesus.

- Venezuelan Christians who go as missionaries to other countries.

You can ask God:

- that many people in Venezuela will decide to follow Jesus.

- that rich people who are Christians will help the poor and support missionaries.

- to help people understand that promises made to dead saints can't help them, but that Jesus is alive and is always ready to help anyone who trusts in him.

- to show people the foolishness and danger of trusting in charms.

Contrasting buildings in Caracas

tell these people more people about Jesus. So now I live in an Indian village in the rain forests in the southwest of the country. I'm just one of the many Venezuelan Christians there. We often use Christian recordings in the different Indian languages to tell people about God's love, and we've translated the New Testament into some of their languages. Some of the Indians are fierce and warlike, but others are peaceable and gentle. A lot of them know nothing of the world beyond their thatched houses, small vegetable plots and the wild pigs, monkeys and plumed birds that live in the forest."

Telling the good news

"That must be a lot different from life in the city," Jim said.

"That's right," Jacinto said. "From the time it was discovered by Christopher Columbus in 1498 until it became independent in 1830, Venezuela belonged to Spain. Because of this, almost everyone believes in God and Jesus. At Easter time people parade through the city streets carrying statues of Jesus on the cross and singing sad songs, but their religion doesn't seem to make a big difference in their lives. Getting a good job, staying healthy and having plenty of money are so important that a lot of people make promises to dead saints to bargain for such things. Others buy charms when they need help – but they rarely work! Not many people really understand who Jesus is, that he died and rose again and helps everyone who trusts in him.

"Some of the churches have started video clubs. There's one really good video, called the *Jesus* film, that shows the life of Jesus. It's a great way of sharing our faith with others and it's such a powerful story that lots of

> **Do you know?**
>
> In southeast Venezuela, the Caroni River rushes down more than 3,000 feet over Mount Auyantepui to form the Angel Falls, the highest waterfall in the world. The hydroelectric power generated by the Caroni River supplies three-quarters of Venezuela's electricity.

people use the prayer at the end of the video to tell Jesus that they want to follow him.

"Even though the evangelical churches in Venezuela are quite small, we're praying that many more people in our own country and around the world will hear the good news about Jesus. Some of us have become missionaries in other countries too, and we know our churches pray for us, asking God to bring lots more people to know Jesus as their friend."

"We'll pray, too!" promised Jim and Claire.

Vietnam

God is Faithful

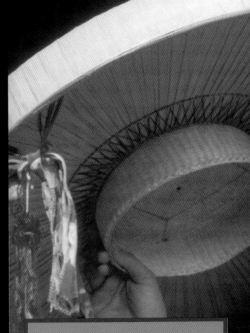

Not afraid!

One by one, and as silently as possible, the montagnard Christians climbed the notched pole into Nai's bamboo and thatch house for the prayer meeting. They knew they would be punished if the agents of the Communist government caught them, but they weren't afraid.

Suddenly, two men burst into the house and grabbed Nai. They marched him away in the darkness, shouting, "You're under arrest. There is no God!" Like shadows, the other Christians slipped away home, wondering who had betrayed them.

Statue of Confucius in a temple in Hanoi

Although the laws of Vietnam say that the people are free to follow whatever religion they choose, the government still persecutes many Christians. Throughout the mountain region of Vietnam thousands of tribal people, or *montagnards*, are becoming Christians. Local government officials have burned their homes and churches and have put many people, even children, in prison. But they haven't been able to make them stop telling others about Jesus.

Vietnamese Christians who live in villages, towns and cities on the coastal plain are sharing the good news of Jesus, too. Pastors who have been put in prison have gone on sharing the good news about Jesus with all the other prisoners – and with their guards as well!

War

France ruled Vietnam from 1858 to 1954. Some Vietnamese people became very rich and lived in magnificent houses in the cities, but most people were poor. Even now, many people in the countryside live in houses made of bamboo and thatch, and some fishermen and their families live on small boats.

The Vietnamese wanted to be free, and in 1954 they defeated the French in a fierce battle. Vietnam was divided into two parts: the

Do you know?

Vietnam is a long, narrow country in southeast Asia. Look at the map and the picture to the right to see if you understand what the Vietnamese mean when they say it looks like a bamboo carrying pole with a basket of rice hanging from each end. The two areas that look like baskets are the Red River Delta in the north and the Mekong Delta in the south. These are the most fertile parts of the country, where they grow most of their rice.

Most westerners find it difficult to learn to speak Vietnamese. This is because there are six tones in the language and the same word can be said six different ways, each with a different meaning. So the word *ma* can mean but, mother, ghost, tomb, a young rice plant or a horse – all depending on the tone!

North, which was under Communist rule, and the "free" South.

The Communists wanted to control the South as well, and they sent guerrilla soldiers to force the people to follow them. America started to help the South, and the North fought

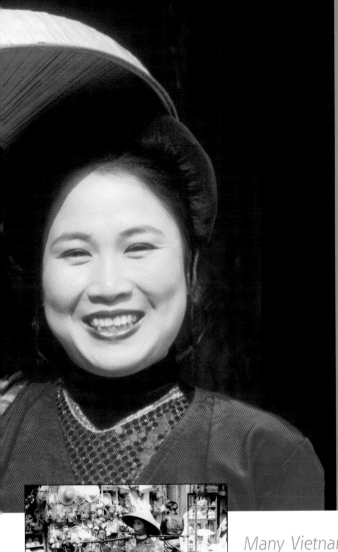

To help you pray for Vietnam

You can thank God for:

- Christians who have followed Jesus faithfully even when they have been persecuted or put in prison.

- the many tribal people living in the mountain areas who are coming to know Jesus and are sharing his love with others.

You can ask God:

- that every tribal group in Vietnam will hear that when Jesus died on the cross, he was the perfect sacrifice for sins and that the sacrifices they make to the spirits will never take away their sins.

- to help boys and girls, as well as grown-ups, talk about Jesus with their friends and families.

- to make it possible for every Christian family to have a Bible.

- that the students who are allowed to study in Bible school will become faithful evangelists and pastors.

- for real peace and freedom so that all the people of Vietnam can worship him without fear of punishment.

Many Vietnamese Christians have suffered for their faith, but the church keeps growing

Carrying vegetables in traditional baskets

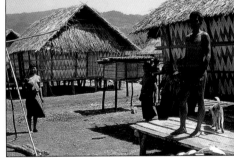

Tribal houses

Fact file

Area: 127,250 sq. mi. (slightly larger than Germany, but it's a long, narrow country)

Population: 79,831,650

Capital: Hanoi

Religions: Buddhism; animism (tribal); Christianity

Language: Vietnamese, but 88 languages are spoken

Chief exports: Oil; fish; rice

Good News
Before the French came to Vietnam, missionaries had started to teach the Vietnamese about Jesus. There were Vietnamese and tribal Christians in towns and villages throughout the land. Their churches are called "Good News" churches. In 1994, the Vietnamese government gave permission for Bibles to be printed again and for a few Christians to be trained as pastors and evangelists.

back. Many people died in this terrible war which ended in 1975 when the government of South Vietnam was overthrown. Once again, North and South Vietnam became one country.

Foreigners, including most missionaries, fled the country. Thousands of South Vietnamese, who were afraid the Communists would treat them badly, tried to escape. Some reached safety and have gone to live in many countries around the world.

Changes
After the war, Christian businessmen and aid organizations went to Vietnam to show the people they were not forgotten. Vietnamese Christians in other countries are going back to Vietnam to help those in need. It's a very beautiful country and is becoming popular with tourists once again.

Although many Christians have suffered for their faith under Communism, the church keeps on growing.

Wodaabe

Beautiful Nomads of the Sahel

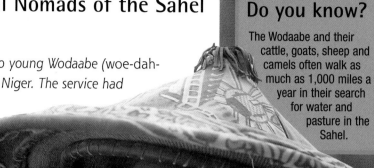

Teach us about Jesus!

One Sunday morning in 1989, two young Wodaabe (woe-dah-bee) men walked into a church in Niger. The service had already started, but they walked right up to the front. Everyone wondered what would happen next. The men looked very poor. Had they come to ask for food? When they reached the front of the church, they turned around. "Will you show us how to follow the Christian way?" they asked. "We want you to teach us and our children about Jesus!"

The people in the church were so excited! Missionaries went with the two men back to their camp and taught the men, their wives and children about Jesus. Some, like the two men, decided to follow Jesus. Now they're telling others about Jesus because they want them to know that Jesus gives joy and hope – especially when life is hard.

Always on the move

And life is often very hard for the Wodaabe. They live in the Sahel, in Niger and Chad. The Wodaabe are nomads, traveling from place to place with their camels, cattle, sheep and goats. During the long dry season, the men often have to walk five hours a day to find water and pasture. When they move their camp, they pack all their

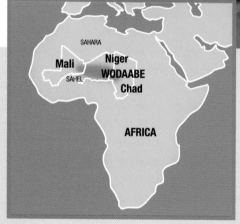

belongings on the backs of their camels. "We're like birds in a bush," a village elder explained. "We never settle down, and we leave no trace of where we've been."

Their food is very simple. They eat porridge made from millet, but milk is the most important part of their diet. If the animals don't have enough food, they become weak and have no milk. Then the people become very hungry and sick. When there's no rain

for several years, the cattle die and the people starve.

Wodaabe taboos

The Wodaabe have many taboos, or things they aren't allowed to do. Some of these might seem strange to us. Wodaabe means "the people of the taboo." How would you feel if you didn't have a name until you were 12 years old? Or if your mother was never allowed to talk to you or call you by name because you were the oldest child in your family?

Wodaabe men parade in an all-male beauty contest

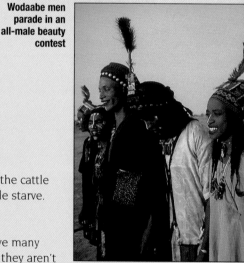

We're taught to look people in the eyes when we talk to them, but the Wodaabe are forbidden to do this. These are just a few of the many taboos that control their lives.

182

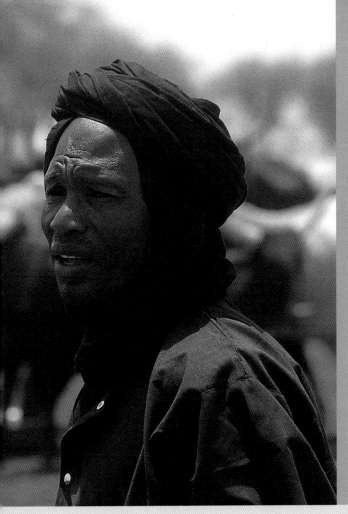

To help you pray for the Wodaabe

You can thank God for:

- each Wodaabe Christian.
- Wodaabe believers in Bible school who want to teach their people about Jesus.

You can ask God:

- that whole families will decide to follow Jesus so they can worship together and help each other as they live and move as a group.
- to help the Wodaabe realize that taboos don't have to control their lives.
- to bring more missionaries to the Wodaabe, and help them as they learn the Wodaabe Fulfulde language.
- to help Wodaabe Christians as they change parts of their culture that aren't pleasing to Jesus.
- that people will see the beauty of Jesus in the lives of believers and will want to follow him too.

Fact file

Countries: Niger; Chad; Mali

Numbers: About 100,000

Language: Wodaabe Fulfulde

Religion: Folk Islam

Occupation: Nomadic herders

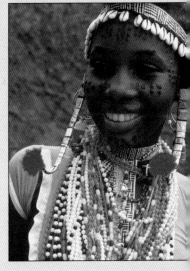

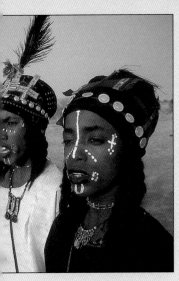

Beauty – inside and out

The Wodaabe think they're the most beautiful people on earth. Every year they hold special celebrations to show off their good looks. Like the other young men, Jebbi wanted to look really handsome on the day of the festival. So he rubbed yellow powder into his skin to make it look lighter. Then he tried to make his eyes and lips look bigger by drawing around them with a black substance called *kohl*. Since a high forehead is a sign of great beauty, he shaved the hair from the front of his head. Finally, he painted a line down his nose to make it look longer. He wanted to be sure he had done everything he could to make himself beautiful, so he hung some little bags of magic powder around his neck. After putting on his lovely hand-embroidered robe, turban, and copper and brass jewelry hung with beads and cowrie shells, he was ready to dance with the other men before their admiring audience.

Like all the Wodaabe, Jebbi wants to be beautiful on the outside. But while we only see what people are like on the outside, God looks at our hearts. He wants us to ask Jesus for forgiveness for all the wrong things we've done. Only then can our hearts be clean and pure and beautiful to him.

Following the nomads

How can you teach people to follow Jesus if they're always moving from place to place? More than 100 Wodaabe people have decided to follow Jesus, and they want others to know him, too. A few have become evangelists, and they move from camp to camp telling people about Jesus. Others are at Bible

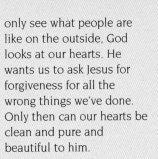

school, learning more about Jesus and how to teach their people. Missionaries and evangelists are praying that whole families will come to know Jesus so that they can learn about Jesus together and encourage one another, especially when life is difficult.

Xhosa

Red-Blanket People of the Transkei

Jill, a missionary in South Africa, made friends with many Xhosa (koh'-suh) children. Here are a few stories she told about some of those she met.

God changes a whole family

Zawa and Sikhono were brothers from a big family in Johannesburg. One day a friend took them to a special meeting for children. At this meeting, they heard for the first time that God loves them. They decided to follow Jesus, and a few weeks later they went to a children's camp to learn more about Jesus.

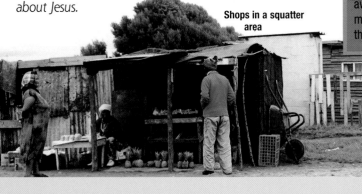

Shops in a squatter area

They had lots of fun at the camp, but they liked the Bible talks the best. They had never realized how special they were to God. When they went home, they talked constantly about all the fun they'd had and all the exciting things they'd learned. Their alcoholic father and tired, overworked mother could hardly believe all that Zawa and Sikhono told them about the way God is always ready to help people who

trust in him.

A few months later, Jill showed a video of the camp at Zawa's and Sikhono's school. When it was over, their father jumped up to say he'd started to go to church because of what his sons had told him. He said he was so happy with God in his life that he didn't want to drink alcohol any more and was giving his wife enough money

to care for the family. Their mother told everyone that Jesus had changed her sons and her husband so much that she, too, had become a Christian. God used two brothers to bring the entire family to follow Jesus, and to change their lives completely!

"Leave me alone, Satan!"

Daniel, a Xhosa boy who lives in the city of Pretoria, decided to follow Jesus at an evangelistic meeting in a big tent. When Jill met him a few days later, he didn't look very happy.

"What's wrong?" she asked him.

"I'm very angry with Satan," he

Do you know?

To speak the Xhosa language, you need to make click sounds by pulling your tongue sharply away from the roof of your mouth or from the teeth at the side of your mouth.

Botswana
Johannesburg
Namibia
XHOSA
Lesotho
South Africa
XHOSA
Cape Town

📋 Fact file

Country: South Africa

Numbers: About 7,500,000

Religions: Christianity; African traditional religions

Languages: Xhosa; English; Afrikaans

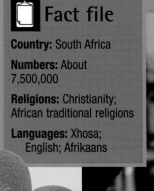

said. "I was just in a store, and Satan told me to steal like I used to."

"Did you?"

"No! But I can't believe he's bothering me like that," he replied. Daniel was very wise, because he realized that Satan was his enemy. He also knew that God would help him to be stronger than Satan.

A bad boy

Bhekinkosi was one of the naughtiest boys in Gugulethu, a poor part of Cape Town. Sometimes he even jumped on the back of moving vans for free rides, but since he was crippled in one leg and couldn't run very fast, angry drivers often caught and beat him. But when he went to a Christian meeting, Bhekinkosi was very serious when he realized how bad he had been. He wanted to be good. Tears were rolling down his face when he prayed, "Lord Jesus, it is I, Bhekinkosi. I'm a bad boy. Please make my heart clean and come and live in me forever."

Life in a township

Most of the seven million Xhosa people live in the Eastern and Western Cape provinces of South Africa. Some of them have been to university and have become teachers, lawyers, businessmen and government officials. Many others are poor and have never been to school. Lots of them live in townships on the edges of big cities where they work as servants or in factories. Others work in the gold or diamond mines, but some have no work at all.

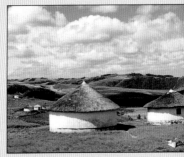

Village life

Life is quite different in Xhosa villages. Families live in beautiful round huts with a fireplace in the center and mud benches built against the walls. Village children work hard. They often have to walk for miles to get water, firewood and food, and little boys know how to look after big herds of cattle. Village women wear black turbans and red blankets, which they dye themselves. They always wear the red blankets when they worship their ancestors. Even though more than half of the Xhosa people say they are Christians, some of them still practice their old traditions as well.

Jill loved to listen to the Xhosa people singing. Even small village schools have choirs. "I'll always remember dancing and singing with some Xhosa Christians on the mountainside at night," she said. "They sang, 'This Jesus of mine, he has power.' I pray that God's power will work in the lives of many Xhosa people."

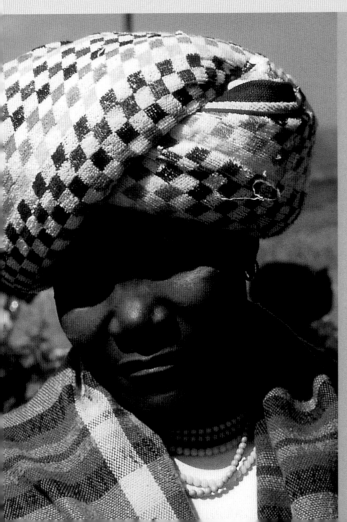

 To help you pray for the Xhosa

You can thank God for:

- every Xhosa who has come to know Jesus as their savior and friend.
- the modern translation of the Bible in Xhosa.
- Xhosa Christians who are part of the new government in South Africa.
- getting rid of the terrible law that separated people of different colors and races in South Africa.

You can ask God:

- to help Xhosa Christians who run Bible camps and Sunday schools, that lots of Xhosa children will be excited as they learn that Jesus loves and cares for them.
- to encourage Xhosa Christians to write Bible songs in their own language.
- that Xhosa Christians will always be ready to share Jesus' love with others.

Xinjiang

Along the Silk Road

Go in but never come out ...

The Takli-Makan (tah-klah mah-kahn) Desert is one of the loneliest and most desolate places on earth. Fierce winds often howl across its huge sand dunes and rocky outcrops, whipping up whirling clouds of sand. In winter it's freezing cold and in summer it's scorching hot and there's almost no water to be found. It's no wonder it's called "the go in but never come out" desert, for that is what its name means. Yet it's an area rich in minerals such as coal, gas, oil, gold and gems, and a number of companies are developing the outer edges of the desert to mine these resources.

Do you know?

The great Chinese inventions of silk, gunpowder, paper making and printing were all carried along the ancient Silk Road, through Xinjiang, to the west.
Nestorian Christians traveled east along this route in the fifth century AD and Buddhism and Islam came to China along this road.

On the way to market

Fact file

Xinjiang is a self-governing region of China

Area: 127,400 sq. mi.

Population: 16,610,000 (60% of the population belong to the nine Muslim peoples of the region. These include Uyghurs, Kazakhs, Kyrgyz, Hui and Tajiks.)

Main city: Urumchi

Products: Silk; cotton; fruit; oil; gas

This huge desert, which is almost as big as Germany, is in Xinjiang (*sin-chi-ang*) in northwest China. But not all Xinjiang is desert. Xinjiang is surrounded by spectacular mountain ranges. Water from these mountains feeds the broad pasture lands for sheep and herds of cattle and horses. There are fertile oases, too, where fruit and vegetables grow in abundance.

Muslims and Christians

Let's visit a Uyghur family in the south of Xinjiang. The family gives us a warm welcome to their flat-roofed home built inside a courtyard. Soon we're nibbling sunflower seeds and drinking tea. As we talk, they tell us, "More than half the people living in Xinjiang are Muslims, and the Uyghur are the largest of the nine Muslim groups living here. The Communist government tried to get rid of all religions, but many Muslims in Xinjiang remained faithful to their beliefs and continued to pray five times a day. The government has a different attitude now and has even given money to rebuild mosques, open an Islamic college and print Muslim books. We're very grateful to Allah."

We ask if there are any Christians in Xinjiang. "Oh, yes, my grandmother told me that about 100 years ago some Uyghurs did become Christians. Most of them were killed or fled to other countries during a time of persecution and violence. I don't think there are any Uyghur Christians now, though. Of course, there are a lot of Christians among the Han Chinese who have been sent here by the government to try to control Xinjiang. Sometimes they try

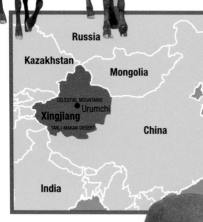

Veiled Uyghur women

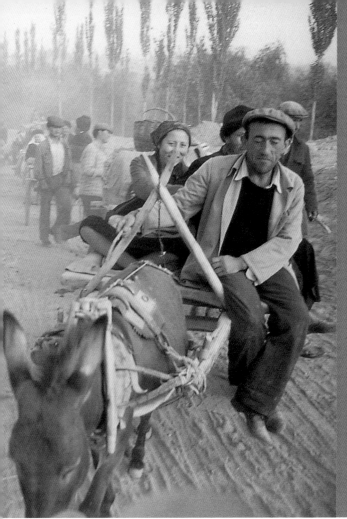

To help you pray for Xinjiang

You can thank God for:

- Christians who have gone to work in Xinjiang so they can share the good news of Jesus' love with the people living there.
- the few Uyghurs who have started to follow Jesus.

You can ask God:

- to break down the barriers of fear, hatred and suspicion between the Muslim peoples of Xinjiang and the Han Chinese.
- that Chinese Christians working in Xinjiang will have courage to share his love with their Muslim neighbors.
- to help Christians who have come from other countries to learn the languages of the local peoples so that they can share with them who Jesus is and why he died.
- that his Holy Spirit will help each Uyghur Christian to read the New Testament, and understand what it means to be a follower of Jesus.
- that many people will tune in to the Christian radio broadcasts in Uyghur and other languages spoken in Xinjiang.

to tell us about the love of someone called Jesus who, they say, is God's Son. But why should we listen to them? After all, they've been sent here to control us!"

A Sunday market

At the western edge of the Takli-Makan Desert is the ancient mud-walled city of Kashgar. Every Sunday morning, Ayshem and her brother Aziz load their flat donkey-cart with fruit and vegetables to take to the market in Kashgar. People come from far and wide, on bicycles, motorcycles, tractors and donkey-carts to sell their produce and buy things to take home.

As soon as they arrive at the friendly, busy, noisy market place, Ayshem and Aziz set out their vegetables on the ground. There's plenty to buy: fruit and vegetables, flowers, knives, Atlas silk cloth, blankets, nan bread, chickens, horses and even camels. Everyone wants a bargain!

Leaving her brother to sell their vegetables, Ayshem wanders off to meet her friends. She's wearing a colorful, knee-length dress, long trousers and embroidered cap. Her long black hair is neatly plaited. She's glad she doesn't have to wear a heavy brown veil like some of the women. The open-air theater is their favorite place in the market. They watch skilled acrobats, dancers and conjurers perform. When Aziz's turn comes to join his friends, he goes to watch the horses as they race along a track.

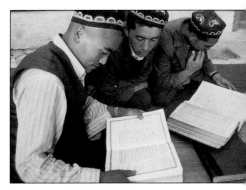

Young men studying the Koran

The Silk Road

Marco Polo, the famous thirteenth-century traveler, passed through Xinjiang along the Silk Road, an ancient trade route that connected Europe and the Middle East with China. Two friars went with him to teach the people the Christian faith. Only a few people have gone to Xinjiang to tell the people about the love of God. Today there are Christians working in Xinjiang, as well as Christian tourists traveling the Silk Road.

Yanomamo

The Children of the Moon

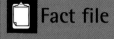
Fact file

Countries: Southern Venezuela; northwest Brazil

Numbers: About 23,000; there are probably 15,000 in Venezuela

Religion: Animism

Occupations: Farming; hunting

Fierce ...

The Yanomamo live deep in the rain forests of South America, in a region called Amazonia on the borders of northwestern Brazil and southern Venezuela. One of their legends says that long ago one of the first living creatures on earth shot the moon with an arrow. The blood of the moon fell to the earth and turned into the first people – the Yanomamo, "Children of the Moon."

Since they were born as a result of this battle with the moon, they call themselves the Fierce People.

The Yanomamo live up to this name. Villages are always fighting other villages, and people are always fighting each other, too. When they're raiding another village, the Yanomamo men cover themselves with charcoal and poison the tips of their arrows.

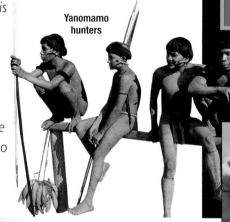

Yanomamo hunters

... but afraid

Although they're fierce, the Yanomamo are afraid of a lot of things: their enemies; evil spirits hiding in the jungle, in the water or the dark; the jaguar living in the forest. They're even afraid to point at the moon in case their fingers rot and fall off.

The medicine man asks the spirits to guard them and to give them help when anyone is sick. He also asks the spirits to hurt their enemies.

Not worth much

Since she learned to walk, Little Girl (she doesn't have a name) went out with her mother to get firewood in a small basket on her back. She was always tired and her legs hurt, but no one noticed. Some girl babies are killed as soon as they're born. Little girls aren't worth much to the Yanomamo.

One day, when she was only four years old, a man from another village asked Little Girl's father if he could have her to be his wife. In exchange, he gave her father a dog. Now Little Girl has to look after the men in her new family, gather the firewood, cook and work in the gardens. She has to work hard, and she's often hungry.

Living in one big house

A Yanomamo village is really like one big circular house with a big courtyard in the middle, and is called a *shabano*. Each family collects trees, vines and thatch from the jungle to help build the *shabano* and cover the roof of their own section. The outside wall of the *shabano* separates the village from the jungle, but there aren't any inside walls. If a Yanomamo person sees that someone

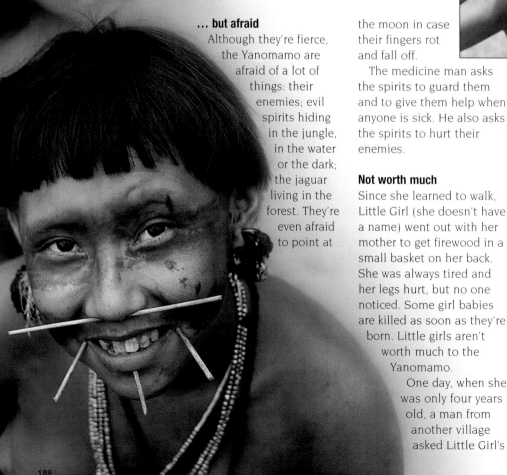

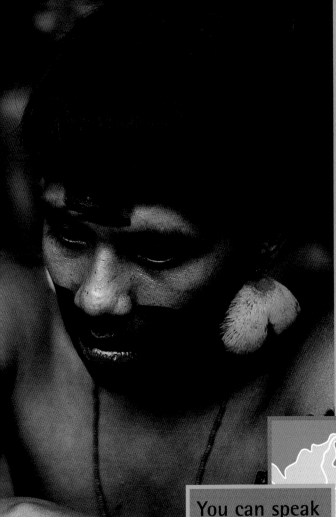

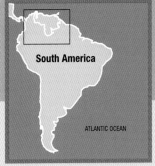
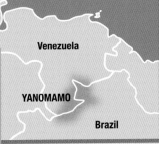

Venezuela

YANOMAMO

Brazil

South America

ATLANTIC OCEAN

You can speak Yanomamo

Where are you going? is "Wedi hami wa huu?"
(we-di ha-mi wa **huu**)

Did you arrive? is "Wa walokei kufawa?"
(wa **wa**-lo-ke ku-fa-wa)

Are you healthy? is "Wa demi tawa?"
(wa **de**-mi ta-wa)

else doesn't want to be disturbed, he acts like a "ghost" (like he's not really there!) to give the other person privacy. People get in and out of the village through little holes left in the outside wall.

Outside the village, the Yanomamo cut down the jungle to make fields for their manioc, plantains, bananas, gourds and sweet potatoes. The men hunt wild pigs, tapir, armadillo and monkeys in the jungle for meat while the women work in the fields.

Help for the Yanomamo

Until the 1940s the Yanomamo didn't have much contact with the outside world, but when they did, a lot of them died from catching "white man's" diseases. More than 1,000 Yanomamo died in the

1980s when mercury, which was used by illegal miners to find gold, poisoned their rivers. Since then, both Brazil and Venezuela have set aside huge areas of the rain forest especially for the Yanomamo so that other people can't hurt them.

When the New Tribes Mission came in 1950 to tell the Yanomamo about Jesus, they found many people who were sick. The missionaries helped them, prayed with them and learned all they could

about them. They also wrote down the difficult Yanomamo language, and now there's a Yanomamo New Testament. At first, only a few Yanomamo people seemed interested in hearing about God, the Great Spirit, who loves them. But God is changing lives, and now there are about 300 Yanomamo Christians in Venezuela and more than 100 in Brazil. Some Yanomamo

Christians are being trained to teach the people in their villages to read and write, and they'll also be part of the government's program to help the Yanomamo. Other Yanomamo, like Maloco, want to tell others about Jesus. He was only eight years old when he decided to follow Jesus. "Don't laugh at me because I'm small," he said. "I want to tell everybody about Jesus."

In a *shabano*

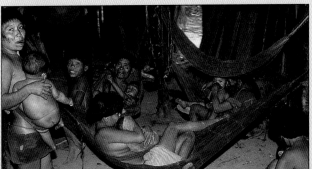

Yao-Mien

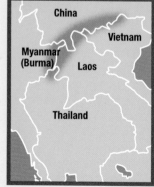

Children of the Dragon-dog

A tribal legend

A strange creature, half-dragon, half-dog, returned from his long journey across the seas. He had killed the enemy of the emperor of China, and now he had come to claim the promised reward, the emperor's beautiful daughter. They had six fine sons and six lovely daughters who, the legend says, were the first ancestors of the Yao.

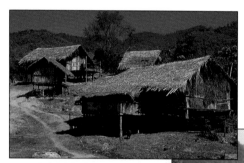

Mountain village

Working in a paddy field

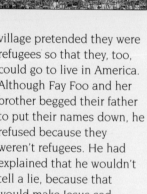

Mountain homes

"Yao" really refers to a number of different tribal groups, each with its own name, that live high up in the mountains of northern Thailand, Laos, Vietnam and southern China. One of these groups is the Yao-Mien.

Let's visit one of their villages in north Thailand. Most of the houses are built from wood, but the poorer families live in houses with bamboo walls, grass roofs and dirt floors. The villagers keep pigs and chickens. We might even see a water buffalo plowing a rice paddy field. The Yao-Mien grow mountain rice and other crops like maize, soya beans and peanuts in fields on the hillsides. The government doesn't allow them to grow opium anymore (although a few people still smoke it).

Sadly, some teenagers have given in to peer pressure from their Thai school friends to take drugs.

A heavenly home

Fay Foo comes to meet us. She is wearing beautifully embroidered clothes and a black turban with a red, fluffy collar around her neck. About ten years ago, refugees from the country of Laos came to stay in their village. Thai officials said that any refugee who wanted to live in America should go to the nearby refugee center. Everyone in the village was excited, and about 80 families from her

village pretended they were refugees so that they, too, could go to live in America. Although Fay Foo and her brother begged their father to put their names down, he refused because they weren't refugees. He had explained that he wouldn't tell a lie, because that would make Jesus sad.

"When we followed the spirits, we thought the most important things in life were money, our fields and our feasts," he said. "When we first left the spirits and did Christian things, the change was only on the outside. Later, we realized that Jesus wanted a change deep

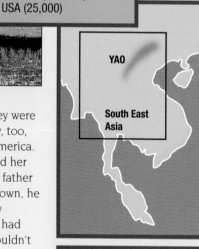

YAO

South East Asia

China
Vietnam
Myanmar (Burma)
Laos
Thailand

190

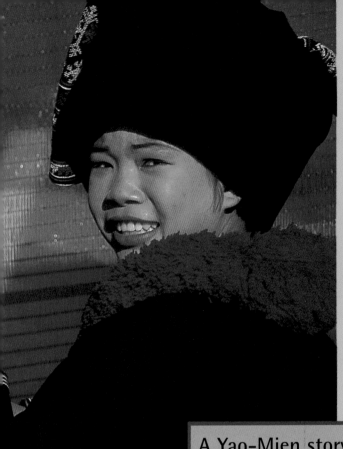

To help you pray for the Yao-Mien

You can thank God for:

● the *Jesus* film.

● the Old Testament translation team.

You can ask God:

● that many people will listen to the Christian radio programs.

● that people will learn to follow Jesus at the new center in Thailand.

● that those who have studied at Bible school will help people understand the Bible.

● for many people to share the good news about Jesus with the Yao-Mien people.

● that Christians will help and encourage Yao people wherever they live.

A Yao-Mien story

Welcoming visitors is very important in Yao-Mien culture. This little story describes the reward of being kind even to a visitor who is unwelcome.

One day, a big snake came to visit two sisters. The older sister refused to invite the snake into the house. She wouldn't give it a seat to sit on, water to wash in, a bed to lie on, or food to eat. The younger sister, however, welcomed the snake and gave it everything it needed. During the night, she discovered the snake was really a handsome prince in disguise.

You can guess the rest of the story!

inside our hearts." He reminded them that Jesus had promised them a home in heaven that was a thousand times more wonderful than America.

It was true – there was a difference between the Christians and the animists in Fay Foo's village. The Christians no longer worshipped the spirits when they were sick. Instead, they prayed to God in Jesus' name. They were always ready to help others and pray for them. Many of the Christians who had never been to school had learned to read so that they could sing songs from the hymnbook and read the New Testament.

Fay Foo is excited that the *Jesus* film is being translated into the Yao-Mien language. She's sure that it will bring many of her people to follow Jesus. She's excited, too, that most of the Old Testament has been translated into her language. Soon the Yao-Mien will have the whole Bible in their language.

Reaching out

The Yao-Mien Christians have saved money to buy a large plot of land in northern Thailand. They plan to build a conference center there, a radio-recording studio and a hostel for the children who have to leave their village homes high up in the mountains to study at high schools in town. The Christians want the hostel to be a happy place where the children will learn to love Jesus and to share his love with their friends.

The Yao-Mien living in other countries are able to listen to Christian radio broadcasts, and some have become Christians and are learning more about Jesus. Some Yao-Mien in America are praying about becoming missionaries to their own people in South East Asia.

Yemen

Land of the Queen of Sheba

An ancient land

Do you remember the Bible story of the Queen of Sheba? In the Old Testament, in the book of 1 Kings 10:1–13, you can read about how she and King Solomon gave each other amazingly expensive gifts. The Queen of Sheba probably came from what is now the Arabian land of Yemen, and the great cities of her kingdom are buried beneath the desert sands. More than 1,500 years after the Queen of Sheba lived, Yemen became a Muslim country.

Curved daggers form part of the traditional dress of Yemen

📋 Fact file

Area: 203,850 sq. mi.

Population: 18,112,066

Capital: Sana'a

Language: Arabic

Religion: Islam

Chief exports: Oil products; cotton; fish

Do you know?

In many parts of Yemen, the mountainsides are terraced to make extra fields where crops can be grown. Some of these terraced fields are more than a thousand years old.

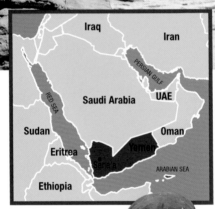

The palace on the rock of Wadi Dhahr

Yemen, at the southern tip of the Arabian Peninsula, was once thought to be one of the most mysterious countries in the world since few people were ever allowed to visit it. It is a beautiful place, with rugged mountain peaks and steep valleys, colorful markets and beautifully decorated houses which are often six or seven storeys high and made of mud. Most of the people in Yemen belong to tribal groups, each with its own leader. There are strong family ties in each tribe and often several generations of one family will all live in the same house.

The country's most important export used to be frankincense, but now it is oil.

Dinner guests

Wearing his white turban and *zanna* (ankle-length cotton tunic), Gadeed watched closely as his father greeted his guests. The Europeans were interested in everything: the mud-walled pen where the goats were tethered, the room storing grain from the harvest, even his sister making bread.

Gadeed also watched as his sister kneaded the dough and slapped it against the sides of the mud oven. A fire blazed at the bottom of the oven, and, unless she was very careful, the flat bread could easily slip off the side into the fire. Later, sitting together on the floor, the men ate chicken, rice and vegetables. Gadeed carefully poured the coffee. After the meal, his father would show the guests his new water pump and vineyard.

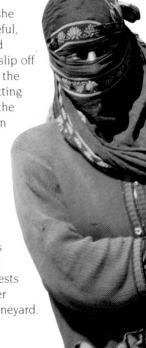

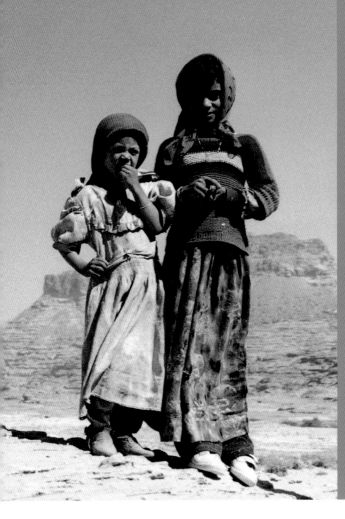

 To help you pray for Yemen

You can thank God for:

- the few Yemeni Christians.
- Christians from other countries who live and work in Yemen.
- the Christian radio broadcasts that are beamed into Yemen.

You can ask God:

- to safeguard the letters that listeners send to the Christian broadcasting company from being opened by Yemeni officials and that the Christian literature sent back to them arrives safely.
- to bring whole families to know and love him so that they can help one another to follow Jesus.
- that as Yemenis read the Koran they will notice what it says about Jesus and will want to find out more about him.
- to use Bibles in Arabic, which are quietly given to Yemenis who ask, to help them understand that the true way to know God is through trusting in Jesus alone.

First, however, Gadeed's father placed a copy of the Koran on a special stand and then read aloud several passages about Isa (the Muslim name for Jesus). Gadeed was sorry when his father put the Koran away and the guests talked about other things: gold, silk and carpets in the souk (market), decorated glass windows and curved daggers.

Suddenly a booming noise from the nearby mosque made the guests jump. Through a loudspeaker, a voice was calling people to prayer. The guests looked around at their Muslim hosts and wished they could tell the veiled women and fierce-looking men that Jesus really is the Son of God, who offers them complete forgiveness and a new life.

North and South

For many years, North and South Yemen were separate countries. South Yemen was Communist, while North Yemen, made up of warring tribes, was strongly Muslim. Then, in 1990, the two countries became one, with Sana'a as its capital. The president wants to unite his 18 million people, but there are many problems and differences between the people.

For a long time, Christians have tried to talk to people in Yemen about Jesus. It's hard because Muslims are proud of their religion and all Yemenis are expected to be Muslims. Because families are very close, it would be unthinkable for one member of the

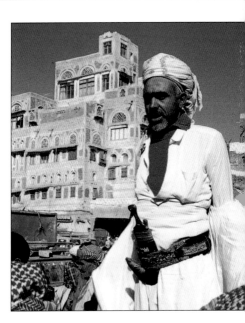

family to choose another religion. Such a person is considered a traitor who deserves to die. There are a few Yemeni Christians. Unfortunately, most Muslims think all foreigners are Christians. So when they see the terrible things people do on foreign TV shows, they have a bad impression of what Christians are like.

Yemenis are Muslims, and they think a person who chooses another religion is a traitor

193

Zimbabwe

Promises and Poverty

Forgiven!

Stephen Lungi couldn't believe his ears. The preacher said, "Some people are so mixed up inside, they'll even kick paraffin stoves!" How did the preacher know that he'd been so mad when his stove wouldn't light that morning that he'd kicked it right across the floor?

Stephen and his friends had gone to the meeting to make trouble. Instead, he was surprised to find that Jesus was real, and that he had to ask him to forgive his sins and change his heart. And what a change there had to be!

When Stephen was a little boy, his mother had left. He stayed with his grandmother, but she was so poor he'd had to scavenge for food. He hated his mother for what she had done to him. But when God forgave him, Stephen knew that he had to forgive his mother as well. One day Stephen did meet his mother again, and he told her how God had helped him to forgive her. She was so sorry for what she'd done, and Stephen helped her to trust in Jesus.

Do you know?

Almost half the population of Zimbabwe is under 15 years of age, and about 600,000 children are orphans. Many of their parents have died from AIDS.

Fact file

Area: 150,804 sq. mi.

Population: 11,669,029

Capital: Harare

Official language: English

Religions: Christianity; traditional religions

Chief exports: Tobacco; gold; nickel; steel; iron alloys

them for teasing him, and he's helping them to improve their farms. "God loves them as much he loves me," he says, "so I can show them his love by helping them."

Christians in Zimbabwe are praying for a new beginning in their country

Helping others

Like Stephen and his mother, a lot of Zimbabweans are finding that Jesus is the friend who is always ready to help them. Some have become strong Christians through the work of organizations like Scripture Union, who meet in schools and run camps for young people. Others are learning to follow Jesus in their churches and through Christian friends.

When Macmillan went to agricultural college, his friends laughed at him. "You're wasting your father's money," they told him. They don't laugh at him any more, because Macmillan's crops always grow better. But Macmillan has forgiven

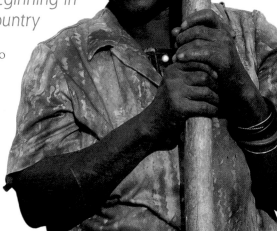

194

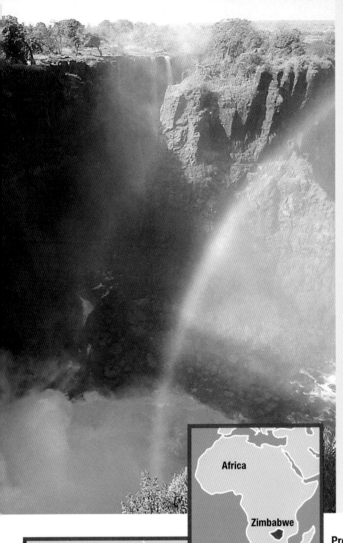

To help you pray for Zimbabwe

You can thank God for:

- every Christian in Zimbabwe.

- Christians who help the poor and care for those who are sick, unemployed or orphans.

You can ask God:

- that he will be with missionaries, evangelists and church workers as they tell others the good news about Jesus.

- that Christians will reach out to the many orphans, giving them love, care and hope in Jesus.

- to give Christians hope and courage to trust him even when they are sick, homeless or have no money.

- to use Christian books, leaflets, radio and TV programs to help Zimbabweans learn more about Jesus.

- for wise leaders who will do what's best for their country and the people.

Africa

Zimbabwe

Victoria Falls

Lioness

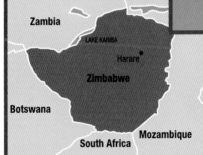

Zambia
LAKE KARIBA
Harare
Zimbabwe
Botswana
Mozambique
South Africa

The smoke that thunders

Some parts of Zimbabwe are quite spectacular. The Zambezi River in the west, which forms the border with Zambia, cascades over the Victoria Falls. There's so much spray and noise that local people call the Falls "the smoke that thunders." Further east, the Zambezi has been dammed to form Lake Kariba. It's one of the largest man-made lakes in the world and provides enough hydroelectric power for both Zambia and Zimbabwe. Zimbabwe's national parks are full of elephants, lions, cheetahs, hyenas and rhinos.

Promises not kept

But Zimbabwe has many problems, and fewer people go there now as tourists. White people ruled Zimbabwe for almost the entire twentieth century. They became wealthy from mining gold and nickel, and some of them owned huge farms. They employed Africans to work in the mines and on the farms. In 1980, after years of fighting, the country gained independence and Africans became the new leaders. The new government promised the people land of their own to farm. The government has divided up some of the big farms, where crops like tobacco used to be grown for sale, and given Africans plots of lands. But the plots are small, and a lot of farmers barely manage to grow enough food for their families to eat. Then, in the year 2000, groups of thugs forced some of the remaining white farmers from their land and destroyed their homes. There are huge areas of land that aren't being used because no one helps poor farmers to settle or learn how to use the land properly. In the towns, too, there is a lot of unemployment and young people find it very hard to get work. Another big problem in Zimbabwe is AIDS, which kills many people – and their children become orphans.

Jesus is our friend

Despite all of these problems, there are Zimbabweans like Stephen and Macmillan who have come to know Jesus and are helping others. They know that Jesus really is alive and ready to help them when they are poor, sick, lonely and afraid. And Christians in Zimbabwe are praying for a new beginning in their country that will bring hope to their people. They want a government that will rule wisely so their country will be a place where everyone has enough and where people can forgive each other for wrong things done in the past.

Zulus

Mighty Warriors of South Africa

Life is changing

The Zulus are famous for their great armies of well-disciplined, highly trained men. They call these armies impis. The Zulu impi is the only African army that has ever defeated the British army. The Zulus still have a king and a royal family, but the glory of their past is now only a memory. The Zulu way of life is changing, and they don't hold their great feasts and ceremonies very often anymore. A lot of Zulu men have left their families and homesteads in the countryside and gone to South Africa's mines and cities to earn a living. Whole families, too, sometimes go to live in townships on the edge of the cities.

Many Zulus call themselves Christians, but a lot of them still worship their ancestors and practice witchcraft. Sadly, even some churches mix up spirit worship with the Christian message.

Most mothers carry their babies on their backs. This little girl learns about rhythm as her mother moves to the music in a church service.

Fact file

Country: South Africa

Numbers: About 8,500,000

Religions: Christianity; African traditional religions

Language: Zulu, also English and Afrikaans

South Africa

ZULUS
Natal

Lesotho

Durban

Africa

Zulu stories

A lady called Jill Johnstone met many children all over the world who didn't know Jesus. She wrote the book *You Can Change the World* because she knew that God would use the prayers of children like you to change the world. She was right! Here are some stories about Zulus she met in South Africa during a week of meetings, held in a big tent, to tell Zulu people about Jesus.

A brave singer

It was cold in the mission tent in Natal, South Africa. Thandiwe, a young Zulu girl, came up to the platform to sing. She was wearing her father's jacket, which nearly touched the floor, with the sleeves rolled up. But she sang bravely into the microphone, her small face shining with happiness.

Jill looked around at all the children singing with such excitement and was so glad to be here as a missionary in Africa. Ever since she was four years old, Jill had wanted to tell African children about Jesus.

After Thandiwe and the other children sang that night, God did some wonderful things! Before long, over 30 Zulu children loved Jesus so much that they started telling everyone they met about him.

Risking his life for Jesus

Beaumont was on his way to the store, thinking about what he would steal this time. Maybe some food? Or a knife? Or something to play with? Then he noticed a big tent he hadn't seen before. He heard some music and a lot of voices coming from inside,

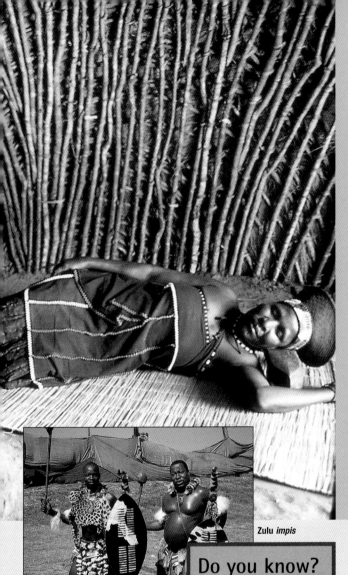

To help you pray for the Zulus

You can thank God for:

- Christian camps where children can learn about him.
- every Zulu Christian who is sharing the good news of Jesus' love with their friends, families and people they meet.

You can ask God:

- to help Zulu pastors and church workers to teach the Bible clearly and to show people how to obey God.
- to show Christians ways in which they can help Zulu boys and girls who have never been to school and find it hard to get jobs.
- to help Christians as they reach out to poor and lonely people, to those who can't get jobs and to people who have been hurt in violent crimes.
- to help Christians of all races in South Africa to love, respect and care for one another, and to work together for the good of their country.
- to help the Zulu leaders guide their people in God's ways and bring peace to South Africa.

Zulu *impis*

Do you know?

Good manners are very important to the Zulus … and having good manners for a Zulu means more than saying "please" and "thank you!" At mealtimes in the homesteads, the people usually sit on grass mats. A woman must kneel to serve a man, making sure that her head is always lower than his, and the man must accept the food with both hands.

so he went in to see what was going on. When he came out again, his life had changed! The man speaking in the tent said that stealing was a sin, that it was wrong. But he also said that Jesus had died to take away the sin of everyone in the world, and that Jesus would give anyone who trusted in him a clean fresh start. Beaumont was so excited to hear that Jesus would also be with him all the time to help him. Beaumont became a Christian, and for four years he told everyone he met about Jesus. He told them outside shops, on buses and while visiting people in their homes. Some bullies got really angry with him. They hated him because he helped so many people to follow God's way. So one day they beat him up and Beaumont died, a martyr for Jesus. We can thank God for Beaumont and his life. Before he went to heaven to be with Jesus forever, he helped lots of other people to know Jesus so that they would go to heaven one day, too.

Killing a chicken

Mrs. Kadebe, who lived near the big tent, was sacrificing a chicken to God when Jill visited her. Mrs. Kadebe told her she was a Christian. "But Jesus died so that we don't have to make sacrifices," Jill told her. "God loved the world so much that he gave his only Son, Jesus, to die on the cross so that our sins can be forgiven. Jesus was God's one and only perfect sacrifice for sin."

Mrs. Kadebe couldn't believe it. Was it really true that she just had to believe that Jesus died for her and ask him to forgive her for all the bad things she'd done? She didn't have to kill chickens or follow any other rituals from other religions? Was that really all there was to it? Mrs. Kadebe didn't sleep for nights as she thought about all she had heard. At last she understood that Jesus died so she could be forgiven and not have to be afraid of evil spirits anymore. She became a great evangelist and traveled to many towns to tell others about God's love and the sacrifice he had made for each one of them.

197

Animism

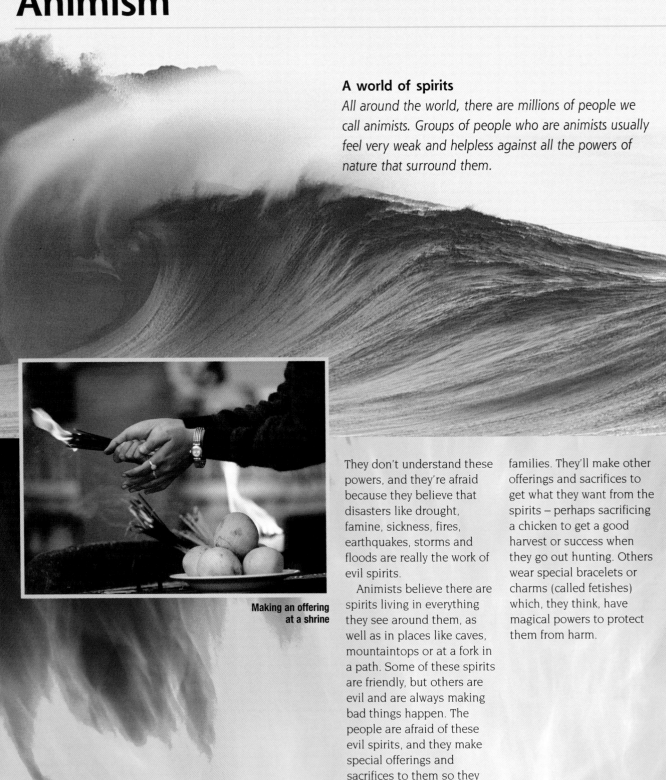

A world of spirits

All around the world, there are millions of people we call animists. Groups of people who are animists usually feel very weak and helpless against all the powers of nature that surround them.

Making an offering at a shrine

They don't understand these powers, and they're afraid because they believe that disasters like drought, famine, sickness, fires, earthquakes, storms and floods are really the work of evil spirits.

Animists believe there are spirits living in everything they see around them, as well as in places like caves, mountaintops or at a fork in a path. Some of these spirits are friendly, but others are evil and are always making bad things happen. The people are afraid of these evil spirits, and they make special offerings and sacrifices to them so they won't hurt them and their families. They'll make other offerings and sacrifices to get what they want from the spirits – perhaps sacrificing a chicken to get a good harvest or success when they go out hunting. Others wear special bracelets or charms (called fetishes) which, they think, have magical powers to protect them from harm.

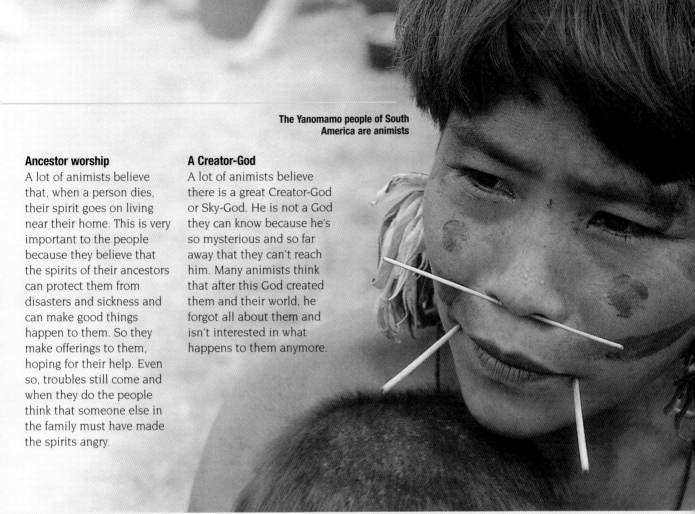
The Yanomamo people of South America are animists

Ancestor worship

A lot of animists believe that, when a person dies, their spirit goes on living near their home. This is very important to the people because they believe that the spirits of their ancestors can protect them from disasters and sickness and can make good things happen to them. So they make offerings to them, hoping for their help. Even so, troubles still come and when they do the people think that someone else in the family must have made the spirits angry.

A Creator-God

A lot of animists believe there is a great Creator-God or Sky-God. He is not a God they can know because he's so mysterious and so far away that they can't reach him. Many animists think that after this God created them and their world, he forgot all about them and isn't interested in what happens to them anymore.

Priests and others

As in any religion, animists have people with special roles. Some of them are known as shamans, medicine men or witch doctors, who have a special knowledge of the spirit world.

Their work is to help their people understand omens and signs and tell them what they must do to keep on the right side of the spirits. Others are priests who look after their shrines and help to organize important festivals and activities.

Some animist peoples

Some of the people we've read about in these books, such as the Bijago, Dogon, Dayak and Yanomamo, are animists. They each have their own ways of reaching out to the spirits and have their own special beliefs and ceremonies. Because animists are afraid of the world of unseen spirits, it's not easy for them to leave their beliefs and turn to another faith. Some who do decide to follow another religion often cling to the power of the spirits and so try to mix the two together. But those who have decided to follow Jesus have discovered that he can set them free from the fear and power of the spirits. Only Jesus is more powerful than any spirit or power.

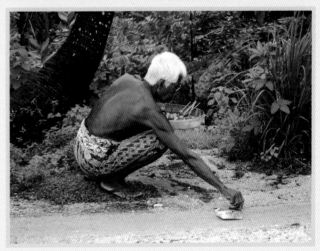
Making a roadside offering

Buddhism

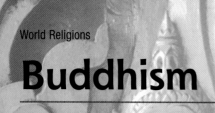

The beginning of Buddhism

Prince Siddharta Gautama lived in India about 2,500 years ago. His wealthy parents didn't want him to see anything that might make him sad. He lived in luxury, got married and had a son, but he felt his life had no meaning.

Young Gautama went on four journeys and saw a man who was sick, a frail old man, the funeral of a dead man and a holy man. It made him sad that people get old, sick and die. He left his parents, wife and child and wandered throughout India for six years, trying to understand the meaning of suffering, life and death.

The Eightfold Path

Gautama spent the rest of his life wandering around and teaching the people who came to him. His followers called him the Buddha, the "enlightened one."

He taught them that only by following the Noble Eightfold Path could they eventually be free from pain and suffering, death and rebirth. They must be kind; not harm any living thing; live in a right way; tell the truth; not think of self; think about others; understand suffering; and meditate. People who follow his teachings are called Buddhists.

Young monk spinning a prayer wheel

Gautama had been taught that everyone dies many times and has thousands of lives. This is called reincarnation. How a person lives in this life affects his next life. If a person has done a lot of good deeds, he or she may be reborn as a wealthy or wise person. People who do bad things will probably be poor and suffer a lot in their next life. Gautama finally decided to seek the answers to his questions through meditation. After a while, he felt that at last he understood the meaning of suffering and the way to be free from it and from endless rebirths. This is called nirvana, or nothingness – the end of the cycle of birth, death and rebirth.

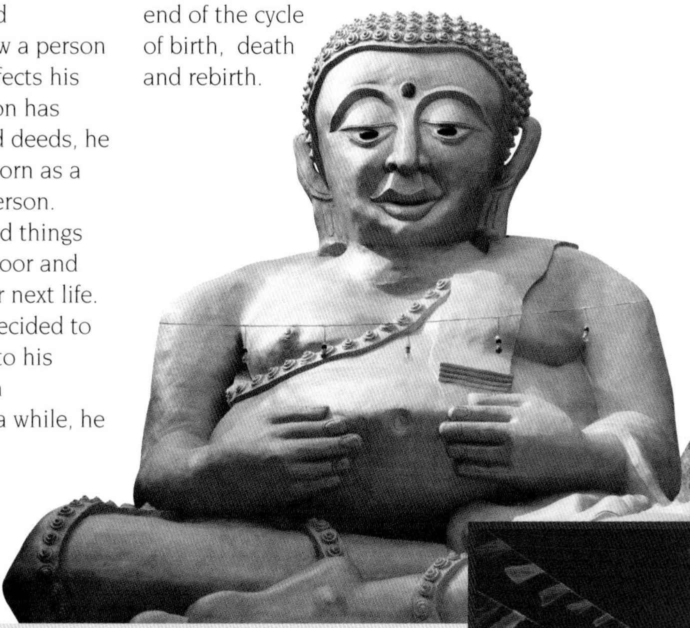

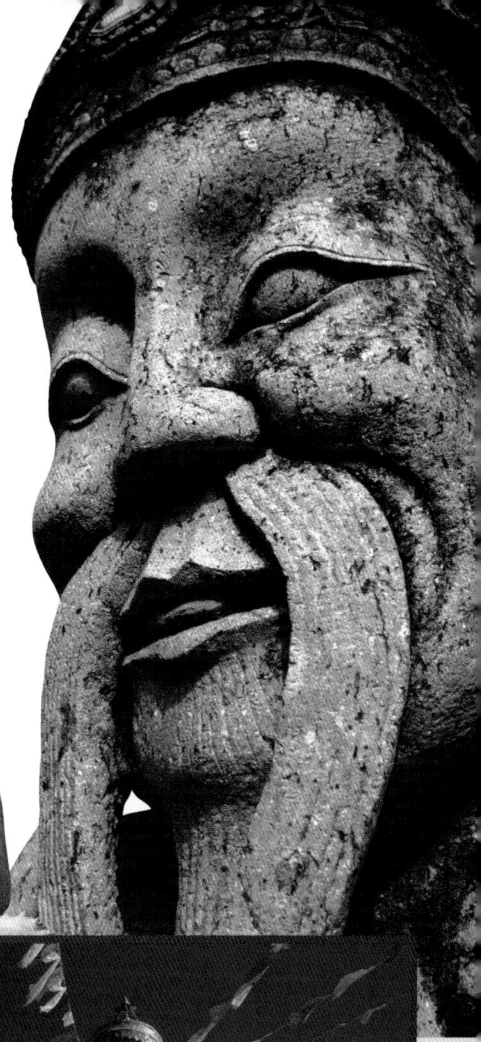

Gaining merit

To reach nirvana, Buddhists try to earn merit by doing good things. Some become monks for a few weeks to gain merit, others for their entire lives. Monks live and dress very simply, usually in a yellow or red robe, and they meditate and teach the laws of the Buddha. Ordinary people try to get merit by giving food to the monks and making offerings in the temples.

Buddhism spread to other Asian countries like Thailand, Burma, Sri Lanka, Tibet, Mongolia, China, Vietnam and Korea. In all these countries there are thousands of Buddhist temples, each with at least one statue of the Buddha. People come seeking merit every day, leaving offerings of flowers, candles or incense in front of the Buddha. They also meditate and pray.

In countries like Tibet, prayer flags flutter from the roofs. People spin small prayer wheels as they walk or sit, and outside the temples are much bigger prayer wheels that people spin as they pass by. On the flags and in the prayer wheels is a mantra, or holy saying, which the people believe carries their prayer to the farthest part of the universe.

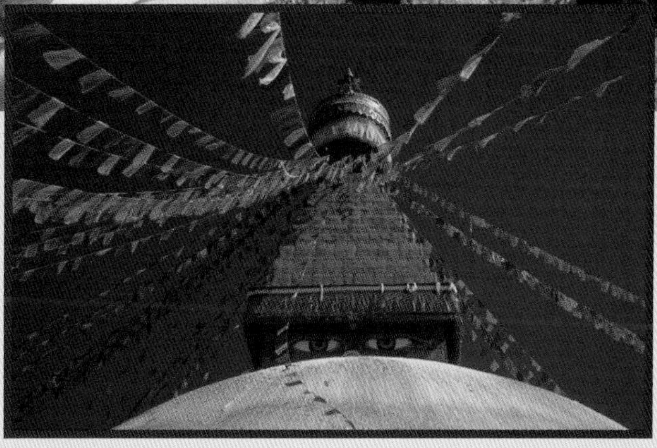

Prayer flags on a Buddhist temple in Nepal

The Dalai Lama

The Dalai Lama, one of Buddhism's greatest leaders and teachers, is reported to have said that Buddhism and Christianity are the same. But they are completely different. Buddhists hope to reach nirvana by their own efforts. Jesus gives new life now – and eternal life – to all who believe in him.

Christianity

Jesus Christ

There are more than 2,000,000,000 people in the world today who call themselves Christians.

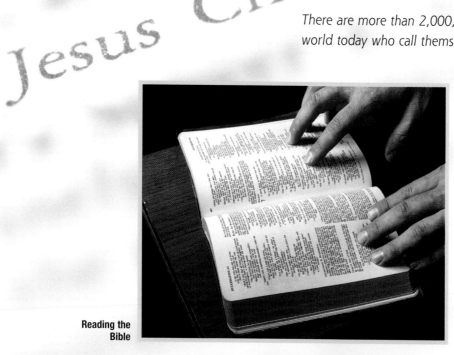

Reading the Bible

Jesus, sent from God

Jesus was born in Bethlehem about 2,000 years ago. God told Mary, his mother, that this baby was God's very own Son, the Messiah (or Savior).

When he was about 30 years old, Jesus chose 12 men to travel with him around the countryside. For three years, wherever they went, Jesus healed the sick and taught people about God's love and the way he wanted them to live. Peter, one of these 12 disciples,

What Christians believe

When God made man and woman, he made them perfect. He wanted them to be his friends and promised to look after them. But because people chose to do what they wanted instead of the good things God wanted, sin came into God's perfect world. Sin isn't just telling lies or stealing. We all want to do things our own way, thinking that God doesn't matter. That's sin, too.

Our sin is like a huge wall that stops us from reaching God. But God loves us very much and wants us to be his friends. So that's why he sent his Son, Jesus, who had never done any wrong, to earth. When Jesus died on the cross, God took all our sins and put them on Jesus. Jesus destroyed that huge wall, so the way to God is open to everyone who trusts in Jesus.

Orthodox church in Eastern Europe

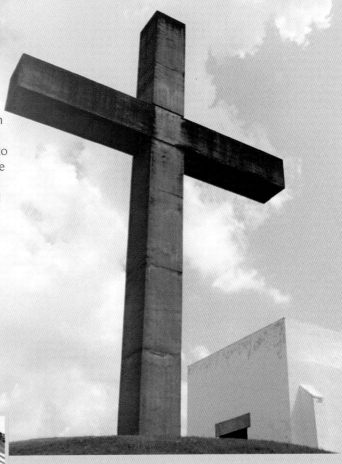

realized that Jesus was the Messiah the Jews had been expecting for many years.

A lot of people loved Jesus, but the Roman rulers thought he was planning a revolt and the Jewish leaders thought he was breaking Jewish laws. They arrested him and accused him of saying things against God!

Jesus was crucified on a big wooden cross. But that wasn't the end. Three days later, Jesus rose from the dead. Over the next 40 days, many people saw him. They believed that Jesus had been raised from the dead by the power of God. Then Jesus returned to his Father in heaven, where he lives forever. Before he went, he promised to send the Holy Spirit to be with his people always.

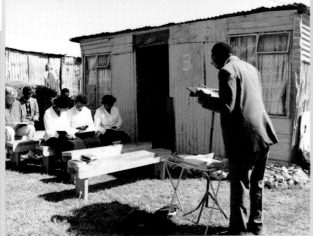

Christians meeting in a South African township

The Bible
The first part of the Bible is called the Old Testament. Many parts of it talk about the Messiah God would send to help his people. Both Christians and Jews read the Old Testament. The four Gospels in the New Testament tell us the story of Jesus' life and his teachings.

Churches
There are many kinds of Christian churches (including Orthodox, Roman Catholic, Protestant and evangelical). Some Christians worship God in huge cathedrals, while others meet in very simple buildings, a room or a hut. But the real church is not the buildings but all the people who have asked Jesus to forgive them and who try to follow his teachings.

Christians know that Jesus is alive today and that he will come back to earth again. They're glad that even though they can't see him, they know he's near and always ready to help them, in hard times as well as good times. They also know that life doesn't end when we die, because Jesus has promised that anyone who believes in him will live forever.

Hinduism

An ancient religion

Hinduism grew out of the way people lived and worshipped in India more than 3,500 years ago. They passed on their beliefs in stories, hymns, poems and prayers. Many of these have been recorded in holy books.

About 80% of the people who live in India are Hindus. India is such a huge country that Hindus who live in different parts of the country worship in different ways and keep different festivals. Temples in the north of India are quite different from those in the south.

Everywhere you go in India you'll see temples and shrines where people worship their gods and goddesses. You'll also see shrines in offices, stores and houses.

There are thousands of Hindu gods, but they're all different forms of one supreme god. Hindus can choose which gods or goddesses they want to worship. Some of the most popular are Vishnu, the protector of the world; Lakshmi, the goddess of wealth and beauty; the fun-loving Krishna who's often thought of as an older brother; and Ganesh, the elephant-headed god of good fortune. Hindus offer their gods food, money and prayers and ask for their help in everything they do.

A Hindu Sadhu

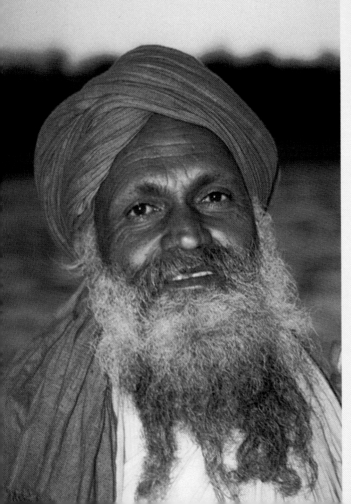

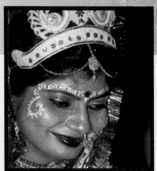

High caste Indian bride

Caste

Every Hindu is born into a group called a caste. A person can't do anything to change caste. Some castes are considered better than others. At the top is the priestly caste, then rulers and soldiers, then merchants and farmers. The people in the lowest castes are usually the servants of the higher castes. The "Untouchables" don't belong to any caste and usually do the jobs nobody else wants to do. Higher caste Hindus don't usually mix with people from the lower castes because they consider them impure.

Life after this life

Hindus believe that when people die, they come back to life again as another person or even an animal. This is reincarnation. They believe in karma, which means that the way people behaved in their past life affects their place in this life, and what they do in this life will decide their place in the next. If they keep the rules of their caste, they believe they'll have a better rebirth. Rebirths may go on forever, as people can never be sure they've done everything the right way. Some Hindus will give up everything – home, family and possessions – to spend their lives in meditation and prayer. They want to become so holy that when they die, they won't be reborn.

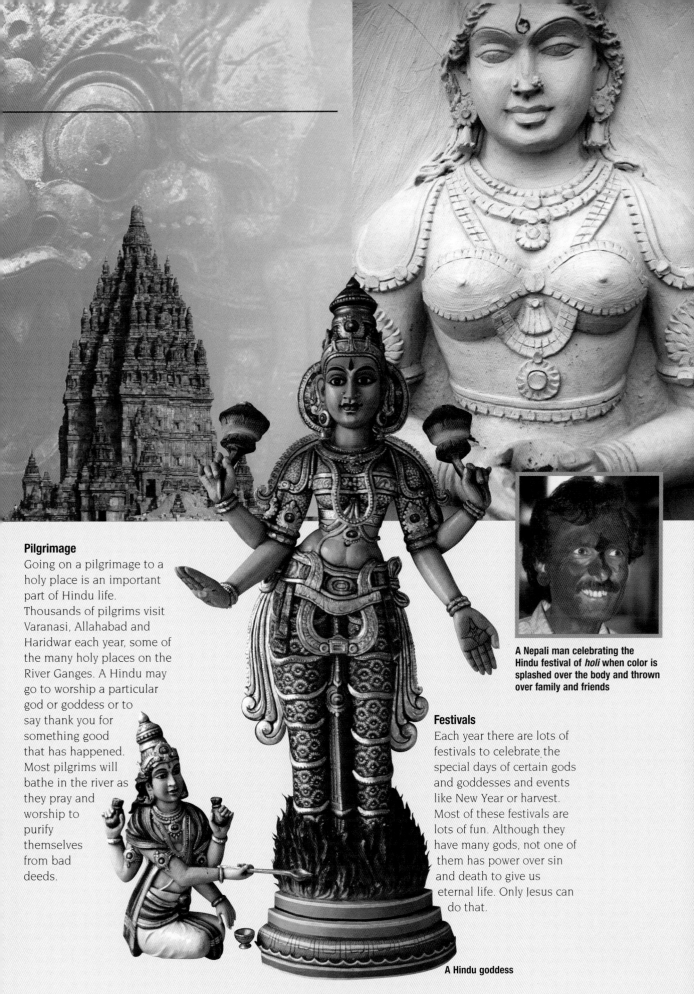

Pilgrimage

Going on a pilgrimage to a holy place is an important part of Hindu life. Thousands of pilgrims visit Varanasi, Allahabad and Haridwar each year, some of the many holy places on the River Ganges. A Hindu may go to worship a particular god or goddess or to say thank you for something good that has happened. Most pilgrims will bathe in the river as they pray and worship to purify themselves from bad deeds.

A Nepali man celebrating the Hindu festival of *holi* when color is splashed over the body and thrown over family and friends

Festivals

Each year there are lots of festivals to celebrate the special days of certain gods and goddesses and events like New Year or harvest. Most of these festivals are lots of fun. Although they have many gods, not one of them has power over sin and death to give us eternal life. Only Jesus can do that.

A Hindu goddess

205

Islam

The prophet Mohammed founded Islam, the religion of Muslims. He was born 1,400 years ago in Mecca, Saudi Arabia. He believed the archangel Gabriel gave him messages from Allah, the Muslim God, which were put together as the Koran, the Muslim's holy book. The Koran describes the way Muslims should live.

There are more than a billion Muslims in our world today. There are two main sects, Sunni Muslims (90%) and Shi'ite Muslims.

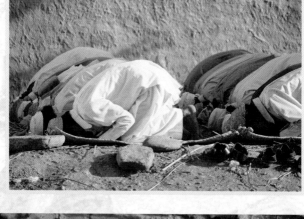

The minaret of a mosque. The call to prayer is made from the upper balcony

Prayers

Muslims worship in mosques, which are often beautifully decorated, but they have no pictures or statues because Mohammed thought people might worship them instead of Allah. Five times every day, the call to prayer "There is no God but Allah, and Mohammed is his prophet" comes from the minaret, the tall tower by the side of the mosque.

Muslims can pray wherever they are, but they have to face towards Mecca, the Muslim's holy city. On Fridays, the Muslim holy day, they pray in the mosques at noon. The men wear a cap and the women a headscarf or veil to show their respect to Allah, and

Muslim men bow down and face Mecca to pray

The Five Pillars of Islam

There are five important duties for every Muslim, called the "Five Pillars of Islam." First, they pray five times every day and declare their faith by repeating the call to prayer. Every year in the month of Ramadan, Muslims fast during the day and only eat and drink between sunset and sunrise. They are to give money to charity. Finally, all Muslims are expected to go to Mecca on a pilgrimage (Hajj), at least once.

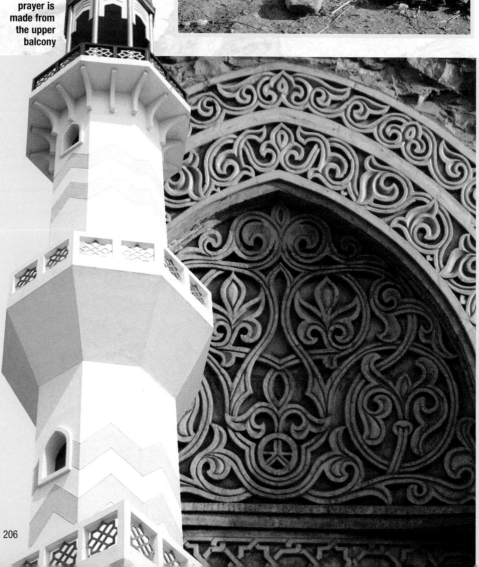

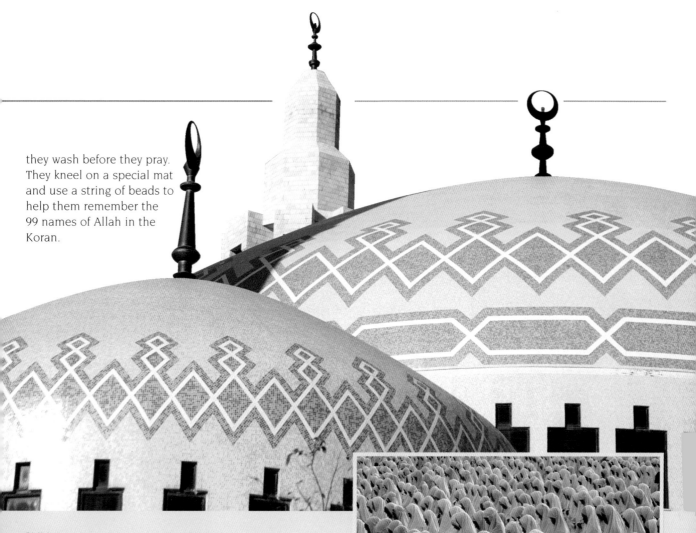

they wash before they pray. They kneel on a special mat and use a string of beads to help them remember the 99 names of Allah in the Koran.

Children

As soon as a baby is born, it's washed and the call to prayer is whispered in its right ear and then in its left, and a little honey or sugar is put on its tongue to make sure it will have a happy life. When they're about seven years old, Muslim children learn to read the Koran in Arabic. They also learn how to pray and how to behave in the mosque. At home they learn what foods they can eat and how to cook them, and how they should behave and dress.

Dress

Muslims are usually modest in their clothing. Neither men nor women would ever wear shorts or tight clothes. Women often wear ankle-length trousers covered by a skirt and a long-sleeved top, or dress, and cover their heads. In some countries women cover themselves in long veils whenever they leave their homes.

Muslims and the Bible

Mohammed taught that there is only one God, Allah. Christians also believe in one God, but Muslims find it hard to understand how God the Father, God the Son and God the Holy Spirit can be one God.

Muslims have a great respect for the Bible and think of Abraham, Moses, David and Jesus as prophets. They're often willing to read the stories about Jesus in the New Testament, which they call the *Injil*. We can tell Muslims about the wonderful things Jesus said and did, and how we can be close to God through him.

Judaism

Judaism, the religion of the Jewish people, is based on the first five books of the Old Testament (the Torah, or teachings).

The Jews believe that God is the creator of everything, that people are created in the image of God, and that the Jews are God's chosen people.

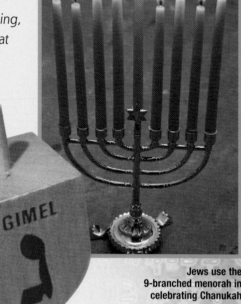

A *dreidel* or spinning top, used in a game played at the festival of Chanukah

Jews use the 9-branched menorah in celebrating Chanukah

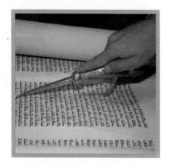

The Hebrew Bible (our Old Testament) is the Jews' holy book. Hebrew is read from right to left

The beginning

God chose Abraham and his family to be his people. He told Abraham to leave his own country (Genesis 12:1–3) and promised him that he would bless him and all the peoples of the world through him.

A chosen nation

Hundreds of years passed, and Abraham's descendants became slaves in Egypt. God chose Moses to lead them out of Egypt to the Promised Land. (You can read the story in Exodus chapters 1–19.) God told Moses that if they obeyed him, they would be his special people. He wanted them to worship him alone and so be different from all the other nations who worshipped lots of gods.

God wanted them to be holy, like himself, so he gave them a set of rules called the Ten Commandments. God promised to bless and help them if they were obedient. If they did not keep God's rules, they would be punished.

Throughout their long history, the Jewish people have seen that everything that has happened to them has been the work of God. He has given them his love and care, guided, helped and punished them. Wherever they have lived and whatever they have suffered – and they have suffered a lot – they have remained Jews.

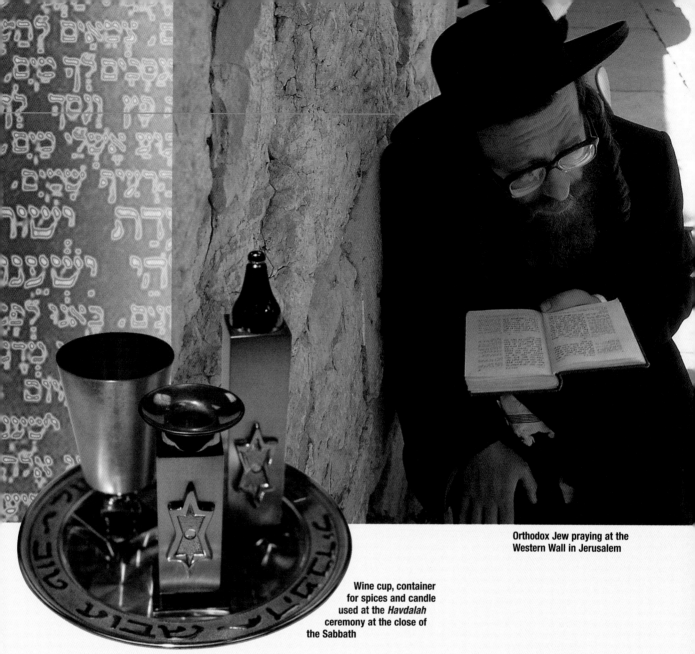

Orthodox Jew praying at the Western Wall in Jerusalem

Wine cup, container for spices and candle used at the *Havdalah* ceremony at the close of the Sabbath

The promised Messiah

The Jews have looked for God's promised Deliverer, or Messiah, to lead them back to their own land and to bring peace and justice on earth. A lot of Jews are still waiting for him to come, but others don't believe in a Messiah at all. Christians, whose beliefs and knowledge of God are based on the Old Testament, are sure that Jesus is the Messiah promised by God.

Worship

The first prayer a Jewish child learns comes from Deuteronomy 6: "Hear, O Israel: the Lord our God is one Lord; and you shall love the Lord your God with all your heart, and with all your soul, and with all your might." They say it every morning and evening.

The Jewish people have lots of festivals during the year that remind them of their history, but every week they keep the Sabbath. The Sabbath starts at sunset on Friday and ends at sunset on Saturday and is very special to Jewish families.

It's their holy day, a day of rest. The family usually goes to a service in the synagogue on Friday evening and again on Saturday morning.

There's always a special Sabbath meal on Friday evenings. Before they eat, the mother lights two candles and blesses God, then the father takes a cup of wine and says a blessing for his family. Everyone eats a piece of bread with salt to remind them of the way God provided his people with manna for food on the way to the Promised Land.

All around the world

There are about 14 million Jews living in countries all around the world. Only 4 million live in Israel, but Jews come from many places to pray at the Western Wall of Herod's Temple in Jerusalem. This is their Holy Land.

What Next?

Get to know Jesus

God has a special purpose for your life and has already planned what he wants you to do. Maybe you're thinking, "I'm not sure if I really know Jesus. So how can I know what he wants me to do?" Jesus knows all about you and wants you to ask him to be your friend! He loves you and died for you because that was the only way to take away all the wrong things that get between God and us. Tell him that you're sorry for all the bad things you've done and that you want to live his way and do what he wants you to do.

Spend time getting to know Jesus. Talk with him and listen to what he says and learn to obey him. Read the Bible and know what it says. God's Holy Spirit will help you to pray and tell other people about Jesus. You can be sure that he will help you and will start showing you his plan for your life.

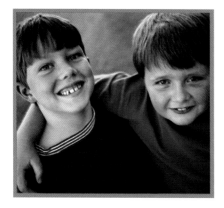

Make friends

- If missionaries come to your church, listen to what they say. Ask them questions and find out how you and your church or Sunday school can help them. If the missionaries have children, make friends with them and write to them.

- There might be people in your church or school who have recently come from another country and might feel very lonely. Be a friend and help them to feel at home.

Pray

Remember that God wants us to share with him in his work through our prayers. Sometimes it's hard for us to keep on praying, but here are a few ideas to help you.

- Choose seven different topics, countries, people groups or individuals. Write them on separate pages in a notebook and pray for one each day of the week.

- When you know a prayer has been answered, write that in your notebook, too.

- Get a world map. Mark on it the places you pray for and add pictures of the people you pray for.

- It helps to pray with someone else – a friend, your family or in Sunday school.

Read

- Get books from your local library about the countries you've read about. Find out how most people make their living; what the government is like; if Christians are accepted in that country or are persecuted. An encyclopedia will answer some of these questions for you.

- There are some exciting missionary biographies that have been written for children. They will help you to understand what it's like to work for Jesus.

Look

- Watch the news and travel programs on TV.

- Look through magazines for pictures of the countries and people you have been learning about.

- Go to the web sites of mission agencies working in the countries you have been learning about. They have lots of interesting information and sometimes they have special pages for children. Countries often have web sites, too. (Remember to ask your parents first.)

Taste

- Ask your parents if you can try food from different countries.

Give

Missions often have special projects. Find out about them and give some of your money to help that project. Your Sunday school and friends might want to help support a project and your teachers will have ideas to help you raise money.

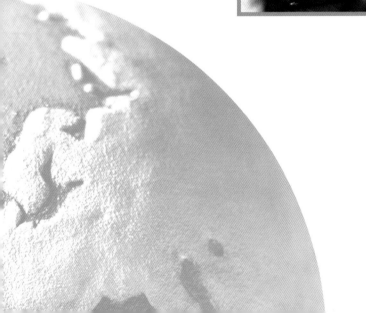

Go!

- Some missionary societies have summer camps for children (for example, WEC International in Britain) where you can have a lot of fun, meet missionaries and learn about their work.

- You or your whole family might even be able to visit missionary friends to find out what it's like to be a missionary.

- When you're on vacation, pray for the people you meet who don't know Jesus.

- Some organizations have special mission trips for teenagers.

Addresses

To Help You Find Out More ...

... on this page are some addresses and web sites of Christian agencies in North America and Britain who may be able to help you. There's also a list of some of the countries they may be able to tell you about. Some agencies, like Gospel Recordings and Wycliffe Bible Translators, have specialized work in many countries all around the world.

If you want to find out more about a people group, first make sure you know which country they live in. Then look for agencies that may have information about that country. If you write to an agency, decide what you want to ask about before you write.

Why not visit the web sites of some of these mission agencies (with your parents' permission) and discover more of what God is doing around the world. Some agencies have lots of interesting and exciting information on their web sites with special pages for children. Agencies marked * have some materials that have been specially prepared for children (general information, activity packs, videos, web pages, pictures, worksheets or books).

... Finding out is fun!

Some North American Mission Agencies

ABWE*
(Association of Baptists for World Evangelism)
USA: P.O. Box 8585, Harrisburg, PA 17105
CANADA: 160 Adelaide Street South, Suite 205, London, Ontario N5Z 3LI
Web: www.abwe.org
(Bangladesh, Central America and the Caribbean, China, Colombia, Japan, Mongolia, Papua New Guinea, Peru, Romania, Spain, Thailand, Uruguay)

American Bible Society
1865 Broadway, New York, NY 10023
Web: www.biblesociety.org/bs-usa.htm
(Worldwide production and distribution of Scriptures)

AmeriTribes*
P.O. Box 27346, Tucson, AZ 85726-7346
Web: www.ameritribes.org
(Native American tribes in USA and Mexico)

Campus Crusade for Christ International*
100 Lake Hart Drive, Orlando, FL 32832
Web: www.ccci.org
(*Jesus* film)

Christian and Missionary Alliance
P.O. Box 35000, Colorado Springs, CO 80935-3500
Web: www.cmalliance.org
(Colombia, Cuba, Guatemala, Guinea, Haiti, Indonesia, Israel, Lebanon, Mongolia, Peru, Russia, Spain, Syria, Thailand, Uruguay, Venezuela, Vietnam)

Christian Literature Crusade
701 Pennsylvania Ave., Fort Washington, PA 19034
Web: www.clcusa.org
(Literature work in 55 countries including Trinidad and Uruguay)

European Christian Mission
110 Juanita Drive, South Zanesville, OH 43701
Web: www.ecmi.org
(Albania, Greece, Romania, Spain)

Gospel for Asia
1932 Walnut Plaza, Carrollton, TX 75006
Web: www.gfa.org
(Bhutan, China, India, Nepal, Russia, Sri Lanka, Thailand, Vietnam)

Gospel Missionary Union*
10000 N. Oak Trafficway, Kansas City, MO 64155
Web: www.gmu.org
(Mali, Morocco, Greece, Russia, Kyrgyzstan, Spain)

Gospel Recordings/Global Recordings Network
122 Glendale Boulevard, Los Angeles, CA 90026
Web: www.gospelrecordings.com
(Recording, producing and distributing audio recordings for evangelism worldwide)

Mission Aviation Fellowship*
P.O. Box 3202, Redlands, CA 92374
Web: www.maf.org/
(Congo, Haiti, Indonesia, Lesotho, Mali, Papua New Guinea, Russia, Venezuela, Zimbabwe)

New Tribes Mission*
1000 E. First Street, Sanford, FL 32771
Web: www.ntm.org/
(Work among people groups in Colombia, Greenland, Guinea, Indonesia, Mongolia, Papua New Guinea, Thailand, Venezuela and in many other countries)

OMF International
10 W. Dry Creek Circle, Littleton, CO 80120
Web: www.omf.org/
(Thailand, Indonesia, Japan)

OMS International
941 Fry Road, Greenwood, IN 46142
Web: www.omsinternational
(Colombia, Haiti, Indonesia, Japan, Russia)

Operation Mobilization, Inc.
P.O. Box 444, Tyrone, GA 30290
Web: www.usa.om.org
(Afghanistan, Bangladesh, India, Kazakhstan, Romania, Russia, Turkey, Uzbekistan. OM works in 85 countries and has two mission ships.)

Rainbows of Hope
P.O. Box 517, Fort Mill, SC 29716
Web:www.wec-int.org/rainbows
(Street children and children in crisis around the world)

TEAM*
(The Evangelical Alliance Mission)
P.O. Box 969, Wheaton, IL 60189
Web: www.teamworld.org/
(Chad, Colombia, Indonesia, Japan, Nepal, Russia, Spain, Trinidad and Tobago, Venezuela, Zimbabwe)

United World Mission
P.O. Box 668767, Charlotte, NC 28270
Web: www.uwm.org
(Bulgaria, China, Cuba, Ethiopia, Greece, Guatemala, India, Mali, Morocco, Nepal, Peru, Romania, Russia, Spain, Uruguay, Uzbekistan, Venezuela, Vietnam)

WEC International*
P.O. Box 1707, Fort Washington, PA 19034
Web: www.wec-int.org
(Albania, Bulgaria, Chad, Greece, East Asia, Guinea, Guinea-Bissau, India, Japan, Spain, Venezuela and other countries in this book)

World Team
1431 Stuckert Rd., Warrington, PA 18976
Web: www.worldteam.org/
(Cuba, Haiti, Indonesia, Peru, Russia, Spain, Trinidad and Tobago, as well as other countries)

Wycliffe Bible Translators
P.O. Box 2727, Huntington Beach, CA 92647
Web: www.wycliffe.org
(Worldwide, helping people put the Bible into their own language for the first time.)

Some Mission Agencies in Britain

Action Partners Ministries
Bawtry Hall, Bawtry, Doncaster, DN10 6JH
Web: www.actionpartners.org.uk
(Chad, Congo, Egypt and North Africa)

Africa Inland Mission International*
2 Vorley Road, Archway, London N19 5HE
Web: www.aim-eur.org
(Chad, Congo, Lesotho, Madagascar, Namibia)

Albanian Evangelical Mission
29 Bridge Street, Penybryn, Wrexham, LL13 7HP
Web: www.albanianmission.demon.co.uk
(Albania)

Arab World Ministries*
P.O. Box 51, Loughborough, LE11 OZQ
Web: www.awm.com
(Middle East and North Africa including Egypt, Lebanon and Syria)

BMS World Mission*
P.O. Box 49, 129 Broadway, Didcot, Oxon.
OX11 8XA
Web: www.bms.org.uk
(Albania, Bangladesh, Guinea, India, Nepal, Sri Lanka, Trinidad and Tobago)

British & Foreign Bible Society
Stonehill Green, Westlea, Swindon, Wilts.
SN5 7DG
Web: www.biblesociety.org
(Production and distribution of Scriptures worldwide)

Church Mission Society*
Partnership House, 157 Waterloo Road, London
SE1 8UU
Web: www.cms-uk.org
(Working in 40 countries in Africa, Asia and Europe)

Church's Ministry Among Jewish People
30c Clarence Road, St. Albans, AL1 4JJ
Web: www.cmj.org.uk

Christian Literature Crusade
Shawton House, 792 Hagley Road West,
Oldbury, B68 0PJ
Web: www.clc.org.uk
(Literature ministry in 55 countries)

Christian Witness to Israel
166 Main Road, Sundridge, Sevenoaks, Kent,
TN14 6EL
Web:www.cwi.org.uk
(Israel, and among Jewish people in other countries)

Crosslinks*
251 Lewisham Way, London SE4 1XF
Web:www.crosslinks.org
(Ethiopia, Greece, India, North Africa, SE Asia, Spain, Zimbabwe)

European Christian Mission (Britain)
50 Billing Road, Northampton, NN1 5DB
Web: www.ecmi.org
(Albania, Greece, Romania, Spain)

FEBA Radio
Ivy Arch Road, Worthing, West Sussex,
BN14 8BX
Web: www.feba.org.uk
(Christian radio broadcasts to more than 30 countries)

Interserve
325 Kennington Road, London S11 4QH
Web: www.interserve.org
(Middle East, North Africa, India, West Asia, Mongolia, East Asia)

Language Recordings, UK
P.O. Box 197, High Wycombe, HP14 3YY
Web: www.gospelrecordings.com
(Recording, producing and distributing audio recordings worldwide)

Latin Link UK
175 Tower Bridge Road, London SE1 2AB
Web: www.latinlink.org
(Colombia, Peru and other South American countries)

Middle East Christian Outreach
22 Culverdon Park Road, Tunbridge Wells, Kent
TN4 9RA
Web: www.gospelcom.net/meco
(Egypt, Lebanon, Syria, Turkey, Yemen)

Mission Aviation Fellowship*
Castle Hill Avenue, Folkestone, CT20 2TN
Web: www.maf-uk.org
(Chad, Congo, Haiti, Indonesia, Lesotho, Madagascar, Mali, Mongolia, Papua New Guinea, Venezuela, Zimbabwe)

New Tribes Mission
North Cotes, Grimsby, DN36 5XU
Web: www.ntm.org.uk
(Colombia, Greenland, Guinea, Indonesia, Mongolia, Papua New Guinea, Russia, Thailand, Venezuela)

Operation Mobilisation (OM)
The Quinta, Weston Rhyn, Oswestry, SY10 7LT
Web: www.uk.om.org
(Afghanistan, Bangladesh, India, Kazakhstan, Romania, Russia, Turkey, Uzbekistan. OM works in 85 countries and has two mission ships.)

OMF International*
Station Approach, Borough Green, Sevenoaks
TN15 8BG
Web: www.omf.org.uk
(East Asia, Indonesia, Japan, Thailand)

OMS International*
1 Sandileigh Avenue, Didsbury, Manchester,
M20 3LN
Web: www.omsinternational.org/uk
(China, Colombia, Haiti, India, Indonesia, Japan, Russia, Spain)

People International, UK
P.O. Box 310, Tunbridge Wells, TN4 8ZJ
(Afghanistan, Kazakhstan, Kyrgyzstan, Turkey, Uzbekistan)

Red Sea Mission Team
P.O. Box 19929, London N3 1WW
Web: www.rsmt.u-net.com
(Djibouti, Mali, Middle East)

SIM UK*
(Society for International Ministries)
Wetheringsett Manor, Wetheringsett,
Stowmarket, IP14 5QX
Web: www.sim.co.uk
(Working in 43 countries in Africa, S. America and Asia)

South American Mission Society*
Allen Gardiner House, 12 Fox Hill, Birmingham,
B29 4AG
Web: www.samsgb.org
(Peru, Spain, Uruguay)

Tearfund*
100 Church Road, Teddington, Middx. TW11 8QE
Web: www.tearfund.org/youth
(Working in 90 countries around the world including Bangladesh, Cuba, Haiti, Mali)

The Leprosy Mission*
Goldhay Way, Orton Goldhay, Peterborough,
PE2 5GZ
Web: www.leprosymission.org/

UFM Worldwide*
47a Fleet Street, Swindon, SN1 1RE
Web: www.ufm.org.uk
(Eastern Europe, Java [Indonesia], Mongolia, Papua New Guinea, Spain)

WEC International*
Bulstrode, Oxford Road, Gerrards Cross, Bucks.
SL9 8SZ
Web. www.wec-int.org
(Albania, Bulgaria, Chad, Greece, East Asia, Guinea, Guinea-Bissau, India, Japan, Spain, Venezuela and other countries in this book)

Wycliffe Bible Translators*
Horsleys Green, High Wycombe, Bucks.
HP14 3XL
Web: www.wycliffe.org.uk
(Worldwide, helping people put the Bible into their own language for the first time.)

Youth With a Mission
Highfield Oval, Ambrose Lane, Harpenden,
Herts. AL5 4BX
Web: www.ywam-england.com
(Albania, Thailand, China, India, Kazakhstan and other Central Asian countries, Middle East, North Africa, Russia)

If you have any difficulty in obtaining the information you need, please contact: Children's Resources, WEC International, who will try to help you.

Word List

agnostic: a person who believes that we can't know anything about God or even if he exists.

Allah: the Muslim God.

alpaca: a South American animal that looks like the llama and is related to the camel; usually raised for its fine wool.

altar: 1. the communion table in a church; 2. a flat-topped block of stone for making sacrifices and offerings to God (in Old Testament times) or to gods.

ancestor: anyone from whom you are descended. Your parents, grandparents and great-grandparents are all your ancestors.

animism: see p. 198.

Armenian Church: historic Armenia (including Georgia, eastern Turkey, Syria and northern Iraq and Iran) was the first country in the world to make Christianity its official religion (in the third century). There are still Armenian churches in most of these places.

Ash Wednesday: the first day of Lent (the 40 days before Easter). Some churches put ash on the foreheads of worshippers as a sign that they're sorry for their sin.

atheist: a person who believes that there's no God.

Bible school: a college where people study the Bible. Churches often hold Bible schools for a week or several weeks.

Buddhism: see p. 200.

cacao: the tree and its seed from which cocoa and chocolate are made.

calypso: a West Indian song with an African rhythm. The singer often makes up the words as he or she sings.

caste: a group into which a Hindu person is born. The most important caste is the priestly caste; then leaders and soldiers and traders and storekeepers. There are other lower castes and "outcastes" (untouchables) who have to do things like sweep and wash clothes; they're often servants of the higher castes.

Catholic: the word "catholic" means "universal," and there are Catholic churches all around the world. Like other Christians, Catholics believe that Jesus is the Son of God and the Bible is the word of God. But they also believe that other traditions are important and worship Mary as the Mother of God. They believe that Jesus gave the apostle Peter special authority, which was handed down to the bishops of Rome. The Pope is the Bishop of Rome, the head of the Roman Catholic Church.

charm: something worn to bring good luck.

civil war: a war between groups of people inside the same country.

colony/colonize: an area taken over, settled and ruled by another country. People who colonize a country often bring foreign cultures, religions and values to the people already living there.

Communism: a political movement. The original idea was for a society in which there would be neither very rich nor very poor people but where everyone was equal. This became the form of government in countries like Russia where the state controlled everything.

continent: one of the seven big land masses in the world. The continents are Africa, Antarctica, Asia, Australia, Europe, North America and South America.

correspondence course: a course (on any subject) in which a teacher mails lessons and questions to students, who return their answers in the same way.

coup: a sudden, and often violent, takeover of a government by a small group of people.

cremation: burning the body to ashes after death.

cult: a religious group that has its own objects of worship and its own ceremonies.

culture: the customs, traditions and way of life of a people.

customs: opinions or beliefs passed on from one generation to the next; the usual ways of doing things.

democracy: a system of government in which the adult population of a country elects ordinary people to govern them.

descendant: a person who is descended from another. You are a descendant of your parents, grandparents and great-grandparents.

dialect: the way people in a particular part of a country speak their language. This includes the words they use and the way they pronounce them.

dictator: a ruler who has total power over all that is done in his country.

drought: a long period of time without rain so there is a shortage of water.

drug cartel: a group of people who control the sale and price of illegal drugs.

embassy: the place where an ambassador (someone representing the government of his own country) lives and works in another country.

emigrate: to leave one's own country and live in another.

evangelical: a person who believes that the Bible is God's word and that the four Gospels tell us about Jesus' birth and sinless life, that he died for our sins so God could forgive us, and rose again from the dead. Evangelical Christians believe that only by having faith in Jesus can we be forgiven for our sins and go to heaven. We cannot earn our way to God by doing good things.

evangelical (church): a church that teaches that Jesus died for us and is alive forever, and that it's important for us to know and follow the Bible, which is God's word.

evangelist: a person who tells others the good news of Jesus' love.

evil spirits: a being that can't be seen but that makes bad things happen.

exile: a person sent away from his or her own country and forced to live in another country.

export: anything people in one country grow or make to sell to another country.

famine: a time when food is scarce so that people (and animals) sometimes die from starvation.

to fast: to not eat for a while, often for religious reasons.

fetish: an object that's worshipped.

guerrillas/guerrilla war: members of a rebel army (against the government) who fight a war by ambush or surprise attacks. They may work on their own or in small groups.

Hajj: the Muslim pilgrimage to Mecca, their holy city in Saudi Arabia. All Muslims are expected to go on this pilgrimage at least once in their lifetime.

Hebrew: the language in which the Old Testament was originally written, a modern version of which is spoken in Israel today.

heretic: a person who believes things that are different from the accepted teachings of his or her church.

Hinduism: see p. 204.

Holy Trinity: God the Father, God the Son and God the Holy Spirit together are called the Holy Trinity, three persons in one God. The Father, Son and Holy Spirit are all equally God; they are all eternal and never change. They all took part in the work of creation. Jesus is the Son of God who came to earth to live and die to save us from our sins. After Jesus returned to heaven, God sent the Holy Spirit to work in the lives of Christians and be with them always.

icon: a sacred painting of Jesus, his mother Mary, or a saint.

idol: a statue or image of something which is worshipped as a god.

Islam: see p. 206.

Jain: a member of a small Indian religion. They must not hurt or kill any living thing and are strict vegetarians.

Jehovah's Witnesses: a cult founded in America in 1872. They believe the whole Bible is from Jehovah (God) and tells them exactly what they must believe and do. They don't believe that Jesus is the Son of God. They believe that God's kingdom is the only kingdom, so sometimes they refuse to obey certain laws of the countries in which they live such as serving in the armed forces. They believe that the end of the world is near and that there will be a great battle, called Armageddon, between God and Satan before a new kingdom belonging to Jesus will be set up.

Jesus film: shows the life of Jesus from Luke's Gospel. It's been translated into many languages and millions of people have seen it. It's available on video and is used in many churches and homes all around the world to help people understand who Jesus is. A lot of people have come to know him through watching this film. In these books you can read about some of the countries like Iraq, Mongolia and Syria and people groups like the Buryats, Garifuna and Uzbeks who have the film in their own language.

jinns: spirits with power to appear in human or animal form.

Judaism: see p. 208.

Koran: (or Qur'an) the Muslim's holy book.

legend: a story passed down from one generation to the next about something that happened a long time ago. The story may or may not be true.

Lent: 40 days, from Ash Wednesday to Easter Eve, of fasting and repenting for sin. Many branches of the Christian Church observe Lent. Some people skip one meal a day during Lent, or give up something they really enjoy, like chocolate, and give the money they would have spent to charity.

linguist: a person who studies languages.

looting: stealing things from houses or stores during a riot or battle or other disaster.

malaria: an illness spread by mosquitoes in which a person has very high fevers and chills.

mango: the delicious, yellowish-orange colored fruit of the mango tree. While it's still green, the fruit is often used to make pickles.

manioc: a plant grown in many tropical countries. The thick roots, a bit like potatoes, are used for food.

March for Jesus: a yearly march in which Christians tell others about Jesus, praise God, sing and pray. Since it began in 1987, more than 50 million people in 117 countries have taken part in the marches.

martyr: a person who is killed because of his beliefs.

masquerade: to wear a mask or costume and pretend you're someone else. The same word is used for a party where everyone is in disguise.

Mass: the service of Holy Communion (in the Roman Catholic Church).

medicine man: in animism, this is a person who has powers of healing. This may be through contact with the spirits or through their knowledge of plants and other natural things that can help healing. (See also: witch doctor; Shamanism.)

meditation: thinking deeply about things, often religious matters.

merit, earning: doing something good that will bring a reward in the future. Buddhists believe that if they earn merit they will be reborn into a better life when they die.

Messianic Jews: Jews who are Christians. They believe Jesus is the Messiah sent by God and have accepted him as their Savior.

millet: a very tall cereal plant with small seeds that are very nutritious. (If you have a pet bird you may feed it millet!)

minaret: a tall, slender tower connected to a mosque.

Word List (continued)

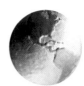

missionary: a person who goes to another place to teach others about his or her faith.

Mohammed: the founder of Islam (see p. 206).

monastery: a building or buildings where monks live, work and study their religion in peace and quiet.

monk: a man belonging to a religious group living in a monastery.

Mormon: a member of a large cult often called the Church of Jesus Christ of Latter-day Saints. Their teaching is based on the Book of Mormon and other writings and uses the Bible as well.

mosque: the Muslim place of worship.

Muslim: a follower of Islam (see p. 206).

noble: a person of high rank by birth such as a duke or duchess.

nomad: a member of a tribe that moves from place to place to find food and pasture for their animals.

offering: something given as a gift and a sign of devotion.

omen: something that happens and is taken as a sign that something else will happen. Some omens mean good things will happen, but others mean bad things will happen.

Orthodox churches: a branch of the Christian Church found in many countries, but mainly in Eastern Europe, Greece and Russia. They base their beliefs on the Bible, the Creed (a statement of faith) and traditions. They have many pictures of saints in their churches. There are no organs or musical instruments, but the services are always sung. Often the only seats in the churches are around the walls, so people stand during the services or move around to pray in front of icons.

papaya (pawpaw): a palm-like tree originally from Central America, now grown in many tropical countries. Its edible fruit is oval, yellow or orange, and can weigh from a few ounces to several pounds.

pastor: a minister in charge of a church.

peasant: a person who lives and works on the land, often as a hired worker.

Pentecost: the day when Christians celebrate the coming of the Holy Spirit (Acts 2). It's sometimes called Whitsun or Whitsunday and takes place on the seventh Sunday after Easter.

persecution: attacking, killing or driving people from their homes because they have different political or religious beliefs.

pilgrimage: a journey to worship at a holy place. People who go on pilgrimages are called pilgrims.

plantain: a kind of large banana that has to be cooked before it can be eaten.

plantation: a large farm or area of land that's planted with trees or crops such as tea, coffee, cotton or sugar. A lot of people are hired to work on plantations.

plateau: an area of high, level ground. It's sometimes called a "tableland."

poncho: a garment, something like a cape, worn in some South American countries. It's made from a piece of cloth with a slit in the middle so it can be put on over the head.

poverty: when someone is very poor and doesn't have enough money to live on.

prayer beads: a string of beads used to help a person repeat prayers. Buddhists and Muslims use them, and in the Christian Church Roman Catholics call it a rosary.

prayer wheels: a tube-shaped box with a prayer written in it. Small ones are held in the hand, but bigger ones are attached to a spindle. It's thought that, as the wheel spins around, the prayer goes out into the universe. They are used by Tibetan Buddhists.

Protestants: members or followers of Christian churches that broke away from the Roman Catholic churches during the Reformation in the sixteenth century.

raid: a sudden attack on another group of people.

Ramadan: a month of fasting during which Muslims don't eat or drink from sunrise to sunset.

to ration: to divide something so that everyone has the same amount; to restrict how much of something someone can have (for example, food during a famine).

rebel: a person who refuses to obey those in authority and fights against them.

refugee/refugee camp: a person who has been forced to flee from his or her home or country because of war, famine or beliefs. Refugees often go to refugee camps where they are looked after until they can go back to their own homes or can settle in another country.

revolt/revolution: a rebellion which overthrows a government.

Russian Revolution: during World War I, a lot of peasants had to join Russia's badly-equipped army. Those who stayed to work on the land were extremely poor. Factory workers were also very poor, and in 1917 they led the revolution against the government and the tsar (king) who stepped down from power. The workers elected councils, helped by a political party called the Bolsheviks who later changed their name to Communists. They seized power and set up "government by the workers." The government took over everything – farms, banks, factories, industries and railways.

Sabbath: the seventh day of the Jewish week, from sunset on Friday to sunset on Saturday. It's the Jews' holy day and day of rest.

sacred: something that's holy and precious to the followers of a religion.

sacrifice: killing an animal as an offering to a god or goddess.

Sahel: sometimes called "the shore of the desert," it's the hot, dry, semi-desert area on the southern edge of the Sahara Desert.

saint: a holy person.

savior: a person who saves another from harm or difficulty. Jesus is our Savior because he died to save us from our sins.

sect: a group of people who have turned their backs on some of the main beliefs of a religion and have formed their own beliefs.

secular: not sacred or holy, but dealing with the ordinary things of this world.

settler: someone who goes to live in a new country, often in an area that hasn't been developed.

Shamanism: a form of animism mainly found in Siberia but also in other parts of Asia and among American Indian peoples. The word "shaman" means "one who knows," and a shaman keeps in touch with the spirits so that he can guide his people to do what the spirits want them to do. (See also: witch doctor; medicine man.)

sheikh: the chief of an Arabian tribe or village.

Shi'ite Muslims: (also called Shi'as) believe that their leaders must be descendants of Ali, Mohammed's cousin and son-in-law.

shrine: a building or place where sacred things are kept.

Sikh: a member of a north Indian religion founded about 500 years ago by a man called Guru Nanak. Sikhs believe in one God and that all people are equally important. Sikh men do not cut their hair but keep it in place with a comb and wear turbans on their heads. Their place of worship is called a *Gurdwara*, and their holy book is the *Guru Granth Sahib*.

slum: an overcrowded and often dirty area of a city. Most people living in slums are often too poor to live anywhere else.

sorghum: a kind of grass grown in dry parts of the world. Its grain (seed) is used to make a kind of bread.

spirit: a supernatural being; ghosts and fairies are spirits.

spiritist: a person who believes that it's possible to make contact with spirits, often with the spirit of a dead person.

Sunni Muslims: Most Muslims belong to the Sunni branch of Islam and closely follow the teachings of the prophet Mohammed. They elect their leaders.

superstition: an idea or action based on a belief in ghosts, lucky and unlucky signs and supernatural happenings.

taboo: something that's forbidden or not acceptable, for religious or social reasons.

tapir: a pig-like animal related to the rhinoceros.

temple: a building used for worship.

terraced fields: level fields made on a hillside, with the outer edge of each field kept in place by a wall. Terraced fields go up a hillside like a series of large steps.

thatch: straw or reeds used to make a roof.

tradition: opinions, ways of doing things or beliefs that have been passed on from one generation to the next.

traditional religion: a religion or way of worship that has been handed down from one generation to another within a tribe or people group.

translate/translation: to put the words of one language into the words of another language so that both mean the same. The person who does this is called a translator. A Bible translation is a Bible put into the words of another language. Bibles translated into hundreds of different languages, then, all say the same thing.

tribe: people belonging to the same race or group and ruled by a chief.

United Nations: a worldwide organization of about 180 countries who want to work together for world peace. It began in 1945 at the end of World War II. It tries to settle quarrels between countries or within a country; to develop friendships between nations; and to help overcome some of the world's problems, like poverty.

visa: an official stamp in a passport that gives someone permission to go in or leave a particular country.

voodoo: a religious system in the West Indies that practices witchcraft.

west, the: can mean the western part of a country or region. We also use it when we talk about the well-to-do countries of western Europe, Great Britain and the United States.

witch doctor: in animism, a person who has contact with the spirits and can understand signs and omens. (See also: medicine man; Shamanism.)

yak: a long-haired Tibetan ox.

Acknowledgements

A great many people and mission agencies have helped in the production of *Window on the World* and I want to thank each of them for the part they have played.

First of all, my thanks to everyone who has prayed for this project. Among them are my own precious grandchildren and their parents as well as friends, colleagues and acquaintances all around the world. They have prayed because they know God hears and answers prayer and are convinced that children have a special part to play in praying for the world in which they live.

Mission agencies and Christian workers all around the world have graciously answered my questions, provided information, stories and pictures, and have checked the results. Their letters have often been a great source of inspiration. Tara Smith, who has edited the material, has been a constant encouragement.

Others have encouraged me as they have told me how much their families, children's groups and churches appreciated the first edition. It gave them a glimpse of a world in need and helped even small children to pray for the world.

The greatest encourager of all is God himself. Time and time again he has given fresh vision, new joy, answers to my prayers and verses from the Bible that have spoken to my heart. And as I have worked, I have discovered that he has answered many of the prayers included in the first edition.

My thanks to each one and may we encourage one another to change our world through prayer.

Daphne Spraggett

218

Picture Acknowledgements

Acknowledgements are given for each spread. Where there is more than one source on a spread the credits are given clockwise from left.

Front Cover
1, 3, 4 & 7 Photodisc, 2 Sarah Errington/Hutchison Picture Library, 5 International Mission Board, 6 Getty Images

Back Cover
All Photodisc

Introduction, pp 8–9
Photodisc
pp 10–11
1 & 2 International Mission Board, 3 Tim Dowley/Three's Company

Afghanistan
1 & 4 Roy Spraggett, 2 & 3 Alex Macnaughton/Impact

Albania
1 Justin Williams/Impact, 2 Material World/Impact, 3 & 4 Howard Sayer/Impact

Azeri
1–3 Caroline Penn/Impact, 4 Danny Isenring

Balinese
1 David Palmer/Impact, 2–4 Dominic Sansoni/Impact,

Baloch
1 Caroline Penn/Impact, 3–5 Roy Spraggett

Bangladesh
1, 2 & 4 Piers Cavendish/Impact, 3 International Mission Board

Beja
All Sarah Errington/Hutchison Picture Library

Bhutan
1, 2 & 4 Alain Le Garsmeur/Impact, 3, N. M. Sture, 5 Material World/Impact

Bijago
All Norman Cuthbert

Bulgaria
1 & 2 Christophe Bluntzer/Impact, 3 Bruce Stephens/Impact, 4 Janet Wishnetsky/Impact, 5 International Mission Board

Buryat
1–4 Judy Starr, 5 Roy Spraggett

Chad
1, 3 & 4 Pauline Wager, 2 International Mission Board

Children of the Streets
1 & 4 Roy Spraggett, 2 & 5 Rainbows of Hope, 3 Wendy Dezan

China
1 & 3–6 Photodisc, 2 Roy Spraggett

Colombia
1 Alexis Wallerstein/Impact, 2 & 4 David Reed/Impact, 3 Robert Gibbs/Impact, 5 Charles Coates

Cuba
1 Tim Dowley/Three's Company, 2 Larry Jerden/United Bible Societies, 3 José López/United Bible Societies/Bible Commission of Cuba, 4 WEC Press

Dai Lu
1, 2 & 4 Mark Henley/Impact, 3 Photodisc, 5 Bruce Stephens/Impact

Dayak
1–3 Robert Francis/Hutchison Picture Library, 4 Michael Macintyre/Hutchison Picture Library

Djibouti
1 Hutchison Picture Library, 2 Trevor Page/Hutchison Picture Library, 3 Timothy Beddow/Hutchison Picture Library, 4 Christina Dodwell/Hutchison Picture Library, 5 Red Sea Team International

Dogon
1 Photodisc, 2 & 3 A. Lorgnier/Cedri/Impact, 4 Joanne Ellington

Druzes
1 & 2 Gail Berrieman, 3 Alan Kedhane/Impact, 4 Roy Spraggett

Egypt
1, 3, 4 & 6 Tim Dowley/Three's Company, 2 David Rudford/United Bible Societies, 5 International Mission Board

Ethiopia
1 & 4 Alice Mason/Impact, 2 Women Material World/Impact, 3 International Mission Board, 5 Material World/Impact

Falashas
1 & 2 Mark Cator/Impact, 3 Jean Cowley/Church's Ministry Among Jewish People

Fiji
1 James Barlow/Impact, 2 & 3 Caroline Penn/Impact, 4 Bhim Singh

Garifuna
All Piers Cavendish/Impact

Gonds
All Stephen Pern/Hutchison Picture Library

Greece
3 & 4 Photodisc, 1, 2 & 6 James McKee, 5 Tim Dowley/Three's Company

Greenland
1 Liv Rognsvåg, 2–4 Eivind Rognsvåg

Guinea-Bissau
1 L. Gaynor, 2–4 Trevor Page/Hutchison Picture Library

Gypsies
1 David Gallant/Impact, 2 & 4 John Cole/Impact, 6 Mark Cator/Impact, 3 & 5 Christian Outreach to Travellers Salisbury Diocese

Haiti
1, 3 & 4 Material World/Impact, 2 Christopher Pillitz/Impact

Hazara
All Andrew McGavin

Herero
1 & 4 Africa Inland Mission, 2 Paul Freestone/Impact, 3 Rhonda Klevansky/Impact

Hui
All Roy Spraggett

Iceland
1, 2 & 6 Piers Cavendish/Impact, 3 V. E. Bowern, 4 & 5 Heather Knight

India
1 Simon Shepheard/Impact, 2 & 6 Material World/Impact, 3 Daniel White/Impact, 4 & 5 Tim Dowley/Three's Company

Indonesia
All Pat Fore

Iraq
1, 2 & 4 Caroline Penn/Impact, 3 Impact

Israel
1 & 3 Roy Spraggett, 2, 4 & 5 Tim Dowley, Three's Company, 6 WEC Press

Japan
1–5 Photodisc, 6 Christophe Bluntzer/Impact

Jolas
All John Hamilton

Kal-Tamashaq
All L. Glover

Kazakhstan
1 & 2 Jin Rice/Impact, 3 Roy Spraggett, 4 Janet Wishnetsky/Impact, 5 Roy Spraggett

Kurds
All Roy Spraggett

Kyrgyz
All Roy Spraggett

Lesotho
1, 3 & 5 Marjorie Froise/*Baptists Today*, 2 Jorn Stjerneklar/Impact, 4 Steve Van t'Slot

Lobi
1, 2 & 4 Jo Parnell, 3 Crispin Hughes/Hutchison Picture Library

Madagascar
1 & 2 Michael Frith, 3 Alain le Garsmeur/Impact, 4 & 5 International Mission Board

Maldives
1 Frontiers, 2–5 Dominic Sansoni/Impact

Mandinka
All Hildegard Damm

Minangkabau
All Pat Store

Missionary Kids
All Jean Barnicoat

Mongolia
All Roy Spraggett

Navajo
1 Heather Knight, 2 & 4 AmeriTribes, 3 & 7 Robin Laurance/Impact, 5 & 6 Sheila Fairmaner

New Zealand
1 David Slimings/Impact, 2 & 6 Simon Grosset/Impact, 3 & 5 S. Fairmaner, 4 Mike McQueen, 7 Louvet/Visa/Cedri/Impact

Newars
1, 5, 6 & 7 Roy Spraggett, 2 & 3 V. E. Bowern, 4 Photodisc

North Korea
All A. Bradshaw/Visions/Impact

Oman
1 J. Rowe, 2 & 4 Alan Keohane/Impact, 3 Robin Laurance/Impact, 5 John Shelley/Impact

Papua New Guinea
1 & 5 Caroline Penn/Impact, 2 Liz Thompson/Impact, 3 Lynn Wood, 4 Grace Fabian

Pygmies
All Brian Woodford

Qatar
1–3 Hutchison Picture Library, 4 Bernard Gerard/Hutchison Picture Library

Quechua
1–3 & 5 A. Donnelly, 4 Charles Coates/Impact

Refugees
1 K. Diagne/UNHCR, 2 R. Chalasani/UNHCR, 3 H. Timmermans/UNHCR, 4 M. Kobayashi/UNHCR

Republic of Guinea
1–3 A. de Bruin, 4 H. Bohl

Riffi Berbers
All Mike Creswell

Romania
1 John Cole/Impact, 2–5 Janet Wishnetsky/Impact

Russia
1 Roy Spraggett, 2 Uba Taylor/Hutchison Picture Library, 3, 4 & 5 Heather Knight

Samoa
All WEC Press

San
1 Marjorie Froise/*Baptists Today*, 2, 3 & 5 David Reed/Impact, 4 V. E. Bowern

Saudi Arabia
1 & 3 Robin Laurance/Impact, 2 Gail McGowan

Spain
1 Tim Dowley/Three's Company, 2 Antonio Gig Binder/Impact, 3 & 4 Peter Stephenson, 5 Roy Spraggett

Sri Lanka
All Roy Spraggett

Sundanese
All Roy Spraggett

Syria
All Alan Keohane/Impact

Tibetans
1 Ian Collinge, 2–6 Roy Spraggett

Trinidad
1 Christophe Bluntzer/Impact, 2 & 4 Mitch de Faria/Impact, 3 & 5 T. Fung

Turkey
1 Roy Spraggett, 2–6 International Mission Board

United Arab Emirates
All Stella Morfey

Uruguay
1 & 2 Robert Gibbs/Impact, 3 & 4 Nick Haslam/Hutchison Picture Library

Uzbeks
All Roy Spraggett

Vagla
All Terry Lobb

Venezuela
1, 3 & 5 Martin Josten, 2 Panayiotis Sofroniou/Impact, 4 Peter Sofroniou/Impact

Vietnam
All Roy Spraggett

Wodaabe
1 Hutchison Picture Library, 2 & 4 Leslie Woodhead/Hutchison Picture Library, 3 Vision Africa

Xhosa
1, 2 & 4 Marjorie Froise/*Baptists Today*, 3 Nancy Durrell McKenna/Hutchison Picture Library

Xinjiang
All Roy Spraggett

Yanomamo
All Símun í Túni

Yao-Mien
1 J. Hitchings/Impact, 2 Piers Cavendish/Impact, 3 & 4 Alain Evrard/Impact

Yemen
1 Michael Good/Impact, 2–6 Roy Spraggett

Zimbabwe
1 & 4 David Reed/Impact, 2 Roger Perry/Impact, 3 S. & D. Stearns

Zulus
1 & 4 Marjorie Froise/*Baptists Today*, 2 Rives/Visa/Cedri/Impact, 3 T. E. Clark/Hutchison Picture Library

World Religions

Animism
1 & 5 Photodisc, 2 Digital Vision, 3 Howard Sayers, 4 Símun í Túni

Buddhism
1–3 Photodisc, 4 Roy Spraggett, 5 N.M. Sture

Christianity
1–3 & 5 Photodisc, 4 Marjorie Froise/*Baptists Today*

Hinduism
1–3 & 5 Photodisc, 4, 6 & 7 Roy Spraggett

Islam
All Photodisc

Judaism
1, 2 , 4 & 5 Photodisc, 3 Tim Dowley/Three's Company

NB Every effort has been made to acknowledge sources accurately. If any inaccuracies have occurred please let us know.

Index

To keep things simple, this index gives just one page number for each two-page spread. For example, 'Afghanistan 12' really means you will find information on Afghanistan on pages 12 to 13.

The index includes names of organizations in the main part of the book, but for these you should also look in the list of addresses starting on page 213.

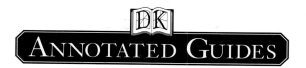

ARCHITECTURE

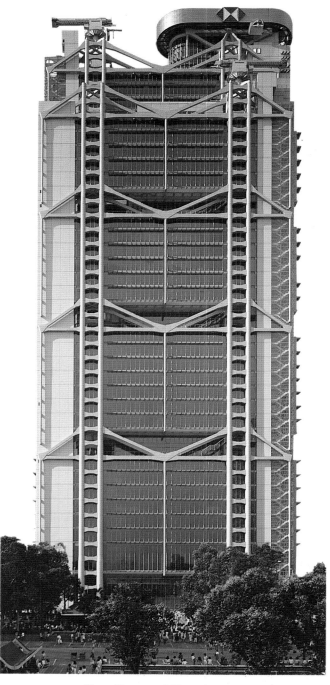

Hong Kong and Shanghai Bank
See page 100

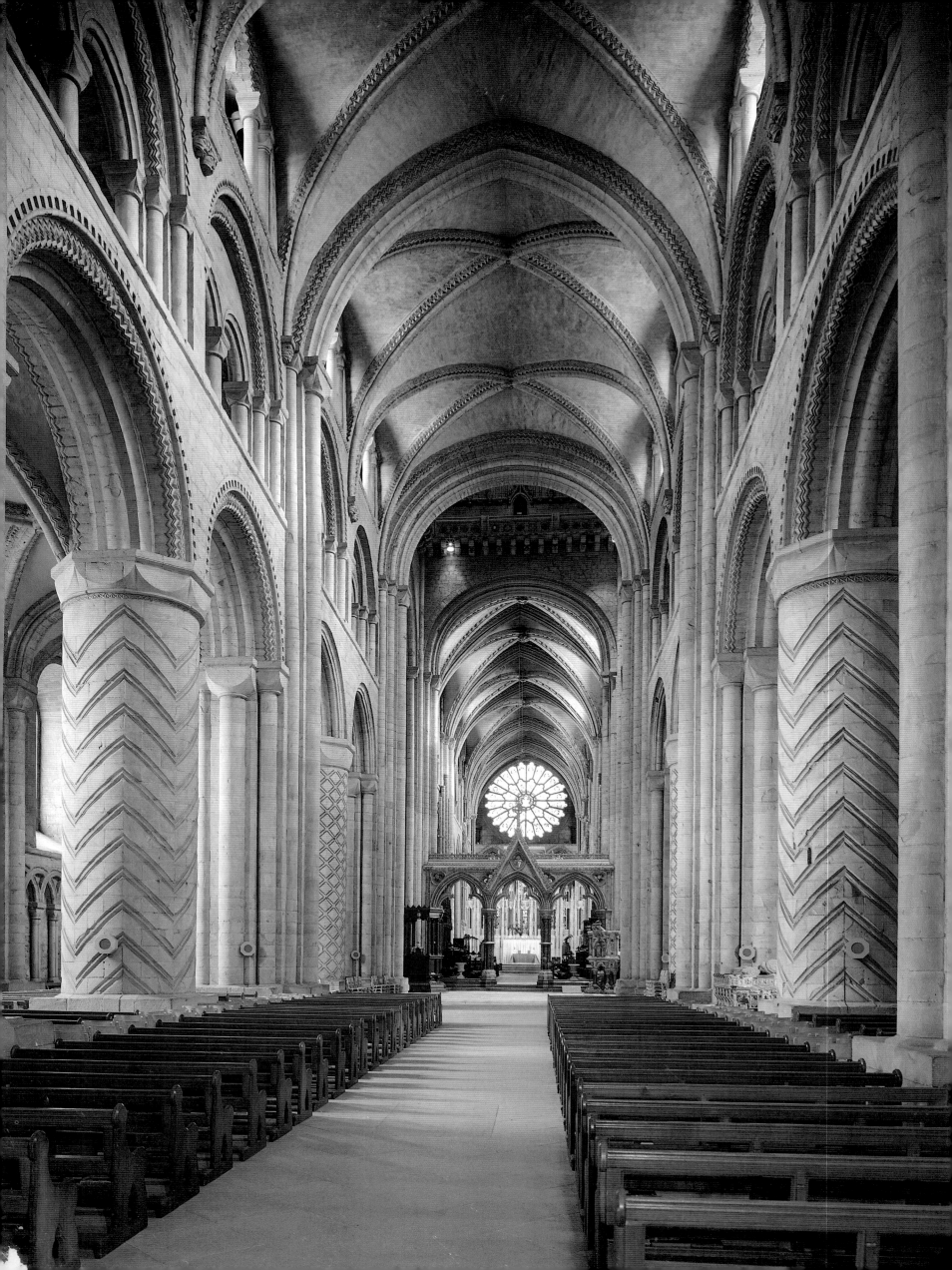

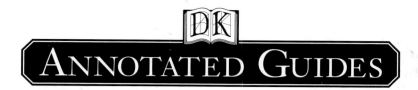

ARCHITECTURE

NEIL STEVENSON

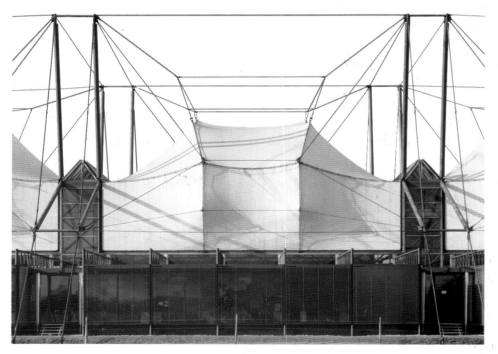

Detail from
*Schlumberger Cambridge
Research Centre*
See page 102

Detail from
Durham Cathedral
See page 26

DORLING KINDERSLEY
London • New York • Sydney • Moscow

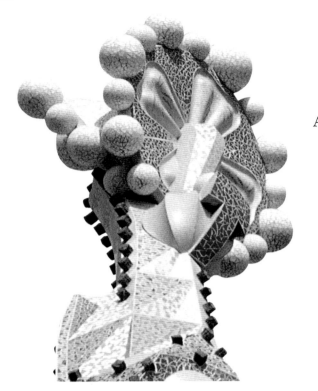

Detail from
Sagrada Familia
See page 72

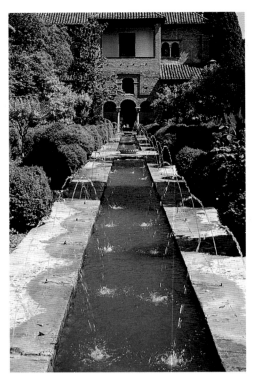

Detail from
The Alhambra
See page 34

![DK logo]

A DORLING KINDERSLEY BOOK

Art Editor Simon Murrell
Project Editor Neil Lockley
Editor Julie Oughton
Managing Editors Gwen Edmonds,
Christine Winters
Senior Managing Editor Sean Moore
Deputy Art Director Tina Vaughan
Production Controller Sarah Coltman
Picture Researcher Deborah Pownall

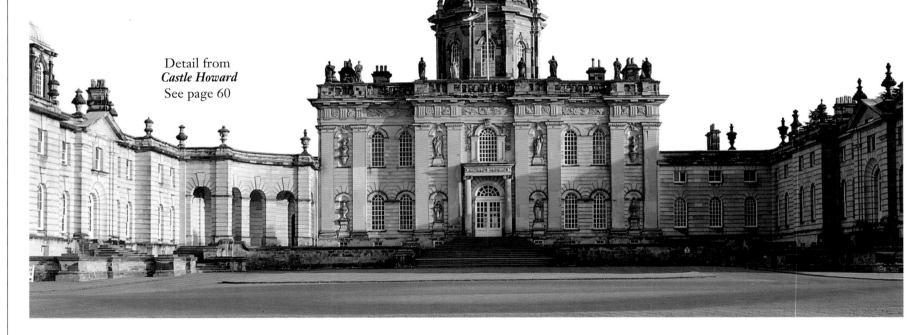

Detail from
Castle Howard
See page 60

First published in Great Britain in 1997
by Dorling Kindersley Limited,
9 Henrietta Street, London WC2E 8PS

2 4 6 8 10 9 7 5 3

Visit us on the World Wide Web at http://www.dk.com

A CIP catalogue record of this book is available
from the British Library

ISBN 0 7513 04468

Colour reproduction by GRB Editrice s.r.l.

Printed in Italy by A. Mondadori, Verona

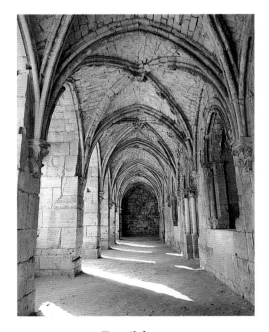

Detail from
Krak des Chevaliers
See page 30

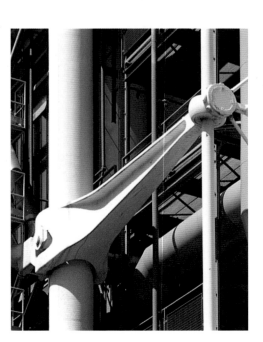

Detail from
The Pompidou Centre
See page 96

CONTENTS

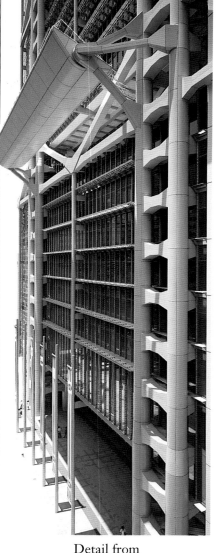

Detail from
Hong Kong and Shanghai Bank
See page 100

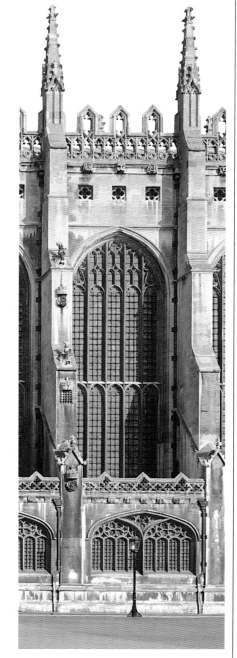

Detail from
King's College Chapel
See page 40

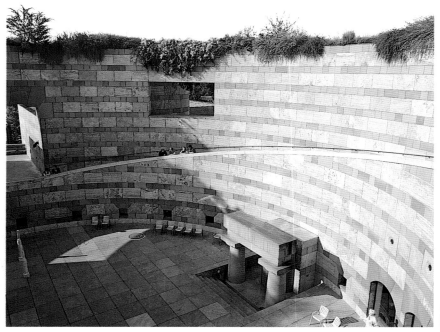

Detail from
Neue Staatsgalerie
See page 98

LOOKING AT ARCHITECTURE

The constant stream of images that pass to us from films, television, books, and magazines, allows us superficial acquaintance with many of the world's great architectural landmarks. Possibilities for international travel – expanded through pilgrimage, trade, and tourism – have brought many of these buildings within reach of a wider audience. The buildings that surround us in our daily lives earn a familiarity of a different kind, however. In both instances, the opportunity to pause and look again, supplemented by some additional information, can be greatly rewarding to our curiosity and general understanding. Making sense of architecture requires some capacity for objective assessment – to stand back from the building and consider aspects of its physical presence.

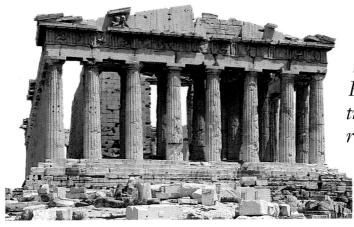

The Parthenon (447–432 BC)
Classical Greek and Roman precedents have exerted a continual influence on western architecture. The Parthenon summarizes the aesthetic refinements of Classical Greece.

Familiarity Throughout this book, consideration is given to form, general organization, materials and methods of construction, principles of structure, and stylistic and decorative features. But few buildings are examples merely of inhabited sculpture, and the *function* and *context* of a building are of fundamental purpose and importance in their appreciation. For this reason, buildings are more easily understood when we see them in use and consider them *in situ*.

Architecture is handed down to us in a "used" condition and is subject to a continual process of evolution. While this may obscure the original work, this process is equally revealing of the developments and cultural preferences of successive generations. On close inspection, buildings can often reveal the results of modification and rebuilding.

To make some sense of the bewildering profusion of historical styles, any study of architecture necessarily has a starting position and a particular sense of direction. The story of western architecture emerged from the reconstructed fragments of ancient Egypt, Classical Greece, and the Roman Empire; western perspectives have traditionally inclined towards Classical architecture and the Greco-Roman model. Until the 19th century, the Gothic period was frequently considered as the product of a dark and uncivilized age. The 19th-century revival of academic interest in the Medieval world produced a categorization of the development of the European Gothic, including a recognition of Byzantine and Romanesque traditions. Modern architecture, developing in the early-20th century from impulses resulting from the Industrial Revolution, polarized attitudes into nostalgic and anti-historic tendencies. While the first idealized Romantic pasts, the second plotted new beginnings on sheets of white paper. Post-modern culture is more pluralistic, however, permitting simultaneously a number of different viewpoints, even when they are taken from the same cultural starting position.

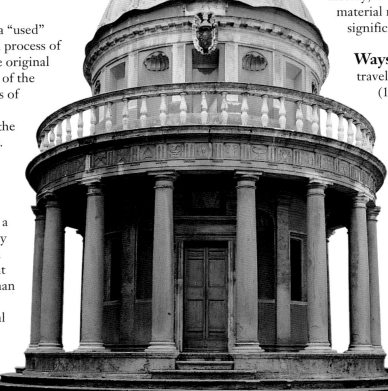

Tempietto San Pietro (1502–10)
Renaissance architecture expanded the Classical architectural vocabulary, seeking a new expression through mathematical order and harmonic proportion.

Surviving Evidence Our interpretation of architectural history is prejudiced by surviving evidence. The priority given to monumental, masonry architecture is, in part, due to the imperishable nature of its construction. Increasingly sophisticated methods of archaeological analysis are giving new insights into other cultures, which use, or have used timber, fabric, mud, and whatever else, to construct their built environments. History, particularly architectural history, is made possible by surviving artefacts – and the material remnants of a society, even when their significance is lost, help to fire our imagination.

Ways of Seeing In the 17th century, the English traveller, scholar, and poet, Sir Henry Wotton (1568–1639), defined architecture as having the prerequisite conditions of "firmness, commodity and delight". "Firmness" here is the method of support and construction, "commodity", the suitability of the design to the purpose, and "delight", the emotional response to its execution. This definition has held up remarkably well, although shifting ground slightly to accompany the pace of western industrial society.

In the late-19th century, the American architect, Louis Sullivan (1856–1924), made the observation that "form follows function", reflecting the search for efficient methods of delivering the new building types required by a rapidly industrialized society. In the 20th century, Le Corbusier (1887–1966) defined architecture as the "masterly, correct, and magnificent play of masses brought together in light", elevating architectural form to a spiritual plane. But society has not always regarded new ideas with such urgency. For example, the slow evolution of ancient Egyptian architecture was related to a spiritual constancy, which developed, and then enshrined, particular architectural types that prevailed for many centuries. Our modern-day perspective is much more immediate. We can see, therefore, that the analysis of construction, function, and form is helpful in tracing architectural development through successive periods. The examples in this book give consideration to these aspects, as they form recognizable characteristics of appearance and provide a means of classification.

While the scrutiny of technology is fascinating and revealing, it disposes a characteristically modern view. The spiritual value of many historic buildings was often of much greater significance to their original constructors than was the means of building them. While technical accounts of ancient building methods are not unknown, architectural prestige rests more with the commissioning client and the commemorative aspects of the building, than with the names or methods of their constructors. The cults of individuals, personal styles, and schools of architecture became more apparent with the rise in status of the artist during the Renaissance, when methods of architecture began to change. Conventional drawings in plan, elevation, and section, accompanied by detailed models, began to conceptualize the building as a unified work, feasibly undertaken for a single client and supervised by a single architect. St Paul's Cathedral (see p. 58) in London was the first major cathedral to be built under such a regime, at the height of the English Renaissance. As construction programmes become increasingly urgent and complex, the method and quantification of such projects becomes more intrusive and influential in the manifestation of the architecture. Ancient practices, which relied on large numbers of people using simple technology, have given way to modern methods involving fewer people with a reliance on sophisticated methods and unique solutions.

The issues of appropriate technology and self-sustainability have a determining influence on the way buildings look and perform. The phenomenal amounts of energy invested in the origination and servicing of buildings has come under close scrutiny. Environmental issues are certain to dominate architectural debate for some time, as are the techniques of designing in a computer-literate world. This reorientation may prove to be a redeeming factor, helping to overcome some of the conservative tendencies prevalent in some societies wishing to preserve everything, irrespective of merit. Elsewhere, it may engender a more appropriate response to climate and culture, working in recognition of context and environment. The imbalance of either condition threatens to blight our contemporary contribution to architectural heritage.

Recurrent Themes

Certain subjects emerge as being particularly instructive to the periodic developments in architecture. The dome, for example, occurs frequently in the architectural vocabulary of many civilizations. It possesses a natural,

Chrysler Building (1928–30)
The skyscrapers of the 1930s were an enduring contribution to monumental architecture. Our modern regard for creativity and technological progress is mirrored in the developments of architecture during the last few decades.

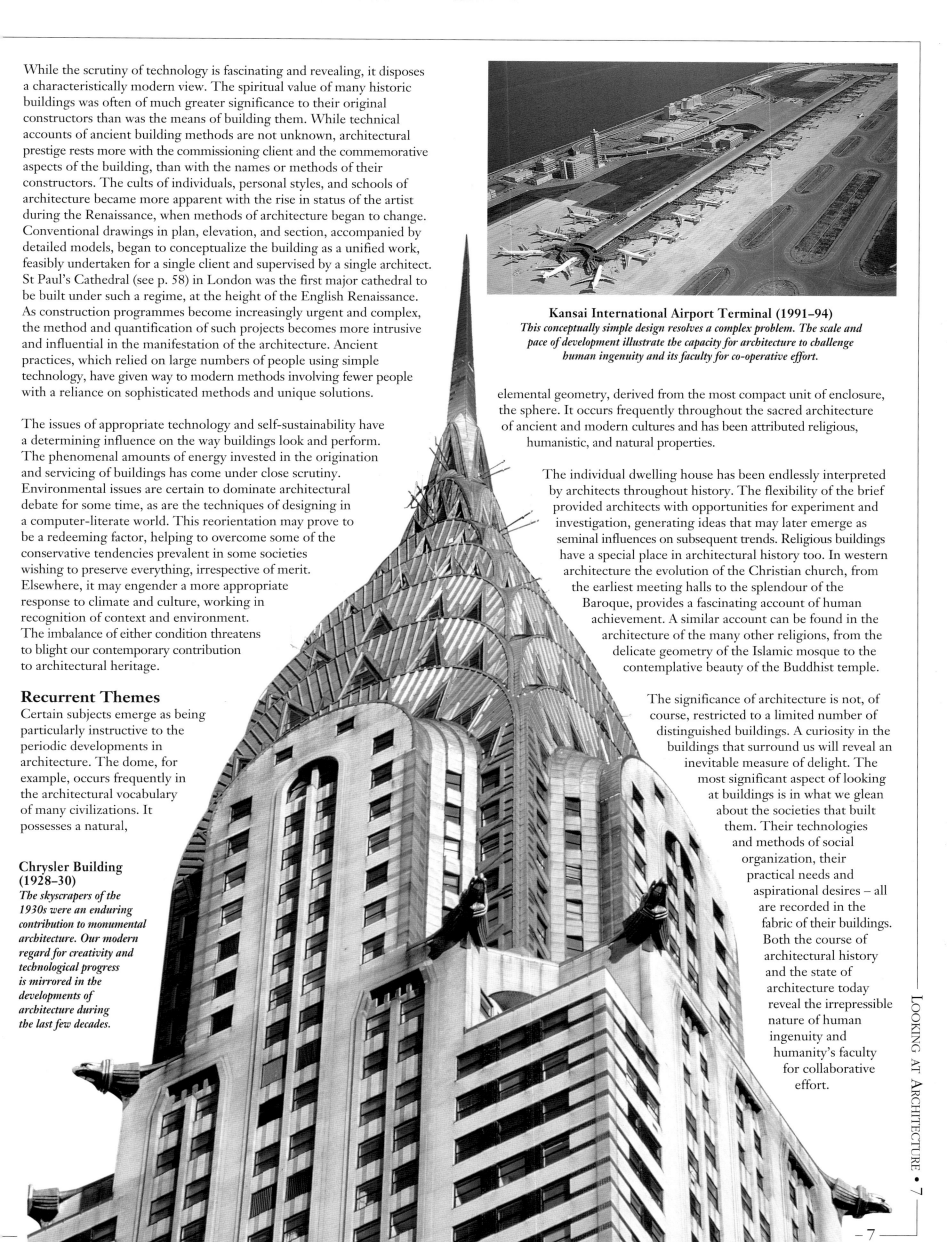

Kansai International Airport Terminal (1991–94)
This conceptually simple design resolves a complex problem. The scale and pace of development illustrate the capacity for architecture to challenge human ingenuity and its faculty for co-operative effort.

elemental geometry, derived from the most compact unit of enclosure, the sphere. It occurs frequently throughout the sacred architecture of ancient and modern cultures and has been attributed religious, humanistic, and natural properties.

The individual dwelling house has been endlessly interpreted by architects throughout history. The flexibility of the brief provided architects with opportunities for experiment and investigation, generating ideas that may later emerge as seminal influences on subsequent trends. Religious buildings have a special place in architectural history too. In western architecture the evolution of the Christian church, from the earliest meeting halls to the splendour of the Baroque, provides a fascinating account of human achievement. A similar account can be found in the architecture of the many other religions, from the delicate geometry of the Islamic mosque to the contemplative beauty of the Buddhist temple.

The significance of architecture is not, of course, restricted to a limited number of distinguished buildings. A curiosity in the buildings that surround us will reveal an inevitable measure of delight. The most significant aspect of looking at buildings is in what we glean about the societies that built them. Their technologies and methods of social organization, their practical needs and aspirational desires – all are recorded in the fabric of their buildings. Both the course of architectural history and the state of architecture today reveal the irrepressible nature of human ingenuity and humanity's faculty for collaborative effort.

TEMPLE OF AMMON, KARNAK

THOUGH WITH ONLY PRIMITIVE TOOLS and an army of enslaved labourers, the ancient Egyptians were among the most prolific builders in history. Through the erection of monumental projects, such as temples, they followed a profound religious conviction to honour and appease the gods. Temples dedicated to the gods and ancestral worship were often the result of successive building phases, periodically remodelled to accommodate grander schemes. At the Temple of Ammon, Karnak, Egypt (1530–323 BC), the buildings are arranged along processional routes connected to the Nile quayside and the nearby temple site of Luxor. The sanctuary is approached through a succession of open courts and the hypostyle hall. The central avenue of this hall was lit by clerestory lighting, with the surrounding columns receding into the vast, dark interior. The inner sanctuary housed the sacred effigy of the creator god, Ammon, attended by the Pharaoh and the priesthood with their secretive rites. The 21.4-hectare (53-acre) precinct was erected over a period of 1,200 years, monumentally recording the Pharaohs dynastic struggle for immortality.

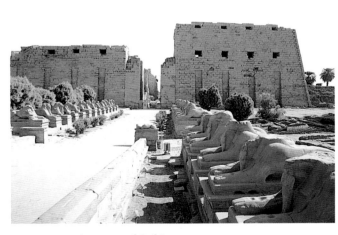

Decoration
The columns and surfaces throughout the hypostyle hall were carved with richly coloured and incised relief designs illustrating dynastic triumphs, scenes from ceremonies, and daily life. Images, statues, and sculpted panels were habitually defaced and identifying hieroglyphics usurped by succeeding Pharaohs seeking to reinforce their own lineage and personality cult.

PYLONS
The pylons were erected by dragging the stone blocks up ramped levels of mud-brick and earth. The outer pylon (centre) was never completed, and part of the ramp structure remains on the inner wall of the south pylons.

The temples were placed at the edge of the fertile Nile valley. Materials were transported by river and brought to Karnak by canal. The tombs of the Pharaohs were located safely away from the flood-plain of the river.

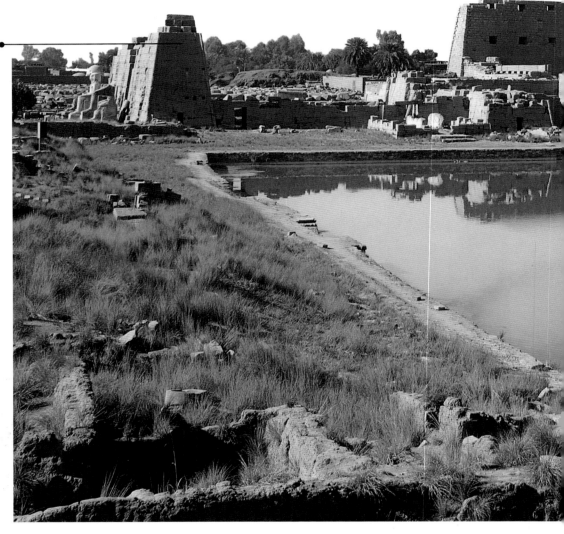

Avenue of Sphinxes
The avenue approaching the outer pylon from the ancient canal quayside is lined with stone sphinxes. The effigy of the god Ammon would have been ceremonially escorted in solemn procession along the avenue on to awaiting barges and taken on a periodic pilgrimage to other sacred temple sites.

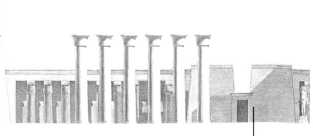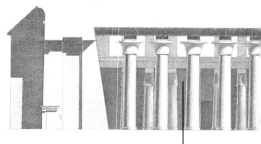

OUTER PYLON
The 42.6-metre- (140-foot-) high outer pylon was once fitted with timber masts bearing immense pennant flags, marking the entrance to the temple.

OUTER COURT
The outer court contains the Kiosk of Taharka, which, used for public ceremonies, marked the limit of public access within the precinct.

HYPOSTYLE HALL
The hypostyle hall consisted of 122 columns, with a central aisle of 12 columns 22 metres (72 feet) high.

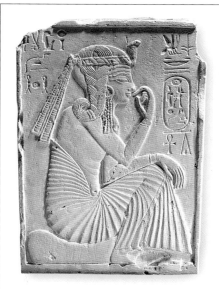

RAMESES II

Rameses II was the third king of the 19th dynasty of Egypt. His 67-year reign (1304–1237 BC) marked the last peak of Egypt's imperial power, and was the second longest reign in Egyptian history. Rameses' reputation as a great king rested on both his fame as a soldier and his prowess in war, and his battle feats were well-documented throughout Egypt and Nubia. Following defeat at the Battle of Kadesh in the early years of his reign, Rameses led many successful attacks, both to recover lost provinces and to conquer new ones. He also undertook a vast building programme, including construction of a number of temples and completion of both the great hypostyle hall at Karnak and two of the six magnificent temples carved out of the cliffside at Abu Simbel, one of which was dedicated to his first and favourite queen, Nefertari.

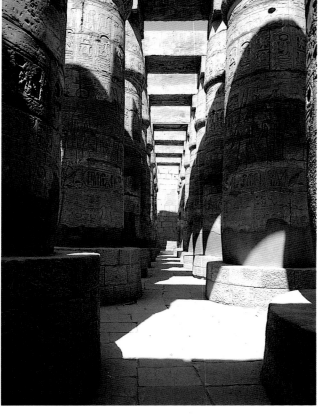

CENTRAL AXIS
The principal halls and courtyards are arranged along a central axis, though the precinct was laterally extended with additional gateways, ceremonial buildings, and commemorative structures.

CONSTRUCTION
The building was gradually filled with earth, providing a platform on which to erect the stone blocks and beams. On completion, the building was then excavated to reveal the internal volume.

Hypostyle Hall
The great hypostyle hall was once covered with a stone roof and lit along a raised, central aisle by clerestory window grills. The aisles are flanked by 12 main columns 3.6 metres (12 feet) in diameter. To either side are seven rows of nine columns, which recede into the darkness, producing an effect of limitless space.

OBELISK OF HATSHEPSUT
The 29-metre- (95-foot-) high obelisk, originally plated with gold, was transported to the site by barge, raised with ramps and levers into a pit of sand, and lowered on to its locating plinth.

Life within the temple was regulated by the rising and setting of the Sun, the cycles of the planets, and the rising of the River Nile. The ceremonial rites, and creation and immortalization beliefs use the imagery of darkness and light, symbolized in the alternation of dark interiors with bright courtyards.

SACRED LAKE
The artificial lake was used for the daily rituals of bathing and ablution undertaken by the priesthood. It also provided a breeding ground for the birds sacrificed as offerings within the temple.

SPECIFICATION

- **Location** — Karnak, Egypt
- **Date** — 1530–323 BC
- **Height of hypostyle hall** — 24 m (78 ft)
- **Building structure** — Stone
- **Building type** — Temple

INNER COURTYARD
Successive pylon gateways, flanked by obelisks, provide access to the inner courtyard.

SANCTUARY
The sanctuary contains the sacred effigy of Ammon, placed in a boat, ritually bathed, anointed, and brought offerings of food.

BOTANICAL HALL
The oldest part of the temple includes the botanical hall of Thutmosis III, with walls decorated with every known species of flora and fauna in his kingdom.

THE PARTHENON

THE PARTHENON (447–432 BC) is situated at the summit of the Acropolis in Athens. Perhaps the greatest monument of the Classical period (650–323 BC), it summarizes the ultimate refinement of the Doric temple. The unusually wide rectangular plan measures 31 x 69 metres (102 x 226 feet). The *peristyle*, the range of 8 by 17 columns surrounding the temple, contains two rooms, enclosed within solid, ashlar walls. The larger room, or *naos*, with its inner, supporting colonnade, accommodated the statue of the patron goddess, Athena. The local, white Pentelic marble provided the perfect medium for the sharpness of detail required for the design and execution of the sculpted relief panels of the frieze and portico. The building was subject to meticulous refinements of proportion and geometry, known as *entasis*, to maintain an appearance of exact alignment. Apparently perpendicular and horizontal lines are, in fact, set out within curved and inclining planes, to correct the optical illusion of perspective distortion.

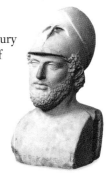

PERICLES

Pericles (*c.* 495–429 BC), the 5th-century Athenian statesman, was the leader of Athens from *c.* 450 until his death. Under Pericles, Greek architecture and sculpture reached their highest point. He is best remembered for his programme of public building, in which he commissioned numerous sacred and public structures.

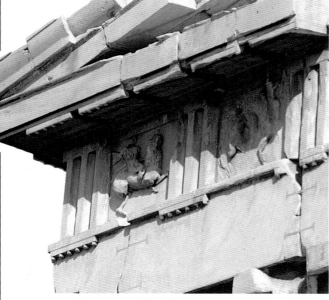

Entablature
The columns are topped by a wide capital and a slab of stone called an abacus, *which helps to relieve the tensile forces in the beam. The Greek form of construction employed a simple post-and-beam (trabeated) arrangement, translated into stone from ancient principles developed in timber construction.*

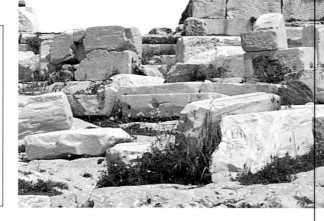

SPECIFICATION

- **Location**   Athens, Greece
- **Date**   447–432 BC
- **Architects**   Ictinus and Callicrates
- **Building structure**   Stone and Pentelic marble
- **Building type**   Temple

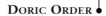

END COLUMNS •
The end columns have a closer spacing and thicker diameter than the main columns and incline diagonally towards the centre of the temple to counteract their appearance of outward inclination. The other columns are inclined inwards, 6 centimetres (2.4 inches) from the vertical.

DORIC ORDER •
The columns have the monumental proportions of the Doric Order. The drums of white Pentelic marble were carved *in situ* to their fluted profiles, which deepen towards the top to emphasize the shadow-lines and volumetric composition.

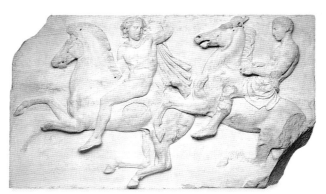

The Parthenon Frieze
The marble panels depict scenes from the procession of the Athenian Knights, contests between the gods and mythical figures, heroic battles of the Greeks and the Amazons, and scenes from the siege of Troy. The frieze's main subject (shown here) is the procession of worshippers on their way to the Acropolis to celebrate the festival called the Great Panathenaea in honour of the goddess Athena. The frieze panels were removed from the building between 1801 and 1803.

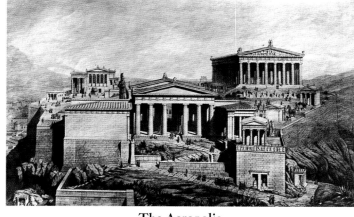

The Acropolis
The sacred and defensive site of the Acropolis contains some of the most impressive monuments of the Greek period. It has served as a model of an idealized civic society for Western architecture.

ENTABLATURE
The entablature is comprised of lintels connected by bow-tie-shaped iron clamps. The lintels have a faceted, curved profile, rising 6 centimetres (2.4 inches) towards the centre.

FRIEZE
The marble frieze was carved along the top of the inner entablature of the *naos* wall just below the peristyle ceiling.

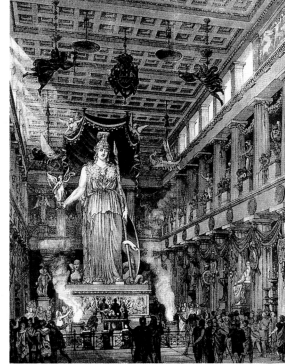

The Statue of Athena
The naos *was dominated by the statue of the patron goddess, Athena, by the sculptor, Phidias. Lit by the rising Sun from the central, east-facing doorway, the statue, constructed from plates of gold and ivory, stood 12.8 metres (42 feet) high.*

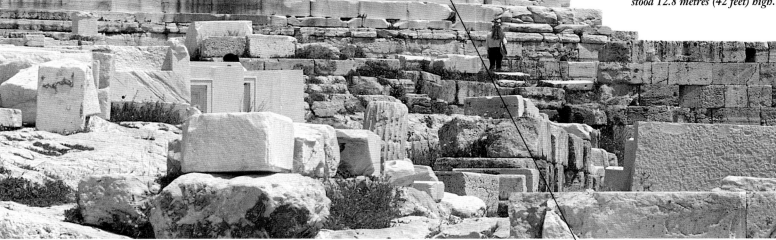

STEPS
The steps have a curved profile, rising towards the centre. The treads are set with a slight upward tilt. The devices of perspective correction produce a complex geometry for construction.

The high-relief sculptures of the frieze are cut more deeply towards the top of the panels to correct the apparent foreshortening when viewed from below.

ENTASIS
The tapering columns are swollen in section, about two fifths of the way up, to correct the illusion of a concave profile that a straight-sided shaft would produce.

THE COLOSSEUM

THE ROMAN EMPEROR VESPASIAN commissioned this vast amphitheatre as a grand civic gesture to satisfy the escalating public appetite for spectacular shows of violent entertainment. The Colosseum (AD 70–82) in Rome proved a public reminder of the power and organization of the Roman Empire. Games were staged in increasingly elaborate spectacles, to which combatants, victims, and animals were imported from across the empire. Up to 5,000 pairs of gladiators and 5,000 animals were slaughtered in a single event before 50,000 spectators. The popularity of Emperors was judged by the success of their games, (which continued until the collapsing Empire lacked the resources to stage them). The Colosseum's rapid programme of construction taxed the organizational skill and ingenuity of the constructors, who used shift work, prefabrication, modular building, elaborate machinery, and a largely skilled workforce in methods not unfamiliar to 20th-century projects.

The name "Colosseum" derives not from the scale of the building but from the nearby colossal statue of Nero, which was erected within the grounds of the pre-existing Golden House of Nero.

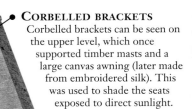

CORBELLED BRACKETS
Corbelled brackets can be seen on the upper level, which once supported timber masts and a large canvas awning (later made from embroidered silk). This was used to shade the seats exposed to direct sunlight.

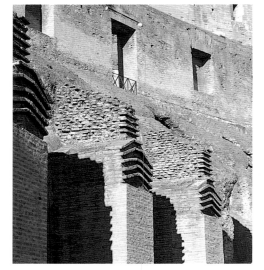

Seating Levels
The tiered structure of the seating levels is supported by load-bearing masonry walls and outer piers radiating from the centre. This system enabled building material to be raised along the inclined sections and supported on scaffolding platforms with workers at each tier, permitting a greater pace of construction.

PIERS
Eighty massive piers support the outer wall, which is connected to the inner piers and walls by concrete vaults.

SPECIFICATION

- **Location**   Rome, Italy
- **Date**   AD 70–82
- **Height**   48 m (157.5 ft)
- **Building structure**   Stone, brick, and concrete
- **Building type**   Civic arena

It has been calculated that the construction of the external walls alone would have required 292,000 cartloads of travertine stone to build – brought along a specially constructed road from Tivoli.

THREE-QUARTER COLUMNS
The three-quarter columns on the outer walls are included purely as decoration, rising through the ascending tiers with their Orders roughly derived from Greek architecture.

In addition to there being gladiatorial combats, criminals were executed under sentence of exposure to wild beasts, and mythological and historical battles were enacted with combatants dressed in theatrical costume.

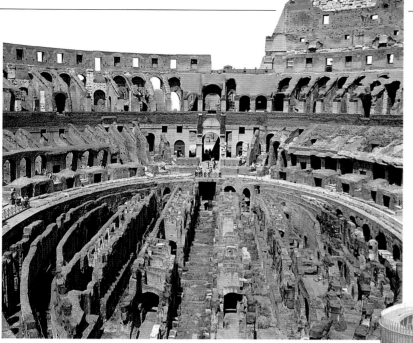

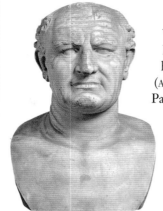

EMPEROR VESPASIAN

Vespasian (Titus Flavius Vespasianus) (AD 9–79) was Roman Emperor from AD 69 to 79. Born in Italy of humble origin, he completed a governorship in Africa (AD 63–66) and also led triumphant campaigns in Palestine (AD 67–68). Following Nero's death in AD 68, Vespasian became founder of the Flavian dynasty and was declared Emperor the following year. His consolidation of the Empire, together with policies of public reform, brought political stability, and he embarked on a vast building programme. In addition to beginning the Colosseum, Vespasian built his Forum and the Temple of Peace (AD 71–79).

Construction Materials
The materials of construction vary according to their imposed loads. Stone of higher strength was used for the piers at the outer walls, with lighter brick and masonry closer to the arena. Concrete (see p. 14) was used extensively for construction of the vaulted floors and encircling corridors.

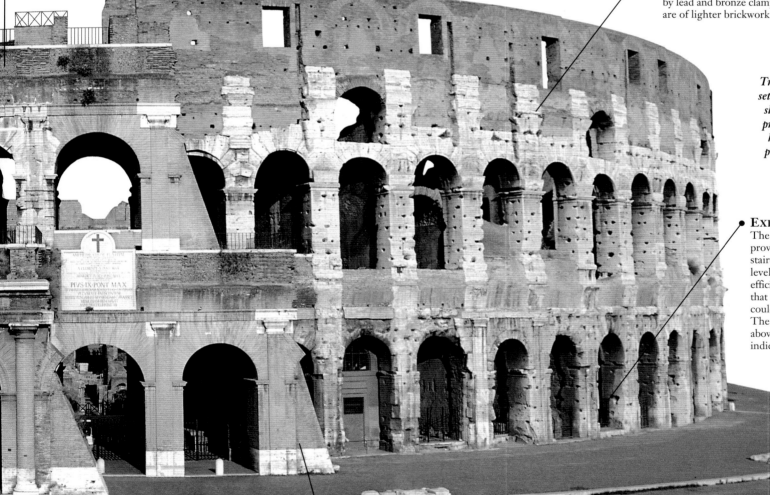

Spectators
The auditorium accommodated 50,000 spectators in rising tiers of seats, which were allocated by ticket in sections according to rank. The arena mirrored the hierarchy of Roman society. The Emperor and his retinue sat in elevated ringside seats; in the upper levels sat slaves, foreigners, and women.

INAUGURATION GAMES
The building was completed in a remarkably short period. The first games were held in AD 80, although the upper storey may have been incomplete.

The immense fabric awning (velarium) was winched into position by gangs of sailors, shading the spectators from the intense summer heat.

WALLS
Originally covered with stucco, the walls reveal their structure of travertine stone blocks laid in courses on mortar beds secured by lead and bronze clamps. The upper sections are of lighter brickwork and tufa limestone.

Travertine stone bollards set into the pavement at a slight incline may have provided anchorage and hauling blocks for the pulley system needed to raise the awning.

EXITS
The many *vomitoria* (exits) provided access to the staircases serving the upper levels. From this remarkably efficient design, it is estimated that a capacity crowd of 50,000 could exit in three minutes. The consecutive numbering above the entrance arches indicates the seat positions.

SITUATION
The Colosseum stands on the site of the lake of the former Golden House of Nero. The lake was drained by a main sewer, discharging into the River Tiber.

COLLAPSED WALLS
Large sections of the walls have collapsed or have been removed. Following the demise of the games, the site was used as a source of building material, reclaimed for many projects throughout Rome.

Sections of floor could be removed to flood the entire arena with water to a depth of 1.5 metres (5 feet) to stage mock naval battles.

THE PANTHEON

THE SUCCESSIVE PERIODS of the Roman Empire provided a continuity of architectural development that advanced techniques in construction and engineering. Though indebted to the established Orders of Greek architecture, the Romans were to find a new form of expression in the range of their building types, their spatial complexity, and a co-ordinated urban planning that achieved cohesion throughout the Empire. The structural potential of the true arch, previously utilized in Etruscan architecture, found its logical conclusion in Roman vaulted and domed structures. These structural developments provided an opportunity for new architectural forms, exceeding the limitations of Greek post-and-beam (trabeated) construction. Systematic engineering methods were used to exploit local resources and to manufacture materials. Domed, concrete-shell construction was used in one of the most impressive surviving buildings of the Roman period, the Pantheon (AD 120–24) in Rome. Uniquely preserved by virtue of its continued use into the succeeding period of Christianity, its astonishing 43.4-metre- (142-foot-) span was unequalled until the 19th century.

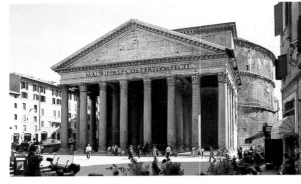

Portico
The temple incorporates part of the portico from a preceding temple. This caused confusion in the dating and attribution of the building. However, suppliers' marks stamped on the Rotunda's brickwork confirmed the construction date as being within the early part of Emperor Hadrian's rule (AD 117–38).

SPECIFICATION

- **Location** — Rome, Italy
- **Date** — AD 120–24
- **Span of dome** — 43.4 m (142 ft)
- **Building structure** — Brick, stone, and concrete
- **Building type** — Temple
- **Construction time** — 4 years

AGGREGATE MATERIAL
The aggregate, layered into the concrete, varies throughout the dome. Lighter pumice stone is used in the upper section to reduce weight in the central area. Heavier material is used at the base, where greater compressive strength is required.

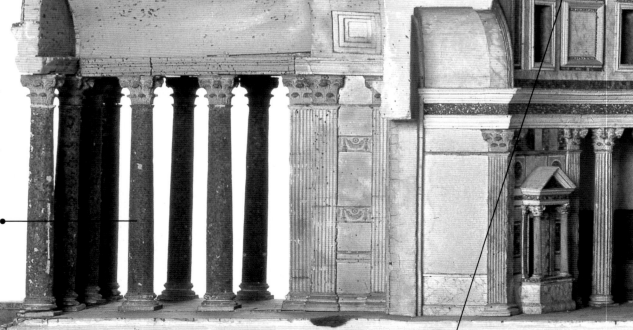

PORCH
The porch comprises a wide triangular stone pediment supported by eight freestanding columns.

Roman concrete construction was economical, fast, and efficient. Small groups of skilled carpenters provided the timber formwork (a temporary casing of woodwork, within which concrete is moulded); the concrete was supplied and layered by large gangs of unskilled labourers.

COLUMNS
The monolithic shafts of Egyptian granite have white marble bases and Corinthian capitals.

The building was originally approached by eight steps. The increase in height of the surrounding area, however, has left the building in a shallow depression.

SPHERICAL VOLUME
The height of the dome above the ground equals the diameter of its plan, describing an internal volume that could contain a perfect sphere – a form with particular cosmological significance.

The form of the building accords with a direct representation of Roman cosmology. The dome represents the celestial vault illuminated by the central source of the Sun.

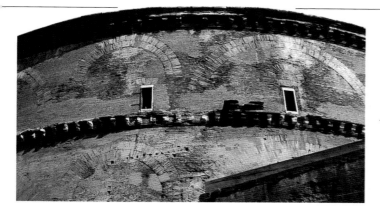

Relieving Arches
Brick arches, embedded in the structure of the wall, act as internal buttresses, distributing the loads from the dome to the walls. Brickwork was commonly used in walls, arches, vaults, and domes. In buildings of importance, the brick was faced with a hard, stucco render and, more lavishly, with a sophisticated arrangement of stone and marble cladding, applied in panels to the brickwork and restrained by bronze cramps and pins.

EMPEROR HADRIAN

Hadrian (AD 76–138) was Roman Emperor from AD 117. He was a great admirer of Greek culture and a patron of the arts. As well as for his political achievements, Hadrian was renowned as a poet and as an architectural designer. Among his buildings were the Villa at Tivoli (AD 124), and the Temple of Venus and Rome (AD 123–35) in Rome, built largely to his own design.

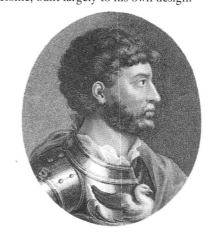

• **COFFERED CEILING**
The form of the coffers emphasizes the lower, recessed mouldings, helping to compensate for the viewers' perspective distortion when viewed from the ground.

• **CONCRETE**
During construction, the dome was supported on timber formwork removed after the concrete had set.

• **ROOF LINE**
The building is a three-tiered cylinder covered by a hemispherical dome. The thickening of material at the dome's perimeter counteracts its outward thrust.

It was the Romans who introduced concrete, a building material that offered the potential for large, spanning, monolithic shell-structures for domes and vaults. Their concrete consisted of lime mixed with volcanic soil, known as pozzolana. This was applied in layers with an aggregate material, such as broken roof tiles, between the faces of brickwork that formed the inner and outer skins. Unlike contemporary concrete, it was not reinforced and required external buttressing, making it unsuitable for restraining tensile loads. Secondly, it was not as fluid when mixed, limiting the complexity of the formwork shapes.

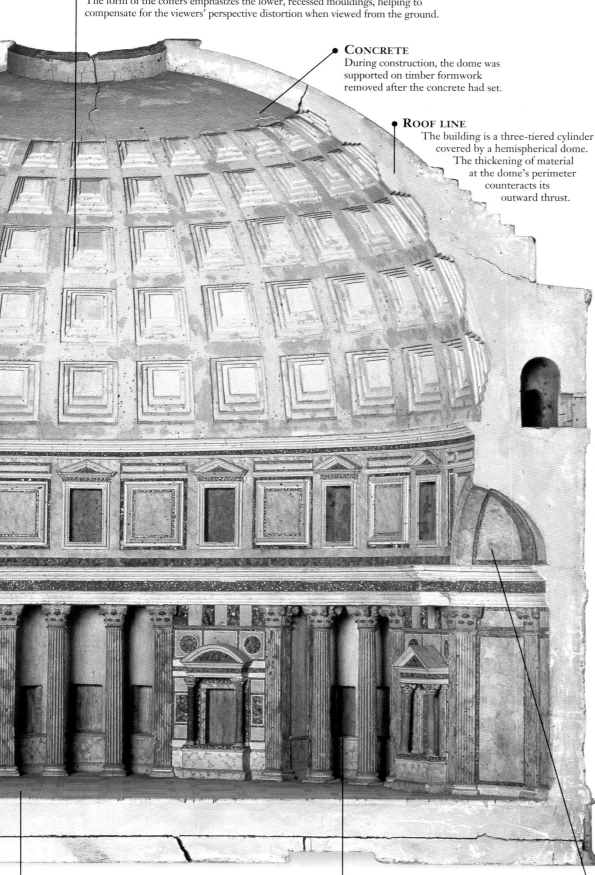

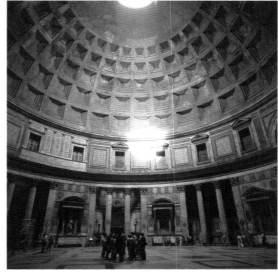

Ocular Window
The interior space is dramatically lit from a single 8-metre- (26-foot-) diameter ocular window in the centre of the dome. This helps reduce the central weight of the construction and obviates the structural difficulty of placing window openings in the perimeter. The effect is dramatic, giving a sense of simplicity and unity.

• **PATTERNED FLOOR**
The floor is paved with coloured flags of marble, porphyry, and granite. The square and circular chequer-board pattern complements the ceiling coffers.

• **NICHES**
Set within the thickness of the wall, niches were dedicated to the five planets known to the Romans, and to the luminaries, the Sun and the Moon.

• **RESTRAINING CUPOLAS**
Above the niches are restraining cupolas, which help relieve the stresses at the edge of the dome and translate the loads vertically, via the walls, to the foundations.

ISE SHRINE

THE SACRED SHRINES at Ise Jingu on Ise Bay, southern Honshu, Japan, preserve the ancient traditions of Japan's indigenous Shinto beliefs. The main complex comprises two separate shrines, each enclosed by four wooden fences. The Imperial Shrine, also known as the Inner Shrine, is dedicated to Amaterasu Omikami, the Sun goddess from whom the Japanese imperial family traces its descent. The Outer Shrine is dedicated to Toyouke Okami, the goddess of farming and harvest. At both shrines, the central enclosure which houses the main shrine, or *shoden*, is flanked by structures that provide storage and accommodation for guardians and officiates. The sacred compound, prohibited from public view, is destroyed and rebuilt on alternating sites at 20 year intervals. Practised since AD 690, this traditional process of renewal, *shikinen sengu*, allows the precise skills of timber joinery in each rebuilding to be undertaken by three successive generations of craftsmen. This remarkable building provides a rare view of the crisp detail and powerful simplicity much admired in Japanese architecture.

With its meticulous and disciplined structure, formal simplicity, and spiritual presence, the Ise Shrine embodies the essence of Japanese architecture in the same way that the Parthenon (see p. 10) can be seen to exemplify western architectural attitudes.

SPECIFICATION
- **Location** — Honshu, Japan
- **Date** — 2nd century AD
- **Building structure** — Timber-frame
- **Building type** — Temple
- **Construction time** — Rebuilt every 20 years

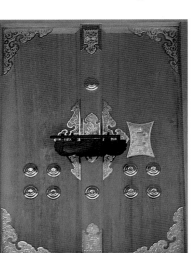

Decorative Fittings
The doors are decorated with metal bracketry, introduced in subsequent rebuilding. Other elements, such as the coloured balls mounted on to the balustrade posts, illustrate Chinese architectural influences arriving with the introduction of Buddhism in the 6th century AD.

WEST AND EAST TREASURY
The western treasury houses ceremonial regalia, while the eastern treasury contains silks and paper. These separate buildings flank the *shinden* in which the ancestral deity is enshrined.

Each compound is reconstructed on alternating adjacent sites at 20-year intervals, allowing each rebuilding to be undertaken by three generations of craftsmen, overseeing, executing, or apprenticed to the construction.

COLUMNS
The supporting columns are embedded in the ground. After the dismantling of the structure for periodic rebuilding, the central "heart pillar", which has a particular spiritual significance, remains *in situ* until reincorporated into the next rebuilding of the site.

SHRINE
The shrine contains objects belonging to the emperor, including a comb and a mirror. His investment ceremony is held within the privacy of the shrine.

SHINTO

The indigenous religion of Japan, Shinto is centred on the worship of nature and the veneration of the spirits of nature – *kami* – found in mountains, rocks, trees, and other natural features. Shinto shrines dedicated to *kami* are found across Japan, particularly in areas of natural beauty. Respect is traditionally shown at these sites by placing offerings, as here at these "meota-iwa" (wedded rocks) near Ise.

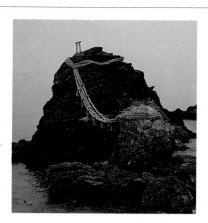

Chigi

The forked finials, or chigi, on the ridge of the frame have become highly stylized, evolving beyond their structural purpose of support into decorative and ritualised elements of construction. The finials are derived from a method of traditional joinery used to secure timber frames. Their use was later restricted to buildings of cultural significance and noble patronage. The building's continuous replication has tended towards an exaggeration of iconographic elements.

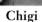

METALLIC CAPS

Embellishing the ends of the frame, metallic caps protect the exposed grain of the timber, which is where it is most vulnerable to moisture penetration and decay.

RIDGE BILLETS

The ridge billets, or *katsuogi*, restrain the ridge boards and help anchor the traditional roof thatch of miscanthus grass. The ridge is supported by two centrally placed cypress posts in a constructional system that has survived from about the 2nd century AD. The shrine is thought to have achieved its final form in the 6th century.

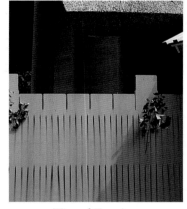

Tiered Fencing

Four concentric fences protect the sacred inner compound from public view. Access for worship is severely restricted to priests, officiates, and members of the Imperial family. Traditionally, the kami had been worshipped within sacred and forbidden areas, such as forests and mountains.

RAISED PLATFROM

The raised platform of the building is derived from the ancient form of rice store houses, which were raised above the ground to protect food from vermin and flooding.

SHODEN

The building is entered by a covered porch. The main *shoden* measures 10.8 x 5.4 metres (35 x 18 feet), comprising a main timber frame of three bays wide and two bays deep.

WALLS

The walls are formed from timber planks, horizontally fitted into rebated channels in the main vertical framing posts. The structure is surrounded by a covered veranda.

SANTA SOPHIA

THE ROMAN METHODS of organized labour and engineering, mixed with the assimilation of indigenous traditions, were celebrated in the scale and magnificence of Santa Sophia (AD 532–37), the most important church of the Byzantine Empire. This monumental building has a vast central nave, measuring 68.6 x 32.6 metres (225 x 107 feet), crowned by a ribbed dome of brick and stone. The domed structure, lined with marbles and glistening mosaics, achieves a remarkable quality of natural lighting. Externally, the building portrays a complex arrangement of piers and cupolas, which are supported by monumental and unadorned bearing walls and buttresses. The minaret towers were added following its conversion to a mosque in 1453. Despite the concealment and disfigurement of much of the original decoration, this awesome structure communicates much of the ethereal mystery and power of the Byzantine world.

Internal Galleries
The internal galleries are supported on columns with monolithic (single-piece) shafts of exotic, coloured marble. The capitals and arcades are highly detailed and carved with tracery motifs incorporating the monogram of the Emperor Justinian I.

PROFILE
The shallow central dome was severely damaged following an earthquake in AD 557 and was rebuilt using a higher profile of greater stability.

MINARET TOWERS
After over 900 years as a consecrated church, in 1453, following the capture of Constantinople by the Turks, the building was converted into a mosque, and minaret towers were added.

"[The dome] seems not to rest upon solid masonry, but to cover the space with its golden dome suspended from Heaven"
PROCOPIUS

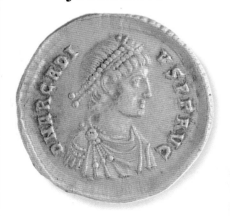

JUSTINIAN I

After the Roman Empire converted to Christianity, Constantinople became the capital in AD 330. Justinian I (c. 482–565) was Byzantine Emperor from AD 527 to 565 and is renowned for his contribution to architecture. In addition to Santa Sophia, Justinian's programme of building included aqueducts, bridges, and fortifications along the frontiers of the Byzantine Empire.

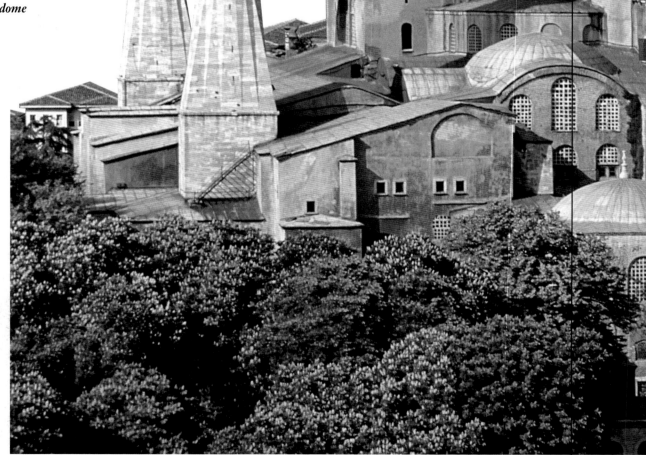

The building was erected in a remarkably short period of 5 years. Two teams of 5,000 workmen competed with each other in the building of the east and west sections.

BUTTRESSING
Earthquakes have created significant movement within the structure, requiring extensive buttressing and additional supportive structures.

Nave Interior
The central section of the nave is spanned by a vast central dome 32.6 metres (107 feet) in diameter. Natural light penetrates apertures at the base of the dome and windows placed within the tympanum wall.

Denied the local availability of pozzolana cement, the Roman constructors were unable to use the technique of concrete construction that had facilitated the building of single-domed structures such as the Pantheon. However, a technique of brick-skin construction, using thickened layers of mortar, produced some of the advantages of speedy construction, deploying large gangs of comparatively unskilled labour.

CONSTRUCTION
The scale of the dome was limited by the precedent of the Pantheon, which had established the constructional limit of a monolithic dome. Following Santa Sophia's collapse, it was rebuilt to a higher profile, and additional height and mass were given to the buttressing towers.

CENTRAL DOME
The central dome is braced by the eastern and western hemispherical domes, which, together, form the main nave.

WINDOWS
The presence of clerestory windows at this point would seem to contradict the requirement for mass to resist the outward thrust of the dome, but this, in fact, reduces the risk of cracking, enabling the dome to perform efficiently as a monolithic shell.

SPRINGING ARCHES
The piers and springing arches provide the primary route of transference to the ground of loads imposed by the main domes.

SPECIFICATION

- **Location**   Istanbul, Turkey
- **Date**   AD 532–37
- **Height**   54.8 m (180 ft)
- **Building structure**   Brick and stone
- **Building type**   Church/ Mosque

TOWERS
Towers abut the north and south elevations either side of the springing arches that support the central dome. The mass of the towers resists the side thrusts exerted from the relieving arches.

TYMPANUM WALL
Beneath the main relieving arches, the tympanum wall is theoretically non-load-bearing and able to provide maximum window area to illuminate the interior.

PIERS
The main piers are constructed from stone, rather than mortar-bonded brick, which requires a substantial curing period before achieving its bonded strength. The use of stone for the initial construction phase enabled work to proceed at a greater pace.

TEMPLE I, TIKAL

RISING ABOVE THE CANOPY OF THE RAINFOREST, the pyramid towers of the Mayan city of Tikal dominate the landscape. The Mayan civilization flourished during the Classic period between AD 300 and 900, but declined abruptly, its great cities abandoned 500 years before the Spanish conquest of South America in the 16th century. Tikal lies in the Petén region of Guatemala in Central America. Excavations have uncovered groups of platforms and stone structures dispersed across a 68.6-square-kilometre (26.5-square-mile) site. At the centre of this city, linked by wide causeways connecting specific building clusters, is a central stucco-lined plaza measuring 85 x 67 metres (280 x 220 feet). Facing each other across this platform are two towers, the largest known as Temple I, or the Temple of the Great Jaguar (c. AD 500). The building groups share a geomantic relationship, suggesting an urban hierarchy and a solar and astral alignment. The interiors of the temples are small and simple. Elevated high above the plaza, they indicate an elitist ceremonial purpose obscured from the assembled crowds below. The urban centre, with an estimated population at its height of around 50,000, was sustained by the support of a wide agricultural empire, which had cultural links with distant cities of the same period. These monuments, now isolated among the dense tangle of undergrowth, communicate silently of a mysterious and lost culture.

ROOF COMB
The temple is surmounted by an intricately carved and painted, crenellated ridge of a much greater height than the temple vault. It rises from the rear wall and provides an imposing silhouette to the structure.

SCULPTURAL DECORATION
The external face of the temple vault carries sculptural decoration depicting a large, seated figure and serpent.

SANCTUARY
The temple sanctuary comprises three connected chambers with a corbel-vaulted roof. The purpose of the chamber is connected with the frequent rites of human sacrifice. The victim's blood ran on to the steps, and the still-beating heart was ripped out and offered to the gods. The inner face of the wooden lintel above the opening is carved with an image of a jaguar.

TERRACES
The pyramid rises in nine tiers to a total height of 47.5 metres (156 feet). The distinct terraces represent the mythical levels of the underworld.

RITUAL ACTIVITIES

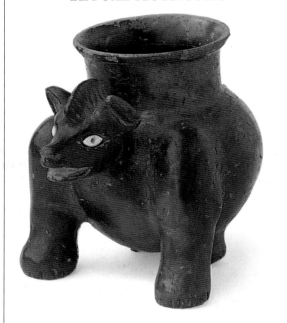

This jaguar-shaped bowl from Guatemala, part of the Mayan Empire, may have been used to collect blood offerings. The drawing of blood from one's body often preceded important ceremonies and sacrifices. These ritual activities were complex and intense, with animals, birds, flowers, jade, and blood being sacrificed in return for divine favour. Special ceremonies took place on the Mayan New Year's Day, with each successive month being devoted to a particular god. Each social group, from priests to fishermen, celebrated its own religious feast.

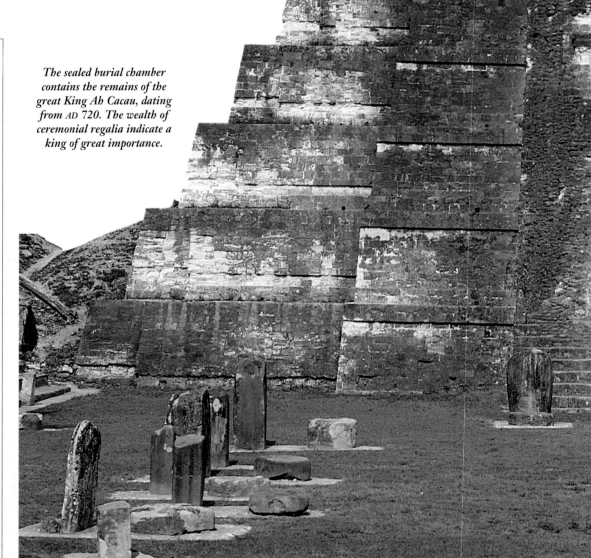

The sealed burial chamber contains the remains of the great King Ah Cacau, dating from AD 720. The wealth of ceremonial regalia indicate a king of great importance.

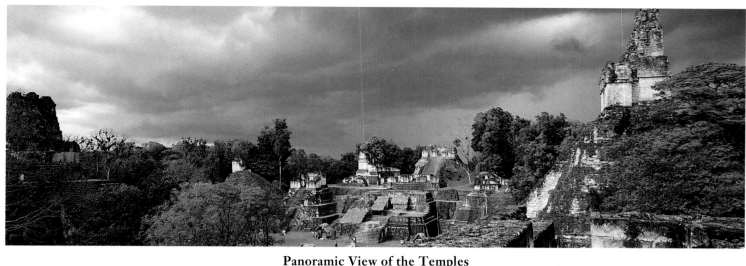

Panoramic View of the Temples

The clusters of pyramidal temples are elevated on high, terraced plinths and arranged around large civic spaces and smaller courtyards. The city lies, roughly, along a broken ridge, connected by a series of causeways,   *which may once have been surrounded by reservoirs, providing food and access to the isolated site. Temple I (right) faces the Temple of the Mask. The northern acropolis and standing stones can be seen in the distance.*

STEPS

The temple is approached by a steep flight of steps. The stairs now visible were used during the construction, the original ceremonial flight (now deteriorated) was much wider.

ASHLAR STONE

The pyramid has a rubble and concrete core faced with blocks of ashlar stone set in regular mortar courses.

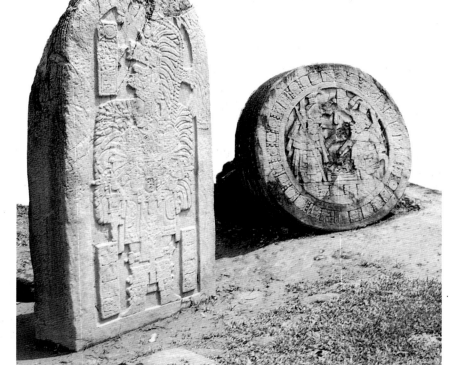

Stone Tablets

Knowledge of Mayan culture has been partly deciphered from the detailed carvings on the upright stone tablets (stellae) found throughout the city, in particular, stones found in an axial arrangement within the Great Plaza. The stellae record a complex and precise calendar of dynastic events. The calendar has a cyclical structure, divided into 20-year intervals; this event was recorded by the construction of a form of pyramid structure.

BALL COURT

Adjacent to the foot of the tower is a ball court for contests between opposing teams. A ball was driven through a stone hoop using elbows and hips.

SPECIFICATION

- **Location**   Tikal, Guatemala, Central America
- **Date**   *c.* AD 500
- **Height**   47.5 m (156 ft)
- **Building structure**   Stone, concrete, and rubble core
- **Building type**   Temple pyramid

KANDARIYA MAHADEV TEMPLE, KHAJURAHO

KHAJURAHO IN CENTRAL INDIA comprises over 80 structures all constructed within the relatively short period between *c.* AD 950 and 1050. The temples, of which only 24 survive, were commissioned by the Chandella kings for their capital city in a style conflating all the temple building traditions of the late Hindu period. The temples, which were once surrounded by irrigated lakes, fell into disuse after the dynastic demise of the 12th century and were abandoned to the encroaching jungle for seven centuries until systematic excavations were undertaken in 1906. Each temple accommodates a devotional image within the darkened, vaulted sanctuary, situated beneath the elaborately carved tower. The sandstone surfaces are suffused with decoration in horizontal, laminated tiers, rising through the adjoining mandapa (hall) to the height of the main sikhara (tower). Continuous friezes of figures carved in deep relief create a highly animated pageant of warriors, dancers, elephants, acrobats, horses, musicians, hunters, and lovers engaged in erotic embrace. The temples at Khajuraho are among the most notable examples of Hindu architecture in Central India.

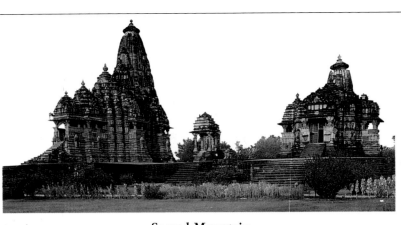

Sacred Mountain
The dominant tower, surrounded by smaller peaks, derives from the sacred image of Mount Meru – the "world mountain". This is a representation of the mountain home of the mythical gods of Indra, which formed the focus of the world's spiritual axis. The Khajuraho temples were shared by the Saiva, Vaishnava, and Jaina sects.

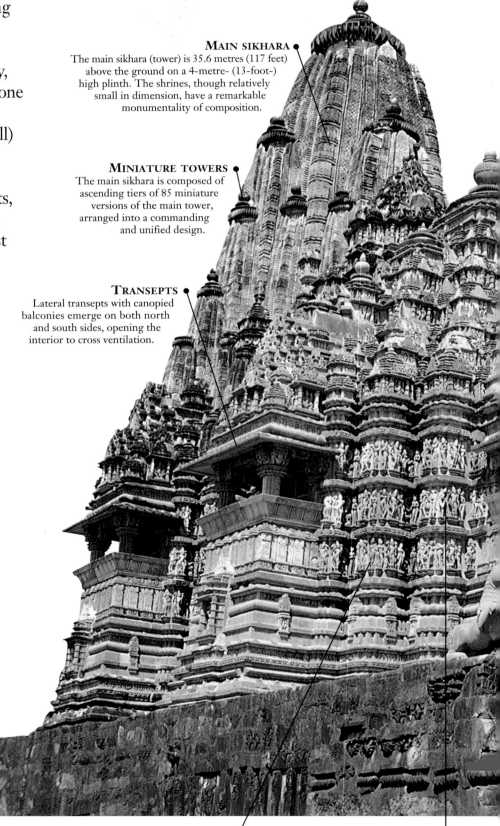

MAIN SIKHARA
The main sikhara (tower) is 35.6 metres (117 feet) above the ground on a 4-metre- (13-foot-) high plinth. The shrines, though relatively small in dimension, have a remarkable monumentality of composition.

MINIATURE TOWERS
The main sikhara is composed of ascending tiers of 85 miniature versions of the main tower, arranged into a commanding and unified design.

TRANSEPTS
Lateral transepts with canopied balconies emerge on both north and south sides, opening the interior to cross ventilation.

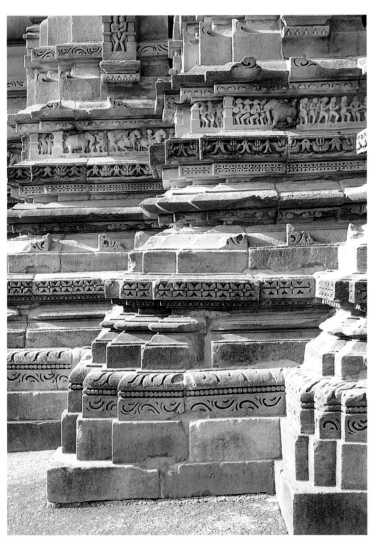

Temple Plinth
The base of the temple is formed from continuous horizontal bands forming a splayed plinth. The rhythmic recession and projection accentuates the light and shadow, adding to the effect of the animated sculptural surface. The tiered bands are decorated with a variety of floral and vegetal mouldings.

FIGURES
Most of the figures are between 75 and 90 centimetres (29–35 inches) high and illustrate an astonishing variety of heavenly and earthly images sculpted in superb movement with minute observation of detail.

SCULPTURES
The three repeated bands of sculptures carry 646 divine and temporal figures carved to the external frieze, with a further 226 figures sculpted internally.

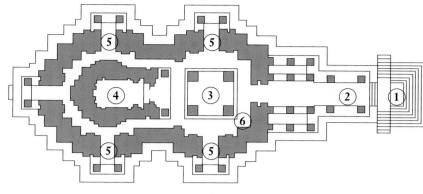

Plan

Each of the temples follows an east-west alignment and is raised upon a platform approached by a steep flight of stairs. The areas distinct within the plan are interconnected and are approached in the following sequence: (1) stairs; (2) entrance porch; (3) Mandapa Hall; (4) sanctuary and sikhara tower; (5) lateral transept with balcony; (6) ambulatory.

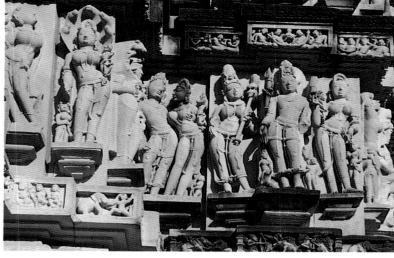

Erotic Figures

The explicitly erotic subjects are presented with a liveliness and delicacy that deeply shocked the English colonial archaeologists who excavated the site in the early-20th century. Guidebooks at that time discouraged visitors to the site for fear of impropriety and moral corruption.

CHANDELLA KINGS

The Chandella kings were the most powerful rulers of northern and Central India from the 9th to the 12th century, achieving their zenith under the rule of Vidyadhara (1004–35). During his reign important temples, including Kandariya Mahadev, were constructed, which show a remarkable stylistic cohesion. Following his death, the Chandella kingdom declined. Temples continued to be built at Khajuraho until the 11th century.

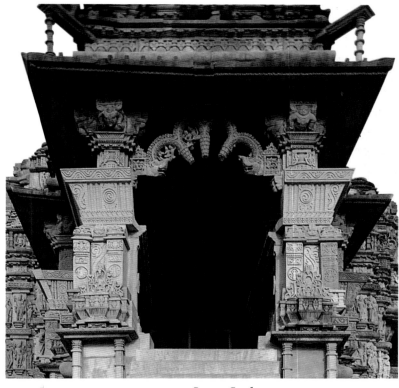

SANDSTONE
The sandstone blocks were shaped and assembled on the ground, then raised individually and carefully positioned. Carving is undertaken both *in situ* and from prefabricated pieces jointed to the main vaulting.

CONSTRUCTION
The constructional details appear to originate from timber building methods using tenoned joints translated into stone.

Stone Sculptures

The entrance porch is flanked by sculptures of crocodiles springing from the diminutive columns and supported by a multitude of smaller figures, each with a profusion of minutely carved details.

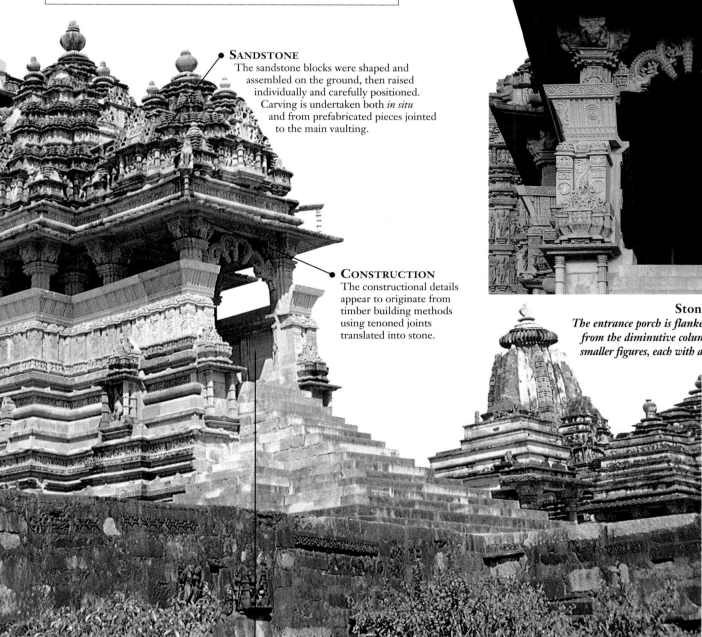

SPECIFICATION

•*Location*	Khajuraho, India
•*Date*	*c.* 950–1050
•*Height*	35.6 m (117 ft)
•*Length*	33.2 m (109 ft)
•*Building structure*	Stone
•*Building type*	Temple

The devotional image is placed within the darkened sanctuary beneath the main tower, which is buttressed by additional towers, entrance vestibule, and hall.

PORTICO
Pilgrims progress from the open portico into increasing darkness within the sanctuary. Light is admitted to the ambulatory via the canopied balconies.

The erotic figures are consistent with the Tantric belief in the primal life energy of sexual coupling, incorporated into religious buildings for its associations with fertility and joy.

PISA CATHEDRAL

THE WEALTH AND PRESTIGE of the established centres of Christian worship during the Romanesque period are reflected in the increasing scale of church building at this time. This is illustrated in the world-famous grouping of cathedral, campanile, and baptistery at Pisa, Italy. Constructional developments in stone vaulting and the use of the peripheral arcade (helping to reduce the thickness of the external wall) are used to explore the possibilities of light and decoration, realized later to great effect in European Gothic architecture. In Italy, the extant remains of Roman architecture provided a source of both architectural material and stylistic precedent. Blended with the influences of Byzantine culture, they provided a measure of continuity between the antique and medieval worlds. The simple, rectangular, basilican form of the early Christian church, dating from the 4th century, has a central nave and side aisles, later adapted to ceremonial practices that required crossing transepts, forming a cruciform plan.

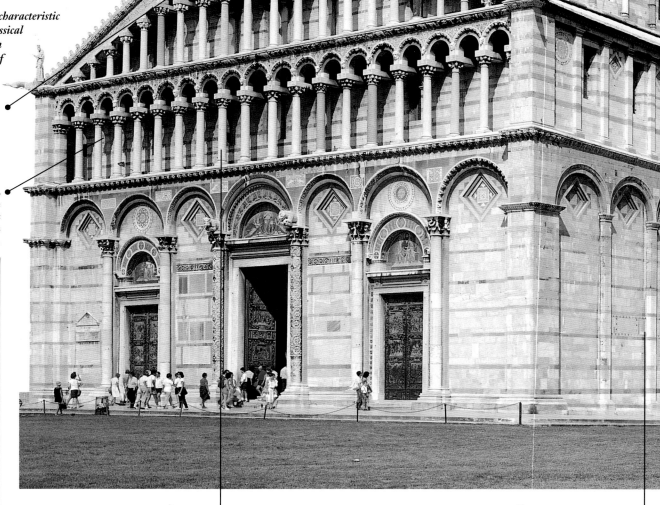

Baptistery
The baptistery (1153–1265) was designed by Dioti Salvi. The unusual profile of the ribbed dome is the product of a composite structural system. The outer dome spans the diameter of the circular baptistery, and an inner cone, which accentuates the height, is supported on an internal colonnade.

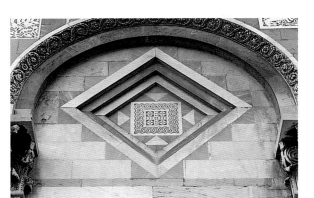

Marble Panels
Polychromatic marble panels provide the characteristic decoration on the façade. The Classical Orders of architecture, with Corinthian capitals, are deployed with a crudeness of detail but a richness of decoration.

COLONNADE
The delicacy and articulation of the arcading in the upper sections of the main façade are characteristic of the Italian Romanesque.

GABLE WALL
The rhythmical arcading of the gable wall, together with the polychromatic marble banding, gives Pisa Cathedral its distinctive character.

ROMANESQUE VAULTING

Developments in techniques of stone vaulting began to open out the nave and aisles, introducing a spatial variation into the strictly rectilinear plan of the basilican church. The nave at Pisa is relatively confined, as the structural limitations of semicircular vaulting had not yet achieved the span and flexibility of the pointed-arch-and-rib vault (see p. 26). The central crossing did not begin to dominate the plan until further developments produced the centralized plan of the Renaissance (see p. 44).

ARCADE
The arches and columns of the peripheral arcade developed as a Romanesque decorative treatment of the Classical façade.

STRUCTURAL FRAME
The arches and columns emerge as distinctive structural elements within the external façade. The repetition of this simple unit reduces the reliance on a uniformly load-bearing wall. This tendency pointed towards the development of a masonry superstructure – the characteristic device of the later Gothic period.

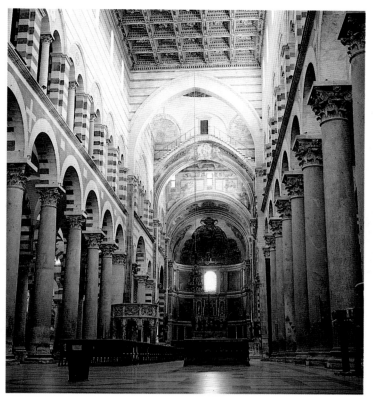

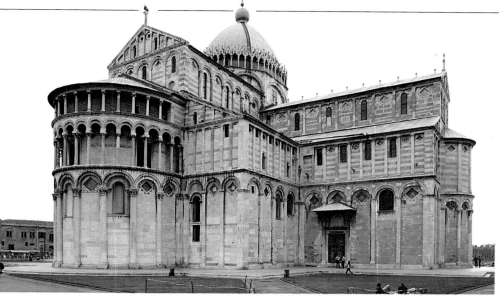

Nave
The nave is flanked on either side by aisles used for the display of religious images and chapels dedicated to the saints. This arrangement is achieved through the use of stone vaulting and a colonnade supporting the nave wall.

Apse and Transept
Developments in Christian worship helped the form of the church evolve towards its characteristic cruciform plan and central tower. The apse, originally a niche at the eastern end of the nave, is enlarged, providing a focus for the rites of Mass. The arms of the cross are extended, providing devotional chapels and the crossing point, which is dominated by a central tower.

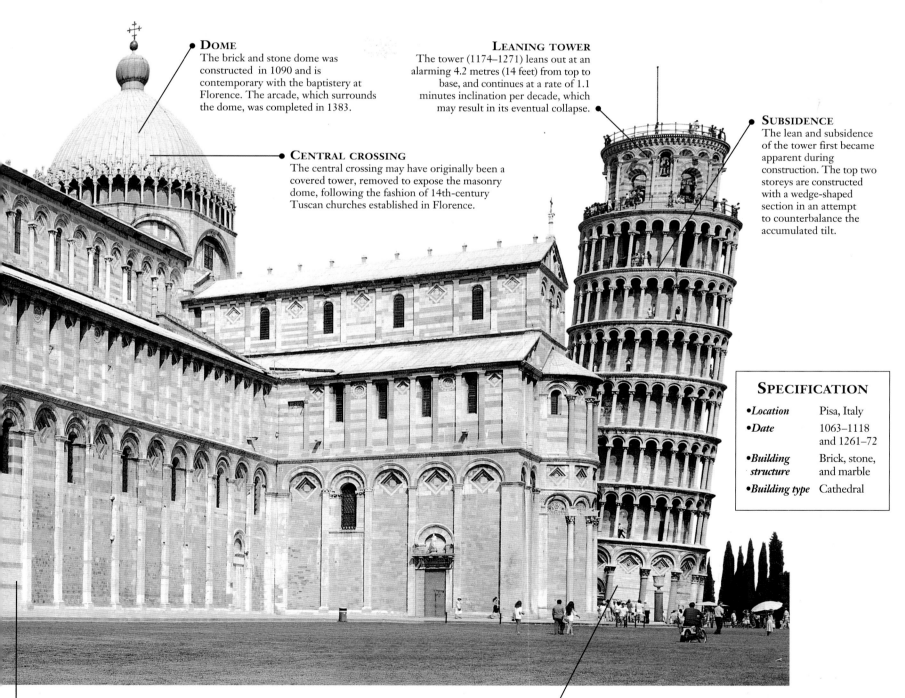

DOME
The brick and stone dome was constructed in 1090 and is contemporary with the baptistery at Florence. The arcade, which surrounds the dome, was completed in 1383.

LEANING TOWER
The tower (1174–1271) leans out at an alarming 4.2 metres (14 feet) from top to base, and continues at a rate of 1.1 minutes inclination per decade, which may result in its eventual collapse.

SUBSIDENCE
The lean and subsidence of the tower first became apparent during construction. The top two storeys are constructed with a wedge-shaped section in an attempt to counterbalance the accumulated tilt.

CENTRAL CROSSING
The central crossing may have originally been a covered tower, removed to expose the masonry dome, following the fashion of 14th-century Tuscan churches established in Florence.

SPECIFICATION

•*Location*	Pisa, Italy
•*Date*	1063–1118 and 1261–72
•*Building structure*	Brick, stone, and marble
•*Building type*	Cathedral

MARBLE BANDING
The cathedral is decorated with horizontal bands of alternate courses of coloured marble, which is characteristic of buildings in central Italy.

Many of the granite columns are of Roman origin. Materials from Classical ruins were frequently incorporated into the construction of new buildings.

BASE
The limited area of the base for the tower's height produced a loading on the foundations that exceeded that of traditional building practices. The tower is subsiding in a rotational movement caused by failure in the clay 10 metres (33 feet) below the surface.

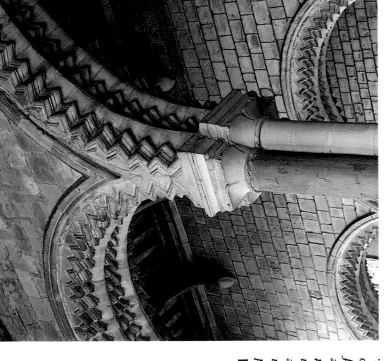

DURHAM CATHEDRAL

ENSHRINING THE HOLY RELICS OF **S**T **C**UTHBERT, the cathedral, monastery, and castle at Durham, England, are situated on a defensive promontory high above a loop in the River Wear. This elevated position, together with the rapid pace of the cathedral's early construction (1093–1104) gives a memorable impression of the power and solidity of Norman architecture and the spirit of the Romanesque in Britain. The holy relics ensured the continued importance and wealth of this northern English outpost as a place of Christian pilgrimage. The monastery and castle reinforced the strategic and military role of the cathedral throughout the Middle Ages until the dissolution of the monasteries (1536–40). The cathedral was the first major structure in England to be vaulted entirely in stone, and the pointed vaults that cross the nave and aisles are the earliest recorded examples of rib vaulting, which was to transform the heavy masonry of the Romanesque into the lightness and soaring verticality of the Gothic. The nave has a powerful and impressive character, which balances the solidity of mass with the lofty proportions of the upper arcade and the verticality of the 22.2-metre- (73-foot-) high vault. The chevron, fluted, reticulated, and spiral motifs of Norman decoration are, for the first time, incised into the broad columns, emphasizing their mass and providing an alternating rhythm that imparts a solemn dignity to this masterpiece of Romanesque architecture.

Galilee Chapel
Added in 1175, the timber roof and five-aisled arcade are supported on slender compound columns of sandstone and Purbeck marble. The simple cushion capital and chevron mouldings that decorate the arch soffits are Romanesque in detail, but, in their lightness of structure, provide a delicate contrast to the monumentality of the nave.

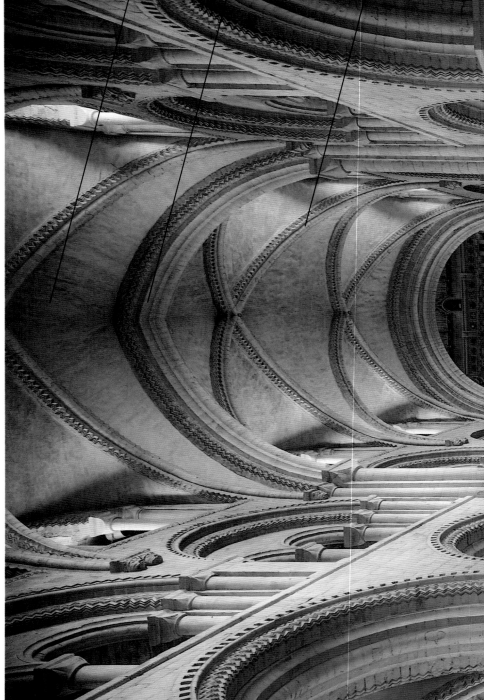

The cathedral was one of 30 churches in England that possessed the right of sanctuary. A criminal seeking refuge was afforded protection within for 37 days. If a pardon had not been obtained within this time the prisoner was sent into exile.

TRANSVERSE RIBS
The transverse ribs occur at alternating positions above the compound columns that divide the nave into rectangular double vaults.

POINTED-RIB VAULT
The nave is vaulted with one of the earliest recorded forms of the pointed-rib vault. The decorated lines of the lofty transverse arches emphasize the size of the nave, enabling a lightness of structure, the style of which was to develop into Gothic vaulting.

DIAGONAL RIBS
Semicircular diagonal ribs spring from twinned corbels below the clerestory. The grinning face of the carved corbelled brackets is in alignment with the alternate positions of the circular columns.

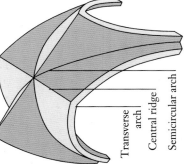

Ribbed Vault
The ribbed vault combines the ease of construction of the semicircular arch with the flexibility of the height and span of the pointed arch. This technique maintains the central ridge height of the nave while freeing the wall for open arcading or clerestory windows, opening out the nave to allow increased natural light.

Transverse arch
Central ridge
Semicircular arch

BUTTRESSES
The thrust of the nave roof is shared between the nave columns and the side-aisles. A premature flying buttress is formed by quadrant arches concealed within the aisle roof structure and thickened piers within the wall.

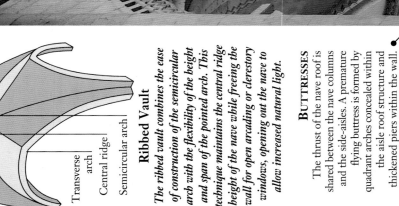

CHOIR

The four bays of the choir at the eastern end of the nave were completed between 1093 and 1104. The vaulting was rebuilt at the end of the 13th century because of structural instability.

A thin line of blue marble, which crosses the nave near the western font, marks the limit of entrance admitted to women during the Middle Ages.

ROSE WINDOW

The rose window at the far eastern end is an addition by the 18th-century architect, James Wyatt, who supervised a number of intrusive modifications, including the stripping of mouldings from the external stonework.

SPECIFICATION

- **Location**: Durham, England
- **Date**: 1093–1133
- **Height**: 44 m (145 ft)
- **Building structure**: Stone
- **Building type**: Cathedral
- **Construction time**: 40 years

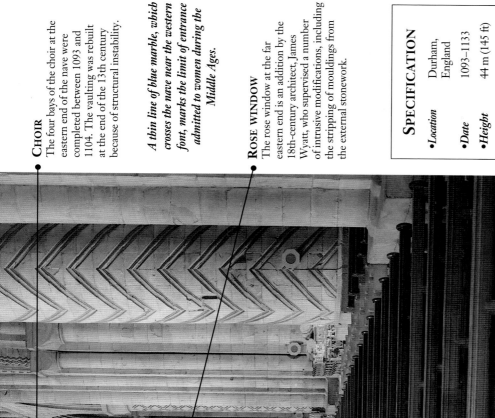
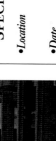

The Chapel of the Nine Altars (1242–80), which once contained the shrine of St Cuthbert, is at the far end of the nave and forms an additional transept at the eastern end. The gilded green marble shrine was broken up after the Dissolution, though the relics of the saint remain buried beneath the chapel floor.

Western Towers

The cathedral is built on a solid foundation of exposed rock high above the River Wear. The western towers adjoin the Galilee Chapel and originate from the 13th century, but were rebuilt in 1487 after being struck by lightning. Rising to 44 metres (145 feet), the towers amplify the massing of the cathedral on its elevated site.

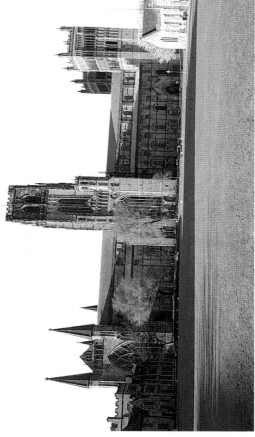

ST CUTHBERT

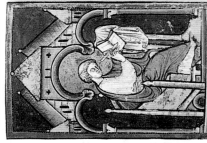

St Cuthbert (c. AD 624–87) is one of the most revered of English saints. After a vision in AD 651 he entered the Northumbrian monastery of Melrose and is attributed with many miraculous events. By AD 685, he had become Bishop of the Abbey of Lindisfarne, where he was later to be buried. His relics were moved to Durham after Viking raids in the 9th century AD, where he was enshrined in the choir and transept of the cathedral, and consecrated in 1104.

COMPOUND COLUMNS

The compound columns continue to support the transverse ribs. They have a sinuous appearance, but are more substantial than the circular columns and carry the greater loads imparted by the ribbed vaulting.

North Facade

Viewed across the Palace Green, the northern façade of the cathedral reveals the full length of the 143-metre (470-foot) nave. The Gothic Chapel of the Nine Altars and the tomb of St Cuthbert are situated at the east end of the cathedral (left). The central tower was completed in 1495 with the addition of a final tier. The towers built above the western end of the nave (right) adjoin the Galilee Chapel, which is perched on the cliff edge.

ANGKOR WAT

THE CITY OF ANGKOR in Cambodia was abandoned to the jungle after periodic occupation as the capital of the Khmer civilization, dating from the 9th century AD to the 13th century. The temple of Angkor Wat is one precinct in a vast site dispersed over a distance of 50 kilometres (31 miles) from east to west. Built on rising ground and surrounded by an artificial moat, the temple is arranged symmetrically on tiered platforms that ascend to the central tower, which rises to a height of 65 metres (213 feet). Long colonnades connect the towers at each stepped level in concentric rings of rectilinear galleries. The site is approached across the moat, via a stone causeway lined with stone figures. The ascending towers represent the spiritual world and mountain homes of the gods and were probably built in homage to ancestral deities. Artefacts taken from the site and large sections cast from the temple buildings were exhibited in Paris in 1867, announcing a great and unknown civilization rivalling in sophistication the western achievements of Classical and Gothic architecture.

VISHNU

The original Khmer builders of the 12th century may have erected the temples in honour of ancestral gods. Vishnu, one of the most important Hindu deities, is revered as the protector of the world and restorer of moral order. He is essentially known through a series of 10 reincarnations, known as *avatars*, which appear to protect good or prevent evil upon the earth. The most important of these are Rama, fearless and noble upholder of the law, and Krishna, who is associated with altruistic love. Vishnu holds in his hands symbols of creation, domination, universal purity, and knowledge of the power of the mind.

SPECIFICATION

- **Location** — Angkor, Cambodia
- **Date** — 12th century
- **Height** — 65 m (213 ft)
- **Building structure** — Stone
- **Building type** — Temple

The Khmer builders accomplished ambitious religious and civil engineering projects with astonishing accuracy. A 65-kilometre- (40-mile-) long canal was built in virtually a straight line, and a 3-kilometre- (2-mile-) long moat deviates by only 5 centimetres (2 inches) from the true alignment.

CENTRAL TOWER
The tower at the centre of the third platform forms the focus of the tiered levels. This central sanctuary is linked to the outer tiers by pavilion towers and covered porticos.

MASONRY BONDING
Despite the competence of Khmer builders, much of the stonework is constructed without offset joints between courses. This lack of simple bonding resulted in the subsequent collapse of the masonry.

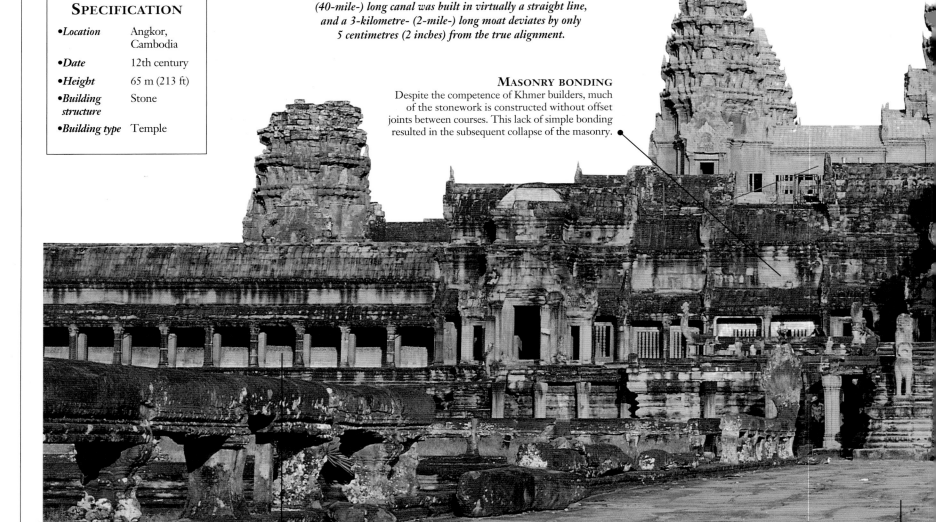

LOW COLONNADES
The long colonnades form peripheral galleries that connect between the main towers. The gallery walls are lined with stone relief carvings depicting female deities and epic scenes.

Though the city of Angkor was abandoned by the Khmer rulers, the temple precinct was continually visited by Buddhist and Hindu pilgrims from as far as Japan, China, and Thailand.

CAUSEWAY
The raised platforms are approached across a wide stone causeway. The form of the balustrade on either side represents the serpent of Hindu mythology – a recurrent image in the myth of creation.

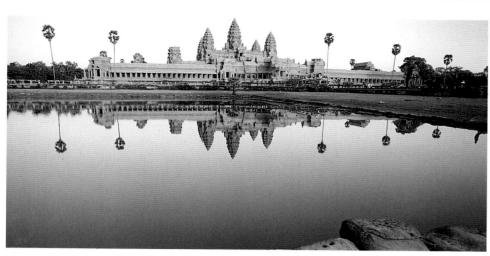

Water
The moat surrounding the temple was supplied by water courses directed from the river and used for irrigating the land. The Khmers' ability to conserve and direct the supply of water ensured the continual productivity of the land, creating a prosperous and organized society.

TOWERS
The stone towers have roofs formed by corbelling stone blocks in successive tiers. The internal soffits are then ground away *in situ* to produce the effect of vaulting. The ceilings were occasionally lined with gilded timber.

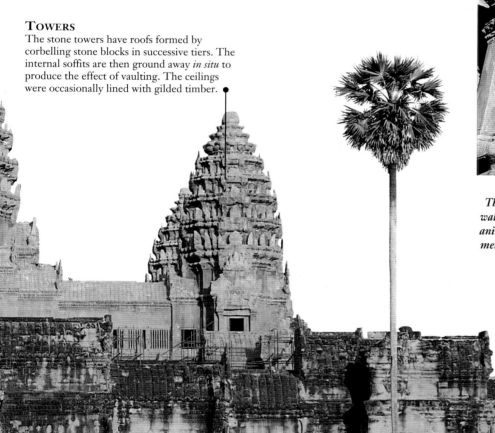

Stone Construction
The buildings are chiefly built in stone with detailed bas-reliefs carved into the walls; the corbelled blockwork and pseudo-vaulted towers are covered with highly animated figures carved into the sandstone and volcanic rock. The constructional methods developed by the Khmers show a change from timber to brick and stone. Decorative motifs, such as roof vaults and wall panels (an imitation of bamboo screens) have petrified earlier forms of construction.

TEMPLE MOUNTAIN
The tiered platforms, culminating in a central tower, conform to the *Linga* or earthly mountain form of temple, representing the sacred Mount Meru of Indian mythology.

STYLISTIC INFLUENCES
In early reconstructions, French archaeologists emphasized the stylistic influences of China, India, and Egypt, wrongly supposing the construction to be by a foreign, rather than an indigenous, civilization.

VAULTED GALLERIES
The curved roof of the galleries is vaulted in corbelled stone blocks, but the form has been carved to imitate the overlapping courses of roof tiles.

KRAK DES CHEVALIERS

HIGH ABOVE THE ORONTES VALLEY, defending the Homs Pass in Syria, the Krak des Chevaliers provided a strategic outpost for the military incursions of the crusading knights. Its formidable situation, along with fortifications undertaken in the early-13th century, made it virtually impregnable to attack. Built on the site of a pre-existing fort, the construction had three lines of defence – two concentric tiers of fortifications and a final donjon tower (a strong, central tower). Though virtually impregnable, its fortification and controlled entrance made it reliant on defensive methods, as it was very difficult to mount a counter-attack. Krak des Chevaliers was occupied from 1142 by the Knights Hospitaller and was besieged 12 times during their occupation, finally being taken by Berber forces in 1271. Rebuilding and further modifications have maintained the castle as an impressive example of medieval military architecture, indebted in construction techniques to the traditions of Norman masons and the historic fortifications of Arab towns. The castle remained in occupation until the resiting of the village that occupied the interior in 1932.

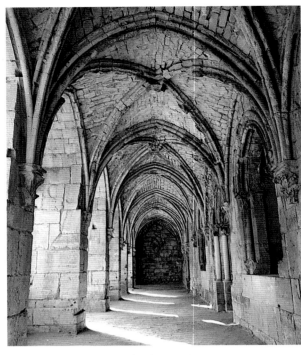

Vaulted Loggia
The inner courtyard has a vaulted loggia running the length of the banqueting hall, providing a shaded retreat from the fierce heat of the day. The courtyard contains the finest rooms in the castle, used as the main apartments of the knights and probably as a refuge from mercenaries garrisoned in the outer walls.

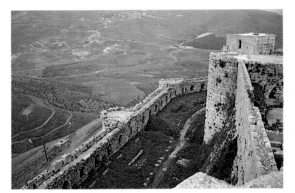

Lines of Defence
Fortifications are arranged in concentric lines of defence – the outer walls defended from the lower ward, and the upper levels of the castle defended from the towers and inner ward. An open moat and cistern within the outer ward were used for water storage. In 1271, Berber forces besieged the castle and gained access to the outer ward but were unable to proceed further. The siege lasted for a further month before the defending troops capitulated.

BUTTRESS TOWERS
The immense stone walls are strengthened along their length by buttress towers which offer concealed positions for surveillance and defence.

MACHIOCOULIS
The parapet of the outer walls has a vaulted gallery equipped at intervals with narrow chambers, cantilevered from the face of the wall. The protected chambers, or *machiocoulis*, are used to drop stones through openings in the floor in order to prevent investing forces from undermining, or scaling, the walls.

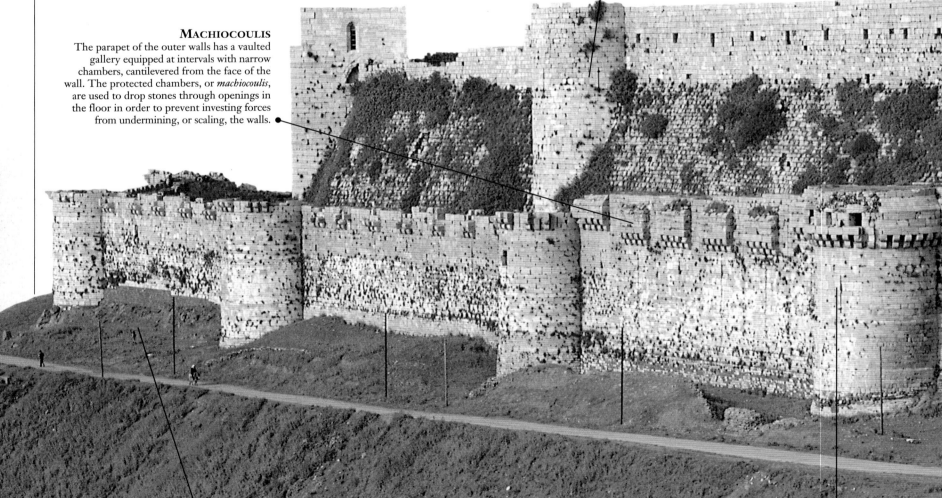

WALL BASE
The thickening at the base of the walls helps protect against attack by sappers charged with excavating lower sections and creating a fire to undermine the structure.

T. E. Lawrence (Lawrence of Arabia), while researching his undergraduate thesis in 1909, undertook a tour of the crusader castles. He described Krak des Chevaliers as "the best preserved and most wholly admirable castle in the world".

SLOTTED OPENING
The slotted openings are less vulnerable to incoming missiles but are given wide internal reveals, increasing the defending archer's scope of fire.

KNIGHTS HOSPITALLER

Krak des Chevaliers was occupied in 1109 and garrisoned by the Knights Hospitaller from 1142, during the crusades undertaken by European Christian forces between the 11th and 14th centuries. These military expeditions were intended to recover the Holy Land (the birthplace of Christ) and the routes of pilgrimage from the possession of Muslim rulers. The successes of the First Crusade and the recapture of Jerusalem were not repeated in later expeditions. Despite the crusaders winning concessions of pilgrimage and access to the Holy Sepulchre, the Holy Land remained under Muslim control.

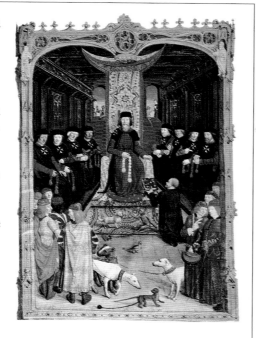

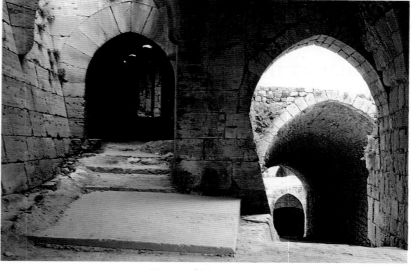

Ramped Entrance
On the outer eastern wall, a gatehouse gives access to the upper levels via a narrow, vaulted ramp. This confined entrance would expose intruders to attack from openings flanking the wall and roof along the length of its steep approach. The dog-leg turn precludes the use of a large battering ram, and the contrast between light and dark adds to the sense of disorientation.

A windmill was positioned on the tower for grinding corn and the castle was equipped to endure long periods of siege. Vaults beneath the upper courtyard contained immense storehouses for provisions.

UPPER TOWERS
The inner ward, defended by the upper towers, contained the dormitories, banqueting hall, store rooms, chapel, and the apartments of the highest-ranking knights.

GLACIS
The upper walls have a glacis (slope) up to 24.3 metres (80 feet) thick, almost as wide as their height. This monumental form of construction provided resistance to earthquakes as well as to assault from undermining and missile attack.

SPECIFICATION

- **Location**   Syria
- **Date**   11th century
- **Architects**   Remodelled by the Knights Hospitaller
- **Building structure**   Stone
- **Building type**   Castle

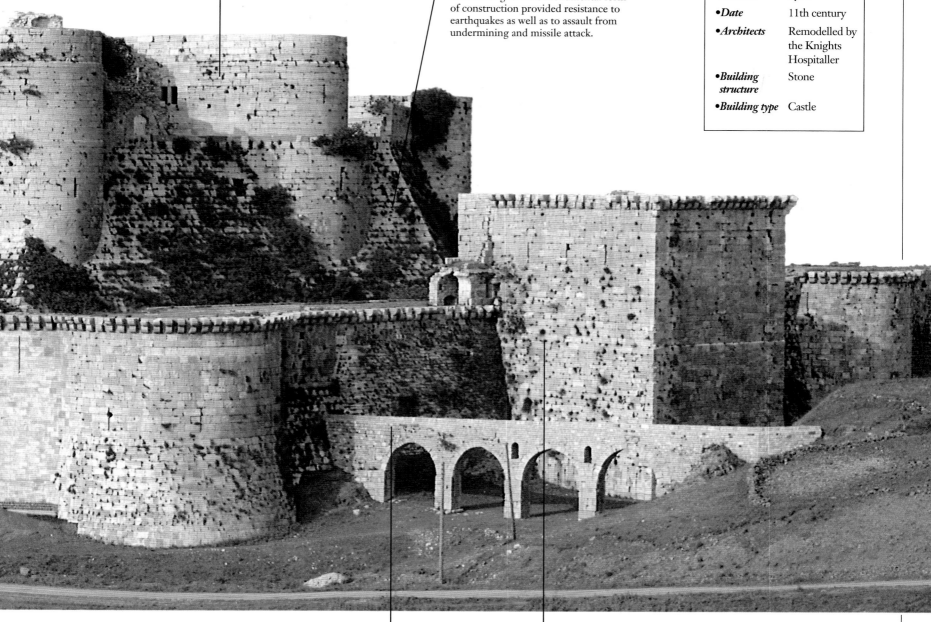

Communication between remote fortifications was made possible by carrier-pigeon. The use of carrier-pigeons was a technique borrowed from Arab practices.

AQUEDUCT
Water was supplied to the castle by an aqueduct. During periods of siege the castle had a reserve contained in subterranean, vaulted cisterns.

SQUARE TOWER
The square tower dates from 1285. It was rebuilt following the damage caused during the siege and capture in 1271. Circular towers, by contrast, offered the advantage of being defendable all around. Their circular walls were also less vulnerable to assault, battering ram, or undermining.

NOTRE DAME, PARIS

THE CRUCIFORM PLAN, elevated nave, transept, and tower of the Gothic cathedral were inherited from 11th-century Romanesque churches. However, it was the structural potential and versatility of the pointed arch and the rib vault (see p. 26) that enabled the early Gothic to exceed all precedents. Notre Dame (1163–*c.* 1250) in Paris is a remarkable illustration of the vision and achievement of the medieval world. The desire for increased height required significant developments in constructional methods. The choir, with a keystone at a height of 33 metres (108 feet), was taller than any previous Gothic structure. As construction began on the nave, the height of the vaults increased a further 2 metres (6 feet), and the method of buttressed support to the side-galleries soon revealed weaknesses in the structure. The remedial means sought by the 13th-century masons resulted in the use of that characteristic device of Gothic architecture, the flying buttress.

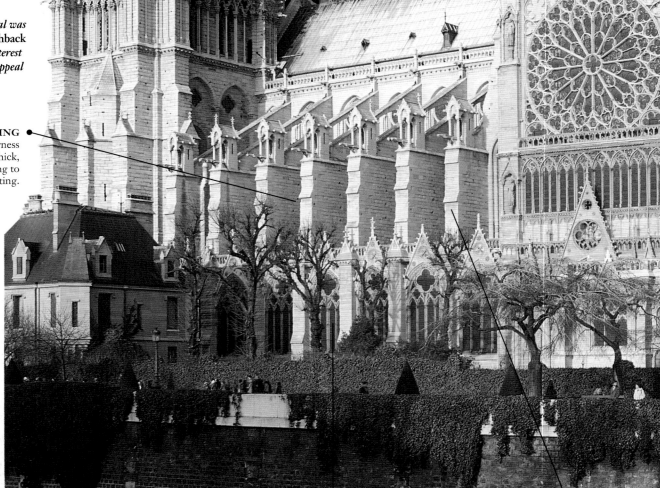

West Facade
The façade balances the verticality of the twin towers, which align to the width of the double side-aisles, with the horizontal banding of the decorated galleries. This produces a simple but powerful western elevation, which dominates the square.

SOUTH-WEST TOWER
The 69-metre- (226-foot-) high south-west tower supported the famous 15th-century bell. The bell was recast in 1686, it is said, with the addition of gold and precious stones, reputedly accounting for the clear resonance of its chime.

The Romantic Gothic image of the cathedral was advanced in Victor Hugo's novel The Hunchback of Notre-Dame (1831). *The revival of interest in the Gothic successfully enabled Hugo to appeal for the cathedral's restoration.*

BUTTRESSING
The height of the nave and the relative slenderness of the wall, an average of 1 metre (3 feet) thick, required supplementary external buttressing to counteract the lateral thrust of the nave vaulting.

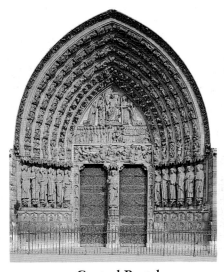

Central Portal
The central portal of the entrance façade is flanked by statues depicting the Last Judgement – the redemption of the pious and the damnation of the wicked.

GLAZING
Gothic structure achieved a remarkable delicacy. The rhythmic structural bays provide the supporting masonry frame, allowing the thin membrane walls to become non-structural and available for large expanses of glazing.

PIERS
Following remedial alterations to the structure, the piers of the buttresses were thickened. The mass of material provides a stability and vertical component to lateral forces transferred from the nave vaulting.

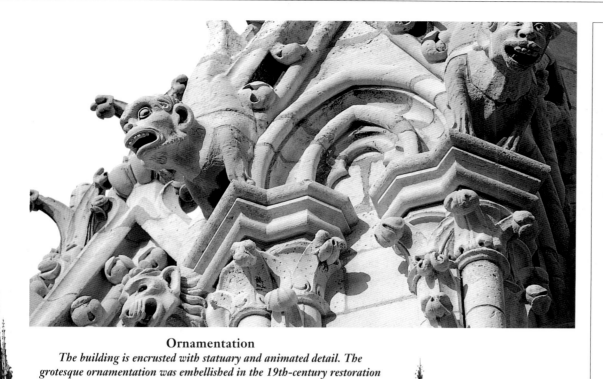

Ornamentation
The building is encrusted with statuary and animated detail. The grotesque ornamentation was embellished in the 19th-century restoration supervised by the famous French architect Viollet-le-Duc. Rather than achieve an authentic rebuilding, the restoration sought to present history as a pastiche of all periods, reflecting the 19th-century taste for Gothic fantasy.

CATHEDRAL BUILDERS

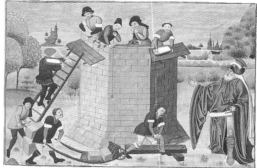

With the aid of only elementary drawings and templates, masons supervised and meticulously directed the construction of the great medieval cathedrals of Europe. The practices of intuitive calculation, largely based on simple mathematical ratios and structural precedent, were closely guarded and passed between successive generations of masons. Specific site conditions and the insatiable demand for higher and lighter buildings provided the impetus for continual development.

The timber spire, 96 metres (315 feet) high, was destroyed during the revolution and completely replaced by the 19th-century restoration (1845–56) conducted by French architect Viollet-le-Duc.

SPECIFICATION

•*Location*	Paris, France
•*Date*	1163–*c.* 1250
•*Height*	90 m (300 ft)
•*Building structure*	Stone and timber
•*Building type*	Cathedral
•*Consruction time*	*c.* 87 years
•*Restored*	19th century

SHALLOW TRANSEPT
The cathedral has a remarkably shallow transept, which, even after extension, does not exceed the line of the outer aisles.

CLERESTORY WINDOWS
The clerestory windows of the original nave were enlarged in the 13th century to supplement natural light to the interior. This was permitted by developments of the structural frame.

FLYING BUTTRESSES
The flying buttresses have two tiers of support. The upper arm contributes to the stability of the wall, counteracting the wind-loading experienced at such height. The main thrust of the wall is supported by the lower arm of the buttress.

THE ALHAMBRA

THE MOORISH CONQUEST OF SPAIN, following their invasions of AD 711, led to a period of occupation lasting for eight centuries, until their final expulsion by Christian forces in 1492. The last bastion of Moorish rule was the city palace of The Alhambra in Granada. The administration of this most western province of Islam emanated from the southern citadels of Granada and Córdoba. Under periods of tolerant rule, Spain became one of the most educated and cultured centres of Europe. The Arab rulers introduced traditional forms of Islamic architecture and irrigation methods into Spain, taming the summer heat to create lush gardens and shaded, airy courtyards. The Alhambra (1238–1358) summarizes the refined pleasures and grace of Moorish culture. Following the expulsion of the Moors and the unification of Spain, Isabella of Castile (1451–1504) and Ferdinand of Aragon (1452–1516) briefly established their palace there. The Alhambra, with its enchanting succession of apartments, exquisitely detailed colonnades, and lush gardens, retains its mysterious charm, a reminder of the rich cultural heritage running parallel to the Christian traditions of the European Gothic.

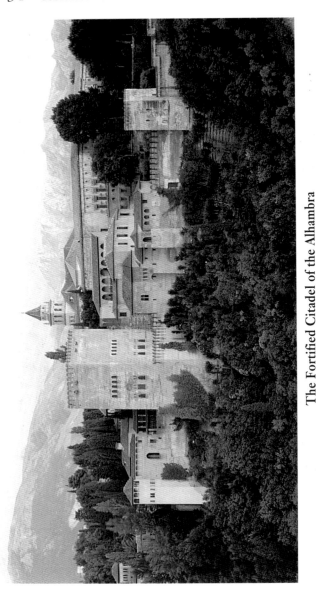

The Fortified Citadel of the Alhambra

The walls of the Alhambra stand out against the mountains of the Sierra Nevada. The palace is essentially a fortified citadel built upon an 11th-century castle. The severity of the external walls contrasts with the decoration of the internal courtyards, which were designed to be viewed from their centre. This characteristic of Islamic architecture is in direct contrast to Classical western composition, which is principally determined by the external view of the façade.

Patio de la Acequia

The rectilinear garden is enclosed by screen walls on the long sides and an arcade at either end. Raised pathways line the central water channel, which is inset with fountains. The courtyard forms part of the Generlife – summer gardens with shaded verandas overlooking the city.

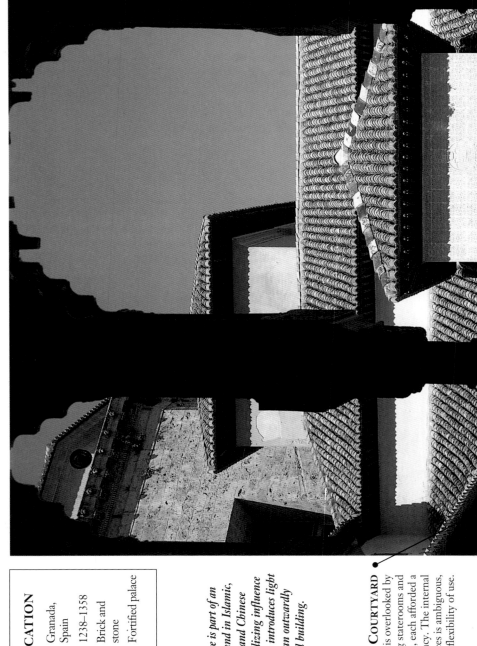

SPECIFICATION

- **Location**   Granada, Spain
- **Date**   1238–1358
- **Building structure**   Brick and stone
- **Building type**   Fortified palace

The courtyard palace is part of an ancient tradition found in Islamic, Classical Roman, and Chinese architecture. The civilizing influence of a recreational space introduces light and planting into an outwardly austere, fortified building.

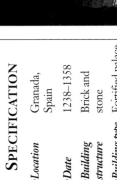

COURTYARD
The courtyard is overlooked by pairs of facing staterooms and private apartments, each afforded a degree of privacy. The internal allocation of spaces is ambiguous, allowing flexibility of use.

TRACERY
The fine tracery of the arcades is carved directly into the stucco applied to the vaulting. The ornate carving produces a raised, decorative design, vividly expressed in the chiaroscuro effects of bright sunlight.

ISLAMIC DECORATION
Islamic decoration is characterized by the proliferation of minutely detailed geometric vegetal and calligraphic motifs, composed into panels, creating a unified field of decoration.

COMPOSITIONAL RHYTHMS
The complex rhythms, established by repeating elements of the arcades, and the arrangement of slender columns into singles, pairs, and groups of three, assist the expansive feel of openness and lightness in the relatively confined courtyard.

LIONS
The stone lions supporting the alabaster basin are an ancient symbol of royal power and are of earlier Romanesque origin.

MUQARNAS
The soffit of the arches is composed by reduplications of the *muqarnas*, the fundamental element of Islamic decoration. These corbelled brackets form the complex geometric vaulting of the honeycombed-domes and arches.

PARADISE GARDEN
The quadrapartite arrangement of the courtyard, divided by water channels, is a characteristic representation of the Islamic Garden of Paradise (see p. 54). The courtyard would originally have been planted with fragrant herbs and flowers.

WATER BASIN
The central water basin is surrounded by 12 stone lions, each fitted with a water spout playing into the circular channel. The spray of water humidifies the dry air, and creates the soothing and cooling effect of moving water.

WATER COURSE
A water course is cut into the stone paving, channelling water from the symmetrical pavilions towards the central basin.

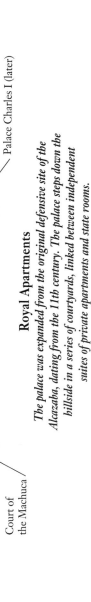

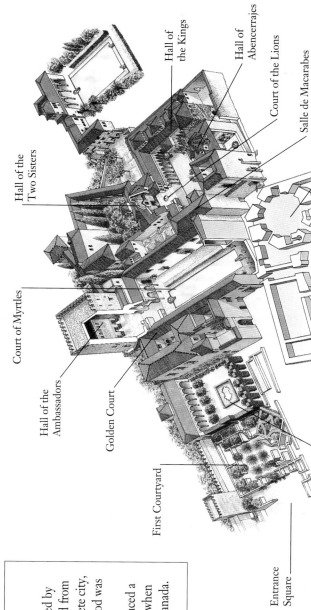

Hall of the Two Sisters

Hall of the Kings

Hall of Abencerrajes

Court of the Lions

Salle de Macarabes

Palace Charles I (later)

Court of Myrtles

Hall of the Ambassadors

Golden Court

First Courtyard

Court of the Machuca

Entrance Square

Royal Apartments
The palace was expanded from the original defensive site of the Alcazaba, dating from the 11th century. The palace steps down the hillside in a series of courtyards, linked between independent suites of private apartments and state rooms.

NASRID RULERS
The Alhambra dates from 1238 and was constructed by the Nasrid kings, principally Yusuf I, who reigned from 1333 to 1354. The fortified walls contained a complete city, which centred on the palace apartments. This period was marked by considerable wealth and political turbulence. The succession of Christian rule produced a rich and unique cultural exchange during a period when Muslim traditions had become concentrated in Granada.

Hall of Kings
The Hall of Kings, on the eastern side of the Court of Lions, is formed by a rhythmic succession of three high-honeycombed-domed, top-lit bays, interspersed with lower, flat-ceiling bays. The wall and ceiling surfaces are decorated with intricate geometric patterns in ceramic tile and carved stucco. Three large alcoves, each with a painted ceiling, open off the linear hallway.

FLORENCE CATHEDRAL

ALSO KNOWN AS SANTA MARIA DEL FIORE, Italy's Florence Cathedral was begun in 1296 in an essentially Gothic style, ornamented with the characteristic inlaid marble panelling of Tuscan Romanesque architecture. Civic rivalry between the Ducal States led to the construction of an ambitious dome, raised to a height above the central nave to exceed that of any church in Tuscany. By 1418, the construction of the nave had already predetermined the octagonal plan arrangement of supporting piers capped by an elevated drum, though the technical means by which to construct the dome had not yet been established. Filippo Brunelleschi's proposal provided a systematic and practical solution, inspired by both the Gothic tradition of stone vaulting and principles of Roman engineering. The cathedral exemplifies the transition between the Gothic world and the new spirit of scientific and aesthetic enquiry. Indeed, Brunelleschi's achievement set the course of the Italian Renaissance, reasserting Italy at the centre of a new cultural empire.

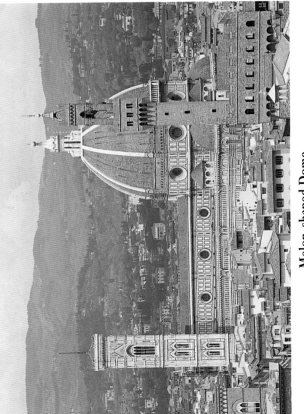

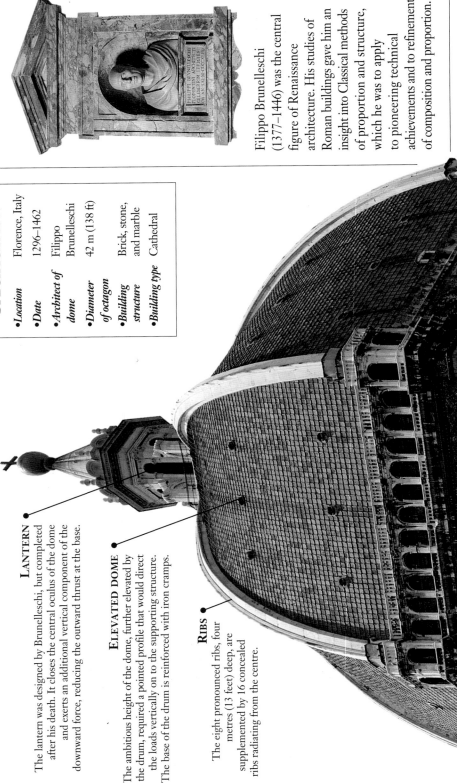

Melon-shaped Dome

The melon-shaped dome dominates the Gothic cathedral. Brunelleschi's success in surmounting the technical problems faced during the dome's construction advanced the prestige of Florence amongst rival cities of Pisa, Sienna, and Lucca.

SPECIFICATION

• *Location*	Florence, Italy
• *Date*	1296–1462
• *Architect of dome*	Filippo Brunelleschi
• *Diameter of octagon*	42 m (138 ft)
• *Building structure*	Brick, stone, and marble
• *Building type*	Cathedral

BRUNELLESCHI

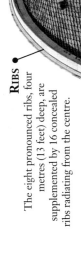

Filippo Brunelleschi (1377–1446) was the central figure of Renaissance architecture. His studies of Roman buildings gave him an insight into Classical methods of proportion and structure, which he was to apply to pioneering technical achievements and to refinements of composition and proportion.

LANTERN
The lantern was designed by Brunelleschi, but completed after his death. It closes the central oculus of the dome and exerts an additional vertical component of the downward force, reducing the outward thrust at the base.

ELEVATED DOME
The ambitious height of the dome, further elevated by the drum, required a pointed profile that would direct the loads vertically on to the supporting structure. The base of the drum is reinforced with iron cramps.

RIBS
The eight pronounced ribs, four metres (13 feet) deep, are supplemented by 16 concealed ribs radiating from the centre.

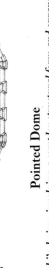

Pointed Dome

Brunelleschi's design, involving a complex structural form and organized method of construction, reconciled the virtues of a self-supporting dome with the plan of the octagonal, segmental vault. The coffered section of the dome reduces the overall weight of the construction. The herringbone bonding of the brickwork and the concentric rings of masonry blocks pioneered a method of construction that dispensed with the need for centring (a temporary framework) – unmanageable at this height and span.

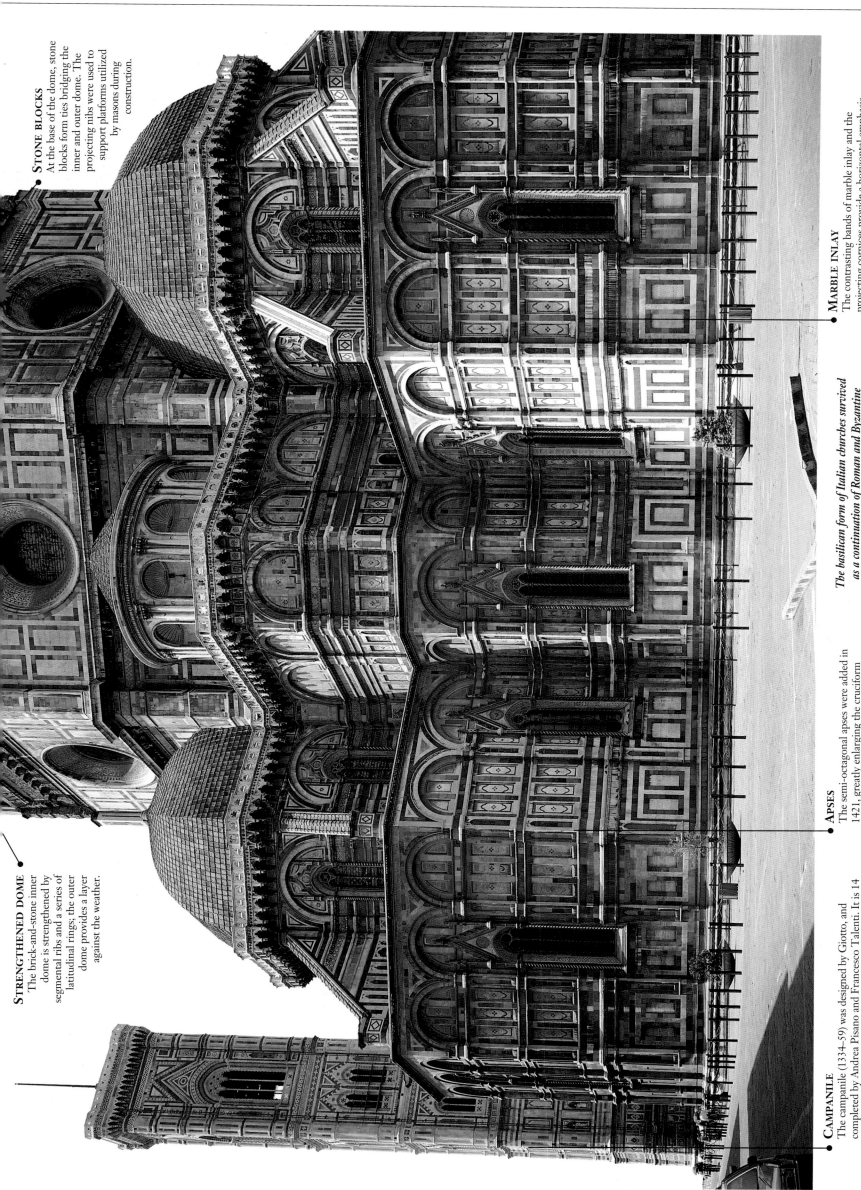

STONE BLOCKS
At the base of the dome, stone blocks form ties bridging the inner and outer dome. The projecting ribs were used to support platforms utilized by masons during construction.

MARBLE INLAY
The contrasting bands of marble inlay and the projecting cornices provide a horizontal emphasis, in contrast to the verticality of the perpendicular styles of northern European Gothic architecture.

STRENGTHENED DOME
The brick-and-stone inner dome is strengthened by segmental ribs and a series of latitudinal rings; the outer dome provides a layer against the weather.

The basilican form of Italian churches survived as a continuation of Roman and Byzantine styles, adapted to the Classically inspired forms of the Renaissance churches.

APSES
The semi-octagonal apses were added in 1421, greatly enlarging the cruciform Gothic plan. They provide additional space for devotional chapels.

CAMPANILE
The campanile (1334–59) was designed by Giotto, and completed by Andrea Pisano and Francesco Talenti. It is 14 metres (45 feet) square and 84 metres (275 feet) high, rising in four successive tiers, and supported without buttresses.

TEMPLE OF HEAVEN

A FUNDAMENTAL PURPOSE OF SACRED ARCHITECTURE is to create a realm that mediates between Humankind and God. Common to all peoples is a cultural connection between fertility and mortality, and instinctively, the expression of this connection is linked with the relationship between day and night, the cyclical movement of the Sun, and the changing seasons. The calibration of these cycles, through observation of the Sun and stars, frequently produces a sacred geometry often used as a determining principle in the layout of religious buildings. In Chinese architecture, this extends to the complete harmonization of a building with its site. The entrance and approach are each determined through the ancient art of *Feng Shui*, with regard to the spiritual influence of environmental features, such as mountains and rivers. The Temple of Heaven in Beijing, China, originating from 1420 (rebuilt 1530 and 1889), is the focus of a ceremony confirming the emperor's temporal power and his authority to intervene with the gods to seek atonement, future providence, and bountiful harvest. The structure of the temple, the raised platform, its relationship with buildings within the sacred precinct and its position within the city are all holistically predetermined in an attempt to harmonize with divine and natural forces.

The orientation of the temple was established with a magnetic compass, in use since the 8th century, pre-dating its use in navigation. The compasses created for the practice of **Feng Shui** *have complex scales that are used to interpret the most providential alignment with environmental features and natural forces. They are able to compensate for periodic variations in polar alignment.*

THIRD MING EMPEROR

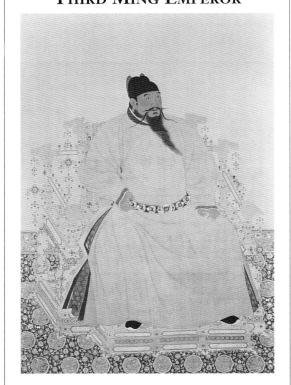

The emperor Yunglo (1360–1424) was the third and most powerful emperor of the Ming dynasty (1368–1644). He founded a new seat of imperial power in Beijing and did much to re-establish China following the collapse of the Yuan dynasty. During his reign, Yunglo led effective campaigns against the Mongols to protect the Great Wall and established his country as a strong maritime nation.

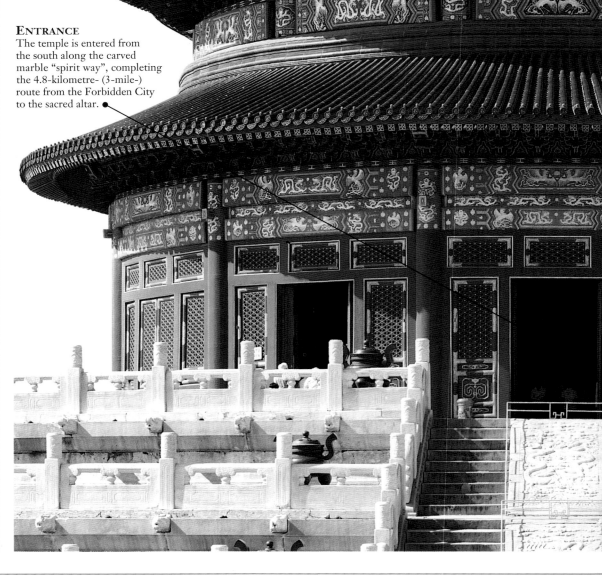

ROOF TILES
The blue of the ceramic roof tiles symbolizes openness to the heavens. On construction, the tiles were laid in a strict rotational sequence, with radiating courses corresponding to auspicious numbers.

ENTRANCE
The temple is entered from the south along the carved marble "spirit way", completing the 4.8-kilometre- (3-mile-) route from the Forbidden City to the sacred altar.

SPECIFICATION

- **Location** Peking, China
- **Date** 1420
- **Height** 38 m (125 ft)
- **Building structure** Timber-frame and stone plinth
- **Building type** Temple

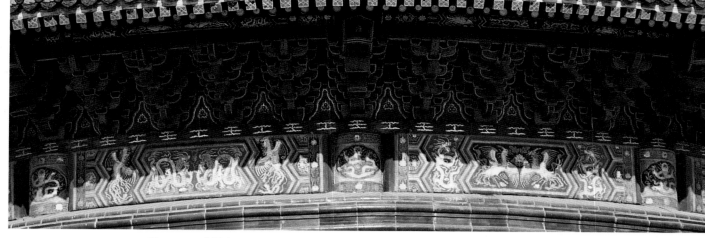

Decorated Frieze

The characters and figures that decorate the frieze and cantilevered timber brackets are of the phoenix and the dragon, invoking a harmonious balance between the forces of Yin and Yang. The dragon is an auspicious symbol of good fortune, while the phoenix, reborn from its own ashes, symbolizes continuity.

CENTRAL TURRET
The temple's dominating roof structure and platform symbolize Heaven, Earth, and the passage of the seasons.

The temple precinct contains three structures: the Altar of Heaven; the Hall of Prayer; and the Hall of Abstinence.

TIERS
The three tiers of the podium correspond to the three-tiered roof, as an expression of an odd number with masculine Yang associations. The temple is 38 metres (125 feet) high and has an internal diameter of 30 metres (99 feet).

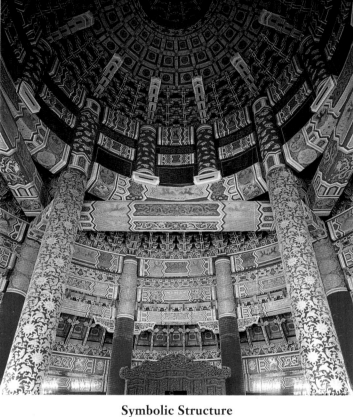

Symbolic Structure

The structural timber frame has three tiers of columns arranged in two concentric rings. The four red columns, 18 metres (59 feet) high, represent the seasons. The 12 outer columns stand for the 12 months, and the 12 gilded, inner columns correspond to the diurnal hourly cycle.

PLATFORM
The temple is raised upon an 8-metre- (26-foot-) high three-tiered platform, emphasizing the temple's mediating connection between Heaven and Earth.

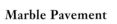

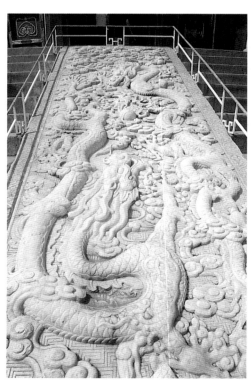

Marble Pavement

The white marble pavement is carved with auspicious symbols and forms the southern approach taken by the emperor when ascending the staircase on a palanquin, a covered litter, carried on poles on the shoulders of his courtiers.

TEMPLE OF HEAVEN • 39

ARCHITECTURE • 39

KING'S COLLEGE CHAPEL

THE CHAPEL OF KING'S COLLEGE, Cambridge (1446–1515) provides a breathtaking conclusion to the perpendicular phase of the English Gothic. The simple rectilinear form, without tower or transept, was intended as one of a group of collegiate buildings arranged around a central courtyard. Internally, the building celebrates the fusion of light, structure, and decoration permitted by the evolution of the Gothic vault. The fluidity of the fan vaulting by the master mason John Wastell and the slenderness of the compound piers provide a structural web of astonishing delicacy. Construction proceeded sporadically in three distinct phases (1446–62, 1477–84, and 1508–15), spanning a pivotal phase in European history. As the foundation stones were laid, Brunelleschi's dome of Florence Cathedral (see p. 36) was already under construction. By the chapel's completion in 1515, the political landscape of the medieval world had changed, unsettling the central position of the Roman Church. While architectural influence was being drawn towards the Renaissance spirit, with an emphasis on secular building, England was on the brink of the Dissolution and Protestant reform. The chapel survived the vandalism wrought on many religious buildings during the period of the Reformation in the 16th century, however, providing an authentic monument to the final phase of English Gothic.

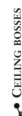

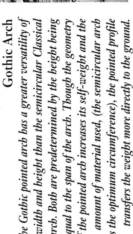

Gothic Arch

The Gothic pointed arch has a greater versatility of width and height than the semicircular Classical arch. Both are predetermined by the height being equal to the span of the arch. Though the geometry of the pointed arch increases its self-weight and the amount of material used, (the semicircular arch has the optimum circumference), the pointed profile transfers the weight more directly to the ground.

Corner Towers

Surmounted by Tudor domes, the corner towers incorporate the Gothic decoration of crockets and pinnacles. The upper tiers have an open fretwork of quatrefoils and cross quarters to accommodate their use as a belfry, there being no tower as in a conventional church.

(see p. 36)

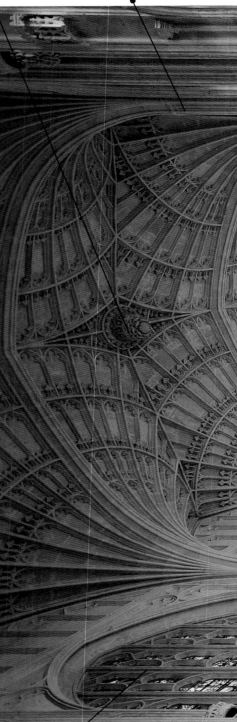

CEILING BOSSES
The inward structural tension directed towards the centre from the radiating fans is relieved by the ceiling bosses. This arrangement reduces lateral thrust towards the outer walls due to the low profile of the vault. The bosses are alternately decorated with the Tudor Rose and the Beaufort Portcullis.

COLUMNS
The columns have multiple shafts, reducing their apparent mass. The structural armature has an amazing fluidity, evaporating within the upper reaches of the vault and providing a perfect metaphorical connection between heaven and earth.

TRACERIED WINDOWS
The upper sections of the traceried windows provide spectacular illumination to the interior. The glazing depicts scenes from both the Old and New Testaments.

The later, and controversial, addition of Rubens' Adoration of the Magi (1634) to the eastern wall beyond the altar completes the perspective view.

HENRY VI

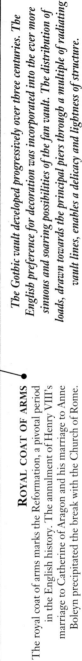

Henry VI (1421–71) was the only son of Henry V and Catherine of Valois. He was king of England from 1422 to 1461 and 1470 to 1471, having been deposed in 1461 during the War of the Roses, a conflict between Yorkist and Lancastrian factions. He founded Eton College (1440–41) and King's College, Cambridge (1441). Henry VI was murdered in the Tower of London.

CHOIR SCREEN

The timber choir screen, completed in 1536, separates the congregation from the clergy. The medieval framing and Classically inspired decoration and arcade record the transition from the Gothic towards the Classical tendencies of the English Renaissance.

SPECIFICATION

- **Location**   Cambridge, England
- **Date**   1446–1515
- **Master mason** John Wastell
- **Building structure**   Brick, stone, and timber
- **Building type**   Church
- **Construction time**   69 years

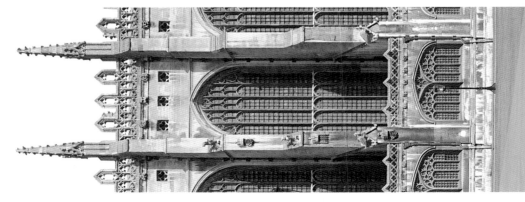

The Gothic vault developed progressively over three centuries. The English preference for decoration was incorporated into the ever more sinuous and soaring possibilities of the fan vault. The distribution of loads, drawn towards the principal piers through a multiple of radiating vault lines, enables a delicacy and lightness of structure.

ROYAL COAT OF ARMS

The royal coat of arms marks the Reformation, a pivotal period in the English history. The annulment of Henry VIII's marriage to Catherine of Aragon and his marriage to Anne Boleyn precipitated the break with the Church of Rome.

WINDOW NICHES

The window niches, with their pedestals and hoods, were intended to receive statues of the saints. The completion of the chapel saw a change in the emphasis of the liturgy, from the commemoration of the dead to the celebration of the living.

SCREEN WALLS

The lower screen walls provide access to the side chapels, which run symmetrically along the length of the nave.

Structural Bays

The chapel was constructed in a sequence of 12 equal bays. The uniformity of structure and the buttressing of the wall piers, anchored at each gable end by corner towers, provide an efficient structural frame. The walls between the piers are relegated to non-load-bearing screens, permitting large areas of glazing.

TEMPIETTO SAN PIETRO

THE CENTRALIZED PLAN held a particular fascination for Renaissance architects, who believed it to be the prevalent form of the Classical temple and to have symbolic associations with divinity, perfection, and unity. This preference for pure form found itself in conflict, however, with the requirements of religious worship and the need for the separation of altar, clergy, and laity. The commemorative shrines of the Christian martyrs offered a variation in the functional requirements of the church and a direct Christian equivalent to the pagan model of the Classical temple. The Tempietto commemorates the place of martyrdom of St Peter, and summarizes, within its modest scale, the striving for harmony and Classical order in the late Renaissance. Here, the central drum, or cella, containing the shrine is surmounted by a simple dome with an external ring of columns, known as a peristyle. The height of the cella is equivalent to the radius, in plan, of the peristyle. The drum is enclosed by 16 Doric columns, in strict proportion according to Classical precedent. The building has a simple unity, derived from a system of harmonious proportion, with each expressed element related to a unified whole.

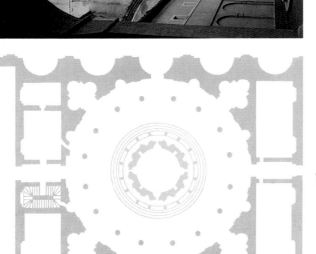
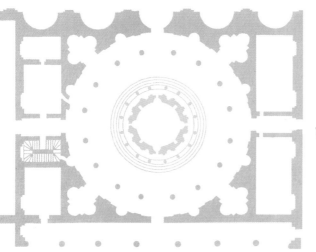

Cloister of San Pietro

Confined within the monastery cloister, the Tempietto carefully manipulates the perspective view of the observer to create an illusion of astonishing monumentality for a building of such modest scale, only 4.5 metres (15 feet) in internal diameter. The form, like that of the Classical temples, is best appreciated from predetermined views.

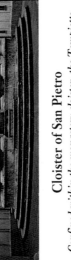

Plan

The Tempietto is enclosed within the cloister of the monastery of San Pietro on the Janiculum hillside overlooking Rome. Bramante proposed a complete reworking of the courtyard. Never executed, it would have extended the systematic, geometrical proportioning of the Tempietto (centre).

DONATO BRAMANTE

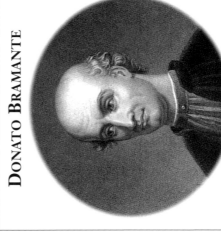

Donato Bramante (1444–1514) was born in Urbino in Italy. He trained as a painter and, from 1477 to 1499, worked in Milan. Under Mantegna's tuition he gained a passion for Classical antiquity and achieved notoriety for his work on the geometry of perspective drawing. In 1499, Bramante settled in Rome. Under the patronage of Pope Julius II he gained the commission for the planning of St Peter's (see p. 44) in Rome.

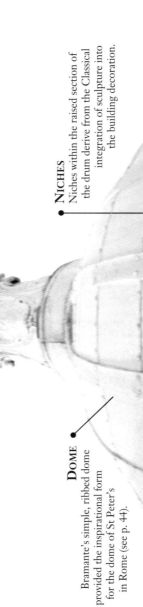

NICHES
Niches within the raised section of the drum derive from the Classical integration of sculpture into the building decoration.

DOME
Bramante's simple, ribbed dome provided the inspirational form for the dome of St Peter's in Rome (see p. 44).

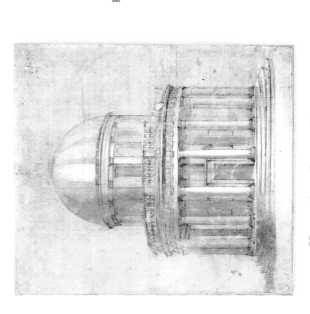
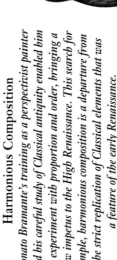

Harmonious Composition

Donato Bramante's training as a perspectivist painter and his careful study of Classical antiquity enabled him to experiment with proportion and order, bringing a new impetus to the High Renaissance. This search for simple, harmonious composition is a departure from the strict replication of Classical elements that was a feature of the early Renaissance.

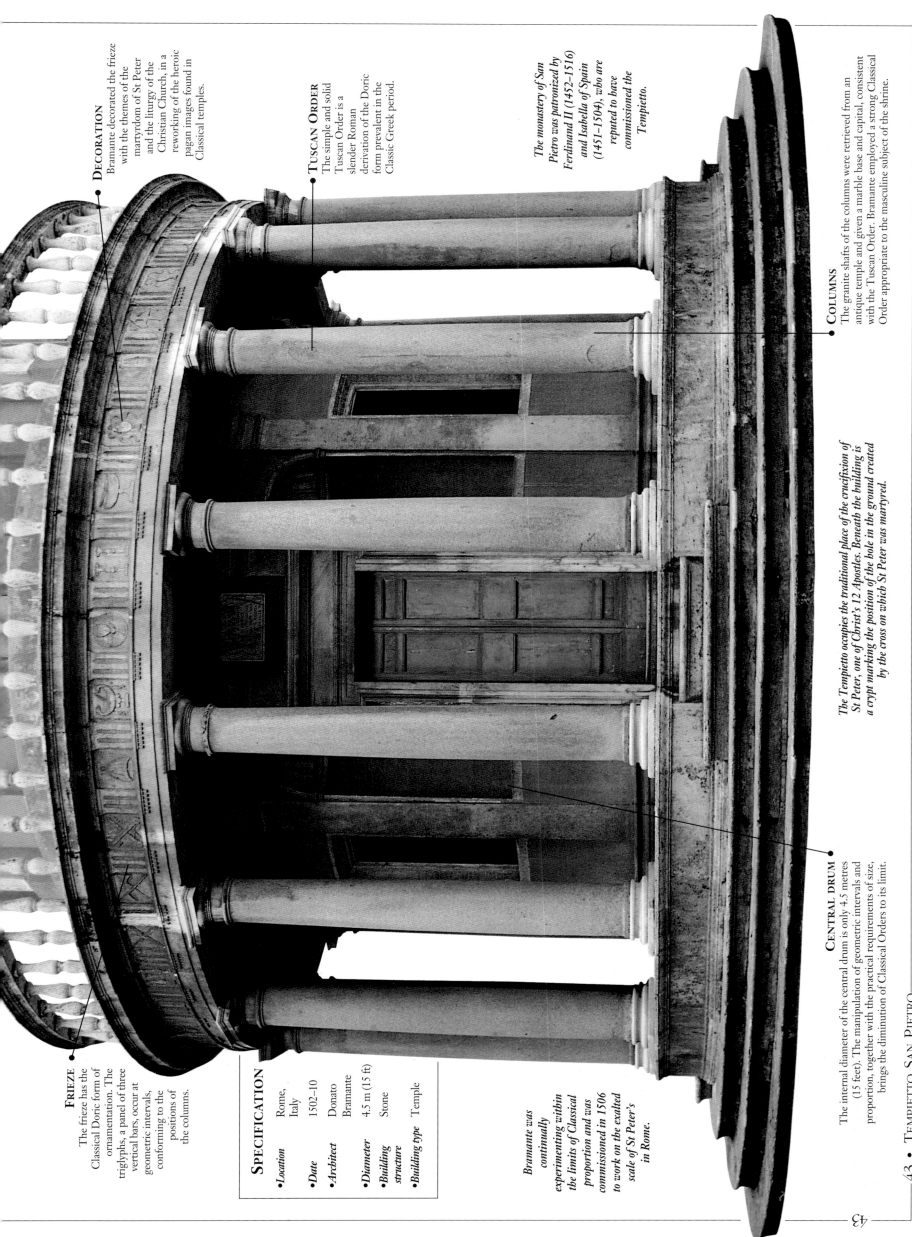

DECORATION
Bramante decorated the frieze with the themes of the martyrdom of St Peter and the liturgy of the Christian Church, in a reworking of the heroic pagan images found in Classical temples.

TUSCAN ORDER
The simple and solid Tuscan Order is a slender Roman derivation of the Doric form prevalent in the Classic Greek period.

The monastery of San Pietro was patronized by Ferdinand II (1452–1516) and Isabella of Spain (1451–1504), who are reputed to have commissioned the Tempietto.

COLUMNS
The granite shafts of the columns were retrieved from an antique temple and given a marble base and capital, consistent with the Tuscan Order. Bramante employed a strong Classical Order appropriate to the masculine subject of the shrine.

The Tempietto occupies the traditional place of the crucifixion of St Peter, one of Christ's 12 Apostles. Beneath the building is a crypt marking the position of the hole in the ground created by the cross on which St Peter was martyred.

CENTRAL DRUM
The internal diameter of the central drum is only 4.5 metres (15 feet). The manipulation of geometric intervals and proportion, together with the practical requirements of size, brings the diminution of Classical Orders to its limit.

FRIEZE
The frieze has the Classical Doric form of ornamentation. The triglyphs, a panel of three vertical bars, occur at geometric intervals, conforming to the positions of the columns.

SPECIFICATION

- **Location** Rome, Italy
- **Date** 1502–10
- **Architect** Donato Bramante
- **Diameter** 4.5 m (15 ft)
- **Building structure** Stone
- **Building type** Temple

Bramante was continually experimenting within the limits of Classical proportion and was commissioned in 1506 to work on the exalted scale of St Peter's in Rome.

ST PETER'S, ROME

THE REBUILDING OF THE **1,100-YEAR-OLD BASILICAN CHURCH** of St Peter's in Rome (1506–1626) was one of the most ambitious projects of the 16th century. Commissioned by Pope Julius II (1443–1513), it employed some of the greatest architects of the late Renaissance, including Bramante, Raphael, Michelangelo, and Bernini. The lengthy and intermittent progress of its construction illustrates the changing course of the High Renaissance towards a break from strict, antique precedent to the freer, eclectic tendencies of High Baroque and Mannerist styles. St Peter's reaffirmed the influence of Rome as the spiritual home of Christianity, which had its architectural origin in Bramante's modest Tempietto (see p. 42). Bramante's original proposal (*c.* 1506) determined the central importance of the dome and, despite modifications by successive architects, was revisited by Michelangelo's definitive design (*c.* 1546) of a centrally planned church, capped by a monumental dome. The cathedral forms the backdrop to the piazza and completes the most memorable formal civic space in Renaissance history.

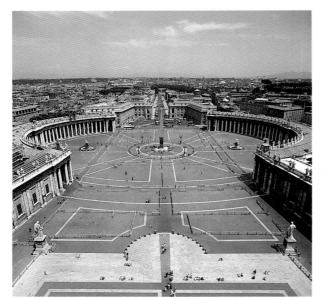

Piazza of St Peter
Viewed in an easterly direction from the roof of the cathedral, the elliptical plan of the piazza encircled by Bernini's Doric colonnade makes a grand sweeping gesture, brilliantly illustrating the High Baroque qualities of axiality, movement, and climax.

CROSS
The brass sphere originally mounted at the pinnacle of the obelisk was said to have contained the ashes of Roman emperor Julius Caesar. This was replaced by the cross, into which a relic purporting to be of Christ's true cross was inserted in 1740. Relics are similarly encased in the cross mounted at the top of the dome.

LANTERN
The 26.5-metre- (87-foot-) high lantern is raised 137.7 metres (452 feet) above the pavement, forming a climax to the sculptural Baroque detail of the church. Paired columns reiterate those at the elevated base of the dome and the façade.

ELEVATION
With an elevational height of 51 metres (167 feet), St Peter's is taller than any other Renaissance church, and provides a spectacular backdrop to the Piazza.

ORIENTATION
The unusual orientation of the church, with the main façade facing east rather than west, was inherited from the form of the Roman basilican church that it replaced.

Raphael's appointment to the cathedral marks the first recorded use of architectural drawings completed to the same representative scale in plan, section, and elevation. This three-part system became the established method for architectural drawing and survives to this day.

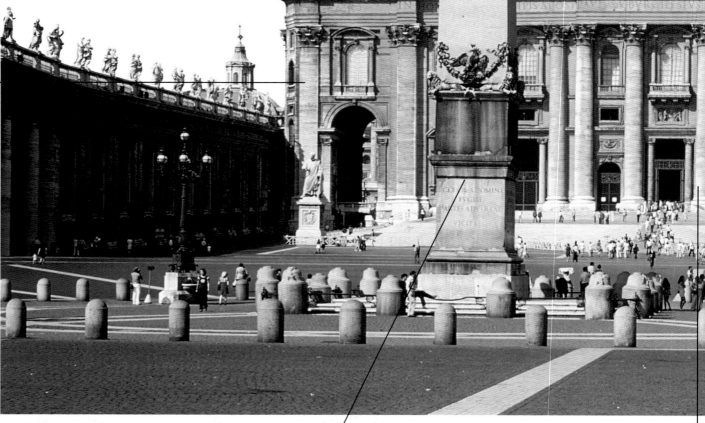

SPECIFICATION

•*Location*	Rome, Italy
•*Date*	1506–1626
•*Main architect*	Michelangelo
•*Height*	137.7 m (452 ft)
•*Building structure*	Stone
•*Building type*	Cathedral

OBELISK
The obelisk, brought to Rome in AD 36 by the Roman emperor Caligula, was moved to its present site in 1586. Raised in complete silence at the Pope's orders by 40 teams of horsemen, its re-erection was seen as a triumph for Christianity over Egyptian and Roman paganism.

FACADE
The completed façade has a gigantic Order of pilastered Corinthian columns, each 27.5 metres (90 feet) high. The attached columns were modified from Michelangelo's proposal for a freestanding colonnaded portico.

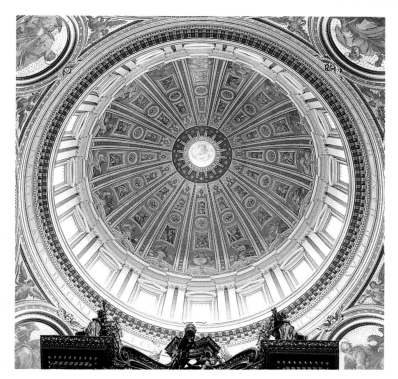

Scale

The scale of the dome is impressive. The pen of St Luke pictured in the top right medallion is 2.3 metres (7.5 feet) in length. Around the frieze of the cupola are inscribed the words of Christ's dedication: "Thou art Peter, and upon this rock I will build my church."

STRUCTURE OF DOME

The dome rests on four pendentives and massive piers, each 18 metres (59 feet) thick. Michelangelo's plan increased the strength and size of the load-bearing structure without destroying the central unity of Bramante's original design.

Classical Dome

The ovoid profile of the dome was changed from Michelangelo's hemispherical design because of fears of instability. The construction is strengthened by 16 radial ribs and a double-layer shell (the inner shell preserves the hemispherical form). The dome is banded by 10 iron chains to resist the outward thrust at the perimeter. The structure achieves an internal span of 42 metres (137 feet), only marginally less than that of the Pantheon (see p. 14), but at a much greater height.

BUTTRESSES

The paired columns that buttress the dome were the result of Michelangelo's original intention to build a hemispherical dome.

PORTICO

Later revisions to Michelangelo's proposal for a deeper, open portico produced a design of lesser sculptural impact when set against the monumental façade.

*The cathedral is maintained by the **Sampietrini** – a hereditary corps of workers continually scaling and inspecting the building's vertiginous surfaces. On St Peter's feast day they stage a dramatic display by illuminating the profile of the cathedral with thousands of torches.*

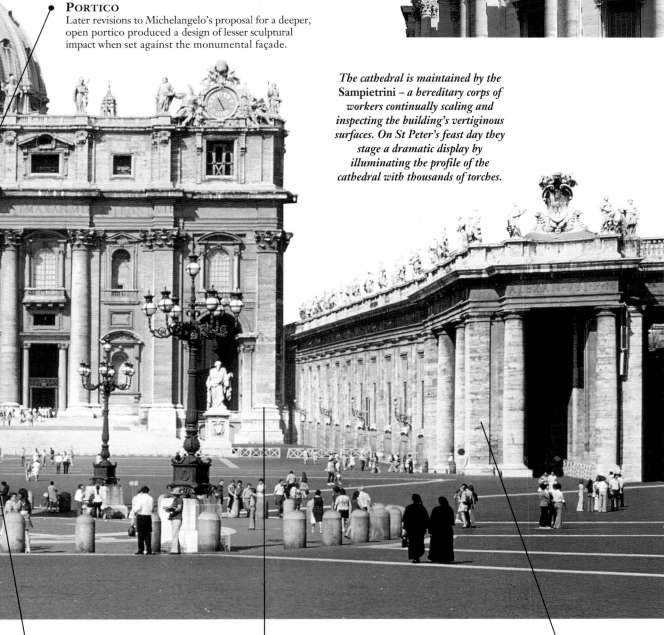

MICHELANGELO

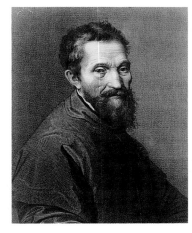

The artistic legacy of Michelangelo di Lodovico Buonarroti (1475–1564) dominated the 16th century, bringing a structural and sculptural clarity to the work of the High Renaissance. At the insistence of Pope Paul III, he succeeded as chief architect of St Peter's in 1546, at the age of 71. Rejecting offers of payment, he undertook the commission "for the love of the saint", and on condition that he would have complete freedom from interference and be without the burden of keeping accounts. St Peter's houses his most famous sculpture, *The Pieta*.

CRYPT

Directly below the dome and the central altar, in a subterranean crypt, is the tomb of St Peter, believed to be founder of the Christian Church in Rome.

INCOMPLETE ELEVATION

The later elevation was intended to have been balanced by the addition of two flanking towers. This design was abandoned after fears of instability in the foundations.

COLONNADE

In his original design, Bernini intended almost completely to encircle the piazza, creating an even greater dramatic contrast when entering from the confinement of the surrounding streets.

ST BASIL'S CATHEDRAL

THE VICTORY OVER THE MONGOL ARMIES at Kazan in 1552 was one of Tsar Ivan IV's earliest campaigns and earned Russia freedom from Tartar rule. St Basil's Cathedral, overlooking Moscow's Red Square, was built to commemorate this victory. Designed by Russian architects Barma and Posnik, the cathedral established the traditional "tent-and-tower" church as a symbol of national unification, and combined the forms of the characteristically helmet-shaped, domed, timber churches of the north with the brick-and-masonry decorative styles of the south. The influence of Renaissance architecture, imported through trading links with Venice, further contributed to this eclecticism. The central "tent" is a separate church dedicated to the Virgin of the Intercession and is surrounded by eight independent chapels, each with their own distinctive tower and onion dome. St Basil, whose name has become synonymous with the unified cathedral, is buried in an additional north-eastern chapel. The fantastically ornate onion domes and profusion of polychromatic tile work are a late-17th-century addition, creating the familiar silhouette associated with Moscow and the Kremlin.

IVAN IV (THE TERRIBLE)

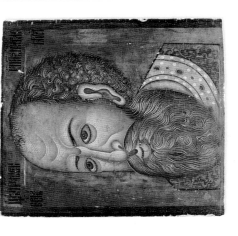

Born in Moscow, Ivan IV (1530–84) was proclaimed grand prince at the age of three, following the death of his father. He was crowned Tsar in 1547, and married the first of his six wives in the same year. Although Ivan is famed for acts of public brutality, his nickname, derived from the Russian word *grozny*, when properly translated means "awe-inspiring". His reign saw the construction of a centrally administered Russian state and moves towards advancing his country into Europe. Ivan remained on the Russian throne until his death in 1584.

Plan

The plan is based on a central church with apse, surrounded by four octagonal chapels on the principal axis, interspersed by four polygonal chapels. The simple plan develops into a complex and highly sculptural composition, rising through the triangulated and arcaded drums towards the billowing domes.

Octagonal chapel

Central church

Chapel of St Basil the Blessed

Polygonal chapel

SPECIFICATION

- **Location** Moscow, Russia
- **Date** 1555–60
- **Architects** Barma, Posnik
- **Building structure** Stone
- **Building type** Cathedral

• **DOMES**
The richly decorated domes are a result of later additions to the forms of the chapels. Originally painted white, the church was refurbished in the 17th century to its multicoloured form.

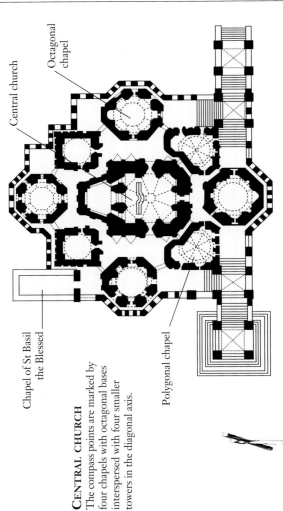

CENTRAL CHURCH
The compass points are marked by four chapels with octagonal bases interspersed with four smaller towers in the diagonal axis.

TENT-AND-TOWER CHURCHES
The tiered composition of "tent-and-tower" churches originates from the timber-framed churches of northern Russia.

SYMBOLIC FORM
The central church, surrounded by independent chapels, has a symbolic association with the hierarchy and centralization of Moscow within the emergent Russian state.

Onion Dome
The true origins of the use of the onion dome in Christian architecture are unclear, although the influence may stem from the church containing the Holy Sepulchre in Jerusalem. The similarities with Islamic forms are remarkable and betray the Eastern influence of Byzantine architecture.

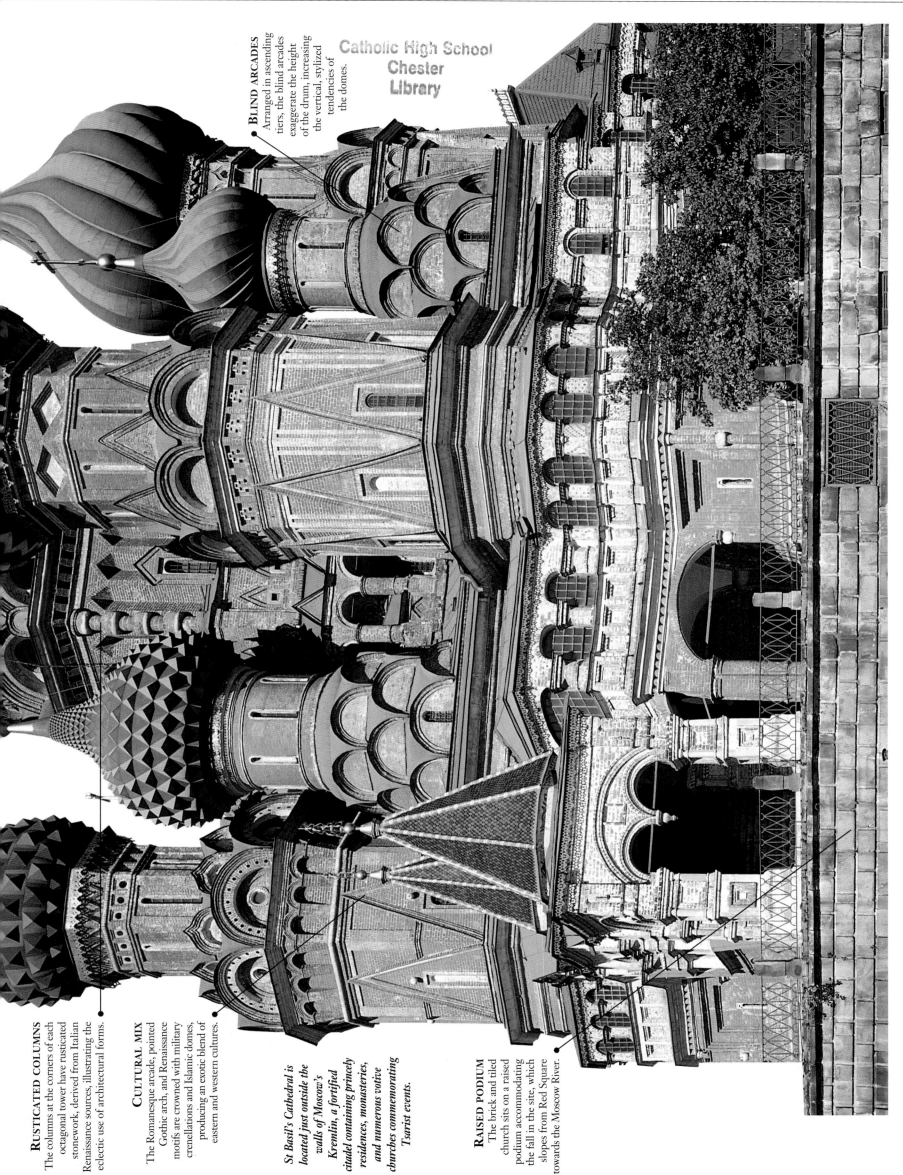

RUSTICATED COLUMNS
The columns at the corners of each octagonal tower have rusticated stonework, derived from Italian Renaissance sources, illustrating the eclectic use of architectural forms.

CULTURAL MIX
The Romanesque arcade, pointed Gothic arch, and Renaissance motifs are crowned with military crenellations and Islamic domes, producing an exotic blend of eastern and western cultures.

St Basil's Cathedral is located just outside the walls of Moscow's Kremlin, a fortified citadel containing princely residences, monasteries, and numerous votive churches commemorating Tsarist events.

RAISED PODIUM
The brick and tiled church sits on a raised podium accommodating the fall in the site, which slopes from Red Square towards the Moscow River.

BLIND ARCADES
Arranged in ascending tiers, the blind arcades exaggerate the height of the drum, increasing the vertical, stylized tendencies of the domes.

Catholic High School
Chester
Library

47 • ST BASIL'S CATHEDRAL

VILLA ROTONDA

THE **HIGH RENAISSANCE** in Italy celebrated artistic endeavour and architectural achievement, with secular architecture enjoying an unprecedented period of patronage in commissions for town houses and rural villas. Antique manuscripts were revived through the new medium of typeset print, popularizing Classical themes. Nature, beauty, and proportion were again studied alongside the poetry of Virgil and Homer, providing an artistic genre for architecture formally set within an "Arcadian landscape". The stylistic excesses of the High Renaissance were to find a perfect foil in the composure and restraint of Andrea Palladio's refined Classicism. The Villa Rotonda (*c.* 1552), Vicenza, brings the Classical elements of temple architecture to the service of a civilized place of rural retreat. This image, in its rustic setting, proved capable of indefinite, subtle variation, providing a subsequent model for the understated grandeur of noble houses from the Georgian mansion to the 20th-century Modernist villa, such as the Villa Savoye (see p. 84).

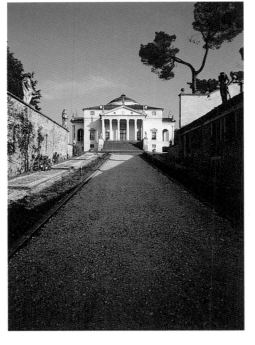

Formal Composition
The building is situated on the brow of a hill, with the advantage of fine views in each direction. The themes of proportion and symmetry, developed in many of Palladio's villas, are extended to the building's plan and the façade of each elevation. The elemental geometry and strictly formal composition are used both to frame views out, taken from within the portico, and those taken towards the building in its landscaped setting.

The rural villa provided a fashionable retreat from the summer heat and the periodic epidemics associated with the increasing density of urban populations.

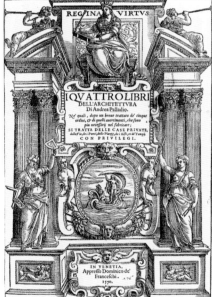

Architectural Theory
Andrea Palladio's architectural treatise, Quattro libri dell'architettura *(1570), records antique buildings, together with a systematic method of proportion, as well as illustrations of his own designs. This followed a trend established by the revival of the principal surviving 1st century work on Classical architecture,* De architectura, *by Vitruvius (first printed edition 1486).*

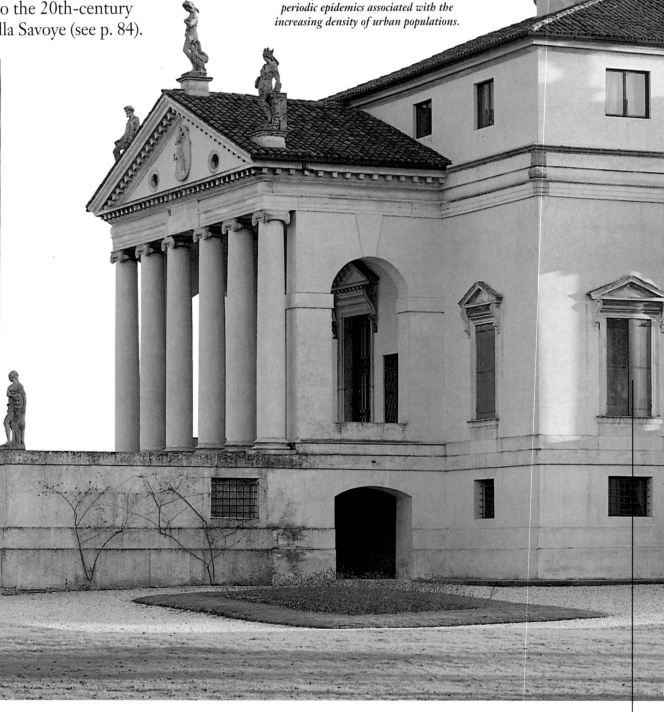

Printed editions of architectural works, such as Leon Battista Alberti's De re aedificatoria *(1485), helped to disseminate the influence of Classicism and the Renaissance throughout Europe.*

PIANO NOBILE
The principal living area, or *piano nobile*, is approached by an external flight of stairs, from which a complete view of the surrounding countryside can be attained.

SPECIFICATION

- **Location**   Vicenza, Italy
- **Date**   *c.* 1552
- **Architect**   Andrea Palladio
- **Building structure**   Brick and stone
- **Building type**   Villa

ANDREA PALLADIO

Andrea Palladio (1508–80) reinvigorated the architecture of the late Renaissance with his freshness and simplicity of approach. He completed many commissions for churches and private villas near his home town of Vicenza in Italy, in the studied and reductive Classical style for which he is most famous. Other commissions include the *Il Redentore* church in Venice. Palladio's influence extended to England and America, where Palladianism became a definitive style of the 18th century.

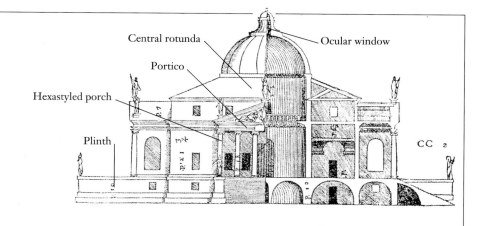

Central rotunda | Ocular window
Portico
Hexastyled porch
Plinth
CC 2

OCULAR WINDOW
The central rotunda is dramatically lit by an ocular window, a device borrowed from Classical Roman architecture (see p. 14).

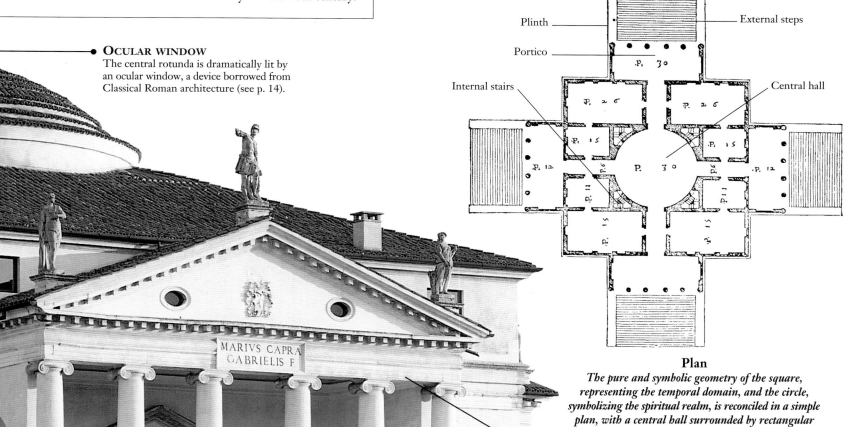

Plinth — External steps
Portico
Internal stairs — Central hall

Plan
The pure and symbolic geometry of the square, representing the temporal domain, and the circle, symbolizing the spiritual realm, is reconciled in a simple plan, with a central hall surrounded by rectangular rooms. The stairs to upper floors are enclosed within the wall that supports the central rotunda.

MARIVS CAPRA
GABRIELIS F

PORTICO
A Classical device, the portico is usually restricted to the main entrance, but here is given to each façade, completing the perceived symmetry and composition of the building, especially when viewed from a distance.

RAISED PLINTH
The raised plinth survives from sacred and fortified buildings, but here serves to emphasize the formal composition of the building, lending a sense of unworldly detachment.

ELEMENTAL FORMS
The cylinder, cube, and sphere – the essential geometric forms – are simply rendered, resolved together without an elaboration of detail, to emphasize their volumetric construction.

CLASSICAL DEVICES
The building skilfully employs the Classical devices of sacred temple architecture – a raised platform, portico, pediment, and rotunda – for the service of a residential building, emphasizing the grandeur of both the setting and its occupant.

The Renaissance period revived the Roman idea of the Villa Surbana, a refuge from the pressures of city life. The search for tranquillity began a romantic genre associated with an idealistic view of nature and the countryside.

HARDWICK HALL

E NGLISH ARCHITECTURE was slow to acknowledge the influence exerted throughout Europe by the Italian Renaissance. The Reformation had provoked a period of cultural detachment, and Queen Elizabeth I refrained from extravagant royal projects, preferring instead to encourage secular building among her courtiers, who vied for her attention and influence. This situation, prompted by the extravagant tours of the royal entourage, stimulated the personality cult of the Queen and a period of conspicuous wealth and construction amongst the gentry. Hardwick Hall (1590–97) blends the traditions and advancements of Gothic church building (the structural possibilities of glass and stone) with the improvements in domestic comfort demanded by a secular patron. A delight in symmetry and novelty is reflected in its architecture and landscape design. The hall survives in a remarkably original condition, providing an example of the authentic character of English architecture before the predominating influence of the late Renaissance.

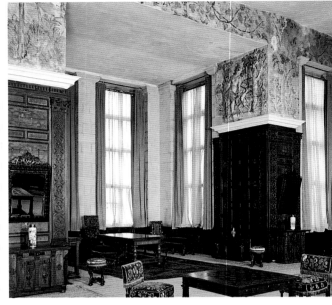

High Great Chamber
The second floor provides the principal room of state, the High Great Chamber, used for banquet receptions and musical entertainments. The plaster frieze, including scenes in the Garden of Eden, is a fine example of English decorative art predating the Italian Renaissance influence.

The writer and biographer Edmund Lodge (1756–1839) described Bess of Hardwick as "a woman of masculine understanding and conduct, proud, furious, selfish, and unfeeling. She was a builder, a buyer, a seller of estates, a money lender, a farmer, and a merchant."

COUNTESS OF SHREWSBURY

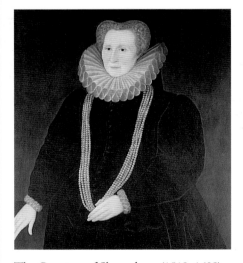

The Countess of Shrewsbury (1518–1608), also known as Bess of Hardwick, directed her wealth and energies into the construction of the New Hall at Hardwick, which, together with its remarkable collection of original tapestries and furnishings, provides a glimpse of the authentic character of Elizabethan architecture. The house was the result of a design by Robert Smythson (1535–1614), who emerged as one of the first English architects to be distinguished from the traditional role of the craftsman-designer. Smythson's designs, executed at Longleat House (1567–80) and Wollaton Hall (1580–88) show a disciplined, conceptual design, with technical competence and a playful measure of artifice and geometrical invention.

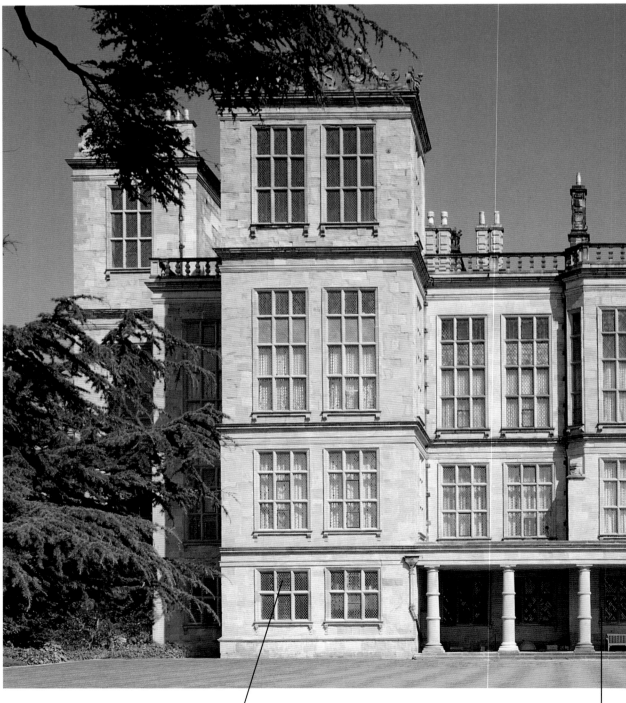

GLAZED ELEVATION
The extravagant use of glass, which was heavily taxed, was a display of wealth and status. Window openings are supported by concealed stone arches and lintels, which transfer the loads to the walls.

HALL
The two-storey-high, centrally placed hall runs from front to back in an unusual arrangement of the plan. This position, rather than the traditional hall running along the length of the plan, permits a flexibility of internal planning and a variety of spatial arrangements within the house.

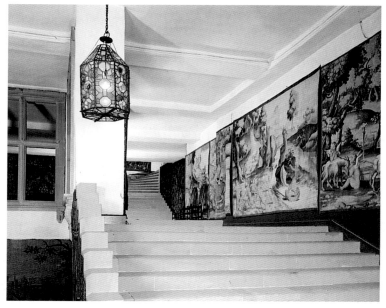

Staircase

The central stair creates a processional route through the house, which was used for the exercise and amusement of family and guests. The delivery of food from the ground-floor kitchen to the second-floor chamber was undertaken with great ceremony.

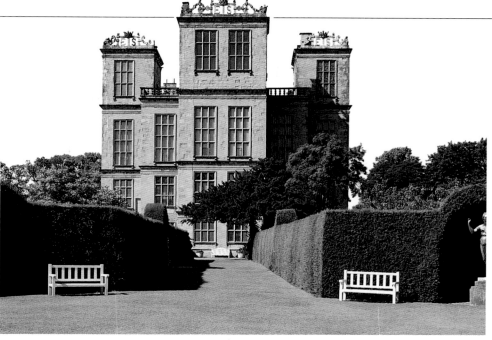

Formal Gardens

Delight in symmetry and novelty was continued into the designs of the formal gardens, laid out to complement the appearance of the house. Floral arrangements and mazes of clipped yew hedges provided diversions during exercise taken in the grounds. Gravel paths were laid out amongst the gardens and orchards.

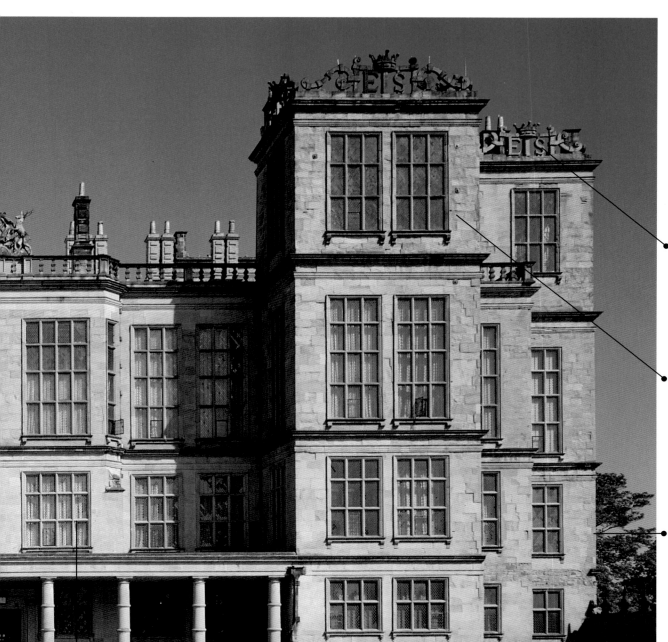

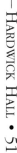

SPECIFICATION

- **Location** — Derbyshire England
- **Date** — 1590–97
- **Architect** — Robert Smythson
- **Building structure** — Brick, stone, and timber
- **Storeys** — 3
- **Building type** — Country house

SCROLL-WORK
The stone scroll-work describes the initials "E S" for Elizabeth of Shrewsbury, and the Countess's coronet. The family coat of arms is displayed upon the parapet above the central entrance.

TOWER ROOMS
On the third floor, the tower rooms are accessible via the stair in the north tower and the flat roof parapets. The rooms were used for relaxation and recreation, and for taking advantage of the fine views.

FALSE WINDOWS
Some side-elevation windows are false, concealing chimney breasts. Here the expression of symmetry overrides practicality. Elsewhere, the chimney flues run up the internal cross walls, freeing the elevations for the maximum amount of glazing.

FIRST FLOOR
The first floor accommodates an informal dining room, known as the Low Great Chamber, an upper gallery to the chapel, and suites of guest rooms connected across the double-height of the main hall, via a mezzanine gallery, to the private family apartments, bed chamber, and maids' room.

SYMMETRICAL FACADE
The house is carefully composed on all four elevations, demonstrating the Elizabethan regard for compact symmetry. The rectangular plan is dominated by six towers advanced from the line of the plan. The elevated proportions of the towers provide an imposing arrangement to the façade.

KATSURA PALACE

THE **KATSURA PALACE** (1620–58) is located near the Katsura river, to the south-west of the imperial city of Kyoto in Japan. The palace and gardens provided a place of seclusion and retreat for a collateral line of the Imperial family, in the cultural epoch of the late-16th century. The main palace is an open, timber-framed construction with simple *tatami* (rice-straw) matted rooms and elevated verandas from which to contemplate the delicate beauty of the changing seasons. The garden arbours and pavilions surrounding the main palace are approached from a sequence of carefully staged routes, recalling the dreamlike and natural landscapes described in Classical Japanese poetry. Throughout these settings, the buildings have an understated simplicity, and the landscape has been subtly manipulated to blur the distinction between artificial and natural environments. Artificial objects, such as fences and paving stones, have been subjected to the forces of nature, such as weathering, while natural features have been clipped, aligned and polished to emphasize their eccentricity and "unnaturalness". The effect is discreet and alluring, contributing to a heightened aesthetic awareness of the architecture and the landscape.

The buildings and gardens fell into decline in the Meiji period (1868–1912), until "rediscovered" by the Modernist German architect, Bruno Taut, who popularized the indigenous forms of traditional Japanese architecture for western viewers. Visitors to Katsura included architects Frank Lloyd Wright, Le Corbusier, and Walter Gropius. They found inspiration in the use of natural materials, simplicity, and a flexible and modulated open plan, suitable for contemporary designs in California and Northern Europe.

OVERHANGING EAVES
The low, overhanging eaves allow rainwater to be thrown clear of the building on to the gravel and stone paths that run around the perimeter. The eaves also provide shade from direct sunlight. Soft, diffused light pours into the interior as it is reflected from the stone paths on to the diffusing screens of the paper covered *shoji* (translucent screens).

PLANTING
Clipped plant displays recede to natural and eccentric forms in the middle distance. The plants create a simple but compelling balance between stillness and movement, between preciseness of form and sheer invention.

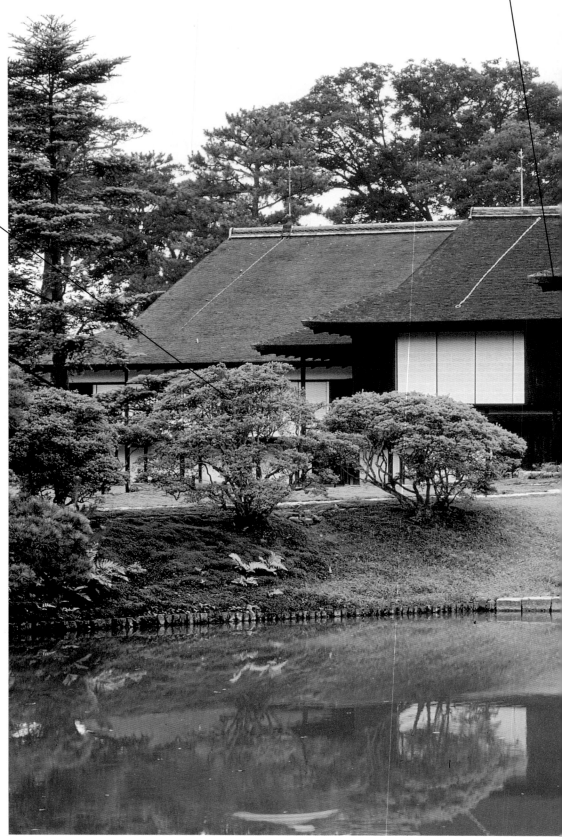

THE SHOKINTEI

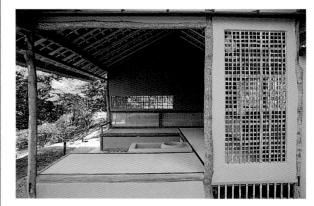

The Shokintei, or Pine-lute pavilion, is the most formal of the tea houses. Approached across a bridge comprising a single stone slab, the path concludes a careful route taken from the main *shoin* (central building). The building has a simple thatched roof and is partially enclosed by rustic screens of timber, paper, and bamboo. A kitchen is provided for the preparation of the tea ceremony, which is taken seated on the *tatami* of the main room. The building, though raised above the ground, has a more direct connection with the exterior than the main *shoin*, and the materials are more rusticated. Some of the outer columns are left unfinished, with their bark intact, but all the timbers are carefully burnished and turned to expose their unique and natural characteristics.

TEA CEREMONY

The gardens at Katsura were used to receive guests for the rituals and discourse of the tea ceremony (*cha-no-yu*), which achieved a particular cultural significance in Japan, inspiring works of poetry, calligraphy, philosophy, and ceramics. The aesthetic refinements of the Imperial Court were, in part, a result of the rise in power of the Shogunate, who imposed restrictive codes confining Imperial influence to artistic and scholarly pursuits.

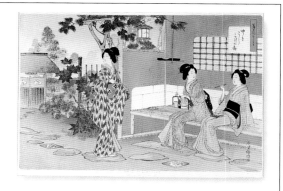

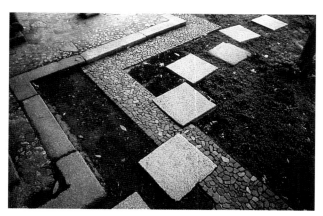

Stones
Stones are set in a grass and moss covered lawn, providing an informal path to the side of the lake and bridging across to the middle islands and the pavilions. Smooth and jagged boulders are carefully selected and juxtaposed to contrast with the shaped edges and formal lines of the paths, which delineate the building's edge.

The nature of the secluded retreat is typified by the translation of the name of one of the tea houses (Shoi-ken) as the Pavilion of Laughing Thoughts. This was inspired by the poet, Li Po, who retired to a hermitage to laugh at the vanity of the world.

● **SHOIN**
The main palace is characterized by the *shoin* style of construction. *Shoin* means a place of study, incorporating *tatami*-matted rooms, a low desk, a *takahoma* (or alcove, for display of art objects or flower arrangements), and a *chigaidana*, a cabinet for books, papers, and calligraphic materials.

● **SEASONAL CHANGE**
The open form of architecture allows unrestricted cross-ventilation during periods of heat and humidity. The lack of insulation and enclosure is inadequate to protect from the wet and cold of the autumn and winter months. The cultural significance of seasonal change – the anticipation of the cherry blossom and the ennui of the autumn leaves – is keenly experienced in such a fragile environment.

● **VERANDA**
The bamboo platform of the veranda and the orientation of the elevation provide the best view of the reflection of the Moon in the lake. The name "Katsura" has poetic associations with the trees, the Moon, and the world of dreams.

● **THE LAKE**
A series of stepping stones leads down to the lake, which is formed from a natural rivulet diverting water from the Katsura river. The lake was used at night by boating parties to view the rising Moon. A pathway encircles the lake, passing each of the miniature landscapes.

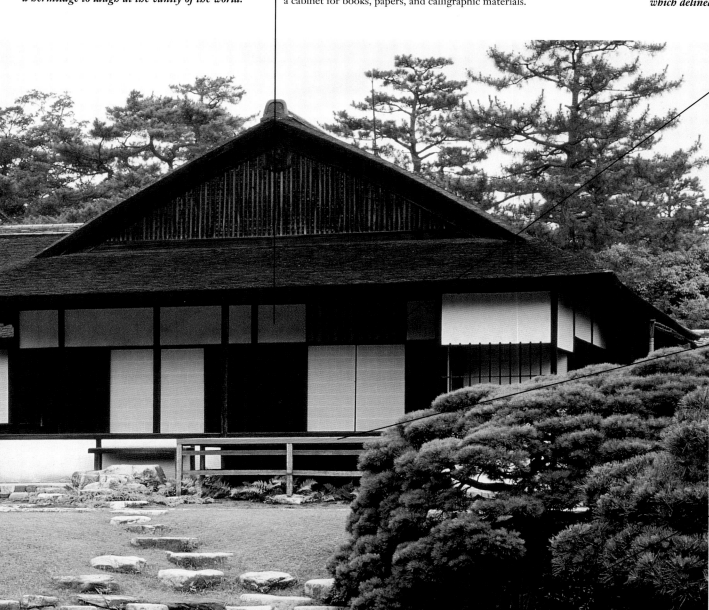

SPECIFICATION

•*Location*	Kyoto, Japan
•*Date*	1620–58
•*Building structure*	Timber-frame
•*Storeys*	1
•*Building type*	Royal residence
•*Construction time*	38 years

THE TAJ MAHAL

THE TAJ MAHAL (1630–53) is situated on the south side of the River Jumna, near Agra, in northern India. The mausoleum, built by the Mogul Emperor Shah Jahan, commemorates his favourite wife, Mumtaz Mahal. The Islamic traditions of architecture were brought to northern India by the Persian invaders of the 11th and 12th centuries and were continued from the 15th to the 18th centuries in the architecture of the Mogul dynasties. The distinctions between secular and religious buildings are less pronounced in Islamic than in Christian architecture. Islamic practice rejects representative images in favour of abstract design, producing a geometrically disciplined architecture. The Taj Mahal achieves a perfect sense of composition and setting. The building housing the tomb is surrounded by the mosque, hall, and gateway, complementing the overall geometry and composition. The effect is unifying, perfect, and complete.

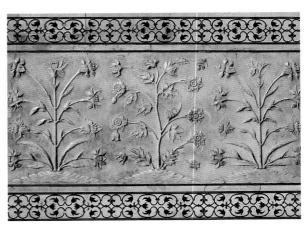

Marble Dado
A dado (decorative band) runs around the building. The white marble is inlaid with precious stones, amber, coral, jade, and lapis lazuli. In Islamic tradition, flowers are seen as symbols of the divine kingdom.

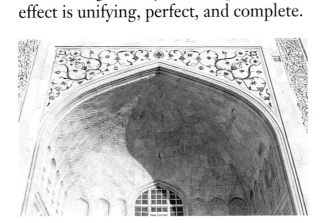

Fine Decoration
The recessed, vaulted openings are framed with flower patterns using semi-precious stone inlay, such as crystal and lapis lazuli, and calligraphic inscriptions in black stone. This detail is continued in the raised relief found in the spandrels and vaults of the interior.

CALLIGRAPHY
Verses of the Qur'an, the holy book of Islam, are recorded in calligraphic inlays of black stone around the openings.

MATERIALS
The building is constructed from a brick and rubble core, veneered with a fine marble secured by metal dowels.

PRAYER TOWERS
The minarets are placed at the edge of the podium, which elevates the whole structure from the surrounding garden.

REFLECTION
The white marble cladding and water landscaping reflect the changing conditions of light, allowing a subtle range of tones that lend the building an ethereal tranquillity.

MAIN BUILDING
The main building is situated alongside the riverbank. The symmetry of this placement, at the edge of the gardens, was to be completed with the construction of a similar mausoleum of black marble, planned on the opposite bank, as the resting place of Shah Jahan.

The pervasive forms of Islamic buildings underline the cultural dominance of the Muslim faith. Islamic architecture is characterized by concise geometry and its use of symmetry and balance. Individual design elements are set within a complex, geometric, unifying field of decoration. Architectural planning is informed by the dominant axis of prayer – oriented towards Mecca, Saudi Arabia, the holiest city of Islam.

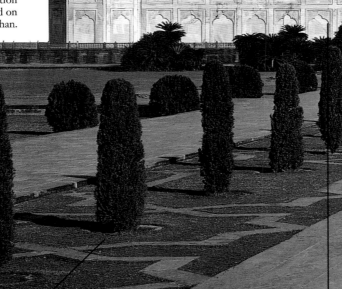

VISION OF PARADISE
The 6.9 hectares (17 acres) of gardens were designed as a vision of an earthly paradise and would originally have been extensively planted with exotic flowers and trees.

MARBLE PLATFORM
The mausoleum is placed on a marble platform that raises it above the river's flood plain. A stone embankment protects the gardens from erosion by the river.

FOUNTAINS
The principal axis of the garden is reinforced with water fountains. Water drawn from the river into subterranean chambers was used to feed the canals and irrigate the gardens.

SHAH JAHAN AND MUMTAZ MAHAL

Shah Jahan (1592–1666), the greatest of the Mogul builders, established the city of Shajahanabad (Old Delhi), enlarging the palace-fortress (1639–48), which contains the magnificent Pearl Mosque (1646–54). His legacy is testament to the power, wealth, and energy of the Mogul dynasties. Mumtaz died in childbirth whilst accompanying the Shah on a military campaign.

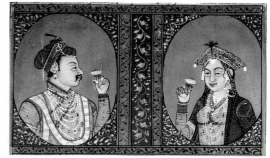

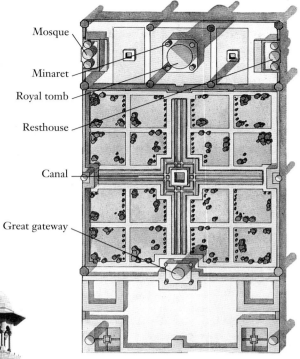

Plan of the Taj Mahal
The principal axis of the garden runs north–south from the gate to the tomb. The intersecting canals (symbolizing the Four Rivers of Paradise), reinforced with fountains and lined with cypress trees, cross at a raised, central lotus pond of white marble. The surrounding hall, mosque, and gateway complement the overall geometry and composition.

Mosque
Minaret
Royal tomb
Resthouse
Canal
Great gateway

● **FINIAL**
The central dome is crowned by a brass finial 17.1 metres (56 feet) high.

" Enter thou among my servants and enter thou My Paradise"
THE QUR'AN, SURA 89

The finest masons were recruited to work on the construction. On completion, Jahan is alleged to have ordered the amputation of the chief mason's hand to prevent replication of such exquisite detail.

● **VAULTED RECESSES**
The vaulted recesses lead to the central space, which contains the displayed cenotaphs, enclosed within a perforated marble screen. The actual tombs lie in a subterranean chamber directly below.

● **COMPOSITION**
The minaret prayer towers are used here for purely compositional effect, off-setting the central composition of the dome.

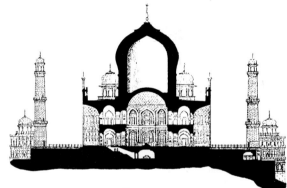

Dome
The main dome, above the central hall, rests on a central drum surrounded by four octagonal towers, each supporting a smaller, domed pavilion. The central, inner dome is 24.4 metres (80 feet) high, surmounted by a raised, outer dome 61 metres (200 feet) high, providing an elongated and slender profile to the outer shell.

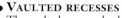

SPECIFICATION

•*Location*	Agra, India
•*Date*	1630–53
•*Height of dome*	61 m (200 ft)
•*Building structure*	Marble-clad brick and rubble core
•*Building type*	Mausoleum
•*Construction time*	23 years

● **WATER**
The use of water for humidification, ritual ablution, and cooling is exquisitely exploited, combining religious metaphor with sophisticated devices for climatic control.

● **CYPRESS TREES**
Cypress trees are used to line the stone paths that run alongside the canal. The trees provide shade and accentuate the lines of the perspective.

The purpose of many Islamic buildings is immediately recognizable by their familiar and standardized forms, such as onion domes and minarets.

POTALA PALACE

THE COUNTRY OF TIBET, high on the Himalayan plateau, has long maintained a distinctive cultural identity, centred on *Vajrayana*, or Tantric Buddhism, which has been practised since the 7th century AD. The Potala Palace in Lhasa enshrines the traditions of this unique history in a vast cultural complex that served as a focus of Tibetan politics, religion, and history. The palace is 400 metres (1,312 feet) long and 13 storeys high. It incorporates the White Palace (1645–90), which was built by the 5th Dalai Lama to mark the re-establishment of the Tibetan capital, and the Red Palace (1690–94), which was constructed following his death in 1682. Replacing an earlier monastery built in the 7th century, the White Palace housed the functions of state, monastic dormitories, and palace apartments, and encircles the Red Palace, which accommodates reliquaries and holy tombs. The building is a poignant reminder of the suppression of Tibetan culture, following the Chinese invasion in 1950, and the subsequent exile of the current 14th Dalai Lama in 1959.

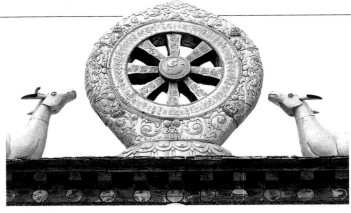

Wheel of Life
The gilded wheel decorating the eaves symbolizes the wheel of life, representing the cyclical nature of life, or rebirth, often used to illustrate Buddhist teaching. The eight spokes represent the eight-fold path towards enlightenment.

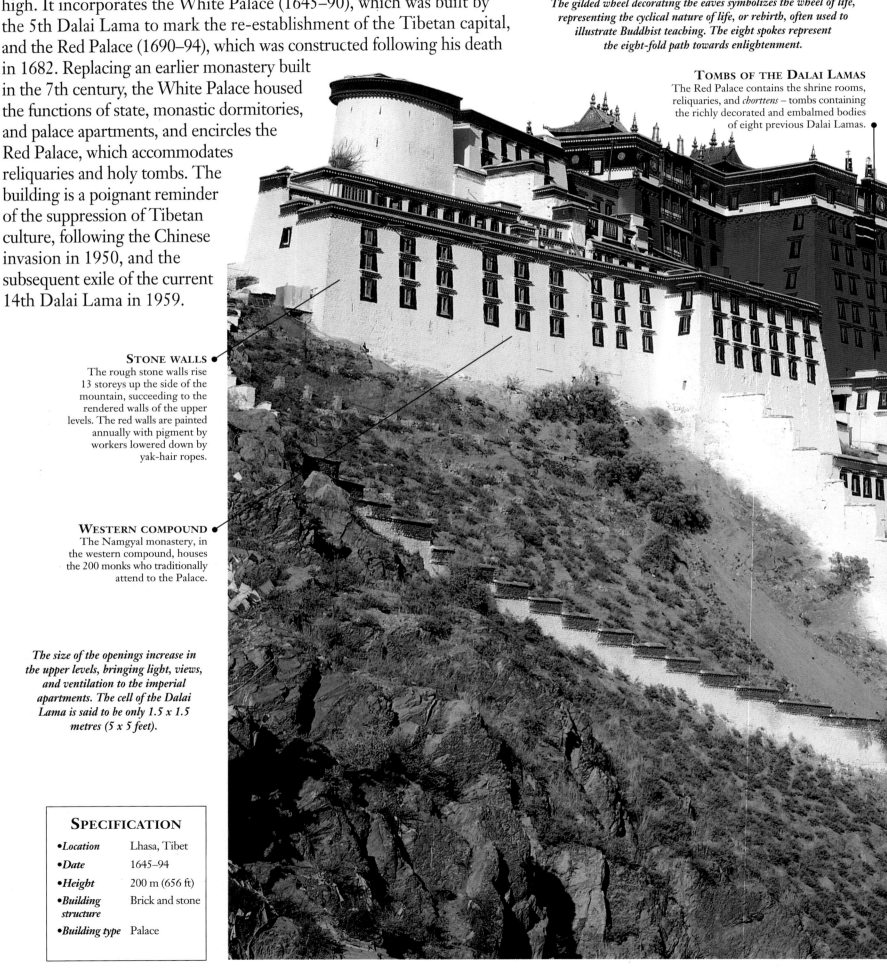

TOMBS OF THE DALAI LAMAS
The Red Palace contains the shrine rooms, reliquaries, and *chorttens* – tombs containing the richly decorated and embalmed bodies of eight previous Dalai Lamas.

STONE WALLS
The rough stone walls rise 13 storeys up the side of the mountain, succeeding to the rendered walls of the upper levels. The red walls are painted annually with pigment by workers lowered down by yak-hair ropes.

WESTERN COMPOUND
The Namgyal monastery, in the western compound, houses the 200 monks who traditionally attend to the Palace.

The size of the openings increase in the upper levels, bringing light, views, and ventilation to the imperial apartments. The cell of the Dalai Lama is said to be only 1.5 x 1.5 metres (5 x 5 feet).

SPECIFICATION

- **Location**   Lhasa, Tibet
- **Date**   1645–94
- **Height**   200 m (656 ft)
- **Building structure**   Brick and stone
- **Building type**   Palace

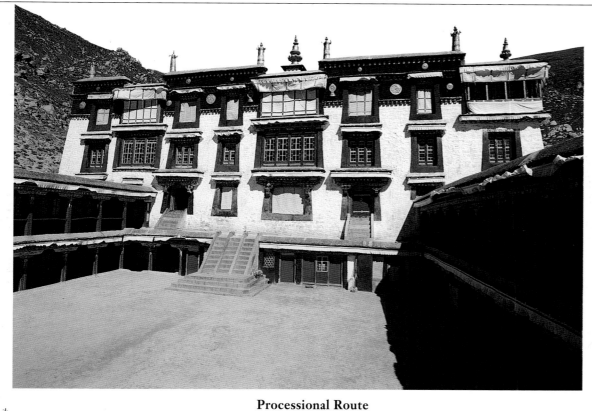

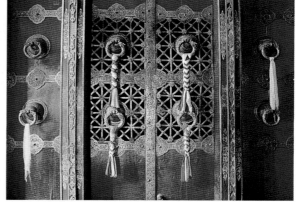

Decoration
The vividly coloured and highly ornate forms of decoration, such as these gilded door-fittings, are derived from Chinese and Indian influences, imported with the introduction of Buddhism, and mixed with the ancient occult traditions of indigenous art and architecture.

Processional Route
The palace is approached by a succession of gateways and courtyards, used to stage religious festivals. The processional route, with its variety of spatial experiences undertaken by all visitors, pilgrims, petitioners, and state visitors alike, is a metaphorical allusion to the successive paths of spiritual enlightenment.

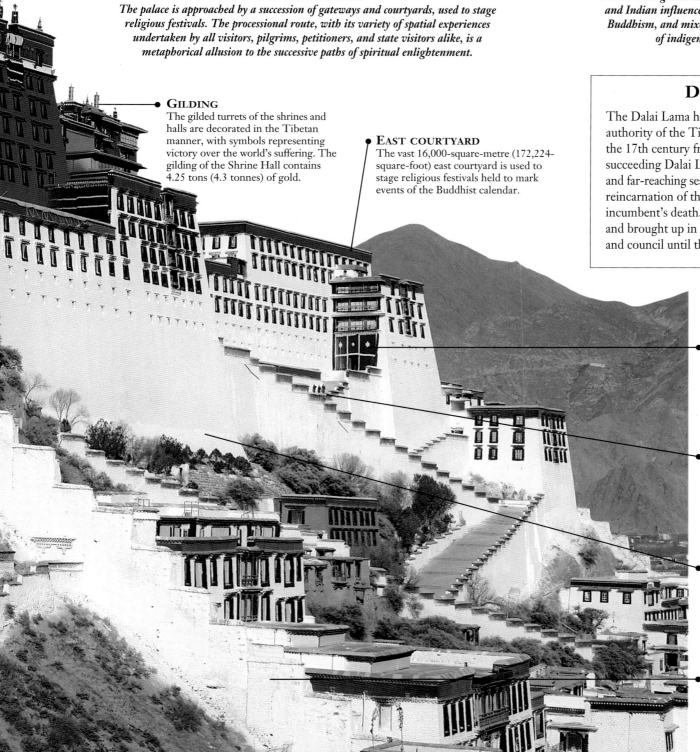

GILDING
The gilded turrets of the shrines and halls are decorated in the Tibetan manner, with symbols representing victory over the world's suffering. The gilding of the Shrine Hall contains 4.25 tons (4.3 tonnes) of gold.

EAST COURTYARD
The vast 16,000-square-metre (172,224-square-foot) east courtyard is used to stage religious festivals held to mark events of the Buddhist calendar.

DALAI LAMA

The Dalai Lama holds the spiritual and temporal authority of the Tibetan people, administered since the 17th century from the palace at Lhasa. The succeeding Dalai Lama is chosen following a long and far-reaching search by senior monks for the child reincarnation of the Lama's spirit, following the incumbent's death. The child is fostered by monks and brought up in the palace, ruled by a regent and council until the age of accession is reached.

SILK AWNINGS
The windows are hung with black yak-hair curtains and bright silk awnings. For particular festivals a gigantic silk banner is unfurled across the steep palace wall.

HIGH PLATFORM
The boundary between the secular and sacred world of the palace precinct is marked by the high platform.

LOWER FLOORS
The lower floors contain underground storage rooms and are said to conceal the darkened Bon shrines of the pre-Buddhist earth cult.

WALLS
The walls are 400 metres (1,312 feet) wide and 200 metres (656 feet) high. They were built up from the cliff face using stones carried long distances by porters and pack horses.

ST PAUL'S CATHEDRAL

OLD ST PAUL'S WAS DESTROYED by the Great Fire of London in 1666. The original scheme for the new cathedral, preferred by the architect Sir Christopher Wren, proposed a centralized Greek cross, without nave or aisles, crowned by an octagonal dome. This was rejected by the church commission, which was unwilling to depart radically from the elongated, Gothic cruciform plan. The plan was remodelled, but the approved design, executed between 1675 and 1710, continued to be developed in accordance with Wren's preference for a Baroque church dominated by an elevated, central rotunda. The cathedral was built on the same site as Old St Paul's. The dome, both internally and externally, is its most striking architectural achievement, rivalling those of St Peter's, Rome (see p. 44) and Florence Cathedral (see p. 36), which it equals in structural innovation. Wren's genius was both as a mathematician and practical architect, able to resolve all elements – from the general form to particular details – into a fluid and balanced design. St Paul's brought a stately magnificence to the London skyline and is the central achievement of Renaissance English architecture.

The Dome

The dome has a triple-layer construction. The external cupola of timber support-bracing and lead-sheathing rests upon the intermediate brick cone, which also supports the weight of the stone lantern, ball, and cross. This cone is strengthened with iron bands, which reinforce the inner brick dome the shell structure. The inner brick dome is fashioned to achieve a lightness of internal decoration.

CLERESTORY WINDOWS
Clerestory light is transmitted directly into the interior through the elevated windows around the drum, and indirectly through ocular windows at the base of the lantern and the apex of the inner dome.

Wren's confident authority, based on a Classical vocabulary, enabled the design to achieve a harmonious unity that exceeds any formulaic adherence to antique precedent.

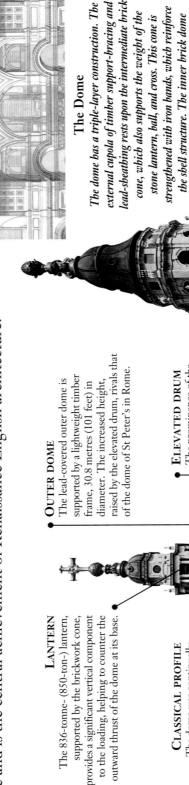

Ocular windows

Lantern

Supporting timber framework

Brickwork cone

Outer dome

Inner dome

Clerestory windows

Elevated rotunda

OUTER DOME
The lead-covered outer dome is supported by a lightweight timber frame, 30.8 metres (101 feet) in diameter. The increased height, raised by the elevated drum, rivals that of the dome of St Peter's in Rome.

ELEVATED DRUM
The prominence of the dome is achieved by an elevated drum, giving the building its characteristic profile.

LANTERN
The 836-tonne- (850-ton-) lantern, supported by the brickwork cone, provides a significant vertical component to the loading, helping to counter the outward thrust of the dome at its base.

CLASSICAL PROFILE
The dome was continually revised in successive designs, developing from a cupola, surmounted by a gothicized spire, into the Classical profile that completes the composition.

ST PAUL
Statues are placed prominently within the façade at elevated positions. The statue of St Paul, above the central portico, is flanked by St John (right) and St Peter (left).

Side Elevation

The false windows and increased height of the side elevation screen the buttressing required by the nave walls of the elongated, Gothic plan. Wren carefully considered the many aspects of the building's elevations, measuring them against its overall appearance as a unified design.

TOWERS
The skilful and restrained handling of the towers, as distinguished, individual elements within the overall design, exemplifies the fluidity of the English Baroque.

Structural science was in its infancy in the late-17th century. In 1638, Galileo published his Dialogue Concerning Two New Sciences, which begins to identify a scientific basis for the strength of materials and the resolution of structural forces. Sir Isaac Newton (1642–1727) had provided a significant advancement in his Laws of Motion. Wren and Robert Hooke (1635–1703), founders of the Royal Society, both undertook systematic enquiry into the theoretical nature of forces.

THE PEDIMENT
The pediment is a Classical device that conceals the pitched roof. Baroque architecture characteristically presents the façade and the main architectural elements as formal compositions, often disguising utilitarian elements of building structure.

The quality and detail of ornamentation lend sufficient animation to the façade without overwhelming the harmony of the overall composition.

COLUMNS
The paired, free-standing columns of the portico, translating to the pilastered columns of the towers, are typical of Wren's command of structural organization.

PEDIMENT SCENE
The portico pediment depicts the scene of the conversion to Christianity of St Paul, following his apocalyptic vision on the road to Damascus.

The cathedral was constructed within 35 years, and was the first to be completed under the direction, and within the lifetime, of a single architect.

WEST FACADE
The principal east-west axis of the church was slightly displaced from that of its predecessor. The congregation faces the position of the Easter morning sunrise in a metaphorical expression of resurrection.

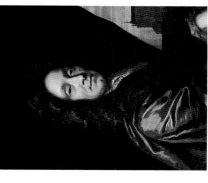
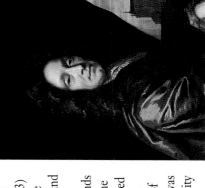

SIR CHRISTOPHER WREN
The architectural contribution made by Sir Christopher Wren (1632–1723) in the rebuilding of London after the Great Fire in 1666, and his background in the scientific enquiry of the time, mark him out as one of the great minds of his age. Wren was appointed as one of three Royal Commissioners charged with replanning the City of London, following the Fire of London. One of his main architectural commissions was the rebuilding of 52 churches in the City of London between 1670 and 1711.

SPECIFICATION

• Location	London, England
• Date	1675–1710
• Architect	Sir Christopher Wren
• Height	111.5 m (366 ft)
• Building structure	Brick and stone
• Building type	Cathedral
• Construction time	35 years

"It seems very unaccountable that the generality of our late architects dwell so much on the ornamental, and so slightly pass over the geometrical, which is the most essential part of architecture"
SIR CHRISTOPHER WREN

Central Crossing
The dome spans the combined width of both nave and aisles, lightening the central crossing and lending grandeur to services and occasions of state. The change to a Latin cross required a skilful handling of the plan, to allow the loads from the dome to be transferred to the ground. This was achieved by bearing the significant weight of the dome and lantern on to piers forming the vestries and stairs.

CASTLE HOWARD

BY THE LATE-17TH CENTURY, the belated influence of the Italian Renaissance had passed into England through the work of Inigo Jones and Sir Christopher Wren (see p. 58), becoming the definitive style for the cultural aspirations of wealthy patrons. This process of assimilation into the temperate English climate and the context of fashionable society provided ample opportunity for stylistic developments of the English Baroque under the distinctive personalities of its patrons, architects, and craftsmen. Castle Howard (1699–1726), in Yorkshire, England, enabled Sir John Vanbrugh, through the considerable wealth and enthusiasm of his patron, Lord Carlisle, to exploit his bold and remarkable architectural vision, carefully staged amidst the dramatic possibilities of its landscape setting. Vanbrugh, in his first major commission, was indebted to the contribution of Wren's former assistant, Nicholas Hawksmoor, whose experience was invaluable to the execution of the scheme. Vanbrugh's facility for grandiose, but lively, formal arrangements, emphasizing mass and monumentality, lends a distinctively theatrical quality to Baroque composition.

Approach
The house is approached by a formal sequence of crenellated gateways, a pyramid, and an obelisk, arranged purposefully within the landscape. The five-mile-long formal axis is diverted in the final sequence, bringing the visitor laterally across the north façade, setting down on the entrance court. The formal gardens and fountain are visible from the principal rooms of the south elevation.

SPECIFICATION

- **Location** — Yorkshire, England
- **Date** — 1699–1726
- **Architects** — Sir John Vanbrugh, Nicholas Hawksmoor
- **Building structure** — Stone and timber
- **Building type** — Country house

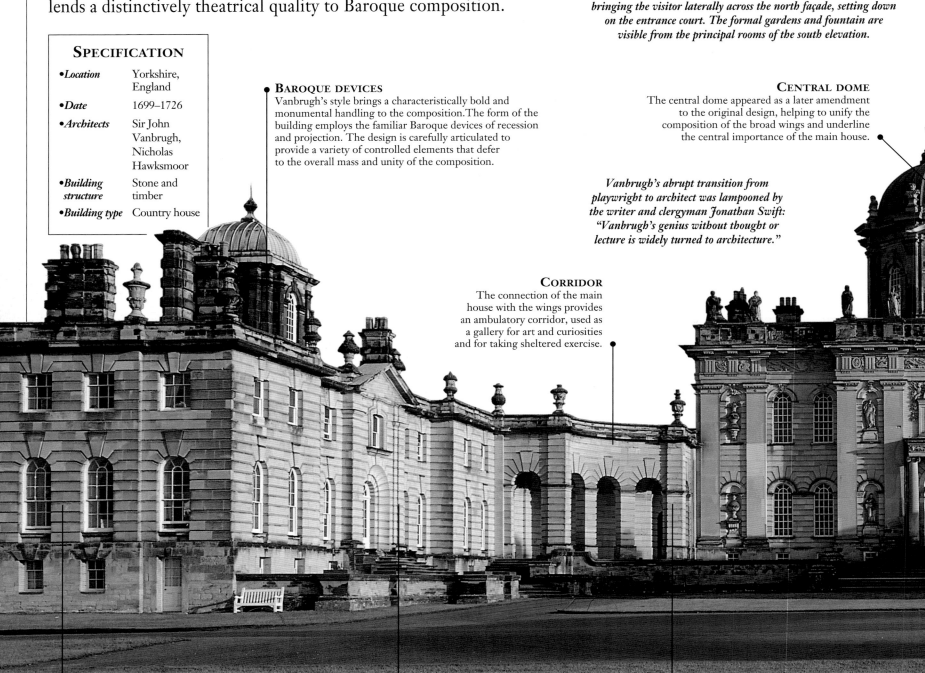

BAROQUE DEVICES
Vanbrugh's style brings a characteristically bold and monumental handling to the composition. The form of the building employs the familiar Baroque devices of recession and projection. The design is carefully articulated to provide a variety of controlled elements that defer to the overall mass and unity of the composition.

CENTRAL DOME
The central dome appeared as a later amendment to the original design, helping to unify the composition of the broad wings and underline the central importance of the main house.

Vanbrugh's abrupt transition from playwright to architect was lampooned by the writer and clergyman Jonathan Swift: "Vanbrugh's genius without thought or lecture is widely turned to architecture."

CORRIDOR
The connection of the main house with the wings provides an ambulatory corridor, used as a gallery for art and curiosities and for taking sheltered exercise.

EAST WING
Construction began with the east wing, which was followed by the main body of the house. Attention was then directed towards the landscaping of the grounds before completion of the west wing.

SERVICE WINGS
Additions to the service wings required the demolition of the former residence, Henderskelfe Castle, from which Castle Howard derives its name.

STONE
The honey-coloured ashlar stone, laid with deeply pronounced coursing lines, was taken from local quarries opened up within the estate.

SIR JOHN VANBRUGH

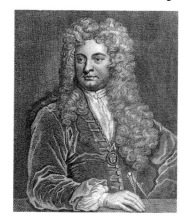

Sir John Vanbrugh (1664–1726) directed his attention to architecture following a career as a commissioned soldier, spy, and writer of Restoration comedies, such as *The Provok'd Wife* (1697). As a wit and eminent Whig, he was able to exploit his social position. Vanbrugh's introduction to Nicholas Hawksmoor (1661–1736) facilitated his aspirations as grand architect to the aristocracy. His appointment as Comptroller at the Office of Works in 1702 and the commission for Blenheim Palace (1705–24) firmly established his reputation and influence within the English Baroque.

THE TEMPLE OF THE FOUR WINDS

Portico — Central rotunda

Elevated base — Symmetrical façade

The Temple of the Four Winds is a miniaturized derivation of Andrea Palladio's Villa Rotonda (see p. 48) and demonstrates Vanbrugh's increasing virtuosity of composition within the confines of a reduced scale. The siting of the temple, and Nicholas Hawksmoor's Mausoleum – a derivation of Bramante's Tempietto (see p. 42) – extends the architecture into the landscape, providing a culminating achievement of the English Baroque. The architectural use of such settings anticipates the poignant beauty of the English Picturesque landscape tradition.

Central Hall
Crowned by an elevated dome, the Central Hall has a typically grand and elaborately detailed Baroque interior. The dome was destroyed by fire in 1940 and largely rebuilt. The ceiling, painted by Giovanni Pellegrini in 1709, depicts the story of Phaeton, who drove Apollo's Chariot of the Sun and fell to earth. The scene parodies Lord Carlisle's own political misfortunes and the recent defeat of the French "Sun" King, Louis XIV, at the Battle of Blenheim in 1704.

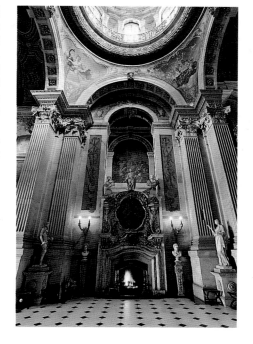

ELEVATION
Vanbrugh's design boldly repositioned the house with the main entrance elevation facing north and the principal rooms facing south, thus providing the best aspect and prominently displaying the house on the ridge of the hill.

SCALE
The extended reach of the wings exaggerates the impression of the scale of the main house. Vanbrugh's plan maintains a controlled sense of movement within a unified composition.

SCULPTURAL SURFACE
The carving of military insignia, cherubs, and sculptures is the work of the French craftsman, Nadauld, whose contribution adds greatly to the fluidity of the façade.

WEST WING
The west wing (1753–59) by Sir Thomas Robinson was completed only after the deaths of Vanbrugh, Hawksmoor, and Lord Carlisle. It is much altered from the proposed scheme and presents inconsistencies in massing and detail with the original building.

PALLADIAN STYLE
The lateral wings connect to the main body of the house. This form, though more compacted, is a derivation of the outstretched plans of Palladian rural villas.

GRANDIOSE PLANNING
The planning of the landscape required the displacement of the existing settlement of Henderskelfe, which was rebuilt at a discreet distance from the main house for the estate workers and their families.

Vanbrugh's commission for Castle Howard in 1699 displaced Lord Carlisle's original architect, William Talman. Vanbrugh's commission continued until his death in 1726.

ROYAL PAVILION

THE ROYAL PAVILION (1815–21) at the fashionable English seaside resort of Brighton, described as "a mad house and a house run mad", was used to host the entertainments of the Prince Regent (later George IV) in the closing chapter of the *ancien régime*. It was transformed from an earlier Palladian style house into a flamboyant palace in the eclectic and whimsical taste of the Picturesque. The oriental style of Mogul Indian architecture used for the exterior and the earlier Chinoiserie of the interior clothe a building that, though thoroughly European in its conception as a royal pleasure house, conveys the Eastern mystical mood of exotic illusion made fashionable in the works of the Romantic poets. The degree of craftsmanship and artifice is astonishing. The architect, John Nash, elaborated on previous schemes by Humphry Repton and James Wyatt, and his designs challenge the boundaries of both good taste and technological achievement of the day. Cast iron, in early structural use, was disguised for the domestic interior as bamboo, and gas lighting was installed to display the interior to its greatest advantage.

JOHN NASH

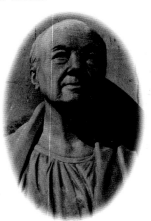

John Nash (1752–1835) was accomplished in a range of architectural styles. The simple geometry and sweeping curves of his town houses epitomized Regency elegance. Their white stuccoed exteriors with restrained Classical detailing are, however, strangely removed from the fantastic schemes devised for grand private commissions.

SPECIFICATION

- **Location** — Brighton, England
- **Date** — 1815–21
- **Architect** — John Nash
- **Building structure** — Brick, stone, cast iron, and timber
- **Building type** — Royal residence

COMPOSITIONAL UNITY
The smaller domes are included purely for the compositional unity of the silhouette, having no function above the drawing rooms adjoining the main saloon.

TURRET STAIRCASE
The Gothic-parapeted, circular staircase in the turret provides access to the upper dome, modified to accommodate three bedrooms, each with windows and fireplaces.

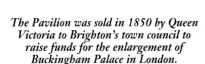

The Pavilion was sold in 1850 by Queen Victoria to Brighton's town council to raise funds for the enlargement of Buckingham Palace in London.

STUCCO FACADES
The façades are faced in stucco, a characteristic feature of Nash's buildings. The domes also were originally rendered and scored with joint lines and coloured to simulate Bath stone.

TRACERY SCREEN
The curved, stone arcade is fitted between the free-standing columns of the exterior. The horseshoe lattice, derived from the Indian *Jali*, (screen) protects the interior from direct sunlight.

Music Room

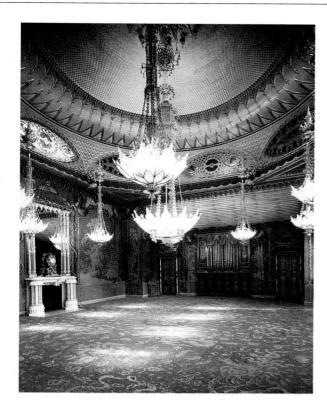

The Music Room is the climax to Nash's fantasy. Pendant gas lights in lotus-leaf-shaded glass lamps light the glittering domes, formed by overlapping tiers of gilded scallop shells. The lower frieze is illuminated by back-lit panels of glass. Flying dragons support the silk and tasselled drapery. Gilded balls, bells, and entwined serpents provide encrusted ornamentation bordering the Chinese scenes painted on the wall panels. The organ, when installed, was the loudest in the country.

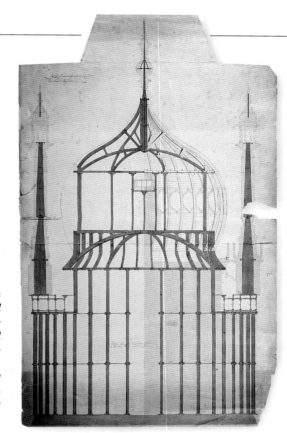

Iron Frame

A cast-iron framework is superimposed over the main saloon, providing the distinctive form of the dome and supporting the Billiard Room inside the turret. Elsewhere, cast iron is used as an exposed finish, creating a "bamboo" staircase and "palm-tree" columns. Nash's advanced technology is the first recorded use of cast iron in a domestic interior.

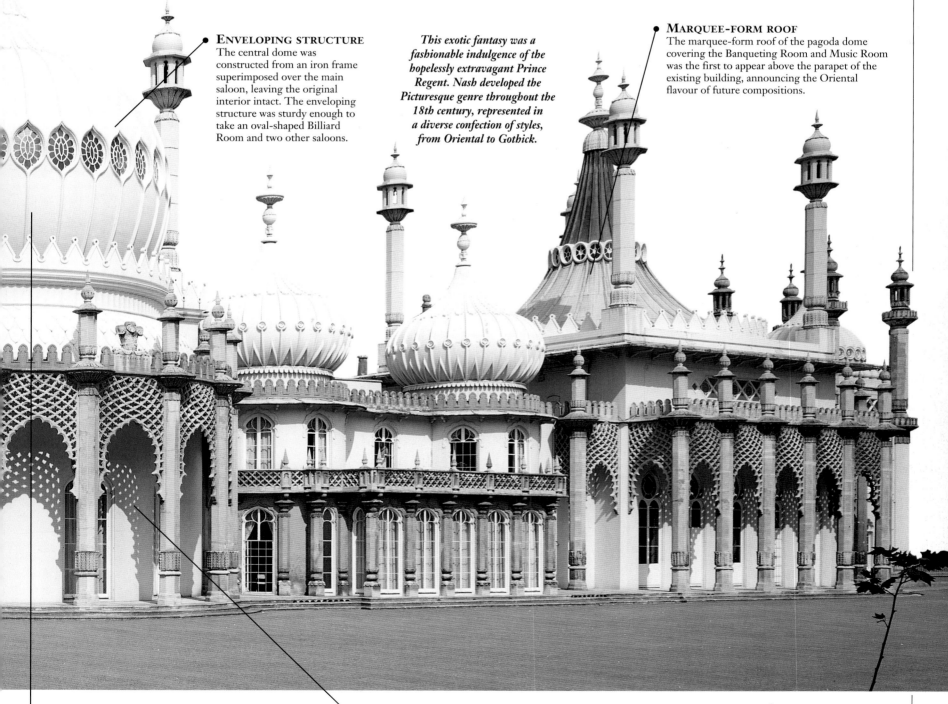

ENVELOPING STRUCTURE
The central dome was constructed from an iron frame superimposed over the main saloon, leaving the original interior intact. The enveloping structure was sturdy enough to take an oval-shaped Billiard Room and two other saloons.

This exotic fantasy was a fashionable indulgence of the hopelessly extravagant Prince Regent. Nash developed the Picturesque genre throughout the 18th century, represented in a diverse confection of styles, from Oriental to Gothick.

MARQUEE-FORM ROOF
The marquee-form roof of the pagoda dome covering the Banqueting Room and Music Room was the first to appear above the parapet of the existing building, announcing the Oriental flavour of future compositions.

ONION DOME
The central onion dome, derived from Mogul architecture (see p. 54), is a visual metaphor, both exotic and familiar, symbolizing the extended reach of the British Empire.

SCREEN WALL
The bow fronts of the earlier Palladian villa remain, but are disguised by a ground-floor screen wall with doors opening on to the lawn.

Having narrowly escaped demolition, the pavilion has since been used for a variety of purposes, including as a hospital during World War Two for invalided Indian soldiers.

ALTES MUSEUM

THE GREEK REVIVAL (1790–1830) saw a continuing fascination with the architectural styles of Classical antiquity, encouraged by archaeological finds in Europe and the Middle East. The restrained, elemental style of Karl Friedrich Schinkel sought a new, Romantic expression of Classicism appropriate to the monumental forms of a progressive city. Placed amongst Berlin's principal civic buildings, the Altes Museum (1824–28) adapts the model of the Greek *stoa* (a detached, open colonnade) for the use of a largely 19th-century invention – the art gallery. The museum faces the royal residence across an open square and is approached via a flight of steps, bringing visitors under the Ionic colonnade and through to the central rotunda. The open staircase lobby of the first floor is used to stage a dramatic panorama, completing Schinkel's romantic vista of the idealized city.

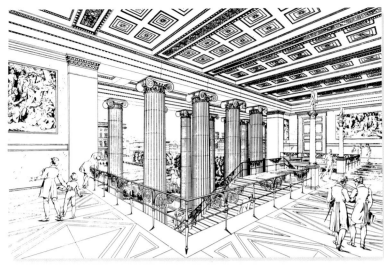

Lobby
The lobby of the main stair, with its double-height colonnade, uses the revelation of a carefully staged vista across the city square to dramatic effect. Schinkel's drawing shows his intention of providing a panorama of the city's monuments; one of the visitors cranes his neck to appreciate this vision.

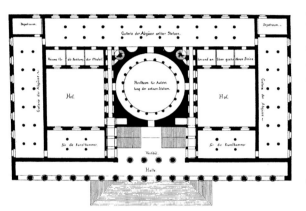

Rectilinear Plan
The rectilinear plan measuring 86 x 53 metres (282 x 174 feet), is arranged around a central rotunda. Schinkel developed the Enlightenment theory regarding honest and legible forms of construction, simple, elemental composition, and an expressive use of materials. These ideas challenge the highly ornamented and degenerate style of the preceding Baroque architecture and begin to investigate fundamental attitudes towards decoration and function – issues that became deeply rooted in architecture of the 20th century.

RAISED PARAPET
The dome of the central rotunda is concealed by the raised parapet. The Prussian eagle decorates the entablature.

STATUES
The rooftop statues symbolize the triumph of civilization over barbarity, a grandiose theme, which Schinkel saw as an essential purpose of art and architecture.

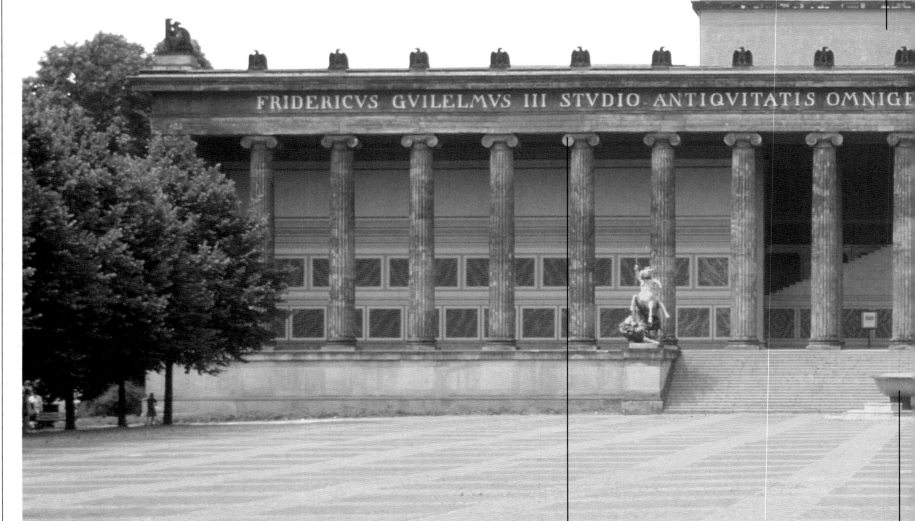

The gallery faces the royal residence and is within sight of Berlin's cathedral and arsenal. The prominence of the art gallery projects Schinkel's vision of cultural institutions being at the heart of the modern city.

IONIC COLUMNS
The long row of 18 Ionic columns is a 19th-century derivation from the Classical form of the *stoa*, a detached, open colonnade used around the Greek *agora* – the central meeting place of a Greek Classical city.

GRANITE VASE
The monumental vase, fashioned from a single piece of Prussian granite, was inspired by an antique design. Originally intended for the rotunda, it turned out to be too large and had to be repositioned in the square.

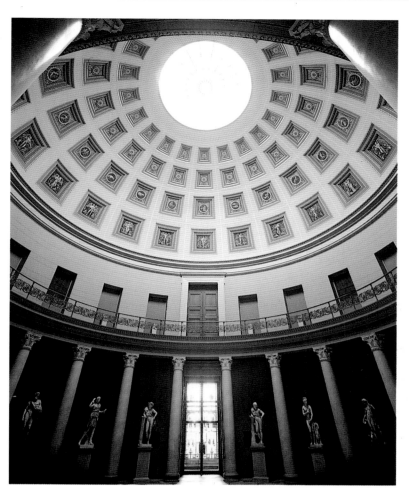

KARL FRIEDRICH SCHINKEL

Karl Friedrich Schinkel (1781–1841) was an architect, draughtsman, and painter who gained an early reputation for theatrical set design in the Romantic style of German Idealism. His influence also extended to urban design and landscape architecture. Early architectural designs employ a range of exotic styles, notably Gothic. Following his travels to Italy, subsequent commissions for the Prussian State were undertaken in the reductive Neoclassical style for which he is famous. For Schinkel, this meant not simply a slavish reproduction of heroic styles, but an idealistic belief in the instructive and civilizing role of architecture and urban design.

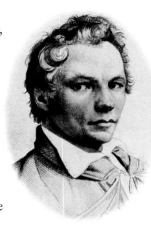

Coffered Dome
The magnificent coffered dome is lit by a central ocular window in a half-scale adaptation of the Roman Pantheon (see p. 14). The rotunda for the display of the statues provides a central focus. The galleries are arranged enfilade *– as a sequence of connected rooms – on two floors around two open courtyards.*

"Architectural detailing and design – the art of architecture – must never hide the larger structural forms"
KARL FRIEDRICH SCHINKEL

SPECIFICATION

- **Location**   Berlin, Germany
- **Date**   1824–28
- **Architect**   Karl Friedrich Schinkel
- **Building structure**   Stone
- **Storeys**   2
- **Building type**   Art gallery
- **Construction time**   4 years

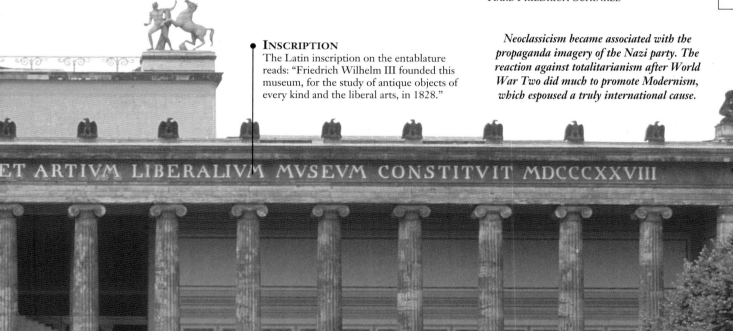

INSCRIPTION
The Latin inscription on the entablature reads: "Friedrich Wilhelm III founded this museum, for the study of antique objects of every kind and the liberal arts, in 1828."

Neoclassicism became associated with the propaganda imagery of the Nazi party. The reaction against totalitarianism after World War Two did much to promote Modernism, which espoused a truly international cause.

ET ARTIVM LIBERALIVM MVSEVM CONSTITVIT MDCCCXXVIII

IMPOSING STEPS
The imposing flight of steps approaching the elevated base are one third the width of the façade and are marked with equestrian statues framing the entrance.

CIVIC SPACE
The siting of the museum as a backdrop to a grandiose civic space underscores Schinkel's interest in the formal role of monumental architecture and urban design.

MURALS
The walls behind the arcade were originally painted with murals (destroyed in 1945) depicting Classical themes, the triumph of Zeus, and the development of the Arts.

THE HOUSES OF PARLIAMENT

THE OLD PALACE OF WESTMINSTER in London was destroyed by fire on 16 October 1834. The building of the New Palace provided an opportunity for a work of national significance – a building that would encapsulate the contemporary interests in Gothic architecture as an authentic national style, appropriate for buildings of religious and civic importance. The design competition, which stipulated a building of Elizabethan or Gothic character sympathetic to the medieval origins of the parliamentary system, was won by Sir Charles Barry in 1836. Barry enlisted A. W. N. Pugin, whose authority on Gothic architecture and skill as a draughtsman were of critical importance in securing the winning entry. Barry's plan incorporated the disparate functions of a complex institution with the pre-existing medieval Great Hall. The unified plan, articulated massing, and carefully composed asymmetry are in keeping with the riverside setting and adjacent medieval towers of Westminster Cathedral. The building is a monument to the High Victorian taste for propriety, whimsy, and nostalgia.

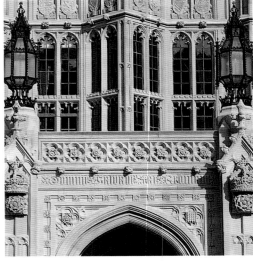

Exterior Detailing
The building is suffused with intricate ornamentation, arising from the Gothic form and Pugin's instinctive talent for balancing decoration and structure.

"There should be no features about a building which are not necessary for convenience, construction, or propriety. All ornament should consist of enrichment of the essential construction of the building"
AUGUSTUS PUGIN

VICTORIA TOWER
When erected, the Victoria Tower was the world's highest square tower at 102 metres (336 feet). The fire-proof construction of stone slabs on brick-and-steel arches is internally supported on cast-iron columns.

The lifting of materials, equipment, and support scaffolding during construction involved numerous technical advances: travelling cranes, climbing scaffolding, and a revolving formwork powered by steam engines and winches.

ROOF VENTS
The roof has cast-iron trusses spanning between the external, load-bearing walls. Cast-iron plates form an external covering to the roof. Smoke and heated air percolated from the underfloor heating through the main chambers and ceilings and escaped through the vents in the roof of the fire-proof construction.

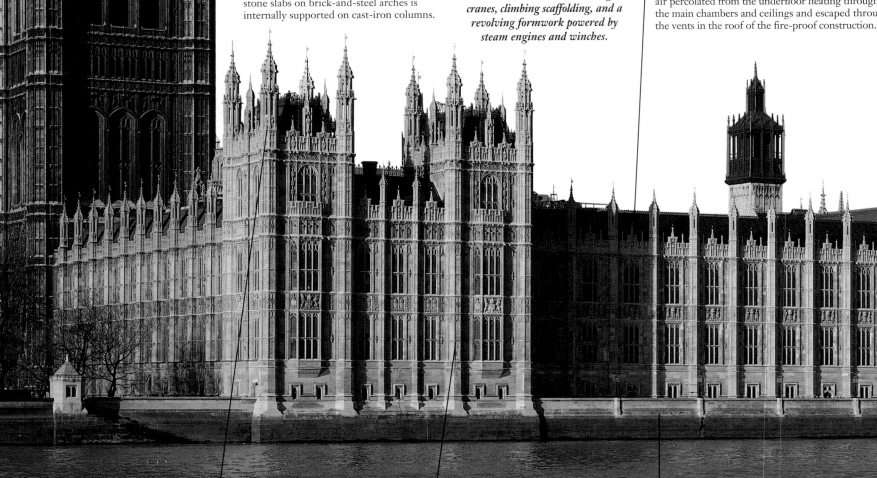

CORNER TURRETS
The polygonal corner turrets, continuous horizontal panelling, and detailing of the parapets were revised during successive stages of the design to emphasize verticality and the skyline.

SUPERSTRUCTURE
The superstructure is of brick and stone load-bearing walls, with cast-iron columns and beams providing internal spans to larger chambers.

BASE
The base rises clear from the water, emphasizing the verticality of the bays. The rhythm of the bays produces what Barry called "tranquillity by the reduplications of similar parts".

FLOORS
The floors are made of brick arches on cast-iron beams, developed from the fire-proof construction of industrial buildings. Construction materials were brought by river and stored on the new embankment.

SIR CHARLES BARRY AND A. W. N. PUGIN

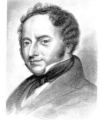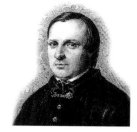

Sir Charles Barry (left) (1795–1860) was an established architect in the Classical style. His Reform Club, London (1837) is a refined Classical design that incorporated the latest technology. A. W. N. Pugin (right) (1812–52) was a champion of the Gothic style, which he pursued in commissions ranging from pattern design to church architecture. His ideas concerning the appropriate character of buildings and their integration of ornament with structure became influential in the Arts and Crafts Movement at the end of the 19th century.

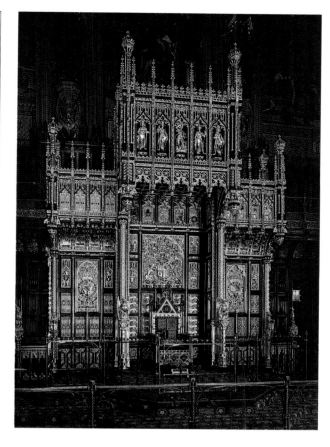

ROYAL THRONE
The Royal Throne, designed by Pugin and modified by Barry, shows a fanatical attention to detail. Pugin's style appropriates Gothic form and ornament for the display of parliamentary pomp and ceremony. The procurement of materials, decorative finishes, furniture, and fittings revived craft traditions and encouraged new techniques exemplary of High Victorian taste.

ORNAMENTATION
The richness of detailing increases progressively with the height above the ground, culminating in the highly ornamented pinnacles, parapets, and towers.

CENTRAL TOWER
The Central Tower, devised by the ventilation engineer, was included contrary to Barry's wishes. The tower ventilates the interior, producing a moving column of air that improves natural circulation.

The choice of limestone and dolomite for the stonework was the result of an investigation into the durability of Gothic construction and its resilience to the effects of coal-burning pollution, particularly destructive in the 19th century.

SPECIFICATION

- **Location** — London, England
- **Date** — 1836–68
- **Architects** — Sir Charles Barry, A. W. N. Pugin
- **Building structure** — Stone and cast iron
- **Building type** — Government building

Clock Tower
The Clock Tower houses the famous Big Ben main chime and four smaller chimes. The main bell was named after Sir Benjamin Hall, the first Commissioner of Works.

FACADE
The three-storey façade is 244 metres (800 feet) long. It contains parliamentary offices, libraries, committee rooms, and refreshment rooms, which conceal the debating chambers of the House of Lords (left) and the House of Commons (right).

EMBANKMENT
The 2.8-hectare (7-acre) site was extended 24–30 metres (80–100 feet) into the river by the construction of an embankment of stone and concrete fill. A coffer-dam constructed from a double layer of timber piles and shoring timbers infilled with clay provided storage space and workshops. The water was pumped out and a retaining wall and terrace for the new building constructed.

CRYSTAL PALACE

THE IMAGE OF LONDON'S CRYSTAL PALACE as the prototypical industrial building in an age of heroic achievement continues to exert its influence within the realm of contemporary architecture. Its history, from its construction in 1851 to its destruction in 1936, provided a premonition of both the beginning and end of the age of Modernism. The story of its construction illustrates the energy and pace of the Victorian era, whose engineering achievements stand aside from the stylistic arguments that dominated the architecture of the period. Indeed, the realization of the building, within both programme and budget, owed more to the methods of engineering and industrial manufacture used than to the conventional process of architecture. The building was designed as a prefabricated structure for temporary erection in London's Hyde Park to house the first international exhibition of industrial design (The Great Exhibition, 1851). It achieved remarkable popularity for such a pioneering design and was re-erected, through public subscription, at Sydenham, England, where it stood until destroyed by fire in 1936.

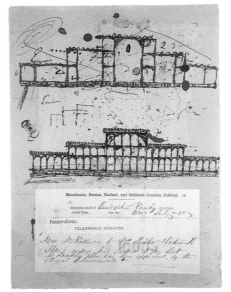

The First Sketch
Architect Sir Joseph Paxton's involvement with the project began with this sketch, which he prepared after hearing that the Exhibition Committee was unable to agree on a winning scheme from the 233 official entries to the competition of April 1850. Paxton made his sketch after visiting the site on 11 June 1850. By 24 June he had prepared drawings for tender by Fox Henderson and Co. The scheme was appointed by the committee on 26 July, and work commenced on 30 July. Construction itself started on 26 September, and the building was ready for occupation on 1 February 1851.

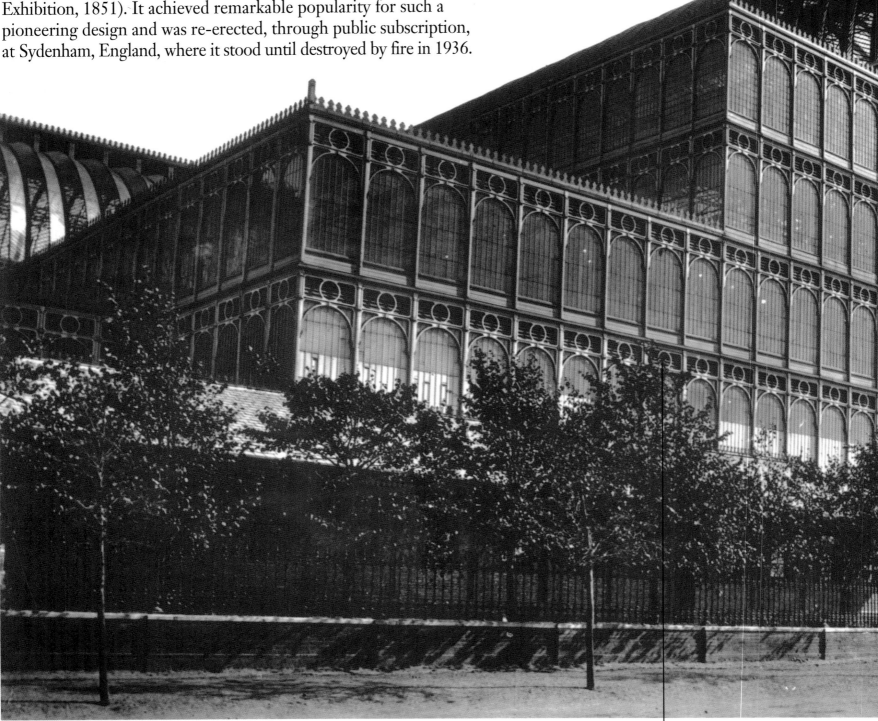

The Paxton gutter was formed by 7.3-metre- (24-foot-) lengths of machine-profiled timber, made into a bow-string truss, with cast-iron brackets and a wrought-iron cord. This supported the roof and formed a gutter that directed rainwater towards the main structural columns, which acted as drainpipes.

STEEL LOUVRES
Horizontal bands of mechanically operated steel louvres allowed a controlled circulation of air. The glazed roof was covered by retractable canvas awnings, sprayed with cool water in hot weather.

GLAZING
Unprecedentedly large sheets of glass, over 1.2 metres (4 feet) long and 25 centimetres (10 inches) wide, were used to glaze the roof and upper sections of the walls.

SPECIFICATION

- **Location**: London, England
- **Date**: 1850–51
- **Architect**: Sir Jospeh Paxton
- **Building structure**: Cast and wrought iron, and timber
- **Building type**: Exhibition hall
- **Construction time**: 6 months

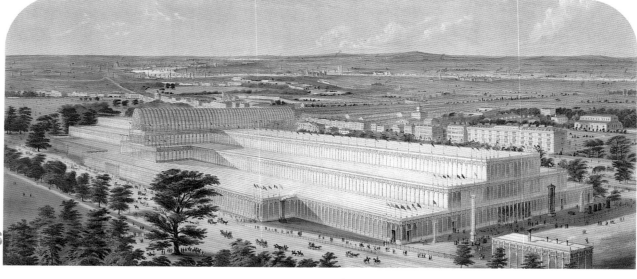

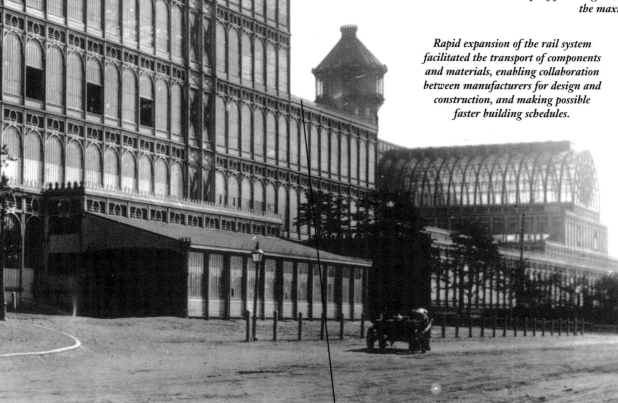

TABLE AND CLOTH
Paxton used the analogy of a table covered by a cloth to explain the internal frame of cast-iron columns and cast- and wrought-iron trusses that provides a rigid "table" over which an external lightweight "cloth" of glass is draped, framed by timber glazing bars.

BARREL VAULT
The timber barrel vault ran the full width of the central transept; its height enabled the retention of elm trees on the Hyde Park site. Further vaults (seen here) were added to the reconstructed building at Sydenham.

The original construction contract was awarded to the contractor on a "recyclable" basis: the budget was £150,000 for the whole building, or £80,000 if ownership reverted to the contractor after the building was dismantled.

FRAMING MEMBERS
The cast-iron, wrought-iron, and timber framing members were assembled from standardized components. Columns, at 7.3-metre- (24-foot-) intervals, ran the full length of the building.

Rapid expansion of the rail system facilitated the transport of components and materials, enabling collaboration between manufacturers for design and construction, and making possible faster building schedules.

The idea of a construction kit of parts brilliantly exploited the potential of industrial production. The advantages of mass production, prefabrication, and systematic site assembly were newly available to Victorian engineers and designers.

DECORATION
Decorative elements were used simply for ornamentation and to regularize the appearance. The arches, circular openings, pinnacles, and trellis around the roof emphasized the rhythm of the structural bays.

The Palace of Industry for all Nations
Prince Albert, husband of Queen Victoria, championed the Great Exhibition, which he heralded as "a true test and living picture of the point of development at which the whole world of mankind has arrived". The exhibition provided an encyclopedic array of industrial and cultural artefacts. Over six million visits (by nearly one in five of the population) were made to the site during the first five months.

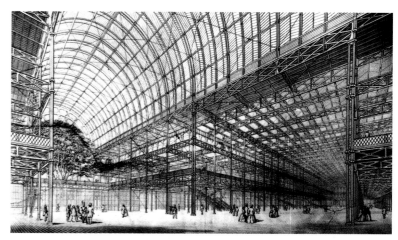

Internal Framework
Internally, the framework was painted in colours co-ordinating the structural trusses. The slender internal structural frame, cloaked with an external envelope of framed glass, provided an economical enclosure that admitted the maximum amount of natural light.

SIR JOSEPH PAXTON

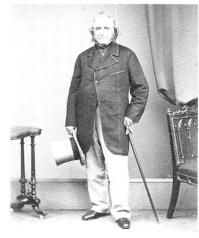

Aged 23, and as head gardener to the Duke of Devonshire, Joseph Paxton (1803–65) landscaped Chatsworth House in Derbyshire, England. He developed the constructional system for the Palm House, which served as a prototype for the design of the Crystal Palace. He also organized botanical expeditions and was involved in the development of many rail projects.

TURBINE BUILDING, MENIER FACTORY

THE INDUSTRIAL TECHNIQUES pioneered in the 19th century responded to a proliferation of new building types that were to influence 20th-century architecture. The early use of iron was largely confined to industrial buildings and engineering structures. In architectural applications, the structural frame was generally disguised with an overcoat of conventional architectural appearance. The Turbine Building (1871–72), at Noisiel-sur-Marne, near Paris, supplied mechanical power to the Menier chocolate firm. Its architect, Jules Saulnier, chose to express the skeletal frame, interpreting the mill building as a bridge spanning masonry piers set into the river bed. The lightweight, wrought-iron frame and thin skin of brickwork are exemplary of the Rationalist integration of structure, function, and decoration championed by the architect and critic, Viollet-le-Duc. With its iron superstructure and thin-walled cladding, the building heralded the arrival of techniques that were to revolutionize 20th-century architecture. Decoratively and technically ostentatious, it is a wonderful reminder of the enterprise of the 19th century.

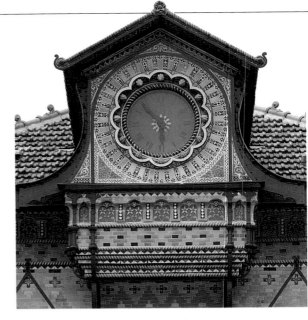

Decorated Surfaces
Nineteenth-century Rationalism sought to integrate structure and ornament with particular relevance to contemporary buildings and industrial materials. Here, the coloured brickwork and ornate mouldings are responsive to the structural form of the building. Identified as the principle of Gothic architecture, this was to develop into a defining principle of Modernism.

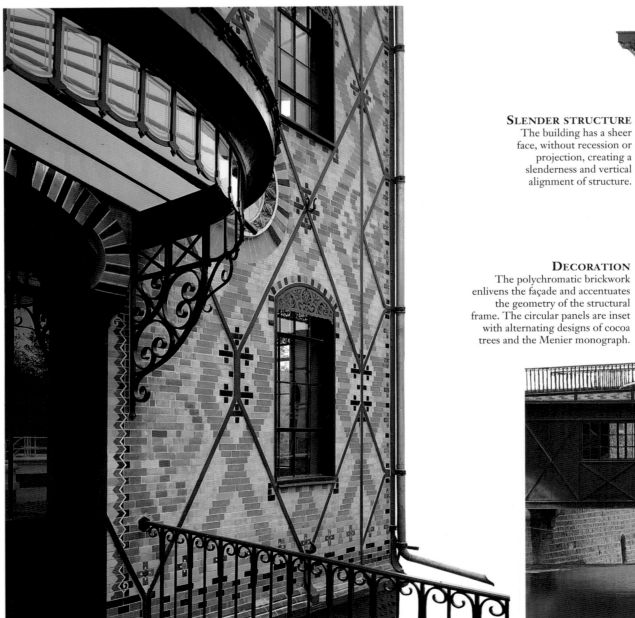

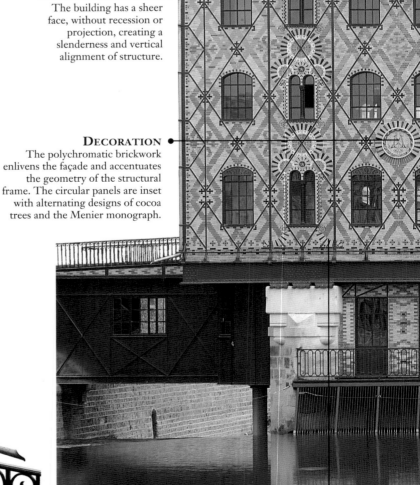

SLENDER STRUCTURE
The building has a sheer face, without recession or projection, creating a slenderness and vertical alignment of structure.

DECORATION
The polychromatic brickwork enlivens the façade and accentuates the geometry of the structural frame. The circular panels are inset with alternating designs of cocoa trees and the Menier monograph.

Curtain Wall
The brick wall makes no contribution to the building structure. This had a particular significance for the future of multi-storey buildings, whose height would preclude the load-bearing support of the external wall. The wall becomes a curtain hung, or held, outside the frame. This device was to become a leitmotiv of the Modern Movement.

CLADDING
The hollow brickwork provides a lightweight panel, infilling the diagonally braced wrought-iron lattice frame.

STRUCTURAL USE OF IRON

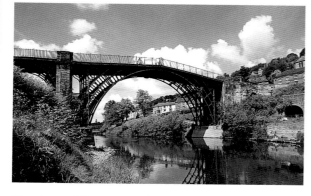

Cast-iron, whilst immensely strong in compression, is brittle and weak in tension. Exploiting its compressive strength, the first cast-iron bridge was erected over the River Severn in Coalbrookdale, England, in 1779. The "puddling" process, patented in 1784, however, introduced wrought iron, which had a greater tensile strength than cast iron, although its use was eventually overtaken by that of steel in 1855.

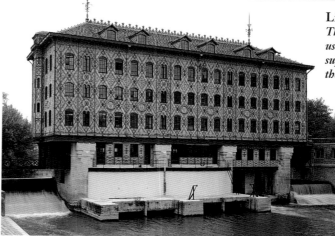

Lightweight Structure
The mill straddles the River Marne, using the water to drive the turbines to supply the power for the process of refining the chocolate. Braced by the diagonal struts, the whole of the wall acts as a gigantic lattice-truss, producing an efficient and lightweight structure. To clear the main production space of columns, the upper floor is suspended from the roof trusses.

• WINDOWS
The skeleton frame allows an increase in the area available for windows and other openings. Industrial processes, before the advent of cheap and safe artificial light, were often reliant on high levels of daylight.

SPECIFICATION
- **Location**   Noisiel-sur-Marne, France
- **Date**   1871–72
- **Architect**   Jules Saulnier
- **Building structure**   Wrought-iron frame and stone piers
- **Building type**   Factory

• EXPOSED FRAMEWORK
The mill structure has an exposed framework, which was probably inspired by the half-timbered framing of the pre-existing mill that Saulnier's building replaced.

• FLOORS
Internally, the floors are constructed from shallow brick vaults spanning on to I-section wrought-iron joints running between the external walls. The second floor uses joists made into a box-section to take the extra weight of machinery.

• BOX BEAM
The hollow-steel box beam, fabricated from wrought-iron plates and angles, spans the stone piers. It forms a composite support with the diagonal struts of the lattice frame.

SAGRADA FAMILIA

THE EXALTED SCALE AND FANTASTICAL IMAGERY of the Expiatory Church of the Holy Family, (the "Sagrada Familia") in Barcelona, Spain, are the vision of the architect, Antonio Gaudí, who directed the project from 1884 until his death in 1926. Gaudí's unique architectural style was fuelled by a deeply held religious conviction. The Sagrada Familia celebrates the Holy Family and the mysteries of the Catholic faith. The fluid manipulation of stone and concrete is achieved by a complex geometry of vaulted structures surrounded by the campanile towers of the main façades, which become increasingly fantastic, rising up to the polychromatic ceramic surfaces of the "pompom" pinnacles representing the Apostles. Though only partially completed, the building rivals in ambition and scale the cathedrals of medieval Europe. The continuation of the work during periods of political and social change symbolizes the vitality of Catalan culture.

SPECIFICATION

- **Location** — Barcelona, Spain
- **Date** — 1884–present
- **Architect** — Antonio Gaudí
- **Height on completion** — 180 m (591 ft)
- **Building structure** — Stone and concrete
- **Building type** — Church

Wire Models
Gaudí used models made from wire and plaster-soaked canvas sheets, suspended with weights, to represent complex (structural) forms. When dry, they were analysed for points of weakness, which could then be reinforced.

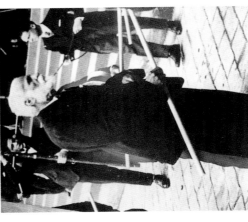

ANTONIO GAUDÍ

Antonio Gaudí (1852–1926) was born in Catalonia. He was inspired by the reawakening of interest in medieval craft guilds amongst the Arts and Crafts Movement, and became associated with the Catalan *Modernista* movement. Gaudí developed his career, notably through commissions from his patron, the textile manufacturer, Don Basilio Güell, such as the Palacio Güell, Barcelona (1886–89), and Parque Güell, Barcelona (1900–14).

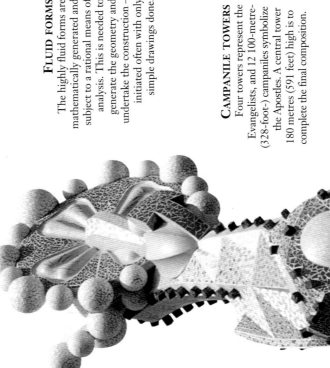

Gaudí had an intuitive genius for structural form, influenced by his knowledge of Gothic architecture and traditional Catalan structures of brick, stone, and ceramic tile.

FLUID FORMS
The highly fluid forms are mathematically generated and subject to a rational means of analysis. This is needed to generate the geometry and undertake the construction – initiated often with only simple drawings done.

CAMPANILE TOWERS
Four towers represent the Evangelists, and 12 100-metre- (328-foot-) campaniles symbolize the Apostles. A central tower 180 metres (591 feet) high is to complete the final composition.

Finials
The highly animated surface of the façade succeeds to the colour and decoration of the upper campaniles, inset with ceramic tiles and figures. This detail of the "pompom" finials of the western transept is symbolic of the Bishop's mitre, ring, and staff.

After Gaudí's death in 1926, the project continued under the direction of his associates. The destruction of the design models and many of the original drawings during the Spanish Civil War (1936–39) halted the construction. By working from retrieved models, architects resumed the project in 1954, which continues with fierce debate as to the nature of the executed design.

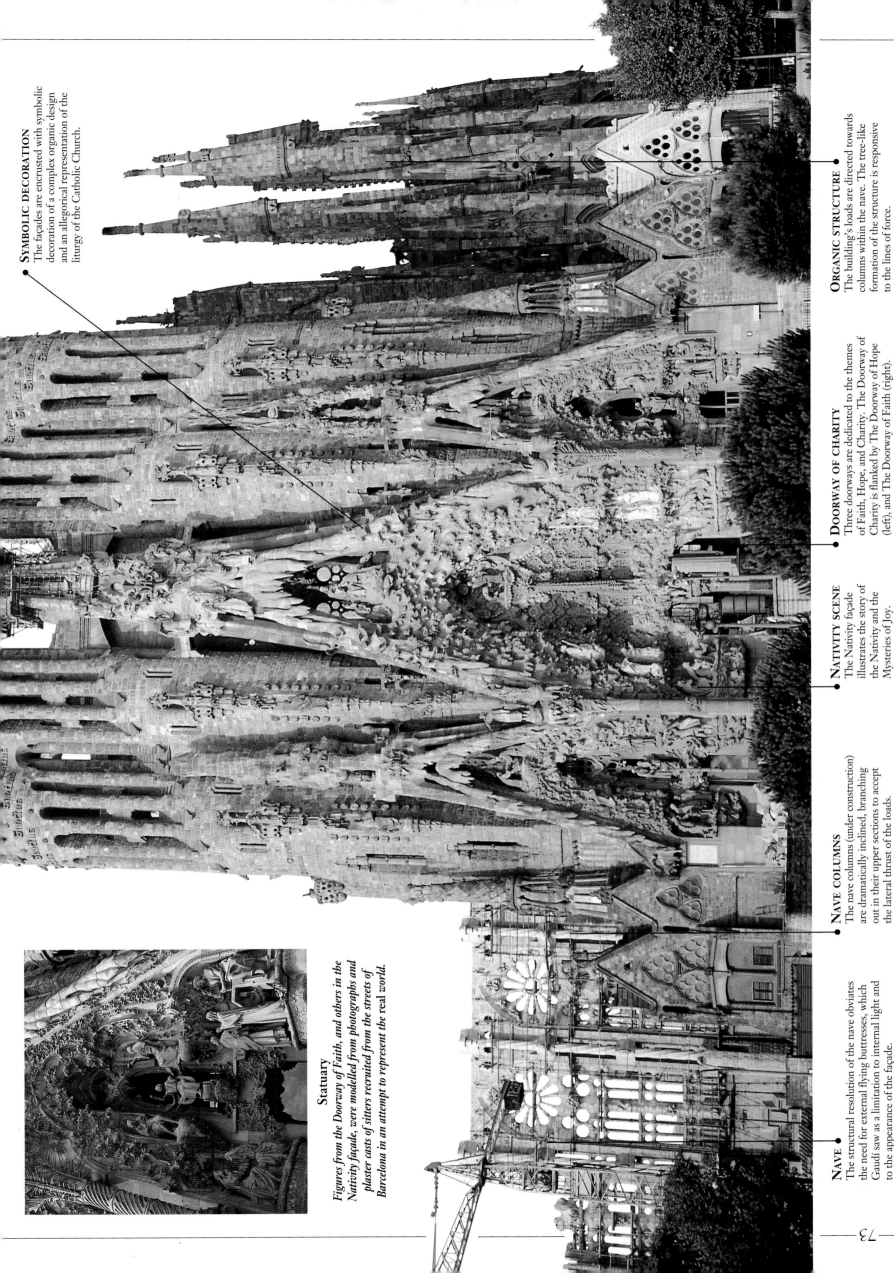

SYMBOLIC DECORATION
The façades are encrusted with symbolic decoration of a complex organic design and an allegorical representation of the liturgy of the Catholic Church.

ORGANIC STRUCTURE
The building's loads are directed towards columns within the nave. The tree-like formation of the structure is responsive to the lines of force.

DOORWAY OF CHARITY
Three doorways are dedicated to the themes of Faith, Hope, and Charity. The Doorway of Charity is flanked by The Doorway of Hope (left), and The Doorway of Faith (right).

NATIVITY SCENE
The Nativity façade illustrates the story of the Nativity and the Mysteries of Joy.

NAVE COLUMNS
The nave columns (under construction) are dramatically inclined, branching out in their upper sections to accept the lateral thrust of the loads.

NAVE
The structural resolution of the nave obviates the need for external flying buttresses, which Gaudí saw as a limitation to internal light and to the appearance of façade.

Statuary
Figures from the Doorway of Faith, and others in the Nativity façade, were modelled from photographs and plaster casts of sitters recruited from the streets of Barcelona in an attempt to represent the real world.

GLASGOW SCHOOL OF ART

THE COMPETITION-WINNING ENTRY by Charles Rennie Mackintosh for a new Glasgow School of Art (1897–1909) produced a work of outstanding originality. Mackintosh's highly personal architectural style blended paradoxical elements of the 19th-century Arts and Crafts Movement and the European avant-garde with a freshness of approach. His ability to integrate a modern design into a historic setting, along with the building's dramatic tension, existing between sensuality and restraint, reduction and enrichment, established Mackintosh's reputation in a work of enduring achievement. Mackintosh submitted designs under the competition rules in 1895 and was appointed as winning entrant for the firm Honeyman, Keppie, and Mackintosh in January 1897. Limited funds required competitors to identify two phases of construction. The first phase (1897–99) terminated at the main entrance tower of the north elevation, and the interval between phases allowed Mackintosh a period of design revision. The west wing (1907–09), with its soaring elevation and magnificent two-storey library, show Mackintosh as a mature and confident designer.

THE GLASGOW SCHOOL OF ART

ELEVATION TO SCOTT STREET

ELEVATION TO DALHOUSE STREET

West and East Elevations
The west elevation (left) combines a powerful formal arrangement with the casual asymmetry of traditional vernacular architecture. The surface of the elevation is skilfully composed, the exploitation of the play of mass against void is used as an articulation of internal function. The modelling of the towers and bays of the east elevation (right) is reminiscent of the baronial houses of Scottish architecture.

SPECIFICATION

• **Location**   Glasgow, Scotland

• **Dates**   1897–99 (Phase 1) 1907–09 (Phase 2)

• **Architect**   Charles Rennie Mackintosh

• **Building structure**   Stone, wrought iron, and steel

• **Building type**   Art school

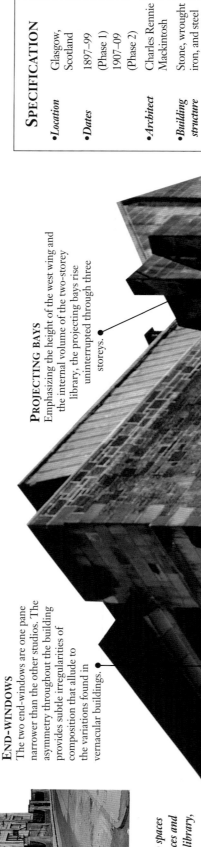

NICHES
The niches within the wall surface were designed to accommodate sculptures depicting the arts. The stone drums were intended for subsequent sculptural decoration, though this omission emphasizes the simple and powerful massing of the façade.

PROJECTING BAYS
Emphasizing the height of the west wing and the internal volume of the two-storey library, the projecting bays rise uninterrupted through three storeys.

END-WINDOWS
The two end-windows are one pane narrower than the other studios. The asymmetry throughout the building provides subtle irregularities of composition that allude to the variations found in vernacular buildings.

North Façade
The building comprises an E-shaped plan with main studio spaces arranged along the long north façade. Further teaching spaces and offices are provided on the east wing, with a lecture theatre, library, and studio spaces on the west façade.

EAVES
The oversailing eaves protect the studio spaces from direct sunlight and establish a strong profile to the roof line.

STUDIO WINDOWS
The large areas of glazing provide ample natural light for the teaching studios. Their appearance in the stone façade evokes both the Elizabethan manor house (see p. 50) and the glazed wall emblematic of the Modern Movement.

INSET WINDOW
Accentuating the thickness and mass of the wall, the tiny window lets light into the life-drawing room.

CONTRASTED STONE
The rough stone of the studio end-walls is contrasted with the dressed course stone around the windows. The junction is subtly demarcated by a horizontal stepped line.

WEST DOORWAY
The fine detail of the door surround relieves the monumentality of the elevation. The doorway has a stepped moulding, which anticipates the motifs of Art Deco.

BRACKETS
The wrought-iron brackets strengthen the slender window mullions and provide support for a window-cleaning platform. The decorative finials recall Celtic motifs and are subtly varied with floral designs.

RAILINGS
The railings carry posts with heraldic Celtic, and Japanese inspired motifs.

NATURAL LIGHT
The façade is set back from the street to admit natural light to the basement.

The main building is 75 metres (245 feet) long and 28 metres (93 feet) deep. The building has five storeys, with an attic storey of studios added in the second phase. The site falls 10 metres (34 feet) towards the south, a condition dramatically emphasized by the verticality of composition on the west elevation.

FACADE
The treatment of the façade is expressive of the internal function and spatial hierarchies within the building, and is characteristic of architecture of the Modern Movement.

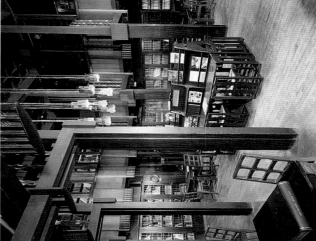

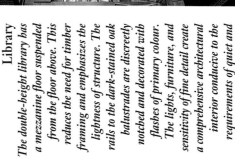

Library
The double-height library has a mezzanine floor suspended from the floor above. This reduces the need for timber framing and emphasizes the lightness of structure. The rails to the dark-stained oak balustrades are discreetly notched and decorated with flashes of primary colour. The lights, furniture, and sensitivity of fine detail create a comprehensive architectural interior conducive to the requirements of quiet and contemplative study.

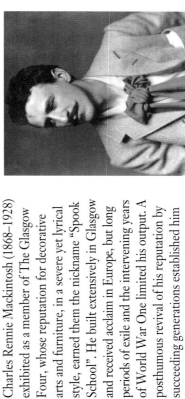

CHARLES RENNIE MACKINTOSH

Charles Rennie Mackintosh (1868–1928) exhibited as a member of The Glasgow Four, whose reputation for decorative arts and furniture, in a severe yet lyrical style, earned them the nickname "Spook School". He built extensively in Glasgow and received acclaim in Europe, but long periods of exile and the intervening years of World War One limited his output. A posthumous revival of his reputation by succeeding generations established him alongside the greatest early-20th-century European architects.

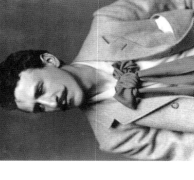

Glass Panel
The coloured glass panel to the ground-floor door shows the characteristic Mackintosh decorative elements: a Tree of Life, emerging as a woman's face with a centrally placed rosebud. The motifs are stylized, sexual, and symbolic, combining the many complex aspects of Mackintosh's personality.

GAMBLE HOUSE

THE ENGLISH ARTS AND CRAFTS MOVEMENT, with its emphasis on dignity in labour and respect for nature, was partly introduced to America through the religious and Utopian communities of the mid-19th century. A crafted use of natural materials and a feeling of closeness to nature prevailed along with a nostalgic pride for the pioneering spirit and middle-class American values of the late-19th-century suburbs. The Californian climate was conducive to this sense of openness, and the traditional form of timber construction was adaptable and accommodating to the rustic image: long, low verandas; sheltering eaves; a centralized hearth; and a direct connection with the garden. Open porches extended the interior from which to enjoy the scented evenings. American architect Frank Lloyd Wright had already popularized the indigenous Shingle Style and imported influences of Japanese *shoin* architecture. In the Gamble House (1908–09), the Greene brothers blended this imagery with the climate, finding a delight in the richness of detail and providing a definitive image of affluence and propriety appropriate to the early-20th century.

GREENE AND GREENE

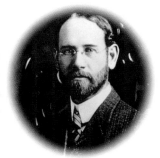 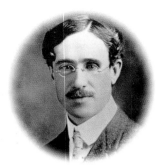

Henry Greene (1870–1954) (left) and Charles Sumner Greene (1868–1957) (right) studied at the Massachusetts Institute of Technology in Cambridge. They were acquainted with the work of the Arts and Crafts Movement through a magazine called *The Craftsman*, which featured the work of many of the English Arts and Crafts studios. But it is perhaps their affinity with Japanese joinery and traditional *shoin*-style architecture that informs the sensitivity to materials and details that distinguishes the Greenes' work. Other examples of their work are the Blacker House (1907), Pasadena, California, and the Pratt House (1909) Ojai, California.

ARTS AND CRAFTS

Inspired by the socialist Utopian William Morris (1834–96) and the architectural writer John Ruskin (1819–1900), the Arts and Crafts Movement of the late-19th century was a response to the deterioration in the quality and design of many machine-made products. It promoted traditional crafts and vernacular building practices and sought to reintroduce the direct relationship between the designer and maker, exploiting the experience of the artisan and emphasizing the innate characteristics of materials.

OVERSAILING EAVES
Shade and protection is provided to the veranda and porches by oversailing eaves. The ends of rafters are exposed, emphasizing the simple arrangement of structure, inspired by vernacular forms and Japanese joinery.

TIMBER FRAME
The lightness of construction and inherent flexibility of timber-framed buildings makes them ideally suited to areas at risk of earth tremors, such as Japan and California.

SLEEPING PLATFORMS
Balconies lead directly from the bedrooms, allowing the occupants to sleep in the open air on summer evenings. The Greenes' father was a respiratory physician who believed in the health-giving virtues of fresh air and cross-ventilation.

CLADDING
The timber frame is clad with redwood *shakes* – large timber tiles with a natural irregularity and pronounced grain – imparting a gentle, weathered finish to the building.

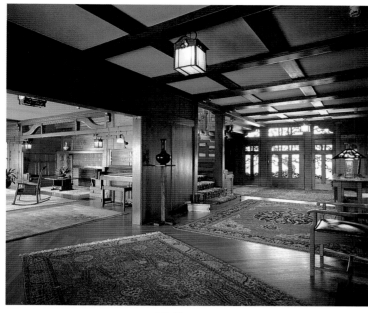

Hallway
The hallway provides a central core for circulation between levels and areas distinct within the floor plan. The richness of materials and attention to detail here are continued throughout the house. Teak-framed entrance doors, with coloured glass panels depicting the outspread arms of an oak tree, wash the interior with light that is then reflected in the hand-polished timber surfaces.

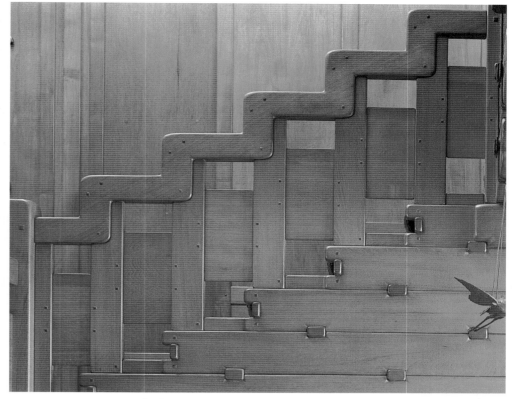

Staircase
The Burmese teak staircase rises from the hallway. The ends of the beams are rounded, and the screwed joints are capped with distinctive dowelled timber heads. The polished finish emphasizes the colour and grain of the timber. The attention to detail and honesty of expression towards materials and construction are characteristic of the Arts and Crafts Movement.

STRUCTURAL FRAME
Traditional Japanese houses use a primary structural frame of larger timbers held by complex joints. American frames could be assembled quickly using a larger number of smaller timbers fixed with nails and screws. The Gamble House uses both principles, expressing, where possible, a simple frame, but using contemporary methods elsewhere.

HORIZONTALITY
The line of the roof provides a low profile for the building. The informal, horizontal composition has a softness that blends with the landscape.

SPECIFICATION
- **Location**   Pasadena, USA
- **Date**   1908–09
- **Architects**   C. S. Greene, H. M. Greene
- **Building structure**   Timber-frame
- **Storeys**   3
- **Building type**   House
- **Construction time**   1 year

PLINTH
The building is placed on a small, terraced plinth, which blurs the edges of the building and provides a subtle transition to the garden.

STRUCTURAL EXPRESSION
The redwood frame emerges on the outside and is similarly exposed within. The simple legibility of the building is prompted by the search for an honesty of expression much used in later modern architecture.

The Gamble House provided an opportunity for a fully integrated design encompassing landscape, fixed and free-standing furniture, rugs, coloured glass, light fittings, and even electrical switches.

ROBIE HOUSE

THE ROBIE HOUSE (1908–10), South Woodlawn, Chicago, Illinois, draws its influence from the flat plains of the American Midwest and epitomizes the domestic style of Frank Lloyd Wright's Prairie House period. These houses are spatially innovative but reassuringly solid, and were well suited to the conservative propriety of their newly affluent suburban owners. The buildings have a strong axiality and openness, with the hearth forming a central feature and pivotal point to the plan. The house is raised above the ground on a substantial plinth; the massing emphasizes the horizontality, using the architectural order of plinth, low elevation, and deeply overhanging eaves. Wright embraced new technology: connective heating, electric lighting, and rudimentary air-conditioning were all adapted to service the domestic interior. Whilst many of the Arts and Crafts architects had rejected the machine, Wright experimented with its potential for precision by incorporating highly finished surfaces, enriched by coloured glass and polished timbers.

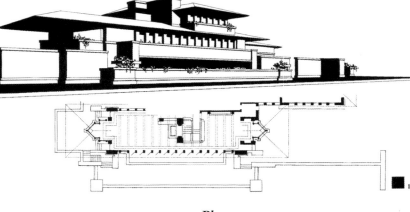

Plan
The principal spaces of the house are essentially open. Independent functions are defined by latticed screens and the central, controlling, position of the hearth and stairs. This relationship produces a subtle differentiation within a sequence of spaces, and is the most dynamic element of Wright's work, contributing to modern architecture's preoccupation with space and volume.

WINDOW BAY
The prow-like form of the window bay has a proudly nautical feel. Wright's style was likened to that of steamships, a dynamic image of the Machine Age that Wright was happy to adopt.

SPECIFICATION

- *Location* — Chicago, USA
- *Date* — 1908–10
- *Architect* — Frank Lloyd Wright
- *Building structure* — Steel-frame and brick
- *Building type* — House

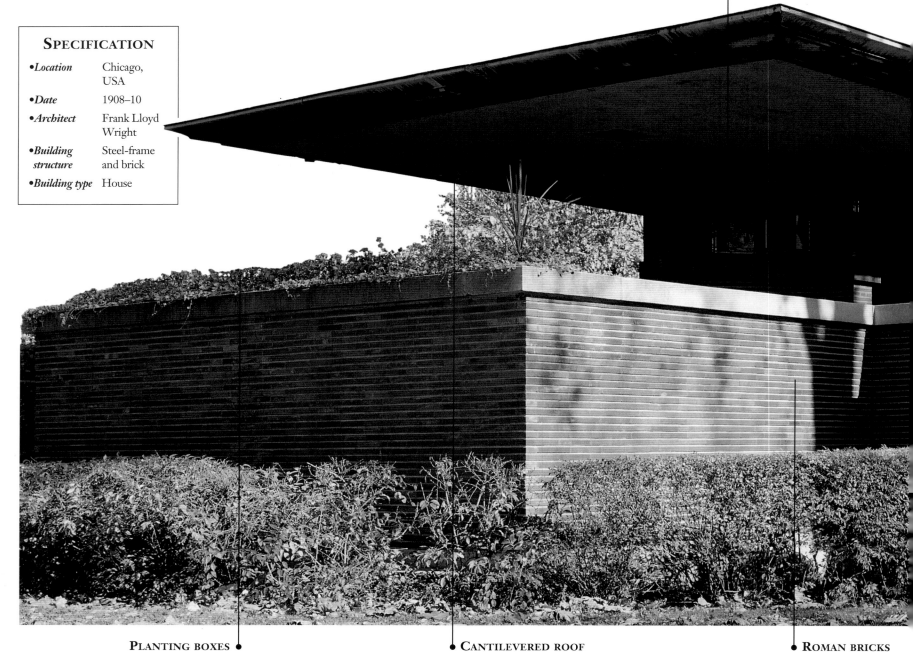

PLANTING BOXES
The planting boxes are discreetly fitted with irrigation sprinklers operated from a central valve – a typical example of Wright's integration of modern technology.

CANTILEVERED ROOF
The cantilever of the entrance porch is supported by steel beams, providing a distinctive silhouette. The reassuring image of the sheltering roof is used for dramatic effect in this reinterpretation of vernacular form.

ROMAN BRICKS
The slender profile of elongated, or "Roman", bricks was originally accentuated by raked mortar courses, which set back the mortar from the face of the brick, creating a shadow-line that reinforced the horizontality of the massing.

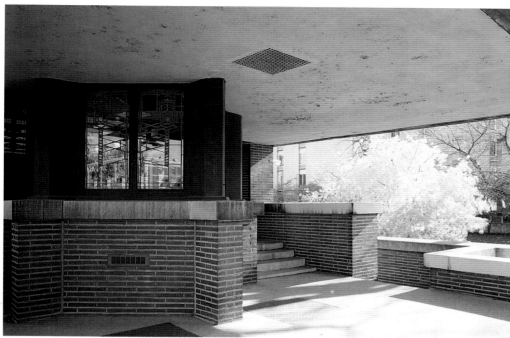

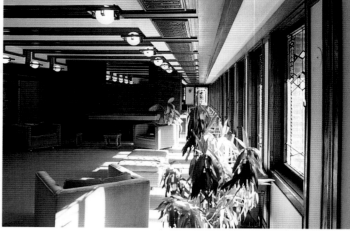

Open Planning
The fireplace divides the living areas of the elevated ground floor and the screen walls provide privacy. The furniture, furnishings, and fittings were specifically designed for the house, and the light-fittings and heating system are integrated into the fabric of the building.

Covered Porch
The covered porch mediates between the building's interior and exterior, expanding the living space of the house. The building is elevated from the street and partially screened; this arrangement provides privacy for the occupants and allows a subtle extension of the external spaces immediate to the house.

FRANK LLOYD WRIGHT

Frank Lloyd Wright (1867–1959) was inspired by a love of nature and the landscape of the Midwest. He began a prolific career with a style that infused vernacular architecture with new technology. Driven by a Utopian spirit, Wright constantly re-invented his style in domestic, commercial, and civic buildings. His astounding variety of work profoundly influenced the course of 20th-century architecture.

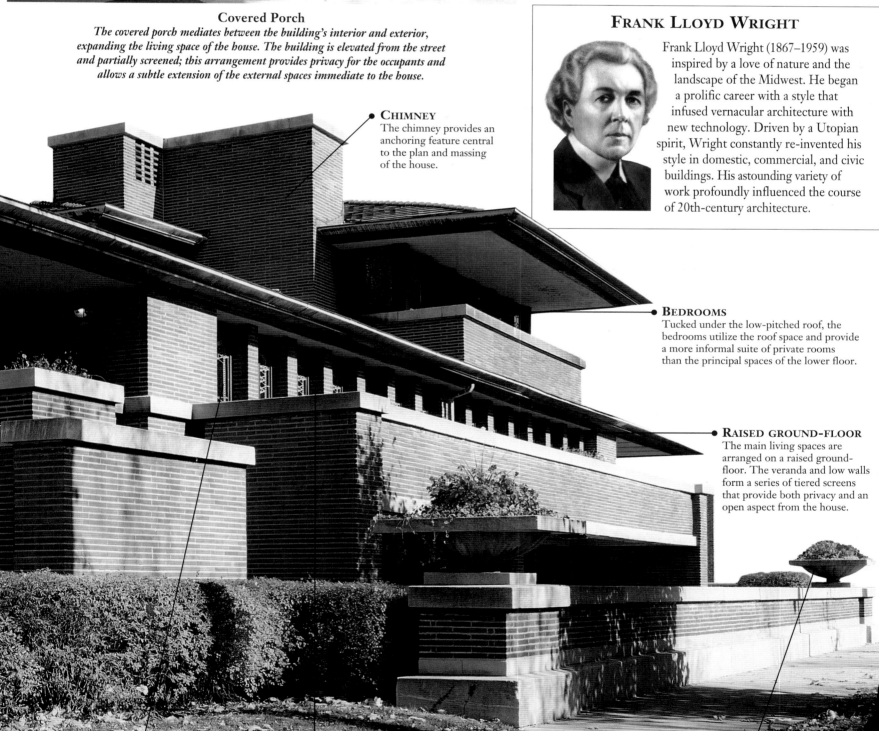

CHIMNEY
The chimney provides an anchoring feature central to the plan and massing of the house.

BEDROOMS
Tucked under the low-pitched roof, the bedrooms utilize the roof space and provide a more informal suite of private rooms than the principal spaces of the lower floor.

RAISED GROUND-FLOOR
The main living spaces are arranged on a raised ground-floor. The veranda and low walls form a series of tiered screens that provide both privacy and an open aspect from the house.

DECORATION
The coloured glass and leaded lights provide a richness of detail and restrained ornamentation, which Wright considered an integral and "constituent" part of the architecture.

BRICK PIERS
The structural arrangement of load-bearing brick piers allows the walls to be inset with opening doors. Light and air permeate the interiors, extending the living space on to porches with views of the garden.

STONE VASES
Stone vases placed on the screen walls define the outer edge of the house under the projecting eaves. They emphasize the horizontality of the massing and visually hold the corners.

CASTLE DROGO

CASTLE **D**ROGO (1910–30) emerges dramatically, like a medieval castle in abstracted, monumental form, from a granite outcrop 61 metres (200 feet) above the River Teign in Devon, England. Designed by Sir Edwin Lutyens, it derives much of its authenticity and boldness of composition from revisions of the original design, which greatly reduced the scale of the project. The omission of additional wings and a central court, which would have balanced the composition of the southern elevation, encourages the illusion of an authentic feudal castle, modified by rebuilding and organically rooted in its site. Lutyens' honesty towards the use of vernacular materials and his willingness to reinterpret traditional forms define a middle ground in contrast to the radical departures of early-20th-century modern architecture. The skilful management of plan and three-dimensional form reconciles a formal grandeur with the intimate spaces of domestic architecture.

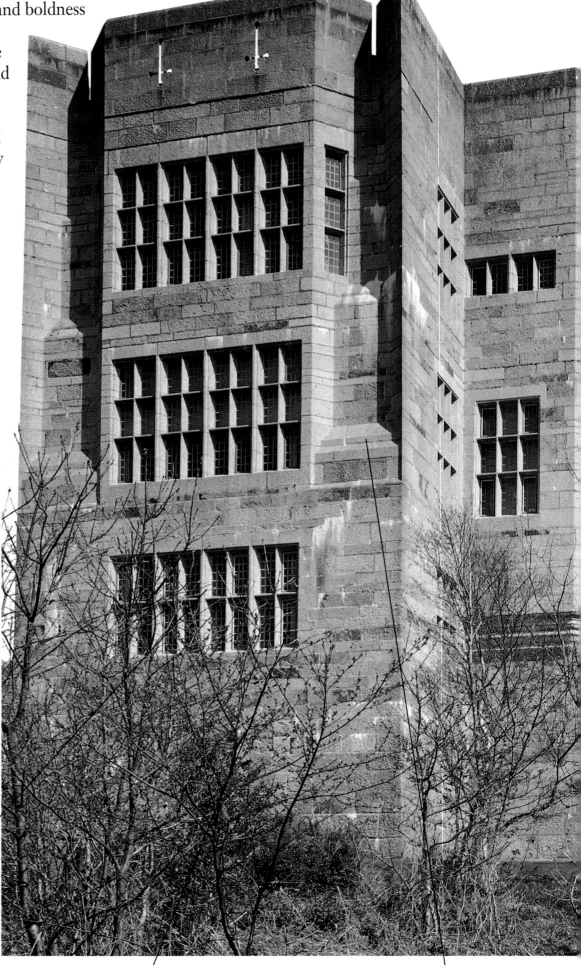

Lutyens had the form of the building partially erected as a timber and canvas mock-up, in order to gauge its completed impact and position on the site. As the original budget of £60,000 began to escalate, the client instructed a curtailment of the scale of the project, requiring continual revisions. The final building constitutes one third of the full proposal.

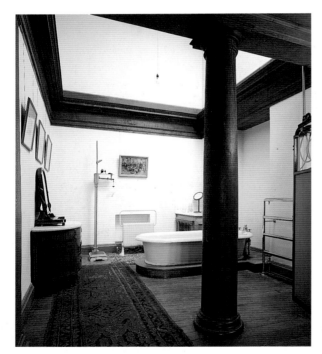

Bathroom
The sky-lit bathroom of the second-floor master bedroom has a Classical simplicity and introduces domestic comforts into an imposing building. The domestic apartments have an intimacy quite apart from the grandeur of the principal reception rooms.

ANGULAR DETAILING
The mass of the 1.2-metre- (4-foot-) thick granite walls is emphasized by angular detailing and the deep recession of the window openings.

SPECIFICATION

- **Location**   Devon, England
- **Date**   1910–30
- **Architect**   Sir Edwin Lutyens
- **Building structure**   Granite and timber
- **Building type**   Castle

MULLIONED WINDOWS
The stone-mullioned windows recall the bays of Elizabethan fortified houses. They carefully order the composition of the façade and command impressive views over the dramatic landscape.

SLOPING WALLS
The upper sections of the walls are inclined, stepping back in tiered courses, giving a distinctive, sculptural definition to the bat-eared towers and parapet detailing. This vernacular device, redeployed for its sculptural effect, is typical of Lutyens' personalization of vernacular forms.

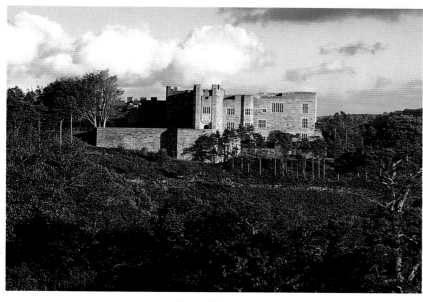

East Elevation

Castle Drogo is prominently positioned on the edge of a steep escarpment and forms a dramatic intermediary between land and sky. The client had sought a medieval romanticism, which Lutyens was able to interpret in rugged detail and sculptural form.

GRANITE WALLS
Rising from the steep escarpment, the granite walls merge the form of the building with the rocky outcrop, culminating in the distinct sharpness of detailing at the skyline.

SECOND FLOOR
The private apartments, guest rooms, and nursery are located on the second floor.

CONSTRUCTION
After the first year of construction, every stone was laid by just two men. These two masons worked under the direction of a master mason in the authentic tradition of medieval construction.

NORTH WING
The splayed north wing follows the contour of the site and houses the bedrooms and lower-ground kitchens.

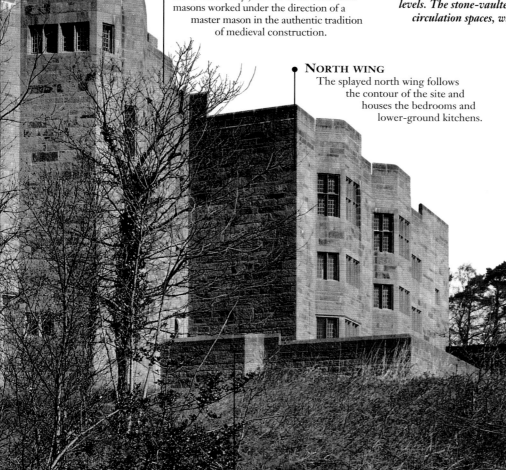

DINING ROOM
The dining room and service wing are on the lower floor, tucked into the slope of the hillside.

STEPPED SECTION
The house is situated on the edge of a steep slope and has a stepped section, with the main entrance and principal rooms on the upper-ground floor, accessible from the court of the entrance elevation.

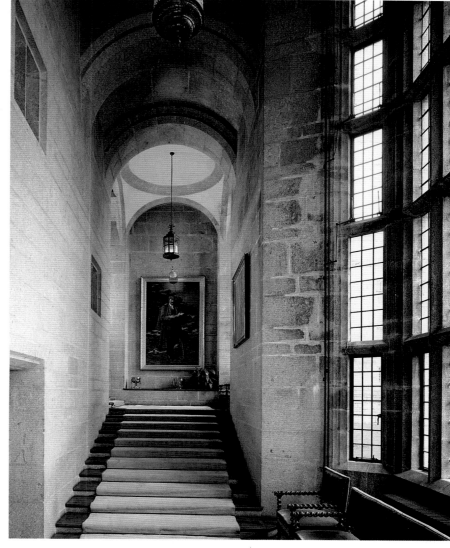

Stepped Levels

Movement throughout the house is carefully managed between the stepped levels. The stone-vaulted corridors and staircases provide a varied sequence of circulation spaces, which gracefully connect principal areas of the house.

SIR EDWIN LUTYENS

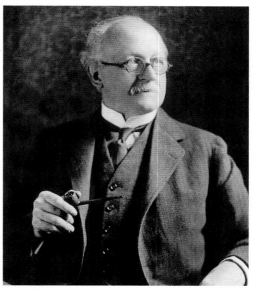

Sir Edwin Landseer Lutyens (1869–1944) developed a highly personal style in his many commissions for private houses completed in the manner of the English Arts and Crafts Movement. Later commissions for civic works, including the Viceroy's House (1912–31) in New Delhi and the Cenotaph (1919) in London, adopted a Neoclassical style suited to the grand plan. Lutyens' work is memorable for its skilful manipulation of the plan, affinity to the site, and versatile architectural vocabulary.

SCHRÖDER HOUSE

THE SCHRÖDER HOUSE (1923–24) IN Utrecht was designed by Gerrit Rietveld and his client, Madame Schröder-Schrader. As with the Villa Savoye (see p. 84) and the Farnsworth House (see p. 90), it provides, within its modest scale (being a two-storey, end-of-terrace house), a succinct essay in some of the defining principles of early Modern architecture. Rietveld was a member of the De Stijl ("the style") group, an influential Dutch tributary to the flood of ideas sweeping Europe in the years following World War One. Its members sought a new mode of expression in geometrical forms. This house is a volumetric composition of sliding and overlapping planes slotted into the co-ordinates of a three-dimensional grid, extending the possibilities explored in artist Piet Mondrian's (1872–1944) abstract use of space and colour. For De Stijl, it was part of a revolutionary package of ideas; for modern architecture, it pointed to the use of architectural elements to delineate, rather than enclose, space. The design challenges the conventional arrangement of static rooms and formal façades, allowing an overlap of functions and a fluid sequence of spaces relevant to the needs of a contemporary house and workspace.

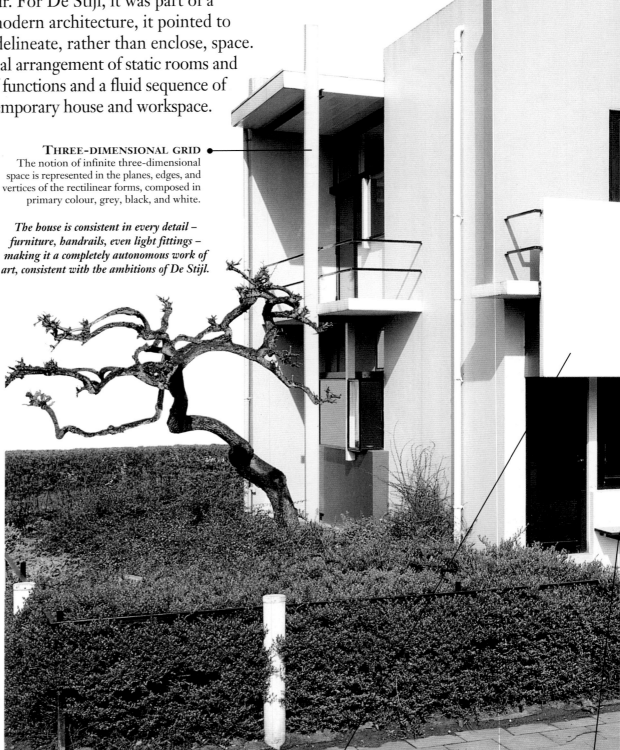

Setting
The house forms the end of an existing terrace in a complete contradiction of its contextual setting. The assertive and revolutionary tone of De Stijl sought to confront rather than defer to established conventions.

DE STIJL

The De Stijl group, formed in Holland in 1917 around the publications of the theorist and architect Theo van Doesburg (1883–1931), sought to liberate art through abstraction and purity of form and colour, as exemplified in the work of its leading painter, Piet Mondrian. Their ideas developed through a period of continuous experimentation, making an important contribution to the debate of the Modern Movement, becoming later absorbed into the teaching of the German Bauhaus. Unlike later Cubist-inspired architecture, it found fewer occasions for architectural realization and is more frequently represented in painting, typography, and furniture design.

THREE-DIMENSIONAL GRID
The notion of infinite three-dimensional space is represented in the planes, edges, and vertices of the rectilinear forms, composed in primary colour, grey, black, and white.

The house is consistent in every detail – furniture, handrails, even light fittings – making it a completely autonomous work of art, consistent with the ambitions of De Stijl.

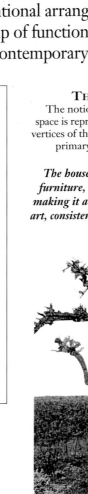

The Red–Blue Chair
Rietveld's Red–Blue Chair (1918) is a clear statement of the principles of spatial abstraction. The overlapping frame, representing a continuous, three-dimensional grid, supports the hovering planes of the seat and back.

PLANAR GEOMETRY
The assembling of perpendicular planes to define the form and delineate spaces deconstructs the conventional cubic volumes of architectural form. The composition gives an impression of the weightless suspension of abstract elements.

PORCH SEAT
The porch seat forms an integral part of the architectural composition, as do all elements of fixed and free-standing furniture.

GERRIT RIETVELD

After apprenticeship to his father as a furniture designer, Gerrit Rietveld (1888–1964) opened his own cabinet-making business in 1911. Rietveld studied architecture and was introduced to Theo van Doesburg and the ideas of the De Stijl group. He collaborated with Madame Schröder-Schrader in a limited output of projects that brought the spatial and abstract concerns of De Stijl to the utilities of domestic living. Though few architectural projects of De Stijl survive, Rietveld's furniture epitomizes the experimental nature of the Dutch school, which exerted a considerable influence on 20th-century art and design.

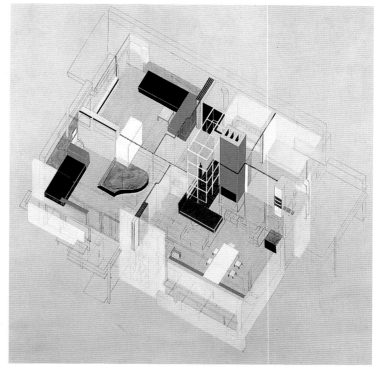

Isometric Projection
The sculptural arrangement is continued throughout the interior. The principal areas for working, relaxation, and sleeping are on the first floor, in an ambiguous and flexible series of spaces temporarily defined by movable partitions. Officially designated an attic, the first floor was not subject to the same statutory building regulations as the ground floor.

ROOF LANTERN
The glazed lantern provides an extruded volume for the central stair shaft, which illuminates the core of the house.

CORNER WINDOW
The windows, when open, are held at angles perpendicular to the frame, expanding the geometrical grid beyond the building envelope. The window, with the structural frame set back from the corner, pivots to reveal a clear opening at the building's defining edge.

STRUCTURAL FRAME
The ad hoc combination of structural systems, load-bearing wall, and steel frame is used for visual effect, lacking the constructional clarity of Le Corbusier's concrete-framed Dom-ino house (see p. 84).

PRIMARY COLOURS
Primary colours are used to distinguish isolated elements of the frame, highlighting them as co-ordinates in an expanding spatial grid. The house has an abstract sculptural composition, destroying the conventions of a rectilinear box.

OVERLAPPING PLANES
Walls meet in a series of overlapping planes, expressing the composition of separate forms.

GROUND FLOOR
More conventional in arrangement than the first floor, the ground floor was dictated by statutory building codes and accommodates a study, kitchen, and two bedrooms.

BALCONY SUPPORT
The steel joist provides necessary support for the concrete slab of the balcony, but is also an integral part of the sculptural composition, extending the frame of the building beyond the external walls.

SPECIFICATION

•*Location*	Utrecht, Holland
•*Date*	1923–24
•*Architects*	Gerrit Rietveld, Mme Schröder-Schrader
•*Building structure*	Steel-frame, load-bearing brick, and concrete
•*Building type*	House

VILLA SAVOYE

BY 1928, LE CORBUSIER'S PUBLICATIONS and early commissions for villas and apartments had found favour amongst the French bourgeoisie, putting him at the centre stage of the avant-garde. His ideas for multi-storey housing, civic buildings, and urban planning were developing into a radical manifesto, consolidating his influence and shaping the course of modern architecture in the years following World War Two. However, it was in the early villa commissions that these ideas were to find expression, in the novel forms and industrial materials to become associated with the Modern Movement. The Villa Savoye at Poissy in France (1928–31), was commissioned as a weekend country house. Unlike with earlier villa commissions, the unrestricted site gave Le Corbusier an opportunity to indulge his preference for the square plan as a pure and natural form. The building expresses his ambition to redefine habitable space, emphasizing volume and natural light. It concluded a period of Purist experimentation, with later projects maturing into the complex sculptural style seen at Ronchamp.

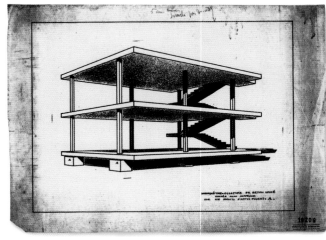

Dom-ino Skeleton
Le Corbusier recognized the architectural possibilities created by the simple skeletal form of framed structures. Concrete slab floors, separated by columns inset from the walls, allowed the plan to develop freely within the structural grid. The walls (solid, glazed, or open) become non-structural, used purely as an envelope to express the Purist form. The Dom-ino system (1914–15) facilitated Le Corbusier's **Five Points for a New Architecture** *(1926): a free plan; pilotis; a free facade; ribbon windows; and a roof garden.*

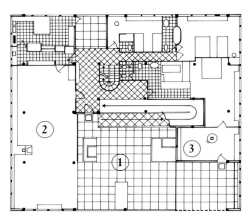

First-floor Plan
The first-floor terrace (1) is enclosed by the screen-wall, glimpsed from the exterior through the ribbon windows continued through the façade. Treated as an outside room, and a clear extension of the living area, the terrace connects to the main living room (2) by sliding, glazed doors. The bedroom (3) also opens on to the terrace, allowing movement between spaces that overlap in use and definition.

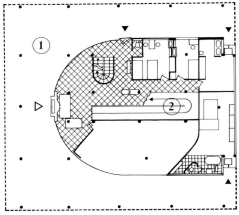

Ground-floor Plan
The U-shaped ground floor-plan of the reception and service areas was designed to accommodate the turning circle (1) of a car delivering occupants to the door, and to continue this flow of movement to the internal ramp (2), which sweeps up through the principal public spaces, terminating at the rooftop sun terrace.

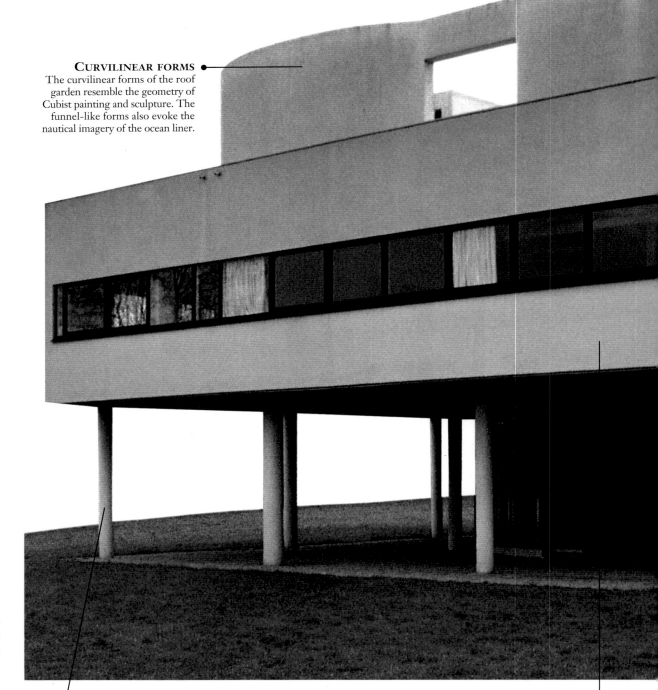

CURVILINEAR FORMS
The curvilinear forms of the roof garden resemble the geometry of Cubist painting and sculpture. The funnel-like forms also evoke the nautical imagery of the ocean liner.

PILOTI
Pilotis are slender columns forming the structural frame, which elevates the main living area above the ground (*piano nobile*).

Le Corbusier celebrated the 20th century and the objects of an industrialized society – the steamship, aeroplane, and car – comparing their engineers to the greatest Classical architects.

PIANO NOBILE
Le Corbusier adopted the *piano nobile* from the palazzos of the Italian Renaissance. This device raises the main living area to above the ground level and provides views from terraces and balconies.

LE CORBUSIER

Le Corbusier (1887–1966) dominated and encompassed the aims of the Modern Movement. The functional requirements of modern society led him famously to offer the analogy of the house as "a machine for living". He was keen to realign construction and design to progressive industrial methods, combining the planar, abstract geometry of Cubist theory with simple and unadorned forms of rendered concrete and plate glass. Later, he pursued sculptural form and poetic simplicity. His buildings demonstrate the potential of simple and radical architecture.

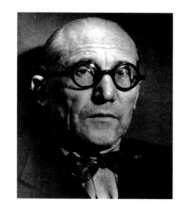

NOTRE-DAME-DU-HAUT

The pilgrimage chapel at Notre-Dame-du-Haut, Ronchamp (1950–54), in the Vosges mountains in France, illustrates the maturity of Le Corbusier's late work – distanced by World War Two from Purism and the machine aesthetic. The hull-like form of the concrete-shell roof is supported in a frame of reinforced concrete, concealed within the curved and tapering walls. The eastern wall, pierced by deeply set, coloured windows, projects to the edge of the roof canopy in a sheltering curve, which protects the altar and pulpit used in the alfresco celebration of Mass. This sculptural device turns the building inside-out, providing a nave of grass and a backdrop of distant views.

ROOF GARDEN
The flat roof emphasizes the planar, Cubist geometry, allowing the roof to become a garden and sun terrace.

WHITE EXTERIOR
The white "ocean-liner" exterior contrasts with the interior spaces, often composed in planes of solid colour.

SPECIFICATION

- **Location** — Poissy, France
- **Date** — 1928–31
- **Architect** — Le Corbusier
- **Building structure** — Concrete-frame
- **Building type** — Villa
- **Construction time** — 3 years

RIBBON WINDOW
Unrestricted by conventional load-bearing walls, the window continues the length of the façade, even turning the corner, allowing a framed view of the horizon and giving a strong horizontal emphasis to the building.

Methods of industrial production and standardized components were considered admirable by Le Corbusier. The "machine" finishes, however, were often achieved through intensive labour skills. In this respect, architectural construction remained far behind the industrial methods common in the automobile industry.

FREE FACADE
The set-back of the perimeter columns from the edge of the wall allows the main, framed structure to be internal. The perimeter wall acts as a *curtain* that can be drawn taut to express the geometry of the cube, or open, to maximize natural light.

"Architecture is the masterly, correct, and magnificent play of masses brought together in light"
LE CORBUSIER

COMPOSITION
The building, when viewed from the edge of the site, is seen as detached and carefully composed, rather like a Palladian villa, such as the Villa Rotonda (see p. 48).

EMPIRE STATE BUILDING

THE EMPIRE STATE BUILDING (1929–31) was designed by R. H. Shreve, T. Lamb, and A. L. Harmon and is an example of the skyscrapers of the glittering interwar era, before the sobriety of post-Depression New Deal America. At 381 metres (1,250 feet) and 102 storeys, it succeeded to the title of the world's tallest building in 1931, previously held by the neighbouring Chrysler Building at 319 metres (1,046 feet) tall. The rapid growth of New York downtown city districts, supported by the growing catchment of a large commuting workforce had increased the density of city development, raising the value of city plots. Improvements in lighting, heating, plumbing, ventilation, mechanical excavation, foundation design, and fire-proofing responded to the demand for increased building height. Clients were greatly attracted to this conspicuous form of construction and competed for prominence in the city skyline. The public was captivated by the excitement of the Jazz Age and the ever increasing confection of architectural style. Completed in the grip of the Great Depression, however, the building remained empty for many years.

Construction

Using new technology and site-management techniques, the building was driven up at a rate of four and a half storeys per week by 3,500 site workers. The construction took 410 days from groundbreak to handover, at one point achieving over 14 storeys in 10 days.

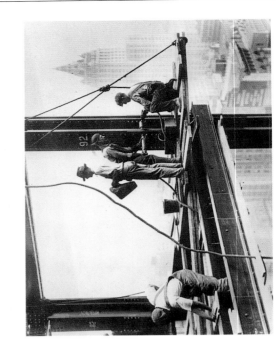

Steel-framed Construction

By the end of the 19th century, engineers were familiar with steel-framed construction for engineering and industrial structures, such as bridges and railway stations. The early-20th century saw the exploitation of this construction method in multi-storey buildings.

MAST TOWER

The mast tower is lit with a changing sequence of coloured lights, marking national holidays and major events. Three thousand visitors a day flocked to the observation room in the initial years of under-occupation, generating a yearly income of $1 million, an important revenue following the Wall Street Crash of 1929.

LANDING STAGE

The 16-storey steel mast houses the observation deck and was designed as a mooring mast for airships. Though used only twice, the progressive image of the skyscraper as a lighthouse reached by airship offered a futuristic image of modernity.

STRUCTURE

The 365,000-tonne- (359,233-ton-) building uses 10 million bricks on a 59,000-tonne- (60,000 ton-) riveted steel structure. The Empire State remained the world's tallest building until 1973, when it was superseded by the World Trade Center.

LIFTS

Technical developments in the speed and increased travel-distance of the passenger-lift enabled practical occupation of multi-storey buildings. The building has a total of 62 lifts, arranged in core clusters.

SPECIFICATION

•Location	New York, USA
•Date	1929–31
•Architects	R. H. Shreve, T. Lamb, A. L. Harmon
•Height	381 m (1,250 ft)
•Storeys	102
•Building structure	Steel-frame
•Building type	Offices
•Construction time	58 weeks

Zoning Laws

The New York Zoning Ordinance Laws of 1916 sought to regulate city development. Buildings were subject to rules that stipulated they be progressively stepped back as they rose higher, thereby improving daylight to ground level and affording better lighting to the ascending floors. Hugh Ferris's drawing (1929) illustrates the maximum permitted volume conforming to the codes.

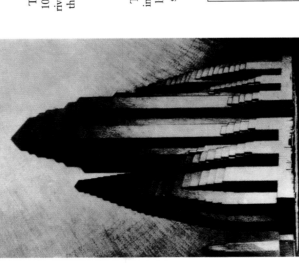

NEW BUILDING TYPE

The unprecedented height of the building by the New York zoning laws exploited the New York zoning laws and attracted publicity because of their conspicuous profile. This entirely novel and exciting building type broke all the formal conventions of architectural order and proportion observed even by the pioneering Chicago skyscrapers. The Modernist decorative elements of the building are influenced by Art Deco styling, but the paring down of the building to provide an efficient functional mass is consistent with reductive Modernist ideas.

MASSING

The massing of the tower was determined by the requirements of light and ventilation. Before the advent of effective air-conditioning, it was a practical necessity for office space to be within 8.5 metres (28 feet) of a window.

ART DECO STYLE

The *Exposition Internationale des Arts Décoratifs et Industriels Modernes*, held in Paris in 1925, created a fashion, known as Art Deco, for a range of forms derived from exotic historical and cultural references, such as, Egyptian and Mayan, in futuristic materials, such as chrome, glass, and plastic.

WINDOWS

The 6,500 windows project from the face of the cladding and are connected by vertical strips of aluminium and stainless steel.

CLADDING

The riveted steel-frame, rather heavy by today's standards, is clad in blocks of grey Indiana limestone highlighted with bands of aluminium.

BASE

The base contains two storeys of galleried shops around the three-storey entrance lobby. The five-storey base of the building occupies the full extent of the site. To minimize the area needed for storage during construction, materials were supplied and erected according to a meticulous schedule. The process of construction resembled contemporary assembly-line methods, enabling the building to be completed at an astonishing pace.

During 1930, the title for the world's tallest building was contested by both the Chrysler Building by William van Alen and the Bank of Manhattan by H. Craig Severance, a former business partner of van Alen. Each building sought permits for additional floors. To achieve the title, van Alen had the Chrysler Building's 56-metre- (185-foot-) high steel spire secretly constructed within the fire shaft. Thus, at 319 metres (1,046 feet) the Chrysler Building exceeded the 282 metres (927 feet) of the Bank of Manhattan. However, within a year, the Empire State Building, at 381 metres (1,250 feet), had taken the title.

VILLA MAIREA

BY THE MID-1930S, the Modern Movement had begun a new phase. Early experimentation with Purist form, new materials, and machine finishes (typified by Le Corbusier's Villa Savoye (see p. 84) and the development of the International Style) had shifted towards establishing regional identities, absorbing local traditions, and responding to specific climatic and cultural preferences. The Villa Mairea (1938–41) was commissioned as a private residence. Set amidst the beauty of the forest at Noormarkku in Finland, it expresses the developing maturity of the Modern Movement. Alvar Aalto brought the Modernist preoccupation with open space, natural light, and sculptural form to a contemporary use of local crafts and building skills. The building achieves a strong sense of connection with its situation and cultural traditions, blending the surviving traditions and vernacular rustication with the simple restraint of Nordic Classicism.

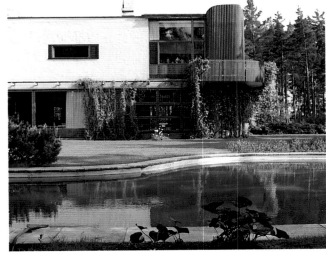

Garden and Pool
The L-shaped plan of the villa shelters the garden and swimming pool to the rear. The glazed screens allow direct connection with the garden terrace and views of the forest. The screens and simple timber detailing illustrate Aalto's interest in Japanese architecture.

COLUMN SPANS
The column spans are varied in order to break away from the monotony of the building grid. In this respect, the building has an informal relationship with structure, unlike Le Corbusier's regulated Dom-ino plan or the disciplined grid of Mies van der Rohe.

TIMBER BOARDS
The studio wing is panelled with vertical boards. The profile of the timber slats emphasizes both the curved volume of the studio wall and the grain of the timber.

HANDRAIL
The "ship's handrail" above the balcony is a familiar Modernist motif, and is detailed in both tubular steel and natural-grained timber.

ALVAR AALTO

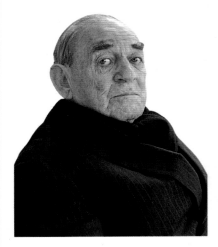

The early designs of Alvar Aalto (1898–1976) established his reputation alongside the major exponents of early International Modernist architecture. His work expresses the Finnish traditions of simple Classicism, an affinity for natural materials, and fine use of indigenous craft skills. His architectural commissions and designs for furniture and glassware consolidated his contribution as one of the most influential of 20th-century architects.

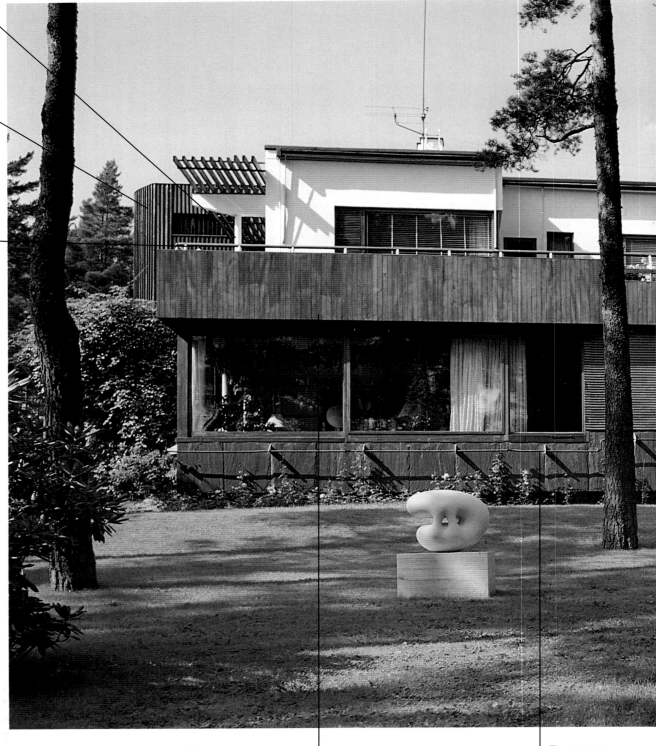

NATURAL MATERIALS
The ground-floor library is clad in teak boards with the lower junctions near the ground panelled in granite. Each has a richly toned self-colour adding to the collage of materials on the façade.

PLANTING
The brackets set between the stone panels support wires for sun screens and a plant-watering conduit. Climbing plants are encouraged as further textural materials in areas of the façade.

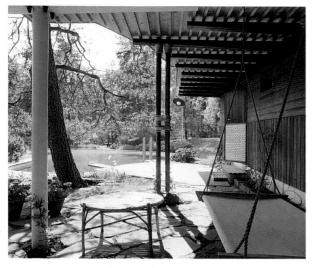

Covered Terrace
A paved terrace, covered by a timber canopy with a turf roof, leads from the main house to the detached sauna. The rustic materials, such as the woven door and wicker binding, create a naturalized, softened edge with the landscape.

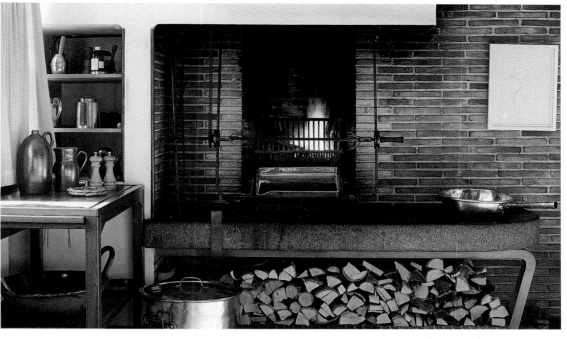

The Fireplace
The hearth provides a simple focus to many of the rooms. The dining-room fireplace, contrasting the exposed brick with white plaster, terminates a view through the open plan of the living areas taken from the entrance porch. The fireplace chimney is shared by an external fireplace to the covered terrace, which backs on to the dining-room.

STRUCTURE
The upper bedrooms are supported on a system of columns and load-bearing walls. The columns vary in material and position, and are chosen with regard to the room size, rather than being determined by the regular intervals of the constructional frame.

BAY WINDOWS
With their triangular plan, the bay windows provide striking views directed towards the landscaped forest approach. The building is adjusted to the site, giving prominence to views out on to the landscape.

TEXTURAL FINISH
The bedroom and studio wings have a white, volumetric form familiar to Modern Movement buildings, but here the smooth white render of modern Cubist architecture is complemented by areas of lime-washed brick, having a textural and rusticated surface.

"Nature, not the machine, is the most important model for architecture"
ALVAR AALTO

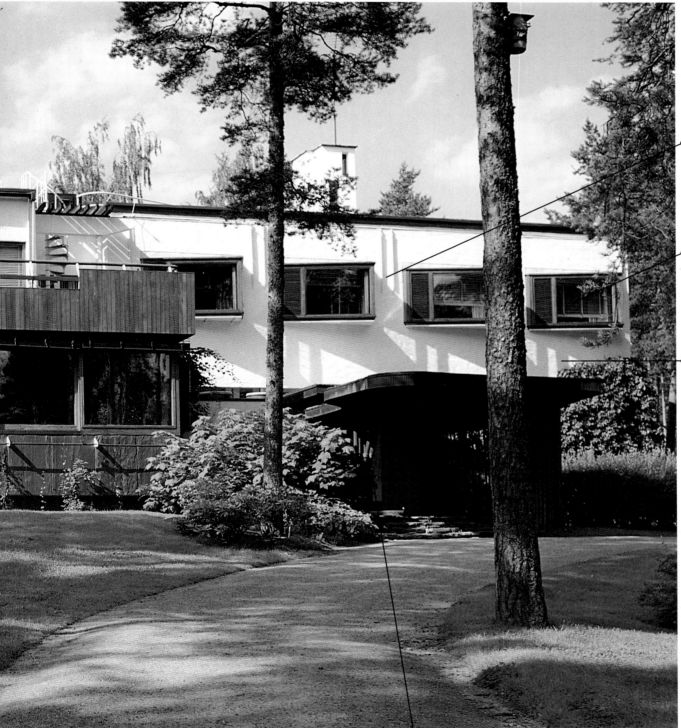

Hand-crafted wood, ceramics, and glass underwrite a characteristic richness and simplicity of Scandinavian design. The skills needed in these crafts, maintained in unbroken tradition, had survived the process of industrialization, becoming absorbed into the rustic tendencies of late Modernism.

ENTRANCE PORCH
The entrance porch has a free-formed timber canopy supported by eccentrically placed columns and a timber screen – in reference to the prevailing image of the sheltering forest.

SPECIFICATION	
•*Location*	Noormarkku, Finland
•*Date*	1938–41
•*Architect*	Alvar Aalto
•*Building structure*	Reinforced concrete, brick, stone, timber, and steel
•*Storeys*	2
•*Building type*	Villa

FARNSWORTH HOUSE

IN CONTRAST TO THE LATER sculptural and rusticated tendencies of Modernist architecture exemplified by Alvar Aalto (see p. 88) and Le Corbusier (see p. 84), Mies van der Rohe was to pursue a disciplined course of Modernism, exploring the minimalist possibilities of the structural steel frame and the transparency of the glass box – an image summarized by his phrase, "less is more". Mies van der Rohe set a trend for the corporate architecture of the high-rise office block, but few exponents achieve the almost abstract beauty of his late work, which combines a rigorous, organizing structure with a fastidious attention to proportion and constructional detail. The Farnsworth House (1945–51), standing on the north bank of the River Fox, 96.5 kilometres (60 miles) from Chicago, Illinois, provides a sophisticated and ascetic place of retreat from urban life, as had Villa Rotonda (see p. 48) four centuries earlier. Like the Villa Rotonda, it shows its lineage from Classical Greek temples, but achieved here in a thoroughly mid-20th-century idiom. The pristine white frame, set amidst the "Arcadian landscape" is a definitive expression of cool Modernism and Classical simplicity.

SPECIFICATION

- *Location*   Chicago, USA
- *Date*   1945–51
- *Architect*   Ludwig Mies van der Rohe
- *Building structure*   Welded steel-frame
- *Building type*   House

PRISTINE FRAME
The zinc-coated steel frame is painted throughout with white enamel paint, polished to a high finish. Thus are covered any marks of fabrication.

ELEVATED STEEL FRAME
The exposed steel frame elevates the floor 1.2 metres (4 feet) above the ground, visually detaching the building from the landscape.

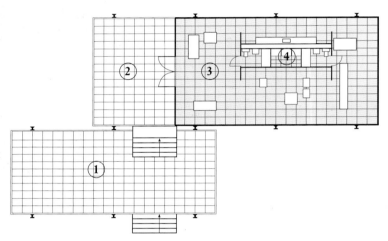

Plan
The plan allows the maximum transparency and views to the landscape. There are three connected areas: an open, raised deck (1); a covered porch (2); and a glazed enclosure (3). The service core (4) contains two bathrooms, kitchen fittings, a fireplace, and a storage unit. The concentration of storage and services into a central core frees the exterior from the interference of pipes and wires, maintaining its simplicity of form.

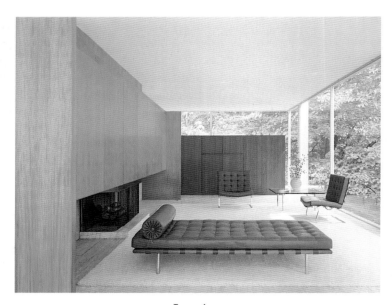

Interior
The bathroom and storage core is concealed behind an arrangement of non-load-bearing partitions, allowing the occupant to presume a life of monastic simplicity. The partitions provide a flexible interior, subtly translating between areas loosely designated for living, sleeping, and eating.

MARBLE SLABS
The marble slabs have a concealed drainage detail, enabling them to be laid completely flat, maintaining the precision and alignment of the horizontal plane.

The house was commissioned by Dr Edith Farnsworth as a weekend retreat. Despite proclaiming dissatisfaction with the finished result, she continued to occupy the house for 17 years.

LUDWIG MIES VAN DER ROHE

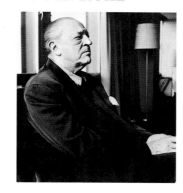

Mies van der Rohe (1886–1969) achieved prominence with his crystalline skyscraper designs in 1919. The Barcelona Pavilion (1928–29) and the Seagram Building (1954–58), New York, exemplify the cool Modernism of the single-storey pavilion and high-rise office block, exerting a lasting influence on the Modern Movement.

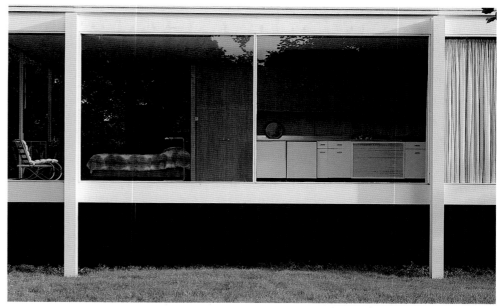

CONCEALED FIXINGS
The steel frame is welded to a high degree of accuracy and workmanship. The welds are meticulously ground off and all other fixings fastidiously concealed.

Minimalism
The understated elegance of the frame and glazing is achieved through careful attention to detail. To maintain this elemental simplicity, all the services, drainage, and fixings must be carefully co-ordinated and controlled. Mies van der Rohe's extremely reductive style helped create the architectural genre known as Minimalism.

PLATE-GLASS WINDOWS
The full-length plate-glass of the windows is set between the structural steel frame secured by a minimal steel glazing bead. Cross-ventilation is provided by the doors and one opening window.

TRANSPARENCY
The addition of silk curtains to screen and shade the interior, following the overlooking of the site by a new road and a river crossing, has resulted in the loss of the transparency of the glazed box.

STAIR TREADS
The travertine marble that is used for the floor deck is also used for the stair treads, which are similarly detailed as hovering horizontal planes.

SYDNEY OPERA HOUSE

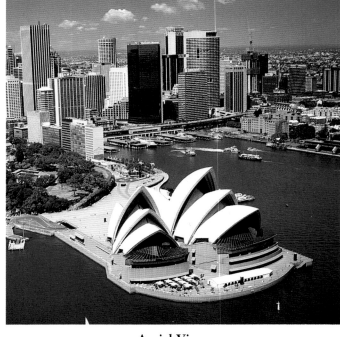

THE OPERA HOUSE ON THE PROMINENT waterfront site of Sydney Harbour has become one of modern architecture's most popular icons. The competition-winning design of 1957, by Jørn Utzon, was awarded on the strength of the conceptual ideas he submitted in outline sketch proposals. The building employs three important elements: a hovering roof structure facilitating public functions; a podium containing the support facilities; and a terraced concourse incorporating the processional routes that link the spaces designed for social gathering. The sail-like, floating roof shells, which rise from the massive, tiered podium, emerge dramatically from the water and are reminiscent of the waterside Gothic churches of Utzon's native Denmark and the yachts in full sail that fill Sydney Harbour. Indeed, it is this last image that succeeds in the executed design – which ultimately overwhelmed the technical problems experienced in matching form to function. Programmatic changes to the brief and protracted delays led to Utzon's resignation. The building was completed – at ten times the original budget – by the team of Hall, Littlemore, and Todd in 1973.

Aerial View
Sydney Opera House stands on the headland of Bennelong Point in Sydney Harbour. The three main clusters of interlocking concrete shells, with an inclined central axis converging toward the landward approach, accommodate two main halls (one for opera and one for concert performances), a cinema (originally a theatre), and a restaurant.

SPECIFICATION

- **Location** — Sydney, Australia
- **Date** — 1959–73
- **Architect** — Jørn Utzon
- **Building structure** — Reinforced concrete vaults with concrete shell covering
- **Building type** — Concert hall
- **Constuction time** — 14 years

GLAZING
The open ends of the shells are enclosed within suspended glazing panels.

SHELLS
The shells are formed with a combination of prefabricated and cast-*in-situ* concrete. The precast concrete ribs are glued together in sections, radiating from the central concrete pedestals. The Y-sectioned ribs are laterally strung together with pre-stressed steel-tie rods and supported at the outward ends by concrete edge beams.

INTERLOCKING SHELLS
The interlocking shell clusters are each generated from segments of a single sphere, providing a common curvature, and helping to simplify the complex resolution of joints and cladding components.

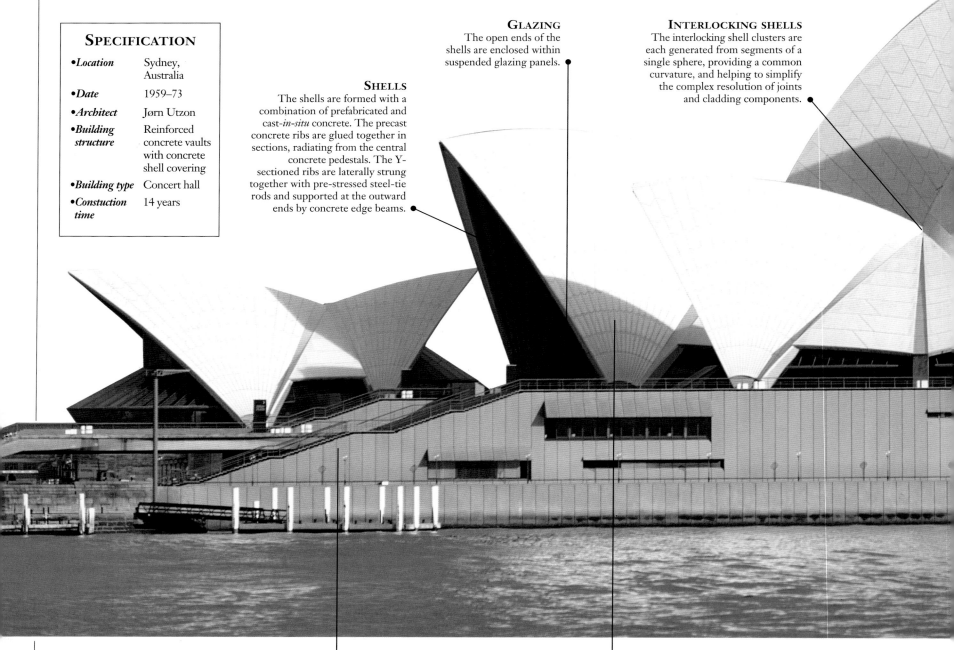

PROCESSIONAL ROUTE
The podium is staged in three tiers, providing a processional route up wide flights of steps towards the entrances for auditoria, which are approached from the main public concourse.

SHELL SEGMENTS
The shell segments, up to 60 metres (197 feet) high, are made from fan-vaulted concrete rib beams with a 5-centimetre- (2-inch-) thick shell wall.

Because scenery is raised from beneath the main stage, the conventional bulk of traditional opera houses, which have large fly towers for scenery changes, is avoided.

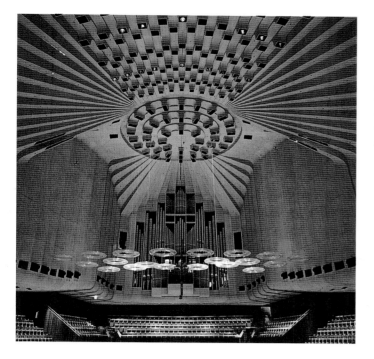

Acoustic Environment
The form of the shell structure posed a number of problems for the functional requirements of the concert hall. Plywood panels line the interior modifying the acoustic environment. Plexiglas panels, seen from above the stage, can be lowered to provide reflective surfaces for sound projection.

*Speaking about the notion of **Additive Architecture** (see box, right), Utzon cited Alvar Aalto's example of cherry blossoms: "each blossom [is] different from its neighbour according to its special position on the branch, but all the blossoms [are] composed of the same elements . . . [this is] the foundation of many of my projects".*

CONCERT HALL
The main concert hall is enclosed within the hightest shell section. Originally, the brief called for a dual-purpose hall that could accommodate both orchesral and operatic performances. The concert hall accommodates 2,900 seats.

OPERA THEATRE
Problems arising from conflicting acoustic and programmatic requirements led to the provision of a separate opera auditoria. This theatre has 1,547 seats.

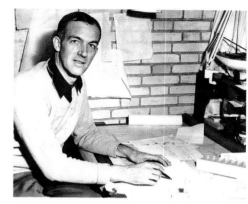

JØRN UTZON

Jørn Utzon (1918–) was born in Copenhagen, Denmark. He worked for two influential modern Scandinavian architects – Gunar Asplund (1885–1940) and Alvar Aalto (see p. 88). Utzon's designs are characterized by clear and conceptual statements that generate simple solutions – often from a "family of related objects". This concept became known as *Additive Architecture.*

Tiles
The precast concrete rib-vaults are clad in a combination of over one million glazed and matt ceramic tiles. The tiles accentuate the radial pattern of the building and glisten in the light like fish scales.

*Utzon uses the device of **served** and **servant** spaces (characteristic of late-modern architecture) in the design of the building. Servant areas within the podium, such as kitchens and offices, house functions that sustain the activities within the prominent served areas of the building, such as the walkways, auditoria, and foyers.*

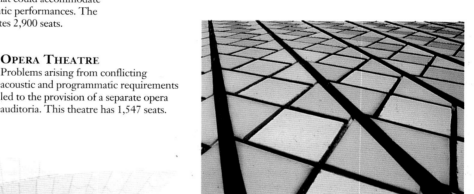

PODIUM
The concrete-framed podium contains all the support facilities, with the main public circulation spaces placed above ground, allowing uninterrupted views across the harbour.

CLADDING
The podium is clad in granite panels, emphasizing its mass, and providing a visually supportive base for the soaring, lightweight roof shells, which are clad in white, ceramic tiles.

The functional requirements of accommodating the shell structure to the form of the interior posed many design problems and required subsequent revisions of the seating capacity.

TOKYO OLYMPIC STADIUM

IN THE SIMPLE, FORMAL, and spiritually resonant qualities of traditional Japanese design, the early-20th-century Modernists were able to recognize a prototype for the language of modern architecture. These intrinsic qualities form part of a national cultural heritage, which Japan continues to exert with influence on contemporary architecture. Designed by Kenzo Tange for the swimming and basketball events of the 1964 Tokyo Olympic Games, the Tokyo Olympic Stadium (1961–64) is a skilful resolution of complex functions demonstrated with disarming simplicity and sculptural clarity. The project has three distinct elements: a large and a small stadium linked by a service building, which uses its flat roof to convey visitors across the site. The dramatic form provides a seamless integration of function and structure and conveys the symbolism and eloquence of traditional Japanese architecture. It succeeds because it goes beyond the realm of mere functionalism. It offers a simple and poetic image to reinterpret the coolly rational principle of "form follows function" and epitomizes Tange's assertion that only something that is beautiful can be truly functional.

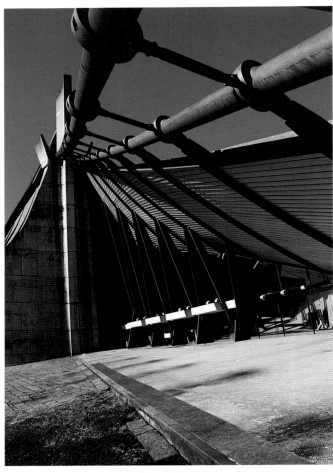

Roof Form
The oversailing canopy of the main stadium expresses an unambiguous and welcoming point of arrival. The form of the roof naturally shelters and funnels spectators into the stadium without disturbing activity within the arena. The articulation of form and function is assisted by the sculptural form of the building.

SPECIFICATION

- **Location**   Tokyo, Japan
- **Date**   1961–64
- **Architect**   Kenzo Tange
- **Building structure**   Reinforced concrete, steel, and tensile structure
- **Building type**   Sports stadium

CONCRETE MAST
The concrete mast forms a cradle supporting the main roof cables. The simple detailing makes a convincing and reassuring display of the means of support of such a dramatic and delicate structure.

CONTEMPORARY EXPRESSION
The forked arms of the concrete mast allude to the crossed rafters of traditional Shinto shrines (see p. 16). Though these references are muted, and intrinsic to the structure, they sufficiently establish their unique cultural heredity.

MAIN TENSION CABLES
The deeply embedded concrete base anchors the massive tension cables, each 33 centimetres (13 inches) in diameter. Tensile structures possess a lightness of appearance, but the forces restrained by the steel cables are immense.

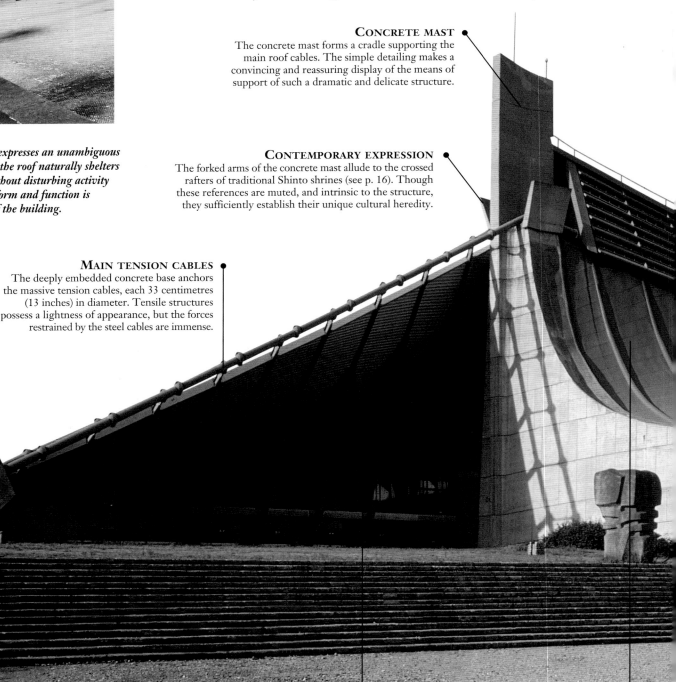

ANCHOR POSTS
The powerful forces of compression and tension, confronted by the concrete and steel, are dramatically conveyed at the junction of the cable and anchor posts.

ENTRANCE CANOPY
The entrance canopy is formed by the dislocation of the elliptical plan along its central axis. The symmetry of the form effortlessly accommodates the function of the plan and has a natural balance of structure.

ROOF LINE
The gentle curve of the roof line makes an oblique reference to the line of traditional Japanese temple roofs.

KENZO TANGE

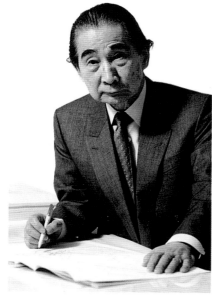

The early career of Kenzo Tange (1913–) established a bridge between European Modernism and Japan's newly emergent culture after World War Two. Tange co-founded the influential Metabolist group, which experimented with radical and flexible solutions to increasing urban density. Tange's career as architect, teacher, and urbanist has earned him an international reputation and inspired a new wave of expressive and original Japanese architecture.

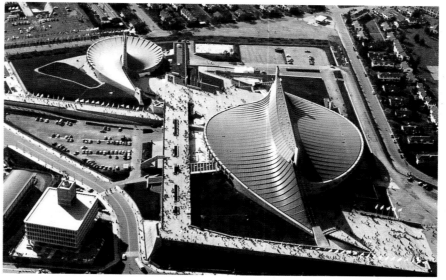

Aerial View
The main stadium is elliptical in plan and seats 15,000 spectators. It contained the swimming and diving events and could also be converted into an ice-skating rink. The smaller, circular stadium, seating 4,000 people, was originally designed for basketball, but hosts other sporting events and conference facilities. The buildings are linked by a support facility housing changing rooms, practice pool, dining hall, and offices. The roof provides a pedestrian causeway across the site for visitors. The elevated walkway has maintained its popularity, to become adopted as a lively space for cultural activities and public promenading.

Suspended Roof Structure
The architecture provides a dramatic backdrop to the international Olympic event without upstaging the function of the building. The pioneering form of the suspended roof provides a lightweight, clear spanning structure. The internal volume dramatically fulfils the promise of its external form, maintaining uninterrupted sightlines and directing the spectators' attention on to the central competition area.

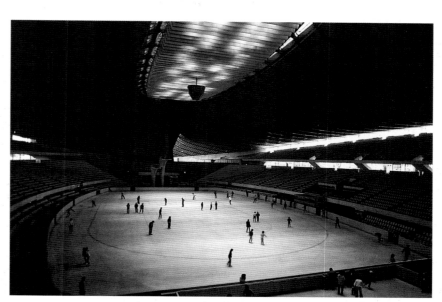

CATENARY ROOF CABLES
The catenary roof cables (hanging freely between two points of support) are tied to the main support cable. A net, produced by the weft of transverse cables, supports the steel plates covering the roof. The shape of the cables describes a complex, but natural, three-dimensional curve to the roof form.

SKYLIGHTS
The tension in the main support cables results in an elliptical opening along the ridge. This has been used to provide a louvered skylight to admit natural light to the interior.

OUTER WALL
The concrete outer wall provides a peripheral restraint to the roof-cable net. Its sculptural curve responds to the forces in the cables. The form is seemingly lifted by the tension in the roof, achieving a taut and natural poise.

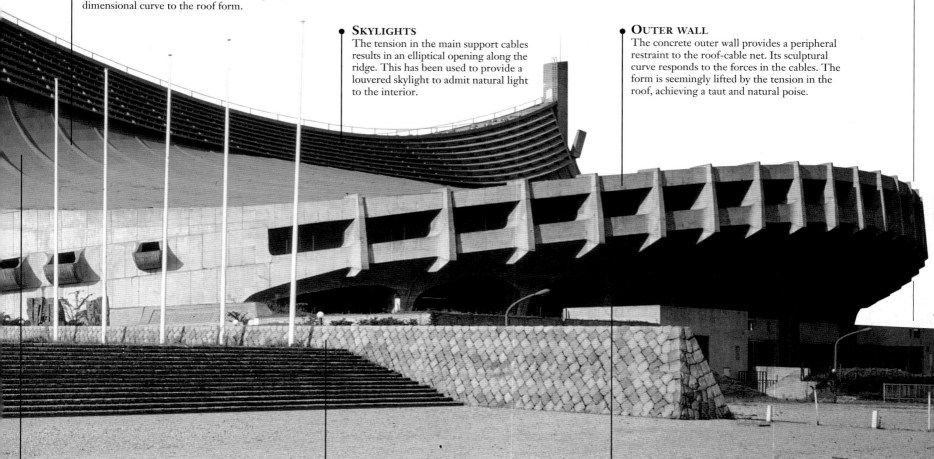

ROOF PROFILE
The undulating profile of the roof is calculated to allow uninterrupted sightlines for spectators within the stadium. The seats are arranged on raked tiers, cantilevered from the concrete piers that support the outer wall.

STONE PLINTH
The stonework of the retaining walls is reminiscent of the massive fortifications of Japanese feudal castles. The landscaping of the terraced levels complements the sculptural form of the stadia.

EXPOSED CONCRETE
The finished quality of exposed concrete is reliant on the precision of the joinery needed to produce the timber formwork, making it a particularly suitable material for the meticulous standards of Japanese construction.

THE POMPIDOU CENTRE

THE POMPIDOU CENTRE (1971–77) is situated in the historic heart of Paris. It has achieved notoriety both for its frank industrial aesthetic (in structure and materials) and for redefining the role of a civic cultural institution. Despite design revisions enforced during its construction, on its completion in 1977, it achieved popular acclaim, receiving six million visitors in its first year. The international competition for its design was won by the young and radical team of Renzo Piano and Richard Rogers, despite the reservations of the architectural establishment. The building was conceived as a large, free-spanning structure, designed to achieve optimum openness and flexibility, while reconciling the requirements of safety, security, and movement for huge numbers of people. The scheme concentrated the accommodation within an underground substructure and an elevated, steel-framed superstructure, releasing the ground-level and providing an open area for public gathering and street entertainment. The building provides gallery space, a library, cinema, and design centre. Power and environmental controls are distributed through vents at floor and ceiling level, creating an uninterrupted, serviced environment. With its lively piazza, it provides a memorable experience for its many visitors, now accustomed to its unconventional appearance and radical design.

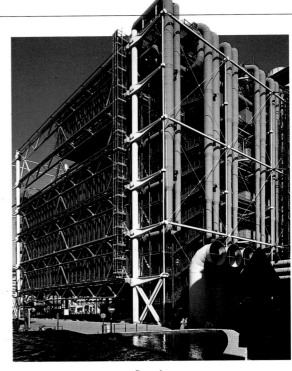

Services
The vertical tubes carrying electricity, water, drainage, and air-handling ducts are placed on the outside of the building. Boldly exposed in coded colours, their position enables accessibility for future modification while allowing flexibility of planning for the interior.

GERBERETTES
Rocker beams, called gerberettes, provide mechanical joints to the steel frame. Gerberettes are cast by spinning molten stainless steel, which allows them to be shaped to the line of forces within the beam. The scale of the span occasioned the unprecedented size of the castings. The structure uses a number of cast connections, lending the component joints a sculptural quality.

PIN-JOINTS
The use of flexible pin-joints within the frame prevents the over-stressing of components that occurs when small movements are locked into a rigid frame.

GLASS WALLS
External glass walls screen the unprotected areas of steel structure from the risk of internal fires. The walls are potentially removable, as they are independent of the building's structure.

PREFABRICATION
Each frame of the bay was constructed from prefabricated components and erected in 10 days. Site connections were screwed and bolted for quick assembly, with very few welded joints.

TRUSSES
Tubular steel floor-trusses provide bracing between the main framing members, spanning front to back.

TIE-RODS
Diagonal tie-rods cross-brace the main structural frames, which comprise 14 vertical six-storey steel frames.

BLINDS
Retractable solar blinds screen glazed façades, providing blackout facilities to gallery spaces.

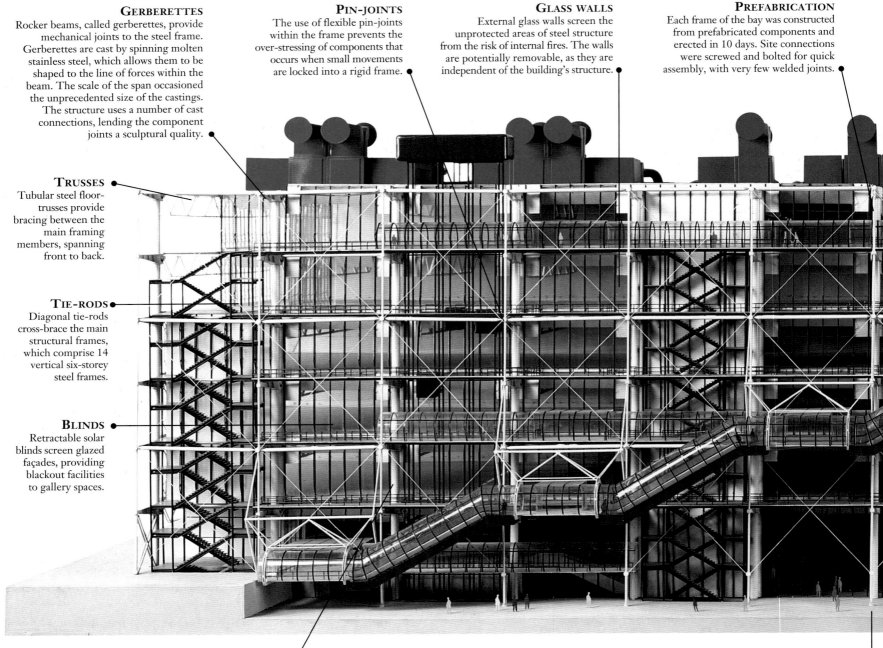

MAIN FRAME
The main frame is set back from the edge of the building, minimizing its impact on the façade and allowing views to and from the building through the delicate layers of structure and building envelope.

Open space for public activity and social gatherings is provided by confining the building to a part of the site that screens traffic noise and pollution from the piazza.

CONCRETE SUBSTRUCTURE
Located beneath the piazza there is underground parking space for up to 700 cars, a cinema, as well as extensive storage space and large areas for plant equipment.

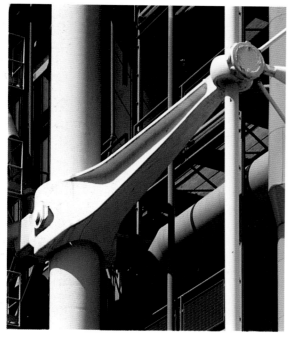

Structural Capabilities

To achieve its long span, the frame fully exploits the structural capabilities of the steelwork. Movement in the rocker-beam, or gerberette, allowed by a pin passing through the main column, puts the hollow column in compression, and the vertical steel rod, gripped at the lever's outer edge, in tension.

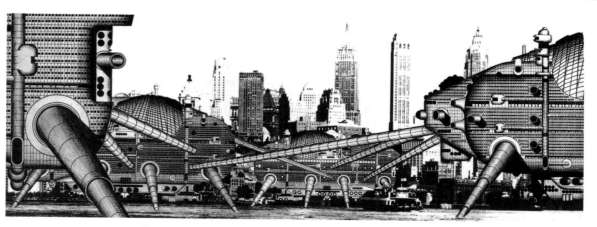

Walking City

The potential for the integration into architecture of advanced technology was explored by an influential group of British architects forming the Archigram group in 1960. The Walking City (1964) by Ron Herron, was one of a series of theoretical projects that used Pop Art and sci-fi imagery to challenge established notions about what buildings did, whom they served, and how they looked. The Pompidou Centre brings a number of these issues into fulfilment.

RENZO PIANO AND RICHARD ROGERS

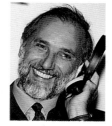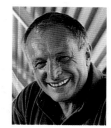

Renzo Piano (above left) (see p. 106) and Richard Rogers (right) (1933–) formed a partnership in 1970 for their competition entry for the Pompidou Centre. In separate careers they have established interests in structural and technological innovation and urban design. They maintain an influential position in contemporary architecture.

ESCALATOR

The 150-metre- (492-foot-) long escalator is suspended within a toughened glass tube, slung like a life-boat from the main structural frame. The escalator provides one of the best free views of the Parisian skyline.

The 48-metre- (157-foot-) span of the frame and the scale of the components required a sophisticated system for relieving stresses in the frame, caused by temperature and settlement movements between materials expanding at different rates.

SPECIFICATION

- **Location**   Paris, France
- **Date**   1971–77
- **Architects**   Renzo Piano, Richard Rogers
- **Building structure**   Steel-frame and concrete
- **Storeys**   6
- **Building type**   Cultural centre

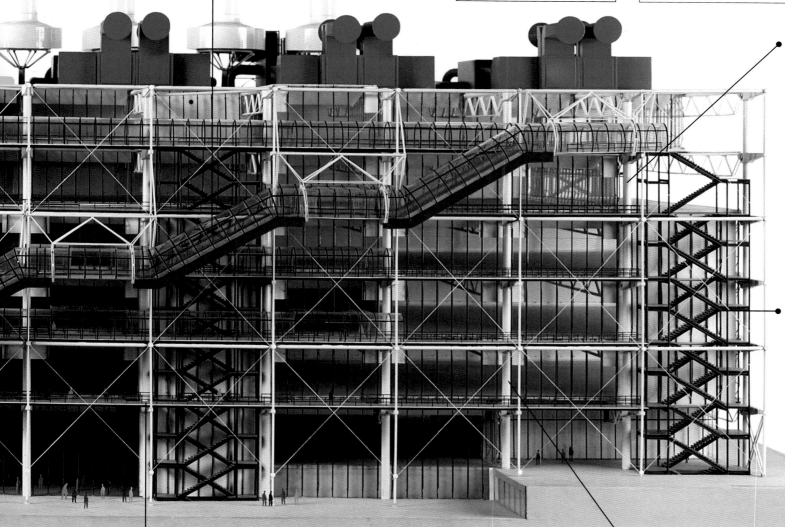

FIRE-PROOFING
Main structural components are protected by fire-proof jackets and over-cladding panels. Water-sprinkler systems, activated in the event of fire, are positioned to cool the structural connections and spray the glass screens.

FIRE-ESCAPE
The eight escape stairs are contained within independent steel towers.

FLOOR BEAMS
The columns, set back 7 metres (23 feet) from the building-face at 13-metre- (43-foot-) intervals, connect to the steel-lattice floor-beams that span the depth of the building.

The glass walls were originally intended to display projected images, incorporating electronic signage, conveying advertising and political messages. These were omitted, however, due to concern that they could be used for propaganda.

MAIN COLUMNS
Water-filled columns cool the building in the event of fire. Open at the top, the columns would allow the water to boil off, preventing the steel from becoming flexible and collapsing.

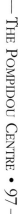

NEUE STAATSGALERIE

THE NEUE STAATSGALERIE (1977–84) in Stuttgart, Germany, by Sir James Stirling (with Michael Wilford) forms an extension to the existing Neoclassical art gallery. It was inspired by 19th-century galleries, notably the Altes Museum (see p. 64), and by the form of the buildings adjacent to the site. The competition brief required a public route through the building and a raised podium to conceal car parking. The galleries are arranged in a U-shaped block, raised on a podium, with administrative buildings to the rear. The central rotunda forms a sculpture court – the focal point of the gallery spaces and the public route through the site. A separate wing provides an experimental theatre. Approached by a ramp from the street, the podium provides access to the free-form lobby, dramatically lit by a curved, glass wall. The building quotes freely from an eclectic architectural vocabulary of Classical and Modernist forms. Stirling's virtuosic composition and rich, spatially innovative style introduce an uncompromising contemporary design in a complex, urban setting.

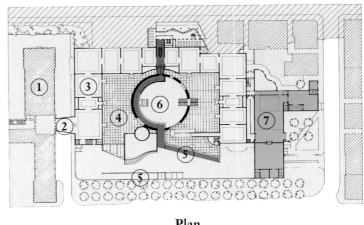

Plan

The building responds formally to the adjacent and facing buildings and to the existing galleries (1), which are connected by a bridge-link (2) to the gallery wings (3) forming a U-shaped plan enclosing the sculpture terrace (4). A sequence of ramps (5) brings visitors up from the street and continues a public route through the central rotunda (6) to the street at a higher level to the back of the site. A separate wing (7) houses an experimental theatre.

SCULPTURE TERRACE
The public terrace flows around the free-formed elements linking the separate parts of the gallery. This collage of sculptural objects is ordered against the simple backdrop of the U-shaped gallery wings.

Stirling exploits the form of the gallery to address fundamental issues of late-20th-century urban architecture – contextuality and urban space.

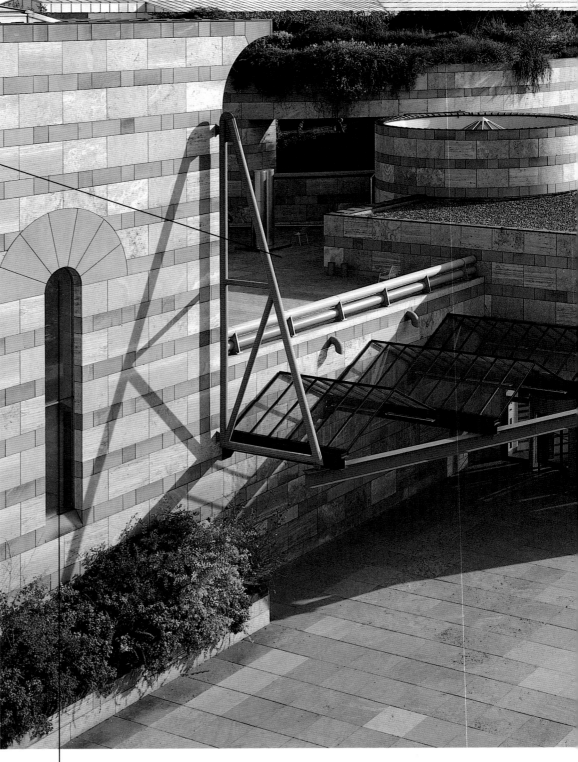

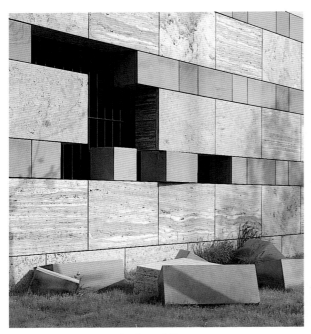

Blocks of Stone
The blocks of stone that appear to have tumbled from the opening in the podium wall – ventilating the car park – are scattered on the lawn. These stones are amongst the few solid blocks in the building, the façade being a thin, cladding veneer. Stirling's witty Mannerism reveals the edges of the building to expose its construction.

ARCHED WINDOWS
The Romanesque arched windows and Egyptian cornices are examples of the many motifs borrowed from a diverse architectural vocabulary.

The controversial competition proposal was criticized as monumental and overbearing, with uncomfortable associations with fascist, Neoclassical architecture. Yet the completed building, while monumental and ironic, is moderated by a skilful – and playful – handling of form and detail.

Central Courtyard
Overlooked by the public route, the central courtyard of the Staatsgalerie provides an active focus for the gallery spaces. The cylindrical form recalls the domed central space of Classical and Renaissance buildings. Though the building was famously criticized as "virtuosity around a void", the rotunda provides a memorable and identifiable civic space. The popularity of the scheme owes much to its architectural image of being both monumental and democratic, retaining a sense of humour that is more readily Mannerist than dogmatically Modernist, or indeed post-modern.

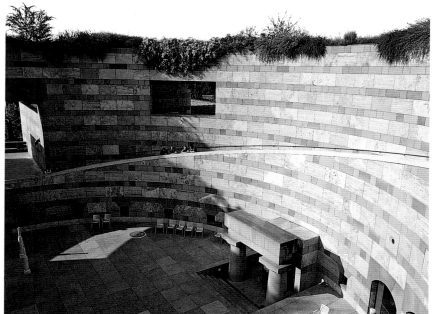

SIR JAMES STIRLING

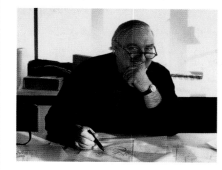

The architecture of Sir James Stirling (1926–92) demonstrates his enthusiasm for structure and technology. His eclectic range of influences are drawn from Modernist and Renaissance sources with great virtuosity and invention. Early buildings, such as Leicester University Engineering Building (1959–63), in partnership with James Gowan (1923–), established his reputation. Other buildings include the Cambridge University History Building (1964–67). Michael Wilford became a partner in 1971 and has continued the practice.

HANDRAILS
The brightly coloured tubular-steel handrails have been whimsically oversized to emphasize the circulation routes of the ramp. Other elements, such as ventilation grills and entrance canopies, have been similarly scaled-up for visual emphasis.

AEDICULE
The steel and glass canopy (aedicule) marks the central line of the building as viewed from the street. However, unlike with a conventional Classical plan, visitors are diverted from what appears to be a centrally placed entrance towards the ramped approach to the first-floor podium and entrance foyer.

The design acknowledges the form of the adjacent buildings (its context) and the precedent of the art gallery as a 19th-century building type, such as Karl Friedrich Schinkel's Altes Museum (see p. 64).

SPECIFICATION

•*Location*	Stuttgart, Germany
•*Date*	1977–84
•*Architect*	Sir James Stirling
•*Building structure*	Masonry, steel, and reinforced concrete
•*Storeys*	2
•*Building type*	Art gallery

ENTRANCE LOBBY
The curved entrance lobby resembles, in plan, the piano-shaped curves of many of Le Corbusier's Modernist buildings. The foyer provides an informal place of assembly for visitors, directing them towards the peripheral circulation routes of the gallery wings.

PODIUM
The podium, which conceals the ground-floor car park, elevates the public space above the noise and pollution of the busy main road.

"In addition to the representational and abstract, this large complex, I hope, supports the monumental and informal; also the traditional and hi-tech"
SIR JAMES STIRLING

HONG KONG AND SHANGHAI BANK

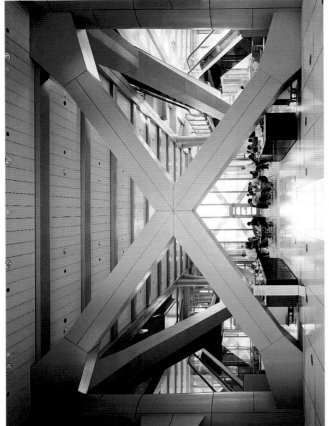

CONSTRUCTED IN FOUR YEARS ON A RESTRICTED SITE, in scale and complexity, this building represents a remarkable technological achievement. Commissioned at a time of political uncertainty, the building is a symbol of confidence in Hong Kong's future as an international centre of finance trading. Foster Associates' initial scheme was based on the concept of "phased regeneration". This would allow flexibility for the constructional phases, keeping the existing banking building on the site in commission until the final phase. The new building, towering over the existing bank, was to be constructed in vertical slices. This concept gave rise to the building's characteristic and identifiable superstructure. The vertical mast towers, which support the floors in tiers of office space, are suspended from the large horizontal steel trusses. Though the idea of phased regeneration was later abandoned in order to utilize the basement levels within the scheme, the positioning of the structural frame at either end of the floor plan allows uninterrupted, flexible planning of the office space. This flexibility is a consistent design philosophy which is used to anticipate future adaptations within the controlling organization of the building's structure.

Main Trusses

Cross-bracing connects the main coat-banger trusses, which occur at eight-storey intervals. The trusses are two storeys high, allowing double-height spaces within staff areas, such as lift lobbies and the restaurant. At the lift lobbies, passengers transfer from the lifts, which connect the main lobby areas, on to escalators to access individual floors. This provides a greater volume of movement within the building and encourages familiarity among company members.

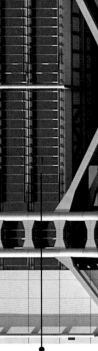

During construction, the loading cranes were mounted on the mast towers to save space on site. During high winds, when typhoon conditions made the site inoperable, the cranes were fitted with wind-vanes, which allowed them to move freely, preventing their collision.

SIR NORMAN FOSTER

The architecture of Sir Norman Foster (1935–) embodies the integral use of technology and new materials, combined with the discipline of structural engineering. Technology is seen as a liberating servant, allowing buildings to meet human needs in a complex and rapidly changing society. Commissions have included office buildings, airports, art galleries, and furniture design. Notable commissions are: the Willis, Faber, Dumas building, Ipswich, England (1975); and the Sainsbury Centre, Norwich, England (1978).

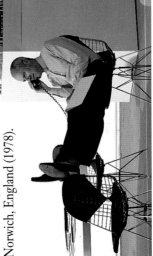

Floor Plan

Eight structural towers, each comprising four columns, are arranged in two rows of four and are positioned at the east and west ends of the building. The service towers, housing lifts and toilets, are grouped at either end and are connected vertically. The diagonal arrangement of the escalators, positioned according to the Chinese practice of Feng Shui, lends a dynamic geometry to the entrance levels and banking hall.

Suspension members
Office floor area
Escalators
Entrance/Lift lobby
Mast towers
Atrium
Service towers

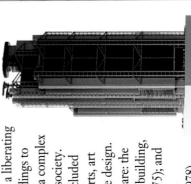

OFFICE PLANNING
Three principles were adopted in the layout of each floor: to use cellular offices to screen points of arrival and passage; to allow the maximum number of occupants views; and to preserve the fluidity and transparency of internal space.

LIFT AND SERVICE TOWERS

Grouped around the main structural frame, lift and service towers containing toilets and local air-conditioning units are positioned at either end of the floor plan. Prefabricated units were hoisted into place in completely assembled modules, reducing site storage and facilitating rapid construction.

MAST TOWERS

The principal vertical loads are supported on the four-column mast towers that rise from the foundation levels. Constructed in prefabricated tubular-steel sections, the masts are sheathed with jackets of concrete, foil, and aluminium panels to protect them from corrosion and fire.

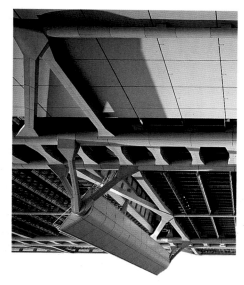

Sunscoop

Externally positioned on the south side of the building, at the upper level of the atrium, the sunscoop tracks the Sun's movement. Using a series of mirrors, it reflects light into the central atrium to the lower levels of the banking hall and the public plaza.

AIR-CONDITIONING

The area allocated for air-conditioning equipment was greatly reduced by cooling the system with seawater provided by an underground tunnel from the bay. It supplies the basement refrigeration plant at a rate of 1,250 litres (275 gallons) per second.

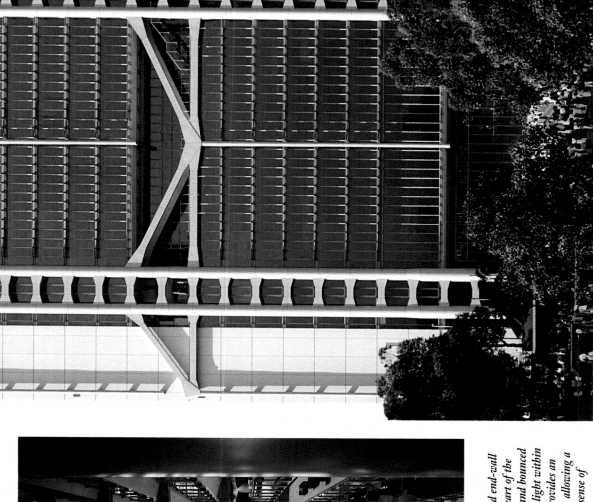

GLAZED PANELS

Made from sandwiched layers of glass and fine mesh, the glazed panels incorporate sunscreen canopies, which control direct sunlight glare and prevent overheating within the work spaces at the perimeter of the building.

CENTRAL SUSPENSION MEMBER

A centrally placed suspension member connects the floors to the coat-hanger trusses.

The scaffolding for the building was made from traditional bamboo poles lashed together with nylon ties. This arrangement produces an economical, light, and flexible temporary structure.

COAT-HANGER TRUSSES

Horizontal trusses positioned at eight-storey intervals suspend the lower tier of floor space. The trusses connect to the vertical load-bearing masts, which transfer the loads to the ground. The two-storey-high trusses give a distinctive rhythm to the façade.

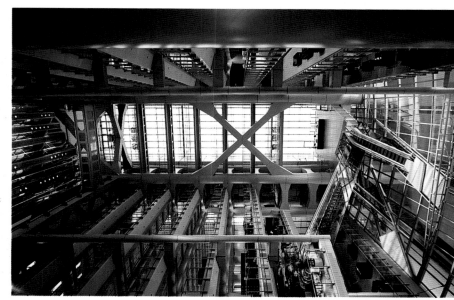

Atrium

The internal 12-storey atrium is lit by the glazed end-wall and by natural light that is reflected into the heart of the building. Sunlight is reflected from the sunscoop and bounced off the ceiling reflectors, to give changing pools of light within the atrium and the public plaza. The atrium provides an active and dramatic internal focus to the building, allowing a deeper plan for office space and promoting a sense of community amongst employees and customers.

SPECIFICATION	
•Location	Hong Kong
•Date	1981–85
•Architect	Sir Norman Foster
•Height	179 m (587 ft)
•Storeys	43
•Building structure	Steel-frame
•Building type	Office
•Construction time	4 years

The mast towers are each supported on four concrete-pile foundations below the four basement levels, cast into shafts manually excavated out of the bedrock.

SCHLUMBERGER CAMBRIDGE RESEARCH CENTRE

THE SCHLUMBERGER Cambridge Research Centre, England (1982–85 and 1990–92), brings a distinctive silhouette to the flat Cambridgeshire landscape. Commissioned as a test-and-research station, the architectural form combines with the pastoral setting of the distant church spires and conveys the excitement of a travelling circus. Accommodating all aspects of industrial research into oil exploration, the design integrates the conflicting spatial requirements of the large-volume industrial test station and staff restaurant, housed under the tented enclosure, with the cellular work spaces and laboratories arranged in wings of single-storey office suites. A second pair of buildings was added to the site in 1992, housing additional laboratories and conference facilities. The commanding spectacle of the mast-and-tented structure, particularly when internally illuminated at night, lends a theatrical image to an industrial building.

SPECIFICATION

- **Location**　　Cambridge, England
- **Date**　　1982–85 (Phase 1) 1990–92 (Phase 2)
- **Architects**　　Michael Hopkins and Partners
- **Building structure**　　Exoskeletal steel-frame, and tensile structure
- **Building type**　　Research centre

FABRIC CANOPY
The Teflon-coated canopy enclosing the test-bay area is lightweight and translucent. Tension in the stretched fabric keeps the tent from flapping in the wind. The structure is designed to prevent uplift – holding the building down as well as up.

WOVEN FABRIC
The fabric, woven from glass fibre, is pattern cut from strips and seamed together by heat welding.

EXOSKELETAL FRAME
The exoskeletal (positioned outside the building envelope) frame supports the building without the additional fire-protecting layers required by internal steel structures exposed to the risk of fire.

WORK AREAS
The work spaces are contained within two single-storey glass-and-steel framed wings. Work stations face outwards; meeting rooms and laboratories face into the courtyard.

Phase Two External Wall
The ground-floor glazed wall is shaded by the oversailing concrete floor slab. This was produced using a combination of precast ferro cement coffers, acting as a framework, and the in situ concrete slab. It has a highly sculptural profile, producing a lightweight section of great strength. The cost of maintaining this quality of finish is offset by savings resulting from lighter foundations, and from leaving the ceiling exposed. The coffered soffit allows for the discreet integration of lighting and an elegant, detailed junction with the column.

Phased Extension
The project was conceived as a research campus accommodating phased expansion. Phase Two comprises a pair of pavilions arranged along the main axis. Developments in computer-research techniques have reduced the need for reliance on the test rig, and the new blocks provide additional computer laboratories connected by a central atrium and reception area. The roof of the atrium is again a tent structure, but here formed by a self-supporting, inflated, three-layer cushion.

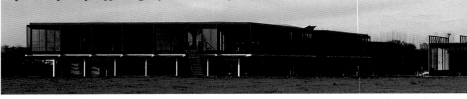

Phase Two section of building

TENSILE STRUCTURE
The canopy is supported by a web of steel cables strung to tubular-steel masts. The wires anchored to the ground counterbalance the load in an efficient structural system that keeps the wire and fabric in tension and the masts in compression.

DRAINAGE
Rainwater runs off the tent membrane and is discharged on to the flat roofs of the single-storey bays, where it is run off into concealed down-pipes.

FIXING DETAILS
The fixing details are clean and direct, inspired both by traditional tented structures and the trimmed sails of hi-tech racing yachts.

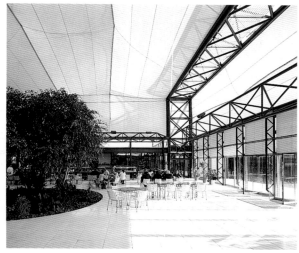

MICHAEL HOPKINS AND PARTNERS

Sir Michael Hopkins (1935–) formed the partnership in 1976 with his wife, Lady Hopkins (left), continuing principles set out whilst in practice with Norman Foster (see p. 100) between 1968 and 1976. The clarity of design and the bespoke use of new and traditional materials combine with a great sensitivity to their contextual setting, earning the partnership widespread acclaim.

INSULATED ROOF
The highly insulated, flat roof of the single storey bays offsets the heat lost through the extensively glazed areas of the façade, which comprise the double-glazed sliding wall panels. Electrically operated blinds reduce glare and solar gain.

Winter Garden and Restaurant
The restaurant and garden are housed under the tensile fabric structure. The test area is separated from the garden and restaurant by a laminated-glass screen wall, which affords protected observation of the test area, thus providing a social space with a direct connection to the research activity of the building.

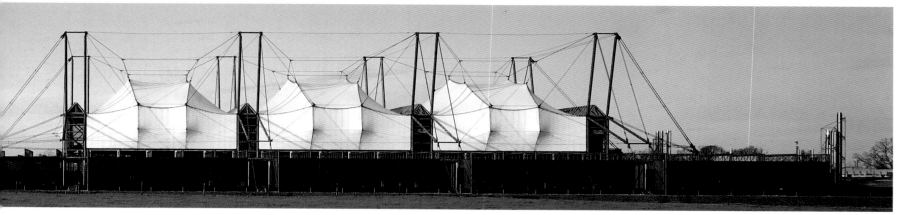

Phase One section of building

THE ARK

SURROUNDED BY AN ELEVATED HIGHWAY and a surface railroad line, the Ark (1989–92) by Ralph Erskine establishes a strong, physical presence in a densely urban environment. The external carapace focuses the building inward toward the large central atrium and protects it from noise and pollution, offering a civilizing social area at the center of this speculatively built office building. The organic, pebble-shaped space increases the rentable area of the mid-level office floors while admitting sunlight onto the island site at the ground-floor entrance level. Erskine's experience with social housing and the inhospitable winter climate of his adopted Sweden are brought to the design of a convivial working environment. The atrium provides interlinking spaces, promoting opportunities for discussion and social interaction. The project is an imaginative, collaborative exercise between the developer and consultant designers – an attempt to introduce an enlightened view of the contemporary workplace into an unprepossessing urban site.

VENTILATION
Computerized controls regulate the supply of air through service ducts, which prioritize natural ventilation through the atrium, reducing the need for mechanical extraction.

The appearance and form of contemporary buildings are increasingly influenced by the choice of materials and methods of environmental control, reducing energy consumption in both manufacture and running costs. About one-half of all the energy produced in Western Europe is currently expended on servicing buildings.

VIEWING TOWER
Whimsical elements break through the building envelope, such as the snorkel-like viewing tower, which provides a panoramic view from the glass-enclosed informal meeting room.

ROOF LIGHT
A glass slot allows natural light into the atrium. In the event of fire, automatically opening vents and ducts would force the discharge of smoke, enabling the office floors to open directly onto the atrium.

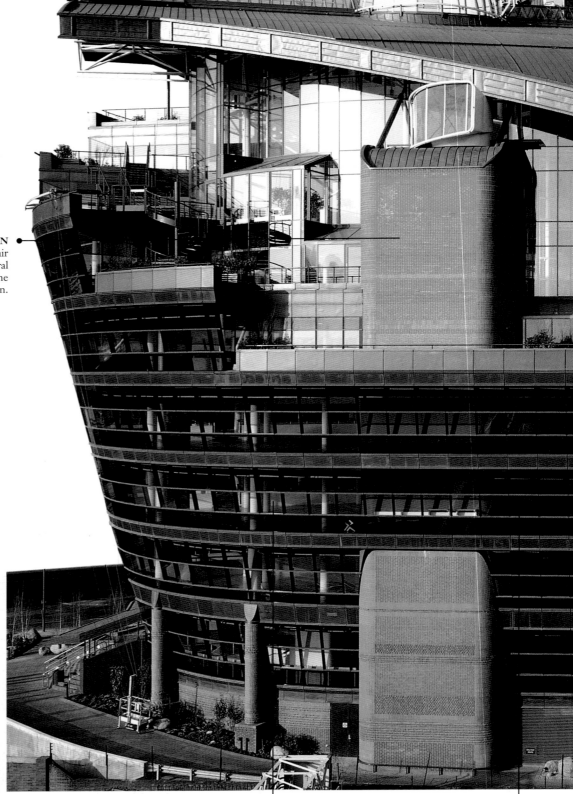

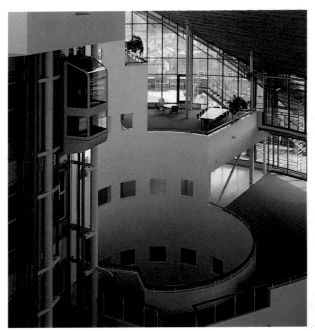

Atrium
Naturally lit, the atrium provides fresh-air ventilation to the open office areas. The area cut out of the floor plates, producing the open atrium, provides spatial variation and direct visual contact across and between levels.

CURVED GLASS
The curved skin inadvertently provides an externally reflective wall, directing traffic noise back to surrounding streets. The building has, therefore, been criticized for detrimentally affecting adjacent sites.

TRIPLE-GLAZED PANELS
Reducing traffic to a mute spectacle, the triple-glazed panels provide an effective barrier to pollution and noise from the surrounding site.

Plan

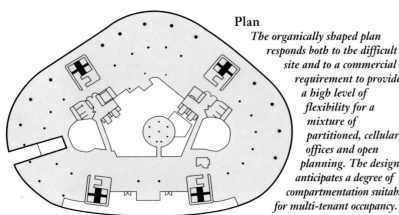

The organically shaped plan responds both to the difficult site and to a commercial requirement to provide a high level of flexibility for a mixture of partitioned, cellular offices and open planning. The design anticipates a degree of compartmentation suitable for multi-tenant occupancy.

RALPH ERSKINE

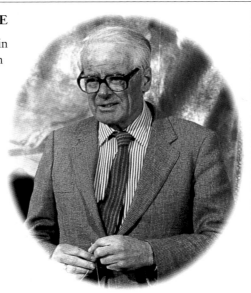

Ralph Erskine (1914–) studied in London and has lived in Sweden since 1939. Many of Erskine's designs are generated in response to climatic conditions and social relationships. His large housing scheme at Byker in Newcastle-upon-Tyne, England (1969–80), uses the form of the building to protect and nurture, providing sheltered spaces for social interaction. This principle has been adopted in a commercial context for the Ark.

TERRACE
The oversailing eaves provide shelter to the terraced areas. Screened from the noise of traffic, the effects of building form, orientation, and position produce specific microclimates that can improve the immediate environment even in inhospitable situations.

Fragmented urban sites, particularly those remaindered around cumbersome transport networks, provide important gaps for future city development. Though commercially undesirable, imaginative ideas are essential if pressure on the city periphery is to be relieved and urban expansion resisted, maintaining an amenable level of open space within urban streets and parks.

COPPER ROOF
The wall panels and copper roof that conceal the ends of the floor slabs are exposed to rain and pollution and will eventually take on a weathered finish.

SPECIFICATION

- **Location** — London, England
- **Date** — 1989–92
- **Architect** — Ralph Erskine
- **Building structure** — Concrete-frame and brick
- **Building type** — Offices

LILLA HUSET
The Lilla Huset (little house), a two-storey building given over to community use, was built within the site boundary. It was provided by the developer as a trade-off against commercial usage of the site. This practice is known as "planning gain".

CONCRETE STRUCTURE
The concrete frame is given additional bracing by the service towers.

Many new buildings now passively reclaim, utilize and store the vast amounts of latent energy previously expelled during cooling and ventilation. Through a variety of active and passive methods, buildings are striving for a level of self-sustainability.

TEXTURAL SURFACE
The bricks used for the cladding of the towers are positioned with the broken edges facing outwards, providing a highly textural surface.

LIFT AND SERVICE TOWERS
The lift and service towers rise through the building, housing stairs and lifts and a pressurized air intake to supply the central atrium.

KANSAI INTERNATIONAL AIRPORT TERMINAL

J APAN'S **KANSAI INTERNATIONAL AIRPORT TERMINAL** (1991–94)
appears to hover like a glider, weightlessly poised at its moment
of landing, above the artificial island in Osaka Bay. Gently curving over
its 1.7 kilometre (1 mile) length, the terminal joins the Great Wall of China
as being one of the two (non-natural) structures discernible from space. Its
building programme required the levelling of three mountains to provide
the land mass, the construction of a transport bridge 5 kilometres (3 miles)
long, and the erection of a building capable of maintaining horizontal
alignment, despite anticipated site settlement of 11 metres (36 feet). The
elegant design solution to the complex activities of a modern airport integrates
structure, function, and environment with a sense of harmony and clarity of
purpose. Its dramatic presence and inspiring sense of technological
achievement make it one of the most impressive
architectural projects of the
20th century.

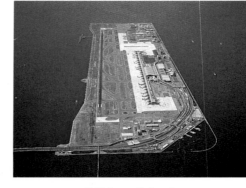

Offshore Island
*The costs and constructional difficulties incurred by
erecting an airport in a typhoon zone 5 kilometres
(3 miles) offshore are outweighed by the advantages
of a site operational on a 24-hour basis, offering
future expansion, and no noise restrictions.*

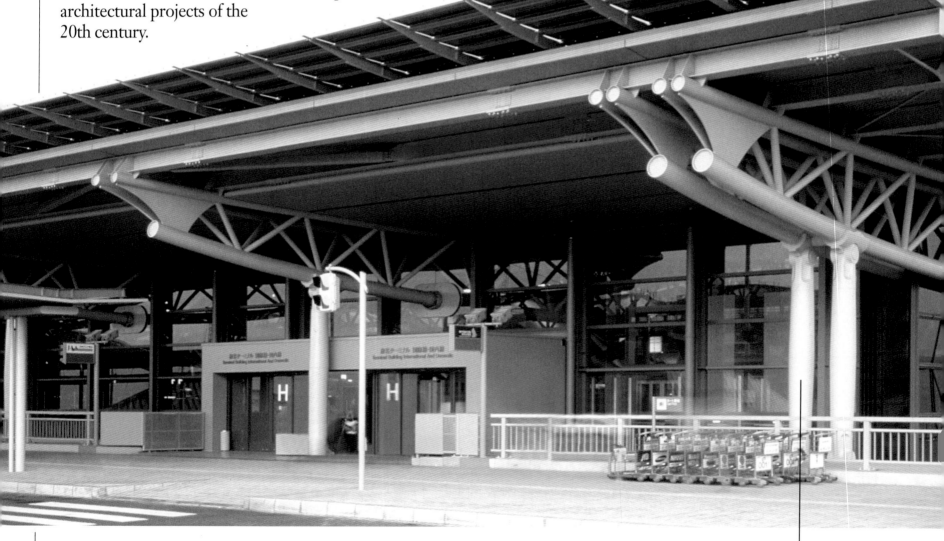

RENZO PIANO

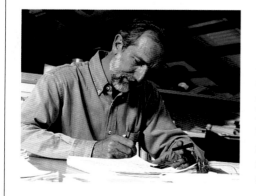

The work of Renzo Piano (1937–) has
continually demonstrated conceptually,
and technically, creative solutions to
architectural, engineering, and urban
design commissions. Piano's continued
collaboration with the engineer, Peter
Rice, has matured the raw hi-tech style of
the Pompidou Centre (see p. 96) through
a process of continual investigation into
new technologies, design methods, and
computer-aided design.

SPECIFICATION

- **Location**   Osaka Bay, Japan
- **Date**   1991–94
- **Architect**   Renzo Piano
- **Building structure**   Steel-frame
- **Building type**   Airport
- **Construction time**   3 years, 2 months

COLUMNS
Each of the 900 supporting columns
is continually adjusted on hydraulic,
computer-controlled jacks to compensate
for continual site settlement.

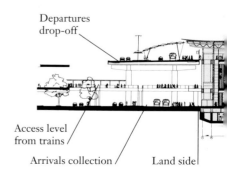

Departures drop-off

Access level from trains

Arrivals collection   Land side

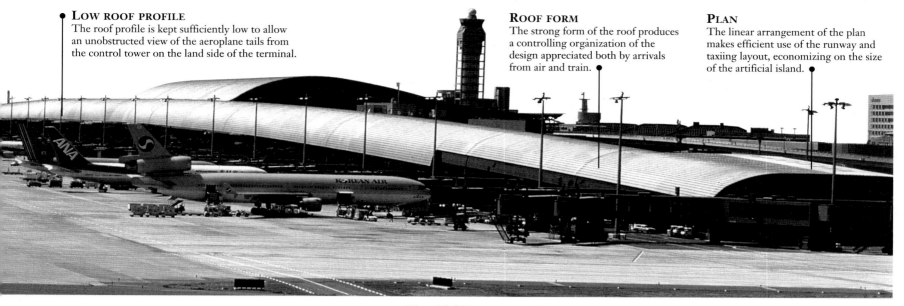

LOW ROOF PROFILE
The roof profile is kept sufficiently low to allow an unobstructed view of the aeroplane tails from the control tower on the land side of the terminal.

ROOF FORM
The strong form of the roof produces a controlling organization of the design appreciated both by arrivals from air and train.

PLAN
The linear arrangement of the plan makes efficient use of the runway and taxiing layout, economizing on the size of the artificial island.

Toroidal Form
The toroidal form of the roof – rather like the segment of a bicycle tyre – curves both across its section and along its 1.7 kilometre (1 mile) length. The 300-metre- (984-foot-) length of the central terminal spans 82 metres (269 feet) on tubular-steel trusses. The symmetrical wings forming the flight lounges are supported on steel ribs of different length but same curvature.

DRAINAGE
Rainwater is drained at the edges of each panel to a waterproof layer beneath. This reduces surface dirt and staining, and maintains the thermal reflectivity and appearance of the roof.

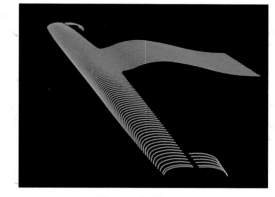

EXPANSION JOINTS
Between the structure and the skin of the building there are expansion joints at sectional intervals, which tolerate seismic and thermal movements.

CURVATURE
The gentle curvature of the roof enables all the 90,000 stainless steel panels to be of identical size, simplifying all joints and components.

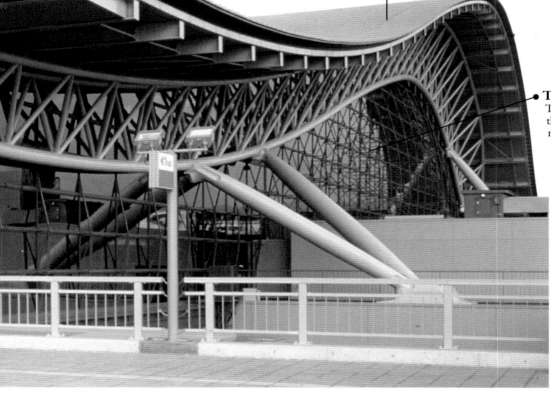

Dynamic Form
The building's form is both symmetrical and directional. The design emphasizes the movement and direction of its passengers in the same elegant and legible way that an aeroplane body and wing shape summarize the dynamics of flight.

TRANSPARENCY
The large areas of glazing allow a transparency throughout the building, helping visitors to orientate themselves and move easily to their destination within the building.

The terminal was divided between two construction teams of 4,000 to 10,000 workers – one working from the north, the other from the south, and meeting in the middle. The project was completed in three years and two months.

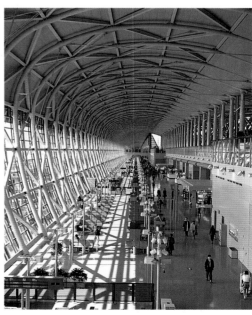

Cross-section
The central terminal has a tiered arrangement allowing passengers to transfer quickly between international and domestic flights. Most passengers arrive, or leave, by mainland trains accessed from the land side of the terminal.

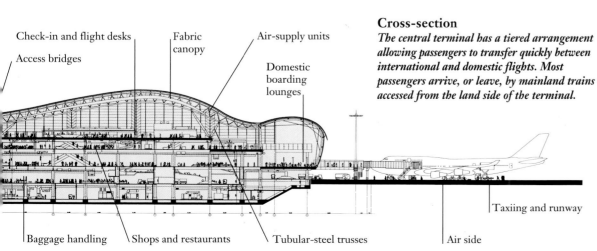

Check-in and flight desks

Access bridges

Fabric canopy

Air-supply units

Domestic boarding lounges

Taxiing and runway

Baggage handling

Shops and restaurants

Tubular-steel trusses

Air side

Curved Roof
The length of the flight lounge wings is visually relieved by the subtly rising curve of the roof and the rhythmical articulation of the structure. The curve of the roof is aerodynamically designed to assist the movement of filtered fresh air, introduced to the space from large, high-level vents.

GLOSSARY

Aedicule Two columns and a pediment framing a shrine. Device used in Neoclassicism to frame a doorway or window opening.

Aisle Lower section of a church, running parallel to the nave, separated from it by columns or a screen wall.

Alberti, Leon Battista (1404–72) Architect and artist, theorist and mathematician, accomplished in many arts and sciences – exemplar of the tradition of Renaissance diversity of interests. Remembered particularly for his architectural treatise *De re aedificatoria* (1485), the first Renaissance systematic theory of proportion, order, and harmony. He defined architectural beauty as being, "the harmony and concord of all the parts, achieved in such a manner that nothing could be added or taken away or altered except to the detriment to the whole."

Apse A large semi-circular or rectagonal recess terminating the chancel at the eastern end of a church.

Atrium Courtyard at the centre of a building that rises through consecutive floors. Derived from Roman courtyard houses, in contemporary use the atrium is often covered, providing natural light and visual contact throughout the building.

Axonometric Three-dimensional drawing projected vertically from a plan that has been rotated through an angle of 45 degrees.

Baroque A form of architecture prevalent throughout Europe during the 17th and early-18th centuries. Developed from the Classically inspired styles of the Italian Renaissance towards distinct national characteristics. Often bold, monumental, decorative, and spatially complex.

Bauhaus German school of art, craft, architecture, and industrial design, originally founded at Weimar in 1906. Led from 1916 by architect Walter Gropius (1883–1969), the school absorbed a number of European avant-garde tendencies, notably De Stijl and Russian Constructivism. Their teachings, which joined together architects, artists, and designers, became a fundamental influence in the development of modern architecture, disseminated throughout the world following its closure by the Gestapo in 1933.

Bow-string truss A composite structural device whereby the load-bearing capacity of the main beam is improved by a lower-tension chord and intermediate vertical or diagonal compression struts in the form of a horizontal bow.

Capital The crowning feature placed on to the shaft of a column, primarily to spread the load transferred from the supported entablature to the column itself. Subject to stylized decoration and often used to identify the classification of architectural Order.

Centring Temporary framework, usually made of timber, used for support during the construction of arches, vaults, and domes.

Chancel Section of the east end of the nave reserved for the clergy and the choir, often separated from the nave by a screen. Also referred to as the choir.

Clerestory The upper part of a building with windows located above adjacent roofs. Found particularly in churches, allowing light to enter the nave and aisles.

Compound column Supporting column comprising multiple attached or detailed shafts. Reduces the visual mass of the support and maintains a large load-bearing cross-sectional area.

Corbel Projecting block of stone used for the support of other structural members, such as beams, or for consecutive courses of projecting stonework to produce a simple vault or dome. Often elaborately carved or moulded.

Crocket Motif or leaf design carved into the projecting ribs that decorate parapets and towers of Gothic buildings and their derivatives.

Curtain wall A lightweight outside wall held off the main structural frame which serves no load-bearing purpose. A requisite of high-rise buildings and a familiar device of modern architecture, allowing a freedom of elevational composition and the use of large areas of glazing in the façade.

Dentil A small, square block projecting from the cornice of a Classical entablature, providing a rhythmical façade.

Enfilade The arrangement of rooms leading from one to another. Connecting doors are often placed in alignment to produce a continuous vista when opened.

Engaged column Column with a shaft attached or incorporated into the thickness of a wall or pier.

Entablature The upper part of an Order of architecture supported by the colonnade.

Finial Crowning ornament placed at the top of a spire or roof pinnacle.

Fluting Concave grooves carved into the shaft of a column, characteristic of Classical Orders. Produces an emphasis on vertical form and volume by creating distinctive shadow lines.

Flying buttress A buttress that stands away from the wall it reinforces, providing support via an arch at the main point of stress.

Geomancy The sacred geometry of architecture. Usually derived from alignment with auspicious groups of star constellations, the Sun or Moon, or axial alignment with distant or adjacent sites.

Hexastyle Classical portico with six supporting columns.

Hypostyle Hall in which the roof is supported by a multitude of columns at close intervals.

Keystone Central closing stone at the top of an arch, constructed from segmental blocks.

Kiosk A light, open pavilion or summerhouse usually supported by pillars.

Latin cross A cross with one long and three short arms. Developed from the plan of the Roman basilican church, the latin cross accommodated lateral transepts

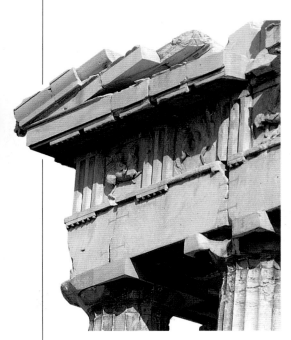

Detail of the entablature from
The Parthenon
See page 10

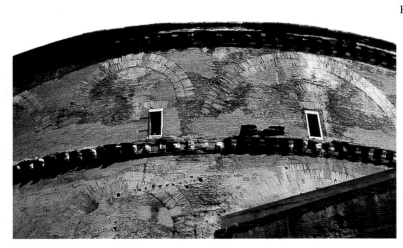

Relieving arches from
The Pantheon
See page 14

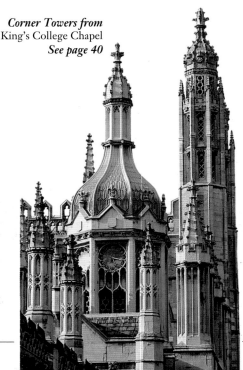

Corner Towers from
King's College Chapel
See page 40

and became the characteristic plan of the Christian church.

Lintel Horizontal supporting beam that spans an opening in a wall or between columns.

Mannerism A stylistic trend of 16th-century Italian architecture, that departed from Classical conventions of Orders and proportion to produce an exaggerated effect by subverting and manipulating architectural forms.

Metope The section of a Classical entablature between triglyphs. Left plain or with carved decoration.

Muqarnas Quintessential form of Islamic decoration and construction using an elaborately molded corbel to create the characteristic honeycomb or stalactite form of arch-and-vaulted structures.

Naos Principal chamber of a Greek temple or the core of a Byzantine church.

Nave The main body of a church to the west of the central crossing. Often flanked by aisles.

Oculus A round window.

Order Used in Classical architecture to describe the base, shaft, capital, and entablature, constituting the architectural form that conforms to prescribed proportion and decorative stylization. Principally Doric, Tuscan, Ionic, Corinthian, and Composite.

Palladianism An architectural style favored in England during the 18th century, derived from the architecture and publications of Andrea Palladio (1508–80). It spread to America in the mid-18th century and became an accepted style for grand residences and civic buildings.

Parapet A low wall screening the roof or protecting the edge of a bridge or quay.

Pavilion An ornamental building placed amid a landscaped setting. Can also be an independently expressed part of a larger building, wing, or façade.

Pediment The triangular section of wall above the entablature surmounting a portico or gable wall.

Pendentive The curved triangular surface formed between the base of the dome and the corners of the supporting structure.

Peristyle A range of columns surrounding a building or courtyard.

Piano nobile The raised floor of a building containing the principal living rooms.

Picturesque A style illustrating the late-18th-century taste for painting and architecture, depicting buildings in a landscape setting.

Pylon The gateway structure to an Egyptian temple comprising massive rectilinear towers with inclining walls.

Rationalism Architectural movement seeking to adopt rationalized and reasoned solutions to design problems, in opposition to historicist and formulaic design traditions. Usually realized through a conscious expression of structural system and constructional materials. The movement emerged through the 18th-century architecture of the French Enlightenment and was championed by French architect and critic Viollet-le-Duc, who interpreted it as an intrinsic quality of Gothic architecture. Developed throughout the 20th century in the teaching of the German Bauhaus, and by architects such as Mies van der Rohe (1886–1969), it became a central principle of Modernism.

Renaissance Derived from the Italian word for rebirth and applied to the artistic movement emanating from Italy in the 15th century. Its influence extended throughout Europe, beginning with a revival of interest in Classical architecture and developing through an extension of the Classical vocabulary into a profusion of national styles. Eventually succeeded by the Baroque period, commencing in the mid-16th century, and continuing with later developments throughout Europe.

Rib Projecting band on a ceiling or vault, often forming the primary structural frame.

Romanesque Prevalent style of architecture in western Europe from the 9th to the 12th century. Characterized by the use of the semicircular arch and simple arcaded and barrel-vaulted structures.

Serlio, Sebastiano (1475–1554) Author of *L'Architettura*, published in six parts between 1537 and 1551, giving a practical account of the Classical Orders of architecture and helping to disseminate the Renaissance throughout Europe.

Stijl (de) A small but highly influential group of architects and artists formed in Utrecht, Holland, in 1917. They sought a radical renewal of society through avant-garde methods of expression that adopted nonrepresentational form and the expansive use of planar geometry and primary colors.

Stoa Detached colonnade found in Classical Greek architecture.

Stucco Plaster work used in imitation of stone, often decoratively incised or elaborately molded.

Trabeated Structural systems comprising posts and beams used for simple support.

Transept The transverse arms joining the main nave or chancel of a church to form the characteristic cruciform plan.

Triglyph Projecting block incised with two vertical grooves, producing a rhythmic decoration on the frieze of Classical buildings.

Tympanum The expanse of wall between the lintel and the supporting arch above. Also used to describe the triangular area enclosed by the form of a pediment.

Vault An arched structure made of stone or brick covering a building. Types inlcude barrel (or tunnel), cross, fan, pendant, and rib.

Vitruvius (Active 46–30 BC) A relatively unknown Roman architect serving under Julius Caesar. Author of *De architectura*, the only surviving work on architecture passed from antiquity. Although obscurely written in ten volumes, it became a major source of reference for Renaissance architects.

Ziggurat A tower structure rising in consecutive and diminishing levels reached by stairs or a ramp.

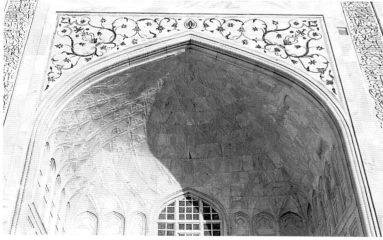

Fine decoration from
The Taj Mahal
See page 54

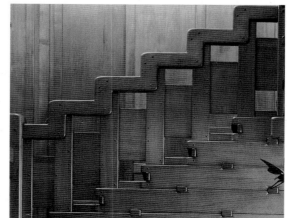

Staircase from
Gamble House
See page 76

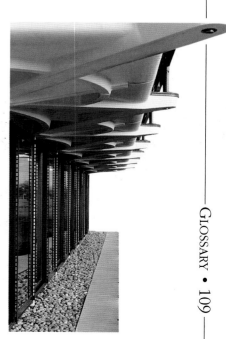

Phase Two external wall from
Schlumberger Cambridge Research Centre
See page 102

INDEX

ACKNOWLEDGMENTS

Author's acknowledgments

I should like to acknowledge Neil Lockley, Simon Murrell, Julie Oughton, Deborah Pownall, Gwen Edmonds, and Christine Winters for their dedication throughout the project; and to thank Sean Moore for his encouragement. In addition,

I would like to thank all at Sagar Stevenson Architects for their patience during my periodic absence while undertaking this work. My thanks also to Melanie and Louis for their constancy and companionship.

Dorling Kindersley would like to thank:

Will Hodgkinson, Karen Homer, Rebecca Munford for editorial assistance; Kathy Gill for the index; Robert Polidori for additional photography, and Deborah Pownall for her splendid picture research.

PICTURE CREDITS

Every effort has been made to trace the copyright holders and we apologize in advance for any unintentional omissions. We would be pleased to insert the appropriate acknowledgment in any subsequent edition of this publication.

Key
t: top, *b*: bottom, *c*: centre, *r*: right, *l*: left

Aerofilms 60*tr*.
AKG/ Eric Lessing 64-5, 65*tl*.
Annan Gallery, Glasgow 75*bc*.
Arcaid back cover *trc*, back cover *br*, back cover *bc*, 4*tl*, 4*c*, 10*cl*, 37*bl*, 46-7, 48*tr*, /**Richard Bryant** 50-1, 51*tr*, /**William Tingey** 53*tr*, /**Clay Perry** 60-1, 66*tr*, 72*bl*, 74*tl*, 75*bc*, 75*br*, 78-9, 79*tl*, 79*tr*, /**Richard Bryant** 80-1, 80*cl*, 84-5, 86-7, /**William Tingey** 94*tl*, 95*cr*, /**Richard Bryant** 98-9, 98*bl*, 100*tl*, 101*bl*, 102-3*b*, 104-5, 104*bl*, 106-7, 108*bl*.
Archigram Archives/ Ron Herron 96*tr*.
Axiom/ Jim Holmes 14*tr*, 16*cl*, 17*tr*, 17*cr*, 29*tl*, 34-5, 45*tr*, 52*cl*.
Bridgeman Art Library 9*tl*, 13*tc*, 13*cr*, 27*tl*, 31*tr*, 33*tl*, 46*tr*, 55*tc*, 59*br*, 68*tr*, 69*t*.

The British Architectural Library, RIBA, London 69*cr*.
British Museum 11*tl*.
Camera Press 72*bl*, 91*tl*, 96*br* both, 105*tr*.
Centraal Museum, Utrecht/Rietveld Schröder Archives back cover *tl*, 82-3, /© **Beeldrecht** 82*bl*, 82*tr*, 83*tl*, 83*tr*.
Corbis 79*cr*, 86*tr*, 86*br*.
Joe Cornish back cover *tr*, 48-9.
James Davis Travel Photography 13*tl*, 15*br*, 28-9, 39*tr*, 44*cl*, 72-3.
Design Press /Lars Hallen 88-9, 88*tr*, 89*tl*, 89*tr*.
Esto Photographics 76-7, 77*tl*, 77*tr*, /**Scott Francis** 90-1, 90*bl*, 91*tr*, 109*bc*.
e.t. archive 10*tr*, 18*bl*, 53*tc*.
Mary Evans 11*cr*, 15*tr*, 41*cr*, 45*cr*, 58*tr*, 61*tl*, 62*tr*, 67*tcl*, 69*br*.
Eye Ubiquitous 73*cl*.
GA Photographers 94-5.
Dennis Gilbert 3, 102-3*tc*, 102*bl*, 103*cr*, 109*br*.
Glasgow School of Art 74*tr*, /**Ralph Burnett** 74-5.
Greene and Greene Library, Pasedena 76*tc*, 76*tr*.
Sonia Halliday 18*tr*.
Robert Harding Picture Library front cover *tl*, font cover *tr*, back cover *cl*, 4*tr*, 4*bl*, 4*br*, 7*bl*, 8*tl*, 9*tr*, 19*tr*, 21*tr*, 23*tr*,

25*tl*, 26*tr*, 28*tl*, 29*tr*, 30*tl*, 31*tl*, 32-3, 32*tr*, 32*cl*, 33*tl*, 36*cr*, 39*br*, 40*tl*, 40*tr*, 45*tl*, 46*tl*, 54*cl*, 54*tr*, 56-7, 57*tr*, 71*tl*, 85*cr*, 88*bl*, 93*cr*, 96*tc*, 108*br*, 109*bl*.
Michael Hopkins and Partners /Richard Davies 103*tr*.
Angelo Hornak 2, 6*c*, 12*cl*, 26-7, 27*bc*, 42-3, 42*tr*, 58*tl*, 66-7, 67*tc*.
Hulton Getty 11*tr*, 49*tl*, 67*tl*, 68-9, 81*br*, 93*tr*.
Kansai International Airport Co Ltd 7*tr*, 106*tr*, 107*t*, 107*br*.
A. F. Kersting front cover *cl*, front cover *c*, back cover *bl*, inside flap *t*, 5*bl*, 6*tl*, 10-11, 30-1, 30*bl*, 36-7, 40-41, 41*bl*, 54-5, 58-9, 59*bl*, 61*tr*, 62-3, 96*tl*.
Ian Lambot back cover *cr*, 1, 5*tr*, 100-1, 100*tr*, 101*tr*.
Le Corbusier Foundation © ADAGP, Paris DACS, London 1997 84*tr*, plans 84*cl*, 84*bl* Le Corbusier re-drawn by Janos Marffy.
Link 17*tl*.
Mansell Collection 42*br*.
Simon Murrell 23*tl*, 46*br*, 90*cl*, 100*cr*, 105*tl*.
Museum of Scotland, Edinburgh 20*bl*.
National Palace Museum, Taiwan 38*bl*.
National Trust Photographic Library 50*cl*, 50*tr*, 51*tl*, 81*tl*, 81*tr*.

Moh Nishikawa front cover *cr*, 16-17, 52-3.
Renzo Piano Building Workshop, Geneva/Stefano Goldbert 106 *bl*, 107*b*, 107*cr*.
Resource Photo/Pankaj Shah 22*tr*, 22*bl*, 23*cr*.
Royal Pavillion Art Gallery and Museums, Brighton 63*tl*, 63*tr*.
Kenzo Tange Associates 95*tl*, 95*tr*.
Trip Photographic Library 21*cr*, 22-3.
Temple Expiatore of the Sagrada Familia, Barcelona 72*tr*.
Scala 42*bl*.
South American Pictures 20-1.
Roger-Viollet 85*tc*.
Michael Wilford and Partners Ltd 98*tr*, 99*tr*.
Frank Lloyd Wright Archives 78*tr*, Frank Lloyd Wright Drawings are copyright © 1997 The Frank Lloyd Wright Foundation.
Zefa back cover *ct*, back cover *cl*, 5*br*, 8-9, 8*bl*, 12-13, 18-19, 24-5, 36*tr*, 38-9, 39*cr*, 44-5, 56, 57*tl*, 67*tr*, 92-3, 92*tr*, 93*tl*, 99*tl*.